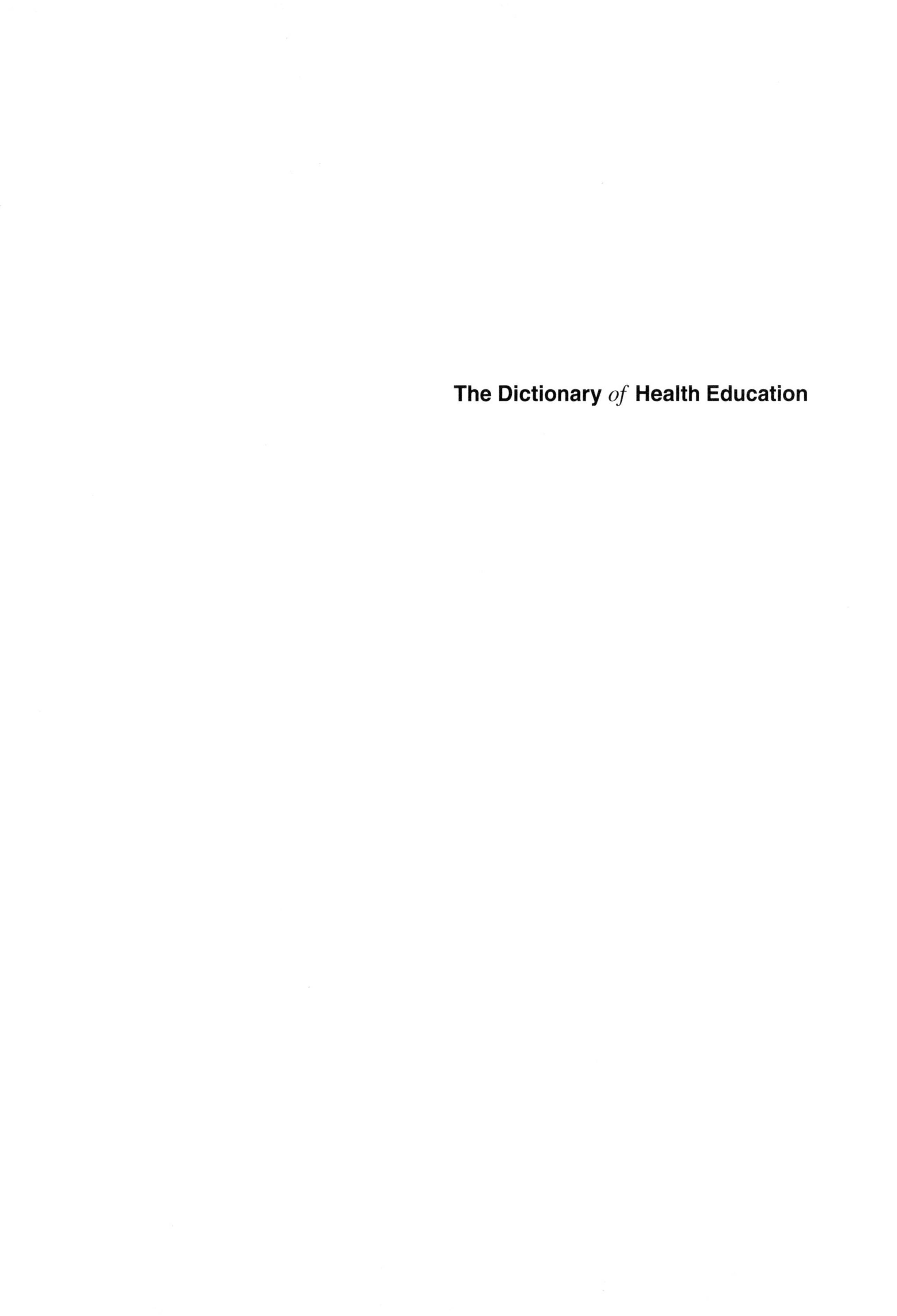

The Dictionary *of* Health Education

The Dictionary *of* Health Education

Edited by

David A. Bedworth, B.S., M.S., Ph.D.

Professor Emeritus, Health Education
The State University of New York
The University of the State of New York

Albert E. Bedworth, B.S., M.S. (1924–2004)

Associate Emeritus, Bureau of School Health Education
The New York State Education Department
The University of the State of New York

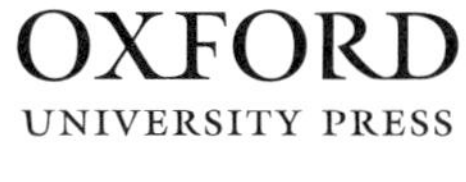

2010

OXFORD
UNIVERSITY PRESS

Oxford University Press, Inc., publishes works that further
Oxford University's objective of excellence
in research, scholarship, and education.

Oxford New York
Auckland Cape Town Dar es Salaam Hong Kong Karachi
Kuala Lumpur Madrid Melbourne Mexico City Nairobi
New Delhi Shanghai Taipei Toronto

With offices in
Argentina Austria Brazil Chile Czech Republic France Greece
Guatemala Hungary Italy Japan Poland Portugal Singapore
South Korea Switzerland Thailand Turkey Ukraine Vietnam

Published by Oxford University Press, Inc.
198 Madison Avenue, New York, New York 10016

www.oup.com

Library of Congress Cataloging-in-Publication Data
The dictionary of health education / edited by David A. Bedworth and Albert E. Bedworth
p. ; cm.
Includes bibliographical references.
ISBN 978-0-19-534259-8
1. Health education—Dictionaries. I. Bedworth, David A. II. Bedworth, Albert E.
[DNLM: 1. Health Education—Dictionary—English.
2. Health Promotion—Dictionary—English. WA 13 D5535 2009]
RA440.D53 2009
613.03—dc22
2008030610

1 3 5 7 9 8 6 4 2

Printed in the United States of America
on acid-free paper

Foreword

ALBERT E. BEDWORTH and I began work on this dictionary in the mid-1980s. At that time, there was no other dictionary of health education on the market; the necessity of such a publication was clear in order to further the development of professionalism among health educators and to clearly identify the language of health education as it is used in the field.

Mr. Bedworth conceived of this project and completed much of the research for it prior to his death in January 2004. I continued work on the dictionary after his passing and was fortunate to have come to an agreement with Oxford University Press to publish it.

The contributions to the field of health education by Mr. Bedworth are numerous. He began working in the field in 1951. He taught health education in several school districts in New York State, most notably teaching in the Ithaca City School district for 17 years. During that time, Mr. Bedworth developed and implemented a regional model for the coordination of school health education, what was to become known as the BOCES health coordinator network in New York State, and which was widely replicated throughout the nation. He served in the New York State Education Department from 1970 until his retirement in 1979.

Mr. Bedworth was the coauthor of four other books in the field of health education, the author of numerous papers in professional journals, and the founding Executive Editor of the *Journal of Drug Education*.

DAVID A. BEDWORTH, PH.D.

Introduction

FORMS OF HEALTH EDUCATION have existed in many cultures throughout the world for centuries. Some of these were intertwined with the political or religious practices of ancient civilizations. Some became traditional childrearing practices within family structures.

Health education was introduced into the schools as a subdiscipline about one hundred years ago. In some instances, it was implemented as a separate discipline, but it was not until the middle 1960s that this approach was more-or-less universally accepted as effective. Health education has also greatly expanded in scope in official and voluntary health agencies, in the workplace, and in clinical settings.

Over the decades, many books have been written about health education. Many have been devoted to the philosophy, problems, and practices of health education. Many of these publications have attempted to define many of the terms used in the health education profession. However, none is complete or useable as a definitive reference. *The Dictionary of Health Education* brings together for the first time in one volume all of the pertinent, important, and vital health education terms and expressions. It clearly defines, explains, and illustrates the entire profession of health education, its professional language, and its technical language. It is the authoritative and definitive source of the language of the profession of health education and all of its subspecialties.

The definitions provided in this book are alphabetically arranged, and the descriptions of terms and expressions are cross referenced where appropriate, and illustrated as needed, for further clarity and understanding. In addition, the dictionary contains tables of important health and medical terms.

The dictionary includes terminology used by health educators and related professions as their foundational language. The terms and expressions presented focus specifically on those that are appropriate to education as they are applied to health education: the principles of learning, the principles of health education methodology, organization, strategies, evaluation, curriculum design, ethics, standards, goals, and objectives. The dictionary also includes technical terms and expressions that health educators must understand to function effectively.

The Dictionary of Health Education is concluded with complete documentation in the form of a bibliography. This section contains a listing of current and classical sources that have used the terms, expressions, and other descriptions contained in this volume.

Editorial Advisory Board

Symbols and Abbreviations Used

cf:	Defined elsewhere. Compared to.
ct:	Defined elsewhere. In contrast to.
e.g.	For example
i.e.	That is
esp.	Especially
ex.	Example
q.v.	Defined elsewhere.
qq.v.	The immediately preceding list defined elsewhere.
~	The term or phrase being defined.

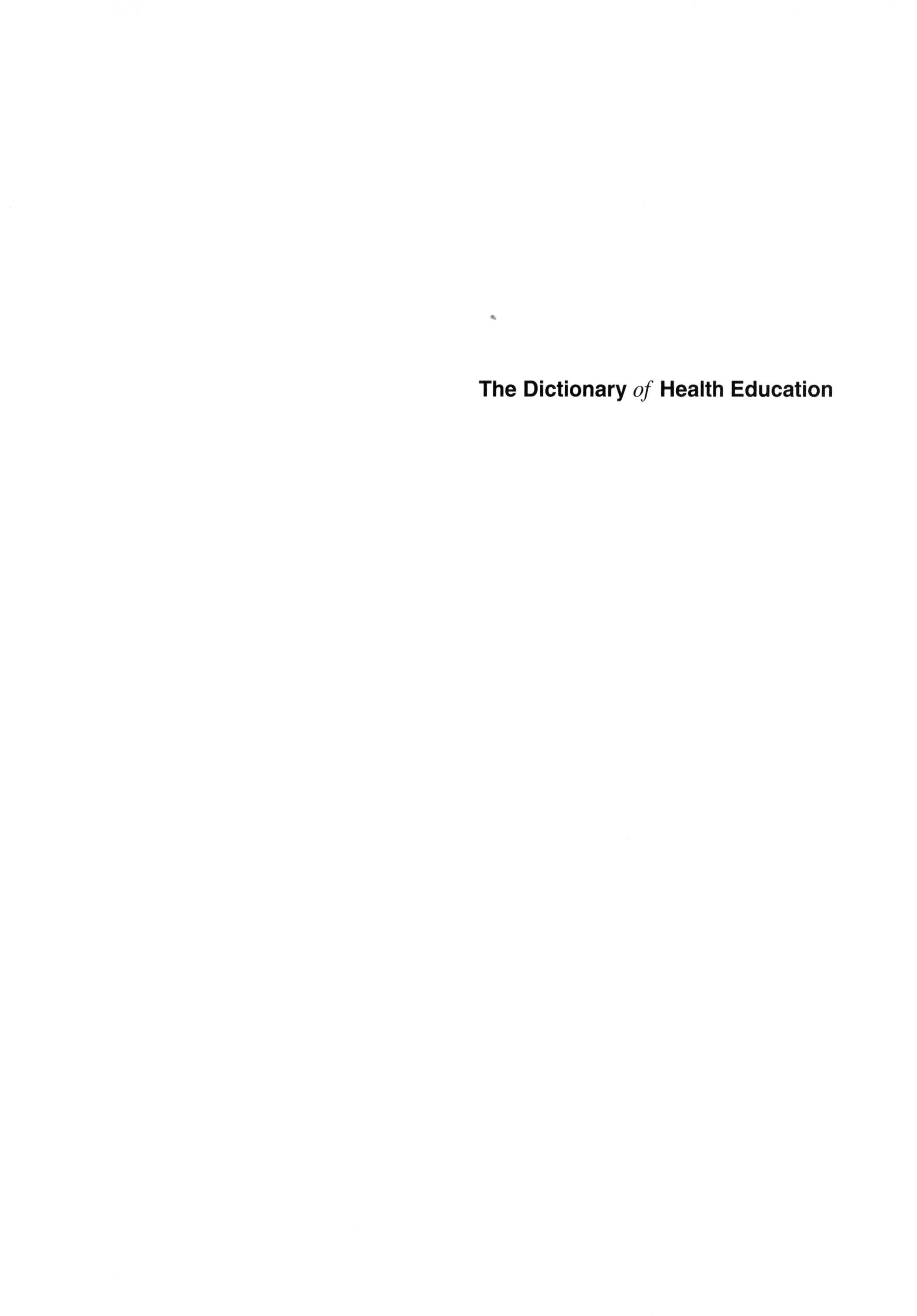

The Dictionary *of* Health Education

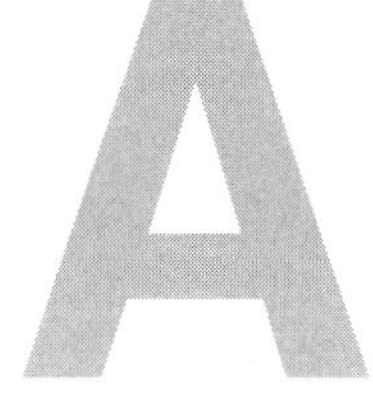

A Angstrom unit *q.v.*

AA An acronym for Alcoholics Anonymous *q.v.*; Addicts Anonymous *q.v.*

AAA An acronym for 1. American Academy of Allergists. 2. American Association of Anatomists. 3. American Automobile Association.

AAAS An acronym for American Association for the Advancement of Science.

AACCN An acronym for American Association of Critical Care Nurses.

AAFP An acronym for American Academy of Family Practice.

AAHB An acronym for American Academy of Health Behavior.

AAIN An acronym for American Association of Industrial Nurses.

AAMA An acronym for American Association of Medical Assistants.

AANA An acronym for American Association for Nurse Anesthetists.

AAP An acronym for American Academy of Pediatrics.

AAPA An acronym for American Academy of Physician's Assistants.

AAPCC An acronym for American Association of Poison Control Centers.

AART An acronym for American Association for Respiratory Therapy.

AASMUS 1. Breathing. 2. Pertaining to asthma *q.v.* related to a physiogenic *q.v.* etiology *q.v.*

AB An acronym for Aid to the Blind.

ABASIA A condition characterized by the inability to walk resulting from motor *q.v.* incoordination *q.v.* or paralysis *q.v.* cf: ataxia.

ABATEMENT In law, the termination of a lawsuit.

ABBEY SCHOOL Monastic school *q.v.*

ABC An acronym for alternative birth center *q.v.*

AB DESIGN In research, a time-series design in which a control phase called the baseline (A) frequently precedes a treatment phase (B).

ABDOMEN 1. The area of the body between the diaphragm *q.v.* and the pelvis. 2. The belly. cf: abdominal cavity.

ABDOMINAL CATASTROPHE The most sudden and severe form of an acute abdominal injury.

ABDOMINAL CAVITY One of the three major body cavities located below the diaphragm *q.v.* and the chest cavity *q.v.* and above the pelvic cavity *q.v.* The ~ contains the stomach, spleen, pancreas, intestines, liver, and gallbladder.

ABDOMINAL MUSCLES The trunk-flexor muscle group that form the supporting wall for the organs of the abdomen *q.v.* and the pelvic *q.v.* regions.

ABDOMINAL PREGNANCY A type of displaced or ectopic *q.v.* pregnancy *q.v.* in which the embryo *q.v.* becomes attached to mislocated endometrial *q.v.* tissue in the abdominal *q.v.* wall.

ABDOMINOPLASTY A surgical procedure for reshaping the abdomen *q.v.*

ABDUCT To move away from the midline. ct: adduct.

ABDUCTION The movement of a body part in the frontal plane *q.v.* away from the midline of the body. ct: adduction.

ABERRATION Deviation from what is common or normal.

ABIC The Adaptive Behavior Inventory for Children, a part of SOMPA *q.v.*

ABIENT The tendency to move away from a stimulus or situation. ct: adient.

ABILITY 1. A pattern of behavioral tendencies responsible for skillful performance in a variety of related tasks. 2. In health, the capacity for self-sufficiency. 3. The present level of performance on some task. ct: aptitude.

ABILITY GROUPING Organizing learners into homogeneous groups based on perceived intellectual ability resulting from intelligence tests *q.v.* and previous performances.

ABILITY TO PAY 1. A theory characterized by a wage determination concept based on the employer's ability to pay certain wage rates. 2. In health, the ability of an individual to pay health/medical expenses given existing health insurance or other means of paying the provider.

ABIOGENESIS 1. Spontaneous generation *q.v.* 2. Obsolete doctrine of the origin of life from lifeless matter.

ABIOSIS The absence of life.

ABLATIVE THERAPY A treatment by the removal or eradication of a body part.

ABNORMAL 1. Deviation from the normal *q.v.* 2. Deviation. 3. Uncommon. 4. In psychology, psychological *q.v.* deviation from the norm or usual; behavior that is detrimental to the person or to the society. 5. Those characteristics that disable a person from functioning in all types of human societies. ct: normal. cf: deviant.

ABNORMAL BEHAVIOR 1. Any behavior *q.v.* that includes at least one of the following characteristics: (a) extreme social deviance *q.v.*, (b) subjective distress, or (c) psychological *q.v.* handicap. 2. Used in the field of psychology to designate behavior that does not meet the criteria of normal *q.v.*

ABNORMAL INTELLIGENCE Pertaining to either unusually low or unusually high intelligence *q.v.*

ABORAL In biology, opposite to the mouth.

ABORTIFACIENT 1. A drug or substance capable of inducing abortion *q.v.* 2. Any substance that causes the pregnant uterus *q.v.* to rid itself of its contents.

ABORTION 1. Terminating a pregnancy *q.v.* 2. The intentional removal (induced) or the spontaneous (natural) expulsion of the fetus *q.v.* or embryo *q.v.* from the uterus *q.v.* before it can survive on its own. 3. Premature expulsion from the uterus of the products of conception *q.v.*: the embryo or a nonviable fetus. ~ may be therapeutic or elective. cf: miscarriage; spontaneous abortion; induced abortion.

ABRADE 1. To wear away by mechanical action. 2. To scrape away the epidermis *q.v.*

ABRASION 1. The scraping off of the superficial layers of the skin. 2. A wound caused when the skin or mucous membrane *q.v.* is scraped off the body.

ABREACTION 1. Catharsis *q.v.* 2. In psychoanalysis *q.v.*, the removal of a suppressed desire or complex *q.v.* by talking it out. 3. Expression of pent-up emotions *q.v.*

ABRUPTION 1. The placenta *q.v.* separates from the uterus *q.v.* during the third trimester of pregnancy *q.v.* 2. A tearing away from.

ABSCESS 1. An inflamed area of the body characterized by swelling and an accumulation of pus *q.v.* 2. An infection *q.v.* restricted to a localized area. 3. A localized collection of pus in a cavity formed by the disintegration of tissues. 4. An ~ of the apex of a tooth.

ABSCISSION 1. In biology, a zone of tissue formed in order that separation may take place. 2. In botany, the dropping of leaves, flowers, fruits, or other plant parts, usually following the formation of a separation layer.

ABSENTEEISM Failure to be in a certain place, e.g., work or class, at a specified time.

ABSOLUTE ALCOHOL One hundred percent alcohol; also called anhydrous alcohol.

ABSOLUTE GLAUCOMA A nonremediable condition of the eye that causes the destruction of the optic nerve *q.v.* and the retina *q.v.*

ABSOLUTE THRESHOLD 1. The lowest intensity of a stimulus *q.v.* that produces a response *q.v.* 2. Detection threshold. 3. The minimal level of stimulation that a person can detect.

ABSOLUTELY REFRACTORY PHASE The period immediately after firing, during which time a neuron *q.v.* is completely unresponsive to a stimulus *q.v.*

ABSOLUTIST ETHIC A system of beliefs in which right and wrong are unchanging and absolute. cf: relativistic; hedonistic ethics.

ABSORBENT An agent that takes up water or fluid and increases in bulk. cf: adsorbent.

ABSORPTION 1. In nutrition, the movement of digested *q.v.* food from the lumen *q.v.* of the intestine *q.v.* into intestinal cells, and from there, into the bloodstream for distribution to other parts of the body. 2. The taking up of a liquid or gas through a mucous membrane *q.v.* or skin. 3. The passage of a substance from the stomach and intestine into the bloodstream, lymph, and cells. 4. Sucking up or imbibing, as a sponge absorbs water.

ABSTENTION 1. Abstinence *q.v.* 2. Voluntarily not engaging in some act.

ABSTINENCE 1. Completely avoiding the use of substances, such as alcohol, tobacco, caffeine, and the like. ~ is also used in other areas of health practices and lifestyles. ~ from sexual intercourse *q.v.* or birth control techniques. 2. A condition of not using a particular substance or refraining from using a drug *q.v.*

ABSTINENCE SYNDROME 1. Withdrawal syndrome *q.v.* 2. Physiological *q.v.* and psychological *q.v.* symptoms *q.v.* that result from an abrupt withdrawal from certain drugs. 3. A set of symptoms that occur together, resulting from withdrawal from alcohol, depressants *q.v.*, and opiates *q.v.*

ABSTRACT IDEAS The concept *q.v.* of creative thoughts that are unsupported or only partially supported by concrete evidence. Things that may not be real or concrete.

ABSTRACT MODELING The act of applying what has been learned to other related situations.

ABULIA 1. Loss of will power. 2. The impairment of the ability to initiate voluntary action and to make decisions.

ABUSE To frequently use improperly or to misuse. cf: child abuse; drug abuse.

ACADEMIC FREEDOM A teaching/learning environment characterized by the freedom and opportunity for a teacher to teach without coercion, censorship, or restrictive interference so long as such teachings are within certain socially acceptable boundaries.

ACADEMIC SUPPORT Generally refers to financial support. ~ includes expenditures for support services that are an integral part of an educational institution's basic functions.

ACADEMIC YEAR The period of time that an educational institution is in session. Pre-college schools usually are in session from late August or early September through June of the next calendar year. Colleges and universities may vary somewhat from this designated year, depending upon their adherence to a semester system.

ACADEMY American secondary school during colonial times which stressed practical subjects.

ACALCULIA 1. Loss of the ability to calculate. 2. Inability to successfully manipulate number symbols.

ACANTHAMOEBA KERATITIS A disease of the eye associated with contact lenses *q.v.* ~ can result in blindness from lesions *q.v.* of the cornea *q.v.*

ACAPNIA A marked decrease in blood carbon dioxide *q.v.* content.

ACCELERATED PROGRAM Educational program established in some schools to make it possible for superior learners to advance more rapidly through the educational program or curriculum *q.v.*

ACCELERATION A process that allows students to achieve at a rate that is consonant with their capacity or ability *q.v.*

ACCEPTANCE The process in qualitative research by which subjects being observed become sufficiently accustomed to the observer that their behavior is normal. cf: qualitative evaluation; qualitative variable.

ACCESS 1. In the health care system, a person's ability to obtain health care. ~ is generally influenced by geographic location of the person or health care providers, social standing, ethnicity, financial status, and psychological *q.v.* and intellectual *q.v.* status. 2. A way or means of approach.

ACCESSIBILITY The degree to which an adaptive specialization *q.v.* in intellectual functioning can be separated from its original function and brought in conscious, deliberate application to other problems for which a similar solution is appropriate.

ACCIDENT 1. An event that happens by chance, or by unforeseen or remote causes. 2. Coincidental happening resulting in tragedy from mild and unimportant to severe. 3. An unintentional, unexpected, avoidable and usually undesirable event. 4. An unplanned happening or circumstance that results in body injury, death, or property damage.

ACCIDENT PRONE A person who experiences a greater number of accidents *q.v.* than would be expected under the circumstances.

ACCOMMODATION 1. The adaptation *q.v.* by the person to the assimilated *q.v.* experience. 2. In health, incorporation of a health fact influencing one's health attitude and subsequent health behavior *q.v.* 3. Complete adaptation *q.v.* to the external environment *q.v.* 4. The way a person changes his or her schemas as he or she continues to interact with the environment. 5. In physiology, the process by which the eye lens is thickened or flattened to focus on an object. 6. A primary cue to depth and distance. 7. In psychology, the tendency to revise an existing schema as the result of a new experience. 8. In sociology, a social process whereby individuals and groups minimize their differences in order to reach adjustment in interactions. 9. The process of intellectual adaptation complementary to assimilation *q.v.*

ACCOMMODATION PROCESS IN SOCIAL EXCHANGE The tendency to engage in relationships so as to provide maximum pleasure and minimal pain to each participant.

ACCOUNTABILITY 1. In education, the requirement that teachers specify objectives *q.v.* at the beginning of a course and present evidence of how well learners have achieved these objectives by the end of the course. 2. Responsibility related to quality of educational programs. 3. Accepting responsibility for one's actions to another. 4. The management philosophy that individuals are held liable or accountable for how well they use their authority and live up to their authority and live up to their responsibility of performing predetermined activities. 5. To furnish justification or detailed explanation of financial activities. 6. To furnish reasons or explanations. account giving. The primary means by which persons make themselves seem intelligible or reasonable to others.

ACCREDITATION 1. Acknowledgment by an outside group that an educational institution or program meets certain standards. 2. The process by which a review agency evaluates an institution. Persons representing the review agency determine whether the institution meets certain predetermined criteria of acceptability. 3. In the case of higher education, students graduating from an accredited school are given the opportunity to become certified *q.v.* 4. Certification *q.v.* by an accrediting agency in accordance with established standards. 5. In reference to hospitals, a voluntary process that indicates that certain minimal standards of institutional care are in effect.

ACCREDITING AGENCY An organization that establishes criteria and standards for judging the quality of an educational institution and its programs. The ~ submits a report concerning the institution's quality.

ACCRETION An increase in size by external addition. ct: intussusception.

ACCRETION AND DELETION OF TEXTURE A dynamic cue that provides information about the relative distance of objects. The cue is created whenever objects move relative to their background.

ACCRETIVE The collection or accumulation of hypotheses derived from scientific investigations that were completed.

ACCULTURATION The process whereby members of a subculture and minorities acquire cultural characteristics such as values, beliefs, language, and acceptable behaviors of the dominant group in the community or society.

ACCUMULATIVE INCIDENCE The occurrence of an event or act by a given time or age.

ACCURACY 1. In testing, the ratio of the number of test items correctly answered to the number of test items attempted. 2. Evaluation *q.v.* related to the number of errors made; the fewer the errors, the greater the ~. 3. In reading or language, the precision in pronouncing words: the exactness of comprehension in reading.

ACCURACY IN REASONING The degree of conformity between an assertion resulting from a reasoning process and an assertion that might logically be deduced from the given premises or from previous assertions.

ACCURATE BODY CONCEPT Pertaining to the ability of a person to evaluate his or her body with accuracy. cf: self-concept.

AC/DC Slang for a bisexual *q.v.* person.

ACENTRIC CHROMOSOME A chromosome *q.v.* fragment lacking a centromere *q.v.*

ACEP An acronym for American College of Emergency Physicians.

ACETABULUM In anatomy, the large cup-shaped depression in the hipbone into which the head of the thighbone (femur) fits.

ACETALDEHYDE 1. A colorless, soluble liquid with the chemical formula C_2H_4O. 2. An organic compound. 3. A toxic breakdown of ethyl alcohol. 4. The chemical product of the first step in the liver's metabolism *q.v.* of alcohol *q.v.* It is normally present only in small amounts, as it is rapidly converted to acetic acid *q.v.*

ACETAMINOPHEN 1. An active ingredient in some nonprescription *q.v.* drugs that relieve pain and reduce fever. ~ is taken for headaches and other pains as a preference to aspirin *q.v.* 2. A substitute analgesic *q.v.* useful for persons who are sensitive to aspirin. 3. A pain reliever. cf: acetylsalicylic acid; ibuprofen.

ACETONE 1. A chemical compound found in the urine in trace amounts. When large amounts are present, it gives off a fruity odor to the urine or breath. This may be present in a diabetic *q.v.* 2. An organic *q.v.* compound in the urine in any condition in which insufficient carbohydrates *q.v.* oxidize in the body.

ACETONE BODIES 1. Ketone bodies *q.v.* 2. Acids *q.v.* formed during the first part of fat catabolism *q.v.* acetoacetic acid, betahydroxybutyric acid, and acetone *q.v.*

ACETOPHENAZINE 1. An antipsychotic *q.v.* drug. Tindal is a commercial preparation of ~.

ACETYLCHOLINE 1. An acetic acid ester *q.v.* of choline *q.v.* that is normally present in many parts of the body and functions in the transmission of nerve impulses *q.v.* 2. A chemical neurotransmitter *q.v.* in many parts of the body, including neuromuscular *q.v.* functions and the nervous system *q.v.* 3. The neurotransmitter secreted by motor nerves *q.v.* to excite skeletal muscles *q.v.* 4. A neurotransmitter in the parasympathetic nervous system *q.v.* 5. Abbreviation Ach. 6. A neurotransmitter that acts as an excitatory transmitter at the synaptic *q.v.* junction between muscle fibers and motor neurons *q.v.*

ACETYLCHOLINESTERASE (AChE) An enzyme *q.v.* that stops the action of acetylcholine *q.v.*

ACETYL COENZYME A (acetyl CoA) An important metabolic intermediate that provides energy *q.v.* for cellular function, and is used for the synthesis *q.v.* of cholesterol *q.v.*, fatty acids *q.v.*, and other biological compounds.

ACETYLSALICYLIC ACID 1. The active ingredient in aspirin *q.v.* 2. A drug that is an anti-inflammatory agent, an antipyretic *q.v.*, and an analgesic *q.v.* 3. Aspirin. cf: acetaminophen; ibuprofen.

ACH Acetylcholine *q.v.*

ACHA Acronym for American College Health Association.

ACHALASIA An obstruction that occurs in the lower esophagus *q.v.* that is thought to be due to a loss of nerve function. The obstruction may be the result of the retention of food in the upper esophagus.

AChE Acetylcholinesterase *q.v.*

ACHIEVED STATUS In sociology, a social position allocated to a person because of his or her achievement *q.v.* or uniquely achieved qualities.

ACHIEVEMENT 1. Reaching a goal *q.v.* 2. Accomplishment or proficiency of performance in a particular skill or in knowledge of a subject. ~ may be categorized into academic, learner, age, quotient, ratio, record of, a scale, score, standards, tests or general.

ACHIEVEMENT AGE The age of a person associated with the level of acquired learning determined by a proficiency test and related to the chronological age of the average with the level of achievement.

ACHIEVEMENT MOTIVATION Behavior that results from the need for achievement, the desire to do something better or more efficiently than it had been done before. cf: achievement motive.

ACHIEVEMENT MOTIVE 1. The desire to meet or exceed some standard of excellence. 2. Techniques used to encourage learners to strive for success. cf: motive; motivation; achievement motivation.

ACHIEVEMENT TEST 1. A device (written, oral, or manipulative) that measures the degree of proficiency already attained in some specific skill or ability (intellectual, social, emotional, or manual). 2. A measure directed toward ascertaining intellectual, social, emotional, or physical skills. 3. In health education, a measure of a learner's level of health knowledge, attitudes, or behavior. 4. An examination that measures the extent to which a person has acquired certain information or mastered certain skills, usually as a result of specific instruction or educational experiences.

ACHILLES TENDON 1. The large tendon *q.v.* at the back of the heel which moves the foot up and down at the ankle joint. 2. The tendon inserted on the calcaneus *q.v.* 3. From Greek mythology, that Achilles' mother held him by the heels when she dipped him in the river Styx, thereby making him invulnerable except in the area of the heel.

ACHLORHYDRIS A lack of hydrochloric acid *q.v.* in the stomach.

ACHONDROPLASIA A condition occurring in fetal life in which cartilage is absorbed during the development of bone tissue resulting in a disproportionate growth of the trunk and extremities producing achondroplastic dwarfism *q.v.*

ACHONDROPLASTIC DWARFISM A peculiar type of dwarfism *q.v.* caused by defective development of the ends of the long bones during fetal development.

ACHROMATIC Colorless visual sensations. cf: rods; cones; retina.

ACHROMATIC VISION Color blindness *q.v.*

ACHROMATIN The substance of the cell nucleus *q.v.* that is not readily stained by staining agents.

ACID Any substance that releases hydrogen ions *q.v.* in solution. The hydrogen ions may be displaced by a metal to form salt. cf: base; alkali.

ACID-BASE BALANCE The ratio of acidity and alkalinity of body fluids.

ACIDOPHIL Eosinophil *q.v.*

ACIDOSIS 1. An elevation in the acidity of the blood. 2. A poisonous chemical imbalance in the blood that may lead to coma and death.

ACID RAIN Rain containing nitric and sulfuric acid, formed when nitrogen and sulfur oxides from motor vehicles and coal-burning power plants and factories react with moisture in the atmosphere.

ACINI The milk-producing glands in the breast.

ACNE 1. A skin disorder occurring naturally in most adolescents and is apparently the result of increased amounts of androgens *q.v.* 2. An inflammatory condition of the oil glands of the skin.

ACOELOMATE In biology, without a body cavity or coelom *q.v.*

ACOUASM A false perception of some sounds such as ringing or hissing.

ACOUMETER An instrument for testing hearing. The Politzer ~ produces a clicking tone that can be heard up to about 45 feet.

ACOUSTIC Pertaining to the sense of hearing or to the science that is concerned with this sense.

ACOUSTIC METHOD Developed by Max A. Foldstein, a method of teaching the deaf. Speech and speech understanding are achieved by training the auditory *q.v.* and tactile *q.v.* senses to recognize sound vibrations produced by the voice or sonorous instruments.

ACOUSTIC BASIS The foundation of phonetic language. The ~ is used to determine the variations in language pronunciations.

ACOUSTICS 1. The science of sound. 2. The science concerned with the cause and characteristics of vibrations resulting in sound.

ACP An acronym for 1. American College of Physicians. 2. American College of Pathologists *q.v.*

ACQUAINTANCE RAPE Rape *q.v.* in which the assailant and the victim know each other. Sometimes involves date rape characterized by a social date ending in unwanted sexual intercourse.

ACQUIRED Characteristics of a person that are not ascribable to heredity *q.v.*

ACQUIRED CHARACTER A modification impressed on an organism by environmental *q.v.* influences during development. cf: acquired traits.

ACQUIRED DRIVE A learned motive *q.v.* cf: primary drive.

ACQUIRED EQUIVALENCE OF CUES In psychology or social science, the tendency to treat persons or object in the same way when they are called by the same name.

ACQUIRED IMMUNE DEFICIENCY SYNDROME (AIDS) 1. The end-stage manifestations of infection *q.v.* with human immunodeficiency virus (HIV) which destroys important components of the human immune system *q.v.* Persons with the disease develop infections that would not occur with normal immunity *q.v.* The Centers for Disease Control and Prevention have strict criteria for a diagnosis of AIDS. These include a positive test for exposure to HIV and certain abnormalities in T-cell *q.v.* ratios, as well as a number of infections and cancers *q.v.* including the following: histoplasmosis *q.v.*, isoporiasis *q.v.*, candidiasis *q.v.*, various forms of pneumonia *q.v.*, esp. Pneumocystis carinii *q.v.*, pneumonia enterocolitis *q.v.*, meningitis *q.v.* esophogitis, encephalitis *q.v.*, chronic mucotaneous herpes simplex *q.v.*, cystome-galovirus infection, chronic progressive multifocal leucoencephalopathy, Hodgkin's disease *q.v.*, non-Hodgkin's lymphoma *q.v.*, Burkitt's lymphoma *q.v.*, liver cancer, cancer of the oropharynx, chronic lymphocytic leukemia, lung cancer *q.v.*, and Kaposi's sarcoma *q.v.* in persons under 60 years. Also included in the Centers for Disease Control and Prevention's definition are central nervous system *q.v.* abnormalities caused by infection with HIV itself. 2. A condition in which the immune system is weakened so that it becomes vulnerable to disease and infection. 3. A disease in which the body's immune system breaks down, leading eventually to death. Because the disease is spread through the mixing of body fluids, it is prevalent in intravenous drug users who share needles. 4. A disease that attacks the body's defense system, gradually rendering it incapable of fighting disease. 5. Also immunodeficiency syndrome *q.v.* A disease believed to be caused by a retrovirus (HIV) and characterized by a deficiency of the immune system. The primary defect is an acquired, persistent, quantitative functional depression within the T4 subset of lymphocytes which often leads to infections caused by opportunistic microorganisms in HIV-infected persons.

ACQUIRED IMMUNITY 1. The major component of the immune system *q.v.* associated with the formation of antibodies *q.v.* and specialized blood cells that are capable of destroying pathogens *q.v.* 2. The potential to resist an infection or disease.

ACQUIRED TRAITS Characteristics developed with growth. cf: acquired character.

ACQUISITION 1. Learning. 2. Assimilation *q.v.*

ACROANESTHESIA A condition characterized by the absence of feeling in the extremities. ct: acroesthesia.

ACROESTHESIA A condition in which there is an increased sensitivity in the extremities, esp. to pain. ct: acroanesthesia.

ACROLEIN 1. A volatile, irritating liquid that results from overheating fat. 2. A decomposition product of glycerol *q.v.*

ACROMANIA A form of manic *q.v.* behavior characterized by extreme motor *q.v.* activity.

ACROMEGALY 1. A progressive disease associated with hyperfunction of the pituitary gland *q.v.* and characterized by enlargement of the skeleton, hands, feet, and face. 2. ~ is characterized by hypertrophy *q.v.* of the bones, and connective tissues *q.v.* of the hands, feet, face, and head. ct: giantism (gigantism).

ACROMELALGIA A disease condition of the extremities, esp. the feet, characterized by pain upon walking. cf: erythromelalgia.

ACROMIO 1. Pertaining to the clavicular joint. 2. The union between the clavicle *q.v.* and the scapula *q.v.* and the supporting ligaments. cf: acromion.

ACROMION 1. The bony process on the superior/lateral region of the scapula *q.v.* 2. The outward extension of the spine of the scapula forming the point of the shoulder. cf: acromio.

ACRONYM A mnemonic device made up of the first letter of a set of several words to be memorized.

ACROPHOBIA 1. An irrational, morbid fear of high places. 2. One of the many human phobias *q.v.*

ACROSOME 1. A chemical reservoir in the head of the spermatozoa *q.v.* 2. The cap-like structure in the head of the sperm *q.v.* that contains chemicals that digest a hole into the ovum *q.v.* allowing penetration of the sperm.

ACROSTIC A mnemonic device made up of a sentence consisting of words that begin with the same letter as a set of words to be memorized.

ACRYLONITRATE A plastic material formerly used as a food container. In 1977, the Food and Drug Administration *q.v.* suspended use of these containers because studies showed that test animals fed ~ had significantly lowered body weight, growths in the ear ducts, and lesions of the central nervous system *q.v.*

ACS An acronym for 1. American Chemical Society. 2. American College of Surgeons. 3. American Cancer Society.

ACSM An acronym for American College of Sports Medicine.

ACT An acronym for American College Testing Program *q.v.*

ACTH An acronym for adrenocorticotropic hormone *q.v.*

ACTING In psychology, to actually do something about a decision that a person values when the opportunity arises. The third step in the valuing process.

ACTING OUT In psychology, manifesting conflicts *q.v.* in overt behavior *q.v.* rather than controlling them through suppression *q.v.* or other defense mechanisms *q.v.* ~ is a characteristic of antisocial *q.v.* personalities *q.v.*

ACTION 1. In law, a lawsuit. 2. An ordinary proceeding in a court by which one party prosecutes another for the enforcement or protection of a right, the redress of a wrong, or the punishment of a public offense. 3. A suit. 4. In sociology or psychology *q.v.*, group action, discussion by two or more people to achieve results or solutions to a problem not likely to occur by actions of one person. Frequently, used in problem solving techniques *q.v.* Also referred to as group action or group problem solving. Used also in group therapy *q.v.* 5. Impulsive ~ is a form of behavior *q.v.* that takes place without conscious deliberation and without regard for the consequences of the behavior. 6. Reflective ~ is a form of behavior occurring after one selects a response to a stimulus *q.v.* Thinking about the consequences of the action taken.

ACTIONABLE 1. In law, that which furnishes legal grounds for action *q.v.* 2. The circumstances are such that there is a ground for court action.

ACTION AT LAW Court action *q.v.* in a law case. ct: equity.

ACTION PLAY Bodily movements associated with verse for the purpose of developing a child's sense of rhythm and large muscles *q.v.* and releasing tensions and stress *q.v.*

ACTION POTENTIAL 1. A brief change in the electrical potential of an axon *q.v.* that is the physical basis of the nervous system impulse *q.v.* 2. A technique for measuring the presence of muscular activity of the speech organs in silent reading by the use of a galvanometer *q.v.*

ACTION PROJECT A school-based activity with specific carryover into the community. ~s are intended to make the learning experience relevant in the social life of learners. Examples include surveying the community, environmental cleanup, and participating in screening programs sponsored by a clinic.

ACTION-SPECIFIC ENERGY In ethology *q.v.*, the proposition that the energy for instinctive behavior *q.v.* is specifically available to certain reactions in the presence of certain stimuli *q.v.* referred to as releasers.

ACTIVATED CHARCOAL Powdered charcoal that has been treated to increase its powers of absorption *q.v.*

ACTIVATING EFFECTS In psychology, influences on the motivation *q.v.* or stimulation of behavior *q.v.* ct: organizing effects.

ACTIVATION 1. Energy mobilization. 2. In reproduction, a series of biochemical changes in the sperm *q.v.* to allow it to fuse with an egg.

ACTIVATOR In chemistry, any substance, usually a particular metal ion *q.v.* that is very low concentration significantly accelerates the speed of a chemical reaction.

ACTIVE COPING In psychology, adjusting that results when people assume they can control their own behavior *q.v.* and patterns of interaction. cf: reactive coping.

ACTIVE EUTHANASIA Direct euthanasia *q.v.*

ACTIVE IMMUNITY 1. The body's immune system *q.v.* is stimulated to develop antibodies *q.v.* to a particular antigen *q.v.* 2. A type of acquired immunity *q.v.* resulting from the body's response to naturally occurring pathogens *q.v.* 3. Protection against a disease resulting from the production of antibodies in a host that has been exposed to a disease-producing antigen.

ACTIVE INGREDIENT 1. In botany, the specific chemical in a plant responsible for the drug action ascribed to the entire plant. 2. In medicine, the chemical or chemicals that affect a reaction in the body.

ACTIVE LEARNING In education, learning *q.v.* situations in which the learner *q.v.* is directly involved in the experiences by doing.

ACTIVE LISTENING 1. In communication theory, paraphrasing what others have said which demonstrates interest and understanding of the conversation. 2. A communication technique that avoids the interference of a listener's judgments. 3. Listening that involves giving complete attention to the communicator as well as reflecting precisely what is being communicated. 4. Critical listening. 5. Evidenced by learners' response to what is being communicated, observed by feedback *q.v.*

ACTIVE METABOLITE In a pharmacological *q.v.* preparation, the chemical substance that is responsible for the effects of a drug or medicine.

ACTIVE-PASSIVE MODEL A model of the practitioner–patient relationship that occurs when the patient is unable, because of a medical condition, to participate in his or her own care and to make decisions for his or her own welfare.

ACTIVE PHASE In psychiatry, the acute phase of schizophrenia *q.v.* in which prominent symptoms *q.v.* such as delusions *q.v.*, hallucinations *q.v.*, and thought disorders are present.

ACTIVE SLEEP 1. REM sleep *q.v.* 2. A stage of sleep during which the EEG is similar to that of waking, during which there are rapid eye movements and during which dreams occur.

ACTIVE STAFF In reference to hospitals, the hospital staff position held by physicians who spend much of their time in the hospital setting admitting patients, serving on hospital committees, and exercising their voting rights relative to hospital policy and operations.

ACTIVE TRANSPORT 1. In physiology, an energy-producing process by which certain nutrients *q.v.* are pumped from one compartment to another against a concentration gradient. 2. The movement of substances across a cell membrane *q.v.* usually against a concentration gradient requiring energy expenditure. 3. Movement across a cellular membrane, dependent upon respiratory energy and upon reactions within the membrane. It may result in accumulation against a diffusion gradient. cf: osmosis; diffusion.

ACTIVITY CURRICULUM A curriculum *q.v.* design in which the interests of, and learning purposes for learners determine the educational program characterized by teachers and learners working together to select goals and objectives and to plan activities.

ACTIVE VOCABULARY The words that a person actually uses in speech. ct: passive vocabulary.

ACTIVISM In educational philosophy, the belief that activity is fundamental to the learning process *q.v.* since it is the basis of reality. Truth is tested through action, and the learner is naturally biologically active. Emphasis is placed on an active learner-centered curriculum *q.v.* cf: pedagogy of action.

ACTIVIST In education, a person who believes that meaning in learning stems from active experience of the learner and that this experience is a continuous flow of complicated and integrated responses to the learning process. cf: activism.

ACTIVITIES 1. In the PERT network *q.v.* ~ are specified sets of behavior within a project. 2. Planned and organized experiences closely related to the curriculum *q.v.* but conducted outside of regular class sessions; such as cocurricular *q.v.*, developmental, and extracurricular ~.

activities alcove. An area of the classroom set aside for individual work on a project. It may contain necessary equipment and supplies for carrying out the project.

ACTIVITIES OF DAILY LIVING (ADL) The skills necessary for independent living.

ACTIVITY Any learning experience designed to allow learners to be actively involved in the learning process *q.v.* An ~ may be designated as cooperative, creative, culminating, curricular, directed, individual, goal-directed, motor, mental, learner-centered, supervised, or random.

ACTIVITY CONCEPT The educational philosophy that activities are necessary for learning to take place.

ACTIVITY MOVEMENT The trend in educational thought to make learning more meaningful by avoiding teacher-centered approaches to learning, such as lectures, and bringing about more learner-centered approaches through implementation of the activity concept *q.v.* including field trip experiences and hands-on experiences.

ACTIVITY RATIOS Ratios used during analysis that indicate how well an organization is selling its products in relation to its available resources.

ACT OF THOUGHT In educational philosophy, thought involves a perception of difficulty, a definition of difficulty, arrival at a solution, mental elaboration of the solution, and testing of the solution. John Dewey defines thinking as "active, persistent, and careful consideration of any belief or supposed form of knowledge in the light of the grounds that support it and the further consequences to which it tends."

ACTUAL FAILURE RATE 1. The rate of failures of a contraceptive method *q.v.* that is due to the failure of the method and failure of correct use. 2. The failure rate of a contraceptive in actual use. The actual failure rate is always higher than the theoretical failure rate *q.v.*

ACTUALITY In philosophy, the mode of being whatever is completely real; the realization of some potentiality (Aristotle). cf: entelechy.

ACTUARIAL PREDICTION Statistical prediction in terms of known probabilities that certain patterns of test behavior *q.v.* are associated with particular signs. cf: clinical prediction.

ACTUARIAN A person trained in statistics who applies probability concepts to practical insurance problems and procedures.

ACUITY 1. In vision, the ability to perceive *q.v.* the details of the visual world. 2. In hearing, the ability to perceive the details of sound. 3. Clarity of discrimination. 4. Perception *q.v.* of finite differences in a sensory stimulus or stimuli *q.v.*

ACUPUNCTURE 1. The insertion of very fine needles into patterned areas of the body for the relief of pain. 2. An ancient Chinese system of healing using needles inserted in body parts based on the concept that disease and pain result from disturbances in a life force (chi). 3. A process that attempts to alter the body's electro-energy fields to cure disease. 4. A method of analgesia *q.v.* in which needles are inserted in the skin at special points and a stimulus applied by twirling, vibrating, or charging them electrically. 5. An ancient Chinese pain control technique in which fine metal needles are inserted under the skin to create stimulation to the peripheral nerves *q.v.*

ACUTE 1. A disease that appears suddenly and usually disappears within a short period of time. Some ~ diseases bring about death very rapidly. 2. Sudden in onset. 3. Generally, sharp. 4. In medicine, rapid. 5. Referring to drugs, the short-term effect or effects of a single administration, as opposed to chronic, or long-term effects of administration. 6. Short-term with severe symptoms *q.v.* ct: chronic.

ACUTE ABDOMEN A serious intra-abdominal condition causing irritation and inflammation *q.v.* of the peritoneum *q.v.* and attended by pain, tenderness, and muscular rigidity.

ACUTE ALCOHOL INTOXICATION A potentially fatal elevation of the blood alcohol concentration, often resulting from heavy, rapid consumption of alcoholic beverages *q.v.*

ACUTE ALCOHOLISM A misnomer, since alcoholism *q.v.* is a chronic condition. The use of the term is inherently contradictory. Generally, ~ is referring to intoxication *q.v.* through the use of alcohol *q.v.* or acute intoxication *q.v.* through the use of alcohol.

ACUTE DISEASE A disease *q.v.* that is characterized by a single episode of a short duration from which the person returns to normal or a previous state of health. It is possible for a person to suffer an acute episode resulting from a chronic *q.v.* disease. cf: acute.

ACUTE EFFECT The immediate, short-term response to a single dose of a drug. ct: chronic effect.

ACUTE LEUKEMIA Cancer *q.v.* of the blood found chiefly in children. ~ responds more readily to treatment than chronic leukemia *q.v.* Treatment consists of chemotherapy *q.v.* and radiation therapy *q.v.* Death usually results from infections *q.v.* or hemorrhage *q.v.*

ACUTE ONSET 1. The sudden occurrence of a disorder or disease *q.v.* 2. Acute *q.v.* 3. Acute disease *q.v.* 4. Acute effect *q.v.*

ACUTE PAIN Pain *q.v.* that lasts less than 6 months.

ACUTE PHASE OF AN ILLNESS (DISEASE) The period of an illness or injury in which the primary concern of both patient and medical personnel is the patient's survival. The person's survival depends on the immediate steps taken to deal with the physical trauma of the disease condition.

ACUTE PSYCHOSIS A sudden, severe behavior or thought disorder of relatively short duration. cf: acute.

ACUTE RHINITIS 1. The common cold. 2. The sudden onset of nasal inflammation *q.v.* associated with a viral *q.v.* infection *q.v.*

ACUTE SITUATIONAL MALADJUSTMENT A superficial *q.v.* maladjustment *q.v.* to newly experienced situations that is especially difficult.

ACUTE STAGE Illness stage *q.v.*

ACUTE STRESS Stress *q.v.* brought about suddenly; usually as a response to a traumatic *q.v.* situation. ct: acute situational maladjustment.

ACUTE TOLERANCE A rapid adaptation *q.v.* to large quantities of a drug or chemical over a short period of time. cf: tolerance; ct: high tolerance.

ACUTE TREATMENT STAGE The first phase of intervention, intended to reduce disorganizing psychotic *q.v.* symptoms *q.v.* and allow the person to reestablish contact with reality.

ACUTE UNDULATING COURSE The course of schizophrenia *q.v.* characterized by the sudden onset of, and rapid recovery from, each or a series of episodes of the disorder.

ACYANOSIS (ACYANOTIC) A defect in the heart that does not allow the mixing of oxygenated unoxygenated blood.

ACYCLOVIR 1. An ointment applied to herpes *q.v.* sores or a tablet to relieve pain, speed healing, and reduce the amount of time live viruses *q.v.* are present in the sores. 2. Also Zovirax, an antiviral drug used in the treatment of herpes 1 and 2 and herpes zoster *q.v.*

ADA An acronym for 1. American Dental Association. 2. American Diabetes Association. 3. American Dietetic Association. 4. Average daily attendance.

ADAA An acronym for American Dental Assistants Association.

ADAMHA An acronym for Alcohol, Drug Abuse and Mental Health Administration.

ADAM'S APPLE The projection in the front of the neck formed by the largest cartilage of the larynx *q.v.*

ADAPIN The brand name of doxepin *q.v.*

ADAPTABILITY 1. Flexibility in meeting changed circumstances. 2. The ability to adapt or adjust to one's environment or to changes in the environment. cf: adaptation.

ADAPTATION 1. Adjustment *q.v.* to physical and social environmental conditions as well as internal stimuli. 2. Essentially, the process of homeostasis *q.v.* 3. In health, emotional, social, and physical adjustment. Healthful attitudes and behaviors as appropriate to the particular situation. 4. The adjustment of the senses to environmental conditions. 5. In intelligence, change of intellectual organization through the complementary process of accommodation *q.v.* and assimilation *q.v.* 6. Changes in the composition of a group of organisms or in the physiology *q.v.* or structure of a single organism resulting in the individual being better fitted to the environment. cf: adjustment.

ADAPTATION BOARD A board containing openings in which a person is to insert pegs to form a particular pattern as instructed by a psychologist *q.v.*

ADAPTATION OF INSTRUCTION 1. The adjustment *q.v.* of teaching methodology *q.v.* to meet individual learner needs, abilities, and interests. 2. Adaptive procedure.

ADAPTATION LEVEL 1. The judgment of the value of a stimulus *q.v.* depends upon the context in which it occurs. 2. Closely related to frame of reference *q.v.*

ADAPTATION MECHANISM A fixed sequence of reactions between the mind and the body. There are three stages: (a) reflex reactions to stimuli *q.v.*, (b) emotional responses, and (c) thought and planning.

ADAPTING APPROACH An approach to planning that is based on the philosophy *q.v.* that effective planning concentrates on helping the organization to change or adapt to internal and/or external variables *q.v.*

ADAPTIVE BEHAVIOR 1. Adjustment *q.v.* 2. A change in one's personality *q.v.* necessary to deal more adequately with environmental stimuli *q.v.* 3. The effectiveness or degree with which individuals meet the standards of personal independence and social responsibility expected for their age and cultural groups. 4. A parameter of classification that pertains to a person's ability to be socially appropriate and personally responsible.

ADAPTIVE ENERGY Body energy reserves that come into play when the body approaches exhaustion.

ADAPTIVE IMMUNITY Acquired immunity *q.v.*

ADAPTIVE REACTION 1. Adaptive behavior *q.v.* 2. A response by a person in an attempt to improve his/her relation to the environment *q.v.*

ADAPTIVE SPECIALIZATION Programs or patterns of adaptive behavior *q.v.* that evolve initially as solutions to particular problems.

ADAPTIVE THERMOGENESIS 1. A physiological *q.v.* response of the body to adjust its metabolic rate *q.v.* to the presence of food. 2. The mechanism in which the brain regulates metabolic activity in accordance with caloric intake.

ADAPTIVE VALUE 1. In biology, the extent to which an attribute increases the likelihood of viable offspring. 2. The unit of inheritance.

ADDITIVE COLOR MIXTURE Mixing colors by stimulating the eye with two sets of wavelengths simultaneously.

ADC Acronym for Aid to Dependent Children

ADD Acronym for attention deficit disorder. This learning disability many or may not be accompanied by hyperactivity *q.v.* cf: ADHD.

ADDICT 1. A person who is dependent upon a drug. 2. One who uses an addicting drug *q.v.* regularly.

ADDICTION 1. Characterized by physiological tolerance *q.v.*, psychological *q.v.* craving, and the presence of the withdrawal syndrome *q.v.* 2. A state of periodic or chronic *q.v.* intoxication *q.v.* produced by repeated consumption of a drug. Its characteristics include as follows: (a) an overpowering desire or need (compulsion) to continue taking the drug and to obtain it by any means; (b) a tendency to increase the drug dose; (c) a psychic *q.v.* (psychological) and generally a physical dependence *q.v.* on the effects of the drug; and (d) an effect detrimental to the individual and to society. 3. Drug dependence, chemical dependence, substance abuse, state of physical and/or psychological need, characterized by compulsive use, tolerance, and physical dependence as manifested by withdrawal sickness. cf: drug dependence; positive addiction.

ADDICTION CYCLE The recurring use of and continued dependence upon a drug because of the perceived effects of the drug, i.e., temporary feelings of enhanced power, confidence, security, and creativity. Without these effects, the person experiences lowered self-esteem *q.v.* and mental pain.

ADDICTION SYNDROME A behavior pattern of compulsive drug users characterized by a preoccupation with acquiring and using drugs.

ADDICTIVE DRUG REACTION A type of drug interaction in which two or more drugs that are similar in their general effects produce a cumulative net effect that is the sum of the effect of the individual substances.

ADDICTIVE DRUGS Drugs that can create a physiological dependence *q.v.* when consumed at a rate greater than the body's ability to metabolize *q.v.* them.

ADDICTS ANONYMOUS An organization consisting of and assisting in the recovery of drug addicts *q.v.*

ADDISON'S DISEASE 1. An endocrine *q.v.* disorder produced by cortisone *q.v.* insufficiency and marked by weight loss, fatigue, a darkening of the skin, anxiety, irritability, lack of motivation, and decreased social ability. 2. A disease *q.v.* of the adrenal glands *q.v.* characterized by an anemic, emaciated condition accompanied by a brownish coloration of the skin. 3. A disease resulting from a deficiency of the suprarenal capsule *q.v.* or to tuberculosis *q.v.* of the adrenal glands causing hypofunction of the adrenal medulla *q.v.*

ADDITIVE 1. A substance added to another substance to improve appearance, increase its nutritional value, or to prolong freshness (preserve), and to improve taste. 2. Unintentional ~s include insecticides, microorganisms, antibiotics; 3. also called incidental ~s.

ADDITIVE EFFECT Combining two or more drugs resulting in effect equal to that of the drugs taken separately. ct: potentiation; synergistic.

ADDITIVE MIXTURE In vision, the mixture of light. ct: subtractive mixture; additive color mixture.

ADDUCT To move toward the midline as in an adductor muscle *q.v.* ct: abduct; cf: adduction.

ADDUCTION The act of drawing toward a center or median line. ct: abduction; cf: adduct.

A-DELTA FIBER A type of nerve fiber that transmits rapidly and leads to the sensation of sharp, prickling pain. cf: C-fiber.

ADENECTOMY The removal or excision of a gland.

ADENINE A purine *q.v.* base found in RNA *q.v.* and DNA *q.v.*

ADENITIS Inflammation *q.v.* and swelling of the lymph glands *q.v.*

ADENOCARCINOMA 1. A rare type of vaginal *q.v.* cancer *q.v.* and associated with women whose mothers took diethylstilbestrol (DES) *q.v.* during pregnancy. 2. A form of cancer that originates in the glands of the body. 3. Cancer involving glandular tissue. 4. A cancer arising from glandular epithelial *q.v.* cells, such as the cells lining the milk duct in the breast.

ADENOHYPOPHYSIS The anterior pituitary gland *q.v.*.

ADENOIDECTOMY Surgical removal of the adenoids *q.v.*

ADENOIDS 1. A lymphoid mass similar to the tonsils *q.v.* containing lymphocytes *q.v.* and located in the nasopharynx *q.v.* 2. Pharyngeal tonsils.

ADENOMA 1. A tumor *q.v.* that resembles a gland in its cellular structure. 2. A benign epithelial tumor *q.v.* of glandular *q.v.* origin.

ADENOPATHY A general enlargement of the lymph glands *q.v.* or any particular area of the body.

ADENOSARCOMA 1. A mixed tumor *q.v.* composed of sarcomatous and glandular elements. 2. Breast cancer.

ADENOSINE A chemical believed to be a neurotransmitter *q.v.* in the central nervous system *q.v.*, primarily at inhibitory receptors. Caffeine *q.v.* may act by antagonizing the normal action of ~ on its receptors.

ADENOSINE DIPHOSPHATE A compound (ester) composed of one molecule *q.v.* each of adenine *q.v.* and D-ribose and two molecules of phosphoric acid. ~ is formed as a result of the breakdown of adenosine triphosphate *q.v.* and is used in the resynthesis of adenine triphosphate. adenosine triphosphatase (ATPase). 1. An enzyme *q.v.* in muscles tissue that catalyzes *q.v.* the hydrolysis *q.v.* of the terminal phosphate group of adenine triphosphate. 2. A chemical compound that stores energy and serves as the cell's power supply.

ADENOSINE TRIPHOSPHATE (ATP) 1. A high-energy compound in metabolic *q.v.* pathways and the electron transport system. ~ is needed for cellular activity. 2. The major source of usable chemical energy in metabolism *q.v.* On hydrolysis *q.v.*, ~ loses one phosphate to become adenosine diphosphate *q.v.* plus usable energy, and on further hydrolysis, it is changed to adenosine monophosphate with further release of energy. 3. An ester *q.v.* composed of one molecule each of adenine and D-ribose and three molecules of phosphoric acid.

ADENOSIS Any disease of a gland, esp. lymph glands.

ADEQUACY A feeling of possessing the ability to cope with one's problems or to achieve a particular goal *q.v.*

ADH Antidiuretic hormone *q.v.*

ADHA An acronym for American Dental Hygienists Association.

ADHESIONS Things that are stuck to each other.

ADHESIVE SEALANT A substance that can be applied to the surface of the teeth to fill in the fissures *q.v.* that are susceptible to decay. ~ was developed in 1970 by the National Institute of Dental Research.

ADIADOCHOKINESIS A condition resulting from cerebellar lesions *q.v.* characterized by the inability to make coordinated successive movement.

ADIENT Tending to move toward a stimulus, characterized by approach responses rather than avoidance responses and characteristic of curiosity, imitation, and aggressiveness. ct: abient.

ADIPOCYTE 1. A cell that stores fat. 2. A fat cell.

ADIPOSE CELL THEORY The number of adipocytes *q.v.* in a person is determined by earliest feeding practices.

ADIPOSE TISSUE 1. Body fat. 2. The body's fat storage deposits located subcutaneously *q.v.* at certain areas. cf: adiposity.

ADIPOSITY The amount of fat in the body. cf: adipose tissue.

ADIPOSAT A center in the brain believed to control eating behavior.

ADJOURNMENT SINE DIE In politics, adjournment with a day. It marks the end of a legislative session because it does not set a time for reconvening.

ADJUSTED RATE In epidemiology, a statistical adjustment to eliminate any effects of a particular variable *q.v.* may have in relation to comparisons that are being made, e.g., adjusted birth rate.

ADJUSTED INDIVIDUAL (PERSON) 1. A person who has adapted to his or her physical, social, and emotional environments. 2. A person who has established an acceptable relationship with self and others. 3. One who is emotionally and socially stable. cf: adjustment.

ADJUSTIVE BEHAVIOR 1. The consistent successful performance of an action or skill in the face of possible unplanned interruption. 2. Behavior *q.v.* by which the person attempts to deal with stress *q.v.* and meet his or her needs *q.v.* 3. Efforts to maintain a harmonious relationship with the environment *q.v.*

ADJUSTMENT 1. Generally, the ability to meet the demands of society and to satisfy basic drives or needs *q.v.* 2. In health, emotional and social ~. 3. Biochemical homeostasis *q.v.* 4. Adaptation *q.v.* 5. The use of behavior *q.v.* necessary to change our environment to one more compatible with our goal achievement or a change in us to the extent that we are able to deal more effectively with our environment. 6. The process of adopting forms of behavior suitable to the physical and social environments or to changes in them. 7. An adaptation to external and internal stimulation. 8. Any form of favorable change: personality, educational procedures, moral, school, social, personal.

ADJUSTMENT ASPIRATION The degree to which a person sets realistic goals as related to personal abilities and the environment.

ADJUSTMENT CASE A situation wherein a learner's problems require analysis and change in the home, school, and community environments.

ADJUSTMENT DISORDER A nonpsychotic disorder in which the person's response to a painful event is more extreme than would ordinarily be expected or considered adequate.

ADJUSTMENT MECHANISM 1. Defense mechanism *q.v.* 2. Behavior of a person for the purpose of adapting to a threatening situation.

ADJUSTMENT TO INDIVIDUAL DIFFERENCES In education methodology, an adaptation *q.v.* of educational methodology *q.v.* and learning environments to the various differences of each learner; biological, social, motor, and intellectual.

ADJUVANT TREATMENT A secondary form of treatment that usually follows surgery and involves chemotherapy *q.v.* or radiation therapy *q.v.*

ADL An acronym for activities of daily living *q.v.*

ADLER'S THEORY Neurosis may develop as a result of emotional conflict regarding real or imagined physical, psychological *q.v.*, or social inferiority.

AD LITUM 1. In law, Latin for the purpose of the suit, usually used when minors are, in fact, the plaintiffs. Because they are minors, they must sue "by next friend", referring to a parent or guardian who is plaintiff for the purpose of the suit. 2. A guardian *ad litum* is one appointed to prosecute or defend a suit on behalf of a party incapacitated by infancy or otherwise.

ADMINISTRATION 1. The head of an organization. 2. The process of administering or conducting according to predetermined plans or policies. 3. The sum total of all those techniques and procedures used in operating the educational organization consistent with its policies and goal achievement.

ADMINISTRATIVE BILL A bill proposed or favored by a governor or president. An administrative hierarchy. An administrative organization of a school district or other organization whose authority levels extend from top to bottom with the greatest authority being upward.

ADMINISTRATIVE STYLE Personal attributes that individuals apply to the management of personnel and programs.

ADMISSION TEST SCORES The results from standardized admission tests or special admission tests that are used to make decisions about admitting students to a school or program.

ADNEXIA The internal female genital organs aside from the uterus *q.v.*

ADOLESCENCE 1. The time period between childhood and adulthood, approximately 12–17 years of age. 2. A sociological and psychological term for the mental and social growth of the child into a young adult. During ~, children mature sexually into young adults. cf: puberty.

ADOLESCENT EDUCATION 1. The educational period beginning with the onset of adolescence *q.v.* and ending with adulthood *q.v.* ~ is generally junior and senior high school *q.v.* beginning with the traditional grade of the seventh year through the twelfth grade and high school graduation. 2. The time from the beginning of middle school *q.v.* (the sixth grade) through high school graduation. ct: adult education; continuing education.

ADOLESCENT EGOCENTRISM The tendency of adolescents *q.v.* to assume that their thoughts and behavior are as interesting to others as to themselves.

ADOLESCENT GROWTH SPURT A period of fast bone growth that usually occurs in the early or middle teens and is caused by the rising levels of the sex hormones *q.v.* of puberty *q.v.*

ADOPTION 1. In psychology, the decision to make full use of a new idea as the best course of available action. 2. In parenting, the legal procedure for obtaining a child to become a member of a family in the same manner as a child who is biologically a member of the family. 3. In politics, approval or acceptance, usually applied to amendments or resolutions to a motion or bill.

ADOPTION STUDIES 1. A method of testing genetic *q.v.* theories of abnormal behavior *q.v.* by studying mental illness *q.v.* in biological *q.v.* and adoptive parents and in adopted children. 2. Studies in which adopted children are compared to members of their adopted families and members of their biological families for the purpose of assessing the relative importance of genes *q.v.* and the environment in individual differences.

ADOPTION HOME An institution providing care for a child until adopted *q.v.* The institution may be an orphanage *q.v.*, foster home, or child custody services facility.

ADP Adenosine diphosphate *q.v.*

ADRENAL ANDROGENS Hormones *q.v.* secreted by the adrenal glands *q.v.* that regulate the development of secondary sex characteristics *q.v.*; particularly associated with masculinity *q.v.*

ADRENAL CORTEX The outer layer of the adrenal glands *q.v.* which secrete the corticosteroids: (a) glucocordicoids *q.v.* (hydrocortisone and cortisone), (b) mineralocorticoids (aldosterone and deoxycorticosterone), and (c) androgens *q.v.* The cells of the cortex, when stimulated by ACTH *q.v.* produce cortisol *q.v.* ct: adrenal medulla.

ADRENALECTOMY The surgical removal of one or both adrenal glands *q.v.*

ADRENAL GLANDS 1. Endocrine glands *q.v.*, one located on the top of each kidney. They secrete hormones *q.v.* from the adrenal cortex *q.v.* and from the adrenal medulla *q.v.* The ~ are the site of epinephrine *q.v.* and cortisol *q.v.* production. 2. Glands near the kidney which produce a variety of substances including estrogen *q.v.*, androgen *q.v.*, and progestin *q.v.* 3. A member of the endocrine system *q.v.* of ductless glands *q.v.* The ~ consist of two major components: (a) a central portion (medulla), which secretes the hormone epinephrine, and (b) an outer portion (cortex), which secretes life-maintaining regulators whose role is to control salt and carbohydrate *q.v.* metabolism *q.v.*

ADRENALINE 1. The hormone *q.v.* produced by the adrenal glands *q.v.* that stimulates the heart and other organs to prepare the body for emergency reactions. 2. A hormone secreted by the adrenal glands whose effects mimic sympathetic nervous system *q.v.* arousal. 3. Epinephrine *q.v.*

ADRENAL MEDULLA The inner portion of the adrenal glands *q.v.* that secrete the hormone *q.v.* epinephrine *q.v.* ct: adrenal cortex.

ADRENARCHE The increase in adrenal androgens *q.v.* that occurs several years before puberty *q.v.* in males.

ADRENERGIC Pertaining to nerves, receptors, or actions that involve the release of epinephrine *q.v.* or norepinephrine *q.v.* Most postganglionic sympathetic nerve fibers are ~.

ADRENERGIC BLOCKER A drug acting at the sympathetic nerve endings to reduce the effectiveness of norepinephrine *q.v.* Different drugs can block the alpha, beta-1, and beta-2 functions selectively.

ADRENERGIC FIBERS Axons *q.v.* whose terminals release norepinephrine *q.v.*

ADRENERGIC SYSTEM All the nerve cells for which norepinephrine *q.v.* and epinephrine *q.v.* are the transmitter substances that consist of the nerve cells activated by acetylcholine *q.v.*

ADRENOCORTICAL HYPERPLASIA An inherited metabolic disorder that results in an excessive production of the androgens *q.v.* by the adrenal cortex *q.v.* During the prenatal *q.v.* period, this condition can cause masculinization *q.v.* of the developing genitals *q.v.* and the brain.

ADRENOCORTICOTROPIC HORMONE (ACTH) A pituitary *q.v.* hormone *q.v.* that regulates the secretion of hormones from the adrenal cortex *q.v.*; stimulates production and release of cortisol *q.v.*

ADRENOGENITAL FEMALES Pseudohermaphrodites *q.v.* cf: adrenogential syndrome.

ADRENOGENITAL SYNDROME An inherited disorder involving an enzyme *q.v.* block in the adrenal glands *q.v.* Females born with this condition frequently have masculinized *q.v.* genitals *q.v.* because of excess androgens *q.v.* exposure prenatally *q.v.* In males, genital appearances are usually unaffected.

ADRIAN PRINCIPLE A law describing the suppression of normal alpha brain waves *q.v.* of the occipital lobe *q.v.* following visual stimulation.

ADSORBENT An agent that binds chemical substances to its surface. ct: absorbent.

ADSORPTION The adhesion of liquid gaseous, or dissolved substances to the surface of a solid body resulting in a concentration of the adsorbed substances.

ADULT 1. In law, an age beyond adolescence *q.v.* This age may vary from state to state: 16 years; 18 years; 21 years are common ages. 2. A specified legal age. 3. In psychology and sociology, a person who has reached maturity *q.v.*; physical (biological), emotional, intellectual, and social.

ADULT DAY CARE 1. The social, recreational, and rehabilitative services provided for persons who require daytime supervision. 2. An alternative between care in the home and in an institution.

ADULT EDUCATION 1. Courses and other organized educational activities usually taken by people who are 17 years of age or older and excludes courses taken by full-time students in programs leading toward a diploma or academic degree and occupational programs of 6 or more months in duration. ~ includes all courses taken for credit by part-time students. Instruction may be provided by public, private educational institutions as well as business, industry, government agencies, private community organizations, and tutors. 2. Also referred to as continuing education *q.v.* or lifelong learning by some agencies.

ADULT EDUCATION CENTER An established area, usually associated with a school, private or voluntary agency, or college, wherein adult education *q.v.* courses are offered for persons who have completed or wish to complete formal educational programs. Frequently, the courses offered in an ~ are for noncredit experiences. Community colleges frequently offer a variety of courses designed to enhance the lives of adults or to provide training in special areas for improving job performance.

ADULTERANT An inexpensive substitute mixed with a pure drug or other substance.

ADULTERATED FOOD As defined by the FDA *q.v.*, food that is defective, unsafe, decomposed, filthy, or produced under unsanitary conditions. cf: adulteration.

ADULTERATION 1. Drug tampering in which inexpensive, inferior, or hazardous substances are mixed with a particular drug. 2. To make impure or inferior by adding inactive or improper substances.

ADULTERER 1. A person who commits adultery *q.v.* 2. One who has voluntary coitus *q.v.* with a person other than his or her spouse.

ADULTERY Sexual relations by a person who is married with someone other than his or her spouse.

ADULT GENDER IDENTITY The developments at puberty *q.v.* that consolidate the gender identity *q.v.* of childhood and integrate a new, adult body image with new secondary sexual characteristics *q.v.* and sexual orientation.

ADULT HEALTH EDUCATION Health education programs *q.v.* designed to meet the health needs of adults in a community *q.v.* cf: community health agencies; health education.

ADULTHOOD 1. A period in life extending from the termination of adolescence *q.v.* to death. 2. One of the stages of the life cycle *q.v.* extending from about 21 years through old age. 3. A period of biological, physical, intellectual, emotional, and social maturity *q.v.* characterized by acceptance of personal and social responsibilities.

ADULT ONSET DIABETES Type 2 diabetes mellitus *q.v.* ct: Type 1 diabetes mellitus.

ADULT RHEUMATOID ARTHRITIS Usually an insidious disease of the joints characterized by swelling, pain, and tenderness. These symptoms are usually most severe in the morning and subside with mild activity, providing fatigue is avoided.

ADVANCED ACCURATE APATHY In psychology, a form of empathy *q.v.* in which the therapist *q.v.* infers concerns and feeling that lie behind what the client is saying. It represents an interpretation. cf: primary empathy.

ADVANCED CANCER 1. Describes the stage of cancer *q.v.* in which the disease has spread from the primary cancer site to other body systems by traveling through the lymphatic system *q.v.* or blood stream and is usually irreversible. 2. Terminal cancer.

ADVANCED PLACEMENT Educational programs provided by high schools in cooperation with community colleges *q.v.* or universities in which certain qualifying students are allowed to pursue college-level courses for college credit while still in high school.

ADVENTITIA 1. The outer coat of a tube-shaped structure such as the blood vessels. 2. Tunica ~. 3. The outermost covering of a structure that does not form an integral part of the structure.

ADVENTITIOUS 1. Not inherent. 2. Acquired. 3. In botany, plant organs produced in an unusual position or at an unusual time of development.

ADVERSARIAL EVALUATION In law, in quasi-legal proceedings, a process whereby teams prepare cases for opposite sides of an issue and present them to a judge or jury in a quasi-judicial proceeding.

ADVERSE DRUG REACTION A drug reaction or effect other than the intended or anticipated one that is unusual, undesirable, discomforting, or life-threatening.

ADVISOR Counselor *q.v.*

ADVISORY ARBITRATION A neutral third party hears both sides of a dispute and renders an award that is not binding on either side.

ADVISORY COMMITTEE A group of people with expertise in some area of health functioning to gather information about a subject and to make recommendations to professional administrators of the health education program *q.v.* cf: health program; health education administrator.

ADVISORY OPINION In law, an opinion rendered by a court when no actual case is before it. State courts may render ~s; however, the United States Supreme Court and lower federal courts do not.

ADVOCACY FOR HEALTH EDUCATION A coordinated effort to influence school administrators, politicians, governmental officials, and others to implement and support comprehensive health education programs.

AEDES MOSQUITO 1. The vector *q.v.* for yellow fever. 2. A species of mosquito.

AELUROPHOBIA 1. A phobia *q.v.* 2. A morbid, irrational fear of domestic cats.

AERATION 1. To expose to air. 2. A process of water purification wherein water is forced into the air with an exchange of gases in the water and the atmosphere.

AERIAL PERSPECTIVE A secondary cue to depth *q.v.* that results from the blurring by the atmosphere of the images of distant objects.

AEROBE 1. Growing or proceeding only in the presence of oxygen. 2. With oxygen.

AEROBIC CAPACITY 1. The maximum amount of oxygen the body can process over a given period of time. 2. Aerobic power *q.v.*

AEROBIC ENERGY PRODUCTION The body's production of energy when the respiratory and circulatory systems *q.v.* are able to process and transport a sufficient amount of oxygen to the muscle cells. ct: anaerobic energy production.

AEROBIC EXERCISE 1. Exercise vigorous enough to improve the rate at which the lungs exchange oxygen. 2. Activities that increase oxygen consumption over an extended period of time. ct: anaerobic exercise.

AEROBIC PATHWAY 1. A metabolic *q.v.* pathway requiring oxygen. 2. The final pathway of carbohydrate *q.v.*, liquid *q.v.*, and protein *q.v.* metabolism *q.v.*, producing carbon dioxide, water, and energy. 3. Also known as the Krebs cycle *q.v.*, tricarboxylic acid cycle *q.v.*, or citric acid cycle *q.v.* ct: anaerobic pathway.

AEROBIC POWER 1. Aerobic capacity *q.v.* 2. The capacity of one's heart, lungs, and vascular system to deliver oxygen to working muscles.

AEROBIC RESPIRATION Respiration *q.v.*

AEROBICS 1. A variety of exercises to increase heart and lung capacity for a time period sufficiently long to produce beneficial changes in the body. 2. Exercises that demand large amounts of oxygen and that last long enough to produce a definite training effect *q.v.* on the cardiovascular, respiratory, and muscular systems. ct: anaerobic exercise.

AEROEMBOLISM A condition produced by a rapid decrease of pressure and characterized by the formation of nitrogen bubbles in the blood and body tissues.

AERO-OTITIS MEDIA Damage to the middle ear due to pressure differences.

AEROSOLS Solid particles or dust held in suspension in the air.

AESTHETE A person who is sensitive to and highly appreciative of the beauty of things; one with artistic taste. cf: aesthetic.

AESTHETIC EXPERIENCE Psychedelic *q.v.* experience marked by sensory aspects, such as fascinating alterations in perceptions *q.v.* and sensations of euphoric *q.v.* illusions *q.v.*, hallucinations *q.v.*, synesthesias *q.v.*

AESTHETIC NEEDS Associated with the beauty of life and the things of living.

AFDC An acronym for Aid to Families with Dependent Children.

AFEBRILE Without fever *q.v.*

AFFECT 1. Priorities, predispositions, and values. ~ influences cognition *q.v.* and performance. 2. Emotion *q.v.* 3. Any experience of emotion or feeling. 4. A subjective feeling or emotional tone often accompanied by bodily expressions noticeable to others.

AFFECTION 1. Love. 2. An emotional state or feeling associated with love or the need to possess.

AFFECTIVE 1. Pertaining to a person's beliefs, values, and predispositions. 2. Moods and emotions. cf: affective disorders.

AFFECTIVE COMPONENT OF EMPATHY In medicine, the component of empathy that involves being sensitive to the patient's feelings and listening to what the patient is saying about those feelings in words, gestures, and actions.

AFFECTIVE DISORDERS 1. A group of severe mental illnesses characterized by unusually deep moods, especially deep depression. 2. Disorders in which there are disabling mood disturbances. 3. Affective reactions *q.v.* 4. A group of mental disorders in which there is a prolonged, pervasive disturbance of mood; either depression or elation. cf: affective; bipolar disorder; depression; mania; unipolar affective disorder.

AFFECTIVE DOMAIN 1. That aspect of learning, especially health education that involves one's interests, attitudes, and values, and the development of appreciations and adequate adjustment. 2. Attitudinal and emotional areas of learning, such as gestures and actions. cf: affective learning; affective teaching; affective education.

AFFECTIVE-EXPERIENTIAL LEARNING 1. Pertains to learning associated with learner's beliefs, values, and emotions. Affected by learner involvement in the learning process and experiences. ~ is related to the affective domain *q.v.* focusing on emotional content in contrast to cognitive *q.v.* content. 2. Learning to do by doing. cf: affective learning.

AFFECTIVE LEARNING 1. Learning taking place within the affective domain *q.v.* 2. Pertains to learning associated with beliefs, appreciations, and values wherein learners are emotionally and actively involved in the learning experiences. 3. The acquisition of feelings, tastes, emotions, will, and other aspects of social and psychological development gained through feeling rather than through intellectualization *q.v.*

AFFECTIVE OBJECTIVES 1. Learning outcomes that stress feelings, attitudes, and values. 2. Objectives *q.v.* geared to the affective domain *q.v.* of learning.

AFFECTIVE REACTION 1. Any emotional reaction. 2. Manic-depressive reaction *q.v.* 3. Affective disorder *q.v.*

AFFECTIVE TEACHING Affective education *q.v.*

AFFERENT NEURON 1. A neuron *q.v.* that conducts impulses toward the central nervous system *q.v.* 2. Afferent nerves *q.v.* ct: efferent neuron.

AFFERENT NERVES Sensory nerves that carry impulses to the brain. ct: efferent nerves.

AFFILIATIVE The desire to join or associate with another person or group.

AFFINITY In pharmacology, the attraction and consequent interaction between a particular drug and a receptor.

AFFIRM In law, to approve or uphold a lower court's judgment.

AFFIRMATIVE ACTION 1. Activities to ensure the job success of minorities, women, and the handicapped. 2. The regulation that federal government contractors are required to give job opportunities to members of minority groups. 3. A plan by which personnel policies and hiring practices do not discriminate and women and members of minority groups.

AFFIRMATIVE ACTION PROGRAM (AAP) 1. A program to ensure the equal treatment of women and minorities. The program takes measures to see that they are recruited, hired, promoted in accordance with their abilities. 2. In the area of equal employment opportunity, programs whose basic purpose is to eliminate barriers and increase opportunities for the purpose of increasing the use or underuse of minorities and disadvantaged persons.

AFFIRMING THE CONSEQUENT An error by which, if A causes B on one occasion, it is assumed that A is the cause when B is observed on any other occasion.

AFRICAN SLEEPING SICKNESS A condition or disease caused by the bite of the tsetse fly *q.v.*

AFT And acronym for American Federation of Teachers *q.v.*

AFTERBIRTH The placenta *q.v.* and other associated tissues that are expelled from the uterus *q.v.* following the birth of a child.

AFTERCARE 1. Outpatient treatment of formerly institutionalized persons within their communities. 2. In drug or alcohol treatment programs, the long-term follow-up or maintenance support that follows a more intense period of treatment.

AFTEREFFECT OF EMOTION Any sensation that follows the perception *q.v.* of emotion *q.v.*

AFTER-THE-FACT NATURAL EXPERIMENTS 1. In research, studies in which the data are assembled after the presumed cause and effect have occurred in an attempt to demonstrate a causal relationship. 2. Ex post facto studies. 3. Causal comparative studies.

AGAMMAGLOBULINEMIA A genetic *q.v.* disease that results in the body's inability to manufacture antibodies *q.v.*

AGAMOGENESIS 1. A form of reproduction as in budding. 2. Asexual reproduction *q.v.* 3. Parthenogenesis *q.v.*

AGAPE 1. Unselfish love that is considered only with the welfare of the beloved. 2. Selfless, charitable love. 3. The Greek form of love most similar to generosity.

AGAR In bacteriology and microbiology, a gelatinous substance obtained from red algae that is used as a solidifying agent in preparation of nutrient media for growing microorganisms *q.v.* and for other purposes.

AGE COHORT Pertains to a group of people defined in terms of the period of time in which they were born.

AGED The state of being old. A person may be defined as ~ on the basis of having reached a specific age. Sixty-five is usually used for social or legislative policies, while 75 is used for physiological *q.v.* evaluation.

AGED MOLESTER An elderly person who molests children. Generally, these people have few social contacts with people in their age group.

AGE EFFECT The consequences of being a given chronological age. ct: cohort effects.

AGEISM 1. Prejudice and discrimination on the basis of age. 2. Prejudicial attitudes toward old people. 3. ~ implies a broader meaning than gerontophobia *q.v.* ~ was coined by Robert N. Butler, M.D., the first director of the National Institute on Aging.

AGENCY 1. In psychology, the feeling on the part of a person that he or she can control his or her own behavior. 2. Personal ~. 3. A tax supported governmental organization at the federal, state, or local level. 4. A donations-supported organization at the national, state, or local level. 5. An organization usually designated as governmental, official, voluntary, professional, or semiofficial.

AGENCY BILL In politics, a bill proposed by an executive agency *q.v.*

AGENCY'S CURRENT GOOD MANUFACTURING PRACTICE REGULATIONS A regulation set up by the FDA *q.v.* providing manufacturers of drugs with guidelines for the composition and manufacture of drugs.

AGENCY SHOP In labor law, though a worker is not required to join a union, he or she must pay his or her share of the cost of negotiating and servicing the master contract to the union, usually the equivalent of the union's dues. cf: closed shop; union shop.

AGE NORMS Standards of correct or appropriate behavior according to age.

AGENSIA Failure of an organ to develop or grow properly.

AGENT 1. One sector or element of the public health model of drug abuse prevention, specifically relating to various drug substances, their content, formulation, distribution, prescription, and availability. 2. In epidemiology, the causative factor of the disease. 3. In insurance, a representative of the insurance company.

AGENTS OF SOCIALIZATION People from whom one learns sexual and other values. cf: sexual values.

AGE OF CONSENT The minimum legal age a person must have attained in order to legally give permission for sexual intercourse *q.v.* ct: statutory rape.

AGE OF REASON In education, ~ marks the beginning of the modern period of educational thought that emphasizes the importance of reason *q.v.* The writings of Voltaire strongly influenced this movement and formed the basis for rationalism.

AGE SCALE A type of intelligence *q.v.* test in which items are arranged in order of difficulty and credit for passing is assigned in age units. ct: point scale.

AGE SEGREGATION The separation of people based on age; as in retirement communities or senior citizens' centers.

AGE-SPECIFIC RATE In epidemiology, the rate of an outcome calculated for a particular age group.

AGE SPOTS 1. Liver spots. 2. Senile lentigines. 3. ~ are dark brown and resemble large freckles. Although these spots appear in older people, aging is not their primary cause. Instead, ~ develop from exposure over many years to the sun's ultraviolet radiation.

AGGLUTINATION A clumping together of cells.

AGGLUTINATION TEST 1. Clumping test. 2. A pregnancy test in which the presence of the chorionic gonadotropic hormone *q.v.* is detected in the urine of a pregnant *q.v.* woman.

AGGLUTININ 1. Antibodies that function with homologous antigens *q.v.* to form lumping or agglutination *q.v.* 2. An antibody in blood plasma *q.v.* that brings about clumping of blood cells carrying an incompatible agglutinogen *q.v.* 3. Antibodies that cause a clumping of microorganisms *q.v.*

AGGLUTINOGEN 1. An antigen *q.v.* in red blood cells which reacts with a specific agglutinin *q.v.* in the plasma *q.v.* to cause a clumping of the cells. 2. A specific antigen when injected into an animal body, stimulates the production of corresponding antibody *q.v.*

AGGRAVATED ASSAULT A legal term referring to an attack by one or more persons on another for the purpose of inflicting bodily injury.

AGGRESSION 1. To attack. 2. A physical, verbal, or symbolic attack on a person, object, or situation. ~ may be realistic and self-protective or unrealistic and unprovoked. ~ may be directed outward to other things or directed inward, toward the self. 3. Standing up for personal basic rights but at the expense of someone else's basic rights. 4. Behavior designed to produce negative outcomes in other people.

AGGRESSIVE-AIM RAPIST A rapist *q.v.* whose assaults express pent-up anger and rage toward women.

AGILITY The ability to move quickly and with ease.

AGING 1. The process of growing old. 2. Aging process *q.v.* 3. The changes that occur normally in plants and animals as they grow older. Some age changes begin at birth and continue until death. Other changes begin at maturity and end at death. cf: aging research.

AGITATION 1. In psychology, marked restlessness and psychomotor *q.v.* excitement. 2. In chemistry and physics, to stir or mix vigorously.

AGNOSIA 1. Loss of comprehension of auditory *q.v.*, optic *q.v.*, or tactile *q.v.* senses, although the sensory sphere is intact. 2. The inability to recognize an object. 3. A serious disturbance in the organization of sensory information produced by lesions *q.v.* in certain cortical *q.v.* association areas. 4. A condition in which the person receives information but is unable to comprehend or interpret it. 5. Inability to recognize objects, events, sounds, and the like, even though the sense organs are not basically defective. There is usually a specific rather than general ~ : A. form agnosia; form discrimination difficulty, as in geometric forms. B. tactile agnosia; does not recognize common objects by touch alone. C. visual agnosia; difficulty in recognition of objects or people even though they should be easily recognized. D. auditory agnosia: cannot differentiate between common sounds.

AGONIST 1. In pharmacology, a drug that increases the action of another drug or a naturally produced body chemical. 2. A drug that mimics the action of a normally present biological compound. cf: hormone or neurotransmitter.

AGONISTICISM The belief that the nature of ultimate reality is not knowable; that affirmation and denial is not possible; that the existence of an ultimate reality, life beyond this one is inconceivable.

AGORAPHOBIA 1. A phobia *q.v.* 2. An irrational and morbid fear of open spaces.

AGOUTI In zoology, a grizzled color of the fur of animals resulting from altering light and dark bands on the individual hairs.

AGRAMMATISM The inability to speak words in grammatically correct order. This is a symptom of motor aphasia *q.v.* characterized by the omission of related words in a sentence.

AGRANULOCYTOSIS An acute disease in which the white blood cell count drops to extremely low levels and is characterized by high fever and infection, usually of the mouth and throat region.

AGRAPHIA 1. Loss or impairment of the ability to express ideas in writing. 2. The inability to relate a kinesthetic *q.v.* pattern requiring motor movements to a visual image of a word or letter. cf: aphasia.

AGREEMENT (method of). If two situations of a phenomenon under investigation have only one circumstance in common, the instances in which they agree is presumed to be causally related to the phenomenon.

AGRICULTURE DEPARTMENT An agency of government responsible for inspecting and grading meats, poultry, fruits, and vegetables. Also referred to as the Department of Agriculture or U.S. Department of Agriculture. Its broad functions are as follows: (a) agriculture, industry, chemistry; (b) animal industry; (c) dairy industry; (e) extension services; and (f) human nutrition and home economics.

AGUE Malarial or comparable intermittent fever.

AHA An acronym for 1. American Heart Association *q.v.* 2. American Hospital Association.

AID 1. An acronym for artificial insemination *q.v.* with sperm from a donor other than the woman's husband. 2. An acronym for Agency for International Development. ct: AIH.

AIDE 1. In politics, a legislative staff member who performs clerical, technical, or official duties. 2. In health care, one who assists nurses or other health professionals. 3. Nursing aide, also nurse's aide.

AIDS And acronym for acquired immune deficiency syndrome *q.v.*

AIDS-RELATED COMPLEX (ARC) Rarely used today, referring to a variety of chronic symptoms that occur in persons who are infected with Human Immunodeficiency Virus *q.v.* but whose conditions do not meet the Centers for Disease Control and Prevention definition of AIDS *q.v.* ARC symptoms may include unexplained swollen lymph glands *q.v.*, fever, weight loss, fatigue, and persistent diarrhea. Some physicians consider two of these symptoms and two laboratory findings, such as indication of opportunistic infection or some immune abnormality as indicative of ARC.

AIDS VIRUS (HIV) TEST A test used to detect antibodies *q.v.* against the AIDS virus (HIV) *q.v.* in blood samples. This test does not detect AIDS *q.v.* but rather the presence of the virus that can result in AIDS.

AID TO FAMILIES WITH DEPENDENT CHILDREN (AFDC) A government program providing cash support for low-income families with dependent children who have been deprived of parental support due to death, disability, continued absence of a parent, or unemployment.

AID TO THE PERMANENTLY AND TOTALLY DISABLED (APTD) A 1950 amendment to the Social Security Act *q.v.*

AIH Artificial insemination *q.v.* with sperm *q.v.* from a woman's husband. ct: AID.

AIM 1. In education, the mission of the accumulated learning experiences achieved through accomplishing goals, which act as intermediary guideposts. 2. The ultimate end result of all health learning or teaching. cf: learner aim; teacher aim; goal.

AIM-INHIBITED SEX A Freudian term for love as defined as sexual lust that cannot be expressed physically.

AIR CHISEL An air hammer used to cut away car roofs, door panels, or door posts in cases of emergency to release a victim of an automobile accident.

AIR EMBOLISM 1. A condition that results during skin diving when an air bubble occurs in the blood. 2. A condition in which air is released into the blood stream through a faulty intravenous injection or, rarely, through oral sex in which air is blown into the vagina.

AIR HUNGER Distress in breathing characterized by rapid or labored breathing or respiration.

AIR PASSAGE 1. Any of several tubes that convey air from the nose or mouth to the bronchioles *q.v.* 2. Airway. 3. A part of the respiratory system *q.v.*

AIR POLLUTION Pollution *q.v.* of the atmosphere from dumps, dust, odors, pesticides, vehicle exhausts, radiation, smoke, industrial gases, incineration smoke, and ash.

AIR SICKNESS A condition due to overstimulation of the labyrinth *q.v.*

AIR SPLINT A double-walled plastic tube in which a limb can be immobilized when air is blown into the space between the walls. An ~ is used by paramedics to immobilize an injured part of the body.

AIRWAY An anatomic passage for conveying air into and out of the lungs. Generally, the lower ~s that include passage from the epiglottis *q.v.* to the alveoli *q.v.*; and the upper ~s that include passage from the nose, mouth oropharynx *q.v.* and nasopharynx *q.v.* to the epiglottis.

AKATHESIA A side effect of major tranquilizers *q.v.* that causes the person to be restless and possibly unable to sit or to lie down quietly or to sleep.

AKINETIC SEIZURE A seizure that is evidenced by an absence or poverty of repetitive or clonic movements.

AL-ANON A twelve-step offshoot of Alcoholics Anonymous *q.v.* It is an organization of spouses, family, and friends of alcoholics *q.v.* whose purpose it is to acquire insight into the problems associated with alcoholism *q.v.*

ALALIA Delayed speech in childhood. at: aphasia.

ALARM CALL A special genetically controlled cry that impels the members of a species to take cover. ~ suggests a form of altruism *q.v.*

ALARM REACTION The initial stage of the General Adaptation Syndrome *q.v.* in which a person reacts vigorously to stress *q.v.*

ALARM STAGE In the General Adaptation Syndrome *q.v.*, the first stage of stress *q.v.* during which the body is made ready to respond to threat. There is an increase in adrenalin activity as well as cardiovascular *q.v.* and respiratory function.

AL-ATEEN An organization whose program is designed to help teenagers who have one or more alcoholic relative to understand their condition and to learn to cope. cf: Al-anon.

AL-ATOT An organization of children who have an alcoholic *q.v.* parent or sibling. cf: Al-ateen.

ALBINISM 1. The absence of pigment in the skin, hair, and eyes of animals. 2. The absence of chlorophyll *q.v.* in plants. In humans, often associated with photophobia *q.v.*, astigmatism *q.v.*, nystagmus *q.v.*

ALBINO An organism afflicted with albinism *q.v.*

ALBUMIN A water-soluble protein *q.v.* that increases the solubility of fatty acids *q.v.* in the blood, and plays a role in maintaining blood volume.

ALBUMINURIA 1. A condition in which protein *q.v.* appears in the urine. 2. Albumin *q.v.* in the urine.

ALCAPTONURIA An inherited metabolic *q.v.* disorder. Alcaptonurics excrete excessive amounts of homogentisic acid (alcapton) in the urine.

ALCHEMIST During the Middle Ages, a person who practiced alchemy *q.v.*, a form of primitive chemistry. A person who attempted to make gold in the laboratory.

ALCHEMY The practice of chemistry during the Middle Ages associated with magic, the transmutation of base metals into gold, and the development of an elixir for immortality.

ALCOHOL 1. Compounds that contain a hydroxyl group (OH) that is attached to a carbon atom. 2. Ethanol, CH_3CH_2OH or C_2H_5OH. 3. A central nervous system *q.v.* depressant *q.v.* cf: ethanol; ethyl alcohol.

ALCOHOL ABUSE In the DSM *q.v.* III, a pattern of pathological *q.v.* alcohol use that causes impairment of social or occupational functioning. cf: alcohol dependence.

ALCOHOL DEHYDROGENASE An enzyme *q.v.* in the liver that acts upon alcohol *q.v.*, oxidizing it, resulting in the release of energy, carbon dioxide, and oxygen.

ALCOHOL DEPENDENCE A physical and/or psychological compulsion to consume alcohol. This includes tolerance to alcohol and withdrawal symptoms *q.v.* upon the cessation of consumption.

ALCOHOL, DRUG ABUSE AND MENTAL HEALTH ADMINISTRATION Created in 1973 as a branch of the United States Public Health Service *q.v.* which incorporated the National Institute on Alcohol Abuse and Alcoholism.

ALCOHOLIC 1. A person who is unable consistently to choose whether he or she shall drink or not, and who, if he or she drinks, is unable to consistently choose whether he or she shall stop. 2. A person who exhibits the characteristics associated with alcoholism *q.v.* 3. A person who is physically and psychologically dependent on alcohol *q.v.* and who experiences personal and social problems from its consumption. cf: addiction; alcoholism.

ALCOHOLIC ADDICTION 1. A misnomer since alcoholic implies addiction *q.v.* 2. The uncontrolled consumption of beverage alcohol *q.v.* 3. Alcoholism *q.v.*

ALCOHOLIC HALLUCINOSIS Associated with delirium tremens *q.v.* ~ is characterized by auditory hallucinations *q.v.* ~ is distinguished from delirium tremens in that it is a more chronic condition but without the disorientation and panic.

ALCOHOLIC HEPATITIS 1. A forerunner of cirrhosis *q.v.* 2. An inflammatory *q.v.* liver disease characterized by fever, abdominal pain, and jaundice *q.v.* ~ usually subsides when alcohol intake is discontinued.

ALCOHOLIC PERSONALITY Pertains to personality *q.v.* traits, such as immaturity and dependency, that are frequently found in alcoholics *q.v.* in treatment. Many of these traits may be a result of years of heavy drinking rather than being a cause of alcoholism *q.v.*

ALCOHOLICS ANONYMOUS A voluntary fellowship of problem drinkers or alcoholics *q.v.* who desire help in maintaining sobriety. ~ was founded in 1935 in Akron, Ohio. Its program is based essentially upon its 12 steps to sobriety and 12 traditions. cf: Al-anon; Al-ateen; Al-atot.

ALCOHOLISM 1. An uncontrollable craving for alcohol *q.v.* which may take a number of forms for satisfying the craving. 2. A disease characterized by a powerful urge to drink alcohol. There are a number of theories related to the cause of ~ including (a) physiologic; (b) genetrophic; (c) genetic; (d) endocrine; (e) psychological; and (f) sociological. 3. Huss was the first to define this disease in 1849 and giving it the name alcoholismus chronicus *q.v.* 4. Jellinek called it alcoholism with complication and established five classes as follows: (a) alpha; (b) beta; (c) delta; (d) epsilon; (e) gamma. 5. A disease of some drinkers characterized in a variety of ways depending upon the drinker's genetic, psychological, and biological makeup. ~ has little to do with the form in which alcohol is drunk or the amount that is drunk or when it is drunk. It is related to the way that the drinker responds to the alcohol being drunk and the way in which it affects the drinker's behavior. ~ is closely related to why a person drinks rather than to the quantities being drunk. 6. An illness characterized by significant impairment directly associated with persistent and excessive use of alcohol. 7. Drug dependence involving progressive preoccupation with drinking, leading to physical, mental, or social dysfunction. 8. A pattern of alcohol use characterized by emotional and physical dependence as well as a general loss of control over the use of alcohol. 9. Abnormal behavior associated with chronic, excessive use of alcohol. 10. Has many different definitions, and is therefore not a precise term. Definitions may refer to pathological *q.v.* drinking behavior, such as remaining drunk for several days, to impaired functioning, such as missing work or to physical dependence. cf: substance dependence; addiction; habituation.

ALCOHOLISMUS CHRONICUS Alcoholism *q.v.*

ALCOHOL STATES OF CONSCIOUSNESS Various states of altered consciousness during the duration of alcohol's effects, depending on whether the blood alcohol concentration *q.v.* is increasing or decreasing.

ALCOMETER An instrument used to determine the amount of alcohol *q.v.* in the blood by analyzing the breath of the drinker.

ALDEHYDE A group of substances derived from the primary alcohols *q.v.* by oxidation.

ALDOSTERONE 1. An adrenal hormone *q.v.* that plays a major role in the regulation of sodium and potassium metabolism *q.v.* 2. A hormone secreted by the adrenal glands *q.v.* that facilitates retention of sodium, heightens muscle tone, aids adjustment to temperature changes, and disperses wastes.

ALE 1. An alcoholic beverage brewed by rapid fermentation *q.v.* from malt with the addition of hops. 2. A beverage related to beer *q.v.*

ALEXIA 1. The loss of the ability to read or an initial inability to learn to read due to brain damage. 2. A type of aphasia *q.v.* associated with brain lesions causing a loss of motor activity interfering with the person's ability to read. 3. Word blindness.

ALEXITHYMIA The inability to express or describe in words emotions that are felt.

ALGAE 1. A group of simple aquatic plants that range in size from microscopic to fronds hundreds of feet in length. 2. Primitive chlorophyll *q.v.* bearing plants that may serve as a source of food.

ALGEDONIC 1. Related to the pain-pleasure concept. 2. The science of pain and pleasure as goals of human conduct (H.R. Marshall).

ALGORITHM In computer problem solving, a procedure in which all of the operations are specified step by step. cf: heuristics.

ALGESIA The capacity to experience pain. cf: algedonic; ct: analgesia.

ALGOPHOBIA 1. A phobia *q.v.* 2. An irrational and morbid fear of pain.

ALIENATION 1. The condition of being uninvolved in, or estranged from others or society in general. 2. An emotional state of indifference.

ALIENIST 1. In law, a psychiatrist giving expert testimony in a medico-legal trial. 2. A psychiatrist who represents the state in psychiatric public health issues.

ALIMENTARY CANAL 1. The digestive system *q.v.* 2. The system of organs concerned with food and its digestion; the mouth, pharynx, esophagus, stomach, small and large intestines. cf: alimentary tract.

ALIMENTARY TRACT The digestive system as a whole which includes the mouth, esophagus, stomach, and intestines, along with accessory organs.

ALIMENTATION The process associated with nourishing the body which includes mastication *q.v.*, swallowing, digestion *q.v.*, absorption of nutrients, and assimilation *q.v.*

ALIMONY Money that a divorced person receives as directed by the court to be paid by the ex spouse. Payments are made in regular increments under specific conditions.

ALKALI A compound that reacts with acid to form salt and water. ct: acid.

ALKALI RESERVE 1. Bicarbonate salts present in body fluids; mainly sodium bicarbonate. 2. The total amount of alkaline salts in the plasma *q.v.* and corpuscles *q.v.* usable in maintaining the normal alkalinity of the blood.

ALKALINE Pertaining to, or having the characteristics of an alkali *q.v.*

ALKALOID 1. Any one of hundreds of plant products distinguished by basic reactions arising from heterocyclic nitrogen-containing and often complex structures. 2. Any member of a very diverse group of organic compounds containing nitrogen atoms in a ring structure; such as morphine *q.v.*, nicotine *q.v.*, and cocaine *q.v.* The chemically basic molecule is unstable and is usually prepared in the more stable form. 3. An organic compound with alkaline properties, produced by plants. These substances, which constitute the active principles of many drugs and poisons of plants have a bitter taste and are sometimes poisonous. All alkaloids contain carbon, hydrogen, and nitrogen, and most contain oxygen as well. 4. An organic base found in seed plants, usually in mixture with a number of similar alkaloids. ~s are the active chemicals that give many drugs their medicinal properties and other powerful physiological effects.

ALKALOSIS 1. A condition that results when the body loses too much carbon dioxide *q.v.* or acid *q.v.* as the result of forced breathing or severe vomiting *q.v.* 2. Alkaline intoxication *q.v.* 3. A condition in which there is an excessive proportion of alkali *q.v.* in the blood.

ALKYLATING AGENTS 1. Cell poisons used in treating cancer *q.v.* They are believed to disrupt the activity of DNA *q.v.* in the nucleus of the cancer cell. 2. One of a group of highly reactive chemical compounds that represents an important class of anticancer drugs which work by inhibiting cell growth.

ALLANTOIS An early tubular structure that pushes into and lies within the body stalk. Important allantoic (umbilical) blood vessels accompany the ~ and extend to the chorion *q.v.* which becomes vascularized through their branches. The ~ itself disappears by the fourth fetal month.

ALLANTOIS MEMBRANE Tissues that contribute to the development of the placenta *q.v.* cf: allantois.

ALLEGATION In law, statement in pleadings, setting forth what the party expects to prove.

ALLEGE In law, to state, assert, or charge; to make an allegation *q.v.*

ALLEGIANCE 1. Loyalty. 2. Faithfulness. 3. Devoted to a person, group, or country.

ALLELE 1. The pairing of genes *q.v.* 2. One of two or more contrasting characters transmitted by alternate genes. 3. One of the two or more alternative, contrasting genes that may exist at a particular locus on a chromosome *q.v.* An organism may be homozygous *q.v.* for some alleles and heterozygous *q.v.* for others. 4. Alternatives forms of genes. 5. Any one of two or more variants of a gene that can occur at a given chromosomal site.

ALLELES, MULTIPLE A series of alternative forms of a gene *q.v.*

ALLELOMORPH 1. In genetics, homologous *q.v.* genes *q.v.* similarly situated on homologous chromosomes *q.v.*

2. An allelomorphic pair; usually, one being dominant and the other recessive.

ALLERGEN 1. A protein substance that results in an allergic reaction *q.v.* 2. Environmental substances to which a person may be hypersensitive. ∼s function as antigens *q.v.*

ALLERGIC DISORDER Allergic reaction *q.v.*

ALLERGIC REACTION 1. The entrance into the body of allergens *q.v.* resulting in an altered state of tissues. 2. Hypersensitivity to a drug or other substance due to an unwanted immune system *q.v.* response. 3. A reaction that results from extreme sensitivity to a drug or agent and is not dependent on the amount of drug to which one is exposed. These may be classified into: (a) immediate and (b) delayed, based on the time it takes for the reaction to occur.

ALLERGIC RHINITIS An inflammation *q.v.* of the nasal passages, commonly referred to as hay fever *q.v.*

ALLERGY A condition characterized by a sensitivity to an allergen *q.v.* resulting in a tissue change and reaction such as running eyes, nose, and swelling of the eyes and nares *q.v.* cf: allergic reaction.

ALLEY MAZE A maze connecting the walled runways with open and closed paths used in learning experiments with small animals, such as mice. The animal is given a reward of food when it finds its way through the maze. The concept is to determine the speed with which the animal can find the right paths to the food reward.

ALLIED HEALTH PROFESSIONALS Persons with special training in areas related to medicine such as medical social work, and physical or occupational therapy. ∼ work with physicians or other related health care professionals.

ALLNESS 1. A form of behavior characterized by the tendency to assume that what a person knows is all that can be known. 2. The behavior of drawing final conclusions from insufficient data or evidence. 3. Making judgments from one level of abstractions *q.v.* as though they were identical with a lower level of abstractions. Semanticists *q.v.* consider this to be a symptom of inadequate language behavior.

ALLOCHIRIA The condition in which sensations are referred to the opposite side of the body.

ALLOEROTICISM In psychoanalysis, a tendency to love others. cf: autoeroticism; ct: narcissism.

ALLOPATHIC MEDICINE Allopathy *q.v.*

ALLOPATHIC PHYSICIAN A misnomer, referring to a physician possessing the degree of medicine.

ALLOPATHY 1. Conventional medical practice. 2. Literally, different disease. 3. A principle of healing used in medical science that involves the use of drugs to eliminate symptoms of disease. 3. Allopathic medicine. 4. A system of medical practice based on producing a condition that is incompatible with the disease being treated. 5. A form of medicine that treats disease with medications and/or surgery.

ALLOPOLYPLOID 1. In genetics, an organism with more than two sets of chromosomes *q.v.* in its body cells, derived from different species. 2. A polyploid *q.v.* having chromosome sets from different sources, such as different species. 3. A polyploid containing genetically different sets derived from two or more species.

ALLOPSYCHE A person who possesses an extraordinary interest in the outer world rather than in his or her inner life.

ALLOPURINAL A drug used to inhibit the formation of uric acid which decreases the likelihood of uremia *q.v.* developing. ∼ is used in the treatment of Lesch–Nyhan syndrome *q.v.*

ALL-OR-NONE LAW 1. Pertains to the fact that once a stimulus *q.v.* exceeds the threshold *q.v.*, further increases in the stimulus will not increase the amplitude of the action potential. 2. When a neuron *q.v.* fires, the resulting impulse is maximal or there is no impulse at all. 3. The principle that a muscle or nerve cell action states that the magnitude of the neural *q.v.* impulse and the extent of muscle response are independent of the magnitude of the stimulus.

ALLOTETRAPLOID An organism with four genomes *q.v.* derives from hybridization of different species. Usually, in forms that become established, two of the four genomes are from one species and two are from another species.

ALMONRY SCHOOL A charity school common in England during the fourteenth century by which boys could attend a monastic, abbey, or charity school that was supported by donations of food or money (almonry).

ALOGIA 1. The inability to express oneself through speech. 2. Aphasia *q.v.* 3. Logagnosia *q.v.* 4. A negative symptom in schizophrenia *q.v.*, marked by blocking and poverty of speech content. ∼ may be associated with mental retardation.

ALOPECIA 1. Loss of hair. 2. Baldness.

ALOPECIA AREATA Irregular loss of hair on the scalp or body. ct: alopecia totalis.

ALOPECIA TOTALIS General loss of hair over the entire body. ct: alopecia areata.

ALPHA 1. In epidemiology, the probability of rejecting a null *q.v.* hypothesis when it is true. 2. Type I error *q.v.*

ALPHA ALCOHOLISM Alcoholism *q.v.* characterized by the person drinking amounts of alcohol beyond the social norm.

ALPHA ANDROSTENOL A male pheromone *q.v.*

ALPHA BLOCKING The disruption of the alpha rhythm by visual stimulation or by active thought with the eyes closed. cf: alpha waves.

ALPHA COEFFICIENT A measure of internal consistency reliability *q.v.* cf: Cronbach's alpha.

ALPHA ERROR Type I error *q.v.*

ALPHA-KETOGLUTARIC ACID A compound that is common to the metabolic *q.v.* pathways of carbohydrates *q.v.*, fats, and certain amino acids *q.v.*

ALPHA LEVEL The percentage of instances, on the average, that a researcher will conclude that a value is atypical when in fact it is not.

ALPHA RAYS Rays of alpha particles *q.v.* that have the power to penetrate the body.

ALPHA PARTICLE A particle, identical to the nucleus *q.v.* of a helium atom, emitted by some radioactive *q.v.* materials.

ALPHA RECEPTOR Post-junctional receptor *q.v.* site that responds to norepinephrine *q.v.*

ALPHA RHYTHM 1. A rhythm of the electroencephalogram *q.v.* typically obtained from the occipital *q.v.* region of the cortex *q.v.* and has an average frequency of about 10 cycles per second. 2. The dominant pattern in a restful but wakeful adult. cf: alpha waves.

ALPHA WAVES Fairly regular EEG *q.v.* waves, between 8 and 12/s, characteristic of a relaxed, waking state, usually with eyes closed. cf: alpha blocking; alpha rhythm.

ALPRAZOLAM 1. A benzodiazepine sedative *q.v.* 2. Xanax is a brand name.

ALS An acronym for amyotrophic lateral sclerosis *q.v.*

ALTERED STATES OF CONSCIOUSNESS (ASC) Profound changes in mood, thinking, and perception *q.v.*

ALTEREGOISM 1. Possessing a tendency to have sympathy only with others who resemble self. 2. Relating to others who experience similar feelings with self.

ALTERNATE HYPOTHESIS 1. In epidemiology, a statistical statement that expresses a relationship between two or more variables *q.v.* 2. In statistics, the hypothesis *q.v.* that the null hypothesis *q.v.* is false.

ALTERNATION OF GENERATION In genetics, the alternation of gametophytic *q.v.* and sporophytic *q.v.* generations in the life cycle. The sporophyte develops from the zygote *q.v.* and produces spores *q.v.* The gametophyte *q.v.* develops from the spore and produces gametes *q.v.* The cells of the sporophyte generation contain twice as many chromosomes *q.v.* as those of the gametophyte.

ALTERNATION OF NEUROSIS The remission of symptoms *q.v.* of a mental illness *q.v.* during an acute physical disease *q.v.*

ALTERNATIVE BIRTH CENTER (ABC) A hospital setting that is an alternative to home birth and traditional hospital birth.

ALTERNATIVE CERTIFICATION In education, teacher licensure obtained through other than traditional course work in education courses.

ALTERNATIVE CONDITIONS In research, conditions sufficient for an effect to occur, but since the effect may occur in the absence of the conditions as well, they are not necessary.

ALTERNATIVE EDUCATION An educational program consisting of unconventional experiences for learners who are inadequately served or taught in regular classes. Alternatives include schools without walls, street academies, free schools, and second-chance schools. cf: alternative school.

ALTERNATIVE FUTURES A method used by futurists to identify and forecast possible scenarios based on current trends.

ALTERNATIVE HYPOTHESIS A statement of what the statistical hypothesis is designed to measure. The final conclusion if stated in terms of the null hypothesis *q.v.*

ALTERNATIVES 1. In drug education, assuming that there are motives *q.v.* for drug use, such as the need to be accepted by a group, many educational prevention programs teach alternative methods for satisfying those motives. 2. In philosophy, competing courses of action or beliefs in which the person must decide which choice to make. 3. In sociology, the traits in a particular culture shared by several individuals but not common to all and that represent different ways of achieving the same goals or ends. cf: alternative approach.

ALTERNATIVES APPROACH In drug education, techniques of drug abuse prevention that provide persons with attractive, optional nondrug substitutes not only to drugs, but to drug using lifestyles. cf: alternatives.

ALTERNATIVE EXPLANATION Rival explanations *q.v.*

ALTERNATIVE MEDICINE Any field of medicine that does not conform to the principles of traditional medical practice.

ALTERNATIVE SCHOOL A school—private, public, innovative, or fundamental—that provides learners with options or alternatives *q.v.* to the regular public school. cf: alternative education.

ALTITUDE SICKNESS A disturbance resulting from repeated flying at high altitudes with insufficient oxygen intake.

ALTRUISM 1. In sociology, any behavior pattern that benefits individual's who are not one's offspring. 2. Behavior that benefits others and is carried out with no expectations of reward. 3. (Selfishness) behavior in which the welfare of others is internalized as part of the person's own welfare to the degree desired by a given society. The distinction, thus turns on the composition of the self, not whether the action is self-oriented. 4. A system of ethics *q.v.* based on the idea of the ultimate obligation of each person to achieve a selfless devotion to others, society, as opposed to the ethical doctrine of egoism *q.v.* and to the theological doctrines of the individual pursuit of charity beatitude. 5. Generally, the pursuit of the good in others. ct: kin-selection hypothesis; alarm call; reciprocal-altruism hypothesis; hedonism.

ALTRUISTIC SUICIDE 1. Self-destruction intended to serve a social purpose or cause. 2. Self-annihilation that the person feels will serve a social purpose, such as self-immolations practiced by Buddhist monks during the Vietnam War.

ALUMINUM SPLINT Rigid splint *q.v.*

ALURATE 1. Brand name for aprobarbital *q.v.* 2. A commercial preparation of aprobarbital.

ALVEOLAR AIR 1. The air in the alveoli *q.v.* of the lungs. 2. The residual air *q.v.*

ALVEOLAR RIDGES The ridges in either jaw containing cavities or sockets for the teeth.

ALVEOLI 1. The smallest airways in the lungs that contain the membranes through which gases are exchanged with the blood. 2. Thin, sac-like terminal ends of the airways in the lungs. 3. The sites at which gases are exchanged between the blood and the inhaled air. There are between 3 and 4 billion ~ in the lungs. The milk secreting cells in the female breast.

ALVEOLUS A small cavity. cf: alveoli.

ALVINE 1. Pertaining to the intestines. 2. A class of infectious diseases characterized by intestinal discharge, e.g., the dysenteries *q.v.*

ALZ-50 A complex protein found in the brain of persons suffering from Alzheimer's disease *q.v.*

ALZHEIMER'S DISEASE 1. Degeneration of the brain cells. 2. A gradual development of memory loss, confusion, and loss of reasoning. ~ can eventually lead to total intellectual incapacitation, brain degeneration, and death. 3. A pre-senile dementia *q.v.* 4. A dementia involving rapid intellectual deterioration, speech impairment, loss of body control, and death, usually within 5 years of onset. 5. A dementia involving a progressive atrophy *q.v.* of cortical *q.v.* tissue and marked by speech impairment, involuntary movements, occasional convulsions, intellectual deterioration, and psychotic behavior. ~ was first described in 1906 by the German neurologist, Alois Alzheimer.

AMA An acronym for American Medical Association *q.v.*

AMANITA MUSCARIA 1. Brand name for hallucinogenic mushroom. 2. The fly agaric mushroom, widely used since ancient times for its hallucinogenic *q.v.* properties.

AMASTIA Failure of breast development in the female.

AMAUROTIC 1. Blindness resulting from a defect of the optic nerve. 2. Designates absolute blindness from any cause or etiology *q.v.* 3. Amaurosis.

AMOURAOTIC IDIOCY 1. Also, amaurotic familial idiocy. 2. A recessive genetic defect manifested as a progressive degeneration of the brain resulting in blindness, muscle waste, and mental retardation, more frequently found in infancy than in later years.

AMBIDEXTERITY (AMBIDEXTRALITY) The ability to use both hands with equal or near equal skill and ease.

AMBIENT Surrounding.

AMBIGUITY 1. A situation in which a statement has two or more meanings. 2. The quality of a statement being easily influenced by subjective factors; the lack of precision or clarity in the wording of a statement such as a test item. 3. In language, words may possess more than one meaning depending on the context in which they are used, their cultural influence, or historical development.

AMBILATERAL Pertaining to both sides of the body.

AMBISEXUAL 1. Bisexual *q.v.* 2. A person who enjoys sexual relations with members of both sexes. 3. A term used by Master and Johnson to refer to men or women who have no preference over the gender of their sex partners and who accept or reject sexual opportunities based on their own physical needs.

AMBIVALENCE 1. Simultaneous attractions to and repulsion from an object, person, or situation. 2. Perception of both positive and negative aspects occurring in the same thing at the same time. 3. Simultaneous hold of two incongruent ideas or aspirations at the same time. 4. In conflict theory *q.v.*, a reaction toward an object that is simultaneously one of approach and avoidance.

AMBIVALENT TRANSFERENCE Analysis of transference *q.v.*

AMBIVERT 1. In type theory *q.v.*, a person who is both introverted *q.v.* and extroverted (extraverted) *q.v.* 2. A person whose interests are equally divided between personal and environmental factors (ambiversion).

AMBLYOPIA 1. "Lazy eye," the most frequent cause of visual impairment in preschool children. 2. Visual weakness or dimness without associated organic pathology *q.v.* of the eye structure. 3. A dimness of vision. cf: congenital ~; toxic ~; hysterical ~.

AMBLIOPIA EX ANOPSIA 1. A weakness of vision resulting from functional disuse of the eyes. 2. Partial loss of vision caused by an act of inhibition or suppression; a defense mechanism *q.v.*, such as a squint. ct: diplopia.

AMBLYSTOMA A class of salamander used in developmental research esp. associated with prenatal development.

AMBULANCE STRETCHER A carrying device used to transport injured victims to, from, and in an ambulance; usually wheeled.

AMBULATION Walking, or the ability to move about.

AMBULATORY (CARE) Outpatient care that does not require hospitalization.

AMBULATORY SCHIZOPHRENIA Mild schizophrenia *q.v.* that does not require hospitalization while the schizophrenic continues to live and function in the community.

AMEBA (AMOEBA) A protozoan *q.v.* 2. Some ameba (amoeba) produce disease in humans: amebic dysentery *q.v.*

AMEBIASIS 1. An infection *q.v.* with the *Entamoeba histolytica*. 2. Amebic dysentery *q.v.* 3. A parasitic infection of the colon that results in diarrhea *q.v.*

AMEBIC DYSENTERY 1. An intestinal disease caused by a protozoan *q.v.*, the ameba *q.v.* 2. Amebiasis *q.v.* cf: bacillary dysentery.

AMEBOID MOVEMENT 1. Movement that is characteristic of amebae *q.v.* 2. Movement by projections of protoplasm *q.v.* called pseudopodia *q.v.* toward the rest of the cell's protoplasm flows.

AMENDMENT In legislative politics, any alteration made or proposed to be made in a bill, motion, or clause thereof, by adding, changing, substituting, or omitting.

AMENDMENT (CONSTITUTIONAL) In legislative politics, resolution passes by both houses that affects the Constitution. Such ~ requires approval by voters at a general election. cf: referendum.

AMENIA Amenorrhea *q.v.*

AMENORRHEA 1. The absence or abnormal stoppage of menstruation *q.v.* 2. Amenia *q.v.* 3. ~ can be caused by obesity *q.v.* or extreme underweight *q.v.*, a disorder of the hypothalamus *q.v.*, a deficiency of the ovaries *q.v.*, or pituitary gland, or pregnancy *q.v.*, and lactation *q.v.* 4. The absence of menstruation for three or more months when a woman is not pregnant, going through menopause *q.v.* nor breast feeding. Two types are: (a)primary ~; the failure to begin menstruation; and (b) secondary ~; the disappearance of menstruation once it has begun.

AMENT A person lacking in intelligence; a mentally retarded person. cf: amentia.

AMENTIA Inferior mental capacity originating before or shortly after birth. ct: dementia; cf: retardation.

AMERICAN ALLIANCE FOR HEALTH, PHYSICAL EDUCATION, RECREATION AND DANCE (AAHPERD) An organization founded in 1885 as the American Association for the Advancement of Physical Education. It became a department of the National Education Association in 1937.

AMERICAN ACADEMY OF HEALTH BEHAVIOR (AAHB) A professional association of health educators, the primary purpose of which is to foster the advancement of health education through research.

AMERICAN ASSOCIATION FOR HEALTH EDUCATION (AAHE) A division of AAHPERD q.v., whose purpose it is to advance the cause of and to enhance the professionalism of health education.

AMERICAN CANCER SOCIETY An organization founded in 1913 for the purpose of disseminating information relative to cancers, to conduct research, and to compile significant data about cancers.

AMERICAN COLLEGE TESTING PROGRAM (ACT) College entrance examination used by many universities for the purpose of screening college entrance candidates.

AMERICAN DENTAL ASSOCIATION (ADA) An organization founded in 1860 to advance the dental profession.

AMERICAN FEDERATION OF TEACHERS (AFT) A national teachers' organization, historically, second in size only to the National Education Association (NEA), and now affiliated with the NEA, concerned with improving educational conditions and teachers' rights.

AMERICAN HEART ASSOCIATION An organization founded in 1948 as an outgrowth of a scientific and professional organization of physicians interested in heart disease. Its purpose is to prevent and control heart disease through research, education, and community service.

AMERICAN LAW INSTITUTE GUIDELINES Rules proposing insanity to be a legitimate defense plea when during criminal conduct a person could not judge right from wrong or control his/her behavior as required by law. Repetitive criminal acts are disavowed as a sole criterion. cf: M'Naghten rule; irresistible impulse.

AMERICAN LUNG ASSOCIATION An organization founded in 1904 as the National Tuberculosis and Respiratory Disease Association. The first voluntary agency whose primary purpose revolved around education and promotion of health.

AMERICAN MEDICAL ASSOCIATION (AMA) A professional organization founded in 1847 with the objective to promote the art of medicine and the betterment of public health. It serves the interests of medical practitioners.

AMERICAN MEDICO-PSYCHOLOGICAL ASSOCIATION A professional organization founded in 1893 as an outgrowth of the American Medical Superintendents of American Institutions for the Insane.

AMERICAN NATIONAL RED CROSS A voluntary organization founded in 1881; under a charter granted by Congress. The President of the United States is the President of the American Red Cross. It was founded in accordance with the Geneva Treaty of 1864. It basically provides relief services during times of disaster, including war.

AMERICAN PUBLIC HEALTH ASSOCIATION (APHA) A professional organization founded in 1872 concerned with all factors affecting the health of people.

AMERICAN STANDARD A safety device for the outlet valves of large gas-filled cylinders to prevent the attachment of a pressure regulator for one gas to the cylinder of another gas.

AMESLAN Slang for American Sign Language.

AME'S TEST A test used to investigate a chemical's ability to induce genetic *q.v.* damage.

AMETROPIA 1. Hypertropia *q.v.* 2. Myopia *q.v.* 3. Astigmatism *q.v.*

AMHPS An acronym for Association of Minority Health Professions.

AMICUS CURIAE 1. In law, literally, friend of the court. 2. One who volunteers or is requested to give information to the court regarding some matter of law in regard to which the judge is doubtful or mistaken. 3. One who has no right to appear in a case but is allowed to file a brief or enter into the argument because of an indirect interest. 4. Generally, one who has an indirect interest in a case and offers or is requested to provide information to the court in order to clarify particular matters before the court.

AMINIA 1. A condition characterized by the loss of the ability to comprehend gestures or to express them. 2. A form of apraxia *q.v.* when motor functioning is involved; a form of aphasia *q.v.* when sign language is involved.

AMINATION 1. The addition of an amino acid *q.v.* group to a molecule. 2. The process by which the elements of nitrogen in the -3 oxidation state are transferred to organic structures, forming an amine *q.v.* compound.

AMINE 1. A substance that has an NH_2 group in its chemical structure. 2. A chemical compound formed from ammonia by replacement of one or more hydrogen atoms *q.v.* with hydrocarbon groups *q.v.* 3. The chemical group NH_2; also used as a prefix.

AMINO ACIDS 1. Nutrient essentials that are changed into body protein within the cell. However, all essential and nonessential ~ must be present. Proteins are composed of ~. 2. The building blocks of protein. 3. Any one of a large group of organic acids characterized by an amino group (NH_2) and a carboxyl group (COOH). 4. The structural unit of proteins. 5. Any one of a class of organic compounds containing the amino group and the carboxyl group. Alanine, proline, threonine, histidine, lysine, glutamine, phenylalanine, tryptophan, valine, arginine, and leucine are among the common amino acids. cf: essential amino acids (Table A-1).

TABLE A-1 CLASSIFICATION OF AMINO ACIDS*

ESSENTIAL	NONESSENTIAL
Threonine	Glycine
Isoleucine	Alanine
Leucine	Serine
Valine	Tyrosine
Phenylalanine	Hydroxyproline
Tryptophan	Cysteine[b]
Methionine	Aspartic acid
Lysine (infants)	Glutamic acid
Histidine	Hydroxylysine
Arginine[a]	
	Citrulline
	Hydroxyglutamic acid
	Norleucine
	Proline

*Although there are about 80 amino acids that have been identified, there are only about 25 that appear necessary for human growth and metabolism. Of these, at least 9 are classed as *essential* since they must be obtained in the food people eat. There are about 14 classed as *nonessential* since the human body is capable of producing them. It is important to note that before human cells can produce body protein, all of the essential and nonessential acids must be present. These are the building locks of protein production which is the essential ingredient of life.

[a]Arginine is regarded as nonessential for adults, but cannot be formed in infants, therefore, its dietary supply is essential in early life.

[b]Cysteine in the diet may substitute for upwards of 30% of the methionine requirement.

AMITOSIS 1. Division of the chromatin body of the prokaryotic cell. 2. In biology, direct cell division that does not involve the formation of chromosomes *q.v.* or a spindle *q.v.* ct: mitosis.

AMITRIPTYLINE 1. A heterocyclic antidepressant *q.v.* 2. Elavil and Endep are commercial or brand names.

AMMONIFICATION The formation of ammonia by decaying organisms of the soil acting upon proteinaceous compounds.

AMNESIA 1. A defense mechanism. 2. The repression *q.v.* of entire episodes of life as a reaction to extremely painful situations. Usually considered a neurotic reaction *q.v.* 3. Loss of memory usually selective, involving only anxiety-provoking situations. 4. ~ may occur as a result of physical injury or psychological stress as the product of repression *q.v.* 5. Total or partial loss of memory that can be associated with a dissociative disorder *q.v.*, and organic brain syndrome *q.v.* or hypnosis *q.v.* Two major forms: (a) anterograde; loss of memory for events that have just occurred; or (b) retrograde; loss of memory for events immediately preceding a traumatic *q.v.* incident, and sometimes for events extending far back in time. cf: psychogenic amnesia.

AMNIOCENTESIS 1. The withdrawing of a sample of amniotic fluid *q.v.*, culturing the cells shed by the fetus *q.v.*, and examining them for biological and chromosomal *q.v.* defects. 2. Amniotic tap. 3. The analysis of a sample of fluid drawn from the sac surrounding the fetus to detect chromosomal aberrations. 4. A process of withdrawing amniotic fluid during the 14th to 18th weeks of pregnancy for the purpose of monitoring the growth of the fetus. 5. A process of determining the genetic makeup of the fetus to evaluate the potentials for abnormality after birth. cf: chronic villus sampling.

AMNION 1. The membrane *q.v.* that surrounds the embryo *q.v.* within the uterus *q.v.* that secretes amniotic fluid *q.v.* to form a bag of waters *q.v.* 2. The innermost membrane of the uterus enclosing the developing fetus. 3. The fluid-filled membrane in the uterus that protects the fetus during prenatal *q.v.* development.

AMNIOTIC FLUID The fluid secreted by the amnion *q.v.* which immerses the fetus *q.v.* in the uterus *q.v.* prior to birth. cf: amniotic sac.

AMNIOTIC SAC The sac containing the watery fluid that surrounds the developing fetus *q.v.* in the uterus *q.v.* cf: amniotic fluid.

AMNIOTIC TAP Amniocentesis *q.v.*

AMOBARBITAL 1. A barbiturate *q.v.* sedative-hypnotic *q.v.* 2. Amytal is a commercial preparation and brand name.

AMORAL 1. In psychology and sociology, acts, attitudes, or discriminatory judgments that are not moral *q.v.*; the inability to judge right from wrong, good from bad. 2. Morally or ethically indifferent or neutral toward actions.

AMORPH In genetics, a mutant allele *q.v.* that has little or no effect on the expression of a trait *q.v.*

AMPHIBOLY A fallacy of ambiguity *q.v.* because of the way words are arranged in a sentence.

AMPHIMIXIS In sexual reproduction, the mixing or uniting of the germ cells *q.v.* from two different persons.

AMOTIVATIONAL SYNDROME 1. A pattern of personality *q.v.* changes observed in some frequent users of marijuana *q.v.*, marked by apathy, lack of concern for the future, and loss of motivation, persisting beyond the period of intoxication *q.v.* 2. A behavioral pattern characterized by widespread apathy toward productive activities.

AMOXAPINE 1. A heterocyclic *q.v.* antidepressant *q.v.* drug. 2. Asendin is a commercial preparation and brand name.

AMP An acronym for adenosine monophosphate *q.v.* cf: adenosine triphosphate.

AMPHETAMINE 1. The most powerful stimulant *q.v.* known. 2. A colorless, volatile liquid with three basic chemical forms: (a) salts of racemic amphetamine, (b) dextroamphetamine, and (c) methamphetamine. ~ potentiates the effects of norepinephrine *q.v.* ~ releases norepinephrine normally stored in the nerve endings, which concentrates in higher centers of the brain resulting in an increased heart action and metabolism *q.v.* 3. A sympathomimetic *q.v.* 4. Benzedrine is a commercial preparation and brand name. Used medically to relieve depression or to lose weight. Misuse results in tremors, talkativeness, hallucinations, excitability, and paranoid *q.v.* delusions *q.v.* 5. Other common commercial preparations are dexedrine and theadrine.

AMPHETAMINE CHALLENGE A single, small dose of amphetamine *q.v.* given to a schizophrenic person to evaluate probable response to treatment with phenothiazine *q.v.* drugs.

AMPHIARTHROSIS A slightly movable joint.

AMPHIASTER In cytology, a figure formed in mitotic *q.v.* cell division consisting of two asters *q.v.* connected by a spindle *q.v.*

AMPHIBIOUS In biology, an animal that is able to live on land and in water.

AMPHIMIXIS The union of the germplasm of two individuals in sexual reproduction.

AMPHOTERIC 1. In chemistry, having both acidic and basic properties. 2. Amphoterism.

AMPULE 1. A sealed glass container of sterile medication. 2. Ampoule.

AMPULLA 1. The dilated section of a tubular structure. 2. A sac-like dilation of a tube or duct *q.v.* 3. A flask-like widening at the end of a tubular structure or canal. 4. Enlarged area of the vas deferens *q.v.* used to store the sperm *q.v.* 5. The middle part of a fallopian tube *q.v.*

AMPUTATION 1. The cutting off of a limb or any other projecting part by surgical means. 2. The lack of a limb resulting from a congenital *q.v.*, injury, disease, or surgery *q.v.*

AMT An acronym for American Medical Technologists.

AMUSIA A condition characterized by the ability to recognize or to reproduce musical sounds.

AMYGDALE 1. An almond-shaped structure. 2. More specifically, a nuclear complex in the temporal lobe *q.v.* that is important for limbic system *q.v.* function. 3. An area of the brain shoes destruction results in excessive sexual behavior. 4. An obsolete designation for tonsil.

AMYGDALIN A poisonous substance that releases cyanide when acted upon by enzymes *q.v.* in the body. It is an active ingredient of Laetrile *q.v.* an unproven treatment for cancer *q.v.*

AMYL ALCOHOL 1. A form of alcohol *q.v.* that is unfit for human consumption. 2. ~ has a chemical formula of $C_5H_{11}OH$.

AMYLASE 1. Ptyalin *q.v.* 2. An enzyme *q.v.* that hydrolyzes *q.v.* starch in the body.

AMYL NITRATE A drug that relaxes muscle spasms. ~ is sometimes used to prolong or intensify an orgasm *q.v.* cf: amyl nitrite; butyl nitrate.

AMYL NITRITE 1. A prescription drug used in the treatment of angina *q.v.* 2. ~ is used recreationally as a euphoriant *q.v.* and presumed sexual stimulant. 3. A volatile organic compound, which, when inhaled, produces dilation of the blood vessels. cf: amyl nitrate.

AMYOTONIA CONGENITA 1. A relatively rare disease characterized by a pronounced flaccidity *q.v.* of the muscles. Oppenheim's disease *q.v.*

AMYOTROPHIC LATERAL SCLEROSIS (ALS) 1. Lou Gehrig's disease. 2. One of the neuromuscular diseases *q.v.* 3. An incurable, degenerative disease *q.v.* of the nervous system *q.v.*

AMYTAL 1. Commercial preparation of amobarbital *q.v.* one of the barbiturates *q.v.* 2. A barbiturate.

ANA An acronym for American Nurses Association.

ANABOLIC STEROID 1. Ant of the synthetic derivatives of testosterone *q.v.* 2. A steroid hormone *q.v.* that promotes general body growth (anabolism). 3. One of the synthetic androgens *q.v.* 4. Synthetically produced drug that is associated with tissue building. The ~s have masculinizing properties, decrease normal testosterone production, increase fluid retention, cause personality changes, and may increase the incidence of kidney and liver tumors *q.v.*

ANABOLISM 1. A phase of metabolism *q.v.* characterized by a chemical synthesis *q.v.* within the body. 2. The energy-requiring metabolic processes in which body substances are synthesized from simpler substances. 3. Constructive, or synthetic metabolism: photosynthesis *q.v.*, assimilation *q.v.*, and synthesis of body proteins. ct: catabolism.

ANACLISIS 1. In psychoanalysis, a condition characterized by dependence upon another person for care and support. 2. A fixation of development characterized by dependence upon a child and its mother.

ANACLITIC DEPRESSION In psychology, the profound sadness of an infant when separated from its mother for a prolonged period of time.

ANACLITIC IDENTIFICATION Developmental identification *q.v.*

ANACLITIC OBJECT CHOICE In psychology, the choice of a love object similar in nature to those who have cared for him or her in earlier years; usually a mother object.

ANACUSIA 1. A condition characterized by total deafness. 2. Anacusis.

ANAEROBE An organism capable of growing in the absence of atmospheric oxygen. cf: anaerobic.

ANAEROBIC 1. Pertaining to organisms that grow and reproduce without the presence of oxygen. 2. Proceeding the absence of or not requiring oxygen. ct: aerobic.

ANAEROBIC ENERGY PRODUCTION The body's production of energy when needed amounts of oxygen are not readily available. ct: aerobic energy production.

ANAEROBIC EXERCISE Exercise that does not require the lungs to increase the rate at which oxygen is exchanged. cf: anaerobics; ct: aerobics.

ANAEROBIC GLYCOLYSIS Glycolysis anaerobic *q.v.*

ANAEROBIC PATHWAY 1. A set of energy-producing reactions that can proceed in the absence of oxygen. 2. Glycolysis *q.v.* 3. Embden–Meyerhof pathway *q.v.* ct: aerobic pathway.

ANAEROBIC RESPIRATION A type of respiration *q.v.* found only in bacteria *q.v.* in which the hydrogen released in glycolysis *q.v.* is combined with the bound oxygen of inorganic *q.v.* compounds.

ANAEROBICS An activity performed at such a high intensity that there is insufficient time for the use of atmospheric oxygen at the tissue level, and thus oxygen debt is created. cf: anaerobic exercise.

ANAEROBIC THRESHOLD The point at which anaerobic energy begins to supplement the already sizable aerobic *q.v.* contributions.

ANAL Pertaining to the anus *q.v.*

ANAL CANAL The terminal portion of the alimentary canal *q.v.* extending from the rectum *q.v.* to its distal *q.v.* opening, the anus *q.v.*

ANALEPTIC A drug that stimulates the central nervous system *q.v.*

ANAL EROTICISM 1. Pleasurable sensations in the region of the anus *q.v.* 2. In psychoanalytic theory *q.v.*, a fixation of libido *q.v.* at the anal stage of development with persistent attempts to maintain pleasurable sensations in the anal region and with anal character traits of obsessive orderliness, cleanliness, and miserliness.

ANALGESIA 1. Relief of pain. 2. Loss or impairment of pain sensibility. 3. An insensitivity to pain without the loss of consciousness; sometimes found in conversion disorder.

ANALGESIC 1. Pain-relieving preparation. 2. A drug that produces relief from pain without loss of consciousness. 3. A class of pain-relieving drugs. 4. A drug producing a selective reduction of pain. ct: anesthetic.

ANALGESIC (EXTERNAL) A chemical or drug applied topically to relieve pain. cf: analgesic (internal).

ANALGESIC (INTERNAL) 1. A drug taken by mouth in tablet or capsule form to relieve pain. 2. A drug administered internally for the relief of pain. cf: analgesic (external).

ANALINGUS Oral stimulation of the anus *q.v.*

ANALISM A sexual variance *q.v.*

ANALOGOUS Similar in function.

ANALOGUE EXPERIMENT 1. An experimental study of a phenomenon different from but related to the actual interests of the investigator. 2. The attempts to recreate and study, in controlled situations, behavior that is analogous to naturally occurring psychopathology *q.v.*

ANALOGY Similarity that derives from having a common function or structure without regard to evolutionary origins. ct: homology.

ANAL PERSONALITY An adult who, when anal retentive, is found by psychoanalytic theory *q.v.* stingy and sometimes obsessively clean. 2. When anal compulsive, to be aggressive. Such traits are assumed to be caused by fixation *q.v.* through either excessive or inadequate gratification of id *q.v.* impulses during the anal stage *q.v.* of psychosexual development *q.v.*

ANAL STAGE In psychoanalytic theory, *q.v.*, the stage of psychosexual development *q.v.* during which the focus of pleasure is on activities associated with elimination. ct: oral stage; phallic stage; latency stage.

ANAL STIMULATION Anal eroticism *q.v.*

ANAL TRIAD The syndrome *q.v.* of parsimony *q.v.*, pedantry *q.v.*, and petulance *q.v.* assumed in psychoanalytic theory *q.v.* to result from fixation *q.v.* at the anal stage *q.v.* of development.

ANALYSAND A person being psychoanalyzed *q.v.*

ANALYSIS 1. The process of resolving a problem into its component parts. 2. An intellectual process beginning with an assumption of the truth or conclusion followed by the gathering of data to support or reject this conclusion. 3. In psychology, a process consisting of distinguishing the elements that go into making up a complex state of mind *q.v.* 4. In logic, a process of attaining clarity of thought by breaking down the whole into distinguishable parts. 5. The process of determining how parts are related to each other within the whole. ct: synthesis.

ANALYSIS OF COVARIANCE A statistical technique for adjusting the means of groups for the effect of an unwanted variable *q.v.*

ANALYSIS OF RESISTANCE When a person exhibits resistance during free association *q.v.* during psychoanalysis *q.v.*, the therapist must attempt to break down the resistance so that the person becomes conscious of the painful conflict. ct: analysis of transference.

ANALYSIS OF TEACHING A contemporary trend to encourage teachers to critique their own performance in the classroom.

ANALYSIS OF TRANSFERENCE A phase of psychoanalysis *q.v.* characterized by the person developing an emotional attachment to the therapist *q.v.* The attachment may be of admiration or love, and called positive transference; hostility called negative transference; or a combination of these two called ambivalent transference. ct: analysis of resistance.

ANALYSIS OF VARIANCE (ANOVA) Estimates of the population variance are made from the variability between groups, presumed to be affected by the intervention or independent variable of interest, and from the within-group variable, which is not so influenced. Comparison of estimates from these two sources shows whether the former is larger than the latter by a ratio (F ratio) greater than would be expected by the influence of random sampling and chance error.

ANALYST Psychoanalyst *q.v.*

ANALYTE A chemical component of a sample to be determined or measured.

ANALYTIC APPROACH In reading education, a method of diagnosing reading difficulties for the purpose of identifying the specific elements that are weak and need remedial training. The ~ assumes that reading ability consists of specific skills that can be identified.

ANALYTIC EPIDEMIOLOGY That phase of epidemiology *q.v.* that attempts to find significant relationships between the frequency, distribution, and other characteristics of the disease process. cf: descriptive epidemiology; experimental epidemiology.

ANALYTIC INDUCTION In research, finding commonalities and regularities in qualitative data, seeking their explanation, and finding other situations in which to test the generality of that explanation.

ANALYTIC METHOD In reading education, a method of teaching reading wherein the whole is presented first and then broken down into its elements. In phonics *q.v.*, the analysis of a word for pronunciation purposes. ct: synthetic method.

ANALYTIC PLAY THERAPY 1. Play therapy *q.v.* 2. ~ is used most by child therapists when the child is too young to talk out his or her problems or feelings.

ANALYTIC PSYCHOLOGY 1. A school or system of psychology *q.v.* 2. According to Carl Jung, the psychological system consisting of growth, action, food, comfort, and reproduction. 3. The systematic study of human behavior characterized by selecting the major factors, arranging them in a logical order, separating them into their parts and considering their relationship to each other and to the whole of psychological thought.

ANALYTIC-SYNTHETIC METHOD In reading education, combining the methods of analytic and synthetic teaching in which reading is taught by taking each word and breaking it down into its parts and then fusing it back into its whole.

ANALYTIC THEORY (OF PERSONALITY) 1. Emphasizes the importance of one's goals and strivings as well as one's past experiences in the development of the personality *q.v.* This theory is centered around four psychological functions: (a) thinking, (b) feelings, (c) sensing, and (d) intuition 2. ~ was developed by Carl Jung.

ANALYZERS Researchers who see challenging and validating hypotheses as the main business of science. They are like the natural scientists in method and outlook.

ANAMNESIS In psychology, the personal and family history of a case as given by the client. 2. In medical practice, the taking of the family and personal medical history of a patient and an account of the circumstances leading to the present illness. ct: catamnesis.

ANAPHASE 1. A stage in mitosis *q.v.* in which the chromatids *q.v.* of each chromosome *q.v.* separate and move to opposite poles. 2. The stage of nuclear division during which the daughter chromosomes pass from the equatorial plate toward opposite poles of the cell. ~ follows metaphase *q.v.* and precedes telophase *q.v.*

ANAPHRODISIAC 1. A drug or substance that reduces sexual desire. 2. Substances that detract from sexual performance and pleasure. ct: aphrodisiac.

ANAPHYLACTIC SHOCK 1. An extreme drop of blood pressure resulting in inadequate flow of oxygenated blood to body organs. 2. A severe hypersensitive *q.v.* reaction accompanied by shock *q.v.* 3. A serious, often fatal allergic reaction occurring in a previously sensitized person, starting within minutes after administration of a foreign serum or certain drugs.

ANAPHYLAXIS 1. An exaggerated reaction to a foreign substance. 2. An antigen–antibody reaction. This can be of life-threatening proportions. 3. A severe, sometimes fatal, reaction to a drug or allergen *q.v.*

ANAPLASIA Failure of the body cells to function normally. cf: cancer.

ANAPLASTIC 1. Undifferentiated cells. 2. Cancerous cells. 3. Referring to cancers *q.v.* whose cellular structure is so abnormal that they no longer resemble the cells from which they originated, and identification is no longer possible.

ANARTHRIA A condition characterized by the inability to articulate speech sounds as a result of a lesion of the central nervous system *q.v.*

ANASTOMOSE 1. In anatomy, to open one into the other. 2. A term used in connection with blood vessels, lymphatics, and nerves.

ANASTOMOSIS In anatomy, fusing of hollow, tubular structures, especially in blood vessels.

A NATION AT RISK The first major national report that was published by the National Commission on Excellence in Education in 1983, calling for educational reform in the curriculum, expectations, time, and teaching.

ANATOMY The branch of science dealing with the structure of the body.

ANC An acronym of autonomic nervous system *q.v.*

ANCILLARY Assisting in the performance of a service, such as ancillary health services.

ANDROGEN 1. A hormone *q.v.* produced in the testes *q.v.* in the male, chiefly by the adrenal glands *q.v.* in the female, but also by the ovaries *q.v.* It is an important source of sexual motivation. 2. The general class of male sex hormones, e.g., testosterone *q.v.* 3. A steroid hormone that produces masculine sex characteristics and having an influence on body and bone growth, and on the sex drive. 4. A type of hormone that promotes male genitalia *q.v.* development and functioning as well as promoting the secondary characteristics that accompany genetic *q.v.* male maturation *q.v.* cf: steroid hormones; androgenic hormones.

ANDROGENIC ALOPECIA 1. A dominant hereditary *q.v.* trait in which the hair follicles in the center of the scalp have inherited an increased sensitivity to androgens *q.v.* 2. Male pattern baldness.

ANDROGENIC HORMONES Male sex hormones, primarily testosterone, found in varying amounts in both men and women. cf: androgen.

ANDROGEN-INSENSITIVITY SYNDROME 1. Feminization of the male sex organs because of cellular insensitivity to androgen *q.v.* in the prenatal *q.v.* environment. 2. Testicular feminization syndrome *q.v.* 3. A condition in which an individual's genes lack full instruction for building androgen receptors, with the result that fetuses develop normal testes but the external genitals of females. These androgen-sensitive women are sterile, but they have firm feminine gender identities *q.v.* 4. A condition resulting from a lack of androgen receptor sites in the cells of the genetic male (XY) resulting in the development of an XY female. 5. Androgenital syndrome.

ANDROGENITAL SYNDROME Androgen-insensitivity syndrome *q.v.*

ANDROGYNOUS (ANDROGYNUS) A female pseudohermaphrodite *q.v.*

ANDROGYNOUS PERSONALITY A sex role identity that allows people to follow their natural personalities *q.v.* and blend traditional male and female traits.

ANDROGYNE (ANDROGYNY) 1. Having both masculine and feminine qualities.

ANDROMANIA Nymphomania *q.v.*

ANDROSTERONE An androgen *q.v.*

ANECDOTAL METHOD 1. A method of analyzing behavior by reliance on records of isolated occurrences. 2. In education, the technique by which a learner's behavior and responses are recorded as they occur and are used as an aid in analyzing the learner's learning problems. cf: observational method; anecdotal record; anecdotes.

ANECDOTAL RECORD 1. In education, a history or biography of a learner kept by the teacher to observe a learner's behavior. The narrative may reflect both positive and negative health behavior during a specific period of time. 2. In psychology, a type of cumulative record that emphasizes episodes of behavior important in the character or personality. 3. A brief, written report of an individual's exceptional behavior.

ANECDOTES Short, often entertaining, accounts of personal experiences.

ANEMIA 1. Several forms of a disease characterized by loss or destruction of blood or malfunctioning of the blood formation tissues. Loss of blood may be acute *q.v.* or chronic *q.v.* Destruction of blood may result from toxins *q.v.* or other foreign substances or from genetic *q.v.* factors. 2. Faulty blood formation, iron deficiency anemia and inhibition or failure of the bone marrow to produce blood cells. 3. A deficiency in the blood, either in quality or quantity: (a) hyperchromic anemia: a decrease in hemoglobin *q.v.* that is proportionately much less than the decrease in the number of erythrocytes *q.v.*, (b) hypochromic anemia: a decrease in hemoglobin that is proportionately much greater than the decrease in the number of erythrocytes, (c) macrocytic a: a condition in which the erythrocytes are much larger than normal, (d) megaloblastic a: an anemia that results from a severe deficiency of folacin *q.v.* It is characterized by enlargement of the red blood cells and failure of them to mature. It may appear in persons suffering from leukemia *q.v.* and some other diseases. Otherwise it is not common among Americans. ~ is a condition in which there are megablasts *q.v.* in the bone marrow, (e) microcytic 1. An anemia in which the erythrocytes *q.v.* are smaller than normal, (f) nutritional 1. Hypochromic *q.v.* and microcytic *q.v.* anemia due to insufficient iron in the diet, (g) pernicious. 1. A form of anemia characterized by weakness, shortness of breath, and palpitations. Gastrointestinal symptoms include nausea, vomiting, diarrhea, and abdominal pain. ~ usually appears in adult life resulting from a reduced ability for the intestines to absorb cobalamin *q.v.* Symptoms do not usually appear until the anemia is well advanced. cf: chronic macrocytic anemia. 2. Macrocytic and hypochromic anemia due to lack of secretion of the intrinsic factor by the gastric mucous membrane which is essential for the absorption of vitamin B_{12} *q.v.*

ANENCEPHALY A condition in which the person has a partial or complete absence of cerebral *q.v.* tissue.

ANESTHESIA 1. Loss of feeling or sensation. 2. Loss of sensation to pain. Consciousness may or may not be affected. 3. In psychology, an impairment or loss of sensation, usually of touch but sometimes of the other senses, that is often part of a conversion disorder *q.v.*

ANESTHESIOLOGY The study of anesthesia and anesthetics *q.v.*

ANESTHETIC 1. A drug used to induce sleep and to reduce sensitivity to pain. 2. A drug that inhibits pain. 3. A drug that causes insensitivity to pain by depressing the central nervous system *q.v.* ~s are used for surgical procedures. They can be either general of local. A. general ~s are administered to the whole body and generally produce unconsciousness. B. local ~s are used to anesthetize only the region of the body on which surgery is to be performed. ct: analgesic.

ANESTHETIST A trained physician or nurse who administers anesthesia, esp. for general anesthesia.

ANETHOPATH A person possessing a pathological *q.v.* lack of development in the Moral–ethical aspects of the personality *q.v.* cf: psychopath.

ANEUPLOID (HETEROPLOID) In genetics, an organism or cell having a chromosome *q.v.* number that is not an exact multiple of the monoploid *q.v.* or basic number.

ANEURISM 1. A sac formed by dilated wall of an artery or vein and is filled with blood. There are three basic form: (a) fusiform, which is a bulging of the blood vessel due to a weakened wall; (b) sacculated, which is the formation of a sac on the side of the blood vessel; and (c) dissecting, which is characterized by blood flowing between the layers of the blood vessel wall, separating the layers. 2. A ballooning of an artery or vein whose walls have been weakened or damaged.

ANF 1. American Nurses' Federation. 2. American Nurses' Foundation.

ANGER One of the three most powerful emotions *q.v.* ~ is frequently associated with frustration and fear *q.v.* and may be manifest through hostility, verbal, or physical. Watson refers to ~ as rage. cf: displacement of anger.

ANGINA PECTORIS 1. Transient chest pain resulting from coronary atherosclerosis *q.v.* preventing the heart muscle from receiving sufficient oxygen. 2. ~ may also be functional *q.v.* sign of atherosclerosis; also called cardiac neurosis *q.v.* 3. There are two kinds of ~: (a) stable which exists in persons when pain occurs only once in while and as a result of a significant increase in the work of the heart; and (b) unstable, which occurs when occlusion of the vessel is pronounced and the pain is severe and frequent. 4. Severe chest pain caused by inadequate blood supply to the heart muscle, brought about by exertion or excitement. 5. Intermittent chest pain caused by decreased blood flow and oxygen to the cardiac *q.v.* muscle and usually occurs after some physical or emotional exertion, or a brief or incomplete blockage of oxygenated *q.v.* blood to the heart muscle.

ANGIOGENESIS FACTOR Angiogenin *q.v.*

ANGIOGENIN 1. A protein substance found in the body that stimulates the growth of blood vessels. 2. Angiogenesis factor *q.v.*

ANGIOGRAM An X-ray viewing of a blood vessel following injection of a dye.

ANGIOGRAPHY A diagnostic procedure through which the chambers and blood vessels of the heart are examined.

ANGIONEUROTIC EDEMA A condition characterized by hives *q.v.* and swelling of the tissues as a result of allergy *q.v.*

ANGIOSARCOMA A rare form of liver cancer *q.v.*

ANGLE OF LEWIS In anatomy, a bony prominence on the breastbone just inferior to the junction of the clavicle *q.v.* and the sternum *q.v.* and just opposite the second intercostal *q.v.* space.

ANGSTROM 1. Angstrom unit. 2. Used to measure or designate radiation. 3. One hundred-millionth of a centimeter. 4. One ten-thousandth of a micron. 5. 1/10 millionth of a meter. 6. About 1/250 millionth of an inch.

ANGULATION 1. The formation of an angle. 2. An abnormal angle or bend in an extremity or organ of the body.

ANHEDONIA 1. In psychology, a psychophysiological *q.v.* condition characterized by the inability to experience joy. 2. The inability to find any pleasure in life. ct: hedonism.

ANHIDROSIS Decreased or absence of the secretion of sweat.

ANHYDROUS ALCOHOL Absolute alcohol *q.v.*

ANALINGUS In sexology, mouth to anus stimulation.

ANIMA 1. Shadow *q.v.* 2. Latin for soul. 3. Carl Jung refers to ~ as the personality *q.v.*

ANIMALCULES The microscopic organism discovered by Anton van Leeuwenhoek in 1683. Today, we know them as one-celled animals and possibly bacteria.

ANIMAL MAGNETISM A theory of Friedrich Mesmer which stated that hysterical disorders are caused by a universal magnetic fluid in the body.

ANIMAL MODEL An animal, other than human, used as an experimental system in research. cf: experimental model.

ANIMAL PARASITE An animal organism *q.v.* that can live in the body of another animal. cf: parasite.

ANIMAL PHOBIA 1. The fear and avoidance of small animals. 2. Zoophobia. 3. An irrational fear of animals.

ANIMISM (THEORY OF) 1. The belief by Stone Age people that all things, inanimate and living things, possessed a spirit. These spirits could be favorable or unfavorable.

The favorable spirits were worshipped while the unfavorable ones were exorcised or appeased. The unfavorable spirits caused disease. This belief in the causation of disease persists in many parts of the undeveloped and primitive parts of the world today. 2. In philosophy, the view that humans are both body and soul and that the soul is the principle of life. cf: demoniac theory of disease.

ANIMUS Shadow *q.v.*

ANION 1. A negatively charged atom. 2. An atom that has acquired one or more electrons. 3. A negatively charged ion *q.v.* that travels to the positive anode during electrolysis *q.v.*

ANISCORIA Inequality in the size of the pupils of the eyes.

ANISEIKONIA A visual condition characterized by images formed on the retinas *q.v.* of both eyes are unequal in size or shape.

ANISOCYTOSIS A lack of uniformity in the size of the red blood corpuscles *q.v.*

ANISOMETROPIA 1. Different visual acuity of the two eyes. 2. A difference in the refractive power of both eyes.

ANISOPHORIA 1. Heterophobia *q.v.* 2. A visual condition characterized by a variation in the visual angle of the eyes according to the direction of the focus or gaze.

ANKYLOSIS 1. Abnormal immobility and consolidation of a joint resulting from bone union. 2. A fusing of the joints rendering them nonfunctional. 3. A skeletal condition in which the cartilage or bones or a joint have grown together with resulting stiffness or immobility of the joint. This condition may be the result of disease or surgery. cf: arthrodesis; otosclerosis.

ANKYLOSING SPONDYLITIS A degenerative *q.v.*, arthritis-like disease of the spine. cf: ankylosis.

ANNOTATION Notes or commentaries in addition to the principal text. A book is said to be annotated when it contains marginal notes.

ANNOYERS AND SATISFIERS In education, technology used by Thorndike to clarify his law of effect in learning: synonymous with rewards and punishments, failures and successes; pleasantness and unpleasantness; satisfaction and dissatisfaction, as they relate to the learner in and during the learning process *q.v.*

ANNUAL GROWTH RATE 1. The percentage of the population increase over the past year. 2. In general, the growth rate in percentage of a given thing over the period of a year.

ANNUAL INCREMENTS In teaching, standard salary increases related to the number of years of teaching experience.

ANNUAL RATE OF NATURAL INCREASE In vital statistics, the difference between the annual birth rate *q.v.* and the annual death rate *q.v.* when the birth rate exceeds the death rate.

ANNUITANT In insurance, the person on whose life an annuity *q.v.* payable according to an annuity agreement *q.v.* is based and at whose death the payment of the annuity ceases.

ANNUITY A regular payment made according to an annuity agreement *q.v.* Also, an annual allowance or income from an agreement.

ANNUITY AGREEMENT 1. Annuity bond. 2. In insurance, an agreement by which money or other property is made available to an institution on the condition that the institution binds itself to hold and administer the property and to pay to the donor or other person a stipulated amount and which ceases at the time of the annuitant's *q.v.* death.

ANNULAR HYMEN A hymen *q.v.* that has a singular opening. ct: cribriform hymen; imperforate hymen.

ANNULMENT A legal dissolving of a marriage based on the grounds that the marriage was not valid. Laws vary in the different states. A marriage may also be annulled when it is not valid in the view of a particular church or religion. ct: divorce.

ANOETIC 1. In psychology, a state of haziness. 2. Pertains to the fringe of consciousness *q.v.*

ANOMALIE 1. A defective, deformed, or diseased structure. May include genes *q.v.*, chromosomes *q.v.*, cells, tissues, organs, or a combination of these. 2. Also, anomaly. 3. A deviation from the rule, form, or type. 4. Irregularity in development.

ANOMALOUS GAMETES Irregular and usually incompatible gametes *q.v.* with chromosome *q.v.* numbers different from those normally produced by members of the species.

ANOMIA 1. Indicating an absence of moral sense (Benjamin Rush). 2. An amnesic aphasia *q.v.* characterized by the inability to name an object even though it is recognized. 3. Difficulty in recalling names of persons and object. 4. Difficulty with recalling nouns.

ANOMIC SUICIDE Self-annihilation triggered by the person's inability to cope with sudden and unfavorable change in a social situation.

ANOMIE 1. In psychology, without relationship or the feeling of belonging. 2. In sociology, a weakened respect for norms. 3. The absence of norms believed by some sociologists to lead to deviant behavior in persons who cannot gain access to conventional or socially approved routes to success. 4. Personal unrest, alienation, and uncertainty arising from a lack of purpose or ideals. 5. Disintegration of society by widespread cleavage among groups in that society.

ANOPHELES A species of mosquito that carries the malaria parasite *q.v.*

ANOPHTHALMOS An absence of the eyeball.

ANORCHISM The congenital *q.v.* lack of both testicles *q.v.*

ANORECTANTS Substances that reduce or eliminate appetite for food. cf: anorectic.

ANORECTIC Having no appetite.

ANORECTIS In pharmacology, a drug that diminishes appetite or causes an aversion to food. cf: anorectants.

ANOREXIA A condition characterized by a severe loss of appetite. cf: anorexia nervosa.

ANOREXIA NERVOSA 1. A psychiatric disorder characterized by obsessive self-starvation that, when carried to extremes, results in death. ~ is chiefly found among white females between the ages of 13 and 30 years. A profile that has been formulated includes girls who (a) are extremely well-behaved; (b) are high achievers; and (c) are physically hyperactive *q.v.* 2. A condition characterized by a profound aversion to food resulting in extreme weight loss. 3. A personality disorder marked by self-starvation and life-threatening weight loss, usually occurring in young women. 4. Loss of appetite due to a lack of love, affection, and emotional support. 5. A disorder in which a person is unable to eat or to retain any food or suffers a prolonged and severe diminution of appetite. The person has an intense fear of becoming obese, feels fat even when emaciated and refuses to maintain a minimal body weight. ct: bulimia.

ANOREXIANT 1. Anorectant *q.v.* 2. A drug that causes loss of appetite.

ANOREXIC 1. An appetite suppressant drug. 2. A person suffering from anorexia nervosa *q.v.*

ANORGASMIA 1. Classified as primary orgasmic dysfunction or secondary orgasmic dysfunction *q.v.* Also pertains to situational or coital or random orgasmic dysfunction. 2. A sexual dysfunction in women consisting of the inability to reach orgasm *q.v.*

ANOSMIA A conversion disorder *q.v.* marked by loss or impairment of the sense of smell.

ANOVA An acronym for analysis of variance *q.v.*

ANOVOLUTORY 1. Not ovulating *q.v.* 2. Anovulatory cycle: a menstrual cycle during which no ovulation occurs. 3. The state when no eggs are released from the ovaries *q.v.* during the menstrual cycle *q.v.*

ANOXEMIA 1. A diminished or inadequate oxygen concentration in the blood. 2. Deficient blood oxygen content. 3. Deficient aeration *q.v.* of the blood. cf: anoxia.

ANOXIA 1. Generally, lack of sufficient oxygen in the blood. 2. A deficiency of oxygen reaching the tissues severe enough to damage the brain permanently. 3. Without oxygen in the cells of the tissues. cf: anoxemia.

ANSWER An acronym for A Computer Based Information System (ATSDR *q.v.*). National Library of Medicine's Workstation for Emergency Response. This system provides information from the Toxicology Occupational Health, Medicine Treatment, Environmental Series (TOMES *q.v.*), industrial chemical database from the National Oceanic and Atmospheric Administration, and a plume dispersion model that allows the user to assess potential threats to the public from a release of hazardous materials into the air.

ANTABUSE 1. Disulfiram *q.v.* 2. A drug when taken internally, interacts with alcohol causing distressing nausea *q.v.* ~ is sometimes used in aversion therapy *q.v.* to discourage alcoholics *q.v.* from drinking. 3. ~ interferes with the enzyme aldehyde dehydrogenase so that there is a buildup of acetaldehyde *q.v.*, the first metabolic *q.v.* product of alcohol when it is ingested. cf: antabuse syndrome.

ANTABUSE SYNDROME An accumulation of the toxic metabolite of alcohol *q.v.*, acetaldehyde *q.v.* resulting from antabuse, or a genetic deficiency, which causes unpleasant symptoms, including intense throbbing in the head and neck, a pulsating headache, difficulty in breathing, nausea, vomiting, sweating, thirst, and chest pain.

ANTACID 1. A substance used to neutralize hydrochloric acid produced by the stomach. 2. A drug intended to relieve symptoms of heartburn, sour stomach, and acid indigestion.

ANTAGONISM Opposition or contrary action between two drugs, thus preventing the expected action of one drug.

ANTAGONIST 1. A substance that exerts a nullifying or opposing action on another substance. 2. A muscle that opposes another muscle. 3. Things that oppose. 4. A drug that blocks or interferes with the action of a normally present biological compound, such as a neurotransmitter or hormone *q.v.*, or of another drug, such as a narcotic antagonist.

ANTAGONISTIC EFFECT The results produced when one drug nullifies the effects of a second drug. cf: antagonist.

ANTAGONISTIC MUSCLES Muscles that are in direct opposition to each other.

ANTECEDENTS In pharmacology, behaviors or individual characteristics that can be measured before drug use and might therefore be somewhat predictive of the drug use.

These are not necessarily causes of the subsequent drug use.

ANTECUBITAL In anatomy, the front of the elbow.

ANTECUBITAL FOSSA In anatomy, the depression in the skin and soft tissue of the upper extremity anterior to the elbow.

ANTENATAL Prior to birth. cf: antepartum.

ANTEPARTUM Before delivery of the fetus *q.v.* cf: antenatal.

ANTERIOR The front of or ventral part. ct: posterior; dorsal.

ANTERIOR PITUITARY LOBE 1. A part of the pituitary gland *q.v.* 2. An important gland in the control of sexual development by secreting four major hormones: (a) follicle stimulating hormone (FSH), (b) luteinizing hormone (LH), (c) interstitial cell-stimulating hormone (ICSH) in the male, and (d) prolactin in the female. 3. A gland that secretes adrenocorticotropic hormone (ACTH) *q.v.* during the stage of resistance of the General Adaptation Syndrome (GAS) *q.v.* cf: posterior pituitary lobe.

ANTEROGRADE AMNESIA 1. Memory loss resulting from brain damage. 2. The inability to learn and remember any information imparted following the brain damage, but little effect on memory prior to the injury.

ANTHELMINTIC (ANTEHELMINTIC; ANTIHELMINTIC) A drug used to combat infestation *q.v.* with worms.

ANTHROPOGEOGRAPHY A branch of anthropology *q.v.* concerned with the distribution of humans. cf: anthropography.

ANTHROPOGRAPHY That branch of anthropology *q.v.* interested in the distribution of people rather than the physical characteristics of customs, language, and the nature of existing institutions. cf: anthropogeography.

ANTHROPOLOGY 1. The science that studies humans. 2. The study of the relationship of mind and body. 3. The science that studies human social life in a variety of cultural settings. 4. Cultural ~ and social ~ are synonymous. 5. Generally, ~ includes archeology, linguistics, and physical studies and relationships of humans. 6. The science concerned with humans; the study of their physical characteristics, racial, geographical, and historical distributions; their cultural, environmental, and social development and relationships. ~ branches include anthropogeography, anthropometry; anthropogeography, ethnicity, folklore, and comparative religion.

ANTHROPOLOGICAL CHARACTERISTICS Human characteristics including the physical and cultural and their relationships.

ANTHROPOMETRIC MEASUREMENTS Measurements taken, using calipers, of various parts of the body to calculate the proportion of fat tissue in the body. cf: anthropometry.

ANTHROPOMETRY 1. The measurement of the size, weight, and proportions of the body. 2. The study of human body measurement, esp. on a comparative basis, through determination of the dimensions of the body. 3. A branch of physical anthropology *q.v.* concerned with human anatomical *q.v.* measurements for the purpose of gathering information regarding race, growth, evolution, etc.

ANTHROPOMORPHISM The attribution of human characteristics, esp. mental traits, to nonhuman beings such as animals or inanimate objects; or the interpretation of the actions, behavior, and reactions of animals in terms of human psychology *q.v.*

ANTHROPONOMY The branch of anthropology *q.v.* concerned with the study of human behavior as related to psychology *q.v.*

ANTHROPOSOCIOLOGY A branch of anthropology *q.v.* concerned with the study of race and environment *q.v.*

ANTHOXANTHINE Generally, any group of yellow pigments found in an organism, esp. plants.

ANTHRAX An infectious *q.v.* disease in sheep and cattle that can be communicable *q.v.* to humans.

ANTIANDROGENS Drugs that oppose the action of male sex hormones *q.v.*

ANTIANGINAL Drugs that relieve or prevent the chest pain associated with angina pectoris *q.v.* An antianginal increases the oxygen supply to the heart muscle.

ANTIANXIETY DRUGS Drugs used primarily to alleviate anxiety *q.v.*

ANTIAUXIN A substance that inhibits the action of an auxin *q.v.*

ANTIBIOTIC 1. An anti-infective drug that inhibits growth of or destroys microorganisms *q.v.* and is used extensively in treating bacteria-caused diseases. 2. A substance of biological origin that interferes with the metabolism *q.v.* of microorganisms in the body. 3. Organic toxins *q.v.* excreted as waste by many microorganisms. 4. A chemical substance capable of destroying bacteria and other microorganisms.

ANTIBODY 1. A protein produced by blood B-lymphocytes to eliminate specific infectious agents *q.v.* in the body. 2. A specific protein molecule or substance synthesized by the immune system *q.v.* as a defense against invading antigens *q.v.* 3. An immune body. 4. Chemical substances that protect the body from invasion of foreign substances, such as disease-producing organisms *q.v.* 5. A protein produced by the body in response to the presence of a foreign agent called an antigen. ~s are part of the body's natural defense against invasion of foreign substances.

ANTICHOLINERGIC 1. A cholinergic blocking agent including atropine, nicotine, which prevents acetylcholine *q.v.* from stimulating the receptor. 2. Anticholinergic effect *q.v.*

ANTICHOLINERGIC EFFECT The effects resulting from a drug's interference with the action of acetylcholine *q.v.* in the brain and peripheral nervous system *q.v.* Common symptoms of these effects include dry mouth, blurred vision, constipation, and mental confusion. cf: anticholinergic.

ANTICIPATION METHOD In serial rote learning *q.v.* the method in which the learner must respond to each item in a list with the item that comes next. ct: paired associate learning.

ANTICIPATORY ANXIETY The fear of recurrence of a panic attack. This condition may cause a person to avoid leaving his or her home or other perceived safe place.

ANTICIPATORY ERROR In serial rote learning *q.v.*, an error that consists of giving as a response an item that would be correct later in the list. ct: perseverative error; cf: anticipatory method.

ANTICLERICALISM A political movement during the nineteenth century, extending into the twentieth century, occurring in countries that were very hostile to the excessive power of the church. Its goals were to establish supremacy of the state over religions.

ANTICOAGULANT 1. A drug that tends to prevent the blood from coagulating *q.v.* An ~ has a blood thinning effect. 2. A substance that slows the rate of blood clot formation. ~s are used for the management of stroke *q.v.* and heart disease *q.v.*

ANTICONFORMITY 1. In sociology and psychology, behavior in which defiance of a group or an authority is an end in itself. cf: independence.

ANTICONVULSANT 1. A drug used to prevent the appearance of the symptoms of convulsion *q.v.* such as is found in some forms of epilepsy *q.v.* 2. Drugs that slow the electrical activity within the brain that reduces the occurrence of seizures *q.v.*

ANTIDEPRESSANTS 1. Drugs that are administered to alleviate depressing moods in a person. 2. Drugs, such as an MAO inhibitor *q.v.* and a tricyclic compound *q.v.* used to elevate mood and relieve certain types of mental depression.

ANTIDIABETIC A drug that increases blood insulin *q.v.* level or increases the use of insulin by the body.

ANTIDIARRHEAL A drug that prevents or is used to treat diarrhea *q.v.*

ANTIDISCRIMINATION A policy of refusing to use or permit the use of nonrelevant factor, such as race, creed, color, ethnic origin, in the employment of faculty, other staff, or in the admission of students to educational institutions or to any of its programs, activities, services, or facilities.

ANTIDIURETIC HORMONE A hormone *q.v.* secreted by one of the parts of the pituitary gland *q.v.* ~ instructs the kidneys to reabsorb more of the water that passes through them.

ANTIDOTE A preparation that neutralizes a poison.

ANTIDROMIC IMPULSE An impulse from axon *q.v.* to dendrite *q.v.* in a single neuron *q.v.* which is the opposite of the normal direction of nerve conduction.

ANTIEMETIC 1. A drug that is used to prevent or treat nausea and vomiting. 2. Preventing or alleviating nausea and vomiting; an agent having such effects. cf: antinauseant.

ANTIFEMINISM An opposition movement to the practice of those who advocate economic, social, and political equality of the sexes.

ANTIFUNGAL A drug used to prevent or treat fungus *q.v.* infections *q.v.*

ANTIGEN 1. Any substance not normally present in the body and that produces an immune *q.v.* reaction when introduced to the body. 2. A toxin *q.v.* foreign protein, or microorganism that invades the body and induces production of defense antibodies *q.v.* 3. A protein substance that stimulates the body's immune system *q.v.* to produce antibodies. 4. Any substance that elicits an immune response *q.v.* 5. A substance that the body recognizes as foreign to itself. 6. A large molecule *q.v.*, usually a protein or carbohydrate *q.v.* which when introduced into the body stimulates the production of an antibody that will react specifically with the ~ antigenic determinants. Molecular patterns on the antigen *q.v.* to which the antibody *q.v.* reacts.

ANTIGEN-PRODUCING CELLS B cells *q.v.*, cells of the monocyte *q.v.* lineage including morophages *q.v.* and dendritic cells *q.v.* and various other body cells that present antigen *q.v.* in a form that T cells *q.v.* can recognize.

ANTIGRAVITY MUSCLES The larger extensor muscles of the body that give support to the skeletal framework and that combat the pull of gravity.

ANTIHEMOPHILIA GLOBULIN Blood globulin *q.v.* which reduces the clotting time of hemophilic blood. cf: hemophilia.

ANTIHISTAMINE 1. A drug that counters the effect of histamine *q.v.* which is naturally produced by the body.

~ tends to dry up the mucous membranes *q.v.* in the nose and may cause drowsiness. 2. A drug used to combat allergic *q.v.* reactions. 3. A drug that blocks the effects of the allergy chemical, histamine, and relieves sneezing, watery eyes, runny nose, and itching of the nose or throat.

ANTIHYPERLIPIDEMIC A drug that decreases blood lipid *q.v.* and/or cholesterol *q.v.* levels.

ANTIHYPERTENSIVE A drug that decreases blood pressure *q.v.* 2. ~ drugs sometimes produce side effects, particularly in older persons. Some ~s interact with other drugs; both prescription and OTC *q.v.* cf: hypertension.

ANTI-INFECTIVE 1. A drug used to treat or prevent infections *q.v.* 2. ~ drugs are administered for the purpose of inactivating or eliminating invading, disease-producing microbes and includes such categories as antibiotics *q.v.*, antifungals, and antiseptics.

ANTI-INFLAMMATORY 1. A drug that reduces inflammation *q.v.* 2. Treatment for reducing the local heat, swelling, and redness caused by injury or infection *q.v.* Aspirin is an example of an ~ drug.

ANTI-INTELLECTUALISM 1. Tendencies to restrict the processes of open inquiry, the freedom of the mind to inquire, and the freedom to teach accordingly. 2. Used to criticize education, particularly secondary and postsecondary education to the effect that the intellectual content of scholarly disciplines and the pursuit of truth for its own sake have been largely replaced by trivia, practical educational procedures, and isolated bits of information.

ANTIKETOGENIC Inhibiting the formation of ketone *q.v.* bodies.

ANTIMANIC A drug used to prevent or treat mania *q.v.*

ANTIMETABOLIC A drug that interferes with a chemical reaction in cells and prevents growth.

ANTIMETROPIA In vision, a condition in which one eye is nearsighted *q.v.* and the other eye is farsighted *q.v.*

ANTIMICROBIAL A substance that kills microorganisms *q.v.* or inhibits their growth.

ANTIMUSCARINIC An anticholinergic *q.v.* drug that affects the muscarinic *q.v.* type of receptor.

ANTINAUSEANT A drug used to prevent or treat nausea *q.v.* and vomiting. cf: antiemetic.

ANTINEOPLASTIC Any agent that inhibits or prevents the formation or maintenance of tumors *q.v.*

ANTINEURITIC A substance or treatment that relieves inflammation *q.v.* of a nerve. Thiamin *q.v.* is the ~ vitamin *q.v.*

ANTIMONY The existence of mutually contradictory principles or conclusions each of which may be supported by reason, but which cannot both be true. The world cannot be both finite and infinite (Kant).

ANTIOCH PLAN A plan of cooperative education developed at Antioch College. cf: cooperative education.

ANTIOXIDANT 1. A substance that delays or prevents oxidation *q.v.* 2. Also, antioxidant; a substance that inhibits the oxidation of other compounds.

ANTIPARAPHERNALIA LAW A statute or law restricting or forbidding the sale and/or promotion of items related to the use of illegal drugs. Such paraphernalia may include pipes, bongs, roach clips, and others.

ANTIPERSPIRANT 1. A chemical ingredient in some deodorants that tend to prevent a person from perspiring. An example is aluminum chlorohydrate. 2. A product that contains a chemical that inhibits the production of perspiration and may also be a deodorant.

ANTIPRURITIC A substance that prevents or relieves itching.

ANTIPSYCHOTIC 1. Neuroleptic *q.v.* 2. Drugs that produce an effect of emotional quieting and relative indifference to one's surroundings. 3. Major tranquilizers *q.v.* 4. A group of drugs that are used to treat psychotics *q.v.*

ANTIPYRETIC 1. A substance that reduces fever. 2. Fever-reducing.

ANTIRACHITIC A substance opposing the development of rickets *q.v.*

ANTISEPTIC 1. A chemical agent that meets the criteria of a disinfectant *q.v.* and is suitable for topical application. 2. A substance that prevents the multiplication of microorganisms *q.v.*

ANTISERUM Serum *q.v.* portion of the blood that carries the antibodies *q.v.*

ANTISOCIAL 1. Describes behavior or conduct that is in conflict with or disregards existing social institutions or moral codes. 2. Behavior characterized by urges to disrupt social relationships or social institutions. 3. Behavior exemplified by destruction of the existing society and its acceptable conduct. ct: a social; unsocial.

ANTISOCIAL PERSONALITY 1. Psychopath *q.v.* 2. Sociopath *q.v.* 3. Antisocial reaction *q.v.* 4. A personality disorder *q.v.* characterized by impulsivity, inability to profit from experience, and unethical behavior *q.v.* 5. Antisocial personality disorder *q.v.* 6. This person is superficially charming and a habitual liar, has no regard for others, shows no remorse after hurting them, has no shame for behaving in an outrageously objectionable manner, is unable to form relationships and take responsibility, and does not learn from punishment.

ANTISOCIAL PERSONALITY DISORDER 1. Chronic antisocial behavior that violates the rights of others. 2. Antisocial personality *q.v.*

ANTISOCIAL REACTION 1. A behavioral act that is destructive to society or some segment of society. 2. Aggressive behavior directed toward others. 3. Persons exhibiting this are said to be psychopathic personalities *q.v.* 4. Symptoms include inadequate conscience development, irresponsible behavior, establishment of unrealistic goals, lack of guilt feelings, and defective social relationships. 5. Psychopath *q.v.* 6. Sociopath *q.v.* cf: antisocial personality.

ANTISPASMODIC An agent that reduces spasm *q.v.* particularly of the intestinal tract. 2. A drug that relieves spasms of a passage or canal.

ANTI-SUICIDE BUREAU OF THE SALVATION ARMY Established in London, England, in 1905. Its establishment was stimulated by a recognition of the need for primary prevention *q.v.* measures for suicide. It is the first evidence of a response to this kind of need.

ANTITHESIS 1. A proposition opposed to a given thesis *q.v.* 2. The second phase of a dialectical process denying or rejecting the first concept *q.v.* and contributing to the emergence of a synthesis *q.v.* that both blends and transcends the partial truths of the thesis and the ~.

ANTITOXINS Antibodies *q.v.* formed against microbial *q.v.* toxins *q.v.*

ANTITUSSIVE 1. A drug preparation that relieves coughing. 2. A drug that sedates *q.v.* the cough reflex *q.v.* center of the brain. 3. Cough-reducing; narcotics *q.v.* have the effect. OTC *q.v.* ~s generally contain dextromethorphan *q.v.*

ANTIVENIN An antiserum *q.v.* used to neutralize an animal or insect venom.

ANTIVIRAL 1. A drug used to prevent or treat viral infections *q.v.* 2. Against a virus *q.v.* 3. Drugs that destroy or weaken viruses, may be specific or nonspecific.

ANTONYM A word whose meaning is opposite to another word. For example, black is the ~ of white and white is the opposite of black. Hot as the ~ of cold; likewise, cold is the ~ of hot. ct: synonym.

ANTRUM 1. A nearly closed cavity. 2. The nasal sinus *q.v.* just below the eye. 3. The ~ of Highmore. 4. The space in each maxillary bone *q.v.* 5. The maxillary sinus.

ANURIA The absence of urine formation.

ANUS The opening of the rectum *q.v.* located between the buttocks through which feces *q.v.* is excreted from the body.

ANVIL BONE Incus *q.v.*

ANXIETY 1. Apprehensive uneasiness, usually accompanied by fear. 2. A vague, undefined fear of impending change. 3. What a person feels when existence is threatened. 4. A tendency toward tension and uneasiness; concern or worry about a social situation or stressful circumstance. 5. A fearful response attached by conditioning to previously neutral stimuli. 6. A subjective state of apprehension or tension accompanied by physiological arousal. 7. In learning theory, a drive which mediates between a threatening situation and avoidance behavior. ~ can be assessed by self-report, by measuring physiological arousal, and by observing overt behavior. ~ involves a number of symptoms that are related to a sense of impending danger. At pathological *q.v.* levels, these symptoms can constitute debilitating disorders.

ANXIETY-BASED DISORDER A category of behavior patterns in which anxiety *q.v.* is the prominent symptom *q.v.* cf: anxiety disorder.

ANXIETY DISORDER 1. A category of moderately severe mental problems. 2. Neurosis *q.v.* accompanied by tension and restlessness. 3. Phobia *q.v.* 4. Generalized anxiety disorder *q.v.* 5. Obsessive-compulsive disorder *q.v.* 6. A condition that is characterized by excessive fears and anxiety *q.v.* about persons, places, or events. 7. Disorder in which tension is overriding and the primary disturbance. A major category of the *DSM* *q.v.* referred formerly to ~ as neurosis *q.v.* including phobic disorders, the anxiety states, panic disorder, generalized anxiety disorder, obsessive-compulsive disorder, and post-traumatic disorder.

ANXIETY HIERARCHY Systematic desensitization *q.v.*

ANXIETY NEUROSIS 1. Generalized anxiety disorder *q.v.* 2. Panic disorder *q.v.* 3. *DSM IV* term for what is now diagnosed as panic disorder and generalized anxiety disorder. cf: anxiety disorder; anxiety panic reaction.

ANXIETY PANIC REACTION Mental and emotional effects associated with drug use that are perceived as unpleasant or undesirable including panic, paranoia *q.v.*, dependency feelings, hallucinations *q.v.*, fear reactions, distortion of body image, and aggressive urges.

ANXIETY REACTION 1. A type of neurotic behavior characterized by continuous fear or apprehension which results in heightened anxiety *q.v.*, tension, sweating, and fatigue. Causes: (a) a conflict in one's primitive organic and pleasure-seeking impulses (id), and the rational aspects of the personality or the self-concept *q.v.* (ego); (b) the inability for the person to close the gap between the actual self and perception of the ideal self; (c) a result of constraints that prevent a person from attaining self-actualization *q.v.*

ANXIOLYTIC 1. Pertaining to drugs that can reduce tension and anxiety *q.v.* without inducing sleep. 2. A drug used to treat anxiety and its associated symptoms. 3. Literally, anxiety dissolving.

ANXIOUS REACTIVE PERSONALITY A person who views problems as greater than they actually are.

AOA An acronym for American Osteopathic Association.

AOEC An acronym for Association of Occupational and Environmental Clinics.

AOHC An acronym for American Occupational Health Conference.

AORN An acronym for Association of Operating Room Nurses.

AORTA The body's main artery originating from the left ventricle of the heart, extending upward then downward to the pelvis, and which carries oxygenated blood to its branches and hence to the body tissues.

AORTIC ANEURYSM An aneurism *q.v.* of the aorta *q.v.*

AORTIC VALVE The valve that controls the blood flow into the aorta *q.v.* from the left ventricle *q.v.* of the heart.

AOTA An acronym for American Occupational Therapy Association.

AOTF An acronym for American Occupational Therapy Foundation.

APA An acronym for 1. American Pharmaceutical Association. 2. American Physiotherapy Association. 3. American Psychiatric Association. 4. American Psychological Association.

APARTHEID 1. A racial policy aimed at the separation and development of races. 2. The separation of whites and nonwhites within a given society. 3. A racially oriented political structure.

APATHY 1. Lack of interest. 2. In general, a lack of feeling. 3. Extreme ~ may be characterized by a pathological *q.v.* mental condition when the ~ symbolizes exaggerated indifference.

APERTURE An opening.

APEX 1. In dentistry, the end of a root of a tooth. 2. In anatomy, any pointed end of a conical structure.

APGAR 1. A physician's rating of a newly born infant's heart rate, breathing, color, muscle tone, and reflex irritability. cf: apgar score.

APGAR SCORE 1. A rapid assessment of a newborn's condition made immediately after birth and again 5 min later. Named after Virginia Apgar, who devised the test. 2. An evaluation of a neonate's apgar *q.v.* cf: apgar test.

APHA An acronym for American Public Health Association.

APHAGIA 1. Refusal to eat brought about by a lesion of the lateral hypothalamus *q.v.* 2. Inability to swallow.

APHASIA 1. A disorder of language produced by lesions *q.v.* in certain association areas of the cortex *q.v.* A lesion *q.v.* in Broca's area *q.v.* leads to expressive ~, whereas a lesion in Wernicke's area *q.v.* leads to receptive ~. 2. A disturbance of speech. 3. Loss of the ability to use language symbols. 4. Auditory ~ is characterized by the inability to comprehend spoken words and may take the form of (a) receptive ~, or (b) receptive dysphasia *q.v.* 5. Expressive ~ is characterized by the inability to speak, even when the person knows what he/she wants to say. 6. A disorder consisting of an inability to produce or comprehend language. The chief types are nominal, syntactical, verbal, and semantic; expressive, receptive, and expressive-receptive. ~ is believed to be cause by lesions of the inferior gyrus, and the association areas of the dominant hemisphere. cf: agnosia; apraxia.

APHEMIA 1. A form of dysphemia *q.v.* 2. A speech disorder without known etiology *q.v.* characterized by the person knowing what he or she wants to say but is unable to produce the words.

APHONIA 1. Loss or impairment of voice without associated organic pathology *q.v.* 2. A conversion disorder *q.v.* 3. Loss of voice resulting from a peripheral lesion *q.v.* that may be structural, neurological, or psychogenic *q.v.*

APHORISM A short, concise statement (aphoristic). Axiomatic *q.v.*

APHRODISIAC 1. A sexual stimulant. 2. Any substance, drug, food, or device that consistently and safely results in sexual arousal or enhanced sexual performance.

APHRODESIAN 1. A substance claimed to increase sexual stimulation. There is controversy about whether or not such a drug or substance actually exists. 2. Anything, such as a drug or a perfume, that stimulates sexual desire. ct: aphrodisiac.

APICOECTOMY In dentistry, the surgical removal of the apex *q.v.* of the tooth.

APLASIA The failure of an organ to develop resulting from congenital *q.v.* factors or disease *q.v.* in infancy.

APLASTIC ANEMIA A form of anemia *q.v.* in which the bone marrow fails to produce adequate numbers of red blood cells.

APNEA 1. The cessation of breathing, especially without apparent cause. 2. A temporary cessation of breathing caused by an overabundance of oxygen in the blood.

APNEIC Characterized by the absence of respiration. cf: apnea.

APOCRINE GLANDS Sweat glands that produce a milky liquid that is decomposed by bacteria on the skin, producing body odor. ~ have no known function to the body. ct: eccrine glands.

APOENZYME 1. Any protein that forms an active enzyme *q.v.* system by combination with a coenzyme *q.v.* and that determine the specificity of this system for any one substrate *q.v.* 2. The protein portion of the enzyme, which acts in conjunction with the coenzyme to constitute the active enzyme.

APOFERRITIN A protein in the mucosal cells of the small intestine, together with iron, that forms the compound ferritin *q.v.*

APONEUROSIS 1. The end of a muscle where it becomes tendon, serving to connect a muscle with other muscle parts that it moves. 2. One of the types of muscle attachments which takes the form of a fibrous sheet. ~ may invest a muscle.

APOPLEXY 1. Stroke *q.v.* 2. A sudden diminution or loss of consciousness with possible paralysis due to brain hemorrhage *q.v.* 3. A condition resulting from an acute vascular lesion of the brain that may result in coma, paralysis, or aphasia *q.v.* The lesion may result from hemorrhage, thrombosis, or embolism *q.v.*

APOSTAT The appetite *q.v.* control mechanism in the brain.

APOTHECARY 1. A druggist or pharmacist. 2. A place where drugs are compounded and dispensed. 3. One who dispenses drugs.

APPARENT MOTION In psychology and physiology, the perception of motion under conditions where there is no physical movement. cf: phi phenomenon.

APPEAL In education law, an application to a higher court to rectify the decision of a lower court.

APPEAL AUTHORITIES Court or law or educational officials or bodies before which legal appeals may be brought for a decision.

APPEAL TO CUSTOM In law, a method used to arrive at a judgment or a decision by invoking long-established usages and tradition, as contrasted by the appeal to the rules of reason and to overwhelming scientific evidence.

APPEARANCE 1. In philosophy, impressions that come to an observer through common sense and sensory impressions. 2. That which an object or event is observed to be, as opposed to that which it really is.

APPELLANT 1. In education law, the party who brings action in a higher court. 2. The party who takes an appeal from one court to another. The ~ may have been the plaintiff *q.v.* or defendant in the power court action. ct: appellee.

APPELLEE In education law, the party to whom an appeal is taken against. Also referred to as the respondent. ct: appellant.

APPENDECTOMY The surgical removal of the appendix *q.v.*

APPENDICITIS An infection *q.v.* of the appendix *q.v.*

APPENDIX 1. In anatomy, a narrow, closed tube protruding from the beginning of the large intestine. 2. Vermiform appendix *q.v.* 3. In publishing, the matter supplementing the text of a book and not necessarily essential to the content of the text.

APPERCEPTION 1. A process of focusing the perception *q.v.* of or being actively aware rather than being passively aware. 2. The process of relating new learning to one's past experiences and of evaluating it in view of that experience. cf: apperceptive mass.

APPERCEPTIVE MASS A person's total knowledge or experience in relation to new facts or experiences. This concept is related to gestalt psychology *q.v.* cf: apperception.

APPESTAT 1. A center of the brain that controls hunger, appetite *q.v.*, thirst, and emotions. 2. The hypothalamus *q.v.*

APPETITE 1. The desire for food, influenced by external stimuli *q.v.* 2. A desire or longing to satisfy the need for food.

APPETITE SUPPRESSANT 1. A drug referred to as a diet aid that helps a person to control his or her appetite *q.v.* resulting in reduced food intake. 2. Anorectic *q.v.*

APPETITIVE BEHAVIOR In motivation, the behavior that attracts a person to the thing that he or she wants or needs. Searching for food is an ~. ~ may be followed by a consummatory response *q.v.*

APPETITIVE DRUG USE Drug taking behavior motivated by the desire for pleasurable responses and sensations resulting from the dynamics of a drug in the body.

APPETITIVE POWERS 1. Specifically, hunger, thirst, sex, or money-loving appetite (Plato). 2. Those powers of humans that strive for the possession of objects viewed as good or for avoidance of those objects viewed as evil (St. Thomas).

APPLICATION 1. In education, the act of concentrating attention on the material at hand. 2. A kind of activity in a directed study method in which learners attempt to apply what they have learned.

APPLICATION FORM In career counseling, a series of questions to be completed by the applicant to supply personal history and work experience.

APPLIED ANATOMY Using knowledge of human anatomy *q.v.* as an aid in diagnosing and treating illness.

APPLIED KINESIOLOGY A pseudoscience that promotes the idea that muscular imbalance is a major factor in most diseases. ct: kinesiology.

APPLIED RESEARCH 1. Study intended to solve immediate practical problems of a limited nature. 2. An investigative study in which the results are used in actual practice. cf: applied science.

APPLIED SCIENCE The application of discovered laws to the matters of everyday living.

APPOINTIVE BOARD A board whose members are appointed by an official who possesses constituted authority, e.g., a board of education appointed by a mayor. Sometimes such appointments must be approved or rejected by the electors of the school district.

APPOINTIVE OFFICE A person in a school system or health agency filled by appointment by a constituted board rather than by an election. cf: elective office.

APPORTIONMENT The system or plan by which funds, materials, supplies, or services are distributed to the operating units of the organization.

APPRAISAL 1. An accurate determination of values *q.v.* 2. The synthesizing and interpreting of data. 3. Placing a value upon something. 4. In counseling, the process of synthesizing and interpreting information concerning a student or client. 5. In insurance and taxation, the formal valuation of property to determine the amount of insurance to be carried or the amount of taxes to be levied.

APPRECIATE 1. To be fully aware of. 2. To evaluate. 3. To judge with heightened understanding.

APPRECIATION An emotionally tinged awareness of the worth, value, and significance of something.

APPREHEND 1. To perceive *q.v.* 2. To understand. 3. To anticipate, especially with anxiety or fear. cf: apprehension.

APPREHENSION 1. Dread or anticipation of evil or danger. 2. The direct understanding of the meaning and content of an object or act.

APPRENTICESHIP TRAINING In education, a method of teaching skills of a specific trade through a progression of on-the-job experiences supplemented by classroom, correspondence, or electronic instruction.

APPROACH–APPROACH CONFLICT 1. In psychology, a situation in which a person must make a choice between two desired objects or goals, either by rejecting one goal entirely or by making a decision about which of the two goals to achieve first. 2. Conflicting attraction. ct: approach–avoidance conflict; avoidance–avoidance conflict.

APPROACH–AVOIDANCE CONFLICT 1. Attraction–repulsion conflict. 2. A situation in which both a positive (desired) and negative (obstruction) goals are present. The closer a person gets to the positive goal, the more repelled he/she is by the negative goal. ct: approach–approach conflict; avoidance–avoidance conflict.

APPROACH GRADIENT In conflict theory *q.v.*, the concept that the tendency to approach a positive goal increases with nearness to the goal. ct: avoidance gradient.

APPROPRIATE In legislative practice, to allocate funds.

APPROPRIATE HUMAN RESOURCES 1. In educational administration, those persons within the organization who make a valuable contribution to management system goal attainment. 2. In educational practice, persons who can contribute expertise to the issues being taught.

APPROPRIATE TECHNOLOGY In industry, using inexpensive methods and equipment to employ people in meaningful work that is nonpolluting and energy independent.

APPROPRIATION A legislative authorization of money in a specific amount for a specific purpose. Funds are allotted to the agency by the budget agency after the ~ is made by the legislative body.

APPROPRIATIONS RESPONSE The process of providing operating funds for governmental programs. A legislature determines the amount of money available and the conditions for distribution.

APPROVED BY GOVERNOR In politics, the signature of a governor on a bill passed by the legislature.

APPROXIMATION 1. In psychology, shaping *q.v.* 2. A value differing from a true value by an amount that can be neglected. 3. A method for arriving at a value.

APRAXIA 1. The inability to recall skilled movement, usually as a result of brain damage. 2. Loss or partial loss of the ability to move purposefully. 3. Dyspraxia *q.v.* 4. The inability to perform various purposive movements in the absence of paralysis, ataxia *q.v.*, or disturbance in sensation. ~ may take the form of motor, ideomotor, or ideational. cf: aphasia; agnosia.

APROBARBITAL 1. A barbiturate *q.v.* sedative-hypnotic. 2. Alurate is a brand name preparation.

APROSEXIA A condition characterized by difficulty in focusing attention.

APSYCHICAL In psychology, not related to the mental.

APTA An acronym for American Physical Therapy Association.

APTD An acronym for Aid to the Permanently and Totally Disabled *q.v.*

APTITUDE 1. An ability that is potentially related to the skillful performance of some task. 2. The capacity to profit from training is some particular skill. 3. In health education, the potential to behave healthfully. 4. A group of characteristics (native or acquired) deemed to be present within a person as a potential to acquire proficiency in a particular area of endeavor, such as music, art, mathematics, etc. ct. ability.

APTITUDE TEST 1. An evaluation instrument designed to measure a person's potentials to perform or to learn. 2. An examination useful in predicting job success or training success.

AQ An acronym for achievement quotient. cf: achievement age; achievement test.

AQUAFORE An underground water channel or water source.

AQUEDUCT In anatomy, a canal for the conduction of liquid. For example, the cerebral aqueduct of Sylvius *q.v.* connects the third and fourth ventricles of the brain.

AQUEOUS HUMOR A watery fluid within the aqueous chamber of the eyeball.

AQUICULTURE 1. The technique of cultivating and harvesting plants and animal that live in water. 2. Hydroponics *q.v.*

ARACHIDONIC ACID A 20-carbon atom of fatty acid *q.v.* with four double bonds. In the body, it is synthesized *q.v.* from the essential fatty acid, linoleic acid *q.v.*

ARACHNOID 1. Resembling a spider web. 2. A delicate membrane interposed between the dura mater *q.v.* and the pia mater *q.v.* and overlying the brain. 3. One of the meninges *q.v.*

ARBITRARY 1. In education and labor relations, not supported by fair cause and without reason given. 2. Fixed or arrived at by caprice.

ARBITRATION 1. In educational labor relations, a procedure under which a neutral third party (arbitrator) hears both the union's and the administration's side in a dispute and issues an award that is binding upon both sides. 2. Submission of a controversy, usually in labor disputes, for determination. cf: mediation.

ARBITRATOR In educational labor relations, an impartial third party to whom disputing parties submit their differences for a decision.

ARC 1. AIDS-related complex *q.v.* (no longer applicable). 2. Association for Retarded Citizens. 3. Advocacy and Resource Center.

ARCHETYPE In psychology, a recurring theme or pattern with threads of common experience.

ARCHIVAL STUDY A research procedure that depends on historical documents and records for data. This method of study is especially useful in studying the unfolding of social patterns over a period of time or the effects of particular historical events or conditions.

AREA OF RESPONSIBILITY In Role Delineation, a major aspect of the role *q.v.* which encompasses an aggregate of related functions.

AREA VOCATIONAL CENTER A shared-time facility that provides instruction in vocational education within a school system or region. Students attending ∼s receive their academic areas of education in regular schools within the district or region.

AREAS OF PRACTICE IN HEALTH EDUCATION Health education practices *q.v.*

AREFLEXIA Loss or absence of the reflexes *q.v.*

AREOLA The pigmented area on the breast of females surrounding the nipple.

AREOLAE The brownish rings that surround the breast nipples.

ARGON A colorless, odorless, chemically inactive, gaseous element that, because of its inertness, is used for filling fluorescent and incandescent lamps.

ARGUMENTATIVE DISCOURSE In family sociology, a form of family interaction wherein parents openly challenge moral positions held by their children and by each other, discussing the differences between the positions.

ARGYLL-ROBERTSON PUPIL (SIGN) Failure of the papillary reflex to respond to light. A diagnostic sign of general paresis *q.v.*

ARHYTHMIA Arrhythmia *q.v.*

ARIBOFLAVINOSIS A condition caused by a lack of riboflavin *q.v.* characterized by cracking of the corners of the mouth, sore skin, and bloodshot eyes.

ARISTOTELIANISM 1. According to the teachings of Aristotle; a moderate realism *q.v.*, as contrasted to nominalism *q.v.*, that universal thoughts and ideas have no real existence in things, and in contrast to Platonism *q.v.*, that such ideas exist or subsist independently of the mind. ∼ holds that the object of the universal idea is real in nature because it represents the reality of each individual essence, but the universality *q.v.* of the universal idea is mental because the individual essence is itself not universal in nature. 2. The system of thought that follows the principles and teachings of Aristotle. cf: Aristotelian method.

ARISTOTELIAN METHOD 1. The method of revealing relations between the particular and the general by means of investigation of the general through induction *q.v.*, perception *q.v.*, memory, and experience; and by means of determination of the particular from the general through deduction *q.v.*, proof, and explanation. 2. The method of explaining particular facts and phenomena by means of accepted principles and laws.

ARM 1. The upper extremity. 2. That segment of the upper extremity between the shoulder and the elbow.

ARMA An acronym for American Registry of Medical Assistants.

ARMORING OF THE EGO In psychology, an ego defense mechanism *q.v.* that becomes a fixed personality characteristic protecting the self from anxiety *q.v.*

ARMY STRETCHER A folding stretcher *q.v.* made of wooden poles covered with canvas, with short, folding legs.

AROUSAL 1. In psychology, a state of generalized physiological activation manifest in bodily changes such as increased heart rate and palmar sweating. 2. A state of activation, either behavioral or physiological.

ARREST In cardiology, a stoppage of the heart or of respiration, due to the interruption of the nervous impulses controlling these functions. cf: cardiac arrest.

ARRHYTHMIA 1. A complication of myocardial infarction *q.v.* resulting from irregular transmission of electrical impulses to the cardiac muscle *q.v.* 2. Damage to the heart muscle causing transmission of the electrical impulses to be irregular and unpredictable. cf: ventricular fibrillation; cardiac arrhythmia.

AART An acronym for American Registry of Radiologic Technologists.

ARSENAL-OF-WEAPONS APPROACH In labor relations, the management holds the threat of a variety of measures abhorrent to the parties as a deterrent to a strike.

ARSENIC A poisonous element whose chemical symbol is As. ~ residue may be found in tobacco smoke as a result of some pesticides *q.v.* used in the growing of tobacco. ~ has the odor of garlic.

ARSPHENAMINE 1. The first successful treatment for syphilis *q.v.* 2. A drug used to treat syphilis before the discovery of penicillin *q.v.*

ARTANE A commercial preparation of trihexyphenidyl *q.v.*

ARTERIAL BLOOD Oxygenated blood distributed throughout the body in the arteries.

ARTERIAL THROMBOSIS A blood clot *q.v.* within an artery. ~ may result in a heart attack or stroke *q.v.* depending upon where the clot forms.

ARTERIOGRAM An X-ray of a vein or artery that is obtained by injecting a radioactive substance into the blood vessel to be examined.

ARTERIOLES 1. Parts of the blood vessels that open and close within the autonomic nervous system *q.v.* 2. The smallest arteries leading to the capillaries *q.v.*

ARTERIOSCLEROSIS 1. A general term that includes several conditions in which either the inner or middle layers of an artery undergo progressive, damaging changes resulting in decreased flexibility of the arterial wall. This may be the underlying cause of coronary heart disease or stroke *q.v.* 2. Calcification of an artery's wall that makes the vessel less elastic, more brittle, and more susceptible to bursting. 3. Hardening of the arteries. 4. Any disease of the arteries. ct: atherosclerosis.

ARTERY A blood vessel that carries blood away from the heart. cf: vein.

ARTHRALGIA Pain in one or more of the joints.

ARTHRITIC DISORDERS A group of diseases affecting the joints. They include rheumatic arthritis, degenerative arthritis, gout, and bursitis. Although there is no cure for arthritic disorders, there are treatments to help reduce some of the symptoms: administration of hormones, diet, rest, controlled exercise, and others. cf: arthritis.

ARTHRITIS 1. A disease, thought to be at least partly of autoimmune *q.v.* origin, in which the joints become stiff and movement if painful. 2. A general term referring to diseases of the joints. ~ includes over 100 different diseases, often involving aches and pains in the joints and connective tissues. Most forms of ~ are chronic *q.v.*, but proper treatment can frequently reduce symptoms *q.v.* The most common types in older people are osteoarthritis, rheumatoid arthritis, and gout. 3. A disease involving inflammation *q.v.* of the joints due to infections *q.v.*, or constitutional (genetic) causes. cf: arthritic disorders.

ARTHRODESIS 1. The fusing of the surfaces of a joint by surgical means. Artificial ankylosis *q.v.*

ARTHROPLASTY Any operation or surgical procedure designed to reconstruct a joint.

ARTHROPOD 1. An animal in the class Arachnida and Insecta, among others, capable of producing disease in humans. An example of a disease produced by an ~ is scabies *q.v.* 2. An animal having an exoskeleton *q.v.*, paired, jointed appendages, and segmented body. ~s include insects, spiders, and ticks. 3. An insect-like animal.

ARTHROSCOPIC Pertaining to joints.

ARTHROSIS A joint or articulation *q.v.*

ARTHROSTEITIS A joint characterized by inflammation *q.v.* of the bony part of a joint.

ARTICULATION 1. A joint between two bones. ~ may be movable or immovable, but most often refers to the movable joints. 2. In education, the relationship between two or more elements of the educational program. Usually, coordination of curricula and educational procedures. 3. The relationship among curricular offerings, out-of-school programs, and successive levels of the educational system.

ARTICULATION DISABILITIES 1. Speech problems, such as omissions, substitutions, additions, and distortions. 2. Articulation disorder *q.v.*

ARTICULATION DISORDER 1. An abnormality in the speech/sound production process resulting in inaccurate or otherwise inappropriate execution of speaking. 2. Articulation disabilities.

ARTICULUS A joint.

ARTIFACT A factor other than those under investigation that influences the results of an experiment.

ARTIFACTUAL Spurious *q.v.*

ARTIFICIAL AIRWAY A device to provide and maintain free passage of air through the upper airway *q.v.*

ARTIFICIAL IMMUNITY 1. Resistance to disease that is induced by scientific techniques, such as inoculation *q.v.* of antibodies *q.v.* into a person's body. 2. A type of acquired immunity *q.v.* resulting from the body's response to pathogens *q.v.* that are introduced into the body by immunization *q.v.* ct: natural immunity.

ARTIFICIAL INSEMINATION 1. Placing sperm *q.v.* in the uterus *q.v.* by artificial means. 2. The introduction of semen *q.v.* into the vagina *q.v.* or womb *q.v.* of a woman by artificial means. 3. The introduction of sperm into a woman's vagina or cervix *q.v.* by means of a syringe rather than a penis *q.v.* The sperm may be from the woman's husband (AIH) or a donor (AID).

ARTIFICIAL INSEMINATION DONOR AID *q.v.*

ARTIFICIAL INSEMINATION HUSBAND AIH *q.v.*

ARTIFICIAL INTELLIGENCE 1. Aspects of cognitive *q.v.* processing carried out by a computer. 2. Problem-solving computer programs.

ARTIFICIAL KIDNEY A mechanical device so designed that, when connect to a person's circulation, impurities are dialyzed from the blood. An ~ is a temporary substitute for the natural kidney.

ARTIFICIAL PARTHENOGENESIS The artificial activation of an egg to develop without fertilization *q.v.* by a male sperm *q.v.*

ARTIFICIAL RESPIRATION An obsolete term pertaining to a substitute for natural breathing. cf: artificial resuscitation *q.v.*

ARTIFICIAL RESUSCITATION 1. Cardiopulmonary resuscitation *q.v.* 2. Techniques used to force oxygen into the lungs of a person who has stopped breathing. The technique may involve the forcing of air from the lungs of a paramedic into the victim's lungs or the use of machinery to pump air into the lungs of the victim.

ARTIFICIAL VENTILATION Movement of air into and out of the lungs by artificial means. cf: artificial resuscitation.

ARTIOGRAPHY A diagnostic procedure for detecting obstructions in the brain.

ARV An acronym for AIDS-related virus. cf: AIDS-related complex.

ARYTENOID 1. Ladle-shaped. 2. Two small cartilages of the larynx.

ASAFETIDA An offensive gum-resin with garlic-like odor that comes from various Oriental plants and used in Asia as a condiment. ~ is used in veterinary medicine as an animal repellent.

ASC An acronym for altered states of consciousness *q.v.*

ASCARIASIS An infection with an intestinal worm, the Ascaris Lumbricoides.

ASCARIS 1. A roundworm. 2. A metazoan *q.v.*, pathogenic *q.v.* to humans.

ASCENDANCE 1. The tendency to assume a dominant role in personal relationships. 2. The state of being able to command, control, or influence other people. 3. Dominance over others. ct: submissiveness.

ASCENDING RETICULAR SYSTEM The system of ascending nerve fibers that carry impulses from the subcortical areas of the brain to the cerebral cortex *q.v.*

ASCETICISM 1. The doctrine that self-denial and avoidance of pleasure is the most desirable lifestyle. 2. Philosophically centered denial of the importance of the body.

ASCETIC A person who renounces comfort to lead a life of self-denial. cf: asceticism.

ASCH'S THEORY OF SOCIAL PERCEPTION The concept that in the perception of another person, the meaning of each idea used in labeling the person is influenced by the surrounding context. The overall impression is therefore qualitatively different from the simple sum of the person's traits.

ASCITES An accumulation of fluid in the abdominal cavity.

ASCORBIC ACID 1. Vitamin C *q.v.* 2. One of the water-soluble vitamins *q.v.* necessary for healthy tissues, especially the formation of collagen *q.v.* ~ is necessary for the transformation of the amino acids *q.v.* proline and lysine. This vitamin prevents scurvy *q.v.* and is needed to aid in the healing of wounds.

ASCRIBED STATUS In sociology, a social position assigned to a person because of the office or position he/she holds.

ASCRIPTIVE RESPONSIBILITY In sociology, the social judgment assigned to a person who has committed an illegal act and who, it is decided, should be punished for the act. ct: descriptive responsibility.

ASEMIA 1. The loss of the ability to understand or communicate by signs, signals, or gestures. 2. Asymbolia *q.v.*

ASENDIN A commercial preparation of amoxapine *q.v.*

ASEXUAL 1. A person with no interest in sex and who does not engage in any form of sexual activity. 2. Without sex. cf: asexual reproduction.

ASEXUAL REPRODUCTION 1. In some lower animals, a form of procreation *q.v.* or reproduction that comes about by means other than sexual relations. 2. A form of reproduction not requiring both male and female interaction. 3. Any process of reproduction that does not involve the formation and union of gametes *q.v.* from the two sexes. 4. The division of a single organism into two identical organisms. ct: sexual reproduction.

ASEXUALS 1. Homosexuals *q.v.* who have infrequent sexual contacts. 2. People who show no erotic interest. cf: asexual.

ASMT An acronym for American Society for Medical Technologists.

ASOCIAL 1. An attitude or behavior characterized by indifference to social customs, moral codes, or acceptable social relationships. 2. Devoid of social values or meanings. ct: antisocial; unsocial.

ASOCIALITY A negative symptom in schizophrenia *q.v.* marked by the inability to form close relationships and to feel intimacy.

ASOCIAL MOLESTER Antisocial *q.v.* persons with long criminal records who have sexual contacts with children.

ASONIA Tone deafness.

ASPARTAME An artificial sweetener made up of two amino acids *q.v.*

ASPHYXIA 1. Suffocation *q.v.* 2. A condition caused by impaired ventilation and characterized by decreased oxygen and increased carbon dioxide in the blood. 3. Loss of consciousness from deficient oxygen supply. cf: asphyxiation.

ASPHYXIATION 1. A condition resulting from inhaling a poisonous gas such as carbon monoxide. The gas inhaled prevents the absorption of oxygen from the lungs by the red blood cells. 2. Death resulting from a lack of oxygen to the brain. ct: suffocation.

ASPIRATE 1. To remove fluid from a cavity by supplying suction. 2. The substance or material obtained by aspiration. 3. To breathe into the lungs.

ASPIRATION 1. Suction. 2. The removal of fluids by suction.

ASPIRATOR An apparatus for removing fluid or other material by suction from a body cavity or opening.

ASPIRE To breathe toward.

ASPIRIN One of the most frequently used analgesics *q.v.* ~ can relieve pain, lower body temperature, reduce inflammation *q.v.*, and prevent the formation of blood clots. However, ~ sometimes produces adverse effects such as stomach irritation and bleeding. ~ is the common name for acetylsalicylic acid *q.v.*

ASRT An acronym for American Society of Radiologic Technologists.

ASSASSIN Pertaining to a hired killer. The term is derived from a hashish-using cult, the hashishiyya.

ASSAULT 1. A threat or attempt to inflict bodily injury where the victim has reason to believe the injury may be inflicted. 2. An attempt to beat another person, without actual contact. ct: battery.

ASSAY An analysis of a substance to determine its constituents and their proportions.

ASSEMBLY In politics, the legislature made up of a certain number of members elected from districts apportioned on the basis of population.

ASSERTION In psychology, standing up for one's basic rights without violating the basic rights of other. cf: nonassertive. ct: aggressive.

ASSERTION TRAINING 1. Behavior therapy *q.v.* procedures that attempt to help a person express more easily thoughts, wishes, and beliefs, and to legitimate feelings of resentment or approval. 2. Behavioral training that teaches a person how to communicate in an open, straightforward way and to refuse unreasonable requests and stand up for his or her rights. 3. Assertiveness training *q.v.*

ASSERTIVENESS TRAINING 1. Assertion training *q.v.* 2. A semi-structured teaching approach that emphasizes acquiring skills through practice. ~ generally includes: (a) teaching people the difference between assertion and aggression and between non-assertion and politeness; (b) helping people to identify and accept both their own personal rights and the rights of others; (c) reducing existing obstacles to acting assertively; and (d) developing assertive skills through active practice methods.

ASSESSMENT 1. The act of measuring or determining the level of an attribute; such as hearing, vision, achievement. 2. Determining the nature and value of a health condition or situation.

ASSESSMENT CENTER 1. A place that provides programs in which participants engage in and are evaluated on a number of individual and group exercises constructed to simulate important activities at the organizational levels to which these participants aspire. 2. A place that uses multiple exercises to evaluate individuals and to identify promotable candidates.

ASSESSMENT TECHNIQUES Methods of observation and measurement used to profile a person's psychological and behavioral traits. Assessment supports diagnosis, intervention, and research.

ASSIGNMENT 1. The act by a teacher of allotting specific mental or physical tasks to be completed within a specified time line. 2. The work or study allotted to the learner or to a group of learners to be completed in a specified manner and time.

ASSIGN-STUDY-RECITE FORMULA A teaching formula that is subject-centered that emphasizes assimilation *q.v.* of information by the learners and the method of explanation by the teacher which follows this procedure: (a) explanation and assignment *q.v.*; (b) study through reading, research, or written exercises; (c) application. cf: Herbatian steps in learning; Morrison plan; assimilation.

ASSIMILATION 1. In education, the process of internalizing the learning experience as a part of the self. 2. Fitting an experience into one's cognitive *q.v.* structure. 3. In health education, applying relevance to a health fact or facts. 4. In physiology, the incorporation into the biological structure, as to assimilate nourishment. 5. In psychology, the cognitive transforming of an external stimulus into a part of one's personality *q.v.* 6. In social psychology, the tendency to twist the details of an ambiguous stimulus in order to produce a more recognizable structure. 7. The tendency to fit a new experience into an existing one or scheme. 8. In sociology, the process whereby individuals or groups in interaction take on the characteristics of one or more of the interacting parties. 9. In nutrition science, the use of food nutrients *q.v.* by the body in cell activities. 10. One of the steps in the Morrison Plan *q.v.* cf: accommodation.

ASSISTANT PRINCIPAL An administrative position in an individual school that primarily assists the principal *q.v.* in administrative duties.

ASSISTANT SUPERINTENDENT An administrative position in a school district that primarily assists the superintendent *q.v.* in administrative duties.

ASSISTANT-TO An understudy position to develop managers.

ASSOCIATEDNESS OF RACE (OR OTHER ATTRIBUTES) In the development of awareness of racial dimensions of social life, preschool children's tendency to connect race and attributes unrelated to race.

ASSOCIATE DEGREE A degree or award based on less than 4 years of academic education beyond high school, frequently awarded by a community college or junior college.

ASSOCIATE PLAY Play that involves a common activity, but that does not require cooperation among children other than perhaps sharing materials or conversation. The children involved in ~ work independently of each other toward goals of their own choosing.

ASSOCIATE STAFF In health care facilities, a hospital staff position usually held by new, young, or inexperienced physicians.

ASSOCIATION 1. In epidemiology *q.v.*, as one variable *q.v.* changes, there is a change in the quality or quantity of another variable. 2. In psychology *q.v.*, the linkage between two mental processes as a result of past experience in which the two have occurred together. 3. In sociology *q.v.*, social contacts and relationships with individuals and groups. 4. A group of professionals organized for the purpose of promoting their particular goals. 5. A society or federation. cf: correlation.

ASSOCIATION AREAS 1. In anatomy *q.v.*, those parts of the cortex *q.v.* that are not projection areas. ~ tend to be involved with the integration of sensory information or of motor commands. 2. The areas, mainly in the frontal cortex, that are thought to subserve thought and other associative functions. 3. The area of the central nervous system *q.v.* in which experiences are related.

ASSOCIATION BY CONTIGUITY In psychology *q.v.*, a state of functional relationship between two or more stimuli *q.v.*, situations, ideas, or concepts resulting from being experienced in temporal or special proximity so that one will evoke the other.

ASSOCIATION FOR THE ADVANCEMENT OF HEALTH EDUCATION A division of the American Alliance for Health, Physical Education, Recreation and Dance (AAHPERD).

ASSOCIATIONIST 1. S-R psychologist *q.v.* 2. The psychological school of thought that maintains that learning is determined by a link which is created between a stimulus and a response through action on the part of the learner; that is, learning is a process of developing associative connections or bonds.

ASSOCIATION LEARNING Learning that one event is likely to occur in the presence of another event.

ASSOCIATION NEURON In the reflex arc *q.v.*, a neuron *q.v.* that transmits impulses from afferent neuron *q.v.* to efferent neuron *q.v.* cf: association areas.

ASSOCIATION OF COLLEGIATE SCHOOLS OF NURSING An organization founded in 1933 and consolidated with the National League for Nursing in 1952.

ASSOCIATIVE INHIBITION 1. Muller–Schumann paradigm. 2. The idea that when an association *q.v.* has been made between any two items, it is difficult to form any association between either of the two and a third item.

ASSOCIATIVE RESPONSE In mental tasks, the first responses that may spring to a person's mind. ct: cognitive responses.

ASSORTIVE MATING 1. The tendency for people to mate with those who are similar in general characteristics. 2. Homogamy *q.v.*

ASSUMPTION (SCIENTIFIC) 1. The fundamental assertions about the nature of the world that are scientifically studied. Such statements are not empirically testable, for they are the starting point of scientific reasoning. 2. A broad concept to implicate any one of the propositions from which reasoning begins or which is essential to the solution of a problem. ct: hypothesis; postulate; premise; presupposition.

ASSUMPTIVE REALITY The failure to distinguish hypothesis *q.v.* from fact, characteristic of egocentrism *q.v.* associated with concrete operations. cf: cognitive conceit.

ASTASIA–ABASIA The ability to stand or walk without the legs wobbling about and collapsing. There is generally normal control of the legs while sitting or lying, and there is no associated organic *q.v.* pathology *q.v.*

ASTEREOGNOSIS 1. The inability to identify objects or forms by touch. Agnosia *q.v.*

ASTHENIA Bodily weakness. cf: asthenic reaction

ASTHENIC REACTION 1. Neurasthenia *q.v.* 2. A loss of strength, weakness, and chronic *q.v.* fatigue resulting from stress, nervousness, or emotional tension. 3. A psychoneurotic reaction *q.v.* 4. Asthenia *q.v.*

ASTHMA 1. Difficulty in breathing caused by spasm of the bronchial tubes *q.v.* or swelling of the mucous membranes *q.v.* of these tubes. 2. A condition, often of allergic *q.v.* origin, that is characterized by continuous labored breathing accompanied by wheezing, a sense of constriction in the chest, and attacks of coughing and gasping. 3. A chronic *q.v.* reactive respiratory disorder that can cause wheezing, considerable difficulty in breathing, and possible life-threatening respiratory failure.

ASTHO An acronym for Association of State and Territorial Health Officials.

ASTIGMATISM 1. A defect of the refractive surface of the eye that distorts light rays so that they cannot focus on a single point on the retina *q.v.* 2. A refractive condition that occurs when the surface of the cornea *q.v.* is uneven or structurally defective, preventing light rays from converging at one point.

ASTRAGALUS The large bone of the ankle that joins with the two bones of the leg.

ASTRINGENT A substance that contracts tissues of the body.

ASTROCYTE 1. A star-shaped neuralgia *q.v.* 2. Connective tissue cells in the brain and spinal cord.

ASTROLOGY A pseudoscience *q.v.* that formulates general concepts of the universe based on the assumption *q.v.* that there is a relationship between the movement of the sun, moon, and the planets, and movement of life on earth. ct: astronomy.

ASTRONOMY The science that deals with the celestial bodies; that studies their positions, motions, distances, constitution, relationships, history, and formation.

ASYLUM A refuge established in Western Europe in the fifteenth century as a place to confine and provide for the mentally ill. ~s were the forerunners of the present-day mental hospitals.

ASYMBOLIA A condition characterized by the inability to use symbols, as found in mathematics.

ASYMPTOMATIC 1. In regard to AIDS *q.v.*, no apparent symptoms *q.v.* of illness even though the person tests positive for HIV *q.v.* 2. In general, a condition or disease that presents no detectable symptoms.

ASYMPTOMATIC SEROPOSITIVE HIV-positive *q.v.* without signs or symptoms of HIV *q.v.* disease. cf: AIDS; AIDS-related complex.

ASYMPTOTE A limit that a mathematical function approaches but never reaches.

ASYNAPSIS 1. In genetics, the failure or partial failure of pairing of homologous *q.v.* chromosomes *q.v.* during the meiotic prophase *q.v.* 2. Failure of chiasma *q.v.* formation resulting in a high frequency of univalents.

ASYSTOLE 1. Cardiac *q.v.* standstill. 2. Absence of any contraction or electrical activity of the heart.

ATARACTIC 1. Any drug that creates a feeling of calmness. 2. The tranquilizers *q.v.* 3. Drugs used to designate a detached serenity without depression of mental faculties or consciousness.

ATAVISM The recurrence in a descendant of genetic characteristics of a remote ancestor. cf: reversion.

ATAXIA 1. Muscular uncoordination, esp. of the arms and legs. 2. A condition in which central nervous system *q.v.* deficits lead to uncoordinated motor activity, characterized by jerky movements, balance problems, and, occasionally, speech and writing difficulties. 3. A condition in which a person experiences extreme difficulty in controlling fine and gross motor movements. cf: locomotor ataxia.

ATELECTASIS 1. A collapse of the alveolar *q.v.* air spaces of the lungs. 2. Airlessness of the lungs.

ATHEROMA An abnormal mass of fatty material that has been deposited in an artery wall.

ATHEROSCLEROSIS 1. A subset of arteriosclerosis *q.v.* specifically involving the inner lining of an artery. 2. The accumulation of fatty substances on the walls of a blood vessel that sometimes restricts or blocks the flow of blood. 3. A disease characterized by formation of fatty, fibrous lesions *q.v.* in the lining of arteries. The danger of ~ is that the accumulated atheroma *q.v.* can eventually block the flow of blood, triggering a heart attack or stroke *q.v.* 4. A disease process that involves the formation of fatty plaques *q.v.* in the arteries. When the plaques form in the coronary arteries *q.v.*, they obstruct the flow of blood resulting in insufficient oxygen to the cardiac muscle *q.v.* which can result in angina pectoris *q.v.*, cardiac insufficiency *q.v.*, and myocardial infarction *q.v.*

ATHEROSCLEROTIC PLAQUE White patches formed in the inner lining of an artery. cf: atherosclerosis; arteriosclerosis.

ATHETOSIS 1. A recurring, involuntary, tentacle-like movement of the hands and feet, usually associated with brain pathology *q.v.* 2. A type of cerebral palsy *q.v.* characterized by purposeless movements and grimaces.

ATHLETE'S FOOT 1. A fungal infection of the feet characterized by itching, peeling of the skin, esp. between the toes, cracking, bleeding, and oozing of lymph *q.v.* 2. Ringworm *q.v.* of the foot.

AT-HOME-CARE Medical care or treatment for people who are too ill to leave home; generally provided by nurses, rehabilitation therapists, and others.

ATIVAN A commercial preparation of lorazepam *q.v.*

ATLAS The first vertebra of the neck that articulates *q.v.* with the skull.

ATOM 1. The basic structural unit of all substances. ~s consist of protons, neutrons, and electrons. 2. The smallest unit of matter that can take part in the formation of molecules *q.v.*

ATOMIC ENERGY Energy *q.v.* that can be liberated by changes in the nucleus of an atom *q.v.*

ATONEMENT 1. A form of intellectualization in which a person acts to atone for his/her misdeeds, thereby undoing them. 2. Expiation *q.v.* 3. A defense mechanism *q.v.*

ATONIA A condition evidenced by lack of muscle tone.

ATONICITY A lack of normal muscle tone. cf: atony; atonia.

ATONY The loss of tone or response in a muscle. cf: atonicity.

ATP 1. Adenosine triphosphate *q.v.* 2. A molecule *q.v.* of prime importance to cellular energy metabolism *q.v.* cf: ATPase.

ATPase Adenosine triphosphatase *q.v.*

ATRESIA 1. A process of the ovaries which reduces the number of primary oocytes *q.v.* from about 60,000 to 20,000. The absence of a body opening which normally should be present. 3. Congenital absence or pathological *q.v.* closure of a normal opening or passage. 4. Involution *q.v.*

ATRIA 1. The heart chambers that receive oxygen-depleted (deoxygenated) blood. The auricles *q.v.* of the heart.

ATRIAL SEPTAL DEFECT An opening between the atria *q.v.* of the heart.

ATRICHOUS In biology, cells lacking flagella *q.v.*, generally used to refer to originally flagellated cells that have lost their flagella.

ATRIOVENTRICULAR BLOCK 1. Interference with conduction of electrical impulses from upper to lower chambers of the heart and throughout the lower chambers. 2. Heart block.

ATRIOVENTRICULAR NODE In the heart, a small mass of special muscular fibers in the septum between the right atrium *q.v.* and the ventricle *q.v.* that forms the bundle of His *q.v.* which receives electrical impulses from the sinoatrial node *q.v.* of the S.A. node *q.v.*

AT RISK 1. In epidemiology *q.v.*, a person or group capable of experiencing the health factor being studied. 2. The state of being subject to the occurrence of some uncertain event that connotes loss or difficulty.

ATRIUM One of the upper chambers of the heart. The right atrium receives venous blood from the systems of the body while the left atrium receives oxygenated *q.v.* blood from the lungs.

ATROPA BELLADONNA The plant from which atropine *q.v.* is derived.

ATROPINE 1. An alkaloid *q.v.* obtained from atropa belladonna *q.v.* ~ inhibits the action of the craniosacral division of the autonomic nervous system *q.v.* 2. An anticholinergic *q.v.*

ATROPINIZATION A treatment for cataracts *q.v.* that involves washing the eye with atropine *q.v.*, which will permanently dilate the pupil of the eye.

ATROPHY 1. A wasting away of a tissue. 2. A weakened condition of muscle tissue generally characterized by decrease in size and strength.

ATSDR An acronym for Agency for Toxic Substances and Disease Registry. cf: answer.

ATTACHMENT 1. In social psychology, the tendency of a child to stay in close proximity to an adult. 2. Bonding *q.v.* 3. Imprinting *q.v.* 4. Close reciprocal bond that may develop between two people.

ATTACK MECHANISM A form of defense mechanism *q.v.* or adjustment mechanism *q.v.*

ATTEMPTED RAPE In law, an effort to commit forcible rape *q.v.* in which the male does not effect penetration.

ATTENDANCE CENTER In education, an administrative unit consisting of the region from which learners may attend a given school building.

ATTENDING PHYSICIAN A medical doctor who directs a patient's care during a hospital confinement.

ATTENTION 1. All the processes by which people perceive *q.v.* on a selective basis. 2. The tendency to focus activities in a certain direction. 3. The maintenance of a readiness to respond, or focusing on relevant information.

ATTENTION DEFICIT DISORDER (ADD) 1. A group of disorders associated in underachievement and low motivation *q.v.* and classified as (a) minimal brain dysfunction; (b) learning disability syndrome *q.v.*; (c) hyperactive child syndrome *q.v.* 2. A learning disability that may or may not be accompanied by hyperactivity. Most common in male children. 3. A diagnostic label used by the American Psychiatric Association to signify a condition in which a person exhibits signs of developmentally inappropriate hyperactivity, impulsiveness, and inattention. cf: attention deficit disorder with hyperactivity (ADHD).

ATTENTION DEFICIT DISORDER WITH HYPERACTIVITY (ADHD) A developmental disorder in children marked by difficulties in focusing adequately on the task at hand and by inappropriate fidgeting and antisocial *q.v.* behavior.

ATTENTION-PLACEBO CONDITION A study in which the client receives a believable treatment containing many of the nonspecific aspects of the active therapy, but does not receive the supposedly active therapeutic ingredient.

ATTENTIONAL PROCESSES One of the four stages to observational learning *q.v.* influenced by one's needs and desires and the attractiveness of the model activity being observed.

ATTENUATED 1. Weakened. 2. The result of a preparation to weaken microorganisms *q.v.* to be used as a vaccine *q.v.* The process is used, e.g., in the preparation of the BCG vaccine *q.v.*

ATTESTATION In law, the act of witnessing a will by its maker and becoming a signature to the completed will.

ATTITUDE 1. A tendency to respond in a characteristic way to some social stimulus *q.v.* 2. A predisposition or set to respond in some consistent way toward an exogenous *q.v.* stimulus. 3. In health education, a set to respond healthfully; safe behavior, avoiding unhealthful situations regarding nutrition, exercise, using drugs, smoking, use of alcohol, and the like. 4. In sociology, preconceived notions or ideas that affect behavior toward certain groups of people or social programs. 5. An enduring predisposition to react negatively or positively toward an object. 6. An evaluation disposition that tends to make a person think, feel, or act positively or negatively about some person, group or social issue. 7. A hypothetical construct that is used to explain consistencies within a person related to affective *q.v.* reactions. 8. A representation of a person's emotional evaluation of an entity. 9. A state of readiness to exhibit a particular response. cf: affective domain.

ATTITUDE-DISCREPANT BEHAVIOR Actions that are inconsistent with a person's attitudes *q.v.* and that may prompt a person to change attitudes.

ATTITUDE POLARIZATION A situation in which an attitude *q.v.* becomes more positive when initially positive, and more negative when initially negative.

ATTITUDE SALIENCE An awareness of an attitude *q.v.* toward any of a variety of objects.

ATTITUDE SCALE A device for measuring attitude *q.v.* toward any of a variety of objects.

ATTITUDE TEST An evaluation of one's attitudes *q.v.*; that is, beliefs, or predispositions to act or respond in some consistent way to an external stimulus *q.v.*

ATTITUDINAL DEVELOPMENT The progressive acquisition of attitudes *q.v.* beginning at birth, but continuing throughout life as learning situations are experienced and new insights *q.v.* are acquired.

ATTRACTION 1. The way or manner in which people positively or negatively evaluate others. 2. A force that draws people together. 3. An attitude *q.v.* of liking or disliking.

ATTRACTION–REPULSION Approach–avoidance *q.v.*

ATTRACTIVE NUISANCE A condition, instrumentally, machine, or other agency, dangerous to young people because of their inability to appreciate its danger, although they may be expected to be attracted to it. cf: nuisance.

ATTRIBUTABLE RISK In epidemiology, quantifying the amount of risk due to a particular characteristic. It is calculated by subtracting the incidence rate *q.v.* for the group that does not have the characteristic from the rate for the group with the characteristic.

ATTRIBUTION 1. The explanation a person has for his or her behavior. 2. The tendency that people have to ascribe causes to their subjective experiences. The ~ process itself can shape the subjective experience. cf: misattribution; ct: muscular strength.

ATTRIBUTION THEORY 1. The process by which people attempt to explain another person's behavior, relating it to situational factors or to some inferred dispositional qualities, or both. 2. A theory concerned with the way people interpret the causes of events or actions.

ATYPICAL Irregular or not of typical character *q.v.*

ATYPICAL PSYCHOSIS A disorder in which the symptoms *q.v.* do not meet the criteria for any specific psychotic disorder *q.v.*

AUDIENCE CREDIBILITY In research, judgment on the part of the audience of the credibility they are willing to grant the researchers for having made good judgments in the design and implementation of the study, esp. for aspects not directly described in the report.

AUDIO Pertaining to sound waves to which the ear responds.

AUDIOGRAM A graph that shows the ability of a person to hear tones of varying frequencies.

AUDIOLOGIST 1. A nonmedical practitioner who is trained to deal with the rehabilitation of persons with hearing difficulties. 2. A health care professional who is trained to assess auditory *q.v.* function.

AUDIOMETER An electronic device used to detect a person's response to sound stimuli *q.v.*

AUDIOMETRICIAN A person trained in the use of various hearing screening devices and procedures.

AUDIO-VISUAL AIDS In education, sensory media that stimulate the senses and assist in the learning process.

AUDIO-VISUAL KIT Instructional materials, usually in the form of CDs, DVDs, and other audio-visual aids *q.v.* and printed information.

AUDIO-VISUAL MATERIAL Any device by means of which the learning process *q.v.* may be encouraged or carried through the senses, esp. hearing and sight.

AUDIT In administration, a comprehensive analysis of all aspects of personnel work and accounting.

AUDITION In physiology and psychology, the act of hearing or the sense of hearing.

AUDITORY Pertaining to sounds and hearing. cf: auditory projection area.

AUDITORY ACUITY Clarity or sharpness at which a particular sound can be heard.

AUDITORY ASSOCIATION The ability to associate verbally presented information.

AUDITORY BLENDING The act of blending the parts of a word into an integrated whole when speaking.

AUDITORY CANAL In anatomy, a section of the outer ear that carries sound waves to the ear drum.

AUDITORY DISCRIMINATION 1. The ability to distinguish between sounds of varying frequencies and intensity. 2. The act of distinguishing between different sounds.

AUDITORY MEMORY 1. The ability to recall words, digits, and the like in a meaningful manner with memory of meaning. 2. The ability to recall verbally presented material and information.

AUDITORY PERCEPTION The ability to receive sounds accurately and to understand their meaning. cf: perception.

AUDITORY PROJECTION AREA The area within the temporal lobe of the cerebral cortex *q.v.* where fibers of the classical auditory *q.v.* pathway terminates.

AUGMENTERS Persons who characteristically perceive *q.v.* greater environmental stimulation than does the average person. ~ respond to external stimuli *q.v.* directly by trying to do something to deal with them.

AURA 1. A distinctive and often subtle sensory stimulation associated with some epileptic seizures *q.v.* 2. Subjective sensations associated with and preceding an epileptic seizure. 3. A signal or warning of an impending convulsion *q.v.*, taking the form of dizziness or an unusual sensory experience.

AURAL HERPES ZOSTER A viral infection *q.v.* of the ear characterized by pain, impaired hearing, vertigo, and vomiting. Sometimes accompanied by facial paralysis *q.v.*, treatment is symptomatic *q.v.*

AURAL SENSATIONS Perception *q.v.* or awareness of sound.

AURICLES 1. Atria *q.v.* 2. The external ear. 3. One of the two main cavities of the heart which receive blood from a vein. 4. Ear-like appendage. 5. The pinna or flap of the ear. 6. A small pouch forming the upper portion of each atrium.

AUSCULTATION 1. The act of listening for sounds within the body. ~ is employed as a diagnostic method by physicians. 2. The process of detecting physical abnormalities by using the sense of hearing. 3. Using the stethoscope *q.v.*

AUTHENTIC ASSESSMENT A means of evaluating student progress through the use of portfolio development and accumulated evidence documenting achievement.

AUTHENTIC SELF 1. In psychology, a positive self-identity *q.v.* that underlies a person's more temporary mood identities. 2. The most basic self-concept *q.v.*

AUTHENTICITY OF EVIDENCE In research, reassurance that the evidence is what it purports to be. For example, that a test score represents a sample of a particular individual's behavior and not that of someone else.

AUTHOR In politics, the member who introduces a bill in the house of its origin. cf: sponsor.

AUTHORITARIAN A person who assumes that human relations are irrelevant to getting work done, and that people are necessarily indolent, self-centered, and uncooperative; and that they require strong direction and control if discipline is to be maintained. cf: authoritarian leader.

AUTHORITARIANISM 1. A philosophy of encouraging and upholding authority against individual freedom. 2. The power that commands influence, respect, or confidence.

AUTHORITARIAN LEADER A person who behaves toward subordinates in a controlling and dictatorial manner. cf: authoritarianism

AUTHORITARIAN PARENTS Parents who believe children's behavior should be closely regulated and who are likely to use power-assertive discipline methods. ct: permissive parents; authoritative parents.

AUTHORITARIAN PERSONALITY 1. A group of personal attributes *q.v.* and social attributes held to constitute a distinct personality *q.v.* 2. A personality style characterized by identification with and submission to authority, denial of feelings, and cynicism. 3. A personality that finds security in a social hierarchy in which people keep their appropriate position. Traits *q.v.* include rigid thinking and prejudice *q.v.* 4. antidemocratic personality.

AUTHORITATIVE PARENTS Parents who allow their children a great deal of freedom, but at the same time, consistently enforce some rules and standards of conduct. cf: authoritarian parents; permissive parents.

AUTHORITY 1. The right to perform or command. 2. A figure who believably asserts that something is true either without explanation or rationale (dogmatic authority, or with it, reasoning authority).

AUTHORITY STRUCTURE In sociology, those elected officials of a community who are mandated to make decisions on behalf of the people; common council, board of supervisors, board of health, state legislature, mayor, and governor. ct: power structure.

AUTISM 1. In psychology, absorption in fantasy *q.v.* to the exclusion of interest in reality. A symptom of schizophrenia *q.v.* 2. A form of early-onset developmental disorder *q.v.* characterized by discontinuities in the sequence of development, pervasive lack of responsiveness to others, and bizarre responses to various aspects of the environment. 3. Absorption in self or fantasy as a means of avoiding communication and escaping objective reality. cf: infantile autism; autistic thinking; Asperger's syndrome.

AUTISTIC Pertaining to a mentally introverted *q.v.*, self-centered condition in which reality is excluded. ~ children have little affect, showing either no emotional response or very inappropriate response.

AUTISTIC HOSTILITY The strong dislike felt by one group for another.

AUTISTIC THINKING Imaginary gratification of desires in fantasy as contrasted with realistic attempts to gratify them. cf: autism.

AUTOCHTHONOUS Native or endogenous microorganisms to an area, usually referring to soil microorganisms.

AUTOCHTHONOUS IDEA An idea that appears independent of a person's train of thought and which is usually regarded as foreign and thrust upon him or her.

AUTOCLAVE 1. A device used for sterilizing instruments and dressings by means of steam or moist heat under pressure. 2. Essentially, a pressure cooker.

AUTOEROTIC 1. Pertaining to self-stimulation or erotic behavior directed toward one's self. 2. Masturbation *q.v.* cf: autoeroticism.

AUTOEROTICISM 1. Masturbation *q.v.* 2. Self-gratification of sexual desires without the presence of another person. cf: autoerotic.

AUTOGENIC TRAINING 1. A system of physical and mental relaxation that employs self-suggestion to effect a physiological change through changes in the autonomic nervous system *q.v.* 2. A process of learning general body relaxation through the use of imagery and the feeling of heaviness and warmth in the body's limbs.

AUTOGNOSIS A process used in psychoanalysis *q.v.* that results in self-understanding using self-confessions.

AUTOIMMUNE 1. A self-immune *q.v.* response. 2. The condition in which the body produces an immune response to itself.

AUTOIMMUNE DISEASE A disease *q.v.* in which the body produces an immune response *q.v.* against itself. cf: autoimmune.

AUTOIMMUNE RESPONSE 1. Autoimmune disease *q.v.* 2. Autoimmune *q.v.*

AUTOINOCULATION A secondary infection *q.v.* originating from an infection site already present in the body.

AUTOINTOXICANT A poison generated within the body. cf: autointoxication.

AUTOINTOXICATION Poison by some uneliminated toxin *q.v.* generated within the body. cf: autointoxicant.

AUTOKINETIC EFFECT 1. An optical illusion in which a stationary pinpoint of light that is viewed in an otherwise dark room appears to be moving. 2. A form of apparent motion *q.v.*

AUTOLOGOUS 1. To one's self. 2. Donating one's own blood for future transfusion to self.

AUTOLYSIS The process of self-digestion in organs and tissues.

AUTOMATIC ACTION See automatic behavior.

AUTOMATIC BEHAVIOR A nonreflex but unconscious act. cf: invariable behavior; variable behavior; adaptive behavior.

AUTOMATIC HYPERREFLEX An exaggerated response by the autonomic nervous system *q.v.* to the birth process.

AUTOMATIC REACTION An action done without conscious thought.

AUTOMATIC THOUGHTS According to Beck, the things people picture or tell themselves as they make their way in life.

AUTOMATION The use of machines to control machines.

AUTOMATISM 1. The performance of an act without awareness. 2. Drug automatism *q.v.* 3. The performance *q.v.* of repetitious acts of a nonhabitual and nonreflex nature without conscious intent or supervision.

AUTOMATIZATION A process whereby skilled activities are subsumed by a higher order organization and are achieved automatically.

AUTONOMIC 1. Self-governing. 2. Independent.

AUTONOMIC HYPERACTIVITY Physical signs of anxiety *q.v.* including sweating, heart pounding, dry mouth, frequent urination, and diarrhea.

AUTONOMIC NERVOUS SYSTEM 1. That part of the nervous system that regulates the internal organs. In consists chiefly of ganglia *q.v.* connected with the brain stem and spinal cord, and is subdivided into the sympathetic and parasympathetic systems *q.v.* 2. That division of the central nervous system *q.v.* that controls the glands *q.v.* and the smooth and cardiac muscles *q.v.* 3. A division of the peripheral nervous system *q.v.* that connects the central nervous system to the organs of the body cavity, including the heart, stomach, and intestines, and whose nerves function automatically without conscious control. 4. The part of the nervous system that controls the involuntary functions of the body. The sympathetic and parasympathetic branches that activate and deactivate body responses as conditions warrant.

AUTONOMOUS PROFESSIONAL SPHERE The functioning of one of the four health education specialties; school, community, patient, corporate (industrial), in isolation of each other and separate from the basic, fundamental core of the health education profession.

AUTONOMY 1. The state of being clear, or realizing and acting on one's values. 2. Self-reliance. 3. The sense of being an individual in one's own right. 4. The degree to which a person is not controlled by outside pressures but permitted to rule the self.

AUTOPOLYPLOID 1. In genetics, an organism with more than two sets of chromosomes *q.v.* in its body cells, all derived from a single species. 2. A polyploid *q.v.* That has multiple and identical or nearly identical sets of chromosomes. 3. A polyploid species with a genome *q.v.* derived from the same original species.

AUTOPSY An examination of surgically removed tissue after death to determine specific cause of death.

AUTORADIOGRAPHY A record or photograph prepared by labeling a substance with radioactive *q.v.* material and allowing the image to develop on a film over a period of time.

AUTOSEXING A method of distinguishing the sex of young chickens by including marker genes *q.v.* into the breeding stock which produce a conspicuous phenotype *q.v.* on the male or female progeny at an early age.

AUTOSEXUAL BEHAVIOR Autoerotic *q.v.*

AUTOSOMAL A condition caused by non-sex chromosomes *q.v.* cf: autosome.

AUTOSOMAL CHROMOSOMES Non-sex chromosomes. cf: autosome; autosomal.

AUTOSOME 1. Any chromosome *q.v.* other than those that determine sex or gender *q.v.* 2. The 23 pairs of chromosomes that are the same in males and females. cf: sex chromosomes; autosomal.

AUTOTROPH In biology, an organism capable of producing all its protoplasmic need from inorganic sources. cf: autotrophic.

AUTOTROPHIC In biology, organisms able to manufacture all of their own food, as most green plants, and some bacteria. 2. Autotroph *q.v.*

AUXOCHROME A radical that forms a due when combined with a chromophore.

AUXOTROPH 1. A mutant *q.v.* bacterium *q.v.* that will not grow on a minimal medium but requires the addition of some growth factor. 2. A nutritionally deficient bacterium.

AUXOTROPH (DOUBLE) A bacterium *q.v.* nutritionally deficient for two growth substances.

AVAILABILITY HEURISTIC A process used to make probability estimates. What has happened before is likely to happen again. cf: algorithm; heuristics.

AVENTYL A commercial preparation of nortriptyline *q.v.*

AVERAGE 1. A measure of central tendency *q.v.* 2. More commonly, the arithmetic mean *q.v.* 3. Statistical measure of central tendency.

AVERAGE DAILY ATTENDANCE (ADA) The aggregate attendance of a school during a reporting period (normally, a school year) divided by the number of days that the school is in session during this period.

AVERAGE LIFE EXPECTANCY The length of life a person can expect to live based on average age of death.

AVERSION CENTER The nerve center in the brain particularly reactive to noxious stimuli *q.v.* or involved in a noxious experience.

AVERSION CONTROL Behaving in a desired manner in order to avoid something unpleasant or disagreeable.

AVERSION DISORDER Sexual disorder in which people feel revolted by sex. A form of desire disorder. cf: hypoactive sexual desire.

AVERSION STIMULUS A stimulus that elicits pain, fear, or avoidance.

AVERSION THERAPY 1. A form of negative reinforcement *q.v.* 2. A behavior therapy *q.v.* procedure in which stimuli associated with undesirable behavior are paired with a painful or unpleasant stimulus; usually done in hope that the undesirable behavior will be suppressed. 3. A behavior therapy procedure which pairs a noxious stimulus with situations that are undesirably attractive. 4. Behavior modification *q.v.*

AVITAMINOSIS Any disease resulting from a lack of sufficient vitamin *q.v.* intake.

AVOIDANCE In psychology, the tendency to avoid an anxiety-provoking situation.

AVOIDANCE–AVOIDANCE CONFLICT 1. Conflicting avoidance. 2. A situation in which one attempts to avoid unpleasant circumstances but is confronted with a second unpleasant circumstance. cf: approach–approach conflict; approach–avoidance conflict; approach gradient.

AVOIDANCE BEHAVIOR The tendency to withdraw from or to avoid contact with specific anxiety *q.v.* producing situations or objects.

AVOIDANCE CONDITIONING A form of conditioning *q.v.* in which the person learns to behave in a certain way in order to avoid unpleasant stimuli. cf: avoidance learning; aversion therapy.

AVOIDANCE GRADIENT A condition in which the strength of behavior is inversely proportional to the distance from the source of punishment.

AVOIDANCE LEARNING 1. An experimental procedure in which a neutral stimulus is paired with a noxious one so that the person learns to avoid the previously neutral stimulus. 2. Instrumental learning *q.v.* in which the response precludes an aversion stimulus before it occurs. cf: instrumental conditioning.

AVOIDANCE TRAINING Avoidance learning *q.v.*

AVOIDANT DISORDER OF CHILDHOOD A persistent shrinking from strangers and peers despite a clear desire for affection to the extent that social functioning is impaired.

AVOIDANT PERSONALITY 1. Thinking poorly of oneself, these people are extremely sensitive to potential rejection and remain aloof from others even though they very much desire affiliation and affection. 2. Avoidant personality disorder; maladaptive personality marked by low self-esteem *q.v.*, hypersensitivity to criticism, and withdrawal from social interaction due to fear of rejection.

AVOLITION A negative symptom in schizophrenia *q.v.* in which the person lacks interest and drive.

AVULSION The tearing away of a part or tissue of the body.

AWARENESS According to Levinger, the first stage of an acquaintance.

AXILLA The armpit.

AXILLARY 1. In botany, pertaining to buds or branches occurring in the axil of a leaf. In anatomy, referring to the axilla *q.v.*

AXILLARY TEMPERATURE The body temperature measured by a thermometer in the axilla *q.v.* with the arm held close to the body for a period of 10 min.

AXIOLOGY That area of philosophy that focuses on values, and value judgments.

AXIOMATIC THEORY A type of scientific explanation that involves stating premises that are assumed to be true and then logically deducing from those premises relationships that can be empirically tested.

AXIOMS 1. Statements whose truths are taken as self-evident. 2. Accepted principles of law.

AXIOSTYLE A bundle of rhizoplasts *q.v.* that extends from the flagellum *q.v.* into the cytoplasm *q.v.*

AXON 1. A nerve fiber that carries nerve impulses away from the cell body of a neuron *q.v.* 2. An extension from the body of the neuron. The ~ may possess an insulating myelin sheath *q.v.* 3. The portion of a neuron that conducts electrical impulses to the dendrites *q.v.* of adjacent neurons. Neurons typically possess one ~.

AZOOSPERMIA 1. A condition in which the male produces no sperm *q.v.* 2. The absence of sperm in the seminal fluid *q.v.*

AZT An acronym for azathioprine, an immunosuppressant *q.v.* used to prevent rejection of kidney transplants and to control the symptoms *q.v.* of rheumatoid arthritis *q.v.*

AZYGOS 1. Odd. 2. Not one of a pair. 3. An unpaired anatomical structure.

B

B CELL A specialized lymphocyte *q.v.* that, upon stimulation by an antigen *q.v.*, releases a specific antibody *q.v.*, resulting in humoral *q.v.* immunity *q.v.* cf: B lymphocyte.

BABBLING Meaningless vocalization that has a syllabic structure. ~ occurs universally among humans beginning around 6 months of age.

BABY PRO 1. A slang expression pertaining to a prostitute *q.v.* below the age of 16, or who is, at least, very young. 2. Street slang for child prostitute.

BAC An acronym for blood alcohol concentration *q.v.*

BACHELOR'S (FIRST-LEVEL DEGREE) The lowest degree conferred by a college, university, or professional school requiring four or more years of academic work in a specified major discipline.

BACILLARY DYSENTERY An intestinal disease caused by a bacterium *q.v.* cf: amebic dysentery.

BACILLUS FUSIFORMIS A pathogen *q.v.* bacterium *q.v.* that causes gingivitis *q.v.*

BACKBONE SYSTEM In emergency situations, a communication system to integrate a number of strategically located base stations into a regional communications system so that a mobile unit within the service area can communicate with its control center.

BACK-CROSSING 1. In genetics, the crossing of a hybrid *q.v.* with one of its parents or with a genetically equivalent organism *q.v.* 2. Test crossing *q.v.* 3. A cross made to a homozygous *q.v.* recessive *q.v.* to detect gene *q.v.* segregation.

BACKGROUND INVESTIGATION In education management, verifying an applicant's information and obtaining additional information from references and previous employers.

BACK-TO-THE-BASICS 1. Any movement to return to schools, emphasizing basic academic subjects in the curriculum, essentially, reading, writing, and arithmetic. 2. A broad, largely grass roots movement evolving out of concern for declining test scores and student incompetence in math and reading.

BACTEREMIA The presence of viable bacteria *q.v.* in the blood.

BACTERIA Microorganisms *q.v.* some of which may produce disease *q.v.* in humans. There are three general forms: (a) cocci, spherical; (b) bacilli, rod shaped; and (c) spirilla, spiral, or cork-screw shaped.

BACTERIAL PLAQUE Organized clusters or colonies of bacteria *q.v.* that inhabit the gum line of a tooth. If not removed, ~ causes tooth decay, diseased gums, and foul breath.

BACTERICIDE 1. A disinfectant *q.v.* 2. A substance that destroys bacteria *q.v.*

BACTERIOLOGIC TESTS A determination of the number and type of bacteria *q.v.* present.

BACTERIOLOGY The science that studies all aspects of microorganisms *q.v.*, specifically bacteria.

BACTERIOPHAGE A virus *q.v.* that attacks bacteria *q.v.*

BACTERIOSTATIC Controlling the multiplication of microorganisms *q.v.* without destroying them.

BACTERIUM Singular for a microscopic *q.v.* organism composed of a single cell. cf: bacteria.

BAG OF WATER Amnion *q.v.*

BAG-VALUE-MASK A portable, artificial ventilator *q.v.* consisting of a face mask, a valve, and an inflatable bag.

BAL 1. An acronym for blood alcohol *q.v.* level. Also referred to as blood alcohol content. 2. The proportion of the blood that consists of alcohol. A person with a ~ of 0.10% has alcohol consisting of one-tenth of 1% of the blood. Legal intoxication ~ in all the U.S. states is 0.08%.

BALANCE OF INTERNAL VALIDITY (LP) AND EXTERNAL VALIDITY (GP) In research, balancing the study's capacity to link cause and effect with its capacity to show generality of the relationship. Internal validity (LP), linking cause and effect, can be strengthened by tight controls and/or using a laboratory. These characteristics decrease external validity (GP), generally, which is strengthened by using natural, usually field, conditions.

BALANCE STUDY In nutrition, a method of determining the amount of a particular nutrient *q.v.* required by a given individual.

BALANCE THEORY In psychology, a cognitive *q.v.* attitude *q.v.* theory *q.v.* assuming that people prefer consistency to inconsistency in their beliefs and that they will make choices that restore balance.

BALANCED DIET Daily food intake that contains in proper proportions all of the body's required nutrients *q.v.*

BALANCED LETHAL In genetics, lethal genes *q.v.* on the same pair of chromosomes *q.v.* that remain in repulsion because of close linkage of crossover *q.v.* suppression *q.v.* Only heterozygotes *q.v.* survive.

BALANCED POLYMORPHISM In genetics, two or more types of individuals maintained in the same breeding population.

BALANCED SALT SOLUTION Pertaining to a solution *q.v.* of water and salts which is so formulated as to resemble normal human blood serum *q.v.*

BALANITIS Inflammation *q.v.* of the head of the penis *q.v.* usually resulting from infection *q.v.*

BALDNESS Alopecia *q.v.*

BALE'S CLASSIFICATION SYSTEM In sociology, grouping people according to their particular styles of relating to others in a group.

BALL AND SOCKET JOINT 1. Pertaining to the type of joint in the hip or shoulder which can rotate in a wide range of motions. 2. A joint in which a ball-shaped end of a bone fits into a socket. 3. Enarthrosis *q.v.*

BALLISTIC EXERCISE Flexibility exercises employing bouncing and jerking movements at the extreme range of motion.

BALLISTOCARDIOGRAPH A device for recording the stroke volume of the heart and a means of determining the cardiac *q.v.* output.

BALLOTTEMENT The sensation that an object is afloat in the uterus *q.v.*

BAR GIRL A prostitute *q.v.* who solicits clients in bars, taverns, or other establishments that serve alcoholic beverages.

BAR GRAPH A form of frequency distribution *q.v.* in which bars are used to indicate number of cases.

BARBACH'S TECHNIQUE A method of treating orgasmic dysfunction *q.v.* and sexual unresponsiveness centered around exploring and understanding one's own body and its sexually stimulating areas.

BARBITURATE 1. Chemically composed of barbituric acid *q.v.* ~ was synthesized in 1846 by Adolph von Baeyer. The first commercial preparation was Veronal developed in 1903 by Emil Fisher and Joseph von Mering. ~s are prescribed for anxiety *q.v.* (as a sedative), for epilepsy *q.v.* (as an anticonvulsant *q.v.*), to reduce pain, to induce sleep, and as a presurgical anesthetic. Some ~s are short-acting and fast-starting (Nembutal, Seconal, and Delvinal), while others are long-acting and slow-starting (Luninal, Veronal, and Amytal). ~s are addicting *q.v.* and subject to drug automatism *q.v.* 2. Sedative-hypnotic drug *q.v.* derived from barbituric acid and used in medical practice to calm nervous persons and to induce sleep. 3. Addictive central nervous system *q.v.* depressant. 4. A class of depressant *q.v.* drugs.

BARBITURATE DEPENDENCE 1. A psychophysiological *q.v.* need for one or more of the chemical compounds that induce sleep. 2. Habituation *q.v.* and addiction *q.v.* to barbituric acid *q.v.* 3. Severe withdrawal syndrome *q.v.* associated with this drug dependence. 4. The drug is subject to drug automatism *q.v.* 5. Commercial preparations include Veronal, Luminal, Amytal, Nembutal, and Seconal.

BARBITURIC ACID The chemical basis for barbiturates *q.v.* Synthesized in 1846 by Adolph von Baeyer.

BARBITURISM Addiction *q.v.* to, or poisoning by, any of the barbiturate *q.v.* drugs.

BARIATRICIAN A physician who specializes in the study and treatment of obesity *q.v.*

BARIATRICS 1. The medical specialty that is concerned with the problem of overweight and obesity *q.v.* 2. Also, bariatric medical specialist.

BARORECEPTORS 1. Nerve endings in arteries that respond to pressure, such as blood pressure, stretching, and touching. 2. A receptor stimulated by a change in pressure. 3. Pressoreceptors *q.v.*

BARR BODY 1. A mass of DNA *q.v.* visible within the nuclei *q.v.* of normal female cells that is thought to represent an inactivated X chromosome *q.v.* 2. A condensed, inactive X chromosome that distinguishes female cells from male cells.

BARTHOLIN'S GLANDS Two glands in the female located at either side of the entrance to the vagina *q.v.* that secrete small amounts of fluid during sexual arousal.

BASAL BODY TEMPERATURE METHOD (BBT) Basal body temperature is the temperature of a woman recorded immediately upon awakening before any activity. The temperature is taken orally or rectally and recorded on a graph. Observation of the temperature on the graph during a menstrual cycle *q.v.* provides some evidence of ovulation *q.v.*

BASAL CELL CANCER A form of skin cancer.

BASAL CELLS The foundation cells that underlie the epithelial *q.v.* cells. An early keratocyte *q.v.*

BASAL GANGLIA 1. In anatomy, the lower part of the brain that contains putamen, caudate nucleus. 2. Interconnected structures in the forebrain that direct involuntary muscle function that is not under conscious control, including maintenance of muscle tone and posture. Dopamine *q.v.* is probably the neurotransmitter *q.v.* involved. 3. Clusters of nerve cell bodies deep within the cerebral hemispheres *q.v.* They are the lenticular nucleus, the caudata nucleus (the corpus striatum), the claustrum, and the amygdale. 4. Also known as the corpus striatum *q.v.* A part of the brain containing large numbers of dopamine synapses *q.v.* It is responsible for maintaining proper muscle tone as a part of the extrapyramidal motor system *q.v.* Damage to the ∼ produces muscular rigidity and tremors as found in Parkinson's disease *q.v.*

BASAL METABOLIC RATE (BMR) The amount of energy expended for involuntary functions of the body per unit of time: measured under standard conditions, affecting age, sex, size, shape of the body, and physiological *q.v.* state. cf: basal metabolism.

BASAL METABOLISM 1. The amount of energy required to maintain cellular activity and vital functions of respiration and circulation in a resting, fasting body. 2. The energy expenditure of the body while at rest, under controlled environmental conditions, and in the postabsorptive state *q.v.*

BASAL SKULL FRACTURE A fracture *q.v.* involving the base of the cranium *q.v.*

BASE In chemistry, any substance that releases hydroxyl ions *q.v.* in solution and reacts with an acid *q.v.* to form salt and water.

BASE RATE 1. The general probability that an event will occur over time. 2. More broadly, the frequency with which an event takes place in the general population. cf: base rate problem.

BASE RATE PROBLEM A problem sometimes encountered in experimental study involving a difficulty in estimating the frequency of occurrence of some bit of behavior in the absence of the experimental treatment. cf: base rate.

BASE STATION In emergency operations, a station equipped with technological communications apparatus installed at a fixed location and used to communicate with mobile, emergency units.

BASELINE In statistics and evaluation, the state of a phenomenon before the independent variable *q.v.* is introduced, providing a standard against which the effects of the variable can be measured.

BASEMENT MEMBRANE In anatomy, the thin layer of tissue that separates the basal cell *q.v.* of the airway tissue from the underlying connective tissue *q.v.*

BASIC HEALTH INSURANCE An insurance policy that provides for hospital, medical, and surgical expenses. Usually has limitations, exclusions, and deductibles.

BASIC NEED 1. An inborn drive *q.v.* Basic needs are classified as biological *q.v.* (the need for food, air, water) or psychological *q.v.*, also psychosocial, (the need for security, love, belongingness, and achievement). 2. In health, satisfaction of ∼s in appropriate ways is essential for biological, social, and emotional health. 3. Physiological drives *q.v.*, safety, psychological, and emotional. cf: metaneeds; biopsychosocial.

BASIC RESEARCH Original investigation for the advancement of scientific knowledge. An investigator may seek knowledge of any problem regardless of its immediate application or practical use.

BASILAR MEMBRANE In anatomy, a structural component of the cochlea *q.v.* which supports the corti *q.v.*

BASILAR SQUEEZE TECHNIQUE In sexology, treatment for erectile dysfunction in which the male's penis *q.v.* is squeezed at the root. cf: squeeze technique.

BASILIC VEIN In anatomy, the vein *q.v.* at the bend of the elbow commonly used for drawing blood.

BASKET STRETCHER In emergency operations, a device originally designed to remove the injured from the holds of ships and called Stokes basket *q.v.* The ∼ was a long, narrow metal basket covered with chicken wire, but now, made of plastic without the original leg divider.

BASLE NOMINA ANATOMICA A publication of anatomic terminology accepted at Basle by the Anatomical Society in 1895.

BASOPHIL 1. White blood cell that stains readily with basic dyes. 2. Basophilic *q.v.*

BASOPHILIC Literally, base-loving. Cells or cellular components that stain readily with basic dyes.

BATTERY In law, wrongful physical touching of a person. 2. An unlawful beating or other wrongful physical violence inflicted upon another without his or her consent. The offer or attempt to commit a battery is an assault. It is possible to have an assault without battery, and battery is always an assault.

BAYLEY SCALES OF INFANT DEVELOPMENT A standardized set of measures for assessing mental development and psychomotor *q.v.* development during the period of 2 months to 2.5 years of age.

BBT Basal body temperature method *q.v.*

B-CELLS Lymphocytes *q.v.* that arise in the bone marrow *q.v.*, and are present in the blood, lymph, and connective tissue.

BCG VACCINE 1. A freeze-dried preparation of an attenuated *q.v.* strain of tuberculosis bacillus *q.v.* used to stimulate immunity *q.v.* against tuberculosis. 2. The Calmette–Guérin vaccine *q.v.*

B-COGNITION 1. According to Maslow, a type of thinking or knowing that is devoid of immediate needs, roles, and projects. 2. Being cognition. ct: D-cognition.

B-COMPLEX VITAMINS Water-soluble vitamins *q.v.* of the B group, e.g., thiamin, riboflavin, niacin, and others.

BEAM Brain electrical activity mapping, a technique to diagnose brain dysfunction, such as Alzheimer's disease *q.v.*

BEAT In audition, the tendency for two tones of similar pitch *q.v.* to be heard as a single tone that waxes and wanes in intensity. ct: summation tone.

BECK DEPRESSION INVENTORY A test of symptoms *q.v.* and attitudes *q.v.* related to depression *q.v.* used by psychologists *q.v.* to assess the severity of a person's mood disorder *q.v.*

BEDLAM A popular corruption of the name of the early London asylum of St. Mary of Bethlehem to describe a chaotic situation as to the perceived condition of the asylum.

BEEPER In emergency operations, pertaining to a selectively activated paging receiver usually carried on a paramedic's *q.v.* pocket or on a belt. Upon receiving a page specifically directed to it, the receiver (~) emits a beeping sound.

BEER An alcoholic *q.v.* beverage containing 2–6% alcohol by volume, derived from cereal grains through the brewing process.

BEHAVIOR 1. Any internal or external, or observable or nonobservable response *q.v.* of a person to a stimulus *q.v.* or to stimuli. 2. Internal responses such as thinking or feeling may be inferred from observable behavior. 3. In health, responding healthfully: proper nutrition, exercise, rest, relaxation, appropriate use of health providers, and the like. Healthful behavior. 4. An action that has a specific frequency, duration, and purpose, whether conscious or unconscious.

BEHAVIOR CONTROL The shaping and manipulation of behavior *q.v.* by the use of drugs, persuasion, and other strategies.

BEHAVIOR DISORDER 1. Emotional disturbance *q.v.* 2. Pertains to people who cannot care for themselves, are unable to function in society, and/or are a threat to themselves or others because of behavioral excesses or deficits.

BEHAVIOR GENETICS The study of individual differences in behavior *q.v.* that are attributable in part to differences in genetic *q.v.* makeup.

BEHAVIOR HEALTH HAZARD APPRAISAL A questionnaire that attempts to identify the problems of health and survival based on individual lifestyle behaviors *q.v.* Many appraisal forms are computerized and use a database to make projections about a person's health status *q.v.* or health potential.

BEHAVIOR MANAGEMENT PROGRAM In clinical psychology, a therapeutic technique in which a systematic application of reinforcement and possibly punishment is used to reduce the undesirable behavior *q.v.* and encourage more acceptable behaviors.

BEHAVIOR MEDICINE A field concerned with the development of behavioral science *q.v.* Knowledge and techniques relevant to the understanding of physical health *q.v.* and illness, and the application of the knowledge and these techniques to prevention, treatment, and rehabilitation.

BEHAVIOR MODIFICATION 1. Relating, associating, and connecting observable responses *q.v.* and actions to antecedents and subsequent events and stimuli *q.v.* 2. ~ is an application of the connectionist theory of learning *q.v.* 3. A program that focuses on managing human activity by controlling the consequences of performing that activity. 4. A school of psychology *q.v.* based on the assumption that schedules of reinforcement for desired behavior *q.v.* and punishments for undesired behaviors most readily produce behavioral change. 5. Behavioral therapy designed to change learned behavior of a person. 6. Psychological and social techniques used to modify deleterious behaviors. cf: behavior therapy; stimulus–response (S-R) theory; social learning theory.

BEHAVIOR PATTERN 1. A sequence of similar behaviors *q.v.* that is repeated. 2. That group of actions or responses one demonstrates as certain stimuli *q.v.* are presented. 3. One's lifestyle *q.v.* or general actions and reactions to health situations.

BEHAVIOR REHEARSAL A behavior therapy *q.v.* technique in which a person practices new behavior *q.v.* in the therapist's room, often aided by demonstrations of the therapist.

BEHAVIOR SETTING Pertaining to self-regulated sequences of interpersonal events that occur within bounded environments. ~ refers to both activities and the environment in which the activities take place.

BEHAVIOR SEX THERAPY Assumes that sexual dysfunctions have been learned and focuses on teaching the person new ways of behaving and relating sexually.

BEHAVIOR SHAPING Reinforcing approximations of the desired end product so that a child will move toward the desired behavior *q.v.*

BEHAVIOR THERAPY 1. Concerned with eliminating symptoms *q.v.* of maladjustment *q.v.* or unwanted actions with little or no insight *q.v.* into the basic causes of the actions. 2. A form of unlearning. 3. Psychotherapy *q.v.* based on conditioned responses *q.v.* and other concepts of behaviorism *q.v.* primarily directed toward habit *q.v.* change. 4. A branch of psychotherapy narrowly conceived as the application of classical conditioning *q.v.*, and operant conditioning *q.v.* to the alteration of clinical problems, but more broadly conceived as applied experimental psychology *q.v.* in a clinical context. cf: systematic desensitization; implosive therapy.

BEHAVIORAL APPROACH TO MANAGEMENT In educational administration, managing or administrative approaches that emphasize increasing organizational success by focusing on human variables within the institution.

BEHAVIORAL ASSESSMENT In psychology, a sampling of ongoing cognitions, feelings, and overt behavior *q.v.* in their situational context. ct: projective test; personality inventory.

BEHAVIORAL CONTRACT In education and psychology, used in both educational and psychological settings as a written agreement between two parties (teacher and student, or therapist and client) to behave in a prescribed manner.

BEHAVIORAL DEVELOPMENT 1. The progressive acquisition of behaviors *q.v.* beginning at birth, but continuing throughout life. A part of human development. 2. The development or acquisition of actions (behaviors) related to lifestyles, individual responses and actions affecting health status, personal and social interactions. cf: interpersonal relations.

BEHAVIORAL DIAGNOSIS In health education, delineation of the specific health actions that can most likely affect a health outcome.

BEHAVIORAL HEALTH An interdisciplinary field dedicated to promoting the philosophy of health that stresses individual responsibility in the application of behavioral and biomedical science knowledge and techniques to the maintenance of health and the prevention of illness and dysfunction by a variety of self-initiated individual or shared activities.

BEHAVIORAL INTENTION THEORY 1. Fishbein's theory. 2. A conceptual framework in an attempt to combine cognitive and connectionist approaches to learning. ~ is based on the concept that a person's basic knowledge results in beliefs that form the basis for determining a person's attitudes *q.v.*, intentions, and behavior *q.v.*

BEHAVIORAL LEARNING THEORIES Set of principles of learning based on observations of overt behavior *q.v.*

BEHAVIORAL MAKEUP The manner in which a person reacts to social stimuli *q.v.*, inner needs, and a combination of these. Behavior *q.v.* may be (a) innate, such as a reflex *q.v.*, called invariable behavior; (b) an unconscious act, called automatic behavior; or (c) a change in a person's personality *q.v.*, called adaptive behavior.

BEHAVIORAL MANIFESTATION A parameter of classification that focuses on a description of behavior *q.v.*

BEHAVIORAL MEDICINE An area of behavioral therapy procedures that apply to psychophysiological disorders *q.v.*

BEHAVIORAL OBJECTIVE 1. In education, a statement describing precisely what the learner will be doing as a result of a learning experience. A ~ is expressed in measurable terms. 2. Performance objective *q.v.* 3. Instructional objective *q.v.* 4. A statement of desired outcome that indicates who is to demonstrate how much of what behavior by when. 5. A statement from which capabilities can be inferred, listing the exact performance to be demonstrated, the exact conditions under which the performance is carried out. And the criterion (or extent) to which the performance will be measured or evaluated. 6. A precise statement of what the learner must do to demonstrate mastery at the end of a prescribed learning task.

BEHAVIORAL PEDIATRICS A branch of behavioral medicine *q.v.* concerned with psychological *q.v.* aspects of childhood medical problems.

BEHAVIORAL SCIENCES 1. The study of human development, values, and interpersonal relations. The ~ encompass such areas of specialization as psychiatry, psychology, cultural anthropology, sociology, and political science. 2. All of the sciences that collectively are concerned with human behavior *q.v.*

BEHAVIORAL STEREOTYPE In pharmacology, and elicit drug use, the process of being trapped in a meaningless repetition of a simple activity for hours at a time. Characteristic of amphetamine *q.v.* abuse, and in psychiatry, paranoid schizophrenia *q.v.*

BEHAVIORAL THEORY A theory *q.v.* that considers the outward behaviors *q.v.* of learners to be the main target for change.

BEHAVIORAL TOLERANCE 1. The learning of control over some drug effects over a period of time. 2. Probably, a subtype of pharmacodynamic *q.v.* tolerance *q.v.* 3. A person's ability to behaviorally compensate for the effects of a particular drug. 4. Repeated use of a drug may lead to diminished effect of the drug (tolerance). When the diminished effect occurs ~ is present.

BEHAVIORAL TOXICITY When a drug impairs behavior and amplifies the danger level of a particular activity, e.g., driving a car.

BEHAVIORALISM (BEHAVIORISM) 1. A psychological school of thought that believes that human behavior *q.v.* arises in response to the presentation of stimuli *q.v.* 2. Belief that human action is governed by external events.

BEHAVIORALLY ANCHORED RATING SCALE (BARS) 1. Performance appraisal. 2. ~ identifies observable, measurable performance behavior *q.v.* and feeds back observed behavior in order to improve performance. Used in management procedures.

BEHAVIORISM 1. A systematic approach or school of psychology *q.v.* that regards objective, observable manifestations as the key to an understanding of human behavior *q.v.* Consciousness, feeling, and other subjective phenomena are disregarded as unnecessary or as mediating processes between stimulus *q.v.* and response *q.v.* 2. The guiding principle of psychology that all conclusions should be based on observation of actual behavior. 3. The school of psychology associated with John B. Watson, who proposed that observable behavior, not consciousness, is the proper subject matter of psychology. Many psychologists, however, who consider themselves behaviorists, do use meditational concepts *q.v.* providing they are firmly anchored to observables. 4. Behavior represents the essence of a person.

BEHAVIORIST ORIENTATION One of the three major theoretical perspectives in social psychology *q.v.* The ~ emphasizes the exploration of reliable relationships between environmental conditions and social behavior *q.v.* cf: cognitive.

BEING NEEDS Needs associated with self-actualization *q.v.* and spiritual growth.

BEING VALUES Values *q.v.* associated with higher human potential, e.g., truth, beauty, goodness.

BE-IN-THE-CLOSET An expression referring to the concept of keeping one's homosexual orientation a secret.

BELCH 1. To orally eliminate gas from the gastrointestinal tract. 2. Eructation *q.v.*

BELIEF A statement or sense, declared or implied, intellectually and/or emotionally accepted as true by a person or group.

BELL AND PAD In psychology, a behavior therapy *q.v.* technique for eliminating nocturnal enuresis *q.v.* When a child wets at night, an electric circuit is closed and a bell sounds, waking the child.

BELLADONNA 1. A poisonous anticholinergic *q.v.* plant. 2. Refers to *Atropa belladonna*; deadly nightshade. 3. The natural source of atropine *q.v.*

BENDER 1. Slang expression for a drinking binge for several days. 2. Excessive drinking of alcohol *q.v.* over an extended period of time.

BENDS 1. Cramps in the abdomen and limbs due to bubbles of gas in the blood. 2. Caisson disease *q.v.* 3. Decompression sickness *q.v.* Common among skin divers.

BENEDICT'S SOLUTION Alkaline copper solution, which is blue in color. When a few drops of sugar solution or urine containing sugar are added after heating the ~ , a change in color takes place.

BENEFICIARY 1. The designated person or persons who receive life insurance benefits upon the death of the insured. 2. In a retirement plan, a person other than the employee who is eligible to receive benefits under the plan.

BENEFIT–RISK EQUATION 1. A principle that in using a drug, the probability of good effects outweighs the possibility of adverse effects, based on the premise that absolute safety in drug reactions does not exist. 2. Benefit–risk ratio *q.v.*

BENEFIT–RISK RATIO Benefit–risk equation *q.v.*

BENEFITS 1. In management and administration, the necessary items that would otherwise require a cash outlay by the employee. For example, health insurance plan, travel allowance, and others. 2. In health education, valued health outcomes or improvements in the quality of life that there is reasonable evidence to believe are actually caused by health care processes.

BENIGN 1. A neoplasm *q.v.* that grows very slowly. 2. Not cancerous *q.v.* 3. Not malignant *q.v.*, nor likely to recur. 4. Favorable for recovery. 5. Harmless, mild, benign prostatic hypertrophy (BPH). An enlargement of the prostate *q.v.* ~ is caused by the general enlargement of the prostate or by small, noncancerous *q.v.* tumors *q.v.* that grow inside. An enlarged prostate sometimes obstructs the urinary *q.v.* flow, which a prostatectomy can relieve.

BENZEDRINE A commercial preparation of an amphetamine *q.v.*

BENZENE A colorless liquid used as a solvent *q.v.* for fats, resins, and other substances.

BENZODIAZEPINE 1. An antianxiety *q.v.* drug used in medical practice to treat anxiety *q.v.* and various neurotic conditions. 2. The parent compound for the synthesis of numerous psychoactive drugs *q.v.* with a common molecular configuration. 3. A class of sedative-hypnotics *q.v.* that includes diazepam *q.v.* and chlordiazepoxide *q.v.* used as anxiolytics *q.v.* or sedatives *q.v.*

BENZOPYRENE 1. A chemical found in tobacco smoke. 2. A known carcinogen *q.v.*

BENZOYLECGONINE A metabolite *q.v.* of cocaine *q.v.* that can be detected in urine samples.

BENZOYLMETHYL ECOGNINE Cocaine *q.v.*

BENZTROPINE 1. An anticholinergic *q.v.* used to control extrapyramidal *q.v.* symptoms. Cogentin is a brand name.

BEQUEATH In law, to give personal property by the directions provided in a person's will to another person who survives the maker of the will.

BEREAVEMENT The period following the realization of the loss of a loved one.

BERIBERI 1. A dietary deficiency disease *q.v.* that affects the nervous system *q.v.* and is characterized by degeneration of nervous tissue and muscle weakness. Complications include heart disease *q.v.*, edema *q.v.*, and paralysis *q.v.* It is the result of thiamine *q.v.* deficiency. 2. A disease caused by a prolonged deficiency of vitamin B_1 *q.v.* Symptoms include loss of coordination, numbness and tingling in the toes and feet, loss of appetite, depression, irritability, inability to concentrate, fatigue, and loss of motivation.

BERKSON'S FALLACY In epidemiology, nonrepresentative cases since those who seek care are selectively different from those who do not.

BEST An acronym for Board for Environmental Studies and Toxicology, NAS/NDC *q.v.*

BESTIALITY A deviant form of sexual expression; sexual relation with an animal. cf: zoophilia.

BETA 1. Second letter of the Greek alphabet. 2. In epidemiology, the probability of not rejecting a null hypothesis *q.v.* when it is false. 3. Type II error *q.v.*

BETA ALCOHOLISM Characterized by excessive drinking of alcohol *q.v.* sufficiently to cause polyneuritis *q.v.*, gastritis *q.v.*, and liver cirrhosis *q.v.*, but without apparent dependence.

BETA BLOCKERS 1. Drugs that prevent overactivity of the heart which results in angina pectoris *q.v.* 2. A group of drugs that prevent stimulation of certain nerve receptors, thereby decreasing the activity of the heart. ~ are used to treat arrhythmia *q.v.* and hypertension *q.v.*

BETA ERROR Type II error *q.v.*

BETA HYPOTHESIS A technique for helping a person overcome an undesirable habit or behavior *q.v.* by exaggerating the wrong response *q.v.* before learning the right response.

BETA PARTICLE An electron emitted by the nucleus *q.v.* of an atom during radioactive *q.v.* decay. cf: beta rays.

BETA RAYS High-speed electrons given off by a radioactive *q.v.* substance with the power to penetrate the body. cf: beta particles.

BETA RECEPTOR Postjunctional receptor site that responds primarily to epinephrine *q.v.* which is divided into beta-1 and beta-2 types based on the response *q.v.* to sympathomimetic *q.v.* drugs.

BETA RHYTHMS 1. Brain waves of 13–25 cycles/s. The dominant pattern in an alert, awake adult.

BETA SUBUNIT 1. HCG *q.v.* radioimmunoassay. 2. The most frequently used laboratory test to confirm pregnancy *q.v.* BETWEEN-GROUP HERITABILITY. In genetics, the extent to which variation between groups is attributable to genetic *q.v.* factors. cf: heritability; within-group heritability.

BHA Butylated hydroxyanisole *q.v.*

BHANG 1. A drink made from milk or water and marijuana *q.v.* It is drunk in India for its mild hallucinogenic *q.v.* effects, to combat fatigue, or in relation to Hindu religious ceremonies. 2. A preparation of cannabis *q.v.* that consists of the whole plant, dried and powdered. The weakest of the commonly used forms of marijuana used in India.

BHCDA An acronym for Bureau of Health Care Delivery and Assistance.

BHT An acronym for butylated hydroxytoluene *q.v.*

BIA An acronym for Bureau of Indian Affairs; IHS *q.v.*

BIAS 1. A tendency to mislabel observations in a systematic manner. 2. In research sampling, an influence that systematically prevents obtaining a representative sample of subjects to be studied.

BIASED SCANNING 1. In memory, the process of reviewing one's memories and selecting from them only those that support one's arguments. 2. A self-generated form of attitude *q.v.* change.

BICEPS A muscle having two heads of origin, esp. the muscle on the front of the upper arm.

BICETRE An 18th century asylum for male lunatics. It was at this asylum that Philippe Pinel removed the chains and shackles from the mentally ill patients. It was a lunatic asylum for male patients only. cf: Salpetriere.

BICUSPID 1. In dentistry, the teeth used to tear and crush food. 2. Teeth with two cusps located posterior to the cuspids *q.v.* or eye teeth.

BICUSPID VALVE Mitral valve *q.v.*

BIDDER'S LIST A list of qualified organizations *q.v.* maintained by some government agencies and used for informing other groups of potential proposals and inviting them to submit proposals for funding.

BIFOCALS Eyeglasses whose lenses correct for both long- and short-range vision.

BIGAMY 1. A legal term in which a person is married to more than one person at the same time. 2. An illegal practice. 3. An unlawful marriage resulting from a person entering into a second marriage while still legally married to another person.

BILATERAL In anatomy, having two sides, or pertaining to both sides.

BILATERAL TRANSFER The effect of practice with one hand upon learning the same skill with the other hand.

BILE A digestive fluid produced by the liver and stored in the gallbladder *q.v.* that aids in the digestion *q.v.* of fat and its absorption.

BILE ACIDS Substances produced by the gallbladder *q.v.* that aid in the digestion *q.v.* of fats. cf: bile.

BILE DUCTS Any of the ducts *q.v.* conveying bile *q.v.* between the liver and the intestine *q.v.*

BILIARY SYSTEM A ductal system consisting of the gallbladder *q.v.* and the bile ducts *q.v.* connecting the liver to the intestine.

BILIARY TRACT The gallbladder *q.v.* and the ducts *q.v.* leading from the liver to the gallbladder *q.v.* and to the intestinal tract *q.v.* cf: biliary system.

BILINGUAL EDUCATION 1. Educational programs aimed at providing equal opportunities to limited English-speaking students. 2. Educational programs in which both English-speaking and non-English-speaking learners participate in a bicultural *q.v.* curriculum *q.v.* using both languages.

BILIRUBIN 1. A reddish bile *q.v.* pigment. 2. A product of degeneration of hemoglobin *q.v.* which must be eliminated from the body. cf: biliverdin.

BILIVERDIN A green pigment in the bile *q.v.* cf: bilirubin.

BILL 1. In politics, a proposed law presented to the legislature for consideration. 2. In law, a written complaint filed in a court.

BILL (EMERGENCY) A bill *q.v.* to take effect upon signing by a governor or president.

BILL (VEHICLE) In politics, a bill *q.v.* that is introduced by title only. The purpose of this is that some legislation is complicated and may not be ready to file by the filing deadline. For example, legislation relative to school-aid distribution formula. The chair with responsibility for the measure, files the bill under a broad title to ensure its timely introduction.

BILL (WHEN FILED) In politics, bills prepared and filed prior to the opening of the regular legislative session.

BILL ANALYSIS In politics, a brief summary of the purpose, content, and effect of a proposed measure.

BILL FOR THE MORE GENERAL DIFFUSION OF KNOWLEDGE A bill *q.v.* presented by Thomas Jefferson in Virginia that would have made 3 years of elementary education available for all children. Although the bill was defeated, it laid the foundation for public education.

BILL OF RIGHTS The first 10 amendments to the Constitution of the United States.

BILL ROOM In politics, a room where bills may be studied. Other legislative documents for reference purposes are also available.

BILLINGS METHOD Cervical mucous method *q.v.* for estimating the time of ovulation *q.v.* bill of attainder. In law, an act of the legislature inflicting a penalty (essentially, capital punishment) without conviction in judicial proceedings. Generally, it is used to include all legislation imposing a penalty applicable to an act not considered a crime when committed.

BILLS (SPECIAL ORDER OF) In politics, an order by the legislative body to consider and reconsider a matter that has been before the legislative body at one time.

BILLS OF MORTALITY In epidemiology, a part of biostatistics *q.v.*

BIMODIAL DISTRIBUTION 1. In epidemiology, a frequency distribution *q.v.* with two peaks or modes *q.v.* 2. A distribution of observations characterized by a number of observations clustering at two different points on the distribution scale. ct: normal distribution.

BINARY FISSION The division of the cytoplasm *q.v.* of a cell with the plane of division at right angles to the long axis of the cell.

BINDERS In chemistry, chemical substances that hold the molecule of an active drug together. cf: binding.

BINDING In chemistry, the interaction between a molecule *q.v.* and a receptor *q.v.* for that molecule. Although the molecules float onto and off the receptor, there are chemical and electrical attractions between a specific molecule and its receptor so that there is a much higher probability of the receptor being occupied by its proper molecule than by other molecules. cf: binders.

BINET–SIMON MENTAL AGE SCALES Developed in 1908, a psychometric instrument that was to be the first reliable and valid *q.v.* means of determining objectively when a child was in need of special education. The test was widely interpreted to be a measure of individual differences in intelligence.

BINOCULAR CUES Visual cues to depth that are created because our two eyes view the environment from slightly different perspectives.

BINOCULAR MICROSCOPE A microscope *q.v.* that has two eye pieces.

BINOMIAL EXPANSION An exponential multiplication of an expression consisting of two terms connected by a+ or a−; $(a+b)^n$.

BINOMIAL NOMENCLATURE In biology, zoology, and botany, the scientific method of designating organisms by two Latin or Latinized words. The first word indicates the genus *q.v.* and the second word the species *q.v.* cf: binomial system.

BINOMIAL SYSTEM See binomial nomenclature.

BIOASSAY The determination of the activity or potency of a substance by measuring the response of test animals or microorganisms *q.v.* to the substance being tested as compared with their response to a standard substance.

BIOAVAILABILITY 1. The extent to which any nutrient *q.v.* in foods is available for use by the body. 2. A measure of a drug's activity within the body as determined by the quantified levels of that particular drug in the blood. 3. The speed and extent to which a drug becomes biologically active in the body. ~ varies between individuals and within a given person over the course of time. 4. The availability of molecules of a drug at the site of the drug's action in the body. This is an important concept in comparing different brands of the same generic *q.v.* drug because one preparation may dissolve better or be absorbed more readily than the other, thus producing greater ~.

BIOCHEMICAL The chemical reactions that occur within a living organism.

BIOCHEMICAL DEFENSES The body's immune system *q.v.*

BIOCHEMICAL DISORDERS Disorders involving disturbances in the metabolic *q.v.* processes. ct: homeostasis.

BIOCHEMICAL INDIVIDUALITY The unique differences of one person as compared to others relative to basic body chemistry, e.g., blood type, metabolic rate, and others.

BIOCHEMICAL OXYGEN DEMAND (BOD) 1. The quantity of oxygen in a given time frame to satisfy the chemical and biological oxidation *q.v.* demands of sewage. 2. An index of water pollution *q.v.* based on the rate and extent that matter uses up dissolved *q.v.* oxygen from a sample of water.

BIOCHEMISTRY 1. The science concerned with chemical actions of living things. 2. The chemistry *q.v.* of life functions.

BIOCHEMISTRY OF SEX 1. The gonads *q.v.* and pituitary gland *q.v.* are the chief structures that control the ~ which, in turn, influence sexual development. 2. The chemical control of sexual development is initiated by the pituitary gland that secretes hormones *q.v.* directly into the bloodstream. These hormones are follicle-stimulating *q.v.*, luteinizing *q.v.*, prolactin *q.v.*, and interstitial cell-stimulating *q.v.* 3. The graafian follicles *q.v.* in the female ovaries *q.v.* is where the egg matures. The gonads in both sexes secrete sex hormones that influence body biochemistry *q.v.* These hormones are testosterone *q.v.*, estrogen *q.v.*, and progesterone *q.v.*

BIOCIDE An agent that destroys life.

BIODEGRADABLE 1. A substance that is capable of being broken into smaller parts by actions of microorganisms *q.v.* 2. The breakdown and assimilation *q.v.* of organic material.

BIOECOLOGICAL STRESSOR An environmental or nutritional stressor *q.v.*

BIOENERGETICS In psychotherapy, the therapy based on Wilhelm Reich's unorthodox analytic theory that all psychological distress is caused by problems in achieving full sexual satisfaction.

BIOFEEDBACK 1. A relaxation technique consisting of using an electronic device that continuously registers pulse rate, muscle tension, and other body activities. 2. A training program designed to develop a person's ability to control the autonomic nervous system *q.v.* 3. A process whereby signals from the body are registered and amplified to inform the person of when he or she is effecting body changes. 4. The use of a signal, such as muscle tension or brain waves, to control a normally involuntary physiological *q.v.* process. 5. Self-monitoring of physiological processes as they occur within the body. 6. Procedures that provide an individual immediate information on even minute changes in muscle activity, skin temperature, heart rate, blood pressure, and other somatic *q.v.* functions. It is assumed that voluntary control over these bodily processes can be achieved through this knowledge, thereby ameliorating to some extent certain psychophysiological disorders *q.v.*

BIOFLAVONOID Pigmented substances once thought to have vitamin functions. Research to date, gives no evidence that ~s are useful for treating any human conditions. ~s are sometimes referred to as vitamin P.

BIOGENIC 1. Motives *q.v.* originating from biological needs *q.v.* or drives *q.v.* 2. Originating in biological processes. ct: sociogenic.

BIOGENIC LAW The principle that animals repeat in modified form during their embryonic *q.v.* and larval development stages, the evolutionary history of the race. 2. Law of recapitulation *q.v.*

BIOGENIC MOTIVE 1. A drive or biological need *q.v.*; motivation *q.v.* originating from the need for biological *q.v.* survival, e.g., hunger. In health, ~s can be powerful movers toward unhealthful, as well as healthful behavior *q.v.* The goal, for example, of a hungry personal is to satisfy the hunger drive and may be moved to eat foods detrimental to health. A thirsty person may drink contaminated water to satisfy the thirst drive. cf: motives.

BIOGRAPHICAL QUESTIONNAIRE Statistically weighted list of questions about an applicant's personal history.

BIOLOGICAL 1. Pertaining to the science of life. 2. Of or pertaining to life or living structures. cf: biology.

BIOLOGICAL Living materials that hold, or are believed to possess, properties usable in the treatment of disease or illness. cf: biologics.

BIOLOGICAL AGENT Disease-producing organisms associated chiefly with infectious *q.v.* diseases. The common agents are viruses, richettsiae, bacteria, arthropods, helminthes, protozoa, and fungi. ct: chemical agents.

BIOLOGICAL ENVIRONMENT That aspect of the total environment *q.v.* that consists of living things. cf: physical environment.

BIOLOGICAL FITNESS In evolutionary theory, the reproductive success of individual animals.

BIOLOGICAL HALF-LIFE The amount of time required to remove half of the original amount of drug from the body. cf: half-life.

BIOLOGICAL HEALTH 1. Structural and functional health *q.v.* 2. The degree to which the structure and function of the body performs effectively.

BIOLOGICAL INDICATORS OF EXPOSURE STUDY A study designed to use biomedical *q.v.* testing or the measurement of a chemical (analyte *q.v.*), its metabolite *q.v.* or another marker or exposure in human body fluids or tissues in order to validate environmental *q.v.* exposure to a hazardous substance.

BIOLOGICAL LEVEL OF HEALTH 1. Characterized by a person's ability to resist disease, maintain body temperature, and total body (biological) chemistry *q.v.* 2. A level of health *q.v.* maintenance *q.v.* cf: interpretive level of health.

BIOLOGICAL MATURITY Physical maturity *q.v.*

BIOLOGICAL NEEDS Those basic needs *q.v.* associated with biological *q.v.* survival: oxygen, water, food, etc.

BIOLOGICAL SURVIVAL The basic maintenance of life.

BIOLOGICAL TOXINS Poisons *q.v.* produced by microorganisms *q.v.* during the course of an infectious *q.v.* disease.

BIOLOGICAL VALUE An index of protein value or quality that reflects the percentage of absorbed dietary nitrogen used by the body.

BIOLOGICAL VARIABILITY In epidemiology, the difference in assessment of test results, resulting from the natural changeability of individual subjects over a period of time.

BIOLOGICALLY AVAILABLE Pertains to the ability of a particular substance to be used by the body.

BIOLOGICS 1. Biologicals *q.v.* 2. Substances, such as blood, blood products, and vaccines, that are controlled by the Food and Drug Administration *q.v.*

BIOLOGY 1. The science concerned with all forms of living things. 2. The science of life.

BIOMEDICAL The science *q.v.* (or subscience) concerned with human (or animal) biology *q.v.* and with disease, its prevention, diagnosis, and treatment.

BIOMEDICAL AND LABORATORY PRACTICES A specialized area of community health *q.v.* that is concerned with laboratory techniques for diagnosing and treating diseases, and for investigating the conditions affecting human health *q.v.*

BIOMEDICAL INDEXES Measurements reflecting the status of various physiological *q.v.* function, e.g., blood pressure, heart rate, and body temperature.

BIOMEDICAL RESEARCH Research that is concerned with human and animal biology *q.v.*, and with disease and its prevention, diagnosis, and treatment. ct: health services research.

BIOMEDICAL TELEMETRY The transmission of biological *q.v.* data from a living subject to a monitoring point by means of radio or wire circuits, and more recently, through computers' medical information Web sites.

BIOMETRY 1. The application of statistical methods to the study of biological *q.v.* problems. 2. The mathematical study of biological facts relative to a subject.

3. A statistical examination of biological data, e.g., the calculation of life expectancy *q.v.*

BIONOMICS The relations of organisms *q.v.* to their environment *q.v.* cf: ecology.

BIOPHYSICAL SYSTEM As applied by Masters and Johnson, the part of the sexual response *q.v.* system that includes the genitalia *q.v.* and hormones *q.v.*

BIOPSY The removal and microscopic examination of a small sample of tissue for the purpose of diagnosis *q.v.* and prognosis *q.v.* of a disease, esp. tumors *q.v.*

BIOPSYCHOSOCIAL Pertains to the relationship and interaction of the biological *q.v.* self with the psychological *q.v.* self and with the sociological *q.v.* self.

BIOPSYCHOSOCIAL NEEDS Pertains to the interrelationship of all human needs: the biological *q.v.*, psychological *q.v.*, and social needs *q.v.* cf: basic needs.

BIOREMEDIATION A series of techniques in which microorganisms *q.v.* are used to degrade hazardous substances released into the environment *q.v.*

BIORHYTHMS 1. A pseudoscience *q.v.* that purports the theory that human behavior *q.v.* is characterized by regular, predictable body rhythms that begin at the moment of birth. 2. Three biological *q.v.* rhythms concerned with variations in physical, emotional, and intellectual capacities.

BIOSOCIAL NORM Some behavior *q.v.* pattern for which one finds evidence of biological *q.v.* preparedness across many species, including humans.

BIOSPHERE 1. The sphere of living organisms *q.v.* including the land, water, and air. 2. The part of the world's crust where living organisms can survive.

BIOSTATISTICS 1. A specialized area of community health *q.v.* that is concerned with the application of statistical *q.v.* procedures, techniques, and methodologies to investigate health problems and programs. 2. The mathematical techniques of quantifying observed phenomena to describe and analyze epidemiological *q.v.* comparisons. 3. An accounting of the causes of death.

BIOTIC POTENTIAL A birthrate of 50 per 1000 population per year.

BIOTIN One of the B vitamins *q.v.* ~ is necessary for metabolism *q.v.* of carbohydrates *q.v.* and the synthesis and oxidation *q.v.* of fatty acids *q.v.* ~ can be synthesized in the body and is widespread in the foods we eat. A deficiency of this vitamin is almost impossible. ~ was first synthesized in the laboratory in 1943. It is a water-soluble vitamin.

BIOTRANSFORMATION The process of metabolism *q.v.* of drugs in the body, usually the liver. cf: detoxification.

BIOTYPE 1. In genetics, a distinct physiological race or strain within morphological *q.v.* species *q.v.* 2. A population of individuals with identical genetic constitutions. A ~ may be made up of homozygotes *q.v.* or heterozygotes *q.v.*, of which only the former would be expected to breed true.

BIPARTITE STRUCTURE In genetics, a chromosome *q.v.* having two corresponding parts.

BIPOLAR DEPRESSION 1. In psychology, a mood disorder characterized by episodes of depression *q.v.* and mania *q.v.* or hypomania *q.v.* 2. Bipolar disorder.

BIPOLAR DISORDER 1. An affective disorder *q.v.* in which a person swings from one emotional state to another. 2. A manic-depressive *q.v.* mood change. ~ replaces manic-depressive psychosis *q.v.* 3. Bipolar depression.

BIPOTENTIAL GONADS The first stage of development of the embryonic *q.v.* gonads *q.v.* At this point, the tissue can differentiate into either ovaries *q.v.* or testes *q.v.*

BIRAMOUS Consisting of or possessing two branches.

BIRTH 1. The entrance into the external environment of a neonate *q.v.* 2. The birth process *q.v.* 3. Labor *q.v.* 4. Labor is divided into three stages: (a) dilation, expansion of the cervix *q.v.* as a result of contractions of the uterine wall *q.v.*, the mucous plug *q.v.* is expelled and the rupturing of the amniotic sac *q.v.* The cervix is considered fully dilated when the opening measures 10–11 cm; (b) expulsion phase begins when labor contractions are 1–2 min apart and when the head of the fetus *q.v.* gains access to the opening of the cervix, actual birth process takes place; and (c) the placental stage is the final stage and occurs after delivery of the baby and results in expulsion of the placenta *q.v.* from the uterus.

BIRTH CANAL The vagina *q.v.*

BIRTH CATCH-UP The rapid human growth that occurs just after birth. It is assumed that this rapid growth represents catch-up for growth that was denied during the fetus' *q.v.* last weeks in the uterus *q.v.*

BIRTH CONTROL 1. Also called family planning. 2. Any of several methods used to anticipate, calculate, and control the birth *q.v.* of a baby. The common methods are the use of the intrauterine device (IUD) and abortion *q.v.* The use of contraceptive techniques *q.v.* is erroneously thought of as synonymous. ct: contraception.

BIRTH DEFECTS 1. Abnormal structures or functions of an infant due to heredity *q.v.*, prenatal environment *q.v.*, or the birth process. 2. Abnormality of body structure or function, whether genetically determined or the result of environmental influence on the unborn baby, or both. cf: teratology.

BIRTH MARK Nervus (nervos) *q.v.*

BIRTH RATE 1. The number of live births per 1000 in a given year:

$$\frac{\text{number of live births}}{\text{total population}} \times 1000$$

2. The number of babies born for a given population size and time. For example, if 30 babies are born in a population of 1000 people during a given year, the birth rate is 30 per 1000.

BIRTHING CENTER A facility with homelike atmosphere used for delivering babies. cf: birthing rooms.

BISEXUAL 1. In sexology, a person who engages in sexual relationships with both sexes. Most often there is a dominating preference for one sex over the other; it is rarely an equal preference. 2. A sexual preference that includes both sexes. 3. In botany, a flower having both functional stamens *q.v.* and pistil *q.v.* A perianth may be present or absent. 4. Any organism *q.v.* having both sexes. ct: hermaphrodite.

BITOT'S SPOT A lesion *q.v.* on the conjunctiva *q.v.* of the eye caused by a severe deficiency of vitamin A *q.v.*

BIVALENT In genetics, a pair of synapsed or associated homologous *q.v.* chromosomes *q.v.* which may or may not have undergone the duplication process to form a group of four chromatids *q.v.*

BIVALENT CHROMOSOMES Two chromosomes *q.v.*, one from the male and the other from the female, united temporarily.

BLACK DEATH Bubonic plague *q.v.*

BLACKHEAD 1. A comedone *q.v.* 2. A hard, black plug in a skin pore.

BLACKOUT 1. Temporary loss of memory. 2. Loss of consciousness. 3. An early warning sign of alcoholism *q.v.* characterized by alcohol-induced amnesia *q.v.* or memory loss, but not loss of consciousness. 4. The inability to recall events that occur during a period of alcohol use. 5. A period of time during which a person was behaving, but for which there is no memory. The most common cause of this phenomenon is excessive drinking, and ~s are considered to indicate pathological *q.v.* drinking. 6. In aviation, momentary failure of vision in aviators due to diminished circulation to the retina *q.v.* as a result of centrifugal acceleration.

BLACK TONGUE A disease of dogs. Significant in human health since niacin *q.v.* was discovered in 1937 when it was found to cure black tongue in dogs.

BLACKWATER FEVER A fatal infectious *q.v.* malarial fever characterized by destruction of the red blood cells. cf: hemoglobinuria.

BLADDER 1. A musculomembranous sac serving to collect and store urine. 2. The urinary bladder.

BLANCH To become white or pale.

BLANKET DRAG Drag *q.v.*

BLASTOCOELE The hollow segmentation cavity of the blastula *q.v.*

BLASTOCYST 1. The fertilized egg in an early stage of cell division when the cells form a hollow sphere. 2. A group of dividing cells that develops from a fertilized egg and implants in the uterine *q.v.* lining.

BLASTOCYTE The cell mass that forms from the morula *q.v.* and is implanted in the uterus *q.v.* during the first week of pregnancy *q.v.*

BLASTODERM A membrane *q.v.* formed by the repeated segmentation of the blastomeres *q.v.*

BLASTOMERE Any of the cells formed from the first few cleavages in animal embryology *q.v.*

BLASTOMYCOSIS A disease caused by a fungus *q.v.*

BLASTULA 1. The embryonic *q.v.* stage of development when the cells form a single-layered hollow sphere. 2. A form of early animal development of the embryo *q.v.* following the morula stage *q.v.*

BLEB A blister *q.v.*

BLEEDING The escape from the body of blood *q.v.* as from an injured blood vessel (veins, arteries, or capillaries). It may be external and visible or internal and detected only by special diagnostic *q.v.* methods or observations.

BLEEDING TIME The time required for the bleeding from a small puncture wound of the finger to stop under carefully controlled conditions.

BLENDED INHERITANCE In genetics, inheritance *q.v.* in which the characters of two dissimilar parents appear to be blended in the offspring and segregation fails to appear in later generations.

BLEPHARITIS Inflammation *q.v.* of the eyelids.

BLEPHAROPLAST In biology, the basal granule of the flagellum *q.v.*

BLEPHAROPLASTY The surgical procedure to remove excess tissue around the eyes.

BLINDISM A physical mannerism that is frequently unique to and typical of blind persons.

BLINDNESS A defect of the visual structures that prevents light images from being perceived by the visual center of the brain. ~ may be caused by diseases of the eye, e.g., conjunctivitis neonatorum *q.v.*, trachoma *q.v.*, cataract *q.v.*, or from complications of other diseases, e.g., diabetes mellitus *q.v.*; or an injury to the optic nerve *q.v.*, retina *q.v.*, or brain; or from genetic anomalies *q.v.*

BLIND SPOT The optic nerve *q.v.* area of the retina *q.v.* that itself does not have the power of vision. 2. The area of the retina that is incapable of receiving light images.

BLIND STUDY An experimental procedure characterized by the persons being studied are unaware of receiving the experimental treatments or a placebo *q.v.* cf: double-blind study.

BLISTER 1. Bleb *q.v.* 2. A collection of fluid under the epidermis *q.v.* or within the epidermis.

BLOC 1. In politics, a group of legislators who have certain interests in common and who may vote together on matters affecting that interest. 2. Caucus.

BLOCK In physiology, an obstruction in any of the systems of the body.

BLOCK GRANTS The availabilities of federal monies that are consolidated into a broad-purpose fund from categories with limited purpose. ~ provide discretion to state and local agencies that receive them.

BLOCKING 1. In psychology, involuntary inhibition *q.v.* of recall, ideation, or communication. 2. In research, grouping individuals with a similar level on a characteristic perceived to be related to the effect.

BLOCKING OF ALPHA RHYTHM Alpha blocking *q.v.*

BLOOD The fluid that circulates through the heart, veins, arteries, and capillaries carrying nutrients and oxygen to the body cells and waste to various organs of excretion. The ~ consists of a pale yellowish liquid, the plasma *q.v.*, the erythrocytes *q.v.*, the leukocytes *q.v.*, and the thrombocytes *q.v.*

BLOOD ALCOHOL CONCENTRATION (BAC) 1. The ratio of alcohol *q.v.* present in the blood to the total volume of blood, expressed as a percent. 2. Blood alcohol level *q.v.* 3. The proportion of alcohol in a measured quantity of blood.

BLOOD ALCOHOL LEVEL (BAL) The concentration of alcohol in the blood at a given point in time. cf: blood alcohol concentration.

BLOOD ANALYSIS A laboratory procedure directed at a chemical analysis *q.v.* of the various substances contained in a sample of blood. ~ helps to determine changes and possible chemical disturbances in the body.

BLOOD–BRAIN BARRIER 1. A barrier produced by the cells in the walls of the capillaries *q.v.* in the brain. This barrier permits passage of only certain substances. 2. A selective filtering system that permits ready passage of oxygen, glucose *q.v.*, and other nutrients *q.v.* into neurons *q.v.* but largely excludes proteins *q.v.*, ionized *q.v.* molecules, and nonfat-soluble substances. 3. In pharmacology, pertains to the process whereby many substances including drugs that may be present in the blood do not readily enter the brain tissue. The chief structural feature of the ~ is the tightly joined epithelial *q.v.* cells lining the capillaries *q.v.* in the brain. All psychoactive drugs *q.v.* must be capable of crossing the ~ to have their effects on the behavior of people.

BLOOD CLOT 1. A soft, coherent, jellylike mass resulting from the conversion of fibrogen *q.v.* to fibrin *q.v.*. 2. Coagulation of the blood.

BLOOD CLOTTING 1. The process whereby blood clots *q.v.* 2. Blood coagulation *q.v.*

BLOOD COAGULATION Blood clotting *q.v.*

BLOOD COUNT A count made with a microscope *q.v.* and special counting chamber of the number of red and white blood cells in a cubic millimeter of whole blood. Normally, there are approximately 5 million red blood cells/mm^3 and 150,000–400,000 platelets/mm^3.

BLOOD DISEASES The inability of the blood *q.v.* to carry out its specialized functions. ~ may be the result of hereditary anomalies *q.v.*, infections *q.v.*, dysfunction of related organs, e.g., the spleen or the presence of toxic chemicals in the blood.

BLOOD–PLACENTAL BARRIER The placenta *q.v.* excludes ransfer of water-soluble substances to the fetus *q.v.* Most lipid-soluble drugs and many water-soluble drugs will transfer to the fetal blood and may result in damage to the fetus.

BLOOD PLATELET 1. A small, colorless cell about the size of a red blood corpuscle *q.v.* 2. Platelet *q.v.* 3. ~s are essential for aiding in blood clotting *q.v.*, and there are approximately 150,000–400,000/mm^3.

BLOOD PRESSURE Measured in millimeters of mercury, the amount of pressure exerted on the wall of an artery. Normal ~ is considered to be in the range of 120 systolic *q.v.* and 70 diastolic *q.v.* written as 120/70.

BLOOD TRANSFER The act of transmitting blood from one person to another. A concept significant in regard to AIDS *q.v.* with reference to the sharing of needles.

BLOOD TYPE One of the several groups into which all human blood can be categorized: A, B, AB, and O.

BLOOD VESSELS 1. The vascular system *q.v.* 2. The vessels through which blood circulates throughout the body. 3. The arteries, veins, and capillaries.

BLOOD VOLUME The total quantity of blood in the body expressed in liters.

BLOOD VOLUME EXPANDER A synthetic solution administered intravenously *q.v.* to expand blood volume *q.v.* in the treatment of shock *q.v.*

BLOODY SHOW The mucus and blood that are discharged from the vagina *q.v.* when labor *q.v.* begins.

B-LOVE 1. According to Maslow, love characterized by an active concern for the well-being of another person. 2. Being love. ct: D-love.

BLS An acronym for Bureau of Labor Statistics.

BLUE BABY A baby born with a bluish coloration of the skin resulting from insufficient oxygen in the blood.

BLUE CROSS 1. A theoretical nonprofit corporation that enjoys tax exempt status for the purpose of underwriting hospital insurance coverage. 2. One of the major health insurance agencies in the United States. ct: Blue Shield.

BLUE SHIELD 1. A theoretical nonprofit corporation that enjoys tax exempt status for the purpose of underwriting surgical and medical insurance coverage. 2. One of the major health insurance agencies in the United States. ct: Blue Cross.

BLUE VELVET A slang expression pertaining to a mixture of paregoric *q.v.*, a tincture of opium, and tripelennamine (Pyribenzamine), an antihistamine *q.v.*

B-LYMPHOCYTE A kind of white blood cell that produces antibodies *q.v.* in response to stimulation by an antigen *q.v.* ~s proliferate under stimulation from factors released by T-lymphocytes *q.v.* cf: B-cells.

BMA An acronym for British Medical Association.

BMI An acronym for body mass index. BMI = weight (kg)/height (m)^2.

BMR An acronym for base metabolic rate *q.v.*

BNA An acronym for the publication, *Basle Nomina Anatomica.* Anatomical nomenclature adopted by the German Anatomical Society in 1895 at Basil, Switzerland.

BOARD AND CARE HOME A residential treatment center in which the patients live in a hostel-like, supervised environment.

BOARD CERTIFIED A physician who has completed written and oral examinations in a particular medical specialty. cf: Board Eligible.

BOARD ELIGIBLE A physician who has completed additional required training in a medical specialty, usually from 2 to 5 additional years in residency, but has not passed the certifying examinations. cf: Board Certified.

BOARD OF DIRECTORS The elected or appointed body of a health agency. Its function is to establish policy for the agency in accordance with the agency's charter and by-laws.

BOARD OF EDUCATION 1. The legally constituted body for the establishment of educational policies governing a school district. The number of member varies. Members are elected for designated terms by the qualified voters of the school district. 2. A group of citizens at the local and state levels, usually elected but occasionally appointed, that set policies for schools. In some states, the board of education is called the school committee.

BOARD OF TRUSTEES An elected or appointed body of people entrusted to administer policy and funds of an organization.

BOD An acronym for biochemical oxygen demand *q.v.*

BODY In politics, a group of elected or appointed officials who serve as public representatives.

BODY COMPOSITION The major structural components of the human body such as muscle, fat, and bone. ct: body density.

BODY CONCEPT 1. Body image *q.v.* 2. How a person thinks he or she looks. cf: self-concept.

BODY DENSITY Body mass *q.v.* divided by body volume. ct: body composition.

BODY FAT Most of the unmetabolized energy food stored in the body in the form of triglycerides *q.v.*

BODY FAT ANALYSIS A procedure directed toward the determination of the percentage of body tissue composed of fat *q.v.*

BODY IDEAL The body as a person would like it to look, or a conception of how a body should look.

BODY IMAGE 1. The way a person perceives his or her own body. 2. A combination of knowledge of how one's body and position in space relates to other objects in space and how one's movements affect that relationship.

BODY LANGUAGE 1. A form of communicating by the posturing of the body and/or its parts. 2. Body expressions. 3. Nonverbal communication through which one manages to establish one's roles, intent, and affection.

BODY LOUSE 1. Infestation *q.v.* with the louse, *Pediculus humanus corporis*. 2. Pediculosis.

BODY MASS The quantity of matter present in the body measured in kilograms.

BODY STALK A complex connecting structure that attaches the embryo *q.v.* and placenta *q.v.* The ~ later develops into the umbilical cord *q.v.*

BODY SURFACE The total outer area surface of the body expressed in square meters (m^2).

BODY TEMPERATURE 1. The temperature of the body. 2. In cold-blooded animals, the ~ varies with the temperature of the environment. In warm-blooded animals, the ~ is usually constant within a narrow range. In humans,

98.6° F is considered normal for oral temperature, or 99.6° F for rectal temperature.

BODY TYPES Theories that hypothesize that a person's personality can be inferred from physical characteristics. Hippocrates formulated the humoral theory *q.v.* while W. H. Sheldon and Ernst Kretschmer formulated the body structure or somatic-type theories *q.v.*

BODY WEIGHT The gravitational forces exerted on a body by the earth.

BODY WORK A regularly practiced physical activity designed to increase physical, psychological, and spiritual dimensions of health *q.v.*

BODYBUILDING Activities in which the person trains his or her body to reach desired goals of muscular fitness: size, symmetry, and proportion.

BODY-CENTERED SEXUALITY Sexual introduction focused upon the body of the partner rather than the personality of the partner.

BODYMIND A coined term to indicate the inseparability of the organism *q.v.*

BOGUS PIPELINE A technique for measuring attitudes *q.v.* Subjects are led to believe that their true reactions will be revealed by a device that measures physiological responses *q.v.*

BOIL 1. Furunculosis *q.v.* 2. A skin inflammation *q.v.* due to bacteria *q.v.* entering the skin by way of a hair follicle *q.v.* or sweat gland *q.v.* 3. To raise the temperature of a liquid to a level high enough to vaporize the liquid. Water: 212° F or 100° C at sea level.

BOMB CALORIMETER 1. An instrument used to measure the amount of heat produced by a weighted sample of food, and thus the food's energy value. 2. Calorimeter *q.v.*

BONA FIDE OCCUPATIONAL QUALIFICATION In business, the necessity of unequal treatment of employees or applicants.

BONDING 1. In psychology, the close emotional attachment between the mother and a child. 2. Expanded definition of ~ includes emotional attachment between adult and child. 3. The important, initial sense of recognition established between the newborn and those adults on whom the baby will be dependent. 4. The process by which a mother develops a strong attachment to her newborn. This process is alleged to occur in humans and some other mammals and is thought to involve hormone *q.v.* events that are stimulated through sight, hearing, touch, and smell.

BONE The hard form of connective tissue *q.v.* that constitutes most of the skeleton in most vertebrates *q.v.*

BONE MARROW The soft tissue located in the cavities of the bones *q.v.* The ~ is the source of all blood cells.

BONUS In business, extra compensation in addition to wages.

BONY SUTURE The junction of two bones *q.v.* that have grown or fused together.

BOOMERANG EFFECT 1. In communication, the reaction of an audience. This reaction is the opposite of that which is advocated by the message being given. 2. Negative feedback *q.v.*

BOOSTER DOSE An injection of vaccine *q.v.* or toxoid *q.v.* administered at some time after primary immunization *q.v.* in order to maintain immunity *q.v.*

BORDERED PIT Pit *q.v.*

BORDERLINE CASES In research, cases used in conceptual analysis to help define the boundaries of the term or subjects being analyzed.

BORDERLINE PERSONALITY In psychology, a person possessing impulsiveness, unpredictability, uncertain self-image *q.v.*, intense and unstable social relationships, and extreme swings of mood. cf: borderline personality disorder.

BORDERLINE PERSONALITY DISORDER Behavior that is closely related to psychosis *q.v.* but that is shorter and less severe. Symptoms include functional difficulties in interpersonal *q.v.* relationships, impulse control, task performance, expression, and perception *q.v.* cf: borderline personality.

BORRELIA VINCENTII A pathogenic *q.v.* bacterium *q.v.* that causes Vincent's disease *q.v.* (trench mouth).

BOTTOM-UP APPROACH In management, nonmanagerial jobs used as a basis for setting salaries for higher level positions.

BOTTOM-UP PROCESSES In language, the process of resolution of forms that start with the smaller units and builds to the larger units, e.g., words to sentences to paragraphs. ct: top–down processes.

BOTULISM The most toxic *q.v.* form of food poisoning. Caused by the *clostridium botulinum* bacterium *q.v.*

BOULEVARISM In management, negotiating tactic in which the company makes a final offer at an early stage and refuses to accept proposals that increase the cost of the offer.

BOURDON GAUGE A pressure gauge calibrated to record the flow rate of a medical gas from a compressed cylinder.

BOWEL The large intestine *q.v.*

BOWMAN'S CAPSULE The enlarged end of a kidney tubule in which a mass of thin-walled capillaries known as the glomerulus *q.v.* is located.

BP British Pharmacopeia, the standard reference of drugs and their preparation in Great Britain.

BPH Benign prostatic hypertrophy *q.v.*

BRACHIAL Pertaining to the arm above the elbow.

BRACHIAL ARTERY The artery *q.v.* of the arm that is a continuation of the axillary artery *q.v.* which, in turn, branches at the elbow into the radial and ulnar arteries *q.v.*

BRACHIAL PLEXUS A network of nerves consisting of the motor and sensory innervation of the arm. cf: plexus.

BRACHIOPROTIC EROTICISM An aspect of gay sexual behavior whereby one male inserts his hand and forearm into the anus *q.v.* of his partner.

BRADLEY METHOD OF CHILDBIRTH (Also known as husband-coached childbirth.) 1. Emphasizes marital communications, the couple's sexual relationship, and parental roles. 2. Psychoprophylaxis approach to natural childbirth that includes breathing and relaxing techniques.

BRADYCARDIA Slow heart beat, generally, below 60 beats per minute. cf: tachycardia.

BRADYKININ One of a group of naturally present peptides *q.v.* that acts on blood vessels, smooth muscles, and nociceptors *q.v.*

BRAIN 1. The mass of nerve tissue contained within the cranium *q.v.*, consisting of the cerebrum *q.v.*, cerebellum *q.v.*, pons *q.v.*, and medulla oblongata *q.v.* 2. The encephalon *q.v.*

BRAIN CONTUSION Cerebral contusion *q.v.*

BRAIN DAMAGE 1. Any structural damage due to any cause or causes. 2. Brain laceration. 3. Brain insult.

BRAIN DEATH The concept that a person may be considered dead when the brain is no longer functioning as determined by technology.

BRAIN HEMISPHERE The left or right half of the brain *q.v.*

BRAIN IMAGING TECHNIQUES The electronic assessment of the structure and function of the human brain *q.v.*

BRAIN INSULT 1. Brain damage *q.v.* 2. Brain laceration *q.v.*

BRAIN LACERATION 1. Brain injury in which an object pierces the skull and tears brain tissue. 2. Brain insult *q.v.*

BRAIN PATHOLOGY Diseased or a disordered condition of the brain *q.v.* cf: pathology.

BRAIN POTENTIALS 1. Brain *q.v.* waves. 2. Minute electrical oscillations given off by the cerebral cortex *q.v.*

BRAIN STEM 1. All of the brain *q.v.* except the cerebrum *q.v.* and the cerebral cortex *q.v.* The ~ is comprised of the hypothalamus *q.v.*, midbrain *q.v.*, and hindbrain *q.v.* 2. Hindbrain: the enlarged extension of the spinal cord *q.v.* which includes the medulla oblongata *q.v.*, the pons *q.v.*, and the cerebellum *q.v.* 3. The part of the brain connecting the spinal cord with the cerebrum *q.v.* and functions as a neural relay station. The ~ is considered to contain the oldest, in an evolutionary sense, and most primitive control centers for the basic functions of breathing, swallowing, etc.

BRAIN WAVES The rhythmic fluctuations in voltage between the parts of the brain *q.v.* produced by the spontaneous firings of its neurons *q.v.* and recorded by the electroencephalograph *q.v.*

BRAINSTORMING A form of group problem solving *q.v.* in which all possible solutions are listed without discussion followed by an evaluation of each item.

BRAINWASHING 1. An intensive form of propaganda conducted under highly stressful conditions. 2. A technique used to alter drastically those attitudes already established.

BRAN 1. The outer coat or layer of a cereal grain. 2. Fiber *q.v.* 3. Nutrient fiber *q.v.*

BRANCHING PROGRAM In education, a program wherein the sequence of frames examined by the learners may vary due to less capable learners being instructed to examine additional explanations in the event of failure to respond correctly.

BRAND NAME DRUGS 1. An over-the-counter drug *q.v.* 2. A patent medicine. 3. A drug product whose generic *q.v.* name has been assigned a trademarked or patented name by a particular pharmaceutical company for advertising and sale. 4. The name of a given drug by a manufacturer and licensed only to that manufacturer, e.g., Tylenol is the brand name of acetaminophen *q.v.*

BRAXTON HICKS CONTRACTIONS 1. Uterine *q.v.* contractions felt by women during later pregnancy *q.v.* but are not true labor contractions. 2. The painless tightening of the uterine muscles that prepare the uterus for childbirth. 3. False labor.

BREACH OF CONTRACT In labor–management relations, failure without legal reasons to perform part or the whole of a contract.

BREAK-EVEN ANALYSIS In management, a control tool based on the process of generating information that summarizes various levels of profit or loss associated with various levels of production.

BREAK-EVEN POINT In management, that situation wherein the total revenue of an organization equals its total costs.

BREAKTHROUGH BLEEDING 1. Mid-cycle uterine *q.v.* bleeding. 2. Spotting *q.v.*

BREAST AUGMENTATION A surgical procedure to increase the size of the breast.

BREAST CANCER A cancer *q.v.* localized in the breast. Most prevalent in females but also found in males. One of the leading causes of cancer deaths among women in the United States.

BREAST FEEDING Giving a baby nourishment from the breast of the mother.

BREAST SELF-EXAMINATION (BSE) A self-care procedure involving periodic feeling of the breasts for detection of any abnormality. Monthly ~ is recommended for every female.

BREATHALYZER One of several instruments used to determine blood alcohol concentration by measuring the amount of alcohol in a sample of a person's breath. The ~ is usually used on suspected drunk drivers.

BREECH BIRTH 1. The birth *q.v.* of a baby when any part of the baby's body is presented other than the head. 2. A birth of a baby when the feet or buttocks enter the birth canal *q.v.* first. The usual birth position is a head first presentation. 3. Breech presentation *q.v.* 4. Breech position *q.v.*

BREECH POSITION 1. The birth position of a fetus *q.v.* in which the feet or buttocks precede the head out of the uterus *q.v.* 2. Breech birth *q.v.* 3. Breech presentation *q.v.*

BREECH PRESENTATION Breech birth *q.v.*

BREWED LIQUOR A nondistilled alcoholic beverage such as ale, beer, hard cider, or wine.

BRIDEPRICE Bridewealth *q.v.*

BRIDEWEALTH 1. A common marriage custom wherein the groom presents some gifts to the bride's family. 2. Brideprice *q.v.*

BRIEF PSYCHIATRIC RATING SCALE An instrument used to rate a subject's psychiatric symptoms along multiple dimensions such as somatic *q.v.* complaint, depressive *q.v.* mood, anxiety *q.v.*, and motor ability.

BRIEF REACTIVE PSYCHOSIS A disorder in which the person has a sudden onset of psychotic *q.v.* symptoms, such as incoherence, loosening of associations, delusions, and hallucinations, immediately after a severely disturbing event. The symptoms last more than a few hours, but for no more than 2 weeks. cf: schizophreniform disorder.

BRIGHT In tobacco agriculture, light-colored, flue-cured tobacco. cf: burley.

BRIGHT'S DISEASE 1. Nephritis *q.v.* 2. An inflammation *q.v.* of the kidney.

BRIGHTNESS 1. In visual perception *q.v.*, the extent to which visual stimuli appear light or dark. 2. A dimension of visual experience that mainly depends upon the energy of the stimulus *q.v.* ct: hue; saturation.

BRIGHTNESS CONSTANCY The fact that objects retain their relative brightness *q.v.* under various levels of illumination. cf: brightness contrast.

BRIGHTNESS CONTRAST The tendency to perceive *q.v.* a light/darkness difference of two areas that are adjacent to each other. An area appears lighter when adjacent to or upon a dark background. cf: brightness ratio.

BRIGHTNESS RATIO The relationship or ratio between the light reflected by an area and the light reflected by the area that surrounds it. cf: brightness contrast.

BRILL'S DISEASE The epidemic variety of typhus fever *q.v.* spread by the bite of a rat flea.

BRIQUET'S SYNDROME Somatization disorder *q.v.*

BRITISH EMPIRICISM The psychological *q.v.* school of thought that holds that all knowledge comes by way of the senses, by empirical experiences.

BRITISH SYSTEM Pertains to the drug addiction approach in force in Great Britain wherein drug addicts may register and be prescribed legal narcotics *q.v.*

BROCA'S AREA 1. In anatomy, the structure located on the left side of the brain and controls movements of the tongue, lips, vocal cords, or motor speech area. 2. An area in the frontal cortex *q.v.* that is responsible for speech. ct: Wernicke's area.

BROMELIN A protease *q.v.* or enzyme *q.v.* found in the fresh juice of the pineapple.

BROMIDE 1. The first drug introduced as a sedative-hypnotic *q.v.* and used initially as a treatment for epileptic seizures *q.v.* 2. A central nervous system *q.v.* depressant *q.v.* 3. A group of salts with sedative *q.v.* properties.

BROMPTON'S COCKTAIL (MIXTURE) An alcoholic solution of an opioid *q.v.*, usually heroin or morphine *q.v.*, and cocaine *q.v.*, amphetamine *q.v.*, or a phenothiazine tranquilizer *q.v.* used to control severe pain associated with terminal cancer.

BRONCHIAL 1. Pertaining to the bronchus *q.v.* 2. A subdivision of the trachea *q.v.*

BRONCHIAL ASTHMA The common form of asthma *q.v.*

BRONCHIAL TUBES The two air tubes that branch from the trachea *q.v.*, one to each lung.

BRONCHIECTASIS 1. A disease caused by an accumulation of pus *q.v.* in the small pouches that are formed in the bronchi *q.v.* as the secondary result of some infection of the lungs. 2. Dilation of the bronchi. 3. Dilation of the bronchi or of a bronchus characterized by offensive breath, spasms of coughing, and expectoration of mucopurulent material.

BRONCHIOLE One of the smaller subdivisions of the bronchi *q.v.* of the lungs.

BRONCHITIS 1. Inflammation *q.v.* of the bronchi. Cigarette smoking is the most common cause of chronic *q.v.* bronchitis in the United States. 2. Inflammation of the bronchial mucous membrane *q.v.* as a result of irritation and often accompanied by a chronic cough.

BRONCHODILATOR 1. A drug that causes dilation of bronchi *q.v.* within the lungs. 2. A drug that relaxes the muscles of the bronchi and increases their diameter, thereby making breathing easier for asthmatic *q.v.* victims.

BRONCHOGENIC 1. A type of lung cancer developing in the bronchi *q.v.* 2. Bronchogenic carcinoma *q.v.*

BRONCHOGENIC CARCINOMA 1. Cancerous *q.v.* growth, malignant neoplasm *q.v.* that arises in the lining of the bronchial tubes *q.v.* of the lungs. 2. Lung cancer *q.v.*

BRONCHOPNEUMONIA An inflammation *q.v.* of the smallest branches of the bronchial tubes *q.v.*, usually present in both lungs.

BRONCHOSCOPE An instrument used for visually examining the internal surfaces of the larger bronchi *q.v.*

BRONCHOSCOPY An examination of the bronchi *q.v.* using an instrument called the bronchoscope *q.v.*

BRONCHOSPASM A narrowing or constriction of the bronchi *q.v.* that occurs during an asthma *q.v.* attack or from a severe allergic reaction *q.v.*

BRONCHUS One of the main branches of the trachea *q.v.* carrying air into the lungs.

BROTHEL A house of prostitution *q.v.*

BROWN SUGAR Sugar crystals in either molasses syrup with natural flavor and color, or refined white sugar with brown sugar added. ~ is usually 91% to 96% sucrose *q.v.*

BROWNIAN MOVEMENT The vibratory movement of microscopic *q.v.* particles of both organic and inorganic substances when suspended in water or other fluids. The movement is the result of the impact of the molecules *q.v.* of the fluid surrounding the particles. This phenomenon was first described by Robert Brown in 1827.

BRUCELLA ABORTUS An organism that causes brucellosis *q.v.*

BRUCELLOSIS 1. A disease caused by a bacillus *q.v.* (*Brucella abortus* or *Brucella melitensis*). 2. A disease that causes an infection *q.v.* in a cow's tissues, blood, urine, and milk. 3. Undulant fever *q.v.*

BRUISE 1. The leakage of blood into the tissues, resulting in a black and blue appearance as a result of a blow. 2. Hematoma *q.v.*

BRUSH BORDER The collective term for the numerous microvilli that cover the villi *q.v.* and epithelial *q.v.* cells of the small intestine.

BSA An acronym for body surface area *q.v.*

BSC An acronym for Board of Scientific Counselors.

BSE Breast self-examination *q.v.*; self-inspection of the breasts by palpation *q.v.* and observation.

BTU An acronym for British Thermal Unit. The amount of heat necessary to raise the temperature of 1 pound of water from 39°F to 40°F. One BTU is equal to 252 calories.

BUBONIC PLAGUE 1. The black death which ravaged Europe for centuries, coming to a peak about the mid-1300s, but with cyclic severity until the late 1600s. 2. A communicable *q.v.* disease caused by a bacterium *q.v.* usually carried by rats and fleas. The ~ is characterized by enlargement of the lymphatic glands *q.v.* and accompanied by pneumonia.

BUCCAL Pertaining to the cheek or mouth. The buccal cavity, usually referring to between cheek and gum.

BUCCAL SMEAR TEST The scraping and examination of the cells from inside the cheek for the purpose of detecting precancerous *q.v.* changes.

BUCKLEY AMENDMENT A federal law that protects the privacy of information held by an institution or an organization regarding an individual until it is released by the individual or his or her guardian.

BUD 1. In botany, an embryonic shoot. 2. A vegetative growth from a yeast cell.

BUDDING 1. In botany, the method of vegetative reproduction in yeasts. 2. A specialized form of grafting.

BUDDY RATINGS In management, a process whereby coworkers rate each other on particular qualities.

BUDGET 1. In management, a written statement of the money a person or organization has or expects to receive and the expenses anticipated for a specified period of time. 2. A control tool that outlines how funds in a given period of time will be spent as well as how they will be obtained. 3. An itemized list of expenditures and income written as a part of a government proposal. The ~ categories include the following: (a) direct costs, the items directly related to producing the product or service specified in the contract or grant; labor, material items, printing, travel, telephone, office supplies; (b) indirect costs, the cost of items not directly related to producing the product or service, such as costs incurred in maintaining personnel and facilities; overhead, such as rent, equipment, employee fringe benefits, and administrative costs, legal expenses, accounting, preparation of the proposal.

BUDGET (EXECUTIVE) In politics, suggested allocation of state money presented by the governor for consideration by the legislature.

BUDGET AGENCY In politics, an executive agency that prepares the budget *q.v.* document for the governor or president.

BUDGET APPROACH 1. Position pricing. 2. A proportion of total payroll allocated to exempt salaried positions.

BUDGET BILL In politics, a bill *q.v.* specifying the amounts approved by the general assembly for each program of state or federal government.

BUDGET COMMITTEE 1. In politics, a committee of legislators, which acts in an advisory capacity to the budget agency *q.v.* between sessions of the general assembly.

BUERGER'S DISEASE A circulatory disease characterized by coldness, numbness, and tingling in the feet. Phlebitis *q.v.* is common. ~ is most prevalent in smokers, although the specific cause of the disease is unknown.

BUFFER In pharmacology, a mixture of an acid *q.v.* and its conjugate base *q.v.* which, when present in a solution, reduces any changes in pH *q.v.* that would otherwise occur when an acid or alkali *q.v.* is added to the solution. cf: buffering effect.

BUFFERING EFFECT Any factor that reduces the harmful effects of various diseases, drugs, stress-related deficits, and the risk of medical problems. cf: buffer.

BUILD-IN SOCIAL DISPLAYS In psychology, expensive movements *q.v.*

BUILDING LEVEL ADMINISTRATION In education, the administration of individual schools.

BULBAR POLIO The type of polio *q.v.* that affects motor nerves of the medulla oblongata *q.v.*

BULBOCAVERNOSUS MUSCLE 1. The ring of sphincter *q.v.* muscles surrounding the opening of the vagina *q.v.* 2. The muscle surrounding the corpus spongiosum *q.v.* that contracts during orgasm *q.v.*

BULBOURETHRAL GLAND 1. Cowper's gland *q.v.* 2. Two small glands located at the outlet of the male urinary bladder *q.v.* that secretes a clear mucous lubricant that makes up much of the fluid portion of the semen *q.v.*

BULIMAREXIA An eating disorder characterized by uncontrolled binge eating followed by forced vomiting because of fear of getting fat. cf: bulimia; anorexia nervosa.

BULIMIA (BOULIMIA) 1. An abnormal increase in the sensation of hunger. 2. A psychogenic *q.v.* disorder in which binge eating patterns are established, usually accompanied by purging *q.v.* 3. Excessive appetite. 4. A compulsion to eat. 5. An eating disorder in which the person alternatively binges on food and then purges herself or himself by forced vomiting or fasting, the use of laxatives *q.v.*, or amphetamine abuse. ct: anorexia nervosa. cf: hyperphagia.

BULK 1. In conditioning, muscle mass accumulated through strength training. 2. In nutrition, an outdated term pertaining to dietary fiber *q.v.*

BUNDLE OF HIS In anatomy, the atrioventricular bundle. 2. A bundle of special cardiac *q.v.* muscle fibers that originate in the atrioventricular node and that extend by two branches down the two sides of the interventricular septum, continuing as the Purkinje fibers. The ~ acts as a relay for nervous impulses to the ventricles causing them to contract.

BUNDLING 1. Tarrying. 2. A courtship custom among Puritans in which the would-be groom slept in the girl's bed in her parent's home. Both were fully clothed and a wooden bar was placed between them.

BUNION 1. An inflammation or growth on the head of the first or fifth toe. Hallux valgus *q.v.*

BUPHTHALMUS An abnormal distention and enlargement of the eyeball.

BURDEN-OF-PROOF In law, the duty of the party to substantiate an allegation or issue.

BUREAU OF ALCOHOL, TOBACCO, AND FIREARMS Organized within the Treasury Department and is concerned with ingredient labeling of alcohol and safe storage and other precautions for explosives.

BUREAU OF HEALTH EDUCATION Once a component of the Centers for Disease Control and Prevention of the United States Public Health Service within the Department of Health and Human Services. It provided for prevention of disease, disability, and premature deaths on a national scale.

BUREAU OF LABOR STATISTICS A record keeping and reporting agency of the federal government that provides statistical data to help monitor and solve health and safety problems in the workplace.

BUREAUCRACY 1. In government, a management system with detailed procedures and rules, a clearly outlined organizational hierarchy, and mainly impersonal relationships between organization members. 2. An organization characterized by a pyramiding of positions or offices.

BUREAUCRATIC MODEL A type of relationship between a client and an intervener expressing a client-to-professional relationship. In exchange, the client surrenders responsibility to the intervener for those actions that are necessary to change the client.

BURKITT'S LYMPHOMA A form of cancer *q.v.* that is found chiefly among Africans and is associated with the presence of a particular viral *q.v.* infection *q.v.*

BURLEY A dark-colored, air-cured tobacco. cf: bright.

BURNOUT 1. The process of losing interest and motivation in teaching or other occupation. 2. A form of emotional and intellectual fatigue. 3. A state of psychological exhaustion usually attributed to job stress.

BURNS 1. Caused by dry or moist heat. There are four classes: (a) first degree characterized by redness of the skin, (b) second degree characterized by blistered skin, (c) third degree characterized by destruction of the outer layer of the skin, and (d) fourth degree characterized by destruction of all layers of the skin. 2. Damage to the tissues resulting from chemicals, heat, or radiation.

BURSA 1. A small sac of fluid located between tendon and bone that reduces friction and facilitates motion. 2. Fluid containing sac or pouch lined with synovial membrane *q.v.*

BURSITIS 1. Inflammation *q.v.*, causing pain, of the fluid-filled sac between a tendon and a bone. 2. Inflammation of a bursa *q.v.*

BUSINESS PROPOSAL The budget and business aspects of a proposal requested to be separate from the technical and program sections. cf: budget.

BUSING A method used extensively during the 1960s and 1970s for remedying segregation by transporting students to schools that had been racially or ethnically unbalanced in the past.

BUTABARBITAL 1. A barbiturate *q.v.* sedative-hypnotic *q.v.* 2. Butisol *q.v.* is a commercial preparation.

BUTISOL A commercial preparation of butabarbital *q.v.*

BUTTOCK 1. The prominence formed by gluteal muscles on the posterior *q.v.* of either side of the body. 2. The butt.

BUTTON In pharmacology, usually pertains to an immature mushroom before the expansion of the cap.

BUTYL ALCOHOL 1. Butanol. 2. A solvent *q.v.* used in industry. ~ is unfit as a beverage. cf: alcohol; methyl alcohol; ethyl alcohol.

BUTYL NITRITE An analogue of amyl nitrate *q.v.* used recreationally as a euphoriant *q.v.* and presumed sexual stimulation.

BUTYLATED HYDROXYTOLUENE (BHT) An antioxidant *q.v.* used in commercial food processing to prevent or retard fat-containing foods from becoming rancid *q.v.* cf: butylated hydroxyanisole.

BUTYLATED HYDROXYANISOLE (BHA) An antioxidant *q.v.* used as a food additive *q.v.* to prevent or retard fat-containing foods from becoming rancid *q.v.* cf: butylated hydroxytoluene.

BUTYROPHENONES Powerful antipsychotic *q.v.* tranquilizers *q.v.*

BV An acronym for biological value *q.v.*

BYSSINOSIS Brown lung disease. A respiratory disease resulting from the inhalation of cotton dust.

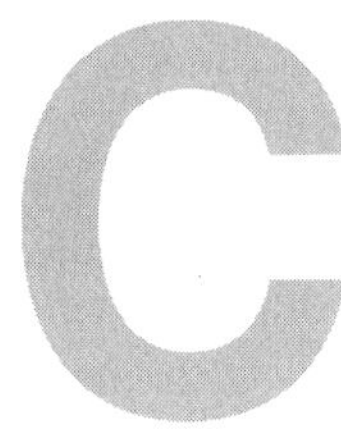

C 1. Chemical symbol for carbon. 2. Symbol for centigrade or Celsius *q.v.* scales. 3. Street slang for cocaine. 4. Symbol for Calorie *q.v.*

CA 1. An acronym for catecholamines *q.v.* 2. An acronym for chronological age *q.v.*

CACHEXIA 1. A severe malnutrition *q.v.* and poor health as a result of a disease or lack of nourishment. 2. Profound and marked state of general ill health and malnutrition.

CACODEMONOMANIA A condition characterized by being possessed by evil spirits.

CACOONING A term introduced during the mid-1980s to describe persons, usually the aged, who have developed a fear of social contacts and who stay at home and go out only as necessary. cf: nesting.

CADAVER A dead body; as one preserved for anatomical study.

CADUCEUS 1. The physician's herald or symbol. 2. The staff of Hermes. The ~ is a winged staff containing two snakes coiled around it.

CAECUM (CECUM) 1. Literally, a blind pouch. 2. The first part of the large intestine. 3. A cul-de-sac. 4. Cecum *q.v.*

CAFFEINE 1. A xanthine (Greek meaning yellow). There are three chief xanthines: (a) caffeine, (b) theophylline, and (c) theobromine. 2. A central nervous system *q.v.* stimulant *q.v.* of relatively low toxicity. The use of ~ may result in a dependence *q.v.* in some people. 3. ~ is an active constituent found in coffee, tea, and many cola and energy drinks. 4. A drug *q.v.* that stimulates the heart, kidneys, and nervous system. 5. A bitter tasting, odorless compound *q.v.* extracted from the fruit of the *Coffea Arabica* plant. 6. An alkaloid obtained from the dried leaves of *Thea sinensis* (tea) used as a diuretic *q.v.* and as a circulatory and respiratory stimulant and to treat headaches. cf: caffeinism.

CAFFEINISM 1. A stimulated *q.v.* condition of chronic *q.v.* poisoning due to overindulgence of caffeine *q.v.*, manifest by mood changes, anxiety *q.v.*, sleep disruption, tremulousness, headache, and ringing in the ears. 2. Habitual use of large amounts of caffeine, usually in the form of coffee or tea.

CAI An acronym for computer-assisted instruction.

CAISSON DISEASE 1. A condition that causes nitrogen in the tissues to surge into the blood stream of deep sea divers who surface too rapidly after being under water at depths of 40 ft or more. 2. Bends *q.v.*

CAL The abbreviation for the large calorie *q.v.* Also symbolized by a capital C.

CALCANEUS 1. The large heel bone at the back of the foot. 2. The heel bone.

CALCAREOUS Of liming composition.

CALCAREOUS DEPOSIT A deposit of calcium or lime in a joint or tissue.

CALCIFICATION The diffuse infiltration of a tissue with calcium. ~ occurs normally in the process of healing of a fractured bone.

CALCIFY To harden.

CALCITONIN 1. Thyrocalcitonin. 2. A polypeptide *q.v.* secreted by the thyroid gland *q.v.* and phosphorous *q.v.* in the plasma *q.v.* 3. A hormone that causes calcium to be absorbed into the bones. 4. A hormone secreted by the parathyroid gland *q.v.*

CALCIUM CHANNEL BLOCKERS Drugs that prevent arterial spasms *q.v.* ~ are used in the long-term management of angina pectoris *q.v.*

CALCULUS 1. A hard substance that may accumulate on the teeth. Kidney stones and gallstones are ~. 2. Tartar on the teeth usually at or below the gum line. 3. Any abnormal concretion occurring in any of the various hollow organs or ducts *q.v.* of the body.

CALCULUS OF POSITIVE SOCIAL ACTION The process by which a person estimates the gains or losses involved in helping other people.

CALENDAR (HOUSE) In politics, a list prepared daily by the Speaker of the bills on second and third readings, which may be acted upon that day.

CALENDAR (SENATE) A daily list of all bills eligible for second and third readings that day.

CALENDAR METHOD A birth control *q.v.* or contraceptive *q.v.* method or procedure whereby the time of the month of greatest fertility is determined by careful observation of a woman's menstrual cycle *q.v.* over an 8-month period and sexual intercourse *q.v.* is avoided during this time. When conception is desired, this method may be helpful in determining the best time for coitus *q.v.* and for fertilization *q.v.* of the ovum *q.v.* to take place.

CALISTHENICS 1. Athletic exercise. 2. Warming-up exercises. 3. Simple gymnastics. 4. Exercises for strength and flexibility that usually do not require equipment.

CALL GIRL An expensive and expert prostitute *q.v.* who entertains clients in her apartment or visits clients in their homes or hotels.

CALLUS 1. Wound tissue, parenchyma tissue formed on or below a wounded surface. 2. Undifferentiated tissue used in tissue culture. 3. A hard skin thickening usually on the sole of the feet or the palms of the hands. 4. An overgrowth and thickening of the horny layers of the skin as the result of prolonged pressure or friction.

CALMETTE-GUERIN VACCINE BCG *q.v.*

CALORIC BALANCE A condition achieved when the calories *q.v.* acquired from food is exactly equal to the calories expended.

CALORIE (CALORIE SPELLED WITH A CAPITAL C) 1. Energy is measured in kilocalories. A kilocalorie is the amount of heat necessary to raise the temperature of 1 kg of distilled water by 1°C (centigrade). A kilocalorie is frequently called a Calorie (spelled with a capital C). 2. A calorie (spelled with a lower case c) is the amount of heat necessary to raise the temperature of 1 g of distilled water by 1°C. 3. 1 kcal = 1 Cal = 1000 cal. 4. A kilocalorie is a nutritional Calorie.

CALORIMETER 1. An instrument for measuring the amount of heat produced by a food when oxidized. 2. Bomb calorimeter *q.v.*

CALORIMETRY 1. The measurement of heat change in a person or system. 2. In nutritional science, the measurement of heat expenditure in the body. cf: direct calorimetry; indirect calorimetry.

CAMELLA SINENSIA The plant from which beverage tea is made.

CAMOUFLAGE In research, a method of control whereby a characteristic that is otherwise prominent is made to become part of the background.

CANALICULUS In anatomy, small channels in bone connecting the lacunae *q.v.* with one another or with the Haversian canals *q.v.*

CANAL OF SCHLEMM In anatomy, a circular canal in the eye through which most of the aqueous humor *q.v.* drains.

CANCER 1. A neoplasm *q.v.* or tumor *q.v.* 2. Unrestrained reproduction of cells more rapidly than is necessary to replace worn-out cells. 3. Reproduction of cells that have no relation to the functions of surrounding tissues. 4. The rapid, unorderly reproduction and spread of cells that interfere with the function of other cells and tissues. 5. ~s are classified according to the characteristics of the healthy cells that make up the tissue from which they arise: (a) sarcomas,; (b) leukemias and lymphomas, and (c) carcinomas.

CANCEROUS Pertaining to cancer *q.v.*

CANDIDA 1. A yeast-like fungus *q.v.* that may infect the vagina *q.v.* or throat. 2. *Candida albicans q.v.* (formerly called monilia).

CANDIDA ALBICANS 1. A yeast *q.v.* (fungus) causing oral, intestinal, vaginal *q.v.*, or skin infections *q.v.* 2. Candidiasis *q.v.* 3. Thrush *q.v.* 4. A yeast that causes whitish patches in the mouth and/or esophagus *q.v.* 5. A fungus; the causative agent of vulvovaginal candidiasis or yeast infection.

CANDIDIASIS 1. A disease characterized by a thrush *q.v.* containing white plaques *q.v.* when the site is the oral cavity *q.v.* 2. Vulvovaginitis *q.v.* is characterized by inflammation *q.v.* and white patches with a discharge when the site is the vagina *q.v.* 3. A fungal infection *q.v.* of the mucous membranes (commonly occurring in the mouth, where it is called thrush) characterized by whitish spots and/or burning or other painful sensations. It may also occur in the esophagus. It can cause a red and itchy rash in moist areas, such as the vagina. cf: moniliasis.

CANKER A lesion *q.v.*, chiefly of the mouth and lips, due to a virus *q.v.* or a vitamin deficiency *q.v.*

CANNABINOID A chemical compound found only in cannabis *q.v.* products, esp. tetrahydrocannabinol (THC) *q.v.*

CANNABIS 1. Marijuana *q.v.* or any preparation from the hemp plant. 2. The dried flowering tops of hemp plants that have euphoriant *q.v.* properties and are prepared as marijuana or hashish *q.v.*

CANNABIS INDICA A variety of the cannabis *q.v.* plant that has a relatively high concentration of THC *q.v.* in comparison to *Cannabis sativa q.v.*

CANNABIS SATIVA 1. The marijuana *q.v.* plant. 2. A hemp plant from which marijuana is obtained. cf: cannabinoid; cannabis; tetrahydrocannabinol.

CANNULA A hollow metal or plastic tube through which materials can be aspired *q.v.*

CANONICAL CORRELATION In research, the prediction of a criterion composed of two or more dependent variables *q.v.* by two or more independent variables *q.v.*

CANTHARIDES A powder made from the bodies of dried beetles causing inflammation *q.v.* of the urinary tract.

CANTHARIA VESICATORIA Spanish fly *q.v.*

CAPACITATION The process by which a sperm *q.v.* becomes capable of fertilizing an ovum *q.v.* after the sperm reaches the fallopian tube *q.v.*

CAPILLARIES 1. The tiny blood vessels that transport blood to tissues and cells. 2. The tiny blood vessels that connect arteries to veins. cf: capillary.

CAPILLARITY The movement of a liquid due to surface forces, esp. observable in capillary *q.v.* tubes.

CAPILLARY 1. The smallest division of the circulatory system *q.v.* 2. A tiny tube where oxygen and nutrients are transferred from the blood to the cells where the waste products of metabolism *q.v.* are transferred from the cells to the blood for excretion *q.v.* 3. Microscopic blood vessels that connect arteries *q.v.* with venules *q.v.* 4. Microscopic lymphatic *q.v.* vessels.

CAPILLARY SOIL WATER In botany, the water held in the soil against the force of gravity and is the chief source of water absorbed by the roots of a plant.

CAPITAL OUTLAY Expenditures for land or existing buildings, improvement of grounds, construction of buildings, additions to buildings, initial or additional equipment, and upkeep.

CAPITATION 1. A method of paying health providers based on the number of patients involved rather than on a fee for service basis. 2. A per capita calculation.

CAPSID In microbiology, the complete protein coat of an animal virus *q.v.* cf: capsomere.

CAPSOMERE A subunit that has been recognized to be made up of protein, esp. in an animal virus *q.v.* cf: capsid.

CAPSULE 1. In botany, a dry fruit that develops from a compound pistil *q.v.* and opens in various ways, allowing the seeds to escape. 2. A slimy layer around the cells of certain bacteria. 3. The spore *q.v.* case in liverworts and mosses. 4. In humans, the fibrous covering of a joint. 5. ~ is also used to denote the covering of certain organs or of a growth in the tissues. 6. In medicine, a solid dosage form in which a drug is enclosed in a soluble container of gelatin that is easily dissolved in the gastrointestinal *q.v.* tract where the drug can be readily absorbed into the bloodstream.

CARAPACE In biology and zoology, the bony or chitinous case or shield covering the back or part of the back of an animal.

CARBAMATE In pharmacology, a salt or ester *q.v.* of carbolic acid. ~ forms the basis for certain hypnotics *q.v.*

CARBAMINOHEMOGLOBIN Carbhemoglobin *q.v.*

CARBHEMOGLOBIN 1. Carbominoglobin. 2. A compound formed by the union of carbon dioxide with hemoglobin *q.v.*

CARBOHYDRATE 1. A nutrient compound consisting of carbon, hydrogen, and oxygen present in foods in the form of starch and sugar. ~s are classified as monosaccharides *q.v.*, disaccharides *q.v.*, or polysaccharides *q.v.* 2. A major nutrient class that provides a chief source of energy in the human diet. 3. A nutrient high in calories *q.v.* 4. Any of the series of compounds whose empirical formula is $(CH_2O)_x$, where x is any integer for simple monosaccharides; for disaccharides, trisaccharides, and higher orders, the formula would have $(n$-1) water molecules *q.v.*

CARBOHYDRATE LOADING A dietary sequence of reduced carbohydrate *q.v.* intake followed by 3 or 4 days of high intake. This loading maximizes the storage of muscle glycogen *q.v.* and is used by long-distance runners in preparing for a race.

CARBOLIC ACID Phenol, an antiseptic first used by Joseph Lister.

CARBON A nonmetallic chemical element with the chemical symbol C. ~ is found in all living tissues.

CARBON DIOXIDE A colorless gas produced in the oxidation of carbon. It has the chemical formula CO_2. ~ in very small quantities may act as a respiratory stimulant *q.v.*

CARBON DIOXIDE PRODUCTION A substance that results from aerobic *q.v.* metabolism *q.v.* While oxygen is being used by the working muscles, a similar volume of carbon dioxide is being produced, transported by blood to the lungs, and exhaled.

CARBONIC ACID The substance formed when carbon dioxide *q.v.* combines with water.

CARBON MONOXIDE 1. A colorless, odorless, and tasteless gas that results from the incomplete combustion of any carbon-containing substance. ~ is absorbed by the red blood cells more readily than oxygen which consequently can result in asphyxiation *q.v.* 2. A gas consisting of one atom of oxygen with the chemical formula CO. 3. A poisonous component of the gas phase of cigarette smoke that combines with the hemoglobin *q.v.* in red blood cells, thus reducing the oxygen-carrying capacity of the blood. 4. An odorless, colorless gas that is toxic *q.v.* in even small amounts and is a major pollutant from automobile exhaust.

CARBON TETRACHLORIDE A colorless liquid used in fire extinguishers, as a cleaning agent, and as an insecticide *q.v.*

CARBONYL GROUP The characteristic group of the ketones *q.v.*

CARBOXYHEMOGLOBIN Hemoglobin *q.v.* that carries carbon monoxide *q.v.*

CARBUNCLE A many-headed boil *q.v.*

CARCINOGEN 1. An environmental agent capable of producing cancer *q.v.* 2. A cancer-causing agent. cf: cocarcinogen.

CARCINOGENESIS The production of a carcinoma *q.v.* cf: carcinogenic.

CARCINOGENIC Related to the production of cancerous *q.v.* changes. The property of environmental agents, including drugs, that stimulate the development of cancerous changes within cells. cf: carcinogen.

CARCINOMA 1. A cancer *q.v.* that arises from the epithelial *q.v.* cells that cover the external and internal surfaces of the body; the skin and membranes *q.v.* 2. A malignant *q.v.* new growth made up of epithelial cells tending to infiltrate the surrounding tissues and metastasize *q.v.* 3. Cancers of the surface tissues or linings of the body.

CARCINOMA IN SITU 1. Noninvasive cancer *q.v.* 2. A cancerous growth remaining at the site of its origin.

CARDBOARD SPLINT Rigid splint *q.v.*

CARDIAC Pertaining to the heart.

CARDIAC ARRHYTHMIA A disturbance of the normal synchronized rhythm of the heartbeat so that the heart does not pump blood. ~ is fatal if not reversed. cf: arrhythmia.

CARDIAC ARREST Any stoppage of the heartbeat.

CARDIAC COMPRESSION External heart massage to restore circulation and the pumping action of the heart. cf: CPR.

CARDIAC DISORDERS Disease of the heart that affects its functioning and output.

CARDIAC DRUG A drug *q.v.* that affects the function of the heart and the blood vessels of the body, including antianginal preparations, antiarrhythmics, digitalis, coronary vasodilators, and vasopressors.

CARDIAC FAILURE 1. Heart failure *q.v.* 2. A condition associated with characteristic signs of disturbed cardiac *q.v.* function, such as raised blood pressure, pulmonary edema *q.v.*, and general peripheral edema *q.v.* 3. Congestive heart failure *q.v.*

CARDIAC GLYCOSIDE A drug related to digitalis *q.v.* that is used to slow the heart rate and to increase the force of the contraction of the cardiac muscle *q.v.*

CARDIAC MUSCLE The muscle *q.v.* of the heart. cf: striated muscle; smooth muscle.

CARDIAC NEUROSIS Functional *q.v.* angina pectoris *q.v.* due to prolonged anxiety *q.v.* or stress *q.v.*

CARDIAC OUTPUT The quantity of blood pumped by the heart measured in a specific unit of time. ~ is equal to the heart rates times the stroke volume.

CARDIAC STANDSTILL Absence of contraction or electrical activity of the heart.

CARDIAC TAMPONADE Compression of the heart muscle caused by the accumulation of fluid within the pericardial sac *q.v.*

CARDINAL DISPOSITION An attribute so pervasive in a person's makeup that it contributes to every action.

CARDINAL PRINCIPLES OF EDUCATION 1. The seven principles established in 1918 by the Commission on the Reorganization of Secondary Schools. They are as follows: (a) health, (b) command of fundamental processes, (c) worthy home membership, (d) vocation, (e) citizenship, (f) worthy use of leisure time, and (g) ethical character. 2. The seven goals for secondary education developed by the National Education Association in 1918.

CARDIOGENIC Of cardiac *q.v.* origin.

CARDIOGENIC SHOCK Extensive damage to the heart muscle resulting in the inability of the heart to pump blood to all parts of the body. ~ is one of the major causes of death among myocardial infarction *q.v.* victims.

CARDIOGRAM A reading of heart and lung function obtained from a cardiograph machine *q.v.*

CARDIOGRAPH MACHINE A device that measures the actions of the heart and records the measurements on a cardiogram *q.v.*

CARDIOLOGIST A physician *q.v.* who specializes in disease of the heart and blood vessels.

CARDIOLOGY 1. The medical subspecialty concerned with the health of the heart. 2. The medical study of the structure, function, and diseases of the heart and blood vessels.

CARDIOMYOPATHY A type of disease affecting the heart muscle, sometimes caused by alcoholism *q.v.*

CARDIOPULMONARY Pertaining to the heart and lungs, particularly to respiration and oxygenation of the blood. cf: cardiorespiratory.

CARDIOPULMONARY ARREST A condition in which blood circulation or breathing has stopped.

CARDIOPULMONARY RESUSCITATION (CPR) A first aid measure to help a victim of heart failure *q.v.* to pump blood to vital organs. It includes the use of artificial resuscitation *q.v.* to force air or oxygen into the lungs and chest pressure to stimulate heartbeat.

CARDIORESPIRATORY Pertaining to the heart and the lungs. cf: cardiopulmonary.

CARDIORESPIRATORY EFFICIENCY The ability of the heart, blood vessels, and lungs to deliver oxygen to all parts of the body. cf: cardiorespiratory endurance.

CARDIORESPIRATORY ENDURANCE The ability of the heart, lungs, and blood vessels to mobilize the body's energy and sustain movement over an extended period of time. cf: cardiorespiratory efficiency.

CARDIORESPIRATORY FITNESS Fitness *q.v.* of the heart and blood vessels and lungs. Generally thought to be best promoted by aerobic exercise *q.v.*

CARDIOSPASM A spasm *q.v.* of the muscle that controls the entrance of food from the lower end of the esophagus *q.v.* into the stomach. This term is considered a misnomer since it does not involve the heart.

CARDIOTOXIC A substance having a poisonous or harmful effect upon the heart.

CARDIOVASCULAR Pertaining to the heart and circulatory system.

CARDIOVASCULAR DISEASE 1. Disease of the heart and blood vessels, including coronary heart disease *q.v.* and atherosclerosis *q.v.* 2. Cardiovascular disorder *q.v.*

CARDIOVASCULAR EFFICIENCY The ability of the heart, lungs, and blood vessels to supply oxygen and nutrients to working muscles while removing waste products created by muscular contractions. cf: cardiorespiratory efficiency.

CARDIOVASCULAR ENDURANCE The ability of the body to process and transport oxygen required by muscle cells so that they can continue to contract. cf: cardiorespiratory endurance.

CARDIOVASCULAR STRESS TEST The use of instruments to measure heartbeat, blood pressure *q.v.*, and electrocardiographic *q.v.* waves to detect the health of the cardiovascular system *q.v.* The test is conducted by gradually changing resistance on a treadmill or stationary bicycle or by increasing walking or pedaling speed. The attached instruments record cardiovascular changes as stress increases. These tests should be conducted by trained physical educators, physiologists, or physicians.

CARDIOVASCULAR SYSTEM The circulatory system; the heart, blood, and arteries and veins.

CAREER 1. An area or field of work for which a person is specially suited or trained. 2. A person's life work. 3. The individually perceived sequence of attitudes and behaviors associated with work-related experiences over the span of a person's life.

CAREER DEVELOPMENT A meaningful progression and achievement of long-term objectives in a person's work or occupation.

CAREER EDUCATION A concept that aims at preparing learners for adulthood with emphasis on careers *q.v.* ~ is frequently infused within existing curricula *q.v.* within a school system.

CAREER GOALS 1. Specific objectives *q.v.* for future positions in an organization. 2. The end result of career planning and development.

CAREER LADDER Pertaining to a number of levels that can be defined within the hierarchy of an organization.

CAREER MANAGEMENT The blending of individual aspiration with organizational needs in formal programs to develop capabilities, allocate human resources, select and place, review accomplishments, and reward desired performance.

CAREER MOLESTER A molester *q.v.* who deliberately and often seeks sexual contacts with children. 2. A pedophiliac *q.v.*

CAREER PATHING Exposure of promotable candidates to a variety of experiences designed to prepare them for replacement positions for which they have been designated.

CAREER PLANNING The individual process of choosing occupations and organizations, planning the route one's career *q.v.* will follow and engaging in appropriate self-development activities.

CARIES 1. In dentistry, dental caries or cavities. 2. Dental decay.

CARING Feeling concern for or about another person or situation.

CARIOGENIC A biological agent *q.v.* that produces tooth decay. cf: caries.

CARNEGIE FOUNDATION REPORT ON SECONDARY EDUCATION The report contends that better teaching is essential to improve secondary education. It also describes the important role teachers have if reform is to be successful.

CARNEGIE REPORT Published by the Task Force on Teaching as a Profession calls for reforms in teacher education, which include competitive salary schedules, incentives for teachers related to student achievement, and the creation of a national board for teaching standards.

CARNEGIE UNIT A unit awarded to a student for successfully completing a high school course that meets for a minimum of 120 clock hours.

CARNIVORE Plants or animals that eat meat as a source of protein.

CARNIVOROUS 1. In biology and zoology, feeding upon other animals. 2. In botany, plants that are able to use protein obtained from trapped animals, chiefly, insects. ct: herbivorous.

CAROTENE The yellow pigment found in various plant and animal tissues that is the precursor of vitamin A *q.v.* An excessive intake of ~ can cause carotenemia *q.v.* cf: carotenes.

CAROTENEMIA A condition in which the skin turns yellow as a result of an excessive intake of vitamin A *q.v.* or carotene *q.v.*

CAROTENES 1. Orange or yellow, unsaturated hydrocarbons, such as provitamin A ($C_{40}H_{56}$) *q.v.* 2. Carotenoids *q.v.*

CAROTENOIDS 1. Yellow or orange or red pigments found in plastids *q.v.* of plants. 2. Carotenes *q.v.* 3. Xanthophylls *q.v.*

CAROTID From the Greek word meaning to plunge into deep sleep. cf: carotid artery.

CAROTID ARTERY One of the main arteries of the neck supplying blood to the head. Pressure on the ~ may produce unconsciousness *q.v.* cf: carotid.

CAROTID ENDARTERECTOMY Surgery used to remove plaque *q.v.* buildup in the carotid artery *q.v.*

CAROTID PULSE The beating of the heart felt in the carotid artery *q.v.* located to the side of the larynx *q.v.*

CARPAL 1. Pertaining to the wrist. 2. The eight bones of the wrist.

CARPAL TUNNEL SYNDROME (CTS) Inflamed tendons and membranes *q.v.* in the wrist and damaged nerves that control finger and hand movement.

CARPEL 1. In botany, a leaf-like organ bearing ovules *q.v.* along the margins. 2. The unit of structure of a compound pistil *q.v.*

CARPOPEDAL SPASM 1. A spastic condition of the hands and feet. 2. The involuntary contraction of the muscles of the hands and feet during sexual arousal.

CARRIER 1. In epidemiology, a human vector *q.v.*; a host who can transmit a disease but who does not necessarily have the symptoms *q.v.* of the disease. 2. In genetics, a person who caries an unexpressed recessive gene. ~s do not have the trait associated with the recessive gene, but are responsible for transmitting it.

CARRIER MOLECULE A specialized protein molecule *q.v.* that enables large molecules to be transported across cell membranes *q.v.*

CARRY 1. Stretcher. 2. A device or method for transporting a person as applied to first aid or emergency treatment of a victim of an accident or sudden illness.

CARRYOVER ACTIVITY In physical education, a physical activity that can be continued in later life with little risk and high fitness value.

CARTILAGE 1. A connective tissue *q.v.* characterized by nonvascularity and a firm texture, consisting of chondrocytes *q.v.*, interstitial substance (matrix), and chondromucoid *q.v.* 2. Fibrous connective tissue between the surfaces of movable and immovable joints.

CARTILAGINOUS Pertaining to or consisting of cartilage *q.v.*

CARNUNCLE 1. A small, fleshy prominence. 2. Carnuncula *q.v.*

CARNUNCULA 1. A small, fleshy prominence. 2. Carnuncle *q.v.*

CARYOSOME In genetics, aggregation of chromatin *q.v.* in an interphase *q.v.* nucleus *q.v.*

CAS Chemical Abstract Service.

CASANOVA COMPLEX Delusion of extraordinary sexual potency and desirability.

CASE–CONTROL METHOD (STUDY) 1. In epidemiology, a method of study that can support and test hypotheses *q.v.* about supposed causes. Data are the past characteristics and events that are analyzed. 2. Retrospective *q.v.* data collection. 3. An epidemiological study design in which individuals with a disease or health problem are matched on a variety of factors with others who do not have the disease or health problem for purposes of comparison. Some matching factors may be age, race, socioeconomic status, occupation, or area of residence.

CASE FATALITY RATE 1. The number of deaths from a specific cause to the number of cases expressed in percentage. The formula is

$$\frac{\text{Number of deaths from a specific cause}}{\text{Number of cases of the cause}} \times 100$$

2. The proportion of persons with a disease who have or are projected to die of that disease. cf: case fatality rate.

CASE FATALITY RATIO In epidemiology, the death rate of specific cases. ~ is calculated by dividing the deaths from a cause by the number at risk *q.v.* cf: case fatality rate.

CASE FINDING A health screening *q.v.* procedure used to identify a specific high-risk health condition in a group of people.

CASE FOLLOW-UP STUDY In epidemiology, the descriptive epidemiology *q.v.* of the natural history *q.v.* of diseases, including recuperation.

CASE HISTORY METHOD In psychology, the investigation of psychological *q.v.* problems through the examination of the biographies of human subjects.

CASEIN Milk protein *q.v.*

CASE SERIES STUDY In epidemiology, a study of cases only, with no control group *q.v.* for comparison.

CASE STUDY 1. The collection of historical or biographical information on a single individual, often including experiences in therapy *q.v.* 2. A report of a unique event usually based on observations that are made of a single person. 3. In education, a teaching method that uses detailed descriptions of expanded situations for analysis and discussion by the learners. 4. A careful, in-depth study of an individual or situation using qualitative research *q.v.* methods; in quantitative research, and application of treatment followed by observation and measurement. 5. A medical or epidemiologic evaluation of a person or small number of persons to determine descriptive information about their health status or potential for exposure through interviews or biomedical *q.v.* testing. cf: case study research.

CASE STUDY RESEARCH 1. A research design that observes and studies a single case or person or situation rather than numerous individuals or situations. 2. An observational study in which one person is studied intensively.

CASH INDEMNITY A cash benefit paid by a health insurance company to the person who is the health insurance policy holder, when there is a loss covered by the insurance policy.

CASPARIAN STRIP (SOMETIMES SPELLED WITH A LOWER CASE C) Strips that seal the radial and transverse walls of the endodermis *q.v.* and prevent diffusion *q.v.* in the walls between adjoining protoplasts *q.v.*

CASSAVA A tropical plant of the spurge family with edible starchy roots.

CAST 1. In botany, a type of fossil that results from the filling of a cavity formed by the decay of plant tissues. 2. In anatomy, mold. ~ may form in renal tubules *q.v.*

CASTE A distinct type or form among a group of organisms.

CASTRATING Pertains to any source of injury to or deprivation of the genitals *q.v.* or, more broadly, to a threat to masculinity *q.v.* or femininity of a person. cf: castration; castration complex.

CASTRATION 1. The surgical removal of the gonads *q.v.* 2. The surgical removal of the testes *q.v.* in the male or the removal of the ovaries *q.v.* in the female.

CASTRATION ANXIETY 1. The fear of harm from fathers assumed to be felt by boys during the Oedipus conflict *q.v.* 2. The fear of having the genitals *q.v.* removed or injured. 3. According to Freud, the unconscious fear in boys about the possible loss of their penis *q.v.* as a terrible form of punishment. cf: castration complex.

CASTRATION COMPLEX 1. In psychology, the unconscious fear centered around an injury or loss of the genitals *q.v.* as punishment for forbidden sexual desires. 2. In males, anxiety about manhood or masculinity *q.v.*

CASUAL CONTACT In epidemiology, day-to-day contact between human immunodeficiency virus-infected *q.v.* (HIV) persons and others at home, at work, or at school. This type of contact does not include sexual or needle-sharing interaction, esp. in regards to AIDS *q.v.*

CATABOLISM 1. A phase of metabolism *q.v.* characterized by a chemical breakdown within the body of foods. 2. The energy-releasing metabolic processes in which body substances are broken down into simpler substances. 3. The destructive or tearing down aspects of metabolism such as respiration and digestion. ct: anabolism.

CATALEPSY A condition in which the muscles are waxy and semirigid, tending to maintain the limbs in any position in which they are placed. cf: catatonic.

CATALYST 1. Any substance that speeds up a chemical reaction without changing its own chemical structure. 2. Any chemical substance that either increases or decreases the rate of a particular chemical reaction without itself being consumed or permanently altered. Enzymes *q.v.* in the human body are special chemical ~s of biological *q.v.* origin. 3. Something that causes activity between two or more entities without itself being affected.

CATARACT 1. Clouding of the lens of the eye. ~ is a major cause of impaired vision in the United States. ~ may be either developmental or degenerative. Developmental ~ occurs congenitally *q.v.* or early in life as a result of heredity *q.v.*, nutritional, or inflammatory disturbances. Degenerative ~ is characterized by loss of transparency in a normally developed lens of the eye and is the result of changes due to aging, or the side effects of heat, X-rays, trauma, disease, or drugs. The major symptom of ~ is a painless loss of vision and is corrected by extraction of the lens and fitting of visual prostheses *q.v.* 2. A cloudiness or opacity that develops in the lens of the eye and results in poorer vision. ~ was previously one of the leading causes of blindness in persons over 60 years, but now, ~ can be surgically removed restoring vision with the aid of corrective lenses.

CATARRH Any inflammation *q.v.* of a mucous membrane *q.v.*

CATARRHAL JAUNDICE Obsolete term for infectious hepatitis *q.v.*

CATASEXUAL Sexual activity with a nonhuman partner.

CATASTROPHIC INSURANCE An insurance policy that provides protection against major medical expenses.

CATASTROPHIC REACTION A severe disintegration *q.v.* of personality organization while under extreme stress *q.v.*

CATATONIA 1. A condition characterized by varying degrees of withdrawal with the person becoming unresponsive to stimuli *q.v.* with possible immobility. 2. A condition of muscular rigidity in which the person remains in whatever position he or she is placed. Occurs in schizophrenia *q.v.*, PCP *q.v.*, and LSD *q.v.* psychosis. 3. Catalepsy *q.v.* 4. Catatonic seizure. 5. A schizophrenic reaction *q.v.* characterized by alteration between stupor and excitement.

CATATONIC 1. Trancelike. 2. Absolute withdrawal from reality. 3. Rigid. 4. Catatonia *q.v.* 5. Catatonic immobility *q.v.*

CATATONIC IMMOBILITY 1. Catatonia *q.v.* 2. Rigidity of posture, sometimes grotesque, maintained for long periods of time with accompanying muscular rigidity, trancelike state of consciousness, and waxy flexibility.

CATATONIC SCHIZOPHRENIA A subcategory of schizophrenia *q.v.* characterized by odd motor behavior, immobility, and catatonia *q.v.*

CATCH UP PHENOMENON In child growth and development, unusually rapid growth following interference with growth in the course of which a child regains some or all of the growth lost during the period of interference.

CATECHOLAMINE 1. A class of biochemical compounds including the neurotransmitters *q.v.* dopamine *q.v.*, norepinephrine *q.v.*, and epinephrine *q.v.* 2. Hormones *q.v.* secreted by the adrenal glands *q.v.*, especially during stress *q.v.* 3. A group of body chemicals that have a strong effect on the nervous system *q.v.* which play an important role in some reactions to drugs taken into the body. 4. Monoamine compounds (NH_2) each having a catechol portion (C_6H_6). ~ known to be neurotransmitters of the central nervous system are norepinephrine and dopamine, while epinephrine is principally a hormone.

CATECHOL-O-METHYLTRANSFERASE (COMT) An enzyme *q.v.* that deactivates catecholamine *q.v.* at the synapse *q.v.*

CATEGORICAL AID Financial assistance provided to a local school district for specific programs or purposes. cf: categorical program.

CATEGORICAL HEALTH EDUCATION APPROACH The process of teaching about health by means of a particular content area. A school curriculum *q.v.* may offer instruction on such topics as disease prevention, physical fitness, sex education, and so forth with each unit standing alone as an educational experience.

CATEGORICAL PROGRAM Programs concerned with only a part of the population or health system.

CATEGORICAL SCALE A scale that divides responses into categories that are numerically related. cf: interval scale; ratio scale.

CATEGORICAL VARIABLE 1. In epidemiology, a variable *q.v.* created by collapsing a larger number of values into a few categories, or one that by its nature is not suited to a long continuum of possible values. 2. Qualitative variable.

CATEGORY TEST A neuropsychological test that assesses abstract concept *q.v.* formation as well as the ability to use positive and negative feedback *q.v.* in solving complex problems.

CATHARSIS 1. A form of emotional release resulting from talking out problems with the aid of a therapist, as applied to psychology. 2. A cleansing. 3. Psychocatharsis *q.v.* 4. Abreaction *q.v.* 5. A sudden, explosive release of pent-up emotions which is believed to have psychotherapeutic effects. 6. An emotional release achieved by reexperiencing and communicating emotions associated with past trauma. cf: frustration-aggression hypothesis.

CATHARSIS THEORY In sexology, a theory that holds that pornography acts as a safety valve for people's unexpressed sexual feelings. cf: modeling theory; null theory.

CATHARTIC 1. A laxative *q.v.* 2. A substance that induces bowel movements. 3. A purgative *q.v.*

CATHARTIC METHOD In psychology, a therapeutic procedure introduced by Breuer in the late nineteenth century whereby a person recalls and relives an earlier emotional catastrophe and reexperiences the tension and unhappiness. cf: catharsis.

CATHETER A piece of plastic or rubber tubing that is inserted into a vein or other hollow structure.

CATHEXIS 1. An investment or an object, idea, or action that has special significance or effect for a person. 2. Concentration of a person's psychic *q.v.* energy on a specific person, thing, or idea.

CATI An acronym for computer-assisted telephone interview. A device used by ATSDR *q.v.* interviews to administer the core questionnaire to people who will participate in a registry.

CATION 1. A positively charged ion *q.v.* attracted to the cathode *q.v.* during electrolysis *q.v.* 2. An atom that has lost one or more of its electrons.

CAT SCAN 1. Computerized axial tomography. 2. An imaging method in which the density of an area of the body is determined with the use of X-rays fed into a computer to create a picture on a screen resembling a cross-sectional photograph. 3. A study of body structures.

CAUDAL Pertaining to the tail of an animal. ct: cephalic.

CAUDETENUCLEUS The mass of gray matter *q.v.* in the corpus striatum *q.v.* of the brain *q.v.* forming part of the floor of the lateral ventricle *q.v.* and separated from the lenticular nucleus *q.v.* by the internal capsule *q.v.*

CAUL 1. An obsolete term used for the sac that encloses the baby before birth and that usually ruptures at the time of delivery. If the ~ does not rupture, it is said that the baby was born with a ~. 2. The great omentum *q.v.*

CAULIFLOWER EAR 1. A deformed, painful ear caused by repeated friction and trauma to the ear. 2. A lay term referring to a deformed ear resulting from continuous trauma characterized by an accumulation of blood and scar tissue in the outer ear. The condition resembles a cauliflower.

CAUSAL 1. Etiology *q.v.* 2. The factor, either alone or in combination with other factors, that is responsible for the onset of disease *q.v.* 3. In epidemiology, inferring from findings that an antecedent leads to the health state under study.

CAUSAL CHAIN The sequence of events that results in an effect.

CAUSAL-COMPARATIVE STUDIES After-the-fact natural experiments *q.v.*

CAUSAL DIAGRAM In sociology, a path diagram. 2. A diagram that presents the causally related variables *q.v.* in time sequence, usually with arrows drawn to indicate the causal direction and showing whether the relationship is positive, negative, or neutral.

CAUSAL INFERENCE In research, a conclusion that indicates that one variable *q.v.* causes another.

CAUSAL MODELING Structural modeling *q.v.*

CAUSATIVE FACTORS In epidemiology, etiological factors *q.v.* The factors, either separately or collectively with others, responsible for the onset of disease or some other health problem.

CAUSE 1. A factor or factors that, when prevented, removed, or eliminated, will preclude the occurrence of a health event; but when permitted, introduced, or maintained, will result in the health event. 2. One or more conditions that are necessary and sufficient for the production of some effect. A necessary condition is one that must occur that is always followed by the effect. A condition may be necessary but not sufficient to produce the effect. A condition may be sufficient but only one of the ways to produce the effect, and thus it is not necessary. Causal analysis *q.v.* is the art of the possible and probable.

CAUSES OF DEATH See leading causes of death.

CAUSE-SPECIFIC MORTALITY The factor responsible for death.

CAUSTIC A substance that burns tissue or causes corrosion.

CAUSTIC POISONS Chemicals that possess properties capable of dissolving other materials.

CAUTERIZE 1. To apply a small electrical current and permanently close a tube or vessel. 2. To burn.

CAUTERY A hot instrument or corrosive chemical used to destroy tissue or to coagulate *q.v.* blood in controlling certain types of hemorrhage *q.v.*

CAVEAT EMPTOR Let the buyer beware. ct: caveat vendor.

CAVEAT VENDOR Let the seller beware. ct: caveat emptor.

CAVERNOUS Pertaining to large hollow cavities that may occur in various tissues normally or abnormally.

CAVERNOUS BODIES The two upper cylinders of erectile tissue that extend the length of the shaft of the penis *q.v.* ct: spongy body.

CBRU An acronym for computer-based resource unit. cf: computerized learning.

CBTE An acronym for competency-based teacher education *q.v.*

CCRIS An acronym for Chemical Carcinogenesis Research Information System *q.v.*

CD 1. An acronym for chemical dependency *q.v.* 2. An acronym for communication deviance *q.v.* 3. An acronym for cluster differentiating type antigens *q.v.* found on T lymphocytes *q.v.* Each ~ is assigned a number such as CD1, CD2.

CDC An acronym for Centers for Disease Control and Prevention.

CECUM (CAECUM) 1. The dilated part of the large intestine into which opens the ileum *q.v.* 2. The first portion of the large intestine into which the small intestine empties. The vermiform appendix *q.v.* is attached to the ~. 3. Literally, blind pouch. 4. Caecum *q.v.*

CEHIC An acronym for Center for Environmental Health and Injury Control; CDC *q.v.*

CEILING EFFECTS In education, a restricted range of test questions or problems that does not permit students to demonstrate their true capacity for achievement.

CELIAC Pertaining to the abdomen *q.v.*

CELSIUS SCALE Centigrade scale *q.v.*

CELIBACY 1. The state of being unmarried. 2. Total abstinence from sexual activity. cf: celibate.

CELIBATE A person who has not and does not engage in sexual behavior with another person or other people. Celibacy *q.v.* may be voluntary or involuntary.

CELL 1. The structural unit composing the bodies of plants and animals. 2. An organized unit of protoplasm *q.v.* in plants, usually surrounded by a cell wall.

CELL BODY The part of the cell *q.v.* that contains the nucleus *q.v.*

CELL CULTURE The growth of cells *q.v.* in vitro *q.v.*

CELL DIVISION The division of the cytoplasm *q.v.* into two equal parts, usually brought about by the formation of a cell plate *q.v.* cf: mitosis; meiosis.

CELL-MEDIATED Refers to the type of immunity *q.v.* produced by T lymphocytes *q.v.* cf: cell-mediated immunity.

CELL-MEDIATED IMMUNITY 1. A defense mechanism in which T lymphocytes *q.v.* (T-cell helper or killer T cells) work together to stimulate immune response *q.v.* and eliminate cells *q.v.* that are infected with infectious agents *q.v.* 2. The reaction to antigenic *q.v.* material by specific defensive cells (macrophages) rather than antibodies. cf: cell-mediated.

CELL PATHOLOGY The process of cell *q.v.* destruction that often accompanies certain diseases *q.v.*

CELL PLATE 1. A membrane-like structure that forms at the equator of the spindle *q.v.* during early telophase in cell division *q.v.* 2. The predecessor of the intercellular *q.v.* layer.

CELL SAP A collective term for the fluid content of the vacuole *q.v.* of a cell *q.v.*

CELLULAR COHESIVENESS A tendency of normal cells *q.v.* to cling or stick together rather than to move independently throughout the body.

CELLULAR HYPOXIA A condition resulting from the disturbed function of cells *q.v.* created by enzyme *q.v.* poisoning.

CELLULAR IMMUNITY A collection of cell *q.v.* types that provide protection against various antigens *q.v.*

CELLULASE An enzyme *q.v.* that hydrolyzes *q.v.* cellulose *q.v.*

CELLULITE 1. A coined term used to describe the dimpled fat present on the thighs of some females. The term is medically recognized. 2. An unscientific term used to describe a special type of body fat.

CELLULOSE 1. The most abundant polysaccharide *q.v.* 2. An indigestible carbohydrate *q.v.* 3. Dietary fiber. 4. A chemical compound that forms the indigestible fiber component within certain foods. 5. A carbohydrate, the chief component of the cell wall in most plants.

CELOM The body cavity of the embryo *q.v.* situated between the somatopleure *q.v.* and the splanchnopleure *q.v.*

CEMENTUM 1. Calcified tissue covering the root and neck of the tooth. 2. The outer covering of the root of a tooth between the periodontal membrane *q.v.* and the dentin *q.v.*

CENSORSHIP 1. In education, the act of censuring materials such as library books and textbooks. 2. In psychoanalytic theory, the functioning of the ego *q.v.* and the superego *q.v.* in preventing dangerous impulses or desires from entering the consciousness *q.v.*

CENSORSHIP IN DREAMS Freud's theory of dreams *q.v.*

CENTENARIAN A person who is 100 years or older.

CENTERS FOR DISEASE CONTROL A branch of the United States public Health Service (USPHS) *q.v.* In 1980, the ~ was reorganized to form six centers: (a) The Center for Prevention Services, (b) The Center for Environmental Health, (c) The National Institute for Occupational Safety and Health, (d) The Center for Health Promotion and Education, (e) The Center for Professional Development and Training, and (f) The Center for Infectious Diseases.

CENTER FOR HEALTH PROMOTION AND EDUCATION A part of the Centers for Disease Control *q.v.* established in 1980, consisting of three divisions: (a) The Division of Nutrition, (b) The Division of Reproductive Health, and (c) The Division of Health Education.

CENTER FOR STUDIES OF SUICIDE PREVENTION A branch of the National Institute of Mental Health *q.v.*, established in 1966. Its purpose was to provide research support, pilot studies, training of personnel, consultation for suicide prevention agencies, dissemination of information, coordination of emergency services, case findings, treatment, and promotion of the application of research findings.

CENTERING In psychology, a term borrowed from Assagioli's system of psychosynthesis based on the process of finding the true self and of allowing that to be the point around which all other elements of the psyche *q.v.* are arranged.

CENTIGRADE SCALE 1. Celsius scale *q.v.* 2. The temperature scale in which the freezing point of water is 0°C and the boiling point of water is 100°C. ct: Fahrenheit scale.

CENTIMETER 1. A unit of measurement equal to about two-fifths of an inch. There are 100 cm–1 m. 2. 1/100th of a meter.

CENTRAL DEAFNESS Loss of hearing caused by damage to the pathways or center of hearing in the brain.

CENTRAL DISPOSITION In psychology, those traits *q.v.* that are uniquely characteristic of a person.

CENTRALIZATION That situation in which a minimal number of job activities and a minimal amount of authority are delegated to subordinates.

CENTRALIZED COMMUNICATION STRUCTURE All communication in a group is directed through one central member.

CENTRAL NERVOUS SYSTEM 1. The brain, spinal cord, and all of the nerves. 2. That major part of the nervous system composed of the brain and the spinal cord. 3. The part of the nervous system which in vertebrates *q.v.* consists of the brain and spinal cord and to which all sensory impulses are transmitted and from which motor impulses pass out. It also supervises and coordinates the activities of the entire nervous system.

CENTRAL NERVOUS SYSTEM DISORDERS Diseases and/or conditions that affect the brain and/or spinal cord.

CENTRAL OFFICE In education, pertains to the district administration level of local school districts.

CENTRAL ORIENTATION Characteristically and relatively unchangeable predisposition to interact in certain ways that shape a person's development. cf: emotional expressiveness reserve; placidity explosiveness.

CENTRAL ROUTE TO PERSUASION When rational processing is employed in response to persuasive messages. cf: peripheral route to persuasion.

CENTRAL SULCUS In anatomy, a major fissure transversing the middle of the top and lateral surfaces of each cerebral hemisphere *q.v.* dividing the frontal lobe *q.v.* from the parietal lobe *q.v.*

CENTRAL TENDENCY In statistics, the tendency of scores in a frequency distribution *q.v.* to cluster around a central value. cf: median; mean; variability.

CENTRAL VENOUS PRESSURE The pressure of the blood in the veins that aids in the return of blood to the heart.

CENTRATION Thinking that is focused on one perceptually obvious feature of a problem to the exclusion of other relevant features so that changes in that feature are not conceptualized in relation to changes in other features, misleading the subject. cf: conservation; egocentrism.

CENTRIFUGAL FORCE 1. The force that tends to impel a thing outward from a center of rotation. 2. A force directed from the axis or center.

CENTRIOLE The central granule in many animal cells *q.v.* that appears to be the active principle of the centrosome *q.v.* and which undergoes duplication preceding the division of the centrosome proper.

CENTRIPETAL A force directed toward the axis. ct: centrifugal force.

CENTROMERE 1. That portion of the chromosome *q.v.* to which the spindle fiber *q.v.* is attached. 2. Kinetochore. 3. The structure that joins each pair of chromatids *q.v.* produced by chromosome duplication.

CENTROSOME 1. A self-propagating cytoplasmic *q.v.* body usually present in animal cells *q.v.* and those of some lower plants, but not present in flowering plants, consisting of a centriole *q.v.* and sometimes a centrosphere *q.v.* or astral rays *q.v.*, located at each pole of the spindle during the process of nuclear division (mitosis). 2. In animals, the area immediately surrounding the centrioles; in plants, the chromogenic area in the nucleus.

CENTROSPHERE Centrosome *q.v.*

CEPHALIC Pertaining to the head. ct: caudal.

CEPHALIC DELIVERY Cephalic presentation *q.v.*

CEPHALIC PRESENTATION Birth position in which the baby is presented head first at birth.

CEPHALIN A lipid *q.v.* released by platelets *q.v.* and injured cells. ~ is important in blood clotting *q.v.*

CEPHALIZATION The development of larger and more elaborate brain and head in higher animals.

CEPHALOCAUDAL From head to tail along the central axis of the body. A ~ gradient is evident in neuromuscular *q.v.* maturation *q.v.* in all vertebrates *q.v.* cf: cephalocaudal sequence.

CEPHALOCAUDAL SEQUENCE A sequence of maturation *q.v.* in which the pattern of development is from the head downward. cf: cephalocaudal.

CEPHALOTHORAX 1. The united head and thorax *q.v.* 2. Pertaining to the head and thorax.

CERCARIA In biology, the fourth larval stage of a fluke usually free-swimming; penetrates the body of a second alternate host of definitive host.

CERCLA An acronym for The Comprehensive Environmental Response, Compensation, and Liability Act of 1980. Also known as the Superfund *q.v.* This is the legislation that created ATSDR *q.v.*

CERCLIS An acronym for Comprehensive Environmental Response, Compensation and Liability Information System.

CEREAL GERM The highly nutritious portion of the cereal grain.

CEREBELLUM 1. That division of the central nervous system *q.v.* postinferior to the cerebrum *q.v.* and above the pons *q.v.* ~ is concerned with coordination of movements and equilibrium. 2. The ~ serves as a reflex center in coordination and integrating skeletal muscle movements.

CEREBRAL Of or relating to the brain or intellect.

CEREBRAL ACCIDENT Stroke *q.v.*

CEREBRAL ANGIOGRAPHY A technique that determines brain death *q.v.* on the basis of whether blood is being circulated to the vital centers of the brain.

CEREBRAL AQUEDUCT A tube that conducts cerebrospinal fluid *q.v.* from the third to the fourth ventricle *q.v.*.

CEREBRAL ATHEROSCLEROSIS A chronic *q.v.* disease impairing intellectual and emotional life, caused by a reduction in the brain's blood supply through a buildup of fatty deposits in the arteries.

CEREBRAL ARTERIOSCLEROSIS Arteriosclerosis *q.v.* of the cerebrum *q.v.*

CEREBRAL CONTUSION A bruising of neural tissue marked by swelling and hemorrhage *q.v.* and resulting in coma *q.v.* ~ may permanently impair intellectual functioning.

CEREBRAL CORTEX 1. The outermost layer of gray matter *q.v.* of the cerebral hemisphere *q.v.* 2. The outer covering of the brain, the site of intellect, memory, thought processes, and rationalization. 3. The thin outer covering of each of the cerebral hemispheres, highly convoluted and made up of nerve cell bodies, which constitute the gray matter of the brain.

CEREBRAL DOMINANCE 1. The concept that one hemisphere *q.v.* of the cerebral cortex *q.v.* controls the person's behavior *q.v.* and thus dominates the other hemisphere. 2. ~ is important to many perceptual motor theorists and the basis for the idea of mixed dominance.

CEREBRAL EMBOLISM A blood clot that breaks loose from its site of origin and lodges in a cerebral artery causing a stroke *q.v.* cf: cerebral thrombosis.

CEREBRAL HEMATOMA A hemorrhage *q.v.* into the substance of the cerebrum *q.v.*

CEREBRAL HEMISPHERES 1. Two structures that comprise the major part of the forebrain and serves as the main coordinating center of the nervous system *q.v.* 2. Either of the two halves which make up the cerebrum *q.v.*

CEREBRAL HEMORRHAGE 1. A cerebral artery that has become diseased, weakened and bursts, depriving the brain cells of sufficient oxygen. 2. When blood comes in direct contact with the brain cells, the waste products in the blood seriously damage the brain cells. This is the cause of stroke *q.v.* 3. Bleeding onto brain tissue from a ruptured blood vessel.

CEREBRAL PALSY 1. A condition that results in a disturbance of motor function. 2. Lack of muscular control arising from brain damage before, during, or after birth.

CEREBRAL SPINAL FLUID (CSF) The fluid surrounding the brain and spinal cord. cf: cerebrospinal.

CEREBRAL THROMBOSIS 1. A clot in a cerebral artery resulting in stroke *q.v.* 2. The formation of a blood clot in a cerebral artery that blocks circulation in that area of brain tissue and produces paralysis, loss of sensory functions, and possibly death. cf: cerebral embolism.

CEREBRAL VASCULAR ACCIDENT (CVA) 1. Apoplectic shock. 2. Stroke *q.v.* 3. A condition characterized by impaired blood supply to some part of the brain. cf: cerebrovascular accident; apoplexy.

CEREBROSPINAL FLUID (CEREBRAL SPINAL FLUID) The fluid contained within the brain and the subarachnoid *q.v.* space about the brain and spinal cord *q.v.*

CEREBROSPINAL MENINGITIS An inflammation *q.v.* of the meninges or membranes *q.v.* covering the cortex *q.v.* of the brain.

CEREBROTONIA 1. An ectomorphy *q.v.* body type. 2. Self-consciousness, overreactiveness, and a desire for privacy. 3. In Sheldon's theory *q.v.*, a personality *q.v.* type characterized by thought rather than action, restraint in social relations, introversion *q.v.*, and the need for privacy. 4. Cerebrotonic *q.v.* ct: viscerotonia; somatotonia.

CEREBROTONIC The temperament originally assumed to be associated with an ectomorphic *q.v.* body build.

CEREBROVASCULAR ACCIDENT 1. Stroke *q.v.* 2. Brain tissue damage resulting from impaired circulation of blood to the brain. 3. Cerebral vascular occlusion *q.v.* 4. The breaking of a blood vessel in the brain. 5. Blockage or rupture of a large blood vessel in the brain resulting in disorientation, cognitive impairment, speech disorders, and transient or permanent paralysis. cf: cerebral vascular accident.

CEREBROVASCULAR DISEASES Illnesses that disrupt blood supply to the brain. cf: stroke; cerebrovascular accident.

CEREBROVASCULAR LESION Release of blood into the brain due to a ruptured blood vessel. cf: cerebrovascular accident; stroke.

CEREBROVASCULAR OCCLUSION A blockage within the arteries supplying blood to the cerebral cortex *q.v.* cf: stroke. ct: cerebrovascular accident.

CEREBRUM 1. The main portion of the brain occupying the upper part of the cranium *q.v.*, the two cerebral hemispheres *q.v.* united by the corpus collosum *q.v.* forming the largest part of the central nervous system *q.v.*

in humans. The ~ consists of derivatives of the mesencephalon *q.v.*, diencephalon *q.v.*, and telencephalon *q.v.* Considered the area of highest intelligence *q.v.* 2. The largest, most complex part of the brain that coordinates and interprets internal and external stimuli. It is the site of higher mental functions, such as memory and reasoning. 3. The convoluted layer of gray matter that forms the largest part of the brain in humans. The ~ is the highest neural center for coordination and interpretation of external and internal stimuli and contains sensory, motor, and association areas *q.v.* cf: cerebral cortex.

CERTIFICATE 1. In law, a document designed as notice that some act has been done, or some event occurred, or some legal formality complied with. 2. Evidence of qualification, as in a teaching certificate.

CERTIFICATION 1. Teacher licensure. 2. The process by which a quasi-governmental agency or association grants recognition to a person who has met certain qualifications specified by that agency. 3. In labor relations, official recognition by the National Labor Relations Board, or a state labor agency, that a labor organization is the duly designated agency for the purposes of collective bargaining.

CERTIFIED HEALTH EDUCATION SPECIALIST (CHES) 1. An individual who is credentialed *q.v.* as a result of demonstrating competence based on criteria established by the National Commission for Health Education Credentialing, Inc. (NCHEC) *q.v.* 2. A person who has met all of the requirements set forth by an agency to receive recognition. 3. A person who has met all of the qualifications of training and experience to practice as a health educator.

CERTIFIED NURSE MIDWIFE (CNM) A nurse who has completed training in pregnancy and birth and who functions in association with a physician.

CERTIORARI 1. In law, proceeding in which a higher court reviews a decision of an inferior court. 2. An action to remove a case from an inferior court. It is most often used when the United States Supreme Court is requested to hear a case from a lower court.

CERULOPLASMIN A plasma *q.v.* copper protein *q.v.* that functions as an enzyme *q.v.* and results in the formation of hallucination *q.v.*-producing products from natural amines *q.v.* cf: ceruplasmin.

CERUMEN 1. Ear wax. 2. A secretion from glands in the outer auditory *q.v.* canal.

CERUPLASMIN 1. A copper-containing protein *q.v.* in blood plasma *q.v.* 2. Alpha-globulin *q.v.*

CERVICAL CANCER 1. Cancer *q.v.* of the cervix *q.v.* 2. Linked to herpes simplex type 2 *q.v.* cf: human papilloma virus (HPV).

CERVICAL CAP 1. A diaphragm *q.v.* that fits over the cervix *q.v.* to act as a barrier to sperm *q.v.* preventing the sperm from reaching the ovum *q.v.* and resulting in fertilization *q.v.* or conception *q.v.* 2. A miniature diaphragm. The ~ may be made of rubber or plastic.

CERVICAL DYSPLASIA Abnormality of the cells *q.v.* of the cervix *q.v.*

CERVICAL MUCUS A thin, watery lubricative secretion produced by the cervix *q.v.* that aids sperm *q.v.* migration from the vagina *q.v.* to the egg in the fallopian tube *q.v.*

CERVICAL MUCUS METHOD 1. The Billings method *q.v.* 2. The natural planning method of contraception *q.v.* 3. A rhythm method *q.v.* of birth control or conception control based on careful monitoring of the consistency of cervical mucus *q.v.* to detect when ovulation *q.v.* occurs and an avoidance of coitus *q.v.* during the time when conception is likely to occur.

CERVICAL OS The opening of the cervix *q.v.*

CERVICAL PLUG Mucus in the mouth of the cervix *q.v.* that prevents bacteria *q.v.* or other foreign substances from entering the uterus *q.v.* and infecting the fetus *q.v.*

CERVICAL SPINE The first seven bones (vertebrae) of the back found in the neck.

CERVICITIS Infection *q.v.* of the cervix *q.v.*

CERVIX 1. Cervix uteri *q.v.* 2. Neck. 3. Any neck-like structure. 4. The neck-like structure that serves as the entrance to the uterus *q.v.*

CERVIX UTERI 1. The lower and narrow end of the uterus *q.v.* 2. The neck of the womb *q.v.* connecting with the vagina *q.v.* 3. The narrow portion of the uterus that projects into the vagina.

CESAREAN BIRTH Cesarean section *q.v.*

CESAREAN (CAESAREAN) SECTION 1. An incision *q.v.* through the abdominal wall and the uterine *q.v.* wall for the delivery of the fetus *q.v.* when birth through the birth canal *q.v.* is impossible or dangerous. The procedure was included in Roman law in 715 B.C. as a means of salvaging the fetus or to provide for separate burial in the event of the mother's death. 2. The surgical removal of the fetus from the uterus through the abdominal wall.

CESSATION The process of stopping, as in ~ of smoking.

CESSPOOL A reservoir for refuse and water with walls sufficiently porous to allow seepage into the surrounding ground.

CESTODE 1. A parasitic *q.v.* worm. 2. Tapeworm.

CEU An acronym for continuing education unit.

C-FIBER A type of nerve fiber that transmits slowly and gives rise to the sensation of dull, diffuse, or burning pain. cf: A-delta fiber.

CHAIN OF INFECTION A series of infections *q.v.* that are directly or indirectly connected to a particular source.

CHAIN OF REASONING The steps in the presentation of a logical argument in support of a knowledge claim.

CHAIN REFERRAL SAMPLING Snowball sampling *q.v.*

CHAIR In parliamentary law, the presiding officer or chairperson.

CHALAZION A small tumor *q.v.* of the eyelid.

CHALONE A hormone *q.v.* that depresses activity.

CHAMBER In politics, the official hall for the meeting of a legislative body, e.g., assembly chamber; senate chamber.

CHALMOMILE A plant from the aster family and formerly popularized as a mild laxative *q.v.*

CHAMPUS Federal insurance program for military dependents and retirees.

CHANCRE 1. A lesion *q.v.*, characteristic symptom *q.v.* of syphilis *q.v.* in its primary stage *q.v.* 2. An open sore or blister produced by syphilis in its earliest stage. 3. A small sore that appears at the point of contact with an infected *q.v.* person.

CHANCROID 1. Soft chancre *q.v.* 2. A sexually transmitted disease *q.v.* characterized by an acute *q.v.*, localized, painful ulceration *q.v.* at the point of entry of the infectious agent *q.v.*, a bacterium *q.v.*, *Hemophilus ducreyi.* ~ is a self-limiting disease. Treatment is by use of sulfonamides *q.v.* 3. A contagious *q.v.* disease characterized by ulcerations at the point of physical contact with an infected person and usually spreads through sexual intercourse *q.v.*

CHANGE AGENT 1. An individual, organization, or group that assists a client or client system to identify issues of concern and the means of dealing with these concerns. Involvement can be intensive or minimal. 2. A role of school administrators related to making and influencing innovations in schools. 3. Anyone inside or outside the organization who tries to modify an existing organizational situation.

CHANGE-OF-ENVIRONMENT METHOD A method of allevating psychopathological *q.v.* symptoms by removing the person from the environment thought to be responsible for the disorder.

CHANGE OF LIFE 1. Climacteric *q.v.* 2. Menopause *q.v.*

CHANGE OF LIFE BABY A baby born to a menopausal *q.v.* woman who, in spite of not menstruating *q.v.* regularly, was ovulating *q.v.*

CHANGING The second of Kurt Lewin's three related conditions or states that result in behavioral change. ~ is the state in which a person begins to experiment with performing new behaviors *q.v.*

CHANGING AN ORGANIZATION In administration procedure, the process of modifying an existing organization to increase organizational effectiveness. cf: change agent.

CHANNEL 1. Frequency. 2. The electronic signal path through which a radiofrequency flows, used esp. by emergency vehicles and corps.

CHAOS A state of complete confusion.

CHAPTER 1 AND CHAPTER 2 FUNDS Federal funds aimed at offering educational support for minority, low-income, and underachieving students (Chapter 1) as well as support for curricular materials (Chapter 2).

CHARACTER 1. A phase of one's personality *q.v.* 2. That part of a person's personality that is determined by social standards. 3. The phenotype *q.v.* of a gene *q.v.* 4. One of the numerous details of structure, form, substance, or function which make up an individual organism. The Mendelian characters represent the end products of development, during which the entire complex of genes interacts within itself and with the environment.

CHARACTER DISORDER 1. A defect of the personality *q.v.* manifest by immaturity *q.v.*, antisocial reactions *q.v.*, asocial reactions *q.v.*, and unsocial reactions *q.v.* ~s are rarely altered by therapy. 2. A personality disorder *q.v.* characterized by developmental defects of a pathological *q.v.* type rather than a decompensation *q.v.* under excessive stress *q.v.* 3. An obsolete term for personality disorder.

CHARAS 1. The unadulterated resin exuded by the flowering tops of the female hemp plant, *Cannabis sativa q.v.* or *Cannabis indica q.v.* 2. A preparation of cannabis or marijuana *q.v.* that is similar to hashish *q.v.* 3. The most potent form of marijuana commonly used in India.

CHARLATAN 1. A person who pretends to have skill in medicine. 2. A quack *q.v.*

CHARLEYHORSE An injury caused by a blow to a contracted or relaxed muscle.

CHASTITY Never having had sexual intercourse *q.v.*

CHATTEL In law, a moveable piece of personal property.

CHD An acronym for coronary heart disease *q.v.*

CHECKUP A routine, but usually, superficial medical or dental examination.

CHEEK The side of the face forming the lateral wall of the mouth.

CHEEKBONE A quadrilateral bone, the zygoma, that forms the prominence of the cheek *q.v.*

CHEILOSIS 1. Sores of the lips. 2. Specifically, sores in the corners of the lips due to a deficiency of vitamin B *q.v.*

CHEMICAL AGENT A liquid, gas, or solid that enters the body through inhalation, ingestion, absorption, or injection that results in disease *q.v.*, disability, or death. cf: biological agent.

CHEMICAL CARCINOGENESIS RESEARCH INFORMATION SYSTEM (CCRIS) An information system that contains scientifically evaluated data derived from carcinogenicity, tumor promotion, and mutagenicity tests on about 2000 chemicals.

CHEMICAL DEPENDENCY (CD) 1. A dependency *q.v.* on drugs including alcohol and tobacco. 2. An inordinate need for tobacco, alcohol, or other drugs.

CHEMICAL EQUATION An equation that uses chemical formulas and their symbols to represent the changes of bonding that occur between atoms *q.v.* involved in a chemical reaction. cf: chemical formula.

CHEMICAL FORMULA The symbol or combination of symbols to represent the composition of an element or compound *q.v.*

CHEMICALLY EQUIVALENT DRUG A drug that contains the same amount of the same active ingredients in the same dosage form as contained in generic *q.v.* or brand name *q.v.* drugs.

CHEMICAL NAME 1. The name used to describe the molecular structure of a drug. 2. For a drug, the name that is descriptive of its chemical structure.

CHEMICAL SCORE An index of protein quality that compares the essential amino acid *q.v.* content of a test protein with that of a standard protein.

CHEMICAL STRUCTURE The arrangement of atoms *q.v.* in a molecule *q.v.* or of molecules in a compound.

CHEMICAL SYMBOL The letter or letters used by chemists to represent an element *q.v.*

CHEMOAUTOTROPHIC Organisms, e.g., bacteria, that are able to manufacture their own basic foods with chemical energy. cf: autotrophic.

CHEMORECEPTOR The distal end of sensory dendrites *q.v.* especially adapted for chemical stimulation.

CHEMORECEPTOR ZONE An area of any cells that are activated by a change in their chemical milieu and that thereby originate a flow of nervous impulses.

CHEMOSURGERY The use of caustic chemicals to remove diseased or unwanted tissue.

CHEMOSYNTHESIS Synthesis *q.v.* of organic compounds from inorganic materials using other chemical reactions as an energy source rather than radiant energy as is found in photosynthesis *q.v.*

CHEMOTHERAPY 1. Treatment of a disease by the use of chemicals or drugs. ~ is especially applicable in the treatment of some forms of cancer *q.v.* 2. The use of drugs to kill or weaken organisms that invade the body or to destroy abnormal cells within the body. 3. The application of chemical therapeutic agents *q.v.* to combat microorganisms *q.v.* 4. The use of chemicals that have a specific and toxic *q.v.* effect on a disease-causing pathogen *q.v.*

CHEMOTROPISM A simple orienting response, either positively or negatively to a chemical or stimulus *q.v.* or stimuli.

CHES An acronym for Certified Health Education Specialist *q.v.*

CHESS An acronym for Council for Health and Environmental Safety of Soils.

CHEST Thorax *q.v.*

CHEST CAVITY Thorax *q.v.* (thoracic cavity).

CHEWING TOBACCO A form of smokeless tobacco that is chewed rather than burned or smoked. cf: snuff.

CHI A Chinese term pertaining to the vital energy in the body.

CHIASM 1. Crossing. 2. A crossing of the optic nerves *q.v.*

CHIASMA A visible change of partners or crossover in two of a group of four chromatids *q.v.* during the first meiotic *q.v.* prophase *q.v.*

CHICKEN 1. Slang for a teenager (male) prostitute *q.v.* 2. Slang for a person who shows cowardice or fear.

CHICKEN PORN A slang expression referring to child pornography.

CHICKEN POX 1. A disease caused by a specific virus. ~ is transmitted by direct and indirect contact with an infected person. It is characterized by general symptoms, low fever, skin eruptions. 2. An infectious *q.v.* disease that usually occurs in childhood. Complications include encephalitis *q.v.* or pneumonia *q.v.* ~ is caused by the Varicella-Zoster (V-Z) *q.v.* virus, the same virus that causes herpes zoster *q.v.* in adults. ~ usually runs its course in 1–14 days and provides life-long immunity.

CHIEF STATE SCHOOL OFFICER The executive head of a state department of education, often referred to as the state school superintendent or the commissioner of education.

CHILBLAIN A chronic *q.v.* injury of the hands or feet characterized by reddish skin, burning, itching, and chapping and ulceration. ~ is caused by repeated or prolonged exposure to damp cold. cf: frostbite.

CHILD ABUSE 1. The cruel and extraordinary harsh treatment of a child by parents, guardians, or caretakers.

2. Void of discipline goals. 3. Punishment without logical reasons. There are three types of ~ : (a) emotional abuse, (b) physical abuse, and (c) sexual abuse. 4. Inflicted, nonaccidental, sexual, physical, and/or psychological trauma and/or injury to the child. 5. An act of either commission or omission that endangers or hinders a child's physical or emotional growth and development. cf: child neglect; child abusers.

CHILD ABUSERS Parents (parents, guardians, or caretakers) who treat children in an unusual and cruel manner. "Punishment" may take the form of kicking, beating, and the use of chains, rods, burning with lighted cigarettes, etc. There is no logical reason for the unusual and cruel punishments; no excuse is evident. ~ may come from any socioeconomic group and are frequently, themselves, victims of child abuse. cf: child neglect.

CHILD ADVOCACY MOVEMENT A movement dedicated to defining, protecting, and ensuring the rights of children.

CHILD BENEFIT THEORY A criterion that is used by the United States Supreme Court to determine whether services provided to public and nonpublic school students benefit children and not the school or religion. If they benefit only the children, the courts have ruled that the services may be funded by public monies.

CHILDBIRTH Birth *q.v.*

CHILD-CENTERED INSTRUCTION Instruction *q.v.* designed for the interests, abilities, and needs of individual students. cf: learner-centered approach. ct: teacher-centered approach.

CHILD-FREE MARRIAGE An alternative term for childless marriage that implies that a couple choose not to have children.

CHILD HEALTH OBJECTIVES The United States set certain objectives for the improvement of child health by the year 1990. Categorically, these objectives included the following: (a) improved health status, (b) reduction in risk factors, (c) increased public and professional awareness, (d) improved services and health protection, (e) and improved surveillance and evaluation systems. cf: Healthy People 2010.

CHILDHOOD Generally, the period of the life cycle *q.v.* from 4 years to the onset of puberty *q.v.* ~ may be further divided into early ~, middle ~, and late ~.

CHILDHOOD ONSET PERVASIVE DEVELOPMENTAL DISORDER A disorder of children older than 30 months but younger than 12 years who indicate little empathy or emotional responsiveness to their peers, who cling to their parents, take particular postures or make stereotyped movements, resist any change, have sudden anxieties and unexplained rages, and may occasionally be self-injurious. (This terminology replaces earlier diagnosis of childhood schizophrenia *q.v.*)

CHILDHOOD SCHIZOPHRENIA 1. A diagnosis that is replaced by childhood onset pervasive developmental disorder *q.v.* 2. A psychosis *q.v.* that generally appears between 5 and 12 years and after a period of normal development, and is characterized by delusions, hallucinations *q.v.*, and thought disorders.

CHILD NEGLECT The failure of parents, guardians, or caretakers to provide a child with the basic necessities of life—food, sanitary environment, clothing, and the like—when they can afford to do so. ct: child abuse.

CHILD PSYCHIATRY The specialized area of medical practice that is concerned with treating mental and emotional disturbances of children. cf: psychiatrist.

CHILD-STUDY MOVEMENT The nineteenth century scientific movement that promoted the collection of normative data on the growth and development of children.

CHILL A feeling of cold with shivering and pallor, accompanied by an elevation of body temperature in the interior of the body. Often an early symptom *q.v.* of an infectious *q.v.* disease caused by invasion of the blood by bacterial toxins *q.v.*

CHIMERA A mixture of tissues or genetically *q.v.* different constitution in the same part of an organism. It may result from mutation *q.v.*, irregular mitosis *q.v.*, somatic *q.v.* crossing over *q.v.*, or an artificial fusion. ~ may be preclinical *q.v.*, with parallel layers of genetically different tissues, or sectorial.

CHIN STRAP In first aid, and emergency care, a strap used to fasten a victim of an injury by the head to a spineboard *q.v.*

CHIROPODIST 1. Generally, an archaic term referring to a nonmedical person who specializes in the minor disorders of the foot. 2. A podiatrist *q.v.* 3. A practitioner of chiropody.

CHIROPRACTIC 1. A pseudoscience *q.v.* based on the belief that most ailments are caused by misaligned vertebrae and can be corrected, cured, treated, and prevented by spinal adjustments. 2. A system of healing based on spinal manipulation to correct disturbances in the nervous system *q.v.* 3. Chiropracty *q.v.*

CHIROPRACTOR A nonmedical *q.v.* person who treats diseases through manipulation of the spinal column *q.v.* cf: chiropractic.

CHIRPRACTY 1. Chiropractic *q.v.* 2. An approach that emphasizes the role of spine placement in physical disorders. cf: chiropractor.

CHI-SQUARE In research, a statistic that helps determine whether the pattern of frequencies found in data assigned to categories is likely due to chance or is atypical. Also used to compare data with a model to determine whether the data's fit is within the typical range of sampling and chance error. Also used to combine the results of independently conducted studies to determine overall statistical significance. cf: chi-square test.

CHI-SQUARE TEST In epidemiology, a statistical test applied to nominal or categorical data. cf: chi-square.

CHIVALRIC EDUCATION During the Middle Ages, young boys were educated in the customs and ideals associated with the duties and privileges of knighthood.

CHLAMYDIA 1. The most common sexually transmitted disease in males and females, caused by *Chlamydia trachomatis q.v.* In females, it may result in infertility *q.v.* 2. A species of bacterium *q.v.*, the causative organism of *Lymphogranuloma venereum q.v.*, chlamydial urethritis and most cases of newborn conjunctivitis *q.v.*

CHLAMYDIA TRACHOMATIS 1. The bacterium *q.v.* causing trachoma *q.v.* and several genital infections *q.v.* 2. Microscopic organisms having features of both viruses and bacteria and are the cause of trachoma and certain sexually transmitted diseases *q.v.*

CHLAMYDOSPORE In botany, a thick-walled asexual *q.v.* thallospore *q.v.* formed by the enlargement of a vegetative cell that assumes an oval shape.

CHLOASMA Brown pigment spots, usually on the face, caused either by birth control pills or hormones produced naturally during pregnancy.

CHLORAL HYDRATE 1. A nonbarbiturate hypnotic *q.v.* drug whose action on the central nervous system *q.v.* resembles that of alcohol *q.v.* 2. Also called knockout drops or Mickey Finn. Got its name prior to 1900 when it was used to shanghai sailors to the orient. When used over an extended period of time, physical dependence *q.v.* develops and a withdrawal syndrome *q.v.* appears when the drug is denied. ~ is a controlled substance under federal law. 3. Noctec is a commercial preparation.

CHLORAZEPATE 1. A benzodiazepine *q.v.* sedative *q.v.* 2. Tranxene is a brand name.

CHLORDIAZEPOXIDE 1. A minor tranquilizer *q.v.* 2. An example of ~ is Librium. cf: meprobramate; diazepam.

CHLORETONE A drug that inhibits movement without disturbing growth.

CHLORINATED 1. The addition of the chemical chlorine to water to kill pathogenic *q.v.* organisms to make the water safe to drink. 2. Decontaminated water.

CHLORINE RESIDUAL Chlorine that remains in water to decontaminate any addition of bacteria in the water system.

CHLOROPHYLLS In botany, green pigments located in plastids *q.v.* necessary to the process of photosynthesis.

CHLOROPLAST In botany, a plastid *q.v.* containing chlorophyll *q.v.*, developed only in cells exposed to light. ~s are the seat of photosynthesis *q.v.* and starch formation. 2. A specialized body in the cytoplasm *q.v.* that contains chlorophyll. 3. Chloroplastid *q.v.*

CHLOROPLASTID 1. In botany, green structure in plant cytoplasm that contains chlorophyll and in which starch is synthesized. A mode of cytoplasmic inheritance *q.v.* independent of nuclear genes *q.v.* has been associated with these cytoplasmic structures. 2. Chloroplast.

CHLORQUINE A synthetic drug used for the treatment of malaria *q.v.*

CHLOROSIS In botany, reduced development or loss of chlorophyll *q.v.*

CHLORPHENIRAMINE An OTC *q.v.* antihistamine *q.v.*

CHLORPROMAZINE 1. Thorazine *q.v.* 2. One of the phenothiazine *q.v.* drugs synthesized in 1950 and first used in the United States in 1954 for the treatment of psychomotor excitement and mania *q.v.* ~ reduces the symptoms of fear and hostility associated with psychosis *q.v.* 2. The generic *q.v.* term for one of the most widely prescribed antipsychotic *q.v.* drugs.

CHLORPROTHIXENE 1. An antipsychotic *q.v.* drug. 2. Teractin is a brand name.

CHOANA Posterior nares *q.v.*

CHOICE SHIFT In sociology, the tendency of a group to choose either a far riskier or a far more conservative solution to a dilemma than any one member of the group would choose. This tendency is the result of the group influence situation. cf: risky shift.

CHOLANGITIS Inflammation *q.v.* of the bile ducts *q.v.* leading from the liver.

CHOLECYSTECTOMY Surgical removal of the gallbladder *q.v.*

CHOLECYSTITIS Inflammation *q.v.* of the gallbladder *q.v.*

CHOLELITHIASIS The presence of stones in the gallbladder *q.v.*

CHOLERA A disease caused by a spirillum bacterium *q.v.* characterized by watery eyes, diarrhea, dehydration, and possible death. It is endemic *q.v.* in Africa and Southeast

Asia, but does occur episodically in other parts of the world.

CHOLESTEROL 1. A fatty substance found naturally in the body. 2. A lipid *q.v.* 3. ~ is an element essential for the construction of cell membranes *q.v.* ~ is thought to be a major contributor to atherosclerosis *q.v.* 4. The chief sterol *q.v.* synthesized in the human body and present in all body tissues. 5. The precursor of steroid hormones and vitamin D *q.v.* Dietary ~ is found primarily in egg yolk, liver, and organ meats. 6. Fat-related substance in alcohol form. 7. Lipid material manufactured within the body as well as derived from dietary sources. 8. An organic alcohol present in bile, plod, and various tissues.

CHOLIC ACID A family of steroids *q.v.* comprising the bile *q.v.* acids. ~s are derived from cholesterol *q.v.*

CHOLINE 1. A lipotropic factor that prevents accumulation of fat in the liver. 2. A transmethylation factor. ~ is found in most animal tissues. 3. ~ is claimed to be a vitamin B complex *q.v.*

CHOLINERGIC A neuron that uses acetylcholine (Ach) *q.v.* as a neurotransmitter *q.v.*

CHOLINERGIC FIBERS Axons *q.v.* whose terminals release acetylcholine *q.v.*

CHOLINERGIC SYSTEM All the nerve fibers for which acetylcholine *q.v.* is a transmitter substance, in contrast to the adrenergic *q.v.* or monoaminergic *q.v.*

CHOLINESTERASE An enzyme *q.v.* that catalyzes *q.v.* breakdown of acetylcholine *q.v.*

CHOLINOCEPTIVE SITE Postjunctional receptor for acetylcholine *q.v.* ~ is also affected by the agonists muscarine *q.v.* and nicotine *q.v.*

CHONDRIOSOME A feebly refractive body found in the protoplasm *q.v.* of a cell. 2. Mitochondria *q.v.*

CHONDROCYTE A cartilage cell.

CHONDRODYSTROPHIC CHILDREN Children with a hereditary abnormality of the bones. cf: chondrodystrophy.

CHONDRODYSTROPHY A trait in humans characterized by abnormal growth of cartilage at ends and along shafts of long bones.

CHONDROMALACIA A roughing of the undersurface of the kneecap producing pain and grating.

CHONDROMUCOID A basophilic *q.v.* glycoprotein present in interstitial *q.v.* substance of cartilage *q.v.*

CHOOSING 1. In values clarification, to freely select from alternatives. 2. The first step in the valuing process.

CHORDEE A downward curvature of the penis *q.v.* that requires corrective surgery. ~ is associated with hypospadia *q.v.* or urethral infection.

CHOREA 1. A pathological *q.v.* condition characterized by jerky, irregular, involuntary movements. 2. Huntington's chorea.

CHOREIFORM Pertaining to the involuntary, spasmodic, jerky movements of the limbs and head found in Huntington's chorea *q.v.* and other nervous disorders.

CHORIOCARCINOMA A rare type of cancer found in the uterus *q.v.*

CHORION A membrane *q.v.* enveloping the fetus *q.v.* of mammals, external to and enclosing the amnion *q.v.* 2. The outermost embryonic *q.v.* membrane, part of which unites with the endometrium *q.v.* to form the placenta *q.v.*

CHORION BIOPSY An alternative to amniocentesis *q.v.* that involves placing a tube into the vagina *q.v.* to the uterus *q.v.* during pregnancy *q.v.* Chorionic *q.v.* tissue that surrounds the embryo *q.v.* is removed and analyzed for the possibility of genetic *q.v.* defects in the developing embryo.

CHORIONIC GONADOTROPIN (HCG) 1. The gonad-stimulating hormone *q.v.* from the embryo *q.v.* 2. A hormone secreted from the underdeveloped placenta *q.v.* that stimulates the corpus luteum *q.v.* to secrete progesterone *q.v.* rather than degenerate. This keeps the endometrium *q.v.* sensitized for blastocyte *q.v.* implantation.

CHORIONIC VILLI Fingerlike projections of the chorion *q.v.* forming the fetal *q.v.* portion of the placenta *q.v.*

CHORIONIC VILLI SAMPLING A procedure in which embryonic *q.v.* cells are removed for the purpose of detecting fetal *q.v.* abnormalities. cf: chorionic villus sampling; chorionic villi sampling.

CHORIONIC VILLUS SAMPLING 1. A technique for prenatal *q.v.* detection of genetic *q.v.* defects that involves removal of some of the villi *q.v.* growing on the outer surface of the chorion *q.v.* and examining their chromosomes *q.v.* 2. A test of fetal *q.v.* cells for the detection of abnormalities in the embryo *q.v.* cf: amniocentesis.

CHOROID 1. The highly vascular membrane *q.v.* situated between the sclerotic coat *q.v.* and the retina *q.v.* of the eye. 2. The thin, pigmented, vascular coat of the eye extending from the edge of the retina to the optic nerve *q.v.* and carrying the blood vessels for the retina. 3. Skin-like.

CHOROIDITIS Inflammation *q.v.* of the choroid *q.v.* ~ is one of the more serious eye diseases.

CHOROIDORETINAL DEGENERATION Deterioration of the choroid *q.v.* and the retina *q.v.* cf: choroiditis.

CHRISTIAN SCIENCE A system of healing and a religion founded my Mary Baker Eddy, which maintains and teaches that disease and sin are caused by mental error.

CHROMATID 1. The parallel threads resulting from chromosome *q.v.* duplication before they separate from each other. 2. One of the two identical strands resulting from self-duplication of a chromosome during meiosis *q.v.* or mitosis *q.v.* One of the four strands making up a bivalent during the later meiotic prophase *q.v.* 3. Optically, single thread of chromatin *q.v.* 4. Prophase chromosomes composed of two chromatids attached to a single centrosome *q.v.* 5. Newly formed chromosomes.

CHROMATIN 1. The nuclear substance which takes basic stain and becomes incorporated in the chromosomes *q.v.*, so called because of the readiness with which it becomes stained with certain dyes. 2. Nuclear materials, primarily nucleoproteins *q.v.* that stain deeply with basic dyes. cf: chromatin body.

CHROMATIN BODY Hereditary *q.v.* material of the prokaryotic *q.v.* cell. cf: chromatin body.

CHROMATOGRAPHIC SCAN 1. A chemical analysis that separates a substance into its components. 2. Chromatography *q.v.*

CHROMATOGRAPHY 1. A method of analyzing and comparing chemicals. 2. Chromatographic scan *q.v.*

CHROMATOPHORE A colored plastid *q.v.* or cell. 2. Chromophore. 3. A colored body in the cytoplasm *q.v.* of cells.

CHROMIDIA Small particles of chromatin *q.v.* outside the nucleus *q.v.* of a cell.

CHROMOCENTER A body produced by fusion of the heterochromatin *q.v.* region of the autosomes *q.v.* and Y chromosome *q.v.* in salivary gland preparations of certain Diptera *q.v.*

CHROMOGEN The color-imparting portion of a dye.

CHROMOMERE 1. One of the linear series of chromatin *q.v.* bodies in a chromosome *q.v.* 2. Chromomeres: small bodies described by Belling which he identified by their characteristic size and linear arrangement on the chromosome.

CHROMONEMA An optically single thread within the chromosome *q.v.*

CHROMOPHORE 1. Chromatophore *q.v.* 2. Color-imparting portion of a chromogen.

CHROMOPLAST A specialized protoplasmic body containing carotenoids *q.v.* or other pigments, with the exception of chlorophyll.

CHROMOSOMAL ABERRATION 1. Defective chromosome *q.v.* 2. Chromosomal anomaly *q.v.*

CHROMOSOMAL ANOMALY A species-atypical chromosomal *q.v.* condition.

CHROMOSOMAL MAP A photograph of the number and arrangement of chromosomes *q.v.* for a given person. Chromosome map.

CHROMOSOMAL SEX Genetic *q.v.* sex usually symbolized by the presence of XX (female) or XY (male) chromosomes *q.v.* of the person and present in all body cells.

CHROMOSOME 1. The hereditary unit that consists of the genes *q.v.* and is the determiner of genetic *q.v.* makeup. 2. The gametes *q.v.* contain 23 ~s while other body cells contain the original 46 ~s. This is accomplished by a process called meiosis *q.v.* 3. A giant molecule of DNA *q.v.* and protein located in all cell nuclei *q.v.* The ~ contains the genes and functions in heredity *q.v.* 4. Microscopic *q.v.* structures contained in the nucleus of all cells which contain the DNA that determines the genetic characteristics of the organism. 5. Rod-shaped bodies found in the nucleus of all cells that contain genes. There are 22 pairs of autosomal *q.v.* ~s which account for all the individual's hereditary traits. Sex is fixed by the 23rd sex-determining chromosomal pair. 6. One of the small bodies, ordinarily definite in number, in the cells of a given species, into which the chromatin *q.v.* of a cell nucleus resolves itself during mitosis *q.v.*

CHROMOSOME ABERRATION Abnormal arrangement of the chromosome *q.v.* complement caused by chromosomal breakage and reunion.

CHROMOSOME MAP 1. The location of genes *q.v.* on chromosomes *q.v.*, as determined by genetic *q.v.* methods. 2. Chromosomal map.

CHRONIC 1. A disease of long duration usually progressive. 2. Marked by a long duration or frequent reoccurrence: constant. 3. Occurring over a long time.

CHRONIC ALCOHOLISM A misnomer since the term is redundant. Alcoholism *q.v.* is a chronic disease.

CHRONIC BRAIN SYNDROME Senile dementia *q.v.*

CHRONIC BRONCHITIS 1. Chronic obstructive lung disease *q.v.* marked by recurring inflammation *q.v.* of the bronchial tubes *q.v.* with excessive mucous *q.v.* production, persistent cough, and reduced normal lung function. 2. Persistent inflammation and infection of the smaller airways within the lungs.

CHRONIC DEGENERATIVE DISEASE A disease that tends to persist for life and that progressively worsens. cf: chronic disease.

CHRONIC DISEASE 1. A pathological *q.v.* condition that persists over a long period of time and progressively worsens unless measures are taken to halt its progress. 2. A disease that results in permanent residual disability; is caused by nonreversible, pathological alteration, requires special training of the person for rehabilitation, or may require a long period of supervision and care. ct: acute disease. cf: degenerative disease.

CHRONIC EFFECT The long-term response to repeated doses of a drug. ct: acute effect.

CHRONIC EXCESSIVE NOISE Constant noise levels that cause personal discomfort, fatigue, or are a health threat.

CHRONIC LEUKEMIA The most common form of leukemia *q.v.* in adults over 40 years. ct: acute leukemia.

CHRONIC MACROCYTIC ANEMIA A category of anemias *q.v.* of a variety of causes and characterized by larger than normal red blood cells among others. cf: pernicious anemia.

CHRONIC OBSTRUCTIVE LUNG DISEASE 1. A slow, progressive interruption of the airflow within the lungs due to pulmonary emphysema *q.v.* and chronic bronchitis *q.v.* cf: chronic obstructive pulmonary disease.

CHRONIC OBSTRUCTIVE PULMONARY DISEASE (COPD) Diseases that restrict the ability of the body to obtain oxygen through the respiratory structures. These diseases include asthma *q.v.*, bronchitis *q.v.*, and emphysema *q.v.* cf: chronic obstructive lung disease.

CHRONIC PSYCHOSIS A pattern of severely disturbed behavior that persists for many years. cf: psychosis.

CHRONIC SCHIZOPHRENIA A psychotic *q.v.* person who had earlier deteriorated over a long period of time and who usually has been hospitalized for more than 2 years. cf: schizophrenia.

CHRONIC SIMPLE COURSE In psychology, the pattern of schizophrenia *q.v.* in which the disorder appears gradually and the recovery is slow and incomplete.

CHRONOLOGICAL Arranged in order of occurrence. For example, ~ age and ~ maturity.

CHRONOLOGICAL AGE (CA) 1. A person's actual age, usually expressed in years or years and months. 2. A person's numerical age dating from the time of birth. ct: conceptual age; functional age. cf: intellectual quotient; mental age (MA).

CHUNK In learning theory, an unrelated bit of information stored in a person's short-term memory. cf: chunking.

CHUNKING 1. The process of recording ideas in memory that permits a number of items to be packed into a larger unit. 2. A memorization technique in which unrelated bits of information are grouped and stored in the memory bank. cf: chunk.

CHYLE 1. The fat containing lymph *q.v.* in the lymphatics *q.v.* of the intestine *q.v.* 2. The milky fluid taken up by the lacteals *q.v.* from food in the intestine after digestion *q.v.* ~ consists of lymph and emulsified fat and passes into the veins by way of the thoracic duct *q.v.*

CHYLOMICRON A particle of emulsified *q.v.* fat present in the lymph *q.v.* ~s are especially numerous after a meal high in fat content. cf: chyle.

CHYME 1. A semifluid, thick mass consisting of food broken down by the digestive action of gastric juices *q.v.* in the stomach and passes into the small intestine. 2. Produced by the action of gastric juices on the ingested food and is passed from the stomach into the duodenum *q.v.*

CIBALITH A commercial preparation of lithium citrate *q.v.*

CICATRIX A scar of heavy formation of fibrous tissue *q.v.*

CIGARETTE A roll of finely cut tobacco or marijuana *q.v.* for smoking, typically enclosed in thin paper.

CIL An acronym for Community Involvement Liaison *q.v.*

CILIA 1. The hairlike structures found in the bronchi *q.v.* 2. The hairlike processes attached to a free surface of a cell. In the respiratory passages, ~ filter out microorganisms *q.v.* and particles before they reach the lungs.

CILIARY FUNCTION Sweeping movements of cilia *q.v.* which sweep mucus and other debris out of the respiratory system into the throat.

CILIATED COLUMNAR EPITHELIAL CELLS Column-shaped cells that line the airways. The cilia *q.v.* on these cells are responsible for moving mucus *q.v.* up the airways to clean lungs of particulate matter.

CILIATOXIC A substance affecting the action of the cilia *q.v.*

CILIUM Singular for cilia *q.v.*

CIRCADIAN Daily. cf: circadian rhythm.

CIRCADIAN RHYTHM The fixed pattern of changes in basic body processes during a 24-h period.

CIRCLE OF WILLIS An anastomosis *q.v.* of certain cerebral *q.v.* arteries.

CIRCUIT The path or course of electricity or other current.

CIRCUIT TRAINING A sequence of exercises or activities performed at individual stations within a given time limit.

CIRCULATORY Pertaining to the heart, blood vessels, and the blood.

CIRCULATORY COLLAPSE Failure of the circulation, either cardiac *q.v.* or peripheral *q.v.*

CIRCULATORY ENDURANCE The ability of the body to perform under stress *q.v.* without undue fatigue. cf: circulorespiratory endurance.

CIRCULATORY HYPOXIA A condition resulting from decreased blood flow caused by blood loss, abnormal blood routes, heart failure, or arterial or venous obstruction.

CIRCULATORY SYSTEM The heart, arteries, veins, and blood functioning as a unit.

CIRCULORESPIRATORY ENDURANCE A measure of how much oxygen is delivered to the tissues of the body by the circulatory and respiratory systems and how efficiently it is used. cf: circulatory endurance.

CIRCUMCISION Surgical removal of the foreskin of the penis *q.v.* cf: superincision; excision.

CIRCUMSTANTIALITY A characteristic of conversation involving the use of many irrelevant details.

CIRRHOSIS 1. A chronic *q.v.*, interstitial *q.v.*, inflammation *q.v.* of any organ. 2. A disease of the liver, marked by progressive destruction of liver cells, accompanied by degeneration of the liver substance and increase of connective tissue *q.v.* 3. Complications, such as hemorrhage and cancer, are always a threat. 4. A chronic disease of the liver often but not always associated with alcoholism *q.v.* 5. Pathological *q.v.* changes taking place in the liver after long-term alcoholism, causing altered liver metabolism *q.v.* that includes decreased testosterone *q.v.* and increased estrogen *q.v.* in the male. 6. Cirrhosis of the liver.

CIRRUS 1. A gelatinous *q.v.* matrix in which ascospores of ascomycetes are shed. 2. Male copulatory structures in some flatworms and roundworms.

CIS Coupling *q.v.*

CIS CONFIGURATION Configuration involving two pairs of linked genes *q.v.* when dominant alleles *q.v.* are on the same homologue and recessive alleles are on the other.

CIS FORM A term indicating that certain atoms or groups of atoms, relative to a double bond between two carbon atoms, are on the same side of a molecule *q.v.*

CISTRON 1. A unit of function. 2. A working definition of a gene *q.v.* One ~ in the DNA *q.v.* specifies one polypeptide *q.v.* in protein synthesis.

CITATIONS In law, references to law books. A ~ includes the book where the reference is found, the volume number, and the section or page numbers. A uniform system of abbreviations in case law has been adopted, but statutory materials differ from state to state according to the official designation accepted by the legislature.

CITRIC ACID CYCLE Krebs cycle *q.v.*

CIVIL ACTION 1. In law, an action brought to recover some civil right to obtain redress for some wrong.

CIVIL COMMITMENT In law, a procedure whereby a person can be legally certified as mentally ill and hospitalized, even against his or her will.

CIVILIAN LABOR FORCE The total of all civilians classified as employed or unemployed.

CIVIL RIGHTS In law, the freedoms and rights that a person has as a citizen that are protected by law and custom.

CIVIL RIGHTS MOVEMENT A social movement that sought equal rights for minority groups.

CLAMMY Damp and unusually cool.

CLAMP CONNECTIONS In botany, structures found on basidiomycete mycelium *q.v.* which function at the time of cell division to reestablish the dikaryotic *q.v.* condition.

CLANG ASSOCIATION 1. In a word association test, a reaction based on the sound of a stimulus *q.v.* word rather than its meaning. 2. A stringing together of words because they are similar in sound, with no attention paid to their meaning.

CLAP Slang for gonorrhea *q.v.*

CLASS In biology, a group of plants or animals ranking above an order and below a division or phylum. 2. In education, a group of pupils or students brought together for the purpose of learning.

CLASS ACTION In law, a lawsuit brought by one or more persons on behalf of all persons similarly situated as to complaint and remedy sought. 2. Also, class action suit.

CLASS BILL (OR SUIT) 1. In law, a case in which one or more in a numerous class, having a common interest, sue on behalf of themselves and all others of the class. 2. Class action *q.v.*

CLASSICAL APPROACH TO MANAGEMENT Managing approach that emphasizes organizational efficiency to increase organizational success.

CLASSICAL CONDITIONING THEORY 1. A subschool of the associationist *q.v.* school of thought. The theory holds that learning occurs as a result of a link established between a stimulus *q.v.* and a response through the use of rewards. In health education, applicable to techniques used in drug withdrawal, treatment of alcoholism *q.v.*, and nutritional abuses. 2. A basic form of learning, sometimes referred to as Pavlovian conditioning *q.v.* in which a neutral stimulus is repeatedly paired with another stimulus (the unconditioned stimulus or UCS) that usually elicits a certain desired response (UCR). After repeated trials, the neutral stimulus becomes a conditioned stimulus (CS) and evokes the same or similar response and is now referred to as the conditioned response (CR). cf: instrumental conditioning.

CLASSICAL ORGANIZING THEORY The cumulative insights of early management theories on how organizational resources can best be used to enhance goal attainment.

CLASSIC PARANOIA A psychotic *q.v.* condition characterized by extreme projection and compensation defense mechanisms *q.v.* The delusional *q.v.* states appear to exist without disintegration *q.v.* of basic drives or emotions. The delusions tend to be progressive, systematic, and logical.

CLASSIFICATION The process of ordering a collection of objects into a set of mutually exclusive and exhaustive classes. The ability to construct such an ordering mentality, and then, to reason about the quantitative relation between classes and their subclasses, first develops in the concrete operational period *q.v.*

CLASSIFICATION SCHEMES In research, schemes that classify events into an organization or a structure that in some way reflects a causal or developmental relationship and thus is a weak form of causal explanation.

CLASSIFICATION VARIABLES The characteristics that subjects bring with them into scientific investigations, such as age, sex, and mental states. ~ are studied by correlational research and mixed designs *q.v.*

CLASSROOM ANALYSIS SYSTEM Clearly defined sets of procedures and written materials that can be used to objectify the interaction between teachers and students.

CLASSROOM CLIMATE The social atmosphere a teacher generates—directive or indirective, democratic or authoritarian—assumed to influence learners' learning and attitudes (research does not yet support this assumption).

CLASSROOM ENVIRONMENT The physical structure, emotional climate, aesthetic characteristics, and learning resources of a classroom.

CLASSROOM MANAGEMENT 1. How teachers organize and structure the flow of activities in their classrooms in order to keep the learners active and minimize disruptions. 2. An area of study in which group behavior is examined and techniques for controlling group behavior are articulated. cf: withitness.

CLASSROOM TEACHER A staff member assigned the professional activities of instructing students, in classroom situations, for which daily student attendance figures for the school system are kept.

CLAVICEPS PURPUREA A fungus yielding the alkaloid, lysergic acid *q.v.*, the active ingredient in LSD *q.v.* Lysergic acid diethylamide was first synthesized by Hofmann in 1938.

CLAVICLE The collar bone that articulates with the sternum *q.v.* and scapula *q.v.*

CLEAVAGE In biology, the division of the zygote *q.v.* into cells.

CLEFT PALATE 1. An opening in the midline of the palate *q.v.* as the result of failure of the two sides to fuse during embryonic *q.v.* development. 2. A gap in the soft palate and roof of the mouth, sometimes extending through the upper lip.

CLERK OF THE HOUSE In politics, the chief administrative officer elected by the members.

CLIENT-CENTERED THERAPY 1. Humanistic psychotherapy *q.v.* 2. Generally, a treatment modality that is centered on the client/patient. 3. Nondirective techniques *q.v.* 4. A humanistic insight therapy developed by Carl Rogers in which the therapist seeks to understand the client's subjective experiences and to create an accepting atmosphere in which the client can actualize his or her potential.

CLIMACTERIC 1. The physical and mental changes occurring at the termination of the reproductive years in the female. 2. A stage in sexual development marked by menopause *q.v.* in women and by reduced sexual function in men. 3. The sum of all the physiological changes that occur as part of the aging process. 4. The aging process of the reproductive system in the female that occurs between 45 and 60 years which involves hormonal changes in the ovaries *q.v.*, pituitary gland *q.v.*, and hypothalamus *q.v.* ~ may also refer to the aging process of the male reproductive system. cf: the change of life; menopause.

CLIMAX 1. Of a disease, its turning point. 2. The crisis. 3. The peak of the disease when signs and symptoms are most intense. 4. In sexology, orgasm *q.v.* 5. In sociology, the terminal community of a succession *q.v.*, which maintains itself relatively unchanged unless the environment changes.

CLINICAL Pertaining to the direct treatment of patients.

CLINICAL DEATH 1. Functional death. 2. When the body systems have stopped functioning. cf: brain death; medical death.

CLINICAL DEPRESSION A severe form of depression *q.v.* characterized by stupor *q.v.* and lack of movement.

CLINICAL ECOLOGIST A medical specialty concerned with the relationship of environment to clinical symptoms *q.v.* cf: environmental medicine.

CLINICAL EPIDEMIOLOGY The application of epidemiology *q.v.* and biostatistics *q.v.* to clinical practice.

CLINICAL EXPERIENCES On-the-job learning experiences built into teacher-training programs, medical training, pharmacy training, etc.

CLINICAL FELLOWS PROGRAM A program est. by ATSDR *q.v.* in environmental health *q.v.* that provides 1–2 years of stipend support for fellows to engage in applied research *q.v.* that helps prevent or mitigate the adverse human health effects and diminished quality of life that may result from exposure to hazardous substances in the nonworkplace environment.

CLINICAL HUNCH In epidemiology, an idea that arises during clinical care that can be a source of epidemiological hypotheses *q.v.* ct: clinical prediction.

CLINICAL INTERVIEW In psychology, a technique introduced by Piaget for discovering what children know and think as a means of studying their cognitive *q.v.* development. The technique allows the interviewer to probe and question.

CLINICAL MANIFESTATION The signs of a disease as they pertain to or are observed in patients.

CLINICAL METHOD A research technique, often used to generate hypotheses that may describe how a particular course of treatment affects a subject. cf: observational method.

CLINICAL MODEL OF HEALTH Medical model of health *q.v.*

CLINICAL PICTURE The total available data concerning a patient, including symptoms *q.v.*, stresses *q.v.*, dynamics *q.v.*, and medical history *q.v.*

CLINICAL PREDICTION Prediction of behavior *q.v.* in terms of hypotheses developed from all available evidence about the dynamics *q.v.* of a particular personality *q.v.* ct: clinical hunch; actuarial prediction.

CLINICAL PROGRAM A plan of formal meetings by professionals outlining schedules, meetings, and other related activities regarding clinical procedures.

CLINICAL PSYCHOLOGIST 1. A person trained in the administration of a variety of psychological tests that aid in the diagnosis and evaluation of a person with mental and emotional problems. A ~ generally uses one or more forms of psychotherapy *q.v.* in treating clients. 2. A specialty concerned with the evaluation and treatment of mental and emotional disorders by nonmedical techniques. 3. An individual who has earned a PhD in psychology and whose training has included an internship in a mental hospital or clinic.

CLINICAL PSYCHOLOGY The special area of psychology *q.v.* concerned with the study of psychopathology *q.v.*, its causes, prevention, and treatment.

CLINICAL RESEARCH CENTER Formerly the U.S. Public Health Service Hospital located in Lexington, KY. Evolved into a major drug research center. cf: United States Public Health Service Hospitals.

CLINICAL STUDIES One phase of the training program for becoming a Medical Doctor (MD).

CLINICAL TRIAL 1. An experimental study to test the efficacy and potential side effects of an intervention such as a drug or vaccine. 2. The systematic investigation of materials and/or methods according to a formal study plan, as a means of determining effect or relative effectiveness, using people with a particular disease or class of diseases.

CLITORAL CIRCUMCISION The surgical removal of the clitoral hood *q.v.*

CLITORAL FORESKIN ADHESION Hooded clitoris *q.v.*

CLITORAL GLANS The tip of the clitoris *q.v.*

CLITORAL HOOD The skin that covers the clitoris *q.v.* cf: hooded clitoris.

CLITORAL ORGASM An orgasm *q.v.* resulting from stimulation of the clitoris *q.v.* Freud viewed ~ as an indication of sexual immaturity or a fixation in early psychosexual development.

CLITORAL SHAFT 1. The body of the clitoris *q.v.* 2. Part of the external female genitals *q.v.*; two small erectile bodies enclosed in a fibrous membrane *q.v.* ending in the glans *q.v.* The ~ corresponds to the corpus cavernosa *q.v.* in the penis *q.v.*

CLITORIDECTOMY Surgical removal of the clitoris *q.v.*

CLITORIS The small, erectile and highly sensitive structure located at the forward juncture of the vulva *q.v.* of the female external genitalia *q.v.* The ~ is highly sensitive to sexual stimulation. cf: clitoral hood; clitoral glans; clitoral shaft.

COACA An opening at the posterior end of the body into which the intestinal, urinary, and reproductive ducts open.

CLOCKLIKE WORLD In research, a conception of causation as resulting from tightly coupled events, such as the meshing of a train of gears.

CLOMIPHENE 1. A synthetic hormone *q.v.* which induces ovulation *q.v.* 2. A drug that stimulates the pituitary gland *q.v.* to secrete gonadotropins *q.v.* that, in turn, induces ovulation.

CLONE 1. A group of organisms *q.v.*, often many thousands in number, that have a common origin and that have been produced only by vegetative means, such as grafting, cutting, or division. The members of a ~ may be regarded as the extension of a single individual. 2. Identical descendents of a single cell. 3. A group of genetically identical cells or organisms descended from a single, common ancestor, or to reproduce identical copies.

CLONIC PHASE The stage of violent contractions and jerking of limbs in a grand mal epileptic seizure *q.v.*

CLONIDINE 1. An antihypertensive *q.v.* drug known to reduce narcotic *q.v.* withdrawal symptoms *q.v.* 2. Catapres is a brand name.

CLONING 1. The process of reproducing a plant or animal identical to one of its kind. 2. The removal of the nucleus from an egg cell and replacing it with a nucleus from a body cell, thus stimulating the egg cell to reproduce a plant or animal identical to that from which the body cell nucleus came. 3. Creating exact duplicates of living things. The first successful attempt was by John Gurdon, a biologist. cf: clone.

CLONUS Rapid oscillatory movements in which muscular rigidity and relaxation rapidly follow each other. Occurs following the tonic phase in a grand mal epileptic seizure *q.v.*

CLOSED-CIRCUIT TELEVISION A form of educational technology using television technology to broadcast a program to a highly defined, limited population.

CLOSED-CLASS MORPHEMES Little words whose function is grammatical in a language. cf: morphemes; open-class morphemes.

CLOSED FRACTURE A fracture *q.v.* which has no communication between the broken bone and the outside environment through the overlying skin. ct: compound fracture.

CLOSED HEAD INJURY A brain trauma *q.v.* in which the skull is not opened by the injury. ct: open head injury.

CLOSED INSTITUTION A closed organization that is set apart from the rest of society, forms an all-encompassing social environment, and serves as the only source of meeting the needs of its members.

CLOSED PANEL HMO An insurance plan that covers limited health and medical services that are provided by specified health and medical practitioners.

CLOSED SHOP A term in labor law meaning that a worker must be a member of the union as a condition precedent to employment. cf: union shop.

CLOSED SYSTEM A system that is not influenced by and does not interact with its environment *q.v.*

CLOSE FRIENDS In regards to sexual activity, swingers *q.v.* who have sexual relations only with a couple to whom they feel very close.

CLOSTRIDIUM BOTULINUM An anaerobic *q.v.* bacterium responsible for causing botulism *q.v.* in people.

CLOSTRIDIUM TETANI The causative agent of tetanus *q.v.*

CLOSURE In psychology, a factor in visual grouping where there is a perceptual tendency to perceive gaps in a figure as being closed or complete.

CLOT 1. A coagulation *q.v.* 2. Thrombus *q.v.* cf: clotting.

CLOTHES DRAG Drag *q.v.*

CLOTTING Coagulation *q.v.* of the blood. cf: clot.

CLOUDLIKE WORLD In research, a conception of causation as resulting from loosely coupled events such as a cloud of gnats always maintaining a cloud rather than dispersing.

CLUB FOOT A genetic defect *q.v.* characterized by an abnormal development of the foot. There are over 150,000 cases in the United States.

CLUSTER FAMILY Separate and distinct nuclear families sharing one household and some duties and responsibilities of family living.

CLUSTER INVESTIGATION STUDY A review of an unusual number—real or perceived—of health events grouped together in time and location. Cluster investigations are designed to confirm case reports, determine whether they represent unusual disease occurrence, an if possible, explore causes and environmental factors.

CLUSTER SAMPLING Random samples of cells in a geographic grid placed over a map, or random samples of units organized on some prior basis such as school rooms.

CLUSTER TESTING A method of identifying new cases of a disease, esp. venereal disease, by interviewing friends of an infected person.

CM The abbreviation of centimeter *q.v.*

CMA An acronym for Canadian Medical Association.

CME An acronym for continuing medical education.

CMV An acronym for cytomegalovirus *q.v.*

CNA An acronym for Canadian Nurses' Association

CNM An acronym for certified nurse-midwife.

CNS An acronym for central nervous system *q.v.*

COA An acronym for coenzyme A *q.v.*

COA An acronym for Children of Alcoholics *q.v.*

COACHING Training technique that incorporates demonstration, practice, encouragement, and strategy by the instructor or coach.

COAGULANT 1. A substance that causes or speeds up the clotting of blood. 2. Coagulant. cf: clotting; clot; coagulation.

COAGULATION 1. The process of changing liquid to a semisolid or solid state. Blood ~. 2. The formation of a blood clot *q.v.* 3. A process of water purification in which chemicals are added to the water to assist in dissolving pollutants.

COAGULATION TIME The time required for a sample of blood to clot *q.v.* under standard controlled conditions.

COALESCE 1. To unite into a whole. 2. To mix. 3. To fuse.

COARCTATION A pressing together or narrowing of a blood vessel, occurring primarily in the aorta.

COBALAMIN One of the vitamin B complex *q.v.* groups of water-soluble vitamins *q.v.* Important for normal functioning of cells, esp. of the nervous system *q.v.*, bone marrow *q.v.*, and digestive tract *q.v.* A deficiency results in pernicious anemia *q.v.*

COBALT A metal element possessing radioactive isotopes *q.v.* used in the treatment of some cancers *q.v.* 2. A metallic element that is found in vitamin B_{12} *q.v.*

COCA 1. Erythroxylon coca. 2. A bush from which the alkaloid cocaine *q.v.* is derived.

COCAINE 1. An anesthetic derived from the coca plant *q.v.* It is often legally classified as a narcotic, but pharmacologically, it is not. Its anesthetic properties were discovered in 1860; between 1885 and 1905, it was extensively used in eye surgery and dentistry. In 1885, Sigmund Freud recommended its use in the treatment of withdrawal symptoms *q.v.* from morphine *q.v.* addiction *q.v.* and as a valuable aid in psychiatry *q.v.* Cocaine numbs a localized area when injected. When injected systemically, however, it stimulates heart action and the central nervous system *q.v.* Large amounts can result in cardiac arrest *q.v.* ~ is a stimulant and addicting drug. 2. A stimulant drug that, when abused, results in excitability, talkativeness, and a reduction of the feeling of fatigue. 3. A powerful central nervous system stimulant of natural origin, extracted from the leaves of the coca plant. 4. A pain-reducing and stimulating alkaloid that increases mental powers, produces euphoria *q.v.*, heightens sexual desire, and in large doses, causes paranoia *q.v.* and hallucinations *q.v.*

COCAINE PSYCHOSIS A severe, relatively rare psychotic *q.v.* reaction characterized by paranoia *q.v.* and hallucinations *q.v.* resulting from prolonged use of cocaine *q.v.*

COCA PASTE A paste derived from the coca *q.v.* leaf in the process of making cocaine *q.v.*

COCARCINOGEN An environmental agent that will activate a carcinogen *q.v.*

COCCUS A spherical bacterium *q.v.*

COCCYGEAL SPINE The lowest segment of the vertebral column, comprising three to five vertebrae which form the coccyx *q.v.*

COCCYX A small bone located at the bottom of the spinal column. cf: coccygeal spine.

COCHLEA 1. A small, snail-shaped organ of the inner ear in which the energy of sound is converted into electrical energy for transmission to the brain. 2. The coiled structure in the inner ear that contains the basilar membrane *q.v.* necessary for auditory reception.

COCURRICULAR ACTIVITIES School-sponsored programs organized and conducted outside of the planned instructional program. Examples include clubs, councils, and sports programs. Also referred to as extracurricular activities.

CODE In law, a compilation of statutes, scientifically arranged into chapters, subheadings, and actions, with a table of contents and index. A ~ supersedes all prior acts on the subject.

CODE ALERT In emergency operations, a means of delivering a specific message or of alerting a particular group or team by signaling with voice, bell, light, pager, or other means.

CODED MESSAGE A component of information theory *q.v.* The stimuli of symbols passing through the communication channel. The use of language is the coded message.

CODEINE 1. A Class B narcotic *q.v.* ~ was first extracted from morphine sulfate *q.v.* in 1832. It is used as an active ingredient in a variety of cough medicines and as an analgesic *q.v.* with only about one-sixth the potency of morphine. It is an addicting *q.v.* drug. 2. An analgesic and antitussive *q.v.* derived from morphine. 3. A naturally occurring narcotic widely used in medical practice, particularly as an antitussive, that is closely related to morphine, but less potent.

CODE OF ETHICS 1. A set of rules for ethical *q.v.* behavior, usually drawn up by a professional organization for the guidance of its members. 2. The moral codes that guide a person, group, or profession in its decisions and behaviors. 3. The philosophy that studies values. 4. Formal statement of appropriate professional behaviors.

CODICIL In law, a supplement to a will that modifies the original will in some respect.

CODIFICATION In law, a process of collecting and arranging the laws of a state into a code *q.v.*

CODING 1. In research, categories of recurring facts, themes, comments, and the like selected from fieldnotes for attention because they are likely to help explain a situation of interest. Once established, new fieldnotes are coded into these categories. 2. A research procedure aimed at placing into clear categories responses obtained on a particular measure. For example, one may ask people how often they go to church and then divide their answers into several categories from zero to every day. This process of creating categories and putting answers into tem is called ~. It is essential for quantitative research.

CODOMINANT GENES In genetics, alleles *q.v.* each of which produces an independent effect in heterozygotes *q.v.*

CODON 1. A three-nucleotide *q.v.* unit that represents the code for the production of a specific amino acid *q.v.* in the process of protein synthesis. 2. A set of bases in DNA *q.v.* which will code one amino acid. 3. A group of three consecutive nucleotides on a DNA molecule *q.v.* that is the information for placing a specific amino acid in a polypeptide chain *q.v.*

COEFFICIENT OF FRICTION An expression of the frictional force developed when two surfaces pass across one another. ~ is useful in predicting the number of feet required to stop a vehicle at a given speed, on a given surface, under specific circumstances.

COELOM 1. A cavity in the mesoderm *q.v.* in the body of higher animals, which arises in the embryo *q.v.* and is lined on all surfaces by a duplicate epithelium *q.v.*, the peritoneum *q.v.* 2. The body cavity. 3. The part of the body in which the organs arise.

COELOMATE Possessing a coelom *q.v.*

CEONOCYTIC 1. Multinucleate, the nuclei are not separated by cross walls. 2. A multinucleated structure without septa *q.v.*

COENZYME 1. A nonprotein compound that functions to activate an enzyme *q.v.* 2. An organic molecule *q.v.* that is required for the activation of an apoenzyme *q.v.* to an enzyme. The ~s are niacin, pyroxidine, thiamin, riboflavin, pantothenic acid, and folic acid *q.v.*

COENZYME A A complex molecule *q.v.* containing pantothenic acid *q.v.* ~ is required for fatty acid *q.v.* oxidation *q.v.* and synthesis *q.v.*, and for the synthesis of cholesterol *q.v.* and phospholipids *q.v.* ~ combines with acetate, and which, in turn, combines with oxaloacetate *q.v.* to form citrate *q.v.* and enter the tricarbolic acid cycle *q.v.* cf: coenzyme.

COFACTOR Any factor, such as stress, malnutrition, or infection by another microorganism *q.v.*, that increases the likelihood of developing a particular disease.

COFFEA ARABICA The plant from which the coffee bean is grown. cf: caffeine.

COFFEE GROUNDS VOMITUS A vomitus *q.v.* having the appearance and consistency of coffee grounds. ~ indicates slow bleeding in the stomach and represents the vomiting of partially digested blood.

CONGENTIN A commercial preparation of benztropine *q.v.*

COGNITION 1. Activities or mental behavior *q.v.* that are not feeling or affectively oriented. 2. Analytical or logical thinking as opposed to emotional thinking. 3. Pertaining to cognitive-behavioral theory *q.v.* to refer to a person's perceptions *q.v.* and interpretations of events. 4. The process of knowing. 5. The thinking, judging, reasoning, and planning activities of the human mind. Behavior is often explained as depending upon the course these processes take.

COGNITIVE Pertaining to the mental processes of comprehension, memory, judgment, and reasoning, as opposed to emotional processes. cf: cognition.

COGNITIVE BALANCE A process characterized by attitudes *q.v.*; going together harmoniously.

COGNITIVE-BEHAVIOR THERAPY A behavioral approach that emphasizes the role of perceptions *q.v.* and interpretations of events as determinants of behavioral disorders *q.v.*

COGNITIVE CONCEIT A common assumptive reality among children that adults are not very bright although the children are. cf: assumptive reality.

COGNITIVE DEVELOPMENT 1. The development of mental processes such as perception *q.v.*, problem solving, reasoning, memory, and the development of knowledge in general. 2. The learner's acquisition of facts, concepts, and principles through intellectualization.

COGNITIVE DEVELOPMENTAL THEORY OF IDENTIFICATION The theory that identification *q.v.* with same sex models is a result of conceptualizing oneself as feminine or masculine, rather than a cause of such conceptualization.

COGNITIVE DISSONANCE 1. An uncomfortable conflict between two realities that do not match and that often leads to the use of the defense mechanism *q.v.*, rationalization *q.v.* 2. Pertains to an inconsistency among some experiences, beliefs, attitudes, or feelings. According to ~, this inconsistency establishes an unpleasant state that people attempt to reduce by reinterpreting some part of their experiences to make them consistent with other experiences. 3. The general proposition that bits of knowledge that fail to fit or harmonize produce a strong negative motive. 4. Those processes by means of which a person becomes aware of objects and situations or represents them to himself or herself and which include learning, reasoning, remembering, imagining, problem solving, and decision making. 5. The tendency to ignore or reject ideas that conflict with an already formed opinion. 6. A conflict between beliefs and behavior.

COGNITIVE DOMAIN 1. In education, that aspect of learning that involves the recall or recognition of knowledge and the development of intellectual abilities and skills. 2. Pertains to the ability to deal with knowledge and factual information from an intellectual perspective. cf: cognitive objectives. ct: affective domain.

COGNITIVE EXPERIENCE 1. In the drug culture *q.v.*, psychedelic experience marked by clearness of thought.

2. Generally, awareness and understanding with clarity of a specific experience.

COGNITIVE FIELD THEORY 1. Cognitive learning theory *q.v.* 2. Explains how people learn human behavior: (a) learning occurs as insights or new meanings are acquired; (b) learning is identified with thought and is purposive, explorative, innovative, and creative.

COGNITIVE IDEOLOGY A life-view that emphasizes the place of intellectual activity and choice in human decision-making.

COGNITIVE INTERPRETATION THEORY OF EMOTIONS A theory which asserts that emotions *q.v.* are an interpretation of the autonomic arousal in view of the situation to which they are attributed.

COGNITIVE LEARNING THEORY 1. The theory that one's characteristics must be taken into account in addition to the various stimuli *q.v.* and responses *q.v.* when explaining learning. 2. A theory that views learning as a process of intellectual development resulting in new insights, discriminations, and associations. 3. Learning is determined by perception *q.v.* 4. According to some psychologists, there are four changes taking place during the learning process: (a) cognitive *q.v.* structure, (b) motivation, (c) group membership, and (d) voluntary muscle control. 5. Learning is a process of making new differentiations and discriminations or reorganizing material into new patterns. 6. Cognitive field theory *q.v.*

COGNITIVELY MEDIATED STRESS Perceived stress *q.v.* that occurs when a person labels something negatively in the mind.

COGNITIVE MAP A segment of a conception of learning that holds that people acquire segments of knowledge of what is where. cf: cognitive theory.

COGNITIVE MONITORING That aspect of metacognition *q.v.* that consists of keeping track of how one is doing on some task and regulating one's behavior accordingly.

COGNITIVE OBJECTIVES In education, learning or instructional outcomes that stress the acquisition of knowledge and intellectual skills. cf: cognitive domain.

COGNITIVE ORIENTATION One of the three theoretical perspectives in social psychology. The cognitive orientation emphasizes the thought processes that organize and interpret the properties of the environment. ct: behaviorist orientation; rule–role orientation.

COGNITIVE PSYCHOLOGY The study of knowledge and awareness, e.g., perception, attention, and information processing. ct: SR learning theories.

COGNITIVE RESPONSE Responses to situations that may require reflection and selection from among strategies. By hypotheses, children must learn to inhibit fast incurring associative responses before they can consistently make cognitive responses.

COGNITIVE RESTRUCTURING 1. Shame aversion therapy *q.v.* 2. A form of therapy in which negative consequences are associated with a particular undesirable behavior by viewing another person engaging in the behavior so that the first person will want to engage in the undesirable behavior less frequently. 3. Any behavior therapy *q.v.* procedure that attempts to alter the manner in which a person thinks about life so that he or she changes his or her overt behavior and emotions.

COGNITIVE SCHEMA Organization of knowledge about a given person, object, or stimulus.

COGNITIVE SET A person's perception of self and others that determines his/her ability to interact effectively. A negative cognitive set is a core feature of depression.

COGNITIVE THEORIES 1. A set of principles of psychology intended to account for intellectual activity resulting from learning. 2. Cognitive learning theories *q.v.*

COGNITIVE THEORY A conception of learning that holds that humans acquire pieces of knowledge. This is in contrast to instrumental learning *q.v.*

COGNITIVE THERAPY 1. An approach to therapy that attempts to change some of a person's habitual modes of thinking. ~ is related to behavior therapy *q.v.* 2. A treatment for mood disorders based on identifying and neutralizing negative cognitions that maintain depressive episodes.

COGNITIVE UNCONSCIOUS All of those adaptive specializations for which an organism is prepared that are specific to a particular function and not accessible for use for other purposes.

COGNITIVE UNIVERSALS The basic attributes of organization and adaptation *q.v.* that apply to all biological *q.v.* characteristics and, therefore, to intelligence *q.v.* as a biological characteristic of humans. cf: organization.

COHABITATION 1. An arrangement in which two or more people live together outside the bonds of marriage. 2. Fornication *q.v.* between unmarried people living together.

COHESIVENESS In social psychology, the degree to which members of a group are attracted to one another and the group as a whole.

COHORT 1. In epidemiology, a group of persons who have characteristics in common and are studied prospectively *q.v.* 2. Generation; all of those persons born at a particular point in time. 3. A group of people who are born at the same period of time or who enter a system at the same time. One type of research design *q.v.* compares

~s to see if there are differences in the way they grow older.

COHORT EFFECT 1. In epidemiology, an age group progressing through life with a high or low rate of a condition and carrying this trait into successive age categories. 2. The consequences of having been born in a given year and having grown up during a particular time period with its own unique pressures, problems, challenges, and opportunities. 3. A cohort *q.v.* difference that shows up as an age difference in a cross-sectional research design. ct: age effects.

COHORT SEQUENTIAL RESEARCH DESIGN A design first used by Schaie that enables developmentalists to separate cohort effects *q.v.* from true developmental changes. To execute the design, the researcher must collect longitudinal data on multiple cohorts *q.v.*

COHORT STUDY In epidemiology, a scientific research design that looks forward in time from baseline data. Health status or characteristics are assessed and later reassessed to determine which characteristics preceded or caused newly developed health conditions. cf: historical cohort study.

COINCIDENCE In genetics, the ratio of observed double crossovers *q.v.* to expected doubles calculated on the basis of independent occurrence and expressed as a decimal fraction.

COINSURANCE An insurance plan or policy that requires partial payment for health and medical services by the policyholder.

COITUS Sexual intercourse *q.v.*

COITUS INTERRUPTUS A method of birth control in which the penis *q.v.* is withdrawn from the vagina *q.v.* just before ejaculation *q.v.* 2. Premature withdrawal. ct: coitus reservatus

COITUS RESERVATUS Suppression of ejaculation *q.v.* by the male during sexual intercourse *q.v.* ct: coitus interruptus.

COKEAHOLIC 1. Cocaine-dependent person who has lost all control over the use of cocaine *q.v.* 2. A coined term to relate to the compulsion created by an addiction *q.v.* "Aholic" is frequently used to show a compulsion or addiction similar to alcoholism *q.v.* even though there is no relation to alcohol.

COLCHICINE An alkaloid *q.v.* from the autumn crocus that is used as an agent to arrest spindle formation and to interrupt mitosis *q.v.*

COLD 1. The common cold. 2. The most common communicable disease caused by a variety of viruses *q.v.*

COLD TURKEY 1. In relation to drug addiction, the process of suddenly stopping the use of a drug. 2. The immediate and total discontinuance of the use of an addictive *q.v.* substance.

COLECTOMY Surgical removal of the colon *q.v.*

COLEMAN REPORT (1981) A major study comparing the effectiveness of public and private schools in the United States.

COLIC 1. A condition found in infants in which gas collects in the stomach and produces distress. 2. Pertaining to the colon *q.v.* 3. Acute abdominal pain.

COLIFORM BACTERIA A group of bacteria *q.v.* whose presence in drinking water is suggestive of fecal *q.v.* contamination *q.v.*

COLITIS An inflammatory disease of the large intestine.

COLLABORATIVE MODEL A type of relationship between a client and an intervener which implies a partnership. The identification of the client's needs is a shared responsibility and the intervention is jointly implemented by client and intervener.

COLLAGEN 1. A comparatively insoluble protein *q.v.* that is found in the skin, tendons, bones, and cartilage. ~ is converted to gelatin by boiling. 2. The substance that binds body cells together. Vitamin C *q.v.* is essential for synthesis of ~.

COLLARBONE The clavicle *q.v.*

COLLATERAL ATTACK In law, an attempt to destroy the effect of a judgment by reopening the merits of a case or by showing why the judgment should not have been given, in an action other than that in which the judgment was given.

COLLATERAL BLOOD VESSELS Blood vessels that develop around a blocked artery. ~ compensate in part for the loss of blood supply to the heart. cf: collateral circulation.

COLLATERAL CIRCULATION Circulation of the blood through nearby smaller blood vessels when a major vessel is blocked or damaged. cf: collateral blood vessels.

COLLECTIVE BARGAINING In labor relations, a continuing institutional relationship between an employer and a labor organization representing a defined group of employees and concerned with the negotiation, administration, interpretation, and enforcement of written agreements concerning joint understandings as to wages, rates of pay, hours of work, and other conditions of employment.

COLLECTIVE BEHAVIOR Ways of feeling, thinking, and acting that are generally spontaneous and unstructured, but largely in agreement.

COLLECTIVE UNCONSCIOUS Refers to that portion of the unconscious *q.v.* that Carl Rogers considered common to all humans.

COLLEGE A postsecondary school that offers general or liberal arts education, usually leading to a first degree. Junior colleges or community colleges are included within this terminology.

COLLEGE BOARD REPORT A report that asserts a set of standards that describe what high school students should master before attending college *q.v.*

COLLEGE WORK-STUDY PROGRAM A program designed to stimulate and promote the part-time employment of students with demonstrated financial need.

COLLENCHYMA 1. Elongated living cells with variously thickened primary cell walls. A flexible, supporting tissue.

COLLES' FRACTURE A fracture *q.v.* of the distal end of the radius *q.v.* ~ may be accompanied by a fracture of a small fragment of the ulna styloid process *q.v.*

COLLOID 1. A dispersal of small particles or very large molecules *q.v.* of one substance in another, e.g., glue in water. 2. Solute *q.v.* particles with diameters of 1–100 μm.

COLLYRIUM A commercial eye lotion preparation.

COLON That part of the large intestine that extends from the cecum *q.v.* to the rectum *q.v.*

COLONIAL PERIOD That period in American education from 1607 to 1788.

COLONY 1. A macroscopic *q.v.* mass of microorganisms *q.v.* growing together, the cells of which have a common origin. Often pertains to bacterial masses growing on a solid medium. 2. In algae, an aggregation of closely associated cells, the units of which function independently of each other but do not usually occur separately. In some colonies, a certain degree of division of labor may be apparent. 3. In regard to bacteria, a mass of individuals, usually derived from cells of a single species. In ecology, pertaining to a group of plants becoming established in a new situation.

COLONY MORPHOLOGY The microscopic *q.v.* appearance of organisms when grown on media. cf: colony.

COLOR BLINDNESS 1. Dichromatism *q.v.* 2. A sex-linked genetic *q.v.* trait affecting more males than females. 3. The inability to distinguish clearly some colors. Generally, one is able to perceive *q.v.* most colors but has difficulty distinguishing between one or two specific colors. cf: color vision.

COLOR CIRCLE A schematic arrangement of colors in which the spectrum *q.v.* is bent back against itself to form a circle.

COLOR SOLID A three-dimensional representation of visual experience.

COLOR VISION The ability to distinguish various colors. ~ is tested by the use of the pseudoisochromatic plates *q.v.* ~ is made possible by the presence of proper functioning of the cones *q.v.* located in the retina of the eye. ct: color blindness.

COLOSTOMY An artificial opening in the abdominal wall through which solid waste products are excreted. A ~ is necessary when a large portion of the colon *q.v.* must be removed because of disease or injury.

COLOSTRUM 1. Mother's milk for the first few days after childbirth. 2. A rather thick, yellowish milk produced by the mother following childbirth.

COLPOSCOPE An instrument used to examine the cervix *q.v.* for abnormalities.

COLPOSCOPY The use of a colposcope to view the cervix *q.v.* for abnormalities in tissue growth.

COMA A state of profound unconsciousness from which a person cannot be aroused.

COMATOSE 1. Affected with coma *q.v.* 2. Exhibiting depressed responsiveness. 3. Unconsciousness.

COMBAT REACTION 1. Transient personality decompensation *q.v.* resulting from the acute *q.v.* stress *q.v.* of battle experience. 2. Combat exhaustion. 3. Traumatic reaction to combat. 4. Battle fatigue.

COMBINATION APPROACH An approach to planning that emphasizes the advantages and deemphasizes the disadvantages of the high probability approach, the maximizing approach, and the adapting approach.

COMBINATION ORAL CONTRACEPTIVE DRUG An oral contraceptive *q.v.* containing small amounts of both female sex hormones *q.v.*: estrogen *q.v.* and progestin *q.v.* Because of negative side effects, removed from the market. cf: combination pill.

COMBINATION PILL A chemical contraceptive *q.v.* in pill form. It contains synthetic estrogen *q.v.* and progestogen, similar to progesterone *q.v.* Both are contained in each pill. The ~ inhibits ovulation *q.v.* and makes the endometrium *q.v.* inhospitable for the implantation of a fertilized egg. Also, the cervical mucus *q.v.* may be altered, becoming a hostile environment for the sperm *q.v.* The combination pill is no longer marketed because of a variety of undesirable side effects. cf: combination oral contraceptive drug.

COMBINATORIAL REASONING The mental process whereby one creates the set of all possible combinations of existing elements. The ability to perform this mental act is associated with formal operational thought.

COMBINED TREATMENT In psychology, a multimodal treatment program that combines drugs with some form of psychotherapy *q.v.*

COME-A-LONG A hand-operated winch of varying capacity used to effect a forceful entry, such as that to free a person trapped in a wrecked vehicle.

COMEDO A pimple.

COMEDONE 1. A blackhead. 2. A sebum plug in the duct from the sebaceous gland *q.v.* to the surface of the skin.

COMING OUT An expression used by homosexuals *q.v.* to describe their acknowledgement of their sexual orientation to themselves and to others. 2. Come out.

COMMAND GROUPS Formal groups that are outlined on the chain of command on an organizational chart.

COMMENSAL 1. In biology, an organism that lives on or in or with another, usually using the same food, but is not truly a parasite. 2. Coexistence.

COMMINUTED 1. Broken into small pieces. 2. Fractures of bones into several small pieces.

COMMISSION 1. A governmental body directed and authorized to carry out a particular task. 2. Pay based on fixed or variable amount per unit sold.

COMMISSION ON HEART DISEASE, CANCER, AND STROKE Established in 1964 by President Lyndon B. Johnson for the purpose of recommending ways the nation might employ in conquering heart disease, cancer, and stroke.

COMMISSION ON POPULATION GROWTH AND THE AMERICAN FUTURE Commission's first report released to President Richard M. Nixon in 1972. The report recommended wide-scale sex education, revised abortion policy, approval of the Equal Rights Amendment, and contraceptive *q.v.* supplies, information, and procedures available on demand. President Nixon rejected the report and its recommendations.

COMMISSURE Bundle of nerve fibers passing from one side to the other side of the brain or spinal cord.

COMMITMENT A legal process for admission to a psychiatric hospital.

COMMITMENT PRINCIPLE A management guideline that advises managers to commit funds for planning only when they can anticipate, in the foreseeable future, a return on planning expenses as a result of long-range planning analysis.

COMMITTEE A task group that is charged with performing some type of specific activity or task.

COMMITTEE (AD HOC) A committee appointed for some special purpose and which automatically dissolves upon the completion of its specific task.

COMMITTEE CHAIR A member appointed to function as the parliamentarian and head of a standing or special committee in the consideration of matters assigned to such committee by the governing body or its leader.

COMMITTEE OF FIFTEEN A committee *q.v.* appointed in 1895 by the National Education Association that reversed the findings of the Committee of Ten *q.v.*

COMMITTEE OF TEN A National Education Association committee established in 1893 to standardize high schools. cf: Committee of Fifteen.

COMMITTEE OF THE WHOLE A parliamentary device by which the entire membership of the legislative body (one house, in Congress) sits as a committee to consider legislation. It reports back its recommendations to the legislative body.

COMMON BILE DUCT The duct *q.v.* formed by the union of the common hepatic ducts *q.v.* and the cystic duct *q.v.* and empties into the duodenum *q.v.*

COMMON COLD An infectious disease *q.v.* of which there are over 120 types of viruses *q.v.* as causative agents. The ~ is transmitted by direct or indirect contact with fluid discharges from an infected person. It is characterized by a sore throat, running nose, chills, mild fever, and muscular aches. The ~ usually lasts from 3 to 5 days, but no autoinfection or relapse is common.

COMMON LAW In law, legal principles derived from usage and custom, or from court decisions affirming such usages and customs, or the acts of Parliament in force at the time of the American Revolution, as distinguished from law created by enactment of American legislation.

COMMON LAW MARRIAGE A marriage effected by an agreement between two people of the opposite sex to live together as husband and wife. A marriage not resulting from a legal or religious ceremony and where no civil license is obtained.

COMMON OWNERSHIP OF INFORMATION A norm of science that states that information is owned by all and is to be shared freely. Researchers have an obligation to share their findings through universally available publications. Data should be shared on request once its use by the researcher is completed. Supporting data for knowledge claims should be open to examination by others.

COMMON SCHOOL A free, publically supported school for all children. A movement that began in the mid-1800s.

COMMON-SOURCE EPIDEMIC In epidemiology, a high level of a communicable disease *q.v.* occurring when a number of people have been exposed to the same agent at the same time. cf: propagated epidemic.

COMMONWEALTH FUND Established in 1918 with the objective to do something for the welfare of humanity.

COMMUNAL FAMILY A group family living arrangement in which all members share household responsibilities and finances. cf: communard.

COMMUNARD A person who supported or took part in the Commune of Paris (1871). cf: communal family

COMMUNE 1. A form of group marriage *q.v.* or economic living arrangement in which income, property, and functions are shared, but each nuclear family *q.v.* held intact. 2. Three or more people living together for the purpose of sharing their lifestyle, and who are not bound by genetics *q.v.*, marriage, or legal ties. cf: communal family.

COMMUNICABLE 1. A disease that can be transmitted from person to person. 2. A disease that is capable of spreading from one person to another person or from one animal to another animal, either by direct contact or by indirect contact. cf: communicable diseases; contagious disease.

COMMUNICABLE DISEASES Diseases *q.v.* that can be transmitted from one person to another person. All communicable diseases are infectious *q.v.*, but not all infectious diseases are communicable. Diseases also vary in their ability to be transmitted; some are more communicable than are others. The chief characteristic are their incubation period, period of communicability, and their signs and symptoms. Before a disease can begin, the biological agent *q.v.* in the infected person (or well person who is a carrier) must find an exit from the host. The agent must then be transported to a susceptible healthy host and gain entry (portal of entry). When the environment in the new host is adequate, the agent must multiply in sufficient numbers to cause an illness that is recognized by the signs and symptoms it produces. Most biological agents have limited adaptive abilities and must exit the infected host and enter the new host directly, others can be transmitted through vectors *q.v.* or fomites *q.v.*, while others need an intermediate host in which to mature sufficiently to cause disease. cf: noncommunicable diseases.

COMMUNICABLE PERIOD The time during which an infectious *q.v.* agent may be transmitted from one host to another host.

COMMUNICATE To talk with other people and to exchange ideas and feelings.

COMMUNICATION 1. The process by which messages are transferred through a channel to a receiver. 2. The transfer of commonly meaningful information. 3. The process of sharing information with other individuals.

COMMUNICATION CHANNEL 1. The mechanism that carries information from its source to its destination. 2. A component of information theory *q.v.* 3. Systems that carry messages from one person or group to another, downward, upward, across, or diagonally.

COMMUNICATION DEVIANCE (CD) Disturbed patterns of expressing thoughts and feelings to others. ~ is hypothesized to be more common in parents of schizophrenics *q.v.*

COMMUNICATION EFFECTIVENESS INDEX Intended message reactions divided by the total number of transmitted messages.

COMMUNICATION MACROBARRIERS Those factors that hinder successful communication and that relate primarily to the communication environment and the larger world in which communication takes place. ct: communication microbarriers.

COMMUNICATION MICROBARRIERS Those factors that hinder successful communication and that relate primarily to such variables as the communication message, the source, and the destination. ct: communication macrobarriers.

COMMUNICATION STRUCTURE The pattern of communication networks that exists among members of a group. Typically, structures are centralized, having one coordinator, or decentralized, having many lines of interaction.

COMMUNICATOR CREDIBILITY The degree to which a communicator is a trustworthy, informed, and unbiased source of information.

COMMUNITY 1. A geographic area that functions as a unit. 2. Standard Metropolitan Statistical Area *q.v.* 3. A group held together by some common interest or goals. 4. A ~ is smaller and less complex than a society *q.v.*, but more complex and complete in its functioning than a neighborhood. 5. Any collection of people sharing a set of common values. 6. In biology, an assemblage of organisms living together and interacting with each other in a characteristic natural habitat. 7. A group of people organized in some way into a unifying body with some aware purpose.

COMMUNITY DEVELOPMENT Approaches and techniques that rely upon local communities as units of action; attempt to combine outside assistance with organized, local self-determination efforts; and correspondingly seek to stimulate local initiatives and leadership as the primary instrument of change.

COMMUNITY HEALTH The collective health status of a community *q.v.*

COMMUNITY HEALTH AGENCY A voluntary or governmental agency functioning in regard to some health issues or problems.

COMMUNITY HEALTH COUNCIL 1. A cooperative body representing all community health *q.v.* interested organizations and agencies. 2. A planning, problem-solving, coordinating body composed of representatives from various agencies melded into one group working for better community health.

COMMUNITY HEALTH EDUCATION 1. All of the methods, techniques, and strategies used by the community health educator *q.v.* to improve the health knowledge, attitudes, and behavior of members of the defined community *q.v.* 2. Health education *q.v.* processes using community organization, intergroup relationships, and communication resources in a specific social system. 3. The application of a variety of methods that result in the education *q.v.* and mobilization of community members in actions for resolving health issues and problems that affect the community. These methods include group process, use of the media, communication skills, planning, and policy making.

COMMUNITY HEALTH EDUCATOR 1. Public health educator. 2. A practitioner who is professionally prepared in the field of community health education *q.v.* who demonstrates competence in the planning, organizing, implementing, and evaluating a broad range of health promoting or health enhancing programs for community groups. 3. A person with professional preparation in public health education, including training in the application of selected content from relevant social and behavioral sciences used to positively influence individual and group learning, mobilization of community health actions, and the planning, implementing, and evaluation of health programs.

COMMUNITY HEALTH ORGANIZATION 1. The voluntary, governmental, and professional agencies, associations, and societies concerned with certain aspects of health *q.v.* 2. Health education *q.v.* processes or methods in which the combined efforts of individuals, groups, and organizations are designed to generate, mobilize, coordinate, use, and redistribute resources to meet unsolved or emerging health problems.

COMMUNITY HEALTH PROGRAM Includes all functions directed toward improving the health of individuals within the community *q.v.* and the health of the community as a whole. Its components are fundamentally the same as those for the school health program, namely, health education, medical and health services, and a healthful environment in which to live.

COMMUNITY HEALTH PROMOTION A combination of educational, social, and environmental supports for behavior conducive to health *q.v.*

COMMUNITY HEALTH SERVICES. PUBLIC HEALTH SERVICES The seven major program emphases are as follows: (a) environmental controls; (b) prevention of disease, disability, and premature death; (c) provision of medical and dental care; (d) collection and analysis of vital statistics and records; (e) provision for public education; (f) health planning and program evaluation; and (g) conducting research into health matters.

COMMUNITY INVOLVEMENT LIAISON (CIL) A position created within the Division of Health Assessment and Consultation. The CIL serves as the agency point person for citizens to directly share their concerns for response and inclusion in the health assessment.

COMMUNITY MENTAL HEALTH The delivery of services to needy, underserved groups through centers that offer outpatient therapy, short-term inpatient care, day hospitalization, 24-h emergency services, and consultation and education to other community agencies.

COMMUNITY ORGANIZATION 1. By this process, a community identifies its needs, develops the abilities and finds the resources to meet these needs, and develops cooperative and collaborative attitudes and practices in the community *q.v.* 2. The process by which a community identifies its needs and objectives, organizes into groups to solve identified problems, develops confidence to work together, takes action in respect to these problems, and develops cooperative attitudes and practices in the community.

COMMUNITY PRODUCING DEVIANCE Behaviors *q.v.* that contribute to a community *q.v.* with deviant *q.v.* behaviors.

COMMUNITY PSYCHOLOGY An approach to therapy which emphasizes prevention and the seeking out of potential difficulties rather than waiting for troubled persons to initiate consultation *q.v.* Professional activities are usually centered in the person's natural surroundings rather than in a professional office. cf: prevention.

COMMUNITY PSYCHIATRY The psychiatric movement toward prevention of emotional disorders *q.v.*, mental health *q.v.* care, provided by the community through public funds. cf: community psychology.

COMMUNITY SCHOOL A school that is intimately connected with the life of the community *q.v.* and tries to provide for the educational needs of all in the geographic locality.

COMPANION CELL In botany, a small, specialized parenchyma cell *q.v.* associated with the sieve-tube elements of flowering plants.

COMPANIONATE LOVE The friendship, caring, and deep attachment of established couples. cf: companion love.

COMPANION BILL 1. In politics and law, two or more bills dealing with related aspects of the same topic. 2. Tie bar.

COMPANION LOVE A form of love characteristic of long-term relationships. ~ involves friendly affection and deep attachment and is less emotionally intense than passionate love *q.v.* cf: companionate love.

COMPANIONSHIP MARRIAGE A marriage *q.v.* that emphasizes mutual consent and agreements above the rules, values, and expectations of society.

COMPANY A profit-making business owned by a single person, parties, or a group of shareholders or stockholders.

COMPARATIVE MANAGEMENT The study of the management process in different countries in order to examine the potential of management action under different environmental conditions.

COMPARISON LEVEL The outcome that individuals feel is appropriate from a relationship, derived from prior experiences as well as the perception of other's satisfaction in similar relationships.

COMPARISON SHOPPING A method by which a person checks out several articles of the same kind for quality, quantity, and price.

COMPARTMENT SYNDROME The shock-like state that follows release of a limb after a long period of compression. ~ is brought about by compression of the arterial blood supply to a muscular compartment.

COMPATIBLE NEEDS The needs *q.v.* of a potential mate that are the same as the needs possessed by the partner. ct: complementary needs.

COMPAZINE A commercial preparation of prochlorperazine *q.v.*

COMPENSABLE FACTORS Certain qualities common to all jobs.

COMPENSATION 1. Usually, a defense mechanism *q.v.* 2. The attempt by a person to disguise an undesirable trait by emphasizing a desirable one. 3. The act of seeking a substitute for something unacceptable or unattainable. ~ may take the form of an unusually high level of development of an originally unattainable trait or skill. 4. The correction of an organic deficit by increasing function of another organ.

COMPENSATION CAFETERIA In labor relations, a flexible compensation package that permits employees to choose the most beneficial form of pay from a variety of alternatives.

COMPENSATION MANAGEMENT In labor relations, the development and implementation of policies to ensure that employees are paid fairly for their efforts.

COMPENSATION POINT In botany, the light intensity at which the rate of photosynthesis *q.v.* and the rate of respiration *q.v.* in the leaf are equal.

COMPENSATORY DAMAGES In law, damages awarded to reimburse the injured party only for the actual loss incurred. Punitive or exemplary damages are not considered compensatory.

COMPENSATORY EDUCATION Enriched or extended educational experiences or services that are made available to children of low-income families.

COMPETENCE 1. In education, the ability to perform a skill or set of skills at a high level or levels determined to be necessary for basic job performance. 2. In psychology, the degree of mastery over one's world. 3. Psychologists' term for what a child knows about a certain subject. 4. The ability one actually has as opposed to the ability that one succeeds in demonstrating. cf: effectance motivation; performance; competency.

COMPETENCY 1. The ability to perform certain skills at appropriate levels. 2. The ability to perform at some predetermined acceptable level of expertise. 3. The demonstrated ability to perform specific acts at a particular level of skill or accuracy. cf: competence.

COMPETENCY-BASED CERTIFICATION The general process by which the state (or agency or organization authorized by the state) provides a credential to an individual. Processes may require individuals to demonstrate a mastery of minimum essential generic and specialization competencies and other related criteria adopted by the certification board through a comprehensive written examination and through other procedures that may be prescribed by the board of educational examiners.

COMPETENCY-BASED EDUCATION Learning based on highly specialized concepts, skills, and attitudes related directly to some endeavor.

COMPETENCY-BASED TEACHER EDUCATION (CBTE) A system of teacher training in which students are required to demonstrate particular competencies *q.v.* in order to qualify for graduation and/or certification *q.v.*, rather than only minimum grade point averages or a minimum number of college credit hours.

COMPETENCY TEST An examination designed to evaluate the quality of a health educator based on predetermined basic skills and responsibilities. cf: competency; competency-based education.

COMPETENCY TO STAND TRIAL In law, a legal decision on whether a person can participate meaningfully in his or her own defense.

COMPETENT BACTERIA The ability of bacteria cells to undergo transduction *q.v.*

COMPETING CUES Stimuli that vie for one's attention, frequently conflictual in nature.

COMPETITION In biology, the effect of a common demand by two or more organisms on a limited supply of food, water, light, mineral, etc.

COMPETITIVE LEARNING A form of learning or a learning process wherein learners compete with each other (or with self) to achieve certain standards of learning. The opposite of cooperative learning *q.v.*

COMPLEMENT 1. In biology, a normal component of mammalian serum which must be present in order for some lysins *q.v.* to function. 2. A series of proteins *q.v.* that aid antibodies *q.v.* in destroying bacteria *q.v.*

COMPLEMENTARITY IN ATTRACTION In sociology, the tendency for people to be attracted to those traits and capacities that complement their own.

COMPLEMENTARY COLORS 1. Colors which, when mixed, produce an achromatic *q.v.* 2. Two colors which, when additively mixed together in the proper proportions, produce the perception of gray.

COMPLEMENTARY GENES In genetics, genes *q.v.* which are similar in phenotypic *q.v.* effect when present separately, but which together interact to produce a different character *q.v.*

COMPLEMENTARY NEEDS The needs of a potential mate that are different from those possessed by the partner. cf: compatible needs.

COMPLEMENTATION 1. In botany, restoration of normal function in an organism that is a hybrid *q.v.* of two defective nonallelic genes *q.v.* 2. In sexology, the process of learning gender-appropriate responses of one's own assigned sex by interacting with a member of the opposite sex.

COMPLEMENT FIXATION A process that helps to make antigen *q.v.*/antibody *q.v.* complexes easier for phagocytes *q.v.* to digest.

COMPLETE CERTAINTY CONDITION The decision-making situation in which the decision maker knows exactly what the results of an implemented alternative will be. ct: uncertainty condition.

COMPLETE PROTEIN FOODS Foods that contain all of the essential amino acids *q.v.* in amounts sufficient for growth and maintenance of body functions.

COMPLETE UNCERTAINTY CONDITION The decision-making situation in which the decision maker has absolutely no idea what the results of an implemented alternative will be. ct: complete certainty condition.

COMPLETION TEST ITEM A test item that evaluates a learner's recall of certain facts. The item is usually constructed as an incomplete statement wherein the learner provides the necessary word or words to complete the statement with factual information.

COMPLEX 1. In psychology, the combination of emotionally toned attitudes, desires, or memories that are partially or totally repressed. 2. A group of symptoms. 3. A syndrome *q.v.* 4. In biochemistry, the combination of a molecule of a drug, hormone, or neurotransmitter *q.v.* with a particular protein, in the blood or in association with a cell. Some complexes function as transport units; in others, the protein changes shape because of the interaction, initiating a metabolic *q.v.* change. cf: protein binding.

COMPLEX CARBOHYDRATE 1. Starches. 2. Compounds composed of long chains of glucose molecules *q.v.* 3. Carbohydrates *q.v.* composed of long molecular chains containing many saccharide *q.v.* units.

COMPLEX INDICATOR In the association word test, an indication of an emotional difficulty associated with the stimulus *q.v.* word. The indication may take the form of an unusual response, a protracted latency, or other evidence of concern or upset.

COMPLIANCE 1. In social psychology, the tendency to yield to group pressure in order to avoid punishment for nonconformity. The outward change is not necessarily accompanied by inward change. 2. Adherence to a prescribed therapeutic or preventive regimen. 3. In education, conformity to education law and/or regulations.

COMPLIANT Willing to follow directions.

COMPONENTS OF THE TOTAL HEALTH PROGRAM The health education program and all of its elements; the medical or health services and all of its functions and the quality of the school/community environment.

COMPOSTING The breakdown of organic garbage and sewage by bacteria *q.v.* into a soil-conditioning, humus-like material.

COMPOUND Any substance composed of two or more different elements.

COMPOUND FRACTURE A break in the bone where the bone protrudes through the skin. ct: simple fracture.

COMPREHENSIVE HEALTH EDUCATION A health education program that is planned and carried out with the purpose of maintaining, reinforcing, or enhancing health-related skills, and health attitudes and practices of people that are conducive to their good health; an educational approach coordinating education, services, and environment as significant influencers of individual and societal health. cf: comprehensive health education approach.

COMPREHENSIVE HEALTH EDUCATION APPROACH An approach to health education *q.v.* that provides learning experiences based on the best scientific information in an effort to promote the understanding, attitudes, behavioral skills, and practices of learners with respect to their health *q.v.* Although the curriculum or program may be made up of individual topics, there is opportunity to show relationships across these topics. ~ also implies that the educator is properly trained or certified as a health educator *q.v.* This is in contrast to the categorical approach *q.v.* in which educators trained or certified in other areas may offer health education programs.

COMPREHENSIVE HEALTH INSURANCE An insurance policy or plan that provides broad health, medical, and surgical coverage; basic health insurance, major medical coverage, and catastrophic coverage.

COMPREHENSIVE HEALTH PROGRAM Includes two broad areas: (a) the community health program and (b) the school health program, which are made up of school/community environment, health education, and medical and health services. cf: comprehensive school health program.

COMPREHENSIVE HIGH SCHOOL 1. Secondary schools *q.v.* that provide a variety of curricular options for students. 2. A secondary school that attempts to cater to the needs of all students by offering more than one course of specialization in its program.

COMPREHENSIVE MAJOR MEDICAL INSURANCE An insurance policy, an integration of basic medical coverage with insurance against catastrophic expenses, forming a single insurance plan.

COMPREHENSIVE SCHOOL HEALTH EDUCATION (INSTRUCTION) Pertains to the development, delivery, and evaluation of a planned curriculum for learners in preschool through grade 12 with achievable goals and objectives, sequential context, evaluation, and methodology related to specific categorical health issues and problems that affect individual and societal health. cf: comprehensive school health program.

COMPREHENSIVE SCHOOL HEALTH PROGRAM 1. The planned, coordinated provision of school health services *q.v.*, a healthful school environment *q.v.* and health instruction (education) for all pupils (and staff) in a school setting, where each of the components complements and is integrated with the others in the total scope of the body of knowledge unique to health education *q.v.* 2. An organized set of policies, procedures, and activities designed to protect and promote the health and well-being of learners which has traditionally included health services, healthful school environment, and health education. The components of these areas include guidance, counseling, physical education, food services, social work, psychological services, and employee health promotion. cf: comprehensive health program.

COMPREHENSIVE SECONDARY SCHOOL A general secondary school offering programs in both vocational and general academic subjects, but in which the majority of students are not enrolled in programs of vocational education.

COMPRESSION In botany, a kind of plant fossil resulting from the weight of accumulated sediments upon plant organs.

COMPROMISE FORMATION A defense mechanism *q.v.* in which an act or a thought expresses two, often, incompatible impulses. cf: compromise reaction.

COMPROMISE REACTION A response to frustration *q.v.* in which a person partially relinquishes his or her original goal. ~ often involves a lowering of one's level of aspiration or the acceptance of substitute goals. cf: compromise formation.

COMPULSION 1. A compelling, irresistible impulse *q.v.* which causes a person to act in a way that may be contrary to his or her good judgment, training, or normal desire. 2. An irresistible tendency to perform some act even though the person realizes it is irrational. 3. A forceful impulse. cf: obsessive-compulsive reaction.

COMPULSIVE PERSONALITY 1. A personality *q.v.* characterized by rigidity, over-inhibition, and over-conscientiousness. 2. The person has an obsessive concern for conformity to standards and the inability to relax. 3. Perfectionistic and work-oriented, rather than pleasure-oriented. People with a ~ have inordinate difficulty making decisions, are overconcerned with details and efficiency, and relate poorly to others because they demand that things be done their way. They are unduly conventional, serious, formal, and stingy with their emotions. 4. Compulsive personality disorder.

COMPULSIVITY The tendency to be systematic and controlled, to cling to familiar routines, and to avoid spontaneity and ambiguity.

COMPULSORY EDUCATION 1. Legally mandated education for all students within certain age groups. 2. School attendance that is required by law on the theory that it is to the benefit of society to educate all the people.

COMPULSORY MEDICAL CARE A plan to provide medical care for all people, required by law and administered by state or national governments.

COMPUTER An electronic device capable of accepting data, interpreting it, performing ordered operations, and reporting on the outcomes of these operations.

COMPUTER-ASSISTED INSTRUCTION (CAI) 1. The use of computers to present learning programs to facilitate and/or evaluate learning. 2. Direct, two-way teaching–learning communication between a student and programmed instructional material stored in a computer *q.v.*

COMPUTER-ASSISTED TELEPHONE INTERVIEWING (CATI) Random digit dialing used to select a sample randomly from among telephone subscribers for interviews. The computer is programmed to determine whether the respondent fits the quota sample, what questions to ask, and in what order. Responses immediately entered directly into the computer *q.v.* are checked for consistency and errors.

COMPUTER-ASSISTED TOMOGRAPHY (CAT SCAN) 1. Brain imaging techniques that pairs sophisticated X-ray techniques with computer technology to obtain three-dimensional images of the structure of the brain. 2. Computer axial tomography *q.v.*

COMPUTER-BASED RESOURCE UNITS (CBRU) Computerized learning *q.v.*

COMPUTERIZED AXIAL TOMOGRAPHY 1. CAT scan *q.v.* 2. An X-ray procedure designed to visualize structures within the body that would not normally be seen through conventional X-ray procedures. 3. Computer-assisted tomography *q.v.* 4. A medical test procedure producing color images, or a map, of the structures of the body being investigated. ~ is a painless procedure. Scans are used in evaluating a person for tumors, a loss of brain tissue, the buildup of calcium deposits in arteries, etc.

COMPUTERIZED LEARNING An electronic method of individualizing learning. This is accomplished by having learners select their own objectives and by identifying their own characteristics, which are then entered into a computer *q.v.* and, in turn, provided suggested learning experiences that can be pursued by the learners to assist them in achieving their objectives. In the early to middle 1970s, the New York State Education Department experimented with its entire health education curriculum for grades K through 12 by developing what was called Computer-Based Resource Units (CBRU). This system of curriculum design was developed by Dr. Robert Harnack at the State University of New York at Buffalo.

COMPUTER-MANAGED INSTRUCTION (CMI) A record-keeping procedure for tracking student performance by using a computer *q.v.*

COMPUTER PROFILES In safety epidemiology, ~ show accident sequences where there are multiple contributing factors.

COMPUTER SCIENCE The study of computers *q.v.* and computer programming.

COMPUTER SEARCH The use of a computer *q.v.* to find specific terms or topics from a search engine.

COMPUTER SOFTWARE Programs, procedures, and associated documentation that instruct the computer *q.v.* to perform certain tasks.

COMT An acronym for catechol-*O*-methyl transferase *q.v.*

CONATIVE Striving; a purposeful act that is related to motivation *q.v.* cf: conative component of attitudes.

CONATIVE COMPONENT OF ATTITUDES A person's orientation toward an object or a class of objects. cf: conative.

CONCEIVED VALUES 1. Beliefs that reflect what we view as ideal. 2. A person's conception of the ideal values *q.v.*

CONCENTRIC CONTRACTION 1. A muscle contraction in which the muscle shortens while overcoming resistance. 2. An isotonic contraction *q.v.* in which the muscle shortens while it produces tension.

CONCEPT 1. A representation of the common properties of distinguished objects. 2. The grouping of a class of objects or ideas on the basis of one or more criteria. In conceptualization *q.v.*, stimuli are grouped together on the basis of common properties. cf: hypothesis testing; natural categories. 3. An idea. 4. A stable impression. 5. A meaning or thought that gives structure to knowledge. 6. According to Woodruft, a relatively complete and meaningful idea in the mind of a person. It is the understanding of something. 7. In health, there are three major components: (a) comprehensive, the quality resulting from total functioning of the person interacting in the environment that enables him or her to achieve a personally satisfying and socially useful life; (b) key: (1) the unity of the individual, (2) health as a quality of life, (3) achievement of a personally satisfying life, and (4) achievement of a socially useful life; and (c) major, the essential factors influencing health and effective living: (1) heredity, (2) growth and development, (3) interaction, and (4) decision making. cf: concept attainment.

CONCEPTACLE A hollow structure containing sex organs.

CONCEPT APPROACH TO CURRICULUM DESIGN Focuses on the attainment of three principles: (a) growing and developing, (b) decision making, and (c) interaction. Learning experiences are directed toward each individual developing health concepts *q.v.* which can be applied to improved daily living. This approach to health education was popularized as a result of the School Health Education Study (SHES) *q.v.* conducted in 1961 and published in 1963. The study was done under the direction of Dr. Elena M. Sliepcevich.

CONCEPT ATTAINMENT A teaching strategy that attempts to develop the thinking process of students around generalizations.

CONCEPT FORMATION The process of categorizing learning experiences in a meaningful way, enabling the learner to appropriately communicate with others. It implies a generalized comprehension as a result of specific learning experiences. Significance and relationships of basic factual information result as concepts *q.v.* are formed.

CONCEPTION 1. Fertilization *q.v.* of an ovum *q.v.* by a sperm *q.v.* cell. 2. Entrance of a sperm into an egg. 3. The beginning of a new life. 4. Impregnation *q.v.* 5. The biological beginning of pregnancy *q.v.*

CONCEPTUAL AGE The age since conception *q.v.* This age provides a more reliable index of developmental status than does chronological age *q.v.* for infants during their first year.

CONCEPTUAL ANALYSIS In research, a process for finding the characteristics that define a term. Especially useful for defining constructs *q.v.* and concepts *q.v.*

CONCEPTUAL APPROACH 1. The use of ideas or concepts *q.v.* as the unifying threads or framework of curricular components. 2. A curriculum *q.v.* organizational plan that employs generalizations or concepts as the framework of its scope. cf: concept approach to curriculum design.

CONCEPTUAL SKILLS The ability to see the organization as a whole.

CONCEPTUS 1. Zygote *q.v.* 2. The product of conception *q.v.* 3. The union between the ovum *q.v.* and the sperm *q.v.* from the moment of contact to the moment of birth. 4. The stages from zygote to fetus *q.v.*

CONCHA In anatomy, a shell-shaped structure.

CONCILIATION The process of getting a party in a dispute to agree.

CONCOMITANT VARIATION (METHOD OF) In research, phenomena that consistently vary together are presumed to be connected to one another, directly or indirectly, through causal relationship.

CONCORDANCE 1. The probability that two people, e.g., identical twins, who stand in a particular family relationship, will both have the same disorder. 2. In behavioral genetics, the similarity in psychiatric diagnosis or in other traits in a pair of twins.

CONCORDANCE RATE The likelihood that when one twin manifests a certain trait, the other twin will also manifest it.

CONCRETE OPERATIONAL PERIOD 1. The developmental period between 7 and 11 years characterized by the capacity to mentally manipulate concrete experiences. 2. Piaget's third period of intellectual growth when children first become capable of using intellectual operations that allow them to think logically about problems that have concrete content; known as classification, seriation, and conservation, which they apply to real objects and their concrete properties. cf: operations; formal operations period.

CONCUBINE In polygamous *q.v.* societies, secondary wives or wives of a lower social status.

CONCURRENCE In politics, action by which one house agrees to a proposal or action that the other house has approved. A proposal may be amended, adopted, and then returned to the other house for ~.

CONCURRENT CONTROL Control that takes place as some unit of work is being performed.

CONCURRENT JURISDICTION In law, two courts having the same authority.

CONCURRENT RESOLUTION In politics, a statement of the attitude or feeling of the two houses, not having the force of law.

CONCURRENT VALIDITY 1. Validity *q.v.* established by the fact that scores on a test correspond to other measures obtained on the same individual at nearly the same time. 2. A measure's relation to other, independent indices of the same phenomenon. cf: construct validity; content validity.

CONCURRING OPINION In law, an opinion written by a judge who agrees with the majority of the court as to the decision in a case, but has different reasons for arriving at that decision.

CONCUSSION 1. A severe impact to the skull causing rupturing of small blood vessels in the brain. 2. A jarring injury to the brain produced by a blow to the head that usually involves a momentary loss of consciousness followed by transient disorientation and memory loss.

CONDENSATION REACTION In chemistry, a chemical reaction in which two or more molecules *q.v.* combine.

CONDENSER In optics and physics, a lens system of one or more elements that gathers light waves, converging them on the subject.

CONDITIONED ANXIETY Perceived stress *q.v.* that results from having learned to fear specific situations.

CONDITIONED INHIBITION The process by which a person is conditioned *q.v.* not to respond to some stimulus *q.v.* that formerly produced a response.

CONDITIONED REFLEX 1. Conditioned response *q.v.* 2. ~ is a somewhat obsolete term used rarely in the literature today. 3. A response brought about by something other than its original, and biologically adequate stimulus is a ~. 4. The term conditioned response is more general than ~ since the term reflex is ordinarily restricted to involuntary and unlearned responses (muscular or glandular) to sensory stimuli. cf: reflex.

CONDITIONED REINFORCER An initially neutral stimulus *q.v.* that acquires reinforcing properties through association with another stimulus that is already reinforcing.

CONDITIONED RESPONSE (CR) 1. The response (behavior) that is evoked by the conditioned stimulus *q.v.* after conditioning has taken place. 2. Conditioned reflex *q.v.* 3. In health, many health behaviors are developed by conditioning usually in early childhood. Examples include some safe behaviors, hygiene practices, eating habits, and others. 4. The response elicited by a given neutral stimulus (CS) after it has become conditioned by repeated contingent pairings with another stimulus (UCS) that naturally elicits the same or a similar response. 5. A learned response to a stimulus not originally capable of arousing the response. cf: classical conditioning theory.

CONDITIONED STIMULUS (CS) 1. The stimulus that is paired with the unconditioned stimulus *q.v.* and subsequently acquires the capacity to evoke a response similar to the one made to the unconditioned stimulus *q.v.* 2. In health, we respond to many stimuli in our environment such as the smell of food cooking. The smell elicits the hunger response. These factors are also referred to as environmental cues *q.v.* 3. In classical conditioning theory *q.v.*, the stimulus that comes to elicit a new response because of pairing with the unconditioned stimulus. 4. A neutral stimulus that, after repeated contingent pairings with another stimulus (UCS) that naturally elicits a certain response (UCR), comes to elicit the same or similar response, called the conditioned response (CR).

CONDITIONING 1. A basic form of learning in which a given stimulus *q.v.* comes to be associated with another stimulus or with a response. 2. A process to produce changes in a response or habit *q.v.* and is achieved by stimulus substitution. 3. A process in which new objects or situations elicit responses that were previously elicited by other stimuli. cf: classical conditioning theory; instrumental conditioning. 4. Physical training. 5. Sports-related exercise program. ct: exercise prescription.

CONDOM 1. A rubber, latex, or animal skin sheath that is placed over the penis *q.v.* to prevent sperm *q.v.* from reaching the egg and resulting in conception *q.v.* 2. A contraceptive *q.v.* device used by males. Slang: rubber; safe. 3. A prophylactic *q.v.* 4. A thin sheath that is rolled over the erect penis before coitus *q.v.* to provide a barrier to sperm that may enter the vagina. 5. Used to prevent the spread of many sexually transmitted diseases.

CONDUCT DISORDER Patterns of excessive disobedience in children, including theft, vandalism, lying, and early drug use; may be precursors of antisocial personality disorder *q.v.*

CONDUCTION The act of transmitting or conveying certain forms of energy from one point to another without evident movement in the conducting body.

CONDUCTION DEFECT In physiology, blocking of nerve impulses that are needed to produce proper heart action.

CONDUCTIVE DEAFNESS Results from an accumulation of excess ear wax (cerumen) which becomes impacted in the external ear canal preventing sound waves from reaching the ear drum (tympanic membrane). ct: perceptive deafness.

CONDUCTIVE HEARING LOSS 1. Conductive deafness *q.v.* 2. A hearing loss resulting from poor conduction of sound waves along the passages leading to the sense organs.

CONDUCTIVITY The power of transmitting or conveying certain forms of energy.

CONDUCTOR Any substance possessing conductivity *q.v.*

CONDYLE A rounded protuberance at the end of a bone forming an articulation *q.v.*

CONDYLOMAS Small lesions *q.v.* sometimes covered with a scab and found around the mouth and in moist folds of the skin such as anus or genitals *q.v.* cf: condylomata acuminatum.

CONDYLOMATA ACUMINATUM Venereal warts *q.v.*

CONES 1. Visual receptors that respond to greater light intensities and give rise to chromatic *q.v.* visual sensations. ~ are located in the retina of the eye. 2. Retinal elements that respond to colors. ct: rods.

CONFABULATION 1. The filling in of memory gaps with false and often irrelevant details. 2. Fabrication of stories in response to questions about situations or events that are not recalled. 3. Filling in gaps in memory caused by brain dysfunction with made-up and often improbable stories that the subject accepts as true.

CONFEDERATE 1. In research, a person allied or in league with an experimenter. 2. A stooge in a scientific investigation.

CONFERENCE COMMITTEE In politics, a bill may be passed by both houses but in different forms. If the house of origin objects to the version passed by the second house, a special committee is appointed by the leadership to reconcile the differences.

CONFERENCE METHOD In education, training through discussion and sharing of experiences and suggestions on a topic.

CONFIDENCE INTERVAL 1. In statistical research, an interval around a sample mean *q.v.* or proportion within which the population mean is likely to fall. The largest value of the interval is 2 standard errors *q.v.* above the mean and the smallest value is 2 standard errors below the mean. 2. An interval constructed around an observed value such as a test score or a mean within which the true value is believed to lie with a confidence expressed by certain odds. The greater the odds (e.g., from 19 to 1 to 100 to 1) and the less reliable the test, the wider the confidence interval.

CONFIDENCE LEVEL In research, the odds we are willing to accept that express our confidence that the population value is contained within the confidence interval.

CONFIDENCE LIMIT One end of a confidence interval. cf: confidence interval; confidence level.

CONFIDENTIALITY 1. A principle observed by lawyers, physicians, pastors, psychologists, psychiatrists, and other professionals that the professional relationships and private relationships with their clients/patients are not divulged to anyone else. 2. Refers to control of access to information obtained during research or obtained for other purposes but made available for research purposes. Assurance is given that none other than persons working on the study will have access to the data without the subject's permission. Typically, in research, identifying information is destroyed as soon as it is no longer needed for research purposes.

CONFIRMATION BIAS The tendency of a researcher to find evidence to support or confirm his or her hypothesis rather than to seek evidence to determine whether the hypothesis is false.

CONFLICT 1. The situation in which there is simultaneous instigation *q.v.* toward two or more incompatible responses *q.v.* 2. Stress characterized by incompatible desires, needs *q.v.*, or environmental demands. 3. A state of being torn between competing forces.

CONFLICT-HABITUAL MARRIAGE A marriage characterized by unending conflict *q.v.* and disagreement.

CONFLICTING-ATTRACTION Approach–approach conflict *q.v.*

CONFLICTING-AVOIDANCE Avoidance–avoidance conflict *q.v.*

CONFLICT OF LAWS An area of law dealing with the clarification of inconsistencies and differences in laws or jurisdictions as they apply to the rights of individuals in particular actions.

CONFLICT RESOLUTION A process used to resolve differences. All parties accept the agreed upon decision and work together toward a solution.

CONFLUENCE MODEL A model devised by Zajonc and Markus for predicting characteristics of one's intellectual growth curve from knowledge about family size, birth order, and spacing.

CONFLUENT The blending together of the intellectual and affective *q.v.* side of humans.

CONFORMITY 1. A change in belief or behavior as the result of real or imagined social pressure. 2. The tendency to respond as others do.

CONFOUNDING Reflecting the fact that two or more variables *q.v.* that might have caused an effect were simultaneously present, so that we do not know to which to attribute the effect. cf: confounding variable.

CONFOUNDING VARIABLE In epidemiology, a factor related to a health condition that is distributed differently in different groups resulting in confusion in making comparisons of the rates of the health condition in the various groups. cf: confounding.

CONFOUNDS Variables whose effects are so intermixed that they cannot be measured separately, making design of the experiment internally invalid and its results impossible to interpret.

CONGENERS 1. Chemical compounds that are the by-products or waste products from the distillation of alcohol *q.v.* 2. Nonalcoholic substances present in minute quantities in all alcoholic beverages, excluding water. 3. Naturally occurring by-products of the fermentation *q.v.* process in alcoholic beverages. Thought to contribute to stomach upset, nausea, and headache. ~ contribute to the taste, odor, and color of distilled spirits.

CONGENITAL A condition occurring during fetal *q.v.* development or at the time of birth.

CONGENITAL ANOMALY An abnormality present at birth.

CONGENITAL DEFECT 1. Any physical abnormality present at birth. 2. Congenital malformation. 3. Congenital anomaly *q.v.*

CONGENITAL HEART DISEASE 1. A defect of the heart that is present at birth. 2. Conditions that ensue for inborn anomalies *q.v.* in heart structure of functioning. cf: congenital defect.

CONGENITAL MALFORMATION Congenital defect *q.v.*

CONGENITAL MICROPHALLUS An unerect penis at birth less than three-quarters of an inch long. This condition may require medical attention.

CONGENITAL POLYPOSIS A congenital defect *q.v.* in which a number of polyps *q.v.* grow in the colon and rectum.

CONGENITAL RUBELLA SYNDROME 1. Infant defects resulting from a woman's infection *q.v.* with the rubella *q.v.* virus during the first trimester of pregnancy *q.v.* 2. Effects on the infant of rubella contracted by the mother during the first trimester of pregnancy which generally include deafness, cataracts, heart disease, retardation, or some combination of these.

CONGENITAL SYPHILIS Syphilis *q.v.* resulting in the transmission of the spirochete *q.v.* from the mother to her unborn baby before or during birth. Incorrectly referred to as hereditary syphilis *q.v.* since syphilis is not caused by any genetic anomaly *q.v.*

CONGESTIVE DYSMENORRHEA A heaviness and aching sensation in the abdomen accompanied by nausea *q.v.*, edema *q.v.*, constipation *q.v.*, headache, backaches, discomfort in the breasts, and psychological *q.v.* uneasiness during menstruation *q.v.*

CONGESTIVE HEART FAILURE The inability of the heart to pump blood efficiently resulting in an accumulation of blood and fluid in certain parts of the body, such as the lungs, liver, kidneys, and legs.

CONGO MATABY An African term for marijuana *q.v.*

CONGREGATE HOUSING Apartment houses or group accommodations that provide health care and support services to functionally impaired older persons who do not need routine nursing care.

CONGRUENCE OF EXPLANATION AND EVIDENCE Evidence that an effect occurred agrees with the explanation advance for the cause-and-effect relationship; a condition strengthening the inference of causation *q.v.*

CONJOINED Joined together as characterized in Siamese twins.

CONJUGAL DELUSION The unfounded conviction that one's spouse is unfaithful.

CONJUGAL FAMILY A nuclear family *q.v.*

CONJUGAL LOVE Realistic love *q.v.*

CONJUGATION 1. Joining of two gametes *q.v.* that are usually not sexually differentiated. 2. Fusing of gametes. 3. Side-by-side association or synapsis *q.v.* of homologous chromosomes *q.v.*, as in meiosis *q.v.* 4. In biology, the joining of Paramecia or other protozoans as a part of the fertilization *q.v.* process. 5. In bacteriology, physical contact, through a conjugation bridge *q.v.*, for transferring genetic *q.v.* material from a donor to a receptor bacterium *q.v.*

CONJUGATION BRIDGE Connection formed between bacteria *q.v.* through which genetic *q.v.* material is transferred.

CONJUNCTIVA 1. The thin and transparent layer of epithelial *q.v.* tissue covering the eye. 2. The mucous membrane *q.v.* that lines the eyelid and covers the eyeball.

CONJUCTIVAL INJECTION Reddened, irritated appearance of the whites of the eyes.

CONJUNCTIVITIS Pertaining to an inflammation *q.v.* of the conjunctiva *q.v.* of the eye.

CONJUNCTIVITIS NEONATORUM An infection *q.v.* of the eye, specifically the conjunctiva *q.v.*, acquired by infants during birth from a birth canal *q.v.* infected with gonococcal, staphylococcal, streptococcal, or pneumococcal *q.v.* bacterial *q.v.* Silver nitrate solution was used to prevent the infection from gonococcal bacterium but has been replaced by other medications, while antimicrobial drugs are used to prevent infection from the other microorganisms *q.v.*

CONNECTEDNESS In sociology, a coined term denoting insight *q.v.* into how one affects or is affected by others.

CONNECTICUT SOCIETY FOR MENTAL HYGIENE Founded on May 6, 1908, by Clifford Beers. It was the forerunner to the establishment of the National Committee for Mental Hygiene in 1909 and the launching of the Mental Health Movement *q.v.*

CONNECTIVE TISSUE A fibrous body tissue with a variety of functions. ~ forms the structural material of some body organs. ~ supports and connects internal organs and attaches the muscles to bones. cf: ligaments; tendons.

CONNECTIONIST THEORY A theory of psychology that is based on the assumption that behavior is triggered by exposure to certain stimuli, or nodes, and that such behavior is predictable based on which stimulus is present.

CONNOTATIVE MEANING The suggestive significance of a word. ~ is distinguished from its explicit reference to physical or other events or relationships.

CONPORNS Jargon for people who are opposed to pornography.

CONSANGUINEOUS FAMILY 1. A group of people whose members are all related by blood or believed to be blood related. 2. Consanguineous relatives *q.v.*

CONSANGUINEOUS RELATIVES 1. Those related by blood as opposed to by marriage or adoption *q.v.* 2. Consanguineous family *q.v.*

CONSCIENCE 1. One's psyche *q.v.* that distinguishes right from wrong. 2. The superego *q.v.* 3. The functioning of a person's system of moral values in the approval or disapproval of his or her own thoughts and actions. 4. A sense of moral responsibility that many believe to be uniquely human. In Freudian theory, the human ~ is represented by the superego.

CONSCIOUS Those aspects of mental function of which a person is aware. cf: conscious action.

CONSCIOUS ACTION 1. Occurring as a result of the perceptive attention of the person. 2. Occurring on purpose. 3. Actions that one is aware of. cf: conscious. ct: automatic; instructive; unconscious action.

CONSCIOUSNESS A state of being aware. cf: conscious.

CONSCIOUSNESS RAISING A technique that aims to sensitize group members to oppressive influences on their lives and to develop a sense of solidarity and a means of collective defense within the group.

CONSENSUAL ADULTERY Adultery *q.v.* in which people agree to their mate's extramarital activity. cf: consensual extramarital sex; consensual sexual behavior.

CONSENSUAL EXTRAMARITAL SEX Sexual activity outside of marriage and according to terms of an agreement between the spouses. cf: consensual adultery.

CONSENSUAL SEXUAL BEHAVIOR 1. Sexual activity in which the persons involved voluntarily participate. 2. Willing participation in sexual activity. cf: consensual adultery.

CONSENSUS In group dynamics, an agreement on a decision by all persons involved in making the decision.

CONSENSUS RULE IN CAUSAL ATTRIBUTION The greater the consensus *q.v.* in other people's response to a stimulus, the greater the attribution of causality to that stimulus.

CONSENT In law, the agreement or rejection by someone considered legally competent to agree or reject participation in an act. cf: informed consent.

CONSENT DECREE OR ORDER In law, a court-approved agreement that has the force of law.

CONSEQUENCES 1. The results or effects of a decision. 2. In the valuing process, when a person chooses a value, he or she must consider the possible effects of each alternative.

CONSERVATION 1. In psychology, the understanding that certain attributes, e.g., substance and number, remain unchanged despite various transformations. 2. The ability to recognize that properties stay the same despite changes in appearance. 3. In ecology, the efforts made to protect the environment from adverse changes.

CONSERVATION MOVEMENT In education, the movement to influence educational programs by conservation groups.

CONSIDERATION BEHAVIOR In group dynamics, leadership behavior that reflects friendship, mutual trust, respect, and warmth in the relationship between the leader and the followers.

CONSIDERATION IN CONTRACTS In law, the inducement, usually an amount of money.

CONSOLIDATION In education, combining smaller school districts into larger districts in order to provide better school facilities and increase educational opportunities.

CONSONANCE OF CHILD ATTRIBUTES WITH SITUATION A close match between a child's attributes and situational features, such as parent attributes or teacher attributes. cf: dissonance of child attributes.

CONSTANT COMPARISON METHOD In research, fieldnotes are coded as the study progresses, and new instances of a dimension or a concept *q.v.* of interest are sought until saturation. These concepts are linked with others to develop a theory or explanation that is constantly compared with new data from the field. Discrepancies call for modification or additions that increase understanding.

CONSTANT DOLLARS In economics, dollar amounts that have been adjusted by means of price or cost indices to eliminate inflationary factors and allow direct comparison across years. ~ are expressed in two ways: (a) according to the calendar year and (b) according to school year.

CONSTANT STIMULI A method of obtaining difference thresholds *q.v.* in which various stimuli are judged with respect to a single standard stimulus *q.v.*

CONSTIPATION 1. Difficulty or inability to have a bowel movement. 2. A decrease in the frequency of bowel movements, usually accompanied by prolonged or difficult passage of stools. Causes include poor diet, decreased fluid intake, or incorrect use of laxatives *q.v.* Normal bowel movements range from two a day to one every 3 days. ct: diarrhea.

CONSTITUENT In politics, a citizen residing within the district of a legislator.

CONSTITUTION 1. In psychology, the relatively constant biological makeup of the person resulting from the interaction of heredity *q.v.* and environment *q.v.* 2. In law, the supreme organic and fundamental law of a nation or state establishing the character and conception of its government; laying the basic principles to which its internal life is to be conformed; organizing the government; regulating, distributing, and limiting the functions of its departments; prescribing the extent and manner of the exercise of sovereign powers.

CONSTITUTIONAL AMENDMENT In law, a change in the provisions of a constitution *q.v.* by modifying, deleting, or adding portions.

CONSTITUTIONAL MAJORITY In politics a bare majority of all members of each house, not merely the members voting on a given issue.

CONSTITUTIONAL PREDISPOSITION A tendency to develop some behavioral attributes more readily than others, perhaps reflecting genetic *q.v.* influences.

CONSTITUTIONAL THEORY OF PERSONALITY 1. According to Sheldon, temperament and physical constitution *q.v.* are correlated. 2. Body type theory *q.v.*

CONSTITUTIVE BACTERIA Bacteria *q.v.* producing specific enzymes *q.v.* in the absence of their substrate.

CONSTRICTION Binding or contraction of a part.

CONSTRICTION OF THINKING A narrowing focus of the mind that is symptomatic *q.v.* of acute *q.v.* suicidal tendencies.

CONSTRUCT 1. An abstract conceptualization such as intelligence, creativity, or dependence, that is inferred from what people do. 2. An entity inferred by a scientist to explain an observed phenomenon. cf: mediator.

CONSTRUCTIONIST THEORY OF PERCEPTION A theory holding that emotions are complex social performances that vary according to historical and cultural context.

CONSTRUCTION THEORY OF PERCEPTION An assertion that visual patterns are constructed based on visual expectation.

CONSTRUCT VALIDITY 1. Validity *q.v.* 2. How accurately a test measures a particular attribute. ct: content validity. cf: face validity; concurrent validity. 3. The extent to which performance on a test fits into a theoretical scheme about the attribute which the test attempts to measure. 4. Validity established by demonstrating that measures obtained on a test function as they should according to some theory *q.v.*

CONSULTATION The process of a third party assisting a person, group, or organization to use internal and external resources to make decisions and affect change.

CONSULTING STAFF Usually, a board-certified *q.v.* specialist with experience and skill whose advice is sought by a hospital's staff of physicians.

CONSUMER One who purchases health products and services.

CONSUMER BILL OF RIGHTS Principles devised by the late President Kennedy that states that consumers have the right to safety, to be informed, to choose, and to be heard.

CONSUMER HEALTH 1. One of the many content areas of the health education program *q.v.* 2. A term used to describe the degree to which a person uses reliable health services and purchases necessary health products. 3. Intelligent decisions pertaining to the purchase and use of products and services that will directly effect one's health.

CONSUMER HEALTH EDUCATION 1. All children, youth, and adults are consumers of health *q.v.* in one way or another. The purposes of ~ are to (a) inform people about health, illness, disability, and ways in which they can improve and protect their health, and more efficient use of the health care delivery system, (b) motivate people to want to change to more healthful practices, (c) help people learn the necessity to adapt and maintain healthful lifestyles, (d) foster teaching and communications skills in all those engaged in educating consumers about health, (e) advocate changes in the environment that facilitate healthful conditions and healthful behavior, and (f) add knowledge through research and evaluation concerning the most effective ways of achieving these objectives. 2. A process that informs, motivates, and helps people to adopt and maintain healthful practices and lifestyles, advocates environmental changes as needed to facilitate this goal, and conducts research to this same end.

CONSUMERISM Consumer *q.v.* advocacy and awareness.

CONSUMER MARKET People who buy and use the products and services of others.

CONSUMER MODEL A type of relationship between client and an intervenor wherein the client is the consumer *q.v.* who enters the marketplace seeking specific services from an intervenor or change agent *q.v.* The consumer purchases the services for a negotiated or agreed upon price.

CONSUMER-ORIENTED EVALUATION An evaluation *q.v.* intended to serve the information needs of consumers *q.v.*

CONSUMER PARTICIPATION IN HEALTH PLANNING The involvement of consumers *q.v.* of health services *q.v.*

in planning the health services they are to receive with the intention of making programs more relevant to their needs.

CONSUMER PRICE INDEX (CPI) 1. An index established by the U.S. Department of Labor for measuring changes in the prices of consumer *q.v.* products using a base year index for comparisons. 2. Statistical measure of changes in the prices of goods and services brought by urban wage earners and clerical workers. It is also called the cost-of-living index. cf: cost-of-living index.

CONSUMER PROTECTION Laws, programs, and agencies whose basic concern is to prevent industries from developing health products and providing health services based on greed or carelessness and unethical or fraudulent practices.

CONSUMER UNIT 1. Pertains to all members of a particular household who are related by blood or legal arrangements. 2. Persons living alone or sharing a household with others. 3. Two or more persons living together who are making joint expenditure decisions. All units are considered financially independent.

CONSUMMATORY BEHAVIOR Behavior *q.v.* that fulfills some motive *q.v.* The consummatory response *q.v.* indicates that the goal has been achieved. cf: appetitive behavior.

CONSUMMATORY RESPONSE 1. Action that represents the completion of goal-seeking activity *q.v.* 2. Behavior that fulfills some motive *q.v.* cf: consummatory behavior.

CONTACT COMFORT The warmth and comfort infants derive from touching their mothers or other caretakers. ~ is an aspect of normal sexual development.

CONTACT DERMATITIS An inflammation *q.v.* of the skin that results from contact with material to which a person is allergic *q.v.*

CONTACT HOUR In education, a unit of measure that represents an hour of scheduled instruction to learners.

CONTACT HYPOTHESIS The hypothesis *q.v.* that bringing conflicting groups together will reduce their antagonism.

CONTACT INHIBITION The ability of a tissue, on reaching its maturity, to suppress additional growth.

CONTAGION 1. In social psychology, the spreading of a behavior pattern through a large number of people. 2. Modeling effect *q.v.* 3. In epidemiology and medicine, nongenetic transmission of a disease-causing organism from one person to another.

CONTAGIOUS A disease that is communicable *q.v.* only on direct contact with an infected *q.v.* person. cf: communicable; communicable disease.

CONTAGIOUS DISEASE 1. An infectious *q.v.* disease *q.v.* transmissible by direct contact. 2. Communicable diseases *q.v.* cf: contagious.

CONTAINMENT THEORY A situation where the internal components in a person and the buffers in the external social structure operate together to prevent social deviancy *q.v.*

CONTAMINATE To soil, or to make inferior by contact or mixture. cf: contamination.

CONTAMINATED Soiled with infectious *q.v.* matter.

CONTAMINATED NEEDLE A needle or works that has been previously used by or among drug addicts *q.v.* with infected blood or blood particles left on the needle and passed on to the next user. This is a significant problem in regards to AIDS *q.v.* transmission.

CONTAMINATED WITH RADIOACTIVE MATERIAL Exposed to or bearing radioactive *q.v.* material on the surface.

CONTAMINATION The presence of pathogens *q.v.* or nonpathogens on inanimate objects. ct: decontamination.

CONTEMPLATION A meditative technique wherein all attention is focused upon a problem, proposition, saying, and so forth, involving thought and observing of the thought process by the core self.

CONTENT 1. In education, the content areas *q.v.* 2. Informational content *q.v.* 3. Subject matter. 4. Facts *q.v.* 5. The subject matter contained in written curriculum guides *q.v.*

CONTENT AREAS Instructional content *q.v.* areas for health education. Although the ~ may vary somewhat, the following areas have been suggested for secondary school: (a) personal health, (b) mental health, (c) emotional health, (d) disease prevention and control, (e) nutrition education, (f) substance use and abuse, (g) safety education, (h) community health, (i) consumer health, (j) environmental health, and (k) family life education. cf: informational content.

CONTENT MEDIATION In group conflict situations, the mediator affects suggestions for compromise or redefining. cf: Process mediation.

CONTENT VALIDITY 1. Validity *q.v.* 2. How well the test items measure what they are intended to measure. 3. Validity established demonstrating that a test provides a measure of the materials for which it was designed. 4. Accuracy of a measure's representation of the variable *q.v.* it attempts to measure. 5. Comparison of the items of the test with a table of specifications or test blueprint to determine whether the items representatively sample the behaviors and content of the subject matter the test is intended to cover. 6. Curricular validity. cf: face validity. ct: construct validity.

CONTEXT THEORY OF MEANING The theory *q.v.* that the meaning of a specific item depends upon the situation in which it occurs.

CONTEXT EFFECTS Top-down processes *q.v.*

CONTIGUITY The togetherness in time of two events that is sometimes interpreted as the condition that leads to association.

CONTINENCE A state of exercising self-restraint, especially in regard to the sex drive.

CONTINGENCY A relationship between events in which one event is dependent upon the other event.

CONTINGENCY APPROACH TO MANAGEMENT Managing approach that emphasizes that what managers do in practice depends upon a given set of circumstances or situation.

CONTINGENCY CONTRACTING 1. A procedure in which treatment or education personnel writes specific agreements with students or clients that specify the amount and kind of behavior necessary to obtain a reward. 2. Education, an agreement between teacher and learner that a particular reward is forthcoming upon the completion of an agreed upon assignment. ct: contract approach.

CONTINGENCY FUND Money appropriated by the respect houses for incidental operating expenses.

CONTINGENCY THEORY There is not one best way to handle a problem. Concerns the determination of technique or approach that will work best under a given set of circumstances.

CONTINGENCY THEORY OF LEADERSHIP A leadership concept that hypothesizes that in any given leadership situation, success is primarily determined by the following: (a) the degree to which the task being performed by the following is structured, (b) the degree of the position power possessed by the leader, and (c) the type of relationship that exists between leader and followers.

CONTINGENT CONDITION In research, a condition that is necessary for an effort to occur but not sufficient to make it appear.

CONTINUATION RATE In family planning, pertaining to the percentage of women who continue to use a contraceptive *q.v.* device after a specified period of time.

CONTINUING EDUCATION 1. In education, college- or university-sponsored programs that range from skills building seminars to a degree program. 2. Extended opportunity for study and training following completion of or withdrawal from full-time school and/or college programs. 3. Often required in professions in order to maintain licensure.

CONTINUITY THEORY In education, the theory *q.v.* that learning occurs gradually and consists of the slow accumulation of increments of a tendency to respond in a particular way.

CONTINUOUS DUTY As applied to emergency communications systems, a rating applied to receivers and transmitters to indicate their capability for use in a continuous duty cycle. ct: intermittent duty.

CONTINUOUS PERFORMANCE TEST (CPT) A test of additional functioning in which the subject is presented with a series of letters at a rapid rate and must respond to the appearance of one particular letter or sequence of letters.

CONTINUOUS REINFORCEMENT In conditioning, reward or punishment administered regularly after each correct response *q.v.* cf: classical conditioning theory; instrumental conditioning.

CONTINUOUS TELEMETRY The transmission of measured data in a continuous uninterrupted fashion as contrasted with short bursts. ~ transmission by radio requires one channel per transmission, whereas burst transmission allows for channel sharing.

CONTINUOUS TRAIT A trait that can be measured in degrees, such as height or intelligence. ct: threshold trait.

CONTINUOUS VARIABLE 1. In epidemiology, a variable *q.v.* or factor that can have an unlimited number of values on a measurable continuum. 2. Variation not represented by distinct classes. ct: discontinuous variable.

CONTINUUM 1. An uninterrupted gradation of characteristics having infinite intermediate degrees. 2. A series in which the discrete parts are united by a common character. 3. A continuous extent.

CONTINUUM APPROACH In psychology, conceptualizing behavior as ranging from effective functioning to severe personality disorganization *q.v.*, used by psychologists to judge the severity of behavioral abnormality.

CONTRACEPTION 1. Methods used to prevent the sperm *q.v.* from entering the ovum *q.v.* or to prevent the ovum from maturing. There are five general techniques used: (a) mechanical devices including the condom and diaphragm; (b) chemicals used in the form of foams, creams, and jellies called spermicides; (c) hormones, for example, the pill; (d) surgical procedures, for example, sterilization *q.v.* by vasectomy or tubal ligation *q.v.*; and (e) natural methods or rhythm method *q.v.*, coitus interruptus *q.v.*, and total abstinence. ~ includes all artificial methods to prevent sperm from fertilizing an egg or to prevent the egg from implanting on the uterine *q.v.* wall. 2. Any method of preventing pregnancy from blocking union of sperm and egg to preventing production of sex cells to preventing sexual intercourse *q.v.*

CONTRACEPTIVE CREAM A cream applied to the vagina prior to intercourse that contains a spermicide *q.v.* that kills sperm on contact.

CONTRACEPTIVE SPONGE A spermicide *q.v.*-filled disposable sponge worn at the cervix *q.v.* to prevent pregnancy *q.v.*

CONTRACT In law, an agreement, upon sufficient consideration, to do or not to do a particular thing; the writing which contains the agreement of the parties and the terms and conditions and which serves as proof of the obligation. Types of contracts include (a) fixed-price contract, (b) cost reimbursement, (c) cost-plus-fixed-fee contract, and (d) sole–source contract.

CONTRACT ACTION In law, an action brought to enforce rights under a contract *q.v.*

CONTRACT APPROACH In education, an agreement between the teacher and a learner stipulating the nature of an assignment, when it is to be completed, and how it will be evaluated. ct: contingency contracting.

CONTRACTION 1. The shortening of a muscle. 2. Tension of the uterine muscle *q.v.* during labor *q.v.*

CONTRACTING OFFICER The official appointed by the sponsoring agency who is responsible for business management aspects of a particular contract *q.v.*

CONTRACTUAL MARRIAGE 1. A marriage *q.v.* in which the partners agree to periodically renew their marriage agreement, adding and subtracting from it or keeping it as it is. 2. A marriage entered into only after a written contract *q.v.* has been drawn up and signed by the partners. The contract is a document beyond traditional marriage vows. Some believe a ~ is a safety device in preparation for the inevitable divorce *q.v.*

CONTRACTURE A progressive stiffening of the muscles, tendons, and ligaments that surround the joints. ~s tend to develop after a stroke or an injury when prolonged immobility has limited the movement of joints.

CONTRACULTURE In sociology, a cultural group whose behavior *q.v.*, norms, and beliefs are contradictory to the larger, established culture.

CONTRAINDICATION 1. In medicine, a situation in which a particular treatment or procedure is medically inadvisable. 2. The presence of factors that make use of a particular drug inappropriate or dangerous for a particular person.

CONTRALATERAL Pertaining to the opposite side.

CONTRARY CASES In research, cases that are sufficiently beyond the boundaries of a term that they help delineate its boundary. Used in conceptual analysis *q.v.* to help establish defining characteristics of a term.

CONTRIBUTING CONDITIONS In research, conditions that make an effect more likely to occur but are neither necessary nor sufficient to cause it to appear. cf: contingent condition.

CONTROL 1. Making something happen the way it was planned to happen. 2. The hallmark of any experiment. 3. To conduct an experiment in such a way as to control the independent variable *q.v.* and all extraneous variables. cf: control condition; control group.

CONTROL CONDITION In research, the condition of subjects whose behavior is not manipulated. Used for purposes of comparison. cf: control.

CONTROL FUNCTION Computer activities that dictate the order in which other computer functions are performed.

CONTROL GROUP 1. The group of people in an experimental study whose conditions remain constant; who are not exposed to the stimulus *q.v.* being studied. 2. A reference group *q.v.* in an experiment. 3. In epidemiology, a group held constant in a case–control or experimental study design against which changes in the group or dependent variable *q.v.* can be measured. 4. The subjects in an experiment for whom the independent variable *q.v.* is not manipulated, thus forming a baseline against which the effects of the manipulation can be evaluated. 5. A group of individuals similar to the test group and used for comparison purposes in scientific experimentation. ct: experimental group. cf: controlled experiment; control condition; control.

CONTROLLED BREEDING STUDIES Studies that use inbreeding or selective breeding in order to determine the relative roles of heredity *q.v.* and environment in creating individual differences.

CONTROLLED DRINKING 1. A pattern of alcohol *q.v.* consumption that is moderate and avoids the extremes of total abstinence and of inebriation. 2. The concept that individuals who have been drinking pathologically *q.v.* may be taught to drink in a controlled, nonpathological manner.

CONTROLLED EXPERIMENT An experiment characterized by a test group and a control group *q.v.* Experimental conditions are identical for both groups except for a single condition or factor. Comparison of results of the test group with those of the control group should reveal the effect (if any) of the test factor or condition. cf: control; control condition.

CONTROLLED OBSERVATION A diagnostic procedure in which the experimenter observes an individual's behavior under standard conditions in the laboratory.

CONTROLLED STUDY A procedure where an assumed cause or related factor is observed while other influences are controlled.

CONTROLLED SUBSTANCE A drug or chemical regulated under the federal Controlled Substances Act of 1970. Its manufacture, distribution, and sale are subject to federal controls. The major criterion for controlling a substance is its potential for abuse and dependence liability.

CONTROLLED VARIABLE A variable *q.v.* whose value is held constant throughout an experiment *q.v.* cf: control; control condition; control group.

CONTROLLING 1. In epidemiology, examining the effect of one variable *q.v.* on a health condition while taking into account the effect of another variable. 2. In educational management, the process that the administrator goes through to control *q.v.*

CONTROL PRACTICES In parenting, procedures parents use to exert their will in situations of parent–child conflict. General categories for ~ include power assertion, love withdrawal, and induction.

CONTROL PROCESSES In memory model, the processes used to transfer, store, and retrieve information.

CONTROL TABLE In epidemiology, a graphic presentation of data relating to two or more variables *q.v.* while illustrating or controlling for the effect of other variables.

CONTROL TOOL A specific procedure or technique that presents pertinent organizational information in such a way that a manager is aided in developing and implementing appropriate control strategy.

CONTUSION 1. A bruise. 2. Rupturing of blood vessels in the skin. 3. Brain bruises caused by compression of neural tissue against the skull which results in loss of consciousness and sometimes permanent impairment. 4. The reaction of body soft tissue to a direct blow characterized by edema *q.v.* and ecchymosis *q.v.* of the tissue.

CONVALESCENCE 1. The period of recovery from a disease. 2. Convalescent stage of a disease *q.v.*

CONVALESCENT STAGE OF A DISEASE Following the decline stage *q.v.*, symptoms have disappeared and the person is entering the recovery period *q.v.*

CONVENIENCE SAMPLE A sample *q.v.* that is not representative of the population about which inferences will be made.

CONVECTION 1. The conveyance of heat in liquid or gaseous form by the movement of heated particles. 2. The loss of body heat to the atmosphere when air passes over the body.

CONVENE In politics, the meeting of the legislature daily, weekly, and at the beginning of the session as provided by the constitution or law.

CONVENTIONAL ADULTERY Adultery *q.v.* in which people hide their extramarital relationships from their mates.

CONVENTIONAL LEVEL OF MORAL REASONING Kohlberg's second level of development of moral reasoning in which judgments are based on doing the right thing as prescribed by social convention.

CONVENTION (CONSTITUTIONAL) The assembling of citizens or delegates for the purpose of writing or revising a constitution *q.v.*

CONVERGENCE 1. The movement of the eyes as they rotate toward each other to focus upon an object. 2. A primary cue to depth and distance provided by kinesthetic *q.v.* stimuli produced by the turning of the eyes to obtain images on both retinae *q.v.*

CONVERGENT EVOLUTION The independent development of similar structures in forms of life that are unrelated or only distantly related.

CONVERGENT LEARNING Learning in which there is only one answer to be learned.

CONVERGENT THINKER A person who tends to respond to questions in a predictable and conventional way. ct: convergent thinker.

CONVERGENT THINKING Thinking that is directed at producing a single, correct answer to a problem. ct: divergent thinking.

CONVERGENT VALIDITY A description of identical results from more than a single method of inquiring into the same research question. cf: replicability; validity.

CONVERSION DISORDERS 1. Conversion hysteria (now obsolete). 2. A condition in which physical symptoms appear to have no physical basis. 3. Conversion reaction *q.v.* 4. A somatoform disorder *q.v.* in which muscular functions are impaired, usually suggesting neurological disease, even though bodily organs are sound.

CONVERSION PRIVILEGES A feature or clause of an insurance plan that allows an insured to change from one type of policy to another as circumstances in life or insurance needs change.

CONVERSION REACTION 1. Changing intense anxiety *q.v.* into bodily functional *q.v.* symptoms. 2. A neurosis *q.v.* characterized by loss of sense or paralysis of some part of the body. 3. Previously called hysteria *q.v.* ~s are controlled by the sensorimotor nervous system *q.v.* 4. An ego defense process by which emotional conflicts *q.v.* are converted into physical illness symptoms. cf: psychophysiological disorders.

CONVERSION THERAPY Treatment for homosexuals *q.v.* who want to become heterosexuals *q.v.* Research shows such initiatives are not very successful.

CONVULSION 1. An involuntary, uncontrollable muscle contraction. 2. Violent and extensive twitching of the body caused by involuntary pathological *q.v.* muscle contractions.

CONVULSIVE THERAPY 1. Treatment used for some forms of psychoses *q.v.* The treatment causes the person to experience controlled convulsions *q.v.* Two methods have been used: (a) electroconvulsive shock treatment *q.v.* and (b) insulin shock treatment *q.v.* 2. A biological therapy which includes convulsions by drugs or electric shock in the hope of affecting beneficial behavior change.

COOING A meaningless vocalization that is purely vocalic consisting of vowel-like sounds.

COOL-DOWN 1. In physiology and exercise, the use of 5–10 min of very light exercise movements at the end of a vigorous workout to slowly cool the body to near normal core temperature. 2. The last phase of an exercise prescription *q.v.* that helps the body to return to its normal metabolic *q.v.* state immediately after exercise.

COOLEY'S ANEMIA A genetic *q.v.* disorder characterized by the inability of the body to produce hemoglobin *q.v.* A person with ~ must have blood transfusions. The disease can be detected by a simple blood test; but the positive diagnosis requires hemoglobin electrophoresis testing *q.v.* cf: Cooley's anemia trait.

COOLEY'S ANEMIA TRAIT A genetic condition when a person has the recessive gene *q.v.* for Cooley's anemia *q.v.* Those with the trait are healthy and will not suffer the symptoms of the disease but may pass the defective gene *q.v.* to their offspring.

COOLIDGE EFFECT The availability of a new sexual partner that stimulates the male's desire to have intercourse with the new partner.

COOLING-OFF PERIOD In labor relations, a provision of law that postpones a strike or lockout action to give mediation agencies an opportunity to settle a dispute.

COOPERATION A social process whereby each person or groups work together to achieve mutually agreed upon goals.

COOPERATIVE EDUCATION 1. A method employed in which learners teach each other or share knowledge of experiences. 2. A system employed by some states in which resources are shared among school districts. cf: Antioch Plan.

COOPERATIVE LEARNING 1. Learning characterized by learners teaching each other or sharing each other's knowledge. 2. Working together to achieve learning goals. The opposite of competitive learning *q.v.*

COOPERATIVE PLAY Play that is organized for some specific purpose and that requires a division of labor. Players are easily distinguished from nonplayers in ~.

COORDINATE REPRESSION In genetics, control of structural genes *q.v.* in an operon *q.v.* by a single operator gene.

COORDINATION The orderly arrangement of a group effort to provide unity of action in the pursuit of a common purpose.

COPE 1. To overcome problems. 2. To deal adequately with frustrations of a person's needs and desires. 3. To adjust *q.v.* When a person copes with a situation, anxiety *q.v.* is reduced. cf: coping.

COPING 1. The ability to deal adequately with an environmental situation or with oneself. 2. Adjustment *q.v.* 3. The process of adjusting or accommodating to the demands of stress *q.v.* and daily living without being overwhelmed so that one's personal and social effectiveness is maintained. cf: coping mechanism; cope.

COPING MECHANISM 1. In psychology, a variety of complex, usually unconscious devices used to handle frustrations or ego threats. 2. In health, also called defense mechanisms *q.v.* These are frequently used as mental attempts to adjust *q.v.* to emotionally or intellectually threatening situations. A term used by psychologists, psychiatrists, social workers, mental hygienists, and others concerned with mental health and some forms of mental and emotional therapy.

COPING SKILLS Techniques one uses for coping *q.v.* cf: coping mechanisms.

COPING STRATEGIES 1. The ways people devise to help prevent, avoid, or control emotional distress. 2. Coping skills *q.v.* 3. Methods of thinking and behaving that are developed in order to deal with a difficult or learned helplessness.

COPOLYMERS Mixtures of more than one polymer *q.v.*

COPROLALIA 1. Sexual arousal through the use of lewd language or of hearing lewd language. 2. Scatologia *q.v.*

COPROPHILIA 1. A sexual variance in which sexual gratification is associated with the act of defecation *q.v.* 2. A morbid interest in feces *q.v.* 3. Sexual arousal from viewing feces or perceiving the odor of feces.

COPULATION 1. Sexual intercourse *q.v.* 2. Coitus *q.v.*

COPULIN A pheromone *q.v.* produced by dogs.

COPY CHOICE In genetics, an explanation for crossing over *q.v.* which assumes that crossing over occurs during the process of chromosome *q.v.* duplication. First suggested by J. Belling in 1930. Duplication or copying proceeds partially alone one homologue and partially along another.

CORACIDIUM In biology, a ciliated *q.v.* free-living stage that emerges from some tapeworm *q.v.* eggs when they hatch.

CORACOID As used in anatomy, like a raven's beak in form or shape.

CORE CURRICULUM In education, required curriculum *q.v.* for all students. Curriculum design in which one subject or group of subjects becomes a focal unit around which all other subjects are correlated.

CORE GENDER IDENTITY The deeply held inner conviction of one's maleness or femaleness that develops in the first few years of life. The sex chromosomes *q.v.* and the gonads *q.v.* a child inherits *q.v.*, the appearance of the child's genitals *q.v.*, and how the child and others see his or her body all influence the formation of ∼.

CORE PROTEINS Proteins *q.v.* that make up the internal structure or core of a virus *q.v.*

CORE TEMPERATURE A body temperature measured centrally as within the rectum *q.v.*

CORIUM 1. True skin. 2. Derma *q.v.*

CORN 1. Medically, heloma *q.v.* 2. Painful foot condition; two types: (a) soft corn, in inflammation *q.v.* of flesh between the toes, and (b) hard corn, hardened, thickened place on the skin, usually the toes, resulting from rubbing or pressure.

CORNEA 1. The clear and transparent membrane *q.v.* covering the anterior part of the eye. 2. The external covering of the eye.

CORNELL MEDICAL INDEX A self-administered medical history form developed at Cornell University Medical School.

CORNERING FORCE The force that results from the steering wheel of an automobile and creating a drag of the tires strong enough to shove the tire over, thereby changing the direction of travel of the car.

CORNIFIED 1. Converted into horny tissue. 2. Keratinized *q.v.* 3. Describing the outmost layer of the epidermis *q.v.*

CORN SYRUP Liquid dextrose *q.v.*

CORONA 1. In anatomy, the ridge at the back of the glans penis *q.v.* 2. The raised rim above the body of the penis that begins the glans penis.

CORONA GLANDIS Corona *q.v.*

CORONAL Of or like a crown.

CORONAL RIDGE 1. The edge of the head of the penis *q.v.* 2. Corona *q.v.* 3. Corona glandis *q.v.*

CORONARY 1. Encircling. 2. In the form of a crown. cf: coronary arteries.

CORONARY ARTERIES The two large arteries that supply blood to the heart muscle. Impairment or blockage of one or more of these arteries can lead to a heart attack *q.v.*

CORONARY ARTERY BYPASS SURGERY A surgical procedure designed to improve blood flow to the heart by providing alternate routes for blood to take around the points of arterial blockage.

CORONARY ARTERY DISEASE A disease *q.v.* resulting from an irregular thickening of the inner layer of the walls of the coronary arteries *q.v.* which conduct blood to the myocardium *q.v.*; the lumens *q.v.* of these arteries are narrowed and the blood supply to the heart muscle is reduced.

CORONARY ATHEROSCLEROSIS A disease process characterized by fatty thickening of the intima *q.v.* of the coronary arteries *q.v.*

CORONARY CIRCULATION That part of the circulatory system *q.v.* that supplies the heart with blood and hence oxygen, food, and the elimination of wastes.

CORONARY DISEASE Inability of the coronary arteries *q.v.* to conduct blood to the heart muscle. cf: coronary heart disease.

CORONARY EMBOLISM A blockage of a coronary artery *q.v.* resulting from a clot.

CORONARY HEART DISEASE (CHD) 1. A condition in which there is a deficient blood supply to the cardiac muscle *q.v.* It is caused by a narrowing of one or more of the coronary arteries *q.v.* resulting in a reduction of blood supply to the cardiac muscle. The obstruction of the flow of blood to the coronary arteries is called ischemia *q.v.* 2. A buildup of cholesterol *q.v.* within the coronary arteries that supply the heart muscle. 3. Angina pectoris *q.v.*, chest pains caused by insufficient supply of blood and thus oxygen to the heart, and myocardial infarction *q.v.* in which the blood and oxygen supply are reduced so much that the heart muscles are damaged.

CORONARY HEART DISEASE RISK FACTORS There are two general classes of risk factors: (a) those that cannot be changed such as age, sex, family history, and personality type and (b) those that each person has some control over such as serum cholesterol level *q.v.*, blood pressure, and smoking behavior.

CORONARY OCCLUSION An obstruction in a branch of a coronary artery *q.v.* that interferes with the flow of blood to parts of the heart muscle.

CORONARY THROMBOSIS 1. The formation of a blood clot on the rough inner surfaces of the atherosclerotic plaque *q.v.* 2. A blood clot in a coronary artery *q.v.*

CORPORA CAVERNOSA The twin cylinders of spongy tissue in the penis *q.v.* that become engorged with blood which results in an erection *q.v.* Also present in the clitoris *q.v.* cf: corpora spongiosa

CORPORAL PUNISHMENT Infliction of physical punishment on the body of a student by a school employee for disciplinary reasons.

CORPORATE HEALTH EDUCATION Occupational health education; those health education programs that are performed for the benefit of employees.

CORPORATION Generally, a large profit-making business or industrial enterprise owned by stockholders and governed by a board of directors.

CORPUS 1. The upper two-thirds of the uterus *q.v.* 2. Body.

CORPUS CALLOSUM A mass of white matter connecting the cerebral hemispheres *q.v.*

CORPUSCLE 1. The red or white cells of the blood. 2. Erythrocyte or leukocyte *q.v.* 3. Very small body or particle.

CORPUS LUTEUM 1. A yellow mass formed in the ovary *q.v.* at the site of the ruptured ovarian follicle *q.v.* When impregnation *q.v.* takes place, the ~ grows and persists for several months. If impregnation does not occur, the ~ shrinks and degenerates. 2. The cellular remnant of the graafian follicle *q.v.* after release of the ovum *q.v.* 3. The ovarian follicle after the discharge of the ovum, persisting as a yellow mass that secretes progesterone *q.v.* and estrogen *q.v.*

CORPUS SPONGIOSUM A spongy body in the penis *q.v.* that contains a network of blood vessels and nerves. 2. A cylinder of spongy tissue in the penis that becomes engorged with blood during erection *q.v.* cf: corpora cavernosa.

CORRECTION FOR ATTENUATION In research, a formula for correcting a correlation coefficient *q.v.* for unreliability in the measures and estimating the size of the relationship if the reliability *q.v.* were perfect.

CORRECTIVE 1. An approach to discipline. 2. Counseling attempts to achieve cooperation. 3. Discipline that is progressive.

CORRECTIVE ACTION A managerial activity aimed at bringing organizational performance up to the level of performance standards.

CORRECTIVE EMOTIONAL EXPERIENCE A therapeutic approach which stresses that past anxieties can be confronted, and strong, blocked emotions must be reexperienced before meaningful relearning is possible.

CORRELATED HEALTH EXPERIENCES Health learning or teaching within the health education program *q.v.* that is associated with learning taking place within another curriculum discipline.

CORRELATED HYPOTHESIS Any of a variety of hypotheses *q.v.* entertained by subjects in experiments on verbal conditioning *q.v.* that attributes reward to some form of behavior other than that being reinforced, but leads to reward more often than would happen by chance because the behavior is somehow related to what is being rewarded.

CORRELATION 1. The tendency of two variables *q.v.* to vary together. 2. The relationship of a change in one variable to a change in other variables. 3. An interdependence existing between two sets of data or quantities such that when one changes the other does also. cf: Pearson product–moment correlation.

CORRELATION ANALYSIS Ascertaining whether or not a relationship exists between two variables.

CORRELATIONAL METHOD A method of psychological *q.v.* investigation in which the attempt is to discover the interrelationships among response measures. cf: correlational studies. 2. A research method involving the measurement of several variables to determine to what extent they are related.

CORRELATIONAL STUDIES 1. Studies dealing with the extent to which two or more variables covary. 2. Investigations that measure the relationship between two or more variables without experimental manipulation. cf: correlational method.

CORRELATION COEFFICIENT 1. A number, referred to as *r*, that expresses both the size and the direction of a correlation *q.v.*, varying from +1.00 through 0.00 to −1.00. Plus 1.00 is perfect, positive correlation, 0.00 is no correlation, while −1.00 is perfect negative correlation. 2. A number that indicates the degree of relationship of two measures obtained on the same unit, usually an individual.

CORRESPONDENCE STUDY Now largely obsolete, in education, learning by written assignments that are mailed to the instructor for grading and comments.

CORROSION The wearing away gradually by pressure or dissolution, as that of tissues distended by a tumor *q.v.* or an aneurysm *q.v.*

CORROSIVE An agent that produces corrosion *q.v.*, such as an acid.

CORROSIVE POISON Acids, alkalis, and petroleum products that burn and inflame body tissues on contact.

CORTEX 1. The outer cells of the human embryo's indifferent gonad *q.v.* These cells may develop into female ovaries *q.v.* 2. The outer part of an internal organ. 3. In botany, the outer primary tissues of the stem or root, extending from the primary phloem *q.v.* to the epidermis *q.v.* composed chiefly of parenchyma cells *q.v.*

CORTI (ORGAN OF) The receptor for hearing which lies within the cochlea *q.v.*

CORTICOID Pertaining to hormones *q.v.* of the adrenal cortex *q.v.*

CORTICOTROPHIN-RELEASING FACTOR A chemical messenger produced by the hypothalamus *q.v.* and released into the closed circulatory pathway shared with the pituitary gland *q.v.* ~ stimulates the pituitary's production of ACTH *q.v.*

CORTIN 1. A hormone *q.v.* from the cortex *q.v.* of the adrenals *q.v.* ~ has been used in treating Addison's disease *q.v.* 2. A hormone secreted by the cortex of the suprarenal gland *q.v.*

CORTISOL 1. A hormone *q.v.* generated by the adrenal cortex *q.v.* ~ influences the body's control of glucose *q.v.*, protein *q.v.*, and fat metabolism *q.v.* 2. Hydrocortisone *q.v.* 3. Compound F *q.v.* 4. A glucocorticoid *q.v.*

CORTISONE A hormone *q.v.* secreted by the adrenal cortex *q.v.*

CORYNEBACTERIUM DIPHTHERIEA The bacillus *q.v.* that causes diphtheria *q.v.*

CORYZA 1. Head cold. 2. A disease caused by an unidentified virus *q.v.* ~ is transmitted by direct or indirect contact with an infected person. It is characterized by nasal discharge, watery eyes, low fever, headache, and cough.

COSMETICS Substances intended to cleanse, beautify, promote attractiveness, or alter appearance. They are applied by rubbing in, pouring on, sprinkling on, or spraying on specific parts of the body, usually to the face area.

COSMIC RADIATION Extremely high energy radiation *q.v.* consisting of both particles and rays that originate in space and bombard the earth.

COSMIC RAYS High velocity particles of enormous energy bombarding the earth from outer space. The primary radiation *q.v.* consists of protons *q.v.* and more complex atomic nuclei which, on striking the atmosphere, give rise to neutrons *q.v.*, mesons, and other less energetic secondary radiating particles.

COSMOS 1. All of the space and matter in the known universe. 2. The spiritual environment.

COSPONSOR In politics, one of two or more persons proposing any bill or resolution.

COSTAL In anatomy, pertaining to the ribs.

COSTAL ARCH In anatomy, the fused costal *q.v.* cartilage of ribs 7–10. The arch forms the upper limit of the abdomen *q.v.*

COST–BENEFIT ANALYSIS 1. In safety epidemiology, the cost of changes made to increase safety as compared to the costs of accidents or illnesses resulting from exposure to the uncorrected hazardous situation. 2. In business, the method to investigate costs and benefits in monetary terms and to find alternatives for which the cost–benefit relationship best satisfies the decision rule that management has decided to apply. 3. Determination of the costs of achieving certain benefits. cf: cost-effective.

COST-EFFECTIVE The degree to which a program is effective in relation to its cost. cf: cost–benefit analysis.

COST-EFFECTIVENESS ANALYSIS 1. Determination of the cost of achieving certain levels of effectiveness. 2. A means of analyzing the extent to which an undertaking accomplishes its objectives in relation to its cost.

COST-OF-LIVING ESCALATORS Pay adjustments geared to increase the Consumer Price Index *q.v.*

COSTO-VERTEBRAL ANGLE The angle by the spinal column *q.v.* and the 12th rib. This is the general anatomic location of the kidneys

COTA An acronym for certified occupational therapy assistant.

CO-TWIN In behavior genetics, research using the twin method *q.v.*, the member of the pair who is tested later to determine whether he or she has the same diagnosis or trait discovered in his or her birth partner, the index case *q.v.* cf: co-twin control.

CO-TWIN CONTROL A method of experimentation on the nature/nurture problem *q.v.* in which the subjects are pairs of twins, one being assigned to the experimental condition and the other being assigned to the control *q.v.* condition.

COUGH MEDICINE A compound that contains chemicals intended to relieve the cough reflex *q.v.*

COUNCIL OF CHIEF STATE SCHOOL OFFICERS An organization representing state education commissioners, superintendents, etc., with respect to all aspects of public education.

COUNCIL FOR EDUCATION IN PUBLIC HEALTH (CEPH) An organization comprised of representatives of the major public health professional organizations that sets standards and procedures for the accreditation for schools of public health and for those public health programs outside schools of public health.

COUNCIL FOR INTERNATIONAL ORGANIZATION OF MEDICAL SCIENCE A branch of the World Health Organization *q.v.* In 1968, the Council established five criteria for determining the presence of death: (a) loss of all responses to the environment, (b) complete lack of any reflexes and the loss of muscle tone, (c) cessation of spontaneous respiration, (d) abrupt drop in arterial blood pressure, and (e) a flat electroencephalogram (EEG) *q.v.*

COUNSELING The process by which a counselor *q.v.* assists a person or group to identify and deal with situations or information related to interactions with others and enables the person or persons to make effective decisions.

COUNSELING SERVICE Activities designed to assist students in making plans and decisions related to their education, career, or personal development.

COUNSELING PSYCHOLOGY A branch of psychology *q.v.* in which the psychologist *q.v.* attempts to help a person solve certain adjustment problems through counseling *q.v.* Problems are usually related to education, occupations, sex, or marriage.

COUNSELOR A person who advises others with relatively normal health problems. Training may be in areas associated with finance, psychology *q.v.*, social interactions, family relations, or religion.

COUNT The most basic quantitative measure in epidemiology *q.v.* Pertains to a notation that X number of people in a particular population have, for instance, developed human immunodeficiency virus (HIV) *q.v.* infection.

COUNTERBALANCE DESIGNS In research, studies designed such that if two or more treatments are administered in sequence, the treatments are administered in all possible sequences so as to reveal and eliminate the effect of ordering. cf: counterbalancing.

COUNTERBALANCING In research, in equivalence reliability *q.v.*, eliminating the effect of the order in which two tests were taken by giving half the group one order and the other half the reverse order and analyzing the combined results. cf: counterbalance designs.

COUNTERCONDITIONING 1. The process for weakening a classically conditioned response *q.v.* by connecting the stimulus *q.v.* that evokes it to a new response that is incompatible with the conditioned response *q.v.* 2. The replacement of one conditioned response by the establishment of an incompatible response to the same conditioned stimulus *q.v.* 3. Relearning achieved by eliciting a new response in the presence of a particular stimulus.

COUNTERIRRITANT Preparation containing an irritant applied to the skin to stimulate sensory receptors *q.v.*, increase blood flow, and induce a sensation of warmth. ~ may have an analgesic *q.v.* effect.

COUNTERIRRITATION An irritation of the skin that is deliberately induced to relieve pain or inflammation *q.v.* elsewhere by reflex action *q.v.*

COUNTERPHOBIA 1. Engaging in the feared activity. 2. Encountering the feared object or activity.

COUNTERSTAIN A background stain applied to stained material to increase contrast.

COUNTERTRANSFERENCE 1. A form of transference *q.v.* recognized by psychoanalytic theory *q.v.* in which the analyst develops strong emotional attachments for his or her patient. 2. Feelings that the analyst *q.v.* unconsciously directs to the analysand *q.v.* but which come from his or her own emotional vulnerabilities and unresolved conflicts.

COUPLING 1. *Cis*-arrangement *q.v.* 2. The condition in linked inheritance *q.v.* in which an individual heterozygous *q.v.* for two pairs of genes *q.v.* received the two dominant members from one parent and the two recessive *q.v.* from the other parent. cf: repulsion.

COURSE OF STUDY A detailed written guide for each grade or developmental level of learners. Such a guide contains all the essential information and components for developing the lesson plan *q.v.*

COURSE OUTLINE A written document containing objectives for each lesson and details the specific material to be covered along with suggested methodology *q.v.* cf: course of study.

COURTESAN A prostitute *q.v.*, especially mistress of noblemen.

COURTESY STAFF A physician who is permitted to admit patients into a particular hospital, but who does little work within the hospital.

COURT OF RECORD In law, a court whose actions are recorded, possessing the authority to levy sanctions.

COUVADE The practice among some cultures wherein the man suffers the same symptoms during pregnancy *q.v.* as those of the partner, the pregnant woman, is experiencing.

COVARIANCE The change of two phenomena in relationship to each other.

COVARIANCE MODELING Structural covariance *q.v.*

COVARIATION PRINCIPLE The rule that an effect will be attributed to the condition that is present when the effect is present or absent when the effect is absent.

COVERT 1. Concealed. 2. Disguised. 3. Not directly observable.

COVERT BEHAVIOR Behavior *q.v.* that is disguised or concealed and not directly observable. cf: covert.

COVERT DESENSITIZATION In psychology, the linking of a previous anxiety *q.v.*-provoking stimulus *q.v.* with rewarding outcomes in fantasy *q.v.* ct: covert sensitization.

COVERT PARTICIPANT OBSERVATION In research, an observation method whereby the observer becomes part of the situation in such a way that individuals are not aware they are being observed. cf: covert behavior.

COVERT SENSITIZATION 1. A behavior therapy *q.v.* technique whereby the person learns to associate negative feelings with the undesirable behavior by thinking of the negative associations. 2. A form of aversion therapy *q.v.* in which the subject is told to imagine the undesirably attractive situations and activities at the same time that unpleasant feelings are being induced by imagery. ct: covert desensitization.

COVERTURE A feudal doctrine adopted into English common law that asserted that after marriage, a woman must turn all her property and money over to her husband. During the 1800s, the laws in the United States gradually rescinded such custom.

COWPER'S GLANDS 1. A pair of small glands *q.v.* located in the lower abdomen *q.v.* of the male that secrete a lubricating fluid into the urethra *q.v.* upon sexual arousal and that contribute a small amount of fluid to the semen *q.v.* 2. The glands that produce the pre-ejaculatory fluid in the male. 3. Glands producing a substance to neutralize the acidity of the urethra in the male before intercourse *q.v.* 4. Bulbourethral glands *q.v.*

CP 1. An acronym for creatine phosphate *q.v.* 2. Cerebral palsy.

CPA An acronym for Canadian Physiotherapy Association. 2. Certified public accountant.

CPI An acronym for consumer price index.

CPR An acronym for cardiopulmonary resuscitation *q.v.*

CPT An acronym for Continuance Performance Test *q.v.*

CR An acronym for conditioned response *q.v.*

CRAB LOUSE 1. Pediculosis. 2. A louse of the *Phthirus pubis* family. 3. The infestation *q.v.* of the ~ is characterized by itching in the genital *q.v.* area with resulting dermatitis *q.v.* 4. Pediculosis pubis *q.v.*

CRADLE CAP A grayish-yellow crusting condition that may appear in infants as a result of inadequate cleansing.

CRAFT UNIONS In labor relations, an organization of workers in a single craft.

CRAMP 1. A painful muscular spasm *q.v.* 2. A gripping pain in the abdominal region. 3. Colic *q.v.*

CRANIAL Pertaining to the cranium *q.v.*

CRANIAL NERVES The twelve pairs of nerves passing from the brain directly to the tissues without traversing the spinal cord. cf: spinal nerves.

CRANIOTOMY 1. A surgical opening made into the skull for the purpose of obtaining surgical access to the brain. 2. Trephining *q.v.*

CRANIUM The skeleton of the head. Includes all of the bones of the head except the mandible *q.v.* and the skeleton of the face.

CRANK A slang term used to identify methamphetamine *q.v.*

CRASH A slang expression originally referring to the rapid emotional descent following a binge of amphetamine *q.v.* use. ~ is characterized by long sleep.

CRASHING A slang expression of a disturbing period of mental depression occurring when a person stops taking a central nervous system *q.v.* stimulant *q.v.* after a period of chronic *q.v.* drug use.

CRAVAT A special type of bandage made from a large triangular piece of cloth, usually muslin or cotton.

CRAVING An overwhelming desire to use a drug or other substances, usually to increase positive feelings and to decrease the negative experience of a withdrawal syndrome *q.v.*

CRAZY A slang and unscientific term pertaining to mental disorders.

CREATION-SCIENCE The study of the development of humanity based on the Bible.

CREATINE 1. A nonprotein nitrogenous substance in muscle tissue. ~ combines with phosphate *q.v.* to form phosphocreatine *q.v.* which serves as a storage form of high-energy phosphate required for muscle contraction. 2. An energy-rich compound that plays a key role in providing instant energy for muscle contraction.

CREATININE 1. A nitrogenous *q.v.* substance in muscles and urine. 2. A nitrogenous compound that is formed as a metabolic *q.v.* end product of creatine *q.v.* ~ is produced in the muscle, passes into the blood, and is excreted in the urine.

CREATIVE ACTIVITIES In education, learner-centered *q.v.* methods or strategies *q.v.* by which learners can acquire insight *q.v.* into the health problems or ways they can assist others to understand the health problem or health issue. ~ are designed to elicit individual potentials for learning.

CREATIVE MODELING In education, combining or relating significant bits of information into innovative concepts *q.v.* and behavioral *q.v.* patterns.

CREATIVE REGRESSION In psychology, deliberate recreating of the psychotic *q.v.* state to facilitate reintegration of the disordered personality *q.v.*

CREATIVITY 1. Innovative ability. 2. Insightful capacity to adapt means to ends. 3. To move beyond analytical logical approaches to experience.

CREDENTIALING A process of identifying individuals who have met established standards of the profession.

CREDIBLE RESULT In research, a summary judgment of the conceptual and empirical evidence for internal validity (LP) together with a judgment of the consistency of the evidence with prior studies. This results in a determination of the internal validity of the study.

CREDIBILITY OF WITNESSES In law, worthiness of belief in testimony of witnesses.

CREDIT In education, recognition of attendance and/or performance in an instructional activity that can be applied by a recipient to requirements for a degree or diploma.

CREDIT BUYING A system of purchasing goods new and paying for them at a later date.

CREDIT COURSE In education, when successfully complete, can be applied toward the number of courses required for achieving a degree, diploma, certificate, or other formal award.

CREDIT HOUR In education a unit of measure that represents an hour of instruction that can be applied to the total number of hours needed for completing the requirements of degree, diploma, certificate, or other formal award. In most institutions, one credit hour is the equivalent to approximately 15 clock hours.

CREDIT UNIONS Employee-operated mutual benefit organizations for savings and low interest loans.

CREMASTER The muscles that elevates the testes *q.v.*

CREMASTER MUSCLE The muscle that extends from the testes *q.v.* into the spermatic cord *q.v.* and controls the proximity of the testes to the body.

CREMASTERIC REFLEX The contraction of the scrotum *q.v.* up toward the pelvis *q.v.* when the inner thigh is stimulated.

CREMATION The incineration of the remains of a dead person.

CRENATION 1. Plasmolysis *q.v.* 2. The shriveling of a cell because of water withdrawal.

CREPITATION A grating sensation felt between the ends of a broken bone.

CREPITUS 1. The grating sensation of the tow ends of a broken bone rubbing together. 2. The bubbly sensation of air palpated in tissues. 3. A specific crackling sound heard in the lung with a stethoscope *q.v.* when pneumonia *q.v.* is present.

CRETINISM 1. A condition caused by thyroid malfunction. ~ typically includes feeble mindedness *q.v.* 2. A mental and physical disorder associated with thyroid *q.v.* deficiency at an early age and usually involves low intelligence *q.v.* 3. A condition beginning in prenatal *q.v.* or early life characterized by mental retardation *q.v.* and physical deformities, caused by severe deficiency in the output of the thyroid gland.

CRF An acronym for corticotrophin-releasing factor *q.v.*

CRIB DEATH 1. Sudden infant death syndrome (SIDS) *q.v.* 2. Unexpected and unexplained death of a well infant.

CRIBIFORM Sieve-like.

CRIBIFORM HYMEN 1. A hymen *q.v.* in which there are three or more openings. A sieve-like covering of the vaginal *q.v.* opening. ct: annular hymen; imperforate hymen.

CRICOID Ring-shaped. cf: cricoid cartilage.

CRICOID CARTILAGE The lowermost of the laryngeal *q.v.* cartilages *q.v.*

CRICO-THYROID MEMBRANE The fibrous portion of the larynx *q.v.*

CRICO-THYROIDOTOMY An incision into the lower airway through the crico-thyroid membrane.

CRICOTHYROTOME A surgical instrument used to make an opening into the trachea *q.v.* through the crico-thyroid membrane *q.v.*

CRIME 1. An act that violates a law. 2. A felony *q.v.* or misdemeanor *q.v.*

CRIMINAL ABORTION Deliberately precipitated abortion *q.v.* A term pertaining to abortion by persons untrained, unlicensed, who perform the procedure purely for profit.

CRIMINAL ACTION 1. In law, a proceeding by which a party charged with a crime *q.v.* is brought to trial, convicted, and punished. 2. A court action, brought by the state, against one charged with an offense against the state. This type of action may result in a fine or incarceration of the defendant.

CRIMINAL BEHAVIOR Antisocial *q.v.* actions that violate some law. A person manifesting criminal behavior may or may not have a psychiatric *q.v.* condition.

CRIMINAL COMMITMENT A procedure whereby a person is confined in a mental institution either for a determination of competency *q.v.* to attend trial or after acquittal by reason of insanity *q.v.*

CRISIS A stressful situation characterized by shock and temporary loss of ability to make decisions.

CRITERIA 1. Predetermined measures against which access, continuity, efficiency, appropriateness, and quality of health education services may be compared. 2. Guidelines.

CRITERIA FOR HEALTH Health criteria *q.v.*

CRITERION 1. Measure to establish to judge proficiency, accomplishment, or success. 2. A standard. 3. A measure generally accepted as valid *q.v.*; a measure to be predicted; a standard to be attained. cf: criteria; criterion-referenced measurement.

CRITERION GROUPS In research, groups whose test performance sets the validity *q.v.* criterion for certain tests.

CRITERION MEASURES In research, measures of behavior *q.v.* against which progress toward goals can be assessed.

CRITERION OF PERFORMANCE Extent of performance *q.v.*

CRITERION-REFERENCED 1. A test to determine an examinee's level of performance in relation to well-defined job-related knowledge and skills. 2. A clear description of a set of skills determined to be essential to performance of a role that can be used in a test situation to determine the person's possession of those skills.

CRITERION-REFERENCED ASSESSMENT Measurement that compares one's performance with an absolute standard, as distinguished from measurement comparing one's performance to that of others.

CRITERION-REFERENCED GRADING A learner's performance is evaluated with reference to specified criteria *q.v.* or to that learner's previous level of performance.

CRITERION-REFERENCED MEASUREMENT A measure designed to yield specific evaluations for the individual learner in terms of clearly defined performance standards.

CRITERION-REFERENCED TEST 1. A test that is designed to assess a student's progress or ability in a particular area. 2. Tests whose scoring is based on meeting the mastery requirements of a content area rather than placing the score in the context of a reference group, such as nonreferenced tests *q.v.*

CRITERION-RELATED VALIDITY 1. Concurrent validity *q.v.* 2. Predictive validity *q.v.*

CRITHIDIA A stage in the life cycle of trypanosomes *q.v.*

CRITICAL-INCIDENT METHOD 1. Performance appraisal. 2. Supervisors list incidents that reflect favorable and unfavorable performance.

CRITICAL PATH That sequence of events and activities within a Program Evaluation and Review Technique (PERT) *q.v.* network that requires the longest period of time to complete.

CRITICAL PERIOD 1. The stage in the development of a person when he or she is especially sensitive to certain environmental influences. Closely related to maturational readiness *q.v.* 2. The period in maturation *q.v.* when the person is physiologically *q.v.* prepared to learn in response to a given type of stimulus *q.v.* 3. Sometimes used in reference to a period of acute stress *q.v.* 4. A period during development when an event must happen or development is forever altered. 5. A period of fixed length during which developmental events have either no effect or a different effect. cf: imprinting; sensitive period.

CRITICAL RATIO In research, a standard score used for testing the null hypothesis *q.v.* ~ is obtained by dividing an obtained mean *q.v.* difference by the standard error *q.v.* so that ~ equals obtained mean difference per standard error.

CRITICAL THINKING One's ability to analyze situations critically.

CRNA An acronym for certified registered nurse anesthetist *q.v.*

CRONBACH'S ALPHA Alpha coefficient *q.v.*

CROP ROTATION The practice of growing different crops in regular succession to aid in the control of insects and diseases, to increase soil fertility, and to decrease erosion.

CROSSBANDING In emergency communications, using VHF equipment to participate in the UHF band of radiofrequencies.

CROSS-BREAK Cross-tabulation *q.v.*

CROSS-CATEGORICAL APPROACH In education, an alternative way of defining and classifying individuals with learning and behavior disorders using descriptors of mild, moderate, and severe or profound multiple problems.

CROSS-COUSIN MARRIAGE A cross-cousin is a child of one's parent's sibling of the opposite gender. There are two forms of ~s: (a) matrilateral cross-cousin wherein the male marries his mother's brother's daughter and (b) patrilateral cross-cousin marriage involves the male child marrying his father's sister's daughter.

CROSS-CULTURAL RESEARCH 1. Ethnographic research. 2. A form of observational research by which investigators study the behavior, customs, and values of people in other cultures. 3. A research method in which people in different societies are compared. cf: observational method.

CROSS-DEPENDENCE 1. In pharmacology, a condition in which one drug can prevent withdrawal symptoms *q.v.*

associated with physical dependence *q.v.* on a different drug. 2. Different drugs may cause physical dependence because of their similar pharmacological activity and can be used interchangeably to prevent withdrawal symptoms.

CROSS-DRESSING Dressing in the clothes of the other sex for sexual arousal.

CROSSING-OVER In genetics, an interchange of parts between the chromatids *q.v.* of two homologous chromosomes *q.v.* at meiosis *q.v.* 2. Mechanism in which a region of one chromosome is replaced by an equivalent region of material from the homologous chromosome. 3. A process inferred genetically by new associations of linked factors and demonstrated cytologically *q.v.* from new associations of parts of chromosomes. It results in an exchange of genes *q.v.* and, therefore, produces combinations differing from those characteristics of the parents. The term genetic crossover may be applied to the new gene combinations. cf: recombination; crossover unit.

CROSS-MATCH A determination of the compatibility of the blood from a donor with that of the recipient before a blood transfusion is conducted. Compatibility is determined by placing red blood cells of the donor in serum *q.v.* from the recipient and red blood cells of the recipient in the serum of the donor. The absence of agglutination *q.v.* indicates that the two blood specimens are compatible.

CROSS-MODEL TRANSFER Being able to make use of information acquired through one sensory modality to solve some problem in another sensory modality. Being able to pick out by touch, for example, some object previously seen but not felt.

CROSSOVER UNIT In genetics, a frequency of exchange of 1% between two pairs of linked genes *q.v.*; 1% of crossing over is equal to one unit on a linkage map. cf: crossing over.

CROSS-POLLINATION In botany, the transfer of pollen *q.v.* from the anther *q.v.* of one plant to the stigma *q.v.* of a flower of another plant.

CROSS-REFERENCES Alternative terms that might also be used to describe a particular word or phrase to which the reader is referred by an abstracting or indexing service.

CROSS-SECTIONAL METHOD 1. In epidemiology, a study design that shows concurrently existing characteristics and health outcomes. 2. Research that assesses patterns of conduct in a population at a given time. 3. Studies in which different age groups are compared at the same time. cf: longitudinal research; cross-sectional research.

CROSS-SECTIONAL RESEARCH 1. Cross-sectional method *q.v.* 2. A design that measures age-related changes by studying the differences between individuals of different ages. 3. Research that involves measuring different groups on the outcome variable and comparing them. ct: longitudinal research.

CROSS-SECTIONAL STUDY 1. Cross-sectional research *q.v.* 2. A research method using subjects of different ages to investigate developmental questions. 3. The study of change that compare current individuals of different age or experience on the variable of interest rather than waiting for change over time.

CROSS-SENSITIVITY A situation in which an allergy *q.v.* to one drug warns of possible similar reactions to other, chemically related substances.

CROSS-SEX TYPING Having interest and attributes stereotypically classed as appropriate for the opposite sex.

CROSS TABULATION 1. In research, tabulation of data in terms of two or more variables *q.v.* For example, respondents' choices of each of five possible answers to a question are tabulated; the tabulations for each response are then categorized by another variable, such as gender. Results would be displayed in a 2 (male, female) × 5 (the number of possible responses) table with the frequency of responses displayed in each cell. 2. Cross beak *q.v.*

CROSS-TOLERANCE 1. A condition in which tolerance to one drug results in a lessened pharmacological *q.v.* response to another drug of the same class even though the person never used this drug before. 2. A tolerance developed for one drug while taking another drug. 3. The development of tolerance to one drug can accelerate the metabolism *q.v.* of, and reduce the nervous system's *q.v.* response to, other drugs that act by the same mechanism.

CROUP A common disease of childhood characterized by spasms *q.v.* of the larynx *q.v.* which interferes with respiration.

CROWDING A stress-related psychological state that may be produced by a perceived high-population density.

CROWNING 1. The presentation of the baby's head at the vaginal *q.v.* opening during the birth process. 2. The point during childbirth when the fetus' head is visible in the birth canal and does not recede with each uterine *q.v.* contraction.

CRTT An acronym for certified respiratory therapy technician.

CRUCIATE Cross-shaped.

CRUDE RATE In epidemiology, the rate of outcome calculated without any restrictions on who is counted. The formula is

$$\frac{\text{Number of persons with the health condition}}{\text{Total population}} \times 1000 \text{ or } 100,000.$$

CRUDE DEATH RATE

$$\frac{\text{Number of deaths}}{\text{Total population}} \times 1000.$$

CRUDE OPIUM Opium *q.v.* extracted from the opium poppy *q.v.* before any processing.

CRUISING 1. Pertains to the homosexual *q.v.* community that refers to a gay *q.v.* person going to a bar, public bath, or party for the purpose of picking up a sexual partner. 2. Searching for a sexual partner.

CRURA Two structures linking the top of the shaft of the clitoris *q.v.* to the public bone. Similar structures link the penis *q.v.* to the pubic bone.

CRURA CEREBRI Fiber tracts of the ventral and lateral regions of the midbrain *q.v.* that connect the spinal cord *q.v.* with the anterior cerebral region.

CRUSHED CHEST Flail chest *q.v.*

CRYOCAPSULE A large thermos-like container in which dead bodies are stored in liquid nitrogen.

CRYONIC SUSPENSION 1. Deep freezing at the time of death to preserve the person until a later date when their diseases or cause of death can be cured. 2. A theoretical process of freezing a person and bringing him or her back to life at a future time.

CRYOSURGERY Destruction of diseased or unwanted tissues by freezing.

CRYOTHERAPY A treatment procedure whereby a cancerous *q.v.* growth is destroyed by freezing.

CRYPT A burial location beneath a church. ct: mausoleum.

CRYPTOCOCCAL MENINGITIS A fungal *q.v.* infection *q.v.* that affects the three membranes (meninges) surrounding the brain and spinal cord. Symptoms *q.v.* include severe headache, vertigo *q.v.*, nausea *q.v.*, anorexia *q.v.*, sight disorders, and mental deterioration.

CRYPTOCOCCOSIS A fungal *q.v.* infectious *q.v.* disease often found in the lungs of AIDS *q.v.* patients. It characteristically spreads to the meninges *q.v.* and may also spread to the kidneys and skin. It is due to the fungus *Cryptococcus neoformans*.

CRYPTORCHIDISM 1. Undescended testicle *q.v.* 2. Failure of the testes *q.v.* to descend into the scrotum *q.v.* 3. Undescended testicles at birth.

CRYPTOSPORIDIOSIS An infection *q.v.* caused by a protozoan *q.v.* parasite *q.v.* found in the intestines of animals. Acquired in some people by direct contact with the infected animal, it lodges in the intestines and causes severe diarrhea *q.v.* It may be transmitted from person to person. This infection seems to be occurring more frequently in immunosuppressed *q.v.* people and can lead to prolonged symptoms *q.v.* that do not respond to medication.

CRYPTOTHERAPY The application of extreme cold to the body cells and tissues.

CRYPTOZOITE A stage in plasmodium *q.v.* life cycle that occurs in the liver.

CRYSTALLINE 1. A substance resembling a crystal. 2. A solid body in which atoms are arranged in a symmetrical pattern.

CRYSTALLINE LENS The transparent structure lying just behind the pupil of the eye that refracts light rays.

CRYSTALLOID Solute particle less than 1 μm in diameter.

CRYSTALLIZED INTELLIGENCE The accumulated information, cognitive *q.v.* skills, and strategies acquired by the application of fluid intelligence *q.v.* to various disciplines. ~ is thought to increase with age.

CS An acronym for conditioned stimulus *q.v.*

CSF 1. An acronym for cerebrospinal fluid *q.v.* 2. The fluid that bathes and cushions nerves in the central nervous system *q.v.* In a spinal tap *q.v.*, ~ is withdrawn.

CTS An acronym for carpal tunnel syndrome *q.v.*

CT SCAN 1. CAT scan *q.v.* 2. A computer-generated cross-sectional image of a part of the body that is produced by specialized X-ray equipment.

CUBITAL Pertaining to the forearm.

CUE In psychology, a stimulus *q.v.* that sets off an internal response to satisfy a drive *q.v.* and external behavior follows. cf: cue function.

CUE FUNCTION An environmental condition that provides the individual with an indication of the direction a behavior response should take.

CUEING Providing clues or evidence to ensure that a person responds to a stimulus.

CUL-DE-SAC The blind alley ending of the vagina *q.v.* just beyond the opening to the uterus *q.v.*

CULDOSCOPY STERILIZATION Cauterization *q.v.* of the fallopian tubes *q.v.* where they join the uterus *q.v.* 2. A method of tubal ligation *q.v.* in which the fallopian tubes are cauterized through incisions at the back of the vagina *q.v.* cf: laparoscopic sterilization.

CULPOTOMY A type of tubal ligation *q.v.* procedure that entails reaching and cutting the fallopian tubes *q.v.* through the vagina *q.v.*

CULTURAL ANTHROPOLOGY A specialized branch of anthropology *q.v.* that compares the similarities and differences among human cultures.

CULTURAL BIAS Accepting one's own cultural values as valid for all.

CULTURAL EVOLUTION 1. The effects of human culture on human evolution *q.v.* 2. The changing pattern in humans that results from the transmission of learned behavior and acquired knowledge.

CULTURAL FAIRNESS OF A TEST The extent to which test performance does not depend upon information or skill provided by one culture but not another. cf: culture fair tests.

CULTURAL FAMILIAL RETARDATION 1. A mild backwardness in mental development with no indication of brain pathology *q.v.*, but evidence of similar limitation in at least one of the parents or siblings. 2. Retardation *q.v.* that has its origins in the general genetic *q.v.* and cultural conditions of families and not any single isolatable cause.

CULTURAL LAG An imbalance or dislocation in a changing culture where one phase lags behind another in rate of change or in status change.

CULTURALLY DEPRIVED Children who are educationally handicapped as a result of their low socioeconomic level and that of their families.

CULTURAL PLURALISM A society composed of many varied cultures *q.v.* forming a unified group.

CULTURAL RELATIVITY An approach to labeling that defines normalcy relative to standards established by a particular social structure.

CULTURAL SCRIPTS Normative statements shared by a group concerning the ways individuals in specific social roles should act, think, and feel.

CULTURAL THEORY OF ALCOHOLISM One of the forms of the sociological *q.v.* theories of alcoholism *q.v.* Specifically, it is thought that as ingestion of alcohol *q.v.* reduces anxiety and tension produced by a society, it is proposed that cultural factors that create these tensions may be responsible for the development of alcoholism.

CULTURAL VALUES 1. Widely held beliefs or sentiment that some activities, relationships, feelings, or goals are important to the community's identity or well-being. 2. What our society expects of us is often integrally related to the values we adopt.

CULTURAL WELL-BEING Interacting with the community. ~ establishes roots in the community and provides a person with a sense of belonging.

CULTURE 1. A pattern set of reaction, habits, customs, and ways of life that are characteristic of a particular group of people. 2. The human aspects of the environment. 3. Shared, relatively stable patterns of belief, thought, and action. Humans alone have culture, and it meshes with biology in the many human arrangements for mating, bearing, and rearing the young. ~ may be viewed as (a) covert, which consists of those shared ways of thinking, feeling, and believing that are usually not directly communicated but whose presence can be detected by long-term residence in a group; or (b) overt, which consists of those elements of ~ that are explicitly stated in obvious ways. 4. The ideas, customs, values, and practices that influence the behavior of a group, organization, or society during a given period of time. 5. In bacteriology, bacteria *q.v.* grown in a growth medium *q.v.*

CULTURE-BOUND The tendency to think that the customs prevailing in one's own culture *q.v.* are the natural and usually superior way of doing things.

CULTURE COMPLEX Culture *q.v.* traits or patterns that combine to achieve a goal.

CULTURE FAIR TESTS Tests designed to be valid *q.v.* for persons from different cultural groups. cf: cultural fairness of a test.

CULTURE-FREE TEST 1. A test designed to reduce or eliminate the influence of different environmental, ethnic, or cultural experiences on test performance. 2. Culture fair test *q.v.* 3. Tests to which a person's responses are presumed to be a fair indication of their abilities regardless of their cultural background. In view of the now recognized interaction of intellect and culture, no longer considered to be a reasonable goal of test development.

CULTURE OF CHILDHOOD The rich repertoire of rituals, activities, traditions, and social codes that children learn from one another rather than from adults.

CULTURE SYSTEM A culture *q.v.* with a high degree of coherence or integration.

CUMULATIVE EFFECTS In pharmacology, drug effects that increase with repeated administrations, usually due to the buildup of the drug in the body.

CUMULATIVE HEALTH FOLDER A form by school health service professionals to maintain records of screening tests, medical examinations, immunizations, illness or disabilities, anecdotal records of health-related behaviors that threaten a pupil's learning ability, and any other relevant information with respect to the education and well-being of a child throughout his or her education.

CUMULATIVE RATE OR INCIDENCE In epidemiology, an incident rate that extends over a given period of time and for which all subjects are followed for this same period of time.

CUNNILINGUS 1. To lick. 2. Oral stimulation of the female genitals *q.v.* 3. The act of using the tongue or mouth in erotic *q.v.* play with the external genitalia.

CURANDERO A specialist in the diagnosis and treatment of illness within the Hispanic folk tradition.

CURARE A drug that is capable of completely paralyzing the skeletal musculature but does not affect visceral *q.v.* reactions.

CURETTAGE The scraping of the interior of an organ or cavity.

CURETTE A metal instrument resembling a spoon with a cup-shaped cutting surface on its end.

CURING In bacteriology, the loss of episomal *q.v.* material from a bacterial *q.v.* population by the inhibition of its further replication.

CURRENS FORMULA An insanity *q.v.* plea following the committing of a crime *q.v.* This is based on the concept that the person committing a crime did not have the capacity to conform to the requirements of the law. cf: McNaghten decision; Durham decision.

CURRENT A stream or flow of fluid, air, or electricity.

CURRENT DEVELOPMENTAL STAGE The development stage that a person is in at a particular point in time. ~ is not necessarily correlated with one's chronological age *q.v.*

CURRENT DOLLARS Dollar amounts that have not been adjusted to compensate for inflation.

CURRENT EXPENDITURES In education, the expenditures for operating public schools excluding capital outlay and interest on school department. The expenditures include such items as salaries for school personnel, fixed charges, student transportation, school books, materials, and energy costs.

CURRENT EXPENSES In education, expenditures that are necessary for daily operation and maintenance.

CURRENT RATIO A liquidity ratio that indicates the organization's ability to meet its financial obligations in the short run. The ratio is determined by:

$$\text{Current ratio} = \frac{\text{Current assets}}{\text{Current liabilities}}$$

CURETTEMENT Dilation and curettage *q.v.*

CURRICULAR DECISIONS The process of establishing educational directions. ~ are based on (a) individuals and organizations, (b) legal agencies, (c) educationists and educators, and (d) students.

CURRICULUM 1. Any and all things that influence in any way the learning or the individual. 2. Usually, some sort of organized and planned procedures for teaching and learning, but may also include those factors and experiences that happen spontaneously. 3. Factors that influence the curriculum are philosophy, goals, mission, society, culture, learners, teachers, educational structure and organization, and learning principles. 4. Planned learning experiences provided by an educational institution. 5. An ongoing continuity of situational school experiences in which teachers are interacting educatively with learners in terms of the cultural conditions, resources, and interactive processes by which learners are actually challenged and zestfully involved. cf: curriculum development.

CURRICULUM DESIGN 1. Planned learning experiences reflecting some pattern of instruction and some framework that organizes appropriate subject matter and content. 2. The format of the curriculum *q.v.* especially in relation to curriculum guide development *q.v.*

CURRICULUM DEVELOPMENT 1. A continuous and planned process embracing initial construction, evaluation, reorganization, experimentation, administration, and all other elements of the school and community that influence the quality of learning and teaching. cf: curriculum. The elements of ~ are (a) goals and objectives, (b) philosophy of health education, (c) organization and administration, (d) teacher competence, (e) learning resources and experiences, (f) program evaluation, and (g) levels of decision making (these levels are societal, institutional, and instructional). 2. That aspect of teaching and administration that designedly, systematically, cooperatively, and continuously seeks to improve the teaching–learning process.

CURRICULUM GUIDE A written plan containing detailed information regarding grade level offerings and other suggestions for the health education program of the school district. It differs from the course of study *q.v.* chiefly in the lack of grade or development level details. The curriculum guide describes overall goals, philosophy, scope, and sequence of the health education program.

CURRICULUM REFORM Movements to change basic curricular options for learners.

CURRICULUM REVISION 1. Changing the nature of the curriculum *q.v.* in view of (a) changed conditions in society, (b) new educational knowledge about the psychology of learning, and (c) new technical knowledge. 2. Changes based on revaluing the curriculum.

CURVATURE OF FIELD In optics, a condition in which the center of the field is in focus but the margins are out of focus.

CUSHING'S SYNDROME An endocrine *q.v.* disorder usually affecting young women, produced by oversecretion of cortisone *q.v.* and marked by mood swings, irritability, agitation, physical disfigurement, obesity, muscular atrophy *q.v.*, and fatigue.

CUSPIDS 1. The teeth used to tear food. 2. The eye teeth. 3. The teeth next to the lateral incisors and before the first bicuspids *q.v.*

CUSTODIAL CHILD A handicapped child below the trainable level for which custodial care is desirable.

CUSTODIAL STUDENT A student who is so limited in mental, social, physical, or emotional development that institutional care or constant supervision at home is required.

CUSTOM A shared way of interacting socially, that has been present in a group for a generation or more.

CUTANEOUS 1. A layer of skin. 2. Pertaining to the skin.

CUTANEOUS BLOOD VESSELS Blood vessels relating to the skin. cf: cutaneous.

CUTICLE 1. A varnish-like layer covering the epidermis *q.v.* 2. The margin of hardened skin around the finger nail or toe nail.

CUT-OFF SCORE A score on a test used for selection below which no person is accepted. The ~ is selected to maximize the number of successes and to minimize the number of failures.

CUT-OFF VALUE The optical density (OD) reading of reference serum in an ELISA test *q.v.* which differentiates a positive from a negative result.

CVA An acronym for cerebral vascular accident *q.v.*

CVD An acronym for cardiovascular disorders *q.v.*

CVS An acronym for chorionic villa sampling *q.v.*

CYANOSIS The presence of a blueness of the skin, especially the lips, caused by an insufficient supply of oxygen in the blood.

CYANOTIC 1. Marked by cyanosis *q.v.* 2. Having a bluish color about the lips or nailbeds.

CYBERNETICS The science that studies the relationship of computer engineering and human neurology *q.v.*

CYCLAZOCINE A synthetic substitute for heroin *q.v.* which reduces the pharmacological *q.v.* effects of heroin. It acts as a narcotic antagonist *q.v.*, produces dependence *q.v.*, withdrawal syndrome *q.v.* ~ produces no further craving for it. Treatment with ~ consists of two steps: (a) use of ~ to reduce craving for heroin, resulting in withdrawal from heroin. Daily injections of ~ obstruct the euphoric *q.v.* effect of heroin and (b) withdraw the addict from ~ which is relatively simple. cf: methadone.

CYCLIC Occurring periodically.

CYCLICAL PSYCHODYNAMICS The reciprocal relations between current behavior and repressed conflicts, such that they mutually reinforce each other.

CYCLOID A personality type *q.v.* characterized by marked mood alterations between elation and depression. cf: cyclothymic personality.

CYCLOSIS The circulatory movement of protoplasm *q.v.* within a cell.

CYCLOTHYMIC 1. A temperament identified by Kretschmer characterized by a person who is jolly, genial, and good-natured but who would fluctuate between elated and depressed moods. ct: schizothymic. cf: cyclothymic personality.

CYCLOTHYMIC DISORDER Chronic mood disturbance characterized by periods of depression and hypomania *q.v.* A milder variant of bipolar disorder *q.v.*

CYCLOTHYMIC PERSONALITY A person characterized by frequently alternating moods of elation and sadness stimulated by internal rather than external events. cf: cyclothymic; cycloid.

CYCLERT A commercial preparation of pemoline *q.v.*

CYST A closed cavity or sac that contains liquid or semiliquid material.

CYSTICERCUS 1. Encysted intermediate stage of a tapeworm formed in the alternate host. 2. The bladder worm or larval stage of certain tapeworms.

CYSTIC FIBROSIS A genetic disorder *q.v.* characterized by a thick, sticky mucus in the respiratory and digestive systems. In the lungs, the mucus interferes with breathing and results is susceptibility to respiratory diseases and lung damage. In the digestive system, the mucus interferes with the secretions of the pancreatic enzymes *q.v.* into the small intestine, resulting in malabsorption of nutrients *q.v.* ~ is caused by a faulty recessive gene *q.v.* ~ can be diagnosed by the sweat test in infants who have a high salt content in their sweat. Treatment consists of (a) postural drainage to expectorate mucus from the lungs and bronchial tubes *q.v.*, (b) the use of aerosol inhalants, (c) medications to prevent infections, (d) diet supplements, and (e) administration of pancreatic enzymes.

CYSTIC MASTITIS Fibrocystic disease *q.v.* characterized by fluid-filled lesions *q.v.* that are tender and that are related to estrogen *q.v.* stimulation.

CYSTINE 1. A sulfur-containing, nonessential amino acid *q.v.* that occurs notably in keratin *q.v.* and insulin *q.v.* In the diet, ~ exerts a sparing effect on methionine *q.v.* 2. A pyrimidine base *q.v.* found in RNA *q.v.* and DNA *q.v.* cf: amino acid.

CYSTITIS Inflammation *q.v.* of the urinary bladder *q.v.* usually characterized by a burning sensation during urination. ~ is often sexually transmitted and afflicts more women than men.

CYSTOCELE In women, a hernia protrusion of the urinary bladder *q.v.* through the vaginal *q.v.* wall.

CYSTOCHROMES Hemoproteins that contain iron. Their principle biological function is electron and hydrogen transport.

CYSTOGENIC 1. Forming cells. 2. Producing cells.

CYSTOGENICS The science of dealing with the study of the structure and function of genes *q.v.* and chromosomes *q.v.*

CYSTOSCOPE An instrument used for visually examining the internal surface of the urinary bladder *q.v.*

CYSTOSCOPY An examination of the interior of the urinary bladder *q.v.* by use of a cystoscope *q.v.*

CYST STAGE The thick-walled resistant stage by means of which parasitic *q.v.* microzoa *q.v.* spread from host to host.

CYTOKINES Powerful chemical substances secreted by cells. ~ include lymphokines *q.v.* produced by lymphocytes *q.v.* and monokines *q.v.* produced by monocytes *q.v.* and macrophages *q.v.*

CYTOLOGY 1. The scientific study of the origin, structure, and functions of cells. 2. The branch of the biological sciences *q.v.* that deals with the structure and processes of protoplasm *q.v.* and the cell.

CYTOLYSIN A substance that destroys cells.

CYTOMEGALOVIRUS (CMV) 1. One of a group of viruses *q.v.* that cause cell enlargement of several internal organs. 2. A member of the herpesvirus group that infects most of humans during childhood or adult life. It can be associated with a congenital *q.v.* infection *q.v.* of infants and infections of bone marrow transplant patients and other patients who have undergone procedures that cause immune *q.v.* suppression. It causes pneumonia and inflammation *q.v.* of the retina, liver, kidneys, and colon in AIDS *q.v.* patients. 3. One of the herpes viruses capable of causing severe damage to a fetus *q.v.* or to a neonate *q.v.*

CYTOMORPHOSIS The series of changes through which cells go in the process of formation, development, and senescence *q.v.*

CYTOPATHIC 1. Cellular destruction. 2. Pertaining to or characterized by abnormal changes in cells.

CYTOPLASM 1. The protoplasm *q.v.* of a cell that does not include the nucleus. 2. The viscous fluid surrounding the cell nucleus *q.v.* and containing cellular organelles *q.v.* 3. The site of most of the chemical activities of the cell.

CYTOPLASMIC Pertaining to or contained in the cytoplasm *q.v.*

CYTOPLASMIC INHERITANCE 1. Hereditary transmission dependent upon the cytoplasm *q.v.* or structures in the cytoplasm rather than the nuclear *q.v.* genes *q.v.* 2. Extranuclear inheritance.

CYTORRHYSIS Wrinkling of the schizophyte *q.v.* cell wall as a result of lacing the cell in a hypertonic solution.

CYTOSOME In biology, an opening into the gullet or cytopharynx of microzoa *q.v.* through which food passes in holozoic nutrition *q.v.* Literally, cell mouth.

CYTOTOXIC Poisonous to cells.

CYTOTOXIC AGENT Chemicals that destroy cells or prevent their multiplication. ~s are used in cancer chemotherapy *q.v.*

CYTOTROPIC Substances having an affinity for cells.

CYTOTOXIC T CELLS A subset of T lymphocytes *q.v.* that carry the T8 marker and can kill body cells infected by viruses *q.v.* or transformed by cancer *q.v.*

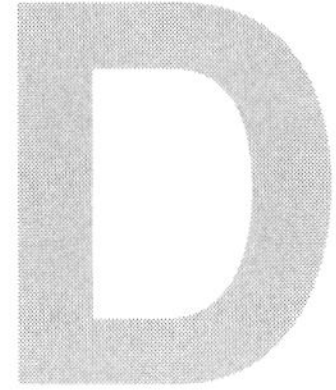

DA An acronym for dopamine *q.v.*

DACRYOCYSTITIS Inflammation *q.v.* of the tear sac of the eye.

DACTYLOGRAM Finger print.

DAGGA South African term for marijuana *q.v.*

DAMAGES In law, pecuniary compensation or indemnity which may be recovered in court by the person who has suffered loss or injury to his or her person, property, or rights through the unlawful act, omission, or negligence of another person.

DAME SCHOOL A low-level primary school in the colonial and early national periods, usually conducted by an untrained woman in her own home.

DANAZOL A drug containing androgens *q.v.* that suppresses production of estrogen *q.v.*

DANDRUFF An infection *q.v.* of the sebaceous glands *q.v.* of the scalp, resulting in flaking of the skin.

DARK ADAPTATION A form of adaptation *q.v.* in which the eye adjusts to low levels of illumination.

DART An acronym for Developmental and Reproductive Toxicology *q.v.*

DARTAL 1. A major tranquilizer *q.v.* 2. A commercial preparation of phenothiazine *q.v.*

DARTH VADAR SYNDROME Fear of a firefighter, especially one who is attired in special firefighting gear. It is especially likely to occur in children during a fire when the firefighter enters the house in which the child is trapped. The child may hide from the firefighter.

DARVON 1. A commercial preparation of propoxyphene *q.v.* 2. Synthetic narcotic *q.v.* closely related to methadone *q.v.* that is used for relief of mild to moderate pain.

DATA (sing.: DATUM) In research, 1. facts and figures, 2. information, and 3. any group of facts from which dedications and conclusions can be made. cf: database; data reduction.

DATABASE A set of facts determined to be adequate for planning or for problem solving. cf: data; data reduction.

DATA REDUCTION Screening out the information that comes to a person through the senses in greater amounts or intensity than can be used in making sense of the environment. cf: data; database.

DATURA 1. In botany, a genus *q.v.* of plants, many of which are anticholinergic *q.v.* 2. The plant genus that includes many species noted for their hallucinogenic *q.v.* properties.

DAUERMODIFICATION 1. A type of acquired characteristic. 2. A characteristic induced by the environment, which persists and appears to be inherited, sometimes for several generations.

DAWN An acronym for The Drug Abuse Warning Network, a federal government system for reporting drug-related medical emergencies and deaths.

DAY-CARE CENTER A place or institution charged with caring for children, typically during normal work hours.

DAY CERTAIN In politics, adjournment with a specific day to reconvene.

DAY HOSPITAL 1. A treatment center providing care for alcoholics *q.v.* or other addicts *q.v.* The person using these facilities has a place to go to at night, but needs assistance during the day. 2. A community-based mental hospital where people are treated during the day, returning home at night. ct: night hospital.

dB An abbreviation for decibel *q.v.*

DBIR An acronym for Directory of Biotechnology Information Resources *q.v.*

DC An acronym for doctor of chiropractic degree. cf: chiropractor.

D&C An abbreviation for dilation and curettage *q.v.*

D-COGNITION 1. According to Maslow, a type of thinking or knowing that is goal oriented, directed toward making sense of the world. 2. Deficiency cognition *q.v.* ct: B-cognition.

DDD SYNDROME Dependency, debility, and dread. The three features of very stressful situations as typified in the procedures used in thought control or brain washing *q.v.*

DDS Doctor of Dental Surgery degree. cf: dentist.

DDST Denver developmental screening test. Designed to detect problems related to the development of children.

DDT 1. An insecticide *q.v.* 2. Dichloro-diphenyl-trichlorethane. 3. A pesticide *q.v.* formerly used to control insect pests, especially on food crops. Its accumulation in the fats of domesticated animals increases the risk of cancer in humans who eat such animals.

D&E Dilation and evacuation method *q.v.*

DEA An acronym for the United States Drug Enforcement Administration, a division of the United States Department of Justice.

DEAF A category for persons who have hearing losses greater than 75–80 dB, who have vision as their primary sensory input, and who cannot understand speech through the ear.

DEAFNESS The inability to perceive sounds. There are two major forms: (a) conductive deafness *q.v.* and (b) perceptive deafness *q.v.*

DEAMINATION 1. The removal of an amino acid *q.v.* from a molecule *q.v.* Some amino acids can be converted to glucose *q.v.* in a process that begins with ~. 2. Elimination of ($-NH_2$) from a carbon skeleton. 3. A chemical reaction by which the amino group, NH_3, is split from an amino acid.

DEATH 1. Cessation of life. 2. A point where life no longer exists. 3. The World Health Organization *q.v.* has established the following criteria to declare that a state of death exists (1968): (a) loss of all responses to the environment, (b) complete lack of any reflexes and the loss of muscle tone, (c) cessation of spontaneous respiration, (d) abrupt drop in arterial blood pressure, and (e) a flat electroencephalogram *q.v.* 4. Recently, the consumption of oxygen by the brain is considered a significant indicator that death has not yet arrived.

DEATH, CAUSES OF See leading causes of death.

DEATH RATE The number of persons who have died in a given period of time and within a specified population size.

DEATH REGISTRATION STATES The states that conform to a uniform death registration system for the purpose of contributing to the national vital statistics system.

DEBATE In politics, discussion of a matter according to parliamentary rules. cf: debates.

DEBATES Learner-centered method typically used to motivate both intellectual and emotional exchange among learners. Through the use of this method, students learn to listen, communicate, and analyze what is being said. It encourages objective thinking and listening.

DEBILITATING A condition that causes weakness and the inability to function adequately under normal environmental conditions. cf: debility.

DEBILITY 1. Weakness. 2. Loss of strength. cf: debilitating.

DEBRIDEMENT The surgical cleansing of a wound by removal of dead, injured, or infected tissue.

DEBRIEFING In research, informing subjects of the true design and purpose of an experiment following their participation in it when partial or deceptive information may have been provided beforehand.

DEBT RATIO A leverage ratio that indicates the percentage of all organizational assets provided by organizational creditors. The formula for calculating ~ is

$$\text{Debt ratio} = \frac{\text{total debt}}{\text{total assets}}$$

DECALCIFICATION The absorption of calcium *q.v.* from a tissue or structure in which it is normally present or is an integral component.

DECARBOXYLATION 1. The removal of a single carbon in the form of CO_2 from a molecule *q.v.* ~ reactions play an important part in the metabolism *q.v.* of glucose *q.v.* 2. The process by which carbon dioxide is eliminated from an organic acid.

DECAY 1. Putrefaction *q.v.* 2. In psychology, a possible factor in forgetting, producing some loss of stored information through erosion of some psychological *q.v.* process.

DECENTRALIZATION The situation in which a significant number of job activities and a maximum amount of authority are delegated to subordinates. cf: decentralized organization.

DECENTRALIZED ORGANIZATION A type of organization in which a great deal of authority is delegated to lower levels of management. cf: decentralization.

DECEREBRATE A condition resulting from brain injury that renders voluntary muscular control and conscious action impossible.

DECIBEL (dB) 1. A unit for measuring the relative loudness of sound on a scale beginning with 1 for the faintest audible sound. 2. The unit of measurement for the volume or intensity of sound. 3. The intensity of any stimulus in ~s is 10 times the logarithm *q.v.* of the ratio of the sound to a standard reference intensity, which is typically in the area of the absolute threshold *q.v.*

DECIDUA The lining of the uterus *q.v.* during pregnancy *q.v.*

DECIDUOUS 1. In botany, the falling parts at the end of a growing period, such as falling leaves in autumn. 2. In anatomy, (a) temporary (b) shedding at a certain stage of growth, as in the ~ teeth *q.v.*

DECIDUOUS TEETH 1. The temporary teeth that appear before the permanent teeth. 2. The baby teeth. 3. The milk teeth.

DECISION 1. A choice made between two or more available alternatives. 2. In law, a conclusion or judgment of a court, as opposed to the reasoning or opinion of the court.

DECISION-DRIVEN EVALUATION Describing an evaluation *q.v.* used to help in the making of a decision *q.v.*, thus influencing both development and implementation.

DECISION MAKING 1. The process by which an individual, organization, community *q.v.*, or society agrees upon a course of action or a solution to an issue. 2. The process of forming probability estimates of events and using them to choose between different courses of action. 3. In health education, a learner-centered method in which learners are given several alternatives and allowed to discover the consequences of each, resulting in the best decision for person health action. cf: decision-making skills.

DECISION-MAKING INTERVIEW Information and related data *q.v.* are gathered, compared to criteria *q.v.*, and a conclusion is drawn or a determination is made.

DECISION-MAKING METHOD In education, a learner-centered method in which the learner is given several alternatives and allowed to discover the consequences of each, resulting in the best decision *q.v.* for personal action.

DECISION-MAKING SKILLS Processes one needs for making decisions *q.v.* based on facts, evidence, consequences, and selection. cf: decision making; decision-making method.

DECISION TREE A graphic decision-making *q.v.* tool typically used to evaluate decisions *q.v.* containing a series of steps.

DECLARATION OF GENEVA A statement adopted by the Second General Assembly of the World Medical Association in 1948. "At the time of being admitted as member of the Medical Profession I solemnly pledge myself to consecrate my life to the service of humanity. I will give to my teachers the respect and gratitude which is their due; I will practice my profession with conscience and dignity; the health of my patient will be my first consideration; I will respect the secrets that are confided in me; I will maintain by all means in my power, the honor and the noble traditions of the medical profession; my colleagues will be my brothers; I will not permit considerations of religion, nationality, race, party politics, or social standing to intervene between my duty and my patient; I will maintain the utmost respect for human life, from the time of conception; even under threat, I will not use my medical knowledge contrary to the laws of humanity. I make these promises solemnly, freely, and upon my honor." cf: Hippocratic Oath; Nightingale Pledge; Prayer of Maimonides.

DECLARATION OF HAWAII The General Assembly of the World Psychiatric Association established the following guidelines for psychiatrists worldwide in 1976:

1. The aim of psychiatry is to promote health and personal autonomy and growth to the best of his or her ability, consistent with accepted scientific and ethical principles, the psychiatrist shall serve the best interests of the patient and be concerned for the common good and a just allocation of health resources. To fulfill these aims requires continuous research and continual education of health care personnel, patients, and the public.

2. Every patient must be offered the best therapy available and be treated with the solicitude and respect due to the dignity of all human beings and to their autonomy over their own lives and health. The psychiatrist is responsible for treatment given by the staff members and owes them qualified supervision and education. Whenever there is a need, or whenever a reasonable request is forthcoming from the patient, the psychiatrist should seek the help or the opinion of a more experienced colleague.

3. A therapeutic relationship between patient and psychiatrist is founded on mutual agreement. It requires trust, confidentiality, openness, cooperation, and mutual responsibility. Such a relationship may not be possible to establish with some severely ill patients. In that case, as in the treatment of children, contact should be established with a person close to the patient and acceptable to him or her. If and when a relationship is established for purposes other than therapeutic, such as in forensic psychiatry, its nature must be thoroughly explained to the person concerned.

4. The psychiatrist should inform the patient of the nature of the condition, of the proposed diagnosis and therapeutic procedures, including possible alternatives, and the prognosis. This information must be offered in a considerate way and the patient be given the opportunity to choose between appropriate methods.

5. No procedure must be performed or treatment given against or independent of a patient's own will, unless the

patient lacks capacity to express his or her own wishes, owing to psychiatric illness, cannot see what is in his or her own best interest or, for the same reason, is a severe threat to others. In these cases, compulsory treatment may or should be given, provided that it is done in the patient's best interests and over a reasonable period of time. A retroactive informed consent can be presumed, and, whenever possible, consent has been obtained from someone close to the patient.

6. As soon as the above conditions for compulsory treatment no longer apply, the patient must be released, unless he or she voluntarily consents to further treatment. Whenever there is compulsory treatment or detention, there must be an independent and neutral body of appeal for regular inquiry into these cases. Every patient must be informed of its existence and be permitted to appeal to it, personally or through a representative, without interference by the hospital staff or by anyone else.

7. The psychiatrist must never use the possibilities of the profession for maltreatment of individuals or groups, and should be concerned to never let inappropriate personal desires, feelings, or prejudices interfere with the treatment. The psychiatrist must not participate in compulsory psychiatric treatment in the absence of psychiatric illness. If the patient or some third-party demands actions contrary to scientific or ethical principles, the psychiatrist must refuse to cooperate. When, for any reason, either the wishes or best interests of the patient cannot be promoted, he or she must be so informed.

8. Whatever the psychiatrist has been told by the patient, or has noted during examination or treatment, must be kept confidential unless the patient releases the psychiatrist from professional secrecy, or else vital common values or the patient's best interest makes disclosure imperative. In these cases, however, the patient must be immediately informed of the breach of secrecy.

9. To increase and propagate psychiatric knowledge and skill requires participation of the patients. Informed consent must, however, be obtained before presenting a patient to a class and, if possible, also when case history is published, and all reasonable measures must be taken to preserve the anonymity and to safeguard the personal reputation of the subject. In clinical research, as in therapy, every subject must be offered the best available treatment. His or her participation must be voluntary, after full information has been given of the aims, procedures, risks, and inconveniences of the project, and there must always be a reasonable relationship between calculated risks or inconvenience and the benefit of the study. For children and other patients who cannot themselves give informed consent, this should be obtained from someone close to them.

10. Every patient or research subject is free to withdraw for any reason at any time from any voluntary treatment and from any teaching or research program in which he or she participates. This withdrawal, as well as any refusal to enter a program, must never influence the psychiatrist's efforts to help the patient or subject. The psychiatrist should stop all therapeutic, teaching, or research programs that may evolve contrary to the principles of this Declaration. cf: Declaration of Geneva.

DECLARATIVE KNOWLEDGE 1. The knowledge of facts and specific bits of information. ct: procedural knowledge. 2. Knowing what as contrasted with knowing how.

DECLARATORY JUDGMENT In law, a judgment establishing the rights of the parties or deciding a point of law without an order for any action.

DECLARATORY RELIEF In law, a judgment that declares the rights of the parties or expresses the opinion of the court on a question of law without ordering anything done.

DECLINE STAGE OF DISEASE When symptoms *q.v.* of the disease *q.v.* disappear and the person feels better but is still sick.

DECLINING ENROLLMENTS In education, a trend where the number of students entering school is less than the number leaving or graduating from school. A trend experienced in the 1980s.

DECODER 1. Destination. 2. That person or people in the interpersonal communication situation with whom the source or encoder *q.v.* attempts to share information.

DECODING A component of information theory *q.v.* consisting of interpretation of the symbols of communication.

DECOMPENSATION 1. In psychology, ego or personality *q.v.* disorganization under excessive stress *q.v.* 2. In physiology, the failure of the heart, as a result of disease *q.v.*, to maintain sufficient circulation of the blood to meet the demands of the body. ct: recompensation.

DECONDITIONING In psychology, the extinction of a learned habit by means of conditioning *q.v.* techniques. cf: classical conditioning theory; instrumental conditioning.

DECONGESTANT A drug that constricts blood vessels and membranes *q.v.* of the respiratory passages to relieve stuffiness or congestion.

DECONTAMINATE To rid clothing, bed linen, a room, or vehicle of dangerous substances—poisonous gases, microorganisms *q.v.*, sputum, feces, or urine—usually in connection with contagious *q.v.* diseases or radioactivity *q.v.*

DECONTAMINATION Killing or removing pathogens *q.v.* from inanimate objects. Methods used for ~ are incineration, drying, ultraviolet rays, or chemicals. cf: disinfection.

DECREASED AWARENESS In psychology, a condition of escaping from reality, problems, physical and emotional pain; desire for total narcosis *q.v.* or insensibility.

DECREASING RADIUS TURN In driving, a curve that becomes increasingly tighter as one drives into it.

DECREE In law, order of court of equity announcing the legal consequences of the facts found.

DECRIMINALIZATION 1. Legal process of reducing the penalty for a particular behavior still restricted by law. 2. The elimination of legal penalties for an act previously considered illegal.

DECUBITUS ULCER 1. Bed sores. 2. Pressure sores. 3. ~ develops when the skin overlying a bony structure is subjected to prolonged, unrelieved pressure. The most common of these ulcers is a long stay in bed without changing the position of the body.

DECUSSATION Crossing over, similar to an X.

DEDICATED CHANNEL In an emergency, a radio channel established between the dispatcher and an EMT *q.v.* that is free from interference by other users.

DEDUCTIBLE A clause in a health insurance policy indicating the amount the insured must pay before the insurance company begins payment for covered medical or health costs.

DEDUCTIVE 1. A type of logical reasoning that starts with a general proposition and derives less general, lower level propositions consistent with it. 2. An essential component of axiomatic theory *q.v.*

DEDUCTIVE LEARNING Assumes certain health facts and premises to be accurate with a conclusion based on "known truths." It is characterized chiefly by memorization of certain health facts presumed to lead to a change in health behavior. ct: inductive learning. cf: deductive reasoning.

DEDUCTIVE REASONING 1. Reasoning in which a person attempts to determine whether a statement logically follows from a certain premise, as in the analysis of syllogisms *q.v.* 2. A system of logic that begins with first principles or generalizations and arrives at secondary principles or specifics. cf: deductive learning. ct: inductive reasoning.

DE-ENERGIZED 1. Render free from electrical current. 2. To become inert.

DEEP KISSING The touching of tongues during kissing.

DEER FLY FEVER Tularemia *q.v.*

DEF An acronym for decayed, extracted, and filled teeth.

DE FACTO 1. In fact; in reality. 2. A state of affairs that must be accepted for all practical purposes, but does not have the sanction of laws behind it. ct: de jure.

DE FACTO OFFICER One who is in actual possession of an office without lawful title. ct: de jure officer.

DE FACTO SEGREGATION In education, the segregation of students by race and/or socioeconomic status resulting from circumstances such as housing patterns rather than from school policy or law.

DEFECATE To discharge excrement *q.v.* from the rectum *q.v.* cf: defecation.

DEFECATION 1. To discharge fecal *q.v.* material from the large intestine and rectum *q.v.* 2. Bowel movement. cf: defecate.

DEFECT THEORIST In the study of mental retardation *q.v.*, a person who believes that the cognitive *q.v.* processes of retardation are quantitatively different from those of normal individuals. ct: developmental theorist.

DEFENDANT In law, the party against whom relief or recovery is sought in a court action.

DEFENDANT IN ERROR In law, defendant in appellate court when the appeal is for review or writ of error.

DEFENSE In law, that which is offered and alleged by the defendant *q.v.* as a reason in law or fact why the plaintiff *q.v.* should not recover.

DEFENSE IDENTIFICATION Identification *q.v.* based on fear of physical harm.

DEFENSE MECHANISM In psychoanalytic psychology, a collective term pertaining to a group of reactions a person may have to lessen anxiety. cf: ego defense mechanism.

DEFENSIVE AVOIDANCE In psychology, the tendency to become increasingly resistant to a persuasive appeal as fear-inducing communications increase.

DEFENSIVE MEDICINE The use of procedures by a physician or dentist for the sole purpose of protecting the physician or dentist from a malpractice law suit. Defensive procedures are generally viewed as essentially unnecessary for diagnosis and treatment, but are done as a defense against malpractice.

DEFERENS Carrying away. cf: vas deferens.

DEFERRED COMPENSATION In labor relations, portion of salary paid to executives and other employees at a specified time after their regular pay ceases, e.g., after retirement.

DEFERVESCENCE A decline in the severity of an infectious disease *q.v.* that follows the fastigium stage *q.v.*

DEFIBRILLATOR 1. A device that emits electrical impulses and is used to treat arrhythmia *q.v.* by overloading the heart with electricity, upsetting the abnormal impulses, and allowing normal impulses to resume. 2. A device used to restart a heart that has stopped beating. 3. Any agent or measures, e.g., an electric shock, used to stop an uncoordinated contraction of the cardiac *q.v.* muscle and restore normal heartbeat.

DEFICIENCY 1. In nutrition, an inadequate dietary intake of one or more nutrients. The effect of dietary ~ depends upon the degree of ~ and on the function of the nutrient in the body. 2. In genetics, absence of a segment of a chromosome *q.v.* involving one or more genes *q.v.* 3. Generally, a lack of, or insufficiency.

DEFICIENCY MOTIVATION In psychology, designing behavior for oneself so that safety is acquired.

DEFICIENCY NEEDS 1. Survival requirements. 2. Needs associated with normal function.

DEFINITIONS There are three types of definitions important in scientific work: (a) nominal definition, which states that we agree to use these particular words to describe some phenomenon; (b) operational definition, which asserts the specific measurements one will use to define a concept; and (c) real definition, which attempts to get at the essence of a phenomenon. Real definitions relate a term that has some shared social meaning to its definition. They assert a proposition and thus can be tested empirically. They have truth value and can be a part of a logical system of inferences.

DEFLORATION The rupture of the hymen *q.v.* in a virgin's first experience with coitus *q.v.*, or through vaginal examination, or other means.

DEFORMITY A deviation from normal shape or size resulting in disfigurement. A ~ may be congenital *q.v.*, genetic *q.v.*, or acquired after birth.

DEGENERATION 1. In neurology, ~ of a neuron *q.v.* following damage. 2. ~ of a tissue. Damage created in one area leads by ~ to damage in cells connecting to the damaged area. cf: degenerative.

DEGENERATIVE A change of tissue to a less active form. cf: degeneration.

DEGENERATIVE DISEASE Characterized by a progressive deterioration of a tissue or tissues resulting in a reduction in the ability to function. cf: chronic disease. ct: acute disease.

DEGLUTITION Swallowing.

DEGRADATION The conversion of a chemical compound to one that is less complex.

DEGREE An award by a college, university, or other postsecondary educational institution as official recognition for successful completion of a program of studies.

DEGREE-SEEKING STUDENTS Students enrolled in courses for credit who are recognized by the institution as seeking a degree or formal award. At the undergraduate level, they include students enrolled in vocational or occupational programs.

DEGREES OF FREEDOM The number of data entries free to vary when their total is fixed.

DEHISCENCE 1. In botany, the opening of an anther *q.v.*, fruit, or other structure, permitting the escape of reproductive bodies contained within. 2. In pathology, the breaking down of a wound, especially of the abdomen.

DEHYDRATION 1. A lack of water in tissues and cells. ~ may be the result of too little intake or the inability of water to pass to the tissues and cells that need it. For example, when the sodium level of the body drops significantly, as in heat exhaustion, water is withdrawn from the cells resulting in ~. 2. Abnormal depletion of fluids from the body. Severe ~ can lead to death. Persons with brain, kidney, or gastrointestinal disease may find it difficult to maintain a normal amount of water in the body without the aid of medication.

DEHYDROEPIANDROSTERONE (DHEA) A hormone *q.v.* formed in the adrenal glands *q.v.* of the fetus *q.v.* and believed to have some influence on the aging process.

DEHYDROGENATION The removal of hydrogen from a molecule *q.v.*, as in cellular oxidation *q.v.*

DEINDIVIDUATION In psychology, a weakened sense of personal identity in which self-awareness is merged into the collective goals of a group.

DE JURE 1. In law, by action of law. 2. By right. 3. A legitimate state of affairs that has the force of law behind it.

DE JURE OFFICER In law, one who has just claim and rightful title to an office although not necessarily in actual possession thereof. ct: de facto officer.

DE JURE SEGREGATION The segregation of students on the basis of law, school policy, or a practice designed to accomplish such separation.

DELAYED SPEECH A deficit in speaking proficiency where the person performs like someone much younger.

DELAY OF REWARD The period of time between the occurrence of a response and the delivery of reinforcement. cf: conditioning.

DELAY OF REWARD GRADIENT The learning theory term for finding that rewards and punishments lose their effectiveness the farther in time they are removed from the response in question. cf: conditioning.

DELEGATE In politics and management, granting authority to conduct a particular function. cf: delegation.

DELEGATION The process of assigning job activities and related authority to specific persons within the organization. cf: delegate.

DELERIANTS Volatile chemicals that include toluene (found in some glues), spot removers, trichloroethane, gasoline, some fluorocarbons (used in some aerosol sprays), benzene, acetone, ether, chloroform, and carbon tetrachloride. Inhalation of ~ can result in death from suffocation *q.v.* and asphyxiation *q.v.* and liver damage, kidney damage, lead poisoning, cardiac *q.v.* disturbance, bone marrow damage, brain damage, and other health problems.

DELINQUENCY 1. Antisocial *q.v.* or illegal behavior by a person under the legal age. 2. In education, absence from school without a legitimate reason during the compulsory school-age period.

DELIQUESCENT 1. In anatomy and botany, dividing onto many branches. 2. A substance that absorbs water from the atmosphere. 3. Mode of branching of a tree in which the trunk divides into many branches, leaving no central axis. 4. Liquefying, or melting away, as of gills in the genus *q.v. Coprinus*.

DELIRIUM 1. A condition of extreme mental and usually motor excitement. ~ is marked by a rapid succession of confused and unconnected ideas, often illusions *q.v.*, and hallucinations *q.v.* 2. Temporary impairment of perception *q.v.*, judgment, concentration, memory, and orientation associated with mental disorders. A ~ may be caused by fever, alcohol or other drug intoxication *q.v.*, head injury, or other medical disorder. Although ~ develops rapidly, it usually can be successfully treated. cf: delirium tremens.

DELIRIUM TREMENS 1. A severe form of the alcohol abstinence or withdrawal syndrome *q.v.* 2. ~ was first described and named by Thomas Sutton in 1813. ~ is characterized by nausea, vomiting, shakes, weakness, hallucinations *q.v.*, and eventually, collapse. ~ occurs in about 5% of alcoholics *q.v.* and lasts from 2 to 6 days following complete abstinence from alcohol use.

DELIVERABLE In business, end product of a contract; specific product that the contractor agrees to deliver within the project period.

DELPHI TECHNIQUE A program of sequential interrogations interspersed with information and opinion feedback.

DELTA ALCOHOLISM Characterized by excessive drinking of alcohol, increased tolerance, withdrawal syndrome *q.v.*, craving, but with the ability to limit the amount within social standards during drinking episodes.

DELTA 9-TETRAHYDROCANNABINOL (THC) The psychoactive chemical found in the marijuana plants, *Cannabis sativa* and *Cannabis indica*.

DELTA RHYTHMS Brain waves *q.v.* of less than four cycles per second; the dominant pattern in a sleeping adult.

DELTOID Triangular. cf: deltoid muscle.

DELTOID MUSCLE The large shoulder muscle.

DELUSION 1. A strong, unshakable belief that has no basis in reality. There are three types of ~s: (a) grandeur, (b) reference, and (c) persecution. 2. Systematized false beliefs. 3. A belief contrary to reality, firmly held in spite of evidence to the contrary. Common in paranoid disorders *q.v.* Characterized by (a) belief that one is being manipulated by some external force, (b) belief that one is an especially important or powerful person, and (c) belief that one is being plotted against or oppressed by others. ct: hallucination.

DELUSIONAL JEALOUSY The unfounded conviction that one's mate is unfaithful. The person may collect small bits of evidence to justify the delusion *q.v.*

DELUSIONS OF PERSECUTION Unjustified belief that one is the target of personal attack or injury. cf: delusion.

DELUSIONS OF REFERENCE The unjustified belief that event, objects, or other persons have exaggerated significance. cf: delusion.

DELUSIONS OF SELF-IMPORTANCE 1. An unrealistic sense of personal importance or power. 2. Delusions of grandeur. cf: delusions.

DELVINAL 1. A barbiturate *q.v.* commercial preparation. 2. A short-acting barbiturate *q.v.* prescribed for sedation *q.v.* 3. The generic name is vinbarbital.

DEMAND CHARACTERISTICS 1. In experimentation, the cues *q.v.* that tell a subject what the experimenter expects of him or her. 2. A cue that makes clear to subjects what the experimenter is attempting to investigate, enabling the subjects to behave in ways that confirm the experimenter's hypothesis. cf: experimental bias.

DEMAND REDUCTION A strategy for preventing drug abuse by reducing or eliminating the actual demand, desire, or need for various drug substances.

DEMAND VALUE UNIT An intermittent positive pressure breathing unit used to assist or control ventilation with a valve connected to an oxygen source that opens in response to a person's inspiratory effort and inflates the lungs until a preset pressure limit is reached. This unit is not acceptable on ambulances unless a manual control is provided.

DEMENTIA 1. A severe mental disorder involving impairment of mental ability. 2. Progressive deterioration of the ability to think abstractly, make judgments, and control impulses. 3. A condition that impairs social and occupational functioning and eventually changes personality. Five to six percent of the U.S. population has ~. Alzheimer's disease *q.v.* causes about one-half of these cases, vascular disorders *q.v.* cause one-fourth, and the other dementias are caused by alcoholism *q.v.*, heart disease, infections, endocrine disorders, toxic reactions to drugs, and other more rare conditions. While impairment from Alzheimer's and vascular disorders are permanent, ~ caused by other disorders can usually be corrected. 4. Chronic mental deterioration sufficient to significantly impair social and/or occupational function, frequently progressive and irreversible.

DEMENTIA PRAECOX 1. An obsolete term for schizophrenia *q.v.* 2. Chosen to describe what was believed to be an incurable and progressive deterioration of mental functioning beginning in adolescence *q.v.* 3. An early term for schizophrenia; connotes early appearance and inevitable progress of the disease.

DEMEROL 1. A commercial preparation that produces analgesic *q.v.* effects. ~ is addicting *q.v.* 2. A synthetic substitute for morphine *q.v.* 3. Meperidine hydrochloride *q.v.* 4. An analgesic, sedative, and antispasmodic that may produce physiologic and psychic dependence.

DE MINIMIS In law, something so insignificant as to be unworthy of judicial attention.

DEMOCRACY A form of government in which the supreme power is given to the people.

DEMOGRAPHER A person who specializes in demography *q.v.*

DEMOGRAPHIC TRANSITION The drop of birth and death rates that accompanies the industrial and technical development of a society.

DEMOGRAPHIC VARIABLE A varying characteristic that is a vital or social statistic of an individual, sample group, or population, e.g., age, sex.

DEMOGRAPHY The study of a population and those variables bringing about change in that population. Variables studied by demographers *q.v.* are age, sex, race, education, income, geographic trends, birth, and death. cf: epidemiology; biometry.

DEMONIAC THEORY OF DISEASE 1. The belief that diseases are caused by evil spirits or demons. 2. The theory of animism *q.v.* 3. Demonology *q.v.*

DEMONSTRATED GENERALITY In research, evidence that the effect appeared in instances where it was expected within the limits of generality provided by the study and did not show where it should not have.

DEMONSTRATED METHOD In education, a learner observational method that is usually teacher-centered or authority-centered. May be effective when students are involved in the planning and conducting phases. It is most effective when the demonstration focuses upon a particular health issue. cf: demonstration program.

DEMONSTRATED RESULT In research, evidence that four conditions were met: (a) the evidence was accepted as authentic; (b) caused preceded or was concomitant with effect; (c) an effect occurred and was sensed—if sensed by inferential statistics—these were correctly applied and interpreted; and (d) the effect was congruent with the expectations created by the explanation, hypothesis, prediction, or model.

DEMONSTRATION PROGRAM In education, an experiment that attempts to demonstrate the viability of a health concept or idea. cf: demonstration method.

DEMULCENT 1. Any substance used to coat the lining of the stomach, administered in cases of accidental or deliberate poisoning. 2. An agent, such as a mucilage or oil, that soothes and relieves irritation, esp. of the mucous membranes *q.v.*

DEMURRER In law, allegation by one party that the other party's allegations may be true, but even so, are not of such legal consequences as to justify proceeding with the case.

DEMYELINATION Destruction of the myelin *q.v.*

DEMYTHOLOGIZATION The transfer of faith from one orientation based on teachings outside of oneself to an orientation developed within oneself.

DENATURATION The disruption of the structural arrangement of the atoms in a protein *q.v.* molecule *q.v.*

DENATURED ALCOHOL Ethyl alcohol *q.v.* that has been made unfit for human consumption by the addition of methyl alcohol *q.v.* and benzene *q.v.*

DENDRITE 1. Nerve fiber that sends impulses toward the cell body of a neuron *q.v.* 2. Extension of the cell body of a nerve cell that receives excitation from a neuron; serves as reception area for signals coming to the neuron from other neurons. 3. That portion of a neuron that receives electrical stimuli from adjacent neurons. Neurons typically have several branches or extensions. 4. Dendron. ct: axon.

DENDRITIC CELLS White blood cells found in the spleen *q.v.* and other lymphoid *q.v.* organs. ~ typically use threadlike tentacles to hold the antigen *q.v.*, which they present to T cells *q.v.*

DENIAL In psychology, a defense or coping mechanism *q.v.* in which a person avoids anxiety *q.v.* by refusing to perceive or accept a stressful situation.

DENIAL OF REALITY Denial *q.v.*

DENITRIFICATION In botany, the process by which nitrogen is released from the soil by the action of denitrifying bacteria *q.v.*

DE NOVO 1. In law, anew. Used to indicate that a court will hear the entire case, not just review the record of the lower tribunal. 2. A proceeding at which all that transpired at prior proceedings is ignored.

DENS Tooth.

DENSIMETRIC METHOD A technique for assessing the proportion of lean and fat tissue in the body by weighing the person first in air, and then again when submerged in water, to determine overall body density in relation to water.

DENTAL CARIES Tooth decay. ~ always begins on the external surfaces of a tooth. No single bacteria has been implicated in the etiology; however, *Lactobacillus acidophilus* and streptococcal bacteria are believed to be responsible.

DENTAL DISEASES Oral diseases *q.v.*

DENTAL EXAMINATION A dental checkup. Consists of visual examination, X-rays, and prophylaxes.

DENTAL FISSURES 1. Imperfections of the tooth enamel *q.v.* 2. Crevasses in the tooth enamel. Fissures may be corrected by application of a dental sealant *q.v.*

DENTAL HYGIENE TEACHER 1. Dental health teacher. 2. A person trained in oral health who is a member of the health services team *q.v.* 3. A person qualified to examine oral structures and to administer oral prophylaxis, and to teach about oral and dental health.

DENTAL HYGIENIST A person trained to assist the dentist, and may work independently. Trained in dental procedures and may perform some of the procedures related to examination and prophylaxis.

DENTAL INSURANCE A policy that provides for dental care. Most have limitations and deductible clauses. Generally, they provide for some coverage for preventive and maintenance care, oral examination, prophylaxis, X-rays, and restorative treatment.

DENTAL LABORATORY TECHNICIAN A person trained in constructing dental prostheses *q.v.* A dental technician makes the dentures according to the directions of the dentist.

DENTAL PATHOLOGY 1. The dental specialty concerned with diseases of the oral cavity. 2. Oral pathology. cf: pathology.

DENTAL PLAQUE A sticky transparent film on the surface of the teeth or other oral structures consisting of colonies of bacteria and sugar as a nutrient for the bacteria. As the bacteria grow and reproduce into large numbers, they produce an acid that attacks the tooth enamel *q.v.*, decalcifying it and resulting in the beginning of a dental carie *q.v.*

DENTAL SCREENING 1. Dental checkup. 2. Dental examination *q.v.*

DENTATE Having toothlike projections.

DENTIFRICE A toothpaste, gel, or powder used to clean and polish the teeth.

DENTIN 1. The hard lining substance of a tooth immediately under the enamel *q.v.* and surrounding the tooth pulp *q.v.* 2. The main part of the tooth.

DENTIST A person who possesses the Doctor of Dental Surgery (DDS) degree, or Doctor of Dental Medicine (DMD) degree, and who is concerned with the prevention of dental disorders and the diagnosis and treatment of dental and oral diseases and restoration of dental defects.

DENTITION 1. Teething. 2. The number, shape, and arrangement of the teeth.

DENTURIST 1. A technician who provides dentures directly to the public without referral or supervision from a licensed dentist *q.v.* Denturism is illegal in most states and is considered to be practicing dentistry without a license. 2. Quack dentists who specialize in prescribing and repairing dentures.

DENVER DEVELOPMENTAL SCREENING TEST DDST *q.v.*

DEODORANT A product that masks body odor or prevents it. Usually, short acting. cf: antiperspirant.

DEONONOLOGY 1. The doctrine that a person's abnormal behavior is caused by an autonomous evil spirit. 2. The demoniac theory of disease *q.v.*

DEONTOLOGY 1. The theory of professional obligations. 2. Medical ethics. cf: ethics.

DEOXYGENATED BLOOD Blood that has lost or been deprived of oxygen.

DEOXYRIBONUCLEIC ACID (DNA) 1. Genetic material composed of the genes *q.v.* that, in turn, make up the chromosomes *q.v.* ~ is self-duplicating. There are four kinds of nitrogenous bases in a single ~ molecule *q.v.*: adenine, cytosine, guanine, and thymine. 2. A large, complex molecule in the cell nucleus *q.v.* that carries the code of genetic information. It is composed of four nitrogen-containing bases, each of which is attached to a pentose (deoxyribose *q.v.*) and to a phosphate. 3. The master chemical that transmits life.

DEOXYRIBOSE A 5-carbon sugar, ribose *q.v.*, reduced by the removal of an atom *q.v.* of oxygen.

DEPARTMENT In organizational structure, a unique group of resources established by management to perform some organizational task.

DEPARTMENTALIZATION In organizational structure, the process of establishing departments *q.v.* within the management system.

DEPARTMENT OF COMMERCE From a health viewpoint, it is concerned with census taking and analysis, and medical services for merchant seamen.

DEPARTMENT OF DEFENSE From a health viewpoint, the federal agency concerned with health services for military personnel.

DEPARTMENT OF EDUCATION 1. The federal, cabinet-level office responsible for education. 2. The federal agency concerned with all aspects of education in the United States. Headed by the Secretary of Education, a cabinet-level position. Formerly a branch of the Department of Health, Education and Welfare *q.v.*, the ~ was reorganized by President Carter in 1979 giving it cabinet status.

DEPARTMENT OF HEALTH AND HUMAN SERVICES (HHS) Established through a reorganization of the Department of Health, Education and Welfare (HEW) in 1979. The Department of Education was removed from HEW.

DEPARTMENT OF HEALTH, EDUCATION AND WELFARE (HEW) Reorganized as the Department of Health and Human Services (HHS) in 1979 *q.v.*

DEPARTMENT OF HOMELAND SECURITY Organized after September 11, 2001, assists in emergency preparedness, with respect to public health.

DEPARTMENT OF LABOR A federal agency concerned with the health of migrant workers, promotion of health in industries, collection and analysis of data relative to health conditions in industries, and health and working conditions of women in industries.

DEPARTMENT OF THE INTERIOR The federal agency concerned with health of miners, fish and wildlife, and the national parks' sanitation.

DEPENDENCY The development of a psychological *q.v.* and/or physical need for a particular drug. cf: drug dependence.

DEPENDENCY RELATIONSHIP The emotional and/or physical need to continue taking a particular drug. cf: drug dependence.

DEPENDENT PERSONALITY A person lacking in self-confidence, those with a ~ passively allow others to run their lives and make no demands on them, lest they endanger these protective relationships.

DEPENDENT PERSONALITY DISORDER A disorder marked by low self-confidence, fear of self-reliance, and inability to function effectively without the help of others.

DEPENDENT VARIABLE 1. In epidemiology, the health condition affected by the effects of other variables. 2. The variable being studied and whose changes are affected by the independent variable *q.v.* 3. The variable in an experiment that is observed and measured. 4. The factor expected to change as a result of the independent variable. 5. In health education, the learner is the dependent variable while learning experiences are the independent variables.

DEPENDING RATIO A comparison between those persons whom society considers economically productive and those it considers economically unproductive. As many people over 65 years of age retire from the work force, this group is usually classified as economically unproductive. Others in this category are children, and the unemployed between the ages of 18 and 64 years.

DEPERSONALIZATION 1. The loss of the sense of personal identity *q.v.*, often with a feeling of being something or someone else. 2. An alteration in perception of the self in which the person loses a sense of reality and feels estranged from the self and perhaps separated from the body. It may be a temporary reaction to stress *q.v.* and fatigue *q.v.*, or part of panic disorder *q.v.*, depersonalization disorder *q.v.*, or schizophrenia *q.v.*

DEPERSONALIZATION DISORDER A dissociative disorder *q.v.* in which the person feels unreal and estranged from the self and surroundings enough to disrupt functioning. The person may feel that the extremities have changed in size or that he/she watches the self from a distance.

DEPILATE To remove hair.

DEPILATORY A substance that removes hair.

DEPO PROVERA 1. A long-acting injectable contraceptive drug containing only progestin *q.v.* 2. Medroxyprogesterone acetate, a synthetic progestinic hormone *q.v.* In sufficient doses, ~ protects women against conceiving for a 3-month period following an injection. The hormone has also been associated with decreased libido *q.v.*

DEPRESSANT 1. Any of several drugs that sedate *q.v.* by acting upon the central nervous system *q.v.* Medical uses include the treatment of anxiety *q.v.*, tension, stress *q.v.*, and high blood pressure *q.v.* 2. The psychoactive *q.v.* drugs that reduce the function of the central nervous system. 3. A drug that slows down the activity of the central nervous system. 4. A sedative *q.v.* that depresses the central nervous system, relaxes, tranquilizes *q.v.*, or produces sleep. ct: stimulant.

DEPRESSED FRACTURE A skull fracture *q.v.* with impaction, depression, or sinking in of the bone fragments.

DEPRESSION 1. A psychotic *q.v.* condition characterized by remorse, sadness, preoccupation with illness and death. ~ may lead to attempts at suicide *q.v.* 2. A feeling of morbidness, sadness, dejection, or melancholy. 3. In physiology, reduction in the rate of functional activity, a slowing down effect. 4. An emotional state marked by great sadness and apprehension, feelings of worthlessness and guilt, withdrawal from others, loss of sleep, appetite, and sexual desire, or interest in usual activities; and either lethargy or agitation. 5. Unipolar depression *q.v.* 6. Major depression *q.v.* It can be an associated symptom of other disorders. ~ is normal and universally experienced, although it can also be a clinical disorder affecting both the physical and mental performance of the person.

DEPRESSIVE REACTION 1. A neurotic *q.v.* condition characterized by a person being more depressed than could reasonably be expected under the circumstances. The duration of depression *q.v.* may be prolonged. ~ is characterized by headache, constipation, anorexia *q.v.*, and fatigue. The person is in touch with reality and often recognizes the source of the depression and frustration but overestimates its significance. 2. A form of psychosis *q.v.* characterized by unhappiness and feelings of worthlessness. cf: depression.

DEPRIVATION DWARFISM 1. Severely retarded growth that is due to parental neglect or emotional upset. 2. Failure-to-thrive syndrome *q.v.*

DEREALIZATION Loss of the sense that surroundings are real. It is present in several psychological *q.v.* disorders, e.g., panic disorder *q.v.*, depersonalization *q.v.*, and schizophrenia *q.v.*

DEREISTIC Thinking in which the person ignores reality and logical organization. A term often applied to irrational schizophrenia *q.v.* fantasies *q.v.*

DERIVATIVE In pharmacology, a substance coming either directly or indirectly from another substance.

DERMABRASION A process that removes the outer layers of the skin for the purpose of improving appearance by removing scars.

DERMAGRAPHIA A highly reactive condition of the skin that causes it to redden and swell wherever it is stroked by a finger.

DERMATITIS Inflammation *q.v.* of the skin. A general term referring to skin irritation regardless of cause. cf: dermatology.

DERMATOLOGY 1. A specialty of medical practice that is concerned with diseases of the skin. 2. The medical study of the structure, function, and diseases of the skin. cf: dermatitis.

DERMATOME The area of the skin supplied by sensory fibers of a single dorsal root *q.v.*

DERMATOPHYTOSIS A disease caused by a fungus *q.v.*, e.g., athlete's foot. cf: dermatitis.

DERMATOSIS A general term pertaining to any skin disease. cf: dermatitis.

DERMIS 1. The thick underlying layer of the skin that contains sweat glands *q.v.*, sebaceous glands *q.v.*, and the hair follicles *q.v.* 2. True skin. 3. Corium *q.v.*

DEROGATORY Expressing a low opinion of someone.

DES An acronym for diethylstilbestrol *q.v.* cf: DES daughters.

DESCRIPTION In research, the perception, naming, organizing, and verbally portraying a situation to highlight its important features, to put those features in context, and to show the interrelations among them.

DESCRIPTIVE ANALYSIS In research, describing the phenomenon being observed in contrast to conducting tests.

DESCRIPTIVE EPIDEMIOLOGY 1. That phase of epidemiology *q.v.* that deals with time, place, and the people affected by a disease. 2. Describing the frequency and relative distribution of health and disease in populations. cf: analytic epidemiology; experimental epidemiology.

DESCRIPTIVE EVIDENCE In research, a set of facts that describe or summarize a phenomenon. Anecdotal evidence that consists essentially of causal impressions rather than recorded data. cf: epidemiological evidence; experimental evidence.

DESCRIPTIVE RESPONSIBILITY In legal proceedings, the judgment that the accused performed an illegal act. ct: ascriptive responsibility.

DESCRIPTIVE RULE Prescriptive rules *q.v.*

DESCRIPTIVE STATISTICS 1. To inform about the characteristics of a particular group. 2. A factual report of what has occurred. 3. Summaries and measurements of behavior within a given group of subjects, often including how often they have behaved in some way. 4. The numerical descriptions of a sample *q.v.* cf: inferential statistics; frequency; incidence.

DESCRIPTIVE STUDY 1. A research approach that describes a phenomenon as it exists or occurs in nature, e.g., case study *q.v.*, survey. 2. A term to describe what is rather that what should or might be.

DES DAUGHTERS Daughters of mothers who were administered DES *q.v.* during pregnancy *q.v.*

DESEGREGATION The process of correcting past practices of racial or any other form of illegal segregation.

DESENSITIZATION 1. In psychology, lowered arousal due to frequent exposure. 2. A therapeutic *q.v.* process by means of which reactions to traumatic experiences are reduced in intensity by repeatedly exposing the person to them in mild form, either in reality or in fantasy *q.v.* 3. Systematic desensitization *q.v.* 4. In allergy, the process of rendering a person clinically less sensitive to various proteins *q.v.* to which he or she would otherwise allergically react. cf: allergy.

DESERTIFICATION Erosion of the soil in a region resulting in climatic changes, drought, and loss of vegetation.

DESERTION In family relations, the act of abandoning a marriage partner.

DESEXUALIZATION 1. Desexualize. 2. To render less sexual.

DESICCATE To remove water. cf: desiccation.

DESICCATION 1. Dried up. A form of mummification in which the body is allowed to dehydrate *q.v.* 2. A drying procedure resulting from the application of a medication or chemical.

DESIGN In research, a translating of questions, hypotheses, or models into choices of subjects, situations, treatments, observations, or measurement, basis for sensing attributes or changes, and procedure so that greater understanding or validation of the former results.

DESIPRAMINE Heterocyclic antidepressant *q.v.* Norpramin is a brand name.

DESIRABLE WEIGHT 1. The range of weights for a particular height as compiled by life insurance companies. 2. The weight range deemed appropriate for persons of a specific gender, age, and frame makeup.

DESIRE To wish for or want some object or condition related to psychobiological needs *q.v.*

DESIRE PHASE A necessary first step in the sequence of human sexual responses. cf: hypoactive sexual desire; satisfaction phase; desire prephase.

DESIRE PREPHASE The second of two prophases to the sexual response cycle *q.v.* during which the person develops a desire for sexual involvement. cf: desire phase.

DESOXYN A commercial preparation of methamphetamine *q.v.*

DESPONDENCY 1. Depression *q.v.* of spirits. 2. Loss of hope. 3. A feeling of uselessness.

DES SYNDROME The occurrence of neoplasms *q.v.* of the vagina *q.v.* in young women whose mothers were given DES*q.v.* during pregnancy *q.v.* cf: DES daughters.

DESTINATION OF MESSAGE In information theory, the point at which information results in some form of reaction; one of the components of the information theory *q.v.* destruction of perception and affect. In psychology, feelings of extreme urgency and anticipation together with the conviction that neutral events have special, personal significance, suggestive of potential psychotic *q.v.* breakdown.

DESUPPRESSION The removal of a mechanism that controls or suppresses a process.

DESYREL A commercial preparation of trazodone *q.v.*

DETAIL REPRESENTATIVE 1. Detail man. 2. Sales persons representing a pharmaceutical company.

DETANE A commercial preparation that may be placed on the glans penis *q.v.* to delay ejaculation *q.v.* There is no scientific evidence that such ointments are effective.

DETECTION THRESHOLD Absolute threshold *q.v.*

DETERGENT A cleansing agent.

DETERIORATION 1. Degeneration of mental abilities due to brain pathology *q.v.* 2. Degeneration of body tissues resulting in reduced ability to function.

DETERIORATION EFFECT In abnormal psychology, a harmful outcome from being in psychotherapy *q.v.*

DETERMINATION In embryology, the process by which embryonic *q.v.* parts become capable of developing into only one kind of adult tissue or organ.

DETERRENT That which deters or prevents action.

DETOXIFICATION 1. The process of making chemical substances nonpoisonous. 2. Removal of a toxic substance from the body. 3. Drying out, the process of clearing the body of a drug completely. 4. The biological *q.v.* process by which toxins *q.v.*, drugs, and hormones *q.v.* are modified into less toxic, or more readily excretable substances, usually in the liver. cf: biotransformation; enzyme induction.

DETOXIFY 1. To render poisons harmless. 2. To remove poisons from the body. 3. To neutralize the poisonous effects of a poisonous substance.

DETRUSOR The muscle fibers of the urinary bladder.

DETUMESCENCE 1. Subsidence of swelling. 2. Subsidence of erection in the genitals *q.v.* following orgasm *q.v.* 3. The flow of blood out of the genital area. 4. The draining of blood from the erect penis *q.v.* Havelock Ellis described ~ as the second stage of sexual response *q.v.* ct: tumescence.

DEUTERANOPIA A form of partial color blindness *q.v.* in which the person is unable to distinguish red and green. ct: protanopia.

DEVELOPMENT 1. Maturation *q.v.* 2. Increase and improvement of the effectiveness of bodily functions.

DEVELOPMENTAL AND REPRODUCTIVE TOXICOLOGY (DART) An information resource focusing on developmental toxicology *q.v.* It replaces the original ETIC *q.v.* file. A bibliographic database covering literature on teratology *q.v.* and DART.

DEVELOPMENTAL APPROACHES 1. Performance appraisal *q.v.* 2. To identify, plan, and activate behavior that will most likely yield desired performance.

DEVELOPMENTAL DISORDERS Childhood disorders characterized by unusually slow progress in attaining developmental milestones or the prolonged demonstration of a behavioral deviance.

DEVELOPMENTAL IDENTIFICATION 1. Identification *q.v.* based on fear of loss of love. 2. Anaclitic identification *q.v.* cf: anaclitic depression.

DEVELOPMENTAL MODEL The theory that a mentally retarded *q.v.* person's learning simply proceeds more slowly, attaining a lower ceiling of performance than that of a normal person.

DEVELOPMENTAL PSYCHOLOGY The scientific discipline concerned with describing age-related changes in the behavior and mental processes of both humans and animals and explaining how nature and nurture through their interaction produce these changes.

DEVELOPMENTAL QUOTIENT (DQ) A measure of development that reflects a person's performance on a standardized test of infant development relative to same-age peers. DQ is not a good prediction of IQ *q.v.*

DEVELOPMENTAL STUDY Research methods, such as cross-sectional *q.v.*, longitudinal, and retrospective *q.v.* studies, used to investigated changes in behavior over a period of time.

DEVELOPMENTAL TASKS 1. Proposed by Robert Havighurst as important achievements each person must go through during various stages of growth and development. The stages suggested are infancy, early childhood, middle childhood, adolescence, early adulthood, middle age, and late maturity. Havighurst believed that as tasks arise, a person must accomplish them, and the degree to which the task is achieved determines the success of a person's achievement of subsequent tasks. 2. Achievements necessary for continued development at various stages of maturity.

DEVELOPMENTAL THEORIST In the study of mental retardation *q.v.*, a person who believes that the cognitive development of retardates has simply been slower than that of normal persons, and not qualitatively different. cf: defect theorist.

DEVELOPMENTAL THEORY Freudian theory that traces the development of personality *q.v.* through five psychosexual stages: oral, anal, phallic, latency, and genital.

DEVELOPMENTAL VIEW In career planning, occupational choice represents an evolving sequence of individual decisions.

DEVIANCE 1. Behavior that differs from a statistical norm. 2. Behavior that is different from established social norms and that social groups take steps to correct. ct: primary deviance; secondary deviance.

DEVIANT 1. Variant. 2. A measure of unacceptable difference.

DEVIANT BEHAVIOR Behavior *q.v.* that deviates *q.v.* markedly from the average or norm. ~ is usually pathological *q.v.* in nature as used in abnormal psychology *q.v.*

DEVIANT BEHAVIOR THEORY OF ALCOHOLISM Based on the way in which society labels alcoholism *q.v.* When society labels excessive use of alcohol as a deviant behavior *q.v.*, the person is forced into playing a deviant role. The deviant behavior may be primary resulting in social norms that label a person as deviant; and secondary, which is the behavior resulting from being labeled deviant. cf: deviant role.

DEVIANT LOGIC Thinking sequences often found in psychotic *q.v.* behavior *q.v.* in which conclusions are drawn that are not logically compatible with the premises or evidence.

DEVIANT ROLE A social role that is substantially different from the majority, and often calls attention of members of the majority to the deviant role player. cf: deviant behavior.

DEVIATED SEPTUM A deviation of the partition between the nares *q.v.* that, when extreme, may interfere with nasal breathing.

DEVIATION 1. Uncommon forms of behavior *q.v.* 2. Unusual actions. 3. As used in statistics, a variation from an expected number. cf: deviant behavior; sexual variance. ct: normal.

DEVIATION IQ A measure of intelligence *q.v.* test performance based on a person's standing relative to his or her age mates. cf: intelligence quotient.

DEVIATION SCORE In statistics, a score that indicates the extent to which one deviates from the average for one's age group on a test. Deviation scores are derived from raw scores using a simple statistical transformation.

DEVITALIZED MARRIAGE A marriage that lacks the vitality or dynamic nature it once possessed.

DEXEDRINE A commercial preparation of amphetamine *q.v.*

DEXTRAN A water-soluble polysaccharide *q.v.* used as a synthetic plasma *q.v.* volume expander in infusion *q.v.*

DEXTRIN 1. A carbohydrate *q.v.* 2. A polysaccharide *q.v.* ~ is digested in the small intestine into glucose *q.v.*, which is absorbed into the bloodstream.

DEXTROAMPHETAMINE A synthetic central nervous system *q.v.* stimulant *q.v.* and one of the three major amphetamines *q.v.*

DEXTROMETHORPHAN 1. A synthetic morphine *q.v.* derivative used as an antitussive *q.v.* agent. It has no central depressant *q.v.* or analgesic *q.v.* action. 2. An OTC *q.v.* cough suppressant *q.v.*

DEXTROSE 1. Glucose *q.v.* or corn sugar. ~ is produced from cornstarch and is often sold blended with sucrose *q.v.* It is about three-fourths as sweet as sucrose. 2. A monosaccharide *q.v.* 3. The principal blood sugar.

DHAC An acronym for Division of Health Assessment and Consultation (ATSDR) *q.v.*

DHE An acronym for Division of Health Education *q.v.* (ATSDR) *q.v.*

DHHS An acronym for Department of Health and Human Services *q.v.*

DHPG An acronym for ganciclovir *q.v.*

DHS An acronym for Division of Health Studies *q.v.* (ATSDR) *q.v.*

DHT An acronym for dihydrotestosterone *q.v.*

DIABETES 1. A disease that prevents the body from properly using sugar. The condition may result from the failure of the pancreas *q.v.* to produce insulin *q.v.* or the body's inability to respond to the insulin it does produce. The most common form in older people is what has been traditionally called adult onset or noninsulin-dependent ~. However, this type has become increasingly common in young people in recent years. 2. A general term pertaining to disorders characterized by excessive urine excretion. cf: diabetes insipidus; diabetes mellitus.

DIABETES INSIPIDUS The constant excretion of large quantities of pale urine of low specific gravity not containing sugar. cf: diabetes mellitus.

DIABETES MELLITUS 1. A disease of metabolism *q.v.* in which the tissues are unable to oxidize *q.v.* sugar. ~ is characterized by hyperglycemia *q.v.*, glycosuria *q.v.*, polyuria *q.v.*, and polydipsia *q.v.* 2. A relative or absolute insulin deficiency and an accelerated probability of vascular disease *q.v.* ~ is a complex, chronic *q.v.*, systemic disorder that interferes with the metabolism and body chemistry. Specific cause is unknown but is related to the inability of the islet cells of Langerhans *q.v.* to produce adequate amounts of insulin. There are two general types of ~: (a) Type 1 (formerly juvenile) diabetes and (b) Type 2 (formerly adult onset or maturity) diabetes. 3. A metabolic disease characterized by a deficiency of insulin production from the pancreas, resulting in a reduced carbohydrate *q.v.* use. 4. A familial constitutional disease *q.v.* characterized by inadequate use of insulin resulting in disordered metabolism of carbohydrates, fats, and proteins.

DIABETIC One who suffers from diabetes *q.v.* cf: diabetes; diabetes mellitus.

DIABETIC COMA 1. A condition resulting from insufficient insulin *q.v.* in the body, characterized by confusion, stupor, sweating, acetone odor on the breath, red lips, thirst, hunger, fever, vomiting, weak pulse, and coma *q.v.* 2. Deep unconsciousness as a result of severe uncontrolled diabetes *q.v.*

DIABETIC KETOACIDOSIS 1. Acidosis *q.v.* 2. Ketoacidosis *q.v.*

DIABETIC PATIENT 1. A person with excessive amounts of sugar in the blood as a result of inadequate secretion or use of insulin *q.v.* in the body. 2. A patient with diabetes *q.v.*

DIABETIC RETINOPATHY A disorder of the blood vessels in the retina *q.v.* ~ develops most often in older diabetic patients *q.v.* who have had the condition for many years. ~ causes blurred vision or it can block vision from broken blood vessels leaking into the retina or it can lead to blindness, although blindness can sometimes be averted through early detection and treatment. cf: diabetes.

DIAGNOSIS 1. The definitive determination of the presence and nature of a disease. 2. Health or behavioral information that designates the problem and its status and information needed for planning and evaluating programs or establishing prognosis *q.v.* A health problem *q.v.* can be a symptom *q.v.* or complaint, an abnormal physical or laboratory finding, a confirmed diagnosis, or a potential or real threat to physical or emotional well-being. 3. The determination that the set of symptoms or problems of a person indicates a particular disorder. 4. Examining the circumstances of a situation in order to make a decision. 5. The process of identifying the nature of an illness. 6. A medical term meaning to identify the cause or causes of, or the characteristics of, or the signs and symptoms of a disease or condition. It is used by other health professionals as an evaluative technique to analyze health issues. In this case, it is call diagnostic evaluation *q.v.* 7. The identification of signs and symptoms of a disease or disorder that, taken together, leads to a conclusion. 8. The identification of a disease by its signs, symptoms, and laboratory findings.

DIAGNOSTIC AND STATISTICAL MANUAL (DSM) A classification system developed by the American Psychiatric Association that specifies behavior criteria for determining a diagnosis *q.v.* based on clinical observation. As of this writing, *DSM-IV* is the latest edition.

DIAGNOSTIC EVALUATION 1. Diagnosis *q.v.* 2. This evaluation serves to make distinctions and characteristics of health issues clear and concise.

DIAGNOSTIC PROBLEM SOLVING The practice of examining ideas by considering opposing forces and the change that is likely to be produced by those forces.

DIAGNOSTIC-RELATED GROUPS (DRGS) Prospective billing categories established by the federal government for Medicare *q.v.* reimbursements to hospitals for patient's illnesses, injuries, and surgical procedures.

DIAGNOSTIC SIGNS Subjective and objective evidence of a person's physiologic state and/or emotional state, and of specific disease processes.

DIAGNOSTIC X-RAY A photograph produced through radiation *q.v.* for the purpose of detecting and diagnosing a disease.

DIAKINESIS In cellular biology, a stage of meiosis *q.v.* just before metaphase I *q.v.* in which the bivalents *q.v.* are shortened and thickened.

DIAL-A-PORN The use of the telephone to convey erotic or pornographic *q.v.* messages.

DIALYSIS 1. The passage of a dissolved substance through a semipermeable membrane *q.v.* 2. A process by which chemical substances may be separated by molecular *q.v.* size and charge, according to their ability to pass through a membrane of specific pore size. Practically speaking, a membrane sac containing a complex mixture that is washed externally with water or other solvent. The low-molecular-weight materials pass through the membrane while the high-molecular-weight materials are retained within the sac. 3. The separation of crystalloids *q.v.* from colloids *q.v.* by the faster diffusion *q.v.* of the former through a membrane.

DIAPEDESIS The passage of blood or of leukocytes *q.v.* through the unruptured walls of the blood vessels.

DIAPHRAGM 1. A contraceptive *q.v.* device that fits over the entrance of the cervix *q.v.* and serves as a barrier to sperm *q.v.* Its effectiveness as a contraceptive is increased when used in conjunction with a spermicidal cream or jelly *q.v.* 2. A method of birth control *q.v.* in which a flexible rubber disc is inserted in the vagina *q.v.* over the cervix to prevent sperm from entering the uterus *q.v.* 3. An anatomy, the domelike muscle that separates the chest or thoracic cavity *q.v.* from the abdominal cavity *q.v.*

DIAPHRAGMATIC Pertaining to the diaphragm *q.v.*

DIAPHYSIS The shaft of a long bone. cf: epiphysis.

DIARRHEA 1. The rapid movement of fecal *q.v.* matter through the intestine. 2. Loose or watery stools and an increase in the number of bowel movements, usually more than two a day. ~ is a common symptom of gastrointestinal disease *q.v.* ct: constipation.

DIARTHROSIS A freely moveable joint.

DIASTOLE 1. Relaxation of the heart in each beat. 2. The dilation, ~ period of dilation, of the heart, especially of the ventricles *q.v.* coinciding with the interval between the second and first heart sounds. 3. The resting period of the heart. ct: systole.

DIASTOLIC BLOOD PRESSURE 1. Pertains to the resting point of the heart beat. 2. The blood pressure in the arteries when the heart relaxes. ct: systolic blood pressure. 3. The blood pressure on arterial walls between heart beats. 4. It is the lower of the two numbers recorded as the blood pressure, e.g., 120/70. 5. Blood pressure against blood vessel walls when the heart relaxes.

DIATHERMY A process of generating heat in tissues by electric currents for medical or surgical purposes.

DIATHESIS 1. Diathesis stress conception *q.v.* 2. A predisposition toward an illness or abnormality. 3. An inherited predisposition to a mental disorder.

DIATHESIS STRESS CONCEPTION The belief that many organic *q.v.* and mental disorders arise from an interaction between a diathesis *q.v.* and some form of precipitating environmental stress. cf: diathesis stress theory; diathesis stress paradigm.

DIATHESIS STRESS PARADIGM A view that, as applied in psychopathology, assumes that individuals predisposed toward a particular mental disorder will be particularly affected by stress and will manifest abnormal behavior. cf: diathesis stress conception; diathesis stress theory.

DIATHESIS STRESS THEORY The theory that mental disorders that emphasizes that both genetic *q.v.* and environmental factors are significant in the development of a number of mental disorders. cf: diathesis stress conception; diathesis stress paradigm.

DIAZEPAM A minor tranquilizer *q.v.* An example is valium. cf: chlordiazepoxide; meprobramate.

DICARYOTIC In cellular biology, a mycelium *q.v.* containing two haploid *q.v.* nuclei in each cell; the result of plasmogamy *q.v.* with delayed caryogamy *q.v.*

DICENTRIC CHROMOSOME In cellular biology, a cell having two centromeres *q.v.*

DICHOTIC LISTENING 1. A procedure by which each ear receives a different message while the listener is asked to focus on only one. 2. An experimental procedure in which a subject hears two recorded messages simultaneously through earphones, one in each ear, usually with the instruction to attend to only one of the messages.

DICHOTOMY The division or forking of an axis into two more or less equal branches.

DICHROMATISM Color blindness *q.v.*

DICK-READ CHILDBIRTH METHOD A method of natural childbirth developed by Grantley Dick-Read.

DICK TEST A skin test that measures sensitivity to scarlet fever *q.v.* toxins *q.v.*

DICTA In law, statements in a judicial opinion not necessary to the decision of the case.

DICTUM In law, a statement of legal principle by the court—this principle is not necessitated by the facts or the law of the case. Because such statements are not directly in point, they are not controlling precedents, though often persuasive.

DIDACTIC In education, instructional methods characterized by lecture or one-way communication. cf: didactic teaching.

DIDACTIC GROUP THERAPY Group therapy *q.v.* consisting of formal group lectures and discussions.

DIDACTIC TEACHING Teaching that uses the lecture method in an information-giving atmosphere. The focus of instructional activity is on the teacher rather than the student. cf: didactic.

DIEFFENBACHIA SEGUINE Dumbcane *q.v.*

DIENCEPHALON 1. The posterior part of the prosencephalon *q.v.* 2. The ~ is located between the forebrain and the midbrain. It includes the hypothalamus *q.v.*, thalamus *q.v.*, and epithalamus *q.v.*

DIET 1. Pertains to the relationship of nutrients in the foods ingested each day over a significant period of time. 2. The food and drink one usually consumes. 3. A food regimen.

DIETARY CHOLESTEROL The cholesterol *q.v.* obtained through food.

DIETARY DEFICIENCY 1. Conditions resulting from prolonged deprivation of some specific nutrient *q.v.* Deficiency of some nutrients may result in clinical symptoms sooner than others. Nutrient deficiency symptoms may result from diets that are restrictive. 2. A state in which a physical disorder appears for a lack of a particular nutrient.

DIETARY GOALS FOR THE UNITED STATES In 1977, the Senate Select Committee on Nutrition and Human Needs released its report recommending that American society strive to meet dietary goals in the areas of carbohydrates, sugar, fat, protein, cholesterol, and salt intake. While revised by various organizations and agencies in the intervening years, these goals established a benchmark for the improvement of nutrition in the United States.

DIETARY RECALL A technique of dietary evaluation in which subjects are asked for specific details of their diets during the preceding 24 h.

DIETHYLPROPION 1. An amphetamine-like appetite suppressant. 2. Tenuate and Tepanil are commercial preparations.

DIETHYLSTILBESTROL (DES) 1. An ingredient in postcoital or morning after contraceptive pill *q.v.* during the 1960s. It is also a chemical used to treat menopausal symptoms on women and prostate gland cancer *q.v.* in men. ~ was also used to prevent miscarriages *q.v.* in women. In 1971, scientists noticed that daughters born to women who took ~ to prevent miscarriage had a greater likelihood of developing vaginal adenosis *q.v.* or a rare type of vaginal cancer *q.v.*, adenocarcinoma *q.v.* In sons, there is a greater likelihood of genital abnormalities, such as undescended testicles *q.v.*, underdevelopment of the testicles, benign cysts *q.v.*, low sperm *q.v.* count, and abnormally developed sperm. 2. A form of the hormone estrogen *q.v.* formerly used to treat pregnant women against spontaneous abortion*q.v.*

DIET OR DIETETIC 1. On food labels. 2. Having the same requirements as low or reduced calories *q.v.*

DIFFERENCE MODEL The theory that a retarded person's learning difficulties result from a cognitive *q.v.* defect, and therefore, the learning processes themselves are qualitatively different from those of normal people.

DIFFERENCES (METHOD OF) In research, a situation in which a phenomenon occurs and one in which it does not occur are exactly alike except for one circumstance in the former. The circumstance in which they differ is presumed to be causally related to the phenomenon.

DIFFERENCE THRESHOLD 1. The amount by which a given stimulus *q.v.* must be increased or decreased so that the person can perceive a just noticeable difference (JND) *q.v.* 2. The smallest difference between two stimuli that can be detected dependably. cf: absolute threshold.

DIFFERENCE TONE A third tone sometimes heard when tones of two widely different frequencies are sounded together. cf: beat; summation tone.

DIFFERENTIAL INTERVENTION PLANNING The planning of the appropriate form of treatment for a distinct disorder.

DIFFERENTIALIST 1. Theory of career planning. 2. Occupational choice is viewed as a matching process that balances satisfaction and stability.

DIFFERENTIALLY PERMEABLE Pertaining to membranes *q.v.* that allow some substances to pass through more readily than others.

DIFFERENTIAL MEDIUM A medium *q.v.* developed to elicit a specific characteristic of an organism or group of organisms.

DIFFERENTIAL PAY In education, extra pay or incentives (added standard increments) awarded to teachers on the basis of merit.

DIFFERENTIAL SOCIALIZATION The ways in which parents and others react differently to children and reinforce different behaviors for the two sexes.

DIFFERENTIATED EDUCATION Instruction and learning activities that are uniquely and predominantly suited to the capacities and interests of gifted students.

DIFFERENTIATED STAFFING Education personnel, selected, educated, and deployed so as to make optimum use of their abilities, interests, preparation, and commitments. It gives them greater opportunity and autonomy in guiding their own professional growth.

DIFFERENTIATION 1. A progressive change from the general to the particular and from the simpler to the more complex, which characterizes embryological *q.v.* development. 2. In psychology, the same pattern relative to the development of behavior following birth. 3. The physiological and morphological *q.v.* changes that occur in a cell, tissue, or organ during development.

DIFFERENTIATION THEORY A theory of perceptual learning that attributes change to increasing sensitivity to properties of stimulus that children learn to differentiate with experience, rather than to learning new responses.

DIFFICULT CHILDREN Children whose temperament patterns include irregularity of timing, withdrawal from new events, unusually intense reactions, frequent expressions of negative mood, and slow adaptability. cf: easy children.

DIFFRACTION The deflection of light waves when passing through narrow slits to form fringes of partial light and dark bands.

DIFFUSED POLLUTION SOURCES 1. Water pollution *q.v.* from large areas. 2. Nonpoint pollution sources.

DIFFUSE PROJECTION The expression in neurological *q.v.* language that stimulation leads to a general state of arousal in the cerebral cortex *q.v.* This effect is produced by the ascending reticular formation *q.v.* and is to be contrasted with the specific representation in the cortex of stimulation in more limited primary projection areas *q.v.*

DIFFUSION 1. In physiology, the passive movement of substances from an area of high concentration to one of low concentration. 2. The movement of substances across a cell membrane *q.v.* 3. The net movement of a substance as a result of the independent motion of its individual molecules *q.v.*, ions *q.v.*, or colloidal *q.v.* particles, from a region of higher diffusion pressure to one of lower diffusion pressure of that substance. 4. In psychology, fixation *q.v.* 5. In sociology, innovations spread to members of a social system by the process of ~.

DIFFUSION PRESSURE The activity of a specific kind of molecule *q.v.* as a result of the combined effects of concentration, temperature, and pressure.

DIGEST 1. In politics, a brief summary of the contents of a bill, which must be attached to the bill before introduction. 2. In physiology and nutrition science, the breaking down of food substances into assimilating particles.

DIGESTION 1. Mechanical and chemical actions required to reduce foods into absorbable substances to be assimilated *q.v.* by the body. Mechanical action begins in the mouth with the chewing of foods and continues throughout the digestive process by the churning action of the gastrointestinal *q.v.* organs. Chemical digestion also begins in the mouth and continues in the stomach and finally in the small intestine. The chemicals of digestion are called enzymes *q.v.* 2. Conversion of complex, usually insoluble foods into simple usually soluble and diffusible forms by means of enzymatic action.

DIGESTIVE SYSTEM One of the 10 body systems consisting of a group of organs responsible for the breakdown and absorption of food substances. The major organs of the ~ are the esophagus, stomach, and intestines.

DIGESTIVE TRACT The passage leading from the mouth to the anus *q.v.* through the pharynx *q.v.*, esophagus *q.v.*, stomach, and small and large intestines *q.v.* cf: digestive system.

DIGITALIS A drug used to stimulate contractions of the heart. ~ is prescribed for certain forms of heart failure, such as congestive heart failure *q.v.*

DIGITALIZATION The process of giving digitalis *q.v.* to the point where the maximum therapeutic *q.v.* effect is obtained without untoward side effects *q.v.*

DIGITAL SUBTRACTION ANGIOGRAPHY (DSA) A technique that uses brain imaging methods to observe the anatomy *q.v.* and functioning of blood vessels, especially in the brain. Computer processing capabilities are paired with X-ray techniques for this assessment method.

DIGITIGRADE Walking on the digits (toes).

DIGIT SPAN The maximum number of digits that can be retained in short-term memory *q.v.* following the oral presentation of a series of digits at the rate of one per second.

DIGLYCERIDE 1. A glycerol *q.v.* ester having two fatty acids *q.v.* 2. A lipid *q.v.*

DIHYBRID 1. In genetics, a cross between parents differing in two pairs of genes *q.v.* 2. An individual that is heterozygous *q.v.* with respect to two pairs of alleles *q.v.* The product of a cross between homozygous *q.v.* parents differing in two respects. 3. ~ inheritance. Inheritance of two trait pairs determined by two nonallelic gene pairs.

DIHYDROCODEINE A narcotic analgesic *q.v.*.

DIHYDROHYDROXYCODEINE 1. A semisynthetic derivative of morphine *q.v.* 2. Oxycodone *q.v.*

DIHYDROTESTOSTERONE (DHT) 1. A hormone *q.v.* synthesized from testosterone *q.v.* that is responsible for the development of the external genitalia *q.v.* of the male fetus *q.v.* 2. A hormone similar to testosterone that stimulates the development of the penis, scrotum, and prostate gland in the embryo *q.v.*

DILATE 1. To expand or widen as dilation of the pupils of the eyes. 2. Expansion of the opening of a vessel or an organ.

DILATED PUPIL A pupil of the eye that is enlarged beyond its normal size.

DILATION A widening of the cervical opening *q.v.* Prior to delivery, the cervix *q.v.* dilates 3.5–4 in.

DILATION AND CURETTAGE (D&C) A common procedure for performing an abortion *q.v.* The cervix *q.v.* is dilated using graduated instruments and the contents of the uterus *q.v.* are scraped away with a curette *q.v.* ct: vacuum aspiration; saline induction; hysterotomy; menstrual extraction; dilation and evacuation.

DILATION AND EVACUATION (D&E) 1. An abortion *q.v.* procedure used in the second trimester *q.v.* that is a combination of a vacuum curettage *q.v.* and dilation and curettage *q.v.* methods. 2. A method of performing an abortion. 3. A procedure for abortion used in pregnancy consisting of opening the cervix *q.v.* and removing the contents of the uterus *q.v.*

DILAUDID HYDROMORPHONE 1. A synthetic drug. 2. A narcotic *q.v.* analgesic *q.v.*

DILDO 1. An artificial penis *q.v.* used by some females (or males) for self-stimulation or masturbation *q.v.* 2. A sexual aid used by some females. 3. Penis substitute.

DIMENSIONS OF HEALTH 1. The aspects of humans that are affected by genetics *q.v.*, environments *q.v.*, and behavior. 2. The dimensions of each person that determine health and effectiveness. They are as follows: (a) the physical dimension, which is associated with the biological aspects of a person; (b) the emotional dimension, which refers to the ability to express feelings adequately and in appropriate ways. It has to do with values and appreciations, as they contribute to worthwhile achievements; (c) the mental dimension, which is related to a person's ability to learn and to behave accordingly. It is associated with rationality, logic, decision making, and wisdom; and (d) the social dimension, which is associated with interpersonal relations. One's social health depends upon the ability to deal effectively with the social environment *q.v.* 3. The interrelated factors of the physical, emotional, mental, and social aspects of each person. cf: three dimensions of health; five dimensions of health.

DIMER 1. In chemistry, a compound having the same percentage composition as another but twice the molecular *q.v.* weight. 2. A compound formed by polymerization *q.v.*

DIMETHOXYMETHYLAMPHETAMINE (DOM) A long-acting psychedelic *q.v.* drug also referred to as STP *q.v.*, an acronym for serenity, tranquility, and peace.

DIMETHYLTRYPTAMINE (DMT) A psychotomimetic *q.v.* agent that produces effects similar to those of LSD *q.v.*, but the onset is more rapid, with greater likelihood of a panic reaction *q.v.*, and is of shorter duration.

DIMORPHISM 1. The condition of a species having two different forms. In animals, those that show marked differences between male and female. 2. Two different forms in a group are determined by such characteristics as sex, size, or coloration.

DIOECIOUS 1. In botany, having only one sex, male or female, present in each individual. 2. Bearing staminate *q.v.* and pistillate *q.v.* flowers or pollen and seed cones of conifers *q.v.* on different individuals of the same species. 3. A unisexual plant, each plant is either a male or a female. ct: monoecious.

DIOPTER The unit of refracting power of a lens.

DIOXIN A powerful and potentially harmful chemical compound found in some herbicides *q.v.*

DIPHASIC A condition in some parasitic *q.v.* fungi in which a mycelial *q.v.* phase alternates with a yeast phase, under environmental change.

DIPHENHYDRAMINE An antihistamine *q.v.*

DIPHOSPHOPYRIDINE NUCLEOTIDE (DPN) Nicotinamide adenine dinucleotide (NAD) *q.v.*

DIPHTHERIA A disease caused by the bacterium, *Corynebacterium diphtheriae*, and transmitted by contact with nose and throat discharges from an infected person. It is characterized by a sore throat, fever, and running nose. Toxins *q.v.* from the bacterium may result in permanent heart or nervous system damage. ~ can be prevented with DPT *q.v.* or TD *q.v.* inoculation.

DIPLEGIA Paralysis of both arms or both legs.

DIPLOBLASTIC Two germ layers; ectoderm *q.v.* and endoderm *q.v.*

DIPLOCOCCUS PNEUMONIAE The causative agent of lobar pneumonia *q.v.*

DIPLOID 1. In genetics, having two sets of chromosomes *q.v.* 2. The nuclear state of an organism in which cells have two of every homologue chromosome. ct: haploid; monoploid.

DIPLOMA MILL An institution not accredited that awards degrees or diplomas without requiring students to meet certain acceptable educational standards.

DIPLOMATE A physician who holds a certificate of the National Board of Medical Examiners or one of the American Boards of the Specialties. cf: Board Eligible; Board Certified.

DIPLONEMA That stage in prophase *q.v.* of meiosis *q.v.* following the pachytene stage *q.v.*, but preceding diakinesis *q.v.*, in which the chromosomes *q.v.* are visibly double, characterized by centromere *q.v.* repulsion of bivalents *q.v.* resulting in the formation of loops.

DIPLOPIA 1. The perception of two images from a single object. 2. Double vision.

DIPSOMANIA Epsilon alcoholism *q.v.*

DIRECT CALORIMETRY The determination of the amount of heat released by the body.

DIRECT CONTACT A means of transmitting a communicable disease *q.v.* directly by touching or being touched by an infected person.

DIRECTED THINKING Thinking that is aimed at the solution of a problem.

DIRECT EUTHANASIA 1. The process of inducing death, often through the injection of a lethal drug. 2. Active euthanasia. cf: euthanasia.

DIRECT HEALTH EXPERIENCES 1. Planned and deliberate health education under the guidance of a trained health educator. 2. Direct health teaching *q.v.*

DIRECT HEALTH TEACHING 1. Direct health experiences *q.v.* 2. Instruction given during regularly scheduled periods, having organized, planned curriculum in equal status with all other basic studies within the school setting. May also occur in nonschool settings.

DIRECTIONALITY Awareness of laterality and verticality, as well as the ability to translate this discrimination within the organism to similar discrimination among objects in space.

DIRECTIONALITY PROBLEM A difficulty in correlational research *q.v.* whereby it is known that two variables are related, but it is unclear which is causing the other.

DIRECTIVE APPROACH In psychotherapy, questions and their sequence are determined in advance of the interview.

DIRECTIVE THERAPY A type of therapeutic approach in which the therapist supplies direct answers to problems and takes much of the responsibility for the progression of the therapy session.

DIRECT-LEASED LAND LINE A point-to-point telephone line to be used only for a specific purpose or service. Generally used in emergency services or situations.

DIRECT METHOD OF AGE ADJUSTMENT A method that uses a standard population and applies the age-specific rates of the population being compared to determine the expected number of events in the standard population.

DIRECTORS OF HEALTH PROMOTION AND EDUCATION An organization of state directors of health promotion and education programs designed to promote the importance of such programs through national leadership.

DIRECTORY An instruction of no obligatory force and involving no invalidating consequences for its disregard.

DIRECTORY OF BIOTECHNOLOGY INFORMATION RESOURCES (DBIR) An information system that contains information on a wide range of resources related to biotechnology. Among these are on-line databases and networks, publications, organizations, and collections and repositories of cells and subcellular elements.

DIRECT TRANSMISSION A manner of transmitting disease organisms in which the agent moves immediately from the infected person to the susceptible person, as in person-to-person contact and in droplets contact.

DIS An acronym for Disease Intervention Specialist *q.v.*

DISABILITY 1. Any temporary or permanent condition of the body or the mind that reduces a person's ability to function at a higher level of effectiveness. 2. More specific than a disorder. Results from a loss of physical functioning or difficulties in learning and social adjustment that significantly interferes with normal growth and development.

DISABILITY INCOME INSURANCE A type of health insurance that replaces the insured's loss of income when he or she is ill or disabled *q.v.*

DISACCHARIDASE One of a group of enzymes *q.v.* that hydrolyze *q.v.* disaccharides *q.v.* ~ is formed in the cells of the brush border *q.v.*

DISACCHARIDES 1. Sugars that must be digested *q.v.* before they can be absorbed by the small intestine. They include sucrose *q.v.*, lactose *q.v.*, and maltose *q.v.* 2. A sugar molecule *q.v.* formed by a condensation reaction *q.v.* between two monosaccharides *q.v.* cf: polysaccharides.

DISAPPOINTMENT In Mowrer's two-factor theory *q.v.*, the state theoretically elected by the presentation of a stimulus *q.v.* that has been paired with the absence or termination of a positive reinforcer *q.v.*

DISCIPLINE 1. Purposeful punishment. 2. Punishment that results in constructive or improved behavior. 3. A broad concept of control by applying teaching or training that may or may not include physical punishment as a technique. 4. Actions in response to inappropriate behavior or actions that prevent inappropriate behaviors. 5. A system of rules or regulations that prescribe a desired behavior.

DISCLOSURE The degree to which a person reveals parts of the self that are not obvious or widely known.

DISCONCERTED To be thrown into a state of confusion or disorder.

DISCONFIRMATION In research, the process of trying to invalidate a proposition. Causal relationships can never be proved; there may always be some as yet untested circumstance under which the relationship does not hold. With each successful test, the relation is said to have escaped disconfirmation.

DISCONTINUOUS VARIATION Distinct categories or classes such as black versus white and tall versus dwarf. ct: continuous variable.

DISCOVERY TEACHING In education, a form of teaching in which the teacher arranges the learning environment so that learners find the answers through discovery.

DISCRETE VARIABLE In epidemiology, a quantitative variable that can assume only a limited set of values no matter how precise measurement techniques are.

DISCRETIONARY FUNDS 1. Federal funding for specific programs granted after specific needs are identified and documented. 2. At the university level, monies that may be spent at the judgment of an administrator, e.g., a department chair or dean.

DISCRIMINATE FUNCTION ANALYSIS In research, determination of the capacity of two or more independent variables to predict correctly the categorization of individuals scaled on a nominal variable.

DISCRIMINATION 1. The behavioral component of prejudice *q.v.* 2. An action that reflects an unfavorable attitude toward a person based solely upon his or her class or category membership. 3. The differential response to different stimuli *q.v.* ~ is produced by reinforcing responses to certain stimuli and extinguishing responses to other stimuli. 4. The tendency for a person to differentiate between two similar stimuli when one is reinforced and the other is not. There are two chief forms of ~: (a) auditory, an identification of likeness differences between sounds; and (b) visual, the ability to recognize differences between similar but slightly different forms or shapes. 5. An illegal practice that uses race, color, religion, national origin, sex, age, or sexual preference as a basis for hiring, firing, or other employment practices. cf: discrimination learning tasks.

DISCRIMINATION LEARNING TASKS 1. Tasks designed to study the processes by which children learn to distinguish among categories of objects. 2. Discrimination *q.v.*

DISEASE 1. Any condition of the body or mind, acute or chronic *q.v.*, that interferes with the person's ability to function effectively under ordinary environmental circumstances. Literally, a lack of functioning. A ~ may be either functional *q.v.*, organic *q.v.*, or both. 2. A scientific, medical, and technical territory that encompasses what is known about biological impairment. 3. Any interference with effective functioning. It is especially applied to pathological *q.v.* conditions. It may affect the whole body or any of its parts. A ~ has characteristic etiology *q.v.* and symptoms *q.v.* 4. The medical concept that distinguishes an impairment of the normal state of the organism by its particular group of symptoms and its specific cause. ~ is to a large extent, defined in terms of social issues. Previously, many ~s were defined as moral or legal issues, e.g., drug abuse, alcoholism, psychosis *q.v.* 5. A condition that interferes with the body's ability to function to its utmost. ~s are classified or categorized according to the parts of the body being affected, according to cause or characteristics (signs and symptoms).

DISEASE AND SYMPTOM-PREVALENCE STUDY A study designed to measure the occurrence of self-reported disease *q.v.* that may in some instances be validated *q.v.* through medical records or physical examinations, and to determine those adverse health conditions that may require further investigation because they were reported at an excess rate. This study can only be considered hypothesis generated.

DISEASE INTERVENTION SPECIALIST (DIS) A person who performs sexually transmitted disease (STD) *q.v.* patient interviewing/counseling and field investigation after initial diagnosis.

DISEASE MODEL Medical model *q.v.*

DISEASE ORIENTATION Health education methodologies *q.v.* that focus attention on diseases rather than health. It implies negative teaching and learning approaches to health rather than positive approaches to health. 2. Pathological orientation *q.v.*

DISEASE PROCESS Involves the interaction of a multiplicity of factors interacting with each other. These factors are the host, agent, and the environment. ~ consists of four stages: (a) the stage of susceptibility, which includes a person's ability to resist the onset of the disease *q.v.* It is the time when a clinical disease has not yet appeared, but when other factors become present; (b) the stage of presymptomatic disease, which is characterized by the onset of disease but with no clinical signs or symptoms as yet apparent; (c) the stage of clinical disease characterized by overt and recognizable clinical signs and symptoms that can be analyzed resulting in diagnosis *q.v.*; and (d) the stage of disability characterized by either residual defects or the onset of death. A composite of the four stages of the disease is referred to as the natural history of the disease *q.v.*

DISEASE REGISTRY An official listing of diseases or serious illnesses found in persons exposed to hazardous substances in the environment.

DISEASES OF ADAPTATION 1. Pathological *q.v.* conditions resulting from severe and prolonged stress *q.v.* 2. Stomach ulcers and other diseases *q.v.* resulting from the stresses of life or when stress is a contributing factor. 3. An illness caused by stress-induced overload on one or more organs. cf: general adaptation syndrome.

DISEMBODIMENT According to Laing, the loss of contact with one's experience; e.g., a sense of separation between one's self and one's body.

DISEQUILIBRIUM In Piaget's theory, a state in which one's available schemas or mental structures are discovered to be inadequate. This state is prerequisite to cognitive *q.v.* advance.

DISIDENTIFICATION In Assagioli's psychosynthesis, a way of reaching one's true self; a process whereby the person carefully and clearly examines those things that normally comprise and/or affect his or her identity.

DISINFECTANT A substance that destroys vegetative cells of microorganisms *q.v.* but not spores *q.v.* in a specified time period. cf: disinfection.

DISINFECTION Killing or removing pathogens *q.v.* or arresting their ability to grow and multiply. A chemical substance that kills bacteria *q.v.* or other microorganisms that can cause infection *q.v.* Examples of ~s are tincture of iodine, argyrols, gentian violet, mercocresols, nitromersol, thimerosal, benzalkonium, and alcohol. ct: sterilization.

DISINHIBITING EFFECT 1. The removal of, or lessening of, inhibitions *q.v.* 2. In drug usage, the effect by which an individual becomes less conscious of the evaluation of others and less concerned with social skills. 3. Disinhibition *q.v.*

DISINHIBITION An increase of some reaction tendency by the removal of some inhibiting *q.v.* influence upon the behavior. cf: disinhibiting effect.

DISINTEGRATION 1. The loss of organization or integration in any organized system. A loss of personality organization *q.v.*

DISINTERESTEDNESS In research, ignoring personal advantage when interpreting data.

DISJUNCTION 1. Separation of homologous chromosomes *q.v.* during anaphase *q.v.* of mitosis *q.v.* or meiosis *q.v.* 2. Separation of synapsed chromosomes *q.v.* occurring during the process of meiosis. cf: nondisjunction.

DISLOCATION 1. In anatomy, a displacement of a bone from its joint. 2. The displacement of the ends of two bones at their joint so that the joint surfaces are no longer in proper contact (Table D-1).

DISMISSAL In law, a final disposition of a suit by a court by sending it out of court without a trial on the issues.

TABLE D-1 TYPES OF DISLOCATIONS

NAME OF DISLOCATION	DESCRIPTION
Closed dislocation	Same as simple dislocation
Complete dislocation	One in which the surfaces of the joint are completely separated
Complicated dislocation	One that is associated with other major injuries
Compound dislocation	One in which the joint extends to the external environment
Congenital dislocation	A dislocation that exists before or as a result of birth
Consecutive dislocation	One in which the luxated bone has changed its position since its first displacement
Divergent dislocation	One in which the ulna and radius are dislocated separately
Habitual dislocation	A dislocation that recurs after reduction
Incomplete dislocation	A slight dislocation
Metacarpophalangeal dislocation	A dislocation of a finger
Monteggia's dislocation	A dislocation of the hip joint in which the head of the femur is near the anterosuperior spine of the ilium
Nelaton's dislocation	A dislocation of the ankle joint in which the talus is between the end of the tibia and the fibula
Old dislocation	A dislocation in which no reduction has been achieved
Partial dislocation	Same as incomplete dislocation
Pathologic dislocation	A dislocation from a paralysis or disease of the joint or supporting tissues involved
Primitive dislocation	A dislocation in which the bones remain as originally displaced.
Recent dislocation	A dislocation recognized at the time it occurs or shortly thereafter
Simple dislocation	A dislocation in which the joint is not penetrating to the outside. No wound occurs
Slipped dislocation	A herniated dislocation
Traumatic dislocation	A dislocation resulting from an injury

DISMISSED FOR WANT OF EQUITY In law, a case dismissed *q.v.* because the allegations in the complaint have been found untrue, or because they are insufficient to entitle complaint to the relief sought.

DISOME Monosomic *q.v.*

DISORDER A disturbance in normal functioning related to mental, physical, or psychological dimensions of humans.

DISORDERS ASSOCIATED WITH IMMATURITY AND INADEQUACY Behavior disorders *q.v.* in which an individual may be exceptionally clumsy, socially inadequate, or easily flustered.

DISORGANIZATION In psychology, the lack of orderly relations.

DISORGANIZED SCHIZOPHRENIC A person with schizophrenia *q.v.* who has rather diffuse and regressive symptoms characterized by silliness, facial grimaces, and inconsequential rituals, and has changeable moods and poor hygiene. There are few significant remissions and eventually considerable deterioration. This from of schizophrenia was formerly called hebephrenia *q.v.*

DISORIENTATION Mental confusion with respect to time, place, or person. cf: disoriented.

DISORIENTED 1. To be confused as to one's relationship with either physical surroundings or with respect to a full grasp of a specific set of ideas. 2. Having lost the sense of familiarity with one's surroundings.

DISPARATE 1. Unequal. 2. Not alike.

DISPATCHER In emergency procedures, one who transmits calls to service units, sending vehicles and EMTs *q.v.* on emergency missions.

DISPLACED AGGRESSION 1. Hostility directed toward a person or object not directly responsible for the frustration *q.v.* that produced it. 2. Displacement *q.v.* 3. Displacement of anger *q.v.* cf: frustration/aggression hypothesis.

DISPLACED REFERENCE A capacity shared by all languages for referring to objects and events that are distant in either time or space.

DISPLACEMENT 1. In psychology, the transfer of hostility *q.v.* from the person or object causing the frustration *q.v.* to a less threatening object or person. 2. A defense mechanism *q.v.* 3. In chemistry, the process whereby one molecule *q.v.* with a greater affinity for a given binding site replaces the existing bound molecule at that site. 4. In psychoanalytic psychology, a redirection of an impulse from a channel that is blocked into another, more available outlet. 5. The transfer of an emotional attitude *q.v.* or symbolic meaning from one object or concept to another. 6. A defense mechanism whereby an emotional response is unconsciously redirected from a perhaps dangerous object or concept to a substitute less threatening to the ego *q.v.*

DISPLACEMENT BEHAVIOR In ethology, the elicitation of instinctive behavior by inappropriate stimuli that resemble the appropriate stimulus.

DISPLACEMENT OF ANGER 1. Releasing anger *q.v.* on a person or object other than the one that is the source of the anger. 2. A transfer of hostility *q.v.* to a person or object that is less threatening than the source of the frustration *q.v.* This tends to lessen the possibility of experiencing an accompanying fear *q.v.* cf: free-floating anger.

DISPLAY In ethology, pertaining to genetically *q.v.* programmed responses that serve as stimuli for the reaction of others and thus serve as the basis of a communication system.

DISPOSABLE DIAPHRAGM A form of contraceptive *q.v.* worn at the cervix *q.v.* and thrown away after an act of sexual intercourse *q.v.* cf: diaphragm.

DISSEMINATION In epidemiology, a scattering or spreading of organisms from host to host or in pathogens *q.v.* from one locus of infection *q.v.* to another.

DISSENT 1. In parliamentary procedure, a difference of opinion. 2. In politics, to cast a negative vote.

DISSENTING OPINION In law, the opinion in which a judge announces his or her dissent *q.v.* from the conclusions held by the majority of the court. Common usage in Supreme Court decisions.

DISSIPATE To scatter or disperse.

DISSOCIAL REACTION 1. Social codes that differ from those of society. 2. Persons with ~ possess strong egos *q.v.* and have no personality disorganization *q.v.*, but whose moral codes go against those of their social environment. 3. ~s are typically exhibited by delinquents and racketeers. 4. Criminal behavior involving distorted values but good ego strength.

DISSOCIATION 1. In psychology, the separation or isolation of mental processes in such a way that they become split off from the main personality *q.v.* 2. The inability of a person to integrate; to see the wholeness of objects. 3. The tendency to see small segments without relation to the total configuration of which a person is a part.

DISSOCIATIVE DISORDERS Dissociative reactions *q.v.*

DISSOCIATIVE REACTION 1. A neurosis *q.v.* caused by overwhelming anxiety *q.v.* characterized by disorganization *q.v.* of the personality *q.v.* ~ is an attempt to repress *q.v.* unacceptable or painful episodes in life. The common forms of ~s are amnesia, fugue, and multiple personality. 2. Disorders in which a whole set of mental events is stored out of ordinary consciousness. 3. A psychoneurotic reaction *q.v.* consisting of splitting of the personality into two or more separate units. 4. Disorders in which the normal integration of consciousness, memory, or identity is suddenly and temporarily altered.

DISSOLUTION OF MARRIAGE Divorce *q.v.* in which there is no fault.

DISSONANCE A feeling of uncertainty that occurs when a person believes two equally attractive but opposite ideas. cf: cognitive dissonance.

DISSONANCE COGNITION Cognitive dissonance *q.v.*

DISSONANCE OF CHILD ATTRIBUTES AND SITUATION A mismatch between a child's attributes and situational features. ct: consonance of child attributes.

DISSONANCE THEORY Cognitive dissonance *q.v.* cf: dissonance.

DISTAL In anatomy, farthest from the center of the median line. 2. In the extremities, farthest from the point of junction with the trunk of the body. ct: proximal.

DISTAL STIMULUS 1. An object or event outside of the person as contrasted to the proximal stimulus *q.v.* 2. The stimulus defined in terms of environmental objects.

DISTAL URETHRA A structure in women homologous to the male's prostate gland *q.v.*

DISTANCING In psychotherapy, a therapeutic process in which the subject learns to recognize the control reality distorting cognitions that cause depression.

DISTENTION 1. The state of being inflated or enlarged, particularly of the abdomen. 2. The act of being distended or stretched.

DISTILLATION 1. Removing water from an alcohol liquid by the process of evaporation and condensation. 2. The process by which alcohol is separated from a weak alcohol solution to form more concentrated distilled spirits. The weak solution is heated and the alcohol vapors are collected and condensed to a liquid form.

DISTILLED SPIRITS 1. Alcoholic beverages containing from 40% to 50% alcohol by volume, made from fermented mixtures of cereal grains or fruits that are heated in a still. 2. Distilled liquor.

DISTINCTIVE FEATURES Particular features or objects or events that enable them to be readily discriminated from other objects or events.

DISTINGUISHABLE HYBRID In genetics, a hybrid *q.v.* in which intermediate inheritance is expressed.

DISTORTION In optics, optical bending of straight lines, thus producing distortion in the appearance of the specimen.

DISTRACTERS In evaluation, words or phrases in a test that are incorrect and require the learner to discriminate in order to correctly complete the test item. An integral part of a multiple-choice question.

DISTRACTIBILITY The tendency to be easily drawn away from any task at hand and to focus on extraneous stimuli of the moment.

DISTRESS 1. Potentially harmful stress *q.v.* 2. Stress that diminishes the quality of life, commonly associated with disease and maladaptation. 3. According to Selye, stress that is inappropriate because of its source or duration and harmful in its effects. cf: eustress.

DISTRIBUTED PRACTICE A system of practice schedules separated by either rest or some activity that is different from the one being practiced.

DISTRIBUTION In pharmacology, circulation of an absorbed drug to all parts of the body by way of the bloodstream.

DISTRIBUTION CURVE In statistics, a graphic representation that reflects the way observations distribute themselves. The frequency of the observations are plotted along a vertical axis *q.v.* and the type of observations are plotted along the horizontal axis *q.v.* cf: normal curve.

DISTRIBUTIVE BARGAINING In labor relations, negotiations whereby the gain of one party represents a loss to the other party.

DISTRICT 1. In politics, the division of the state represented by a legislator, designated numerically or by geographic boundaries. 2. In education, the boundaries constituting a population served by a school and board of education.

DISTURBED-NEUROTIC DELINQUENCY In psychology, an adolescent's adoption of impulsive antisocial *q.v.* behavior as a means of rebelling against the family.

DISULFIRAM 1. Antabuse *q.v.* 2. An antioxidant *q.v.* that interferes with the metabolism *q.v.* of alcohol *q.v.* resulting in an accumulation of acetaldehyde *q.v.* producing flushing, dizziness, heart palpitations, and extreme fear. Used in aversion therapy *q.v.* for alcoholics *q.v.*

DIURESIS 1. Excretion of urine. 2. Commonly denotes production of unusually large amounts of urine.

DIURETIC 1. A drug used to increase the output of urine. 2. A drug that helps the body excrete excess water and salt, causing a sudden and copious flow of urine. 3. Anything that increases the production of urine used for lowering blood pressure *q.v.* Common side effects are dehydration *q.v.* and loss of potassium. cf: hypertension.

DIURNAL Daily.

DIVERGENT LEARNING 1. Extends in different directions. 2. There are multiple acceptable answers to a question.

DIVERGENT THINKER A person who tends to respond to question in unpredictable and unconventional ways. ct: convergent thinker.

DIVERGENT THINKING 1. Thinking that is directed toward producing as many novel but appropriate ideas as possible. 2. An open-ended type of thinking that extends in different directions and considers multiple answers to a question. ct: convergent thinking.

DIVERTICULOSIS 1. An inflammation *q.v.* and ballooning of the intestinal wall in the lower colon. Symptoms include fever, abdominal pain, and constipation or diarrhea *q.v.* 2. An outpouching of some hollow organ.

DIVERTICULUM Outpocketing from a tubular organ such as the intestine.

DIVISIBLE CONTRACT In labor relations, one which can be separated into two or more parts not necessarily dependent upon each other nor intended by the parties to be so.

DIVISION 1. In politics, a method of voting. 2. In botany, the largest category of classification of plants according to the rules of nomenclature, an aggregation of classes. ~ in botany is synonymous with phylum *q.v.* in zoology.

DIVISION OF HEALTH EDUCATION Established in 1980 as a division of the Center for Health Promotion and Education *q.v.* in the CDC *q.v.* Its major programs were as follows: (a) School Programs and Special Projects, (b) Behavioral Epidemiology and Evaluation Branch, and (c) Program Services and Development Branch.

DIVISION OF LABOR The assignment of various portions of a particular task among a number of organization members.

DIVISION OF QUESTION In politics, a procedure to separate a matter to be voted upon into two or more questions.

DIVORCE 1. A legal dissolution of marriage. 2. Legally ending a marriage.

DIZYGOTIC TWINS 1. Twins from two ova *q.v.* 2. Fraternal twins *q.v.* 3. Birth partners who have developed from separate fertilized eggs and who are only 50% alike genetically *q.v.*, no more similar than siblings born from different pregnancies.

DIZZINESS 1. A disturbed sense of relationship to space. 2. A sense of unsteadiness. cf: vertigo.

D-LOVE 1. According to Maslow, love characterized by seeking in another to meet one's own deficiencies. 2. Deficiency love *q.v.* cf: B-love.

D-LYSERGIC ACID DIETHYLAMIDE TARTRATE 25 Lysergic acid *q.v.*, the psychoactive *q.v.* ingredient in LSD *q.v.*

DMD An acronym for Doctor of Dental Medicine degree. cf: DDS.

DMF An acronym for the total number of decayed, missing, and filled teeth.

DMSO An acronym for the controversial drug, dimethyl sulfoxide, originally used by veterinarians *q.v.* to reduce joint inflammation *q.v.* in animals, and presently used by some athletes for joint and soft tissue injuries.

DMT An acronym for a semisynthetic hallucinogen *q.v.*, also known as the business man's trip. 2. Dimethyltriptamine *q.v.*

DNA 1. An acronym for deoxyribonucleic acid *q.v.* 2. A polymeric polynucleotide *q.v.* whose sugar portion is 2-D-deoxyribose and whose principal purine *q.v.*, an pyrimidine *q.v.* base compliment, is made up of adenine, guanine, cytosine, and thymine. 3. An acid found in the nucleus of all cells which carries genetic *q.v.* information.

DNA (DENATURED) An acronym for the chemical and physical state of DNA *q.v.* after melting or after treatment with other chemical or physical agents.

DNA HELIX A coil or spiral containing the DNA *q.v.*

DNase An acronym for the enzyme *q.v.* that hydrolyzes *q.v.* DNA *q.v.*

DNA VIRUSES Viruses *q.v.* that contain DNA *q.v.* as their genetic *q.v.* material.

DO An acronym for Doctor of Optometry. 2. Doctor of Osteopathy.

DOA An acronym for dead on arrival.

DOCTOR 1. One skilled or specialized in a healing art. 2. A scholar or teacher. 3. One who teaches the knowledge and principles of a particular discipline. 4. One who holds the highest academic degree such as the PhD, a doctor of philosophy. cf: doctor's degree.

DOCTOR'S DEGREE The highest academic degree conferred by a university in any field, e.g., doctor of education, doctor of juridical science, doctor of public health.

DOCTRINE OF SPECIFIC NERVE ENERGIES The assertion that qualitative differences in sensory experiences are not attributed to the differences in the stimuli that correspond to different sense modalities, but rather to the fact that these stimuli excite different nervous structures.

DOD An acronym for Department of Defense *q.v.*

DODERLEIN'S BACILLI The bacteria *q.v.* normally present in the vagina *q.v.* cf: *lactobacilli*.

DOE An acronym for Department of Energy *q.v.*

DOGMATIC AUTHORITY One who asserts that something is true without explanation or rationale. ct: reasoning authority.

DOI An acronym for Department of Interior *q.v.*

DOLOPHINE A commercial preparation of methadone *q.v.*

DOM An acronym for a synthetic hallucinogen *q.v.* 2. Also referred to as STP *q.v.* 3. Dimethoxymethylamphetamine *q.v.*

DOMICILIARY CARE FACILITY A nonmedical institution providing room, board, laundry, some forms of personal care, and usually recreational and social services. Licensed by state departments of social services; these facilities are not eligible for Medicare *q.v.* or Medicaid *q.v.* reimbursement. cf: intermediate care facility; skilled nursing facility.

DOMINANCE 1. In genetics, applied to one member of an allelic *q.v.* pair of genes *q.v.*, which has the ability to manifest itself wholly or largely at the exclusion of the expression of the other member. 2. An inherited *q.v.* trait expressed when the controlling gene is either homozygous *q.v.* or heterozygous *q.v.*

DOMINANCE HIERARCHY In social groups, the dominance ranking of their members.

DOMINANT 1. A gene *q.v.* that expresses itself to the exclusion of the expression of its allele *q.v.* 2. A character possessed by one parent of a hybrid that appears in the hybrid to the exclusion of the contrasting character of the other parent. 3. In ecology, a species that to a considerable extent controls the conditions for existence of its associates within an ecosystem *q.v.* The dominance may be due to numbers or to size of the individual dominants.

DOMINANT GENE A genetic material that is expressed even in the presence of a recessive gene *q.v.* When one member of a gene pair is dominant *q.v.* and the other is recessive, the dominant gene will exert its effects regardless of what the recessive gene calls for. cf: chromosome.

DOMINANT RESPONSE TENDENCY The response that is learned most thoroughly.

DOMINATOR UNIT Retinal *q.v.* loci of electrical responsivity to light. ct: modulator unit.

DON JUAN A term sometimes used in psychology *q.v.* to describe a person who possesses the personality *q.v.* of a roué, seducer, and profligate.

DONOVANIA GRANULOMATIS A bacterium that causes granuloma inguinale *q.v.*

DOOR-IN-THE-FACE TECHNIQUE When an extreme request is refused, it is more likely that a second, smaller request will be granted. Used in labor relations.

DOPAMINE (DA) 1. A catecholamine *q.v.* that is a neurotransmitter *q.v.* in various brain structures. Some psychologists *q.v.* believe that schizophrenia *q.v.* is based on the oversensitivity to ~ in some part of the brain. 2. Levodopa *q.v.* 3. A substance that regulates normal body movement. 4. A neurotransmitter substance heavily, but not exclusively, concentrated in the limbic system *q.v.* of the brain that facilitates or inhibits transmission of nerve impulses between neurons *q.v.* cf: dopamine hypothesis of schizophrenia; Parkinson's disease.

DOPAMINE HYPOTHESIS OF SCHIZOPHRENIA The theory that schizophrenia *q.v.* victims are oversensitive to the neurotransmitter dopamine *q.v.* and are therefore in a state of over arousal. Phenothiazines *q.v.* alleviate schizophrenia symptoms acting as a block to ~ transmission.

DO PASS In politics, the affirmative recommendation made by a committee in sending a bill to the floor for additional action.

DOPING The use of ergogenic agents *q.v.* to artificially improve athletic performance.

DORMANCY In botany, a period of inactivity in bulbs, buds, seeds, and other plant organs.

DORSAL 1. Pertaining to the back. 2. The upper surface of the penis *q.v.* 3. The upper surface of the plant body, in botany. 4. Posterior. ct: ventral.

DORSALIS PEDIS ARTERY The artery whose pulse is palpable on the dorsal *q.v.* surface of the foot. The ~ supplies the medial foot and great toe.

DORSAL KYPHOSIS Round upper back. cf: kyphosis.

DORSIFLEXION Turning of the foot or of the toes upward.

DORSIVENTRAL SYMMETRY Having distinct lower and upper surfaces.

DOSAGE A specific, calculated amount of a drug to be taken or administered at a particular time. cf: dose.

DOSE A quantity or amount of a drug taken at a particular time. cf: dosage.

DOSE–RESPONSE CURVE A graph showing the relationship between the size of a drug dose *q.v.* and the size of the response. cf: dose–response relationship.

DOSE–RESPONSE RELATIONSHIP 1. In epidemiology, as the amount of exposure to a risk factor *q.v.* increases, the rate of the effect of the exposure increases. 2. The intensity and character of a response to a drug depends upon the amount administered and individual variability. 3. The relationship between the amount of a drug taken and the intensity of its effects. cf: effective dose; threshold dose; time action function; dose–response curve.

DOT 1. An acronym for *Dictionary of Occupational Titles*. 2. An acronym for Department of Transportation *q.v.*

DOUBLE APPROACH/AVOIDANCE CONFLICT In psychology, conflict *q.v.* instigated by the necessity of making a choice between two objects neither of which is wholly desirable or undesirable.

DOUBLE-BARRELED QUESTION In research, two questions rolled into one, making it impossible to determine to which question the respondent is responding.

DOUBLE BLIND 1. In social psychology, a situation characteristic of the relationship in the families that produce schizophrenics *q.v.* The child is punished for the expression of affection and simultaneously blamed for not expressing it. 2. A situation in which a person will be disapproved for performing a given act and equally disapproved when he or she does not perform it. 3. An interpersonal situation in which an individual is confronted, over a long period of time by mutually inconsistent messages to which he or she must respond, believed by some theorists to cause schizophrenia.

DOUBLE BLIND DESIGN A procedure for comparing the effectiveness of a drug with that of a placebo *q.v.* Neither the subjects nor the experimenter know which of the agents the subjects are given, the actual drug or the placebo. cf: double blind technique.

DOUBLE BLIND PROCEDURE 1. A method for reducing the biasing effects of the expectations of subject and experimenter. Neither is allowed to know whether the independent variable *q.v.* of the experiment is being applied to the particular subject. 2. Double blind design *q.v.* 3. Double blind technique *q.v.*

DOUBLE BLIND STUDY Double blind design *q.v.*

DOUBLE BLIND TECHNIQUE 1. A method of investigation in which neither the subject nor the investigator knows what treatment the subject is receiving. 2. A conflict setup in a person who is told one thing while simultaneously receiving the message that what is meant is the opposite. cf: double blind design; double blind procedure. ct: placebo effect.

DOUBLE CROSS In genetics, a cross involving four inbred strains.

DOUBLE FERTILIZATION In genetics, the fusion of the egg and the sperm, resulting in a $2n$ fertilized egg, and the fusion of the second gamete *q.v.* with the polar nuclei *q.v.*, resulting in a $3n$ primary endosperm nucleus *q.v.*

DOUBLE HEMIPLEGIA Paralysis that involves both sides of the body, with one side being more greatly affected.

DOUBLE INDEMNITY An insurance policy containing a clause that calls for a doubling of benefits when certain types of accidents occur, usually related to death benefits.

DOUBLE STANDARD 1. Within a particular culture, the application of different standards of behavior to members of the two sexes. 2. The judging of the same act by two different standards for two different groups. ct: single standard. 3. A cultural situation in which a behavioral standard is applied to one sex but not the other sex. 4. Generally refers to greater sexual permissiveness of male sexual behavior than of female sexual behavior.

DOUBLE TRACK 1. Duel-track. Refers to salary progression. 2. Two distinct parallel ladders of compensation progression for managerial and professional/technical personnel.

DOUBLING RATE The time required for a cell to divide into two identical cells. cf: mitosis.

DOUBLING TIME The period of time required for a total population to double in size.

DOUCHE 1. A vaginal *q.v.* rinse. Sometimes used as a contraceptive *q.v.* measure, but is ineffective as it may force sperm *q.v.* farther into the vagina thus increasing the likelihood of conception *q.v.* 2. A stream of fluid directed into the vagina to wash away sperm or for hygienic purposes.

DOUCHING Rinsing the vagina with water or a cleaning solution. cf: douche.

DOWER In some states, refers to the wife's right to one-third or one-half interest in her husband's real property following his death.

DOWN SYNDROME 1. A birth defect *q.v.* related to faulty chromosomes *q.v.* Chromosomal aberrations *q.v.* are of three types: (a) trisomy 21, (b) translocation, or (c) mosaicism. 2. Previously called mongolism *q.v.* 3. ~ is characterized by mild to severe mental retardation *q.v.* accompanied by recognizable physical features and is one of the most common forms of mental retardation. It may be detected and diagnosed during prenatal *q.v.* development by the use of amniocentesis *q.v.*

DOWNWARD ORGANIZATIONAL COMMUNICATION Communication that flows from any point on an organizational chart downward to another point in the organizational chart.

DOWRY Goods or money given by a bride's family to the family of her intended.

DOXEPIN 1. A heterocyclic antidepressant *q.v.* 2. Sinequan and Adapin are brand names.

DP An acronym for Doctor of Pharmacy or Doctor of Podiatry.

DPM An acronym for Doctor of Podiatric Medicine.

DPN An acronym for diphosphopyridine *q.v.*

DPT An acronym for a triple vaccine *q.v.* for the prevention of diphtheria, pertussis, and tetanus.

DQ An acronym for developmental quotient *q.v.*

DRAG In rescue operations, a general term referring to methods of moving a victim without a stretcher or litter. Usually employed by a single rescuer. There are three types of ~s: (a) blanket drag, by which one EMT *q.v.* encloses a victim in a blanket and drags him/her to safety; (b) clothes drag, by which one EMT can drag a victim to safety by grasping his or her clothes; and (c) fireman's drag, by which one EMT crawls with the victim by looping his or her tied wrists over his or her neck to support the victim's weight.

DRAG FORCE The force that causes a scrubbing action or drag of the tire on the road surface when a vehicle is turned, thus slowing the speed of the vehicle.

DRAG QUEENS Homosexual men who habitually dress as women.

DRAINAGE In medicine, the creation of an opening through which accumulated pus can escape, especially in purulent *q.v.* infections.

DRAPE 1. In surgery, a sterile covering used about an operative site to decrease the chance of contamination from the surroundings. 2. The act of placing a sterile covering about an operative site.

DRAW A PERSON TEST A projective test *q.v.* in which the subject, who is usually a child, draws a person, then draws one of the opposite sex. The results can be scored for cognitive development *q.v.* or for psychotherapy *q.v.*

DREAD DISEASE POLICY An insurance policy that protects a person against a specific disease.

DREAM ANALYSIS 1. The attempt by a psychotherapist *q.v.* to interpret a person's dreams to reveal symbolic meaning to dream episodes. 2. A key psychoanalytic technique in which the unconscious meanings of dream material are uncovered.

DRESSING 1. Sterile gauze or compresses of various sizes applied and fixed in position for the protection of a wound. 2. A bandage.

DRG An acronym for diagnosis (diagnostic)-related groups *q.v.*

DRIFT 1. Random genetic drift *q.v.* 2. Change in gene *q.v.* frequency in small breeding populations due to chance fluctuations. 3. Sewall Wright effect *q.v.*

DRIFT ANGLE The angle that is formed when the steering wheel of a car is turned and the center line of the front tires heads away from the direction in which the vehicle is traveling.

DRIVE 1. A condition or state of the individual that activates or directs behavior, hunger, thirst, etc. ~s are powerful motivational forces. 2. Biological need *q.v.* 3. A biological mechanism that initiates activity or behavior in a person. 4. A construct *q.v.* explaining the motivation of behavior or an internal physiological tension impelling an organism to activity.

DRIVE REDUCER A condition or set of circumstances that act to lessen physiological arousal or need state.

DRIVE-REDUCTION THEORY 1. The precept that all built-in rewards are responsible for some noxious body state.

This theory tends to ignore motives *q.v.* 2. A theory of reinforcement that holds that reinforcement consists of the reduction of a motive. cf: drive-stimulus reduction theory.

DRIVE STIMULUS A stimulus associated with a drive *q.v.*

DRIVE-STIMULUS REDUCTION THEORY The version of drive-reduction theory *q.v.* that maintains that it is the reduction in the intensity of the drive stimulus *q.v.* that provides the basis for reinforcement.

DRONES Slang term for gay men who dress in leather and other very masculine fashions and who favor sadomasochism *q.v.*

DROPLET CONTACT 1. A means of indirectly transmitting a communicable disease *q.v.* by droplets in the spray from an infected person's coughing or sneezing. 2. Droplet infection *q.v.*

DROPLET INFECTION 1. A means of spreading disease whereby tiny droplets of saliva containing the microorganisms *q.v.* are spread by coughs or sneezes. 2. Droplet contact *q.v.*

DROPLET NUCLEI Minute particles from the evaporation of droplets of moisture.

DROPLET SPRAY Organisms that are projected in droplets of water when an infected person coughs or sneezes and are received in the eyes, nose, or mouth of a nearby person.

DROPOUT In education, a student who leaves school before graduation.

DROPPING Engaging *q.v.*

DROPSY Excessive accumulation of fluids in a cavity or the tissues.

DROWN To suffocate by submersion, especially in water.

DRPH An acronym for Doctor of Public Health.

DRUG 1. Any medical substance possessing the qualities that will aid in the diagnosing, treating, curing, or preventing disease or maintaining health. 2. A chemical substance other than food that speeds, slows, or interferes with the system(s) of the body.

DRUG ABUSE 1. The use of legal drugs in a manner or amount contrary to their intended dosage or purpose and the use of illegal drugs for the purpose of bringing about a change in feelings, mood, or behavior. 2. The self-administration of any drug(s) for nontherapeutic purposes. 3. Taking a drug to such a degree as to impair the ability of the individual to cope with a particular circumstance or to increase risk to self or others.

DRUG ABUSE EPIDEMIC The sudden increase in a disease condition (drug abuse *q.v.*) in a particular population or locality.

DRUG ADDICTION Continual use of and physiological *q.v.* dependence *q.v.* upon certain drugs. cf: addiction; drug habituation; drug abuse.

DRUG AUTOMATISM 1. A state of confusion following the taking of a drug resulting in repeated ingestion of the drug. An overdose is often the result. 2. Some authorities question the existence of ~ because it cannot be measured and refer to this phenomenon as distorted perception.

DRUG BEHAVIOR One's attitudes and practices regarding the use of drugs and medicines. cf: drug abuse.

DRUG COMBINATIONS The use of a variety of drugs at one time. ~ can produce unwanted and undesirable side effects *q.v.*

DRUG CULTURE 1. A sociological subgroup consisting chiefly of persons who are drug addicts or semiaddicts whose primary concern is in seeking familiar or new drug experiences. 2. A subculture consisting of drug users, abusers, addicts, suppliers, usually involving illegal drugs.

DRUG DEPENDENCE 1. Habituation or addiction *q.v.* to a drug or drugs. 2. A state arising from repeated administration of a drug on a periodic or continuous basis. Its characteristics vary with the agent involved. This is made clear by designating the particular type of drug dependence in each specific case, e.g., ~ of the morphine type, ~ of the cocaine type, etc.

DRUG DISPOSITION TOLERANCE 1. The state in which enzyme *q.v.* systems in the liver increases their capacity to metabolize *q.v.* a drug, so the body disposes of the drug faster. 2. The reduced effect of a drug that may result from more rapid metabolism or excretion of the drug. 3. Tolerance *q.v.* to a drug that occurs via the process by which the drug increases the number and rate of action of the microsomal enzymes in the liver.

DRUG ENFORCEMENT ADMINISTRATION (DEA) The principal federal agency for enforcement of drug laws pertaining to drug trafficking, investigation, drug intelligence, and regulatory control, administered within the United States Department of Justice.

DRUG FAMILIES The major categories or types of drugs that share important characteristics in terms of chemical composition or actions within the body.

DRUG HABITUATION A psychological dependence *q.v.* on the effects of a drug without a withdrawal syndrome *q.v.* upon denial.

DRUG INTERACTION 1. Potentiation *q.v.* 2. When a drug action is modified by another substance, it may add to, inhibit, or be enhanced.

DRUG LAG The charge that drug testing procedures required by the government regulations result in a delay in the introduction of new prescription drugs for marketing and use in the United States.

DRUG MISUSE Unintentional or inappropriate use of prescribed or OTC *q.v.* drugs resulting in impaired physical, mental, emotional, or social well-being of the user.

DRUG POTENCY The amount of a drug that must be taken to produce the desired effect. The smaller the amount needed, the more potent the drug.

DRUG RECEPTOR The specific area on or within a particular neuron with which a drug must interact or attach itself before any change in cell function occurs.

DRUG REINFORCER Any short-term effect of using a drug that is perceived as beneficial, which increases the likelihood of repeated drug use.

DRUGS OF ABUSE Drugs, almost always mood altering drugs, that are taken to help cope with stress *q.v.*, to relieve pain, to enhance pleasure, and are thus taken too often and on too large a dosage.

DRUG SYNERGISM Synergism *q.v.*

DRUG THERAPY 1. Chemotherapy *q.v.* 2. The use of a drug or drugs in an effort to treat an illness.

DRUG-USE INDICATORS Descriptions of or statistics on the incidence and prevalence of drug use in a particular area or in a specific population.

DRUNKENNESS A state of intoxication *q.v.*

DRY-DRUNK PHENOMENON An alcoholic's typical state of mind when not drinking, marked by a lack of insight, exaggeration of self-importance, overestimation of abilities, insensitivity to others' needs and feelings, rigid judgmental outlook, impatience, and dissatisfaction with life.

DRY ORGASM Sexual climax in the male without apparent ejaculation of semen *q.v.* Often an instance of retrograde ejaculation caused by some anomaly within the prostate *q.v.* in which semen is ejaculated backward into the posterior urethra *q.v.* and urinary bladder *q.v.* rather than out the penis *q.v.* Removal of the prostate often is the cause of ~.

DRY WEIGHT Moisture-free weight obtained by drying at high temperatures for a sufficient period of time.

DSA An acronym for digital subtraction angiography *q.v.*

D SLEEP REM sleep *q.v.*

DSM The *Diagnostic and Statistical Manual* of the American Psychiatric Association. It categorizes mental disorders and their descriptive characteristics to assist in their diagnosis. It is now in its fourth edition (DSM-IV).

DT An acronym for Division of Toxicology *q.v.* Also, ATSDR *q.v.*

DTS Delirium tremens *q.v.*

DUAL CAREER MARRIAGE A marriage in which both partners seriously pursue professional careers. Now largely thought to be the rule rather than the exception.

DUAL CODING HYPOTHESIS The hypothesis that concrete objects or words are to be remembered more readily than abstract objects or words because they are encoded as images and as verbal labels.

DUALISM 1. The Persian philosophy that the spirit and the flesh are in conflict with one another. 2. Philosophical doctrine that a human being is both mental and physical and that these two aspects are separate but interacting. ~ was advanced in its most definitive statement by Descartes. ct: monism.

DUAL PERSONALITY Multiple personality *q.v.*

DUAL SPORTS Physical activities that require two participants, e.g., wrestling.

DUAL WORLD PROSTITUTE A prostitute *q.v.* who identifies with her family and has middle class values.

DUCT Any tube that conveys the secretion of any gland from one point to another.

DUCTLESS GLANDS The glands of internal secretion *q.v.*, the glands of the endocrine system *q.v.* whose hormones *q.v.* are secreted directly into the vascular system *q.v.*

DUCT SYSTEM 1. The body's collection system of tubes and canals. 2. The collection or system of tubes within the embryo *q.v.* that eventually gives rise to various reproductive structures. cf: duct.

DUCTUS ARTERIOSUS A small vessel connecting the pulmonary artery with the descending aorta *q.v.*

DUE PROCESS 1. In law, a legal term referring to the regular administration of the law wherein no person may be denied his or her legal rights. 2. In education, procedural safeguards afforded to students, parents, and teachers that protects individual rights. 3. The exercise of the powers of government in such a way as to protect individual rights. Denial of this right is prohibited by the Fifth and Fourteenth Amendments to the United States Constitution.

DUES CHECKOFF In labor relations, the arrangement whereby employers deduct union dues from the wages of employees and transmit them to the union.

DUMBCANE 1. A tropical American herb that, when chewed, causes the tongue to swell. The reaction can be severe enough to cause obstruction of the airway. 2. *Dieffenbachia seguine*.

DUODENUM The first part of the small intestine.

DUPLICATION In genetics, the occurrence of a segment more than once in the same chromosome *q.v.* or genome *q.v.*

DUPLICITY Inconsistency between a person's beliefs and actions.

DUPLICITY THEORY OF VISION The theory that has essentially the status of fact, that vision involves two separate senses. cf: rods; cones.

DURA MATER 1. A tough, fibrous membrane *q.v.* covering the brain. 2. Literally, strong and hard mother. 3. Outermost layer of the meninges *q.v.*

DURATION 1. In exercise, the length of time one needs to exercise at the target heart rate to produce the training effect *q.v.* 2. One of the chief variables of exercise prescription *q.v.*

DURHAM DECISION 1. An insanity *q.v.* plea following the commitment of a crime. This is based on the concept that a person committing a crime is not responsible if the crime resulted from a mental disease or defect. cf: Currens formula; McNaghten decision. 2. A 1954 American court ruling that an accused person is not ascriptively responsible *q.v.* if his or her crime is judged attributable to mental disease or defect.

DUROPHET A commercial preparation of 12.5-mg capsules of amphetamine *q.v.*

D_5W A solution of 50 g of dextrose *q.v.* in 1000 ml of sterile water. cf: D_{10}W.

D_{10}W A solution of 100 g of dextrose (glucose) *q.v.* in 1000 ml of sterile water. cf: D_5W.

DWARFISM Caused by a combination of genetic *q.v.* and endocrine factors characterized by a shortness in stature that results from premature ossification *q.v.* of the epiphysis *q.v.* of the long bones.

DYAD In sociology, a two-person group.

DYADIC Between two partners.

DYING, STAGES OF Theoretical emotional phases that a person passes through when faced with imminent death: (a) denial and isolation, (b) anger, (c) bargaining, and (d) acceptance.

DYNAMIC 1. In a state of change. Health is dynamic in the sense that it is influenced by factors from both within and outside of the person. 2. A pattern of interactive factors underlying a particular event or condition.

DYNAMIC CONTRACTION 1. Isotonic contraction *q.v.* 2. A type of muscle contraction in which the muscle fibers shorten and movement is involved.

DYNAMIC CURES Visual cues to depth that are created by movements of either the viewer or the objects in the visual field of the viewer.

DYNAMICS Moving moral or physical forces of any kind.

DYNAMISM 1. An ego defense mechanism *q.v.* 2. A device used to protect ego integrity.

DYSARTHRIA Interference with the proper articulation of speech.

DYSCALCULIA 1. Acalculia *q.v.* 2. May mean partial or less severe acalculia.

DYSCRASIA 1. An abnormal condition. 2. A general term pertaining to any disease of the blood.

DYSENTERY 1. An intestinal disease characterized by diarrhea *q.v.* and abdominal cramps. ~ is caused by bacteria, protozoa, or viruses.

DYSFUNCTION 1. Malfunction. 2. Inadequate, excessive, abnormal function of an organ, tissue, or other body structure. 3. Impaired function. 4. Harmful function. 5. An impairment or disturbance in the functioning of an organ, organ system, behavior, or cognition.

DYSFUNCTIONAL A part of a social system that disrupts the operation of another part of that system.

DYSFUNCTIONALS Homosexuals who live alone, have many sexual contacts, and encounter many adjustment problems.

DYSGENIC In genetics, a situation that tends to be harmful to the hereditary *q.v.* qualities of future generations. cf: eugenic.

DYSGRAPHIA 1. An impaired ability to write because of ataxia *q.v.*, tremors *q.v.*, or similar conditions. 2. The inability to express ideas in writing even though motor ability is present.

DYSKINESIA Poor coordination, clumsy, inappropriate movements in a person without detectable cerebral palsy *q.v.*

DYSLEXIA 1. A perceptual dysfunction *q.v.* characterized by the inability to clearly distinguish words and letters in the way and order presented. 2. The reversing of letters in a word. 3. A disturbance in the ability to read, one of the learning disabilities *q.v.* or specific developmental disorders *q.v.* 4. Reading difficulty not attributable to ordinary causes; generally, but not always, attributed to some sort of brain impairment. Though some would make the case for differences in meaning between alexia *q.v.* and ~, in practice they are often used interchangeably. Some authorities would delineate as many as 8–10 types of ~, including congenital *q.v.*, constitutional, affective *q.v.*, and partial.

DYSMENORRHEA 1. A menstrual *q.v.* irregularity characterized by pain just above the pelvic bone and abdominal region. 2. Menstrual pain. 3. Discomfort associated with the menstrual cycle *q.v.* 4. Menstrual cramps.

DYSPAREUNIA 1. Painful sexual intercourse *q.v.* 2. Coitus *q.v.* that is difficult and painful, especially for a woman. 3. Painful or difficult sexual intercourse usually being caused by infection *q.v.* or a physical injury, such as torn ligaments in the pelvic region. 4. Painful sexual intercourse resulting from vaginal dryness and a thinning of the vaginal walls resulting from menopause *q.v.*

DYSPEPSIA Indigestion.

DYSPHASIA 1. Aphasia *q.v.* 2. Interference with the act of swallowing.

DYSPHORIA 1. Depression. 2. A lack of sense of well-being or excitement. 3. A feeling of unpleasantness or discomfort. cf: euphoria.

DYSPHORIC 1. An emotional response to an antipsychotic tranquilizer *q.v.* characterized by a drop in mood or slowed thought process. 2. A sad mood state. cf: dysphoria. ct: euphoria.

DYSPLASIA An abnormal development of a tissue.

DYSPNEA Difficult, rapid breathing.

DYSPRAXIA Apraxia *q.v.*

DYSRHYTHMIA 1. Disturbance in rhythm. 2. Irregular or chaotic brain-wave sequences.

DYSSOMNIA A sleep disorder characterized by chronic sleeplessness when sleeping should occur.

DYSTHYMIC A chronic *q.v.* disturbance of mood involving either depressed mood or loss of interest, but not of sufficient severity and duration to meet the criteria for a major depressive episode. Dysthymic disorder.

DYSTOCIA Any abnormality of the normal process of birth.

DYSTROPHY 1. Faulty nutrition. 2. Progressive weakness. 3. Progressive atrophy *q.v.*

DYSURIA Painful urination.

EAA Essential amino acid.

EARLY CHILDHOOD EDUCATION Any systematic effort to teach a child before the normal period of schooling begins.

EASY CHILDREN In psychology, children whose temperament patterns include a positive mood, low to mild intensity of reaction, a positive approach to new events, and adaptability *q.v.* ct: difficult children.

EATING DISORDERS Conditions that include abnormal fears regarding eating, significant weight loss from not eating or from regurgitating food, binge eating, and eating nonnutritive substances. cf: anorexia nervosa; bulimia.

EATON TEST 1. A diagnostic technique of X-raying the breast for detection of cancer. 2. Mammography *q.v.*

EBV An acronym for Epstein–Barr virus.

ECCENTRIC CONTRACTION 1. A muscle contraction in which the muscle gradually lengthens while combating the pull of gravity. 2. An isotonic contraction *q.v.*

ECCHYMOSIS 1. Diffusion of blood into the tissue spaces. 2. A discoloration of the skin resulting from subcutaneous *q.v.* and intracutaneous *q.v.* hemorrhage *q.v.* Bluish color in the early stages changing to a greenish yellow because of chemical changes in the pooled blood. 3. Bruise *q.v.* 4. Hematoma *q.v.* cf: ecchymotic.

ECCHYMOTIC 1. Black and blue areas of the skin. 2. Bruise *q.v.* 3. Hematoma *q.v.* cf: eccymosis.

ECCRINE GLANDS Sweat glands that produce a clear, colorless liquid to prevent the body from overheating. ct: apocrine glands.

ECDYSIS The losing or shedding of an outer structure.

ECF An acronym for extracellular fluid *q.v.*

ECHOCARDIOGRAPHY A method using ultrasonic waves to study the structure and movement of the heart.

ECHOLALIA 1. Meaningless repetition of words by a person, usually of whatever is said to him or her. 2. The immediate and sometimes pathological *q.v.* repetition of the words of others. A speech problem often found in autistic *q.v.* children. In delayed ~, this inappropriate echoing takes place hours or weeks later. cf: echopraxia.

ECHOPRAXIA An automatic imitation by a person of another person's movements or mannerisms. cf: echolalia.

ECLAMPSIA 1. A condition characterized by convulsions *q.v.* and coma *q.v.* that may occur in a woman during pregnancy *q.v.* or immediately following childbirth. 2. The occurrence of one or more convulsions not attributable to other cerebral *q.v.* conditions, such as epilepsy *q.v.* or cerebral hemorrhage *q.v.* in a woman with eclampsia. 3. A toxic condition of unknown etiology *q.v.* associated with some pregnancies. cf: toxemia.

ECLECTIC LEARNING THEORY A learning theory that includes a combination of the major learning theories. cf: eclecticism.

ECLECTIC THERAPY Psychotherapy *q.v.* based on elements from various theories or procedures. cf: eclecticism.

ECLECTICISM 1. In psychology, the view that more is to be gained by employing concepts from various theoretical systems than by restricting oneself to a single psychological theory or school of thought. 2. Eclectic therapy *q.v.* 3. In education, drawing elements from several educational philosophies or methods.

ECOLOGIC FALLACY In epidemiology, an error in interpreting associations between ecologic *q.v.* indices. It is not necessarily accurate to assume that because a majority of a group has a particular characteristic, the characteristic is associated with the health condition that is common in the group. ct: ecologic index.

ECOLOGIC INDEX In epidemiology, a system of classification that applies the majority of characteristics of an entire group to all individuals within the group irrespective of individual characteristics.

ECOLOGICAL Pertaining to ecology *q.v.*; the interaction of people with their environment *q.v.* The interaction of all living things with the environment and segments of one environment with other segments.

ECOLOGY 1. The interaction of people with their environment. 2. The interaction of all living things with the environment and segments of one environment with other segments. 3. The study of the relationship between an environment and the social behavior of organisms in the environment. cf: human ecology.

ECONOMY (PRINCIPLE OF) In psychology, the theory *q.v.* that the person meets stress *q.v.* in the simplest way possible.

ECOSYSTEM 1. The study of the relationship between organisms and their environments. 2. The interacting system of one to many living organisms and their nonliving environment. cf: ecology.

ECT 1. Electroconvulsive shock therapy *q.v.* 2. A procedure in which an electric current is passed through the head, resulting in an epileptic-like seizure *q.v.* Although this procedure is now used less frequently than in the past, it has recently undergone a resurgence in popularity and is considered by many to be the most effective and rapid treatment for severe depression.

ECTODERM 1. The outermost layer of differentiated cells in the embryo *q.v.* from which the nervous system, sense organs, oral cavity, and skin eventually develop. 2. The primary tissue comprising the surface layer of cells in the gastrula *q.v.*

ECTOMORPHY One of the three body types indentified by Sheldon as indicative of one's temperament: characterized by one who is fragile, thin and tall, and whose temperament is cerebrotonic *q.v.*, i.e., asocial *q.v.*, unamiable, lacks desire for exercise, and nonadventurous. cf: endomorphy; mesomorphy.

ECTOPIC 1. Pertains to being in an abnormal place. 2. Displaced. cf: extrauterine pregnancy; ectopic pregnancy.

ECTOPIC PREGNANCY A pregnancy in which the fertilized egg becomes implanted outside the uterus.

ECTOPLASM 1. The outermost portion of the cytoplasm *q.v.* of the microzoan *q.v.* cell, consisting of jellylike plasmagel *q.v.* that is hyaline *q.v.* and relatively free of granules. 2. The outer layer of cytoplasm of a cell.

ECTOTHRIX Infection of the hair where sporulation *q.v.* is outside the hair.

ECTROPION A contraction of the eyelid, usually the lower lid, so that it is turned outward and becomes easily irritated.

ECZEMA A skin condition characterized by red, scaly, swollen areas on the skin, which contain clear fluid.

EDC 1. An acronym for expected date of confinement *q.v.* 2. The due date for a normal pregnancy usually determined by Nagele's rule *q.v.*

EDEMA 1. Accumulation of water in the tissues. 2. Tissue swelling caused by an excess of fluid in the interstitial *q.v.* space, seen in thiamin and protein deficiency *q.v.* and other health conditions. 3. The presence of abnormally large amounts of fluid in the body, characterized by swelling or puffiness.

EDP An acronym for electronic data processing *q.v.*

EDUCABILITY EXPECTATION A parameter of classification that represents a predictable expectation of educational achievement.

EDUCABLE CHILD 1. A child able to benefit from academic instruction at some level. 2. A child of borderline or moderately severe mental retardation who is capable of achieving only a limited degree of proficiency in basic learning and who usually must be instructed in a special class. ct: trainable child.

EDUCATED CITIZENRY A goal of society according to which all members of society participate intelligently in its direction and development.

EDUCATION A complex process of experiences that influence the way a person perceives him or herself in relation to the social and physical environments. It is a purposeful process for expediting learning *q.v.* although it does take place in other contexts.

EDUCATION MAJOR A student whose program of studies gives primary emphasis to subject matter in an area of education and who, according to his or her institutional requirements, concentrates on a minimum number of courses or semester hours of college credit in the specialty of education.

EDUCATION PROGRAM The organized learning environment, integrating and coordinating all elements that are intended to expedite learning. cf: educational process.

EDUCATION TRENDS Forecasted patterns in education *q.v.*

EDUCATIONAL AIDS Materials, technology, and other resources that enhance the quality of the educational experience.

EDUCATIONAL ATMOSPHERE 1. The degree to which conditions in a particular classroom favors effective instruction. 2. The quality of the learning environment.

EDUCATIONAL DIAGNOSIS The delineation of factors that predispose, enable, and reinforce a particular health behavior.

EDUCATIONAL EFFORT The amount spent for education in relation to taxable income, or potential for school support.

EDUCATIONAL LEADERSHIP That action or behavior among persons or groups that causes both the individual and the groups to move toward educational goals that are increasingly mutually acceptable to them.

EDUCATIONAL MALPRACTICE Culpable neglect by a teacher or school administrator in the performance of his or her duties as an educator.

EDUCATIONAL MATERIALS See educational aids; educational tools.

EDUCATIONAL PARK A large campus-like school plant containing several units with a variety of facilities, often including many grade levels and varied programs and often surrounded by a variety of cultural resources.

EDUCATIONAL PROCESS The systematic arrangement of the learning environment that purposely expedites learning *q.v.* cf: education programs.

EDUCATIONAL PSYCHOLOGY The application of psychological *q.v.* principles to education *q.v.*

EDUCATIONAL RESEARCH 1. Any systematic striving for understanding, actuated by a need or sensed difficulty toward some complex phenomenon or more than immediate personal concern stated in problematic form. 2. Any scientific effort to understand the nature or problems associated with the educational process or the learning process.

EDUCATIONAL STRATEGY The general approach to the organization of any educational program, including curriculum *q.v.* arrangement, instructional techniques, and goals and objectives *q.v.*

EDUCATIONAL TECHNOLOGY 1. Technology applied to educational practices, primarily instruction. 2. Scientific application of knowledge of educational institutions for purposes of instruction or institutional management.

EDUCATIONAL TELEVISION (ETV) 1. Educational programs broadcast by either commercial television or specialized educational networks that emphasize educational subjects. 2. Educational programs in the broadest sense—cultural, informative, and instructive—that are usually telecast by stations outside the school setting and received on standard television sets by the general public.

EDUCATIONAL TOOL Any material designed to aid learning and teaching primarily through sight and sound. cf: educational aids; educational materials; audiovisual aids.

EEG 1. An acronym for electroencephalogram *q.v.* 2. Electroencephalograph *q.v.*

EEG PATTERNS Patterns reflecting the type and extent of electrical activity occurring in the cerebral cortex *q.v.* cf: electroencephalogram.

EEOC An acronym for Equal Employment Opportunity Commission *q.v.*

EESS An acronym for Emergency Event Surveillance System *q.v.*

EFA An acronym for essential fatty acids, essential fats *q.v.*

EFFACEMENT 1. Flattening and extension of the cervix *q.v.* 2. Thinning of the cervix during labor *q.v.*

EFFECT MODIFIER In epidemiology, a variable that changes or influences the effect; the disease or health outcome.

EFFECT SIZE In research, the average size in standard deviation units of an effect as determined by data combined from several studies.

EFFECTANCE MOTIVATION Behavior deliberately focused toward increasing tension and creating conditions that provide suspense and excitement.

EFFECTIVE DATE In law, a law becomes binding, either on a date specified in the law itself or in the absence of such date, within a certain number of days specified by the constitution or other law.

EFFECTIVE DOSE 1. The dose that is effective therapeutically. 2. Therapeutic index *q.v.* 3. The dose level of a drug that produces the desired effect. ED_{50} means that the dose given causes the desired response in 50% of the test animals used in researching the drug.

EFFECTIVE ENVIRONMENT That part of the external environment to which a person is responding. ct: noneffective environment.

EFFECTIVE STIMULUS A stimulus *q.v.* that affects an appropriate receptor *q.v.* in detectable strength. ct: distal stimulus. cf: proximal stimulus.

EFFECTIVE TEACHING A movement to improve teaching performance based on the outcomes of educational research. Also referred to as effective schools.

EFFECTIVENESS 1. A person's dynamism *q.v.* 2. The degree to which a person is able to achieve within genetic *q.v.* potentials and environmental constraints. 3. The extent to which benefits that could be achieved under optimal conditions are achieved in practice. Sometimes equated with a person's level of health *q.v.* 4. Efficiency *q.v.* in achieving realistic goals. 5. The degree to which diagnostic, preventive, and therapeutic actions achieve the intended result.

EFFECTOR 1. A muscle or gland that carries out responses to nervous stimuli *q.v.* or impulses *q.v.* 2. An organ of action. 3. An organ capable of producing a response.

EFFERENT Carrying from. ct: afferent neurons. cf: efferent nerves.

EFFERENT NERVES Nerves that carry messages to the effectors *q.v.* ct: afferent nerves.

EFFERENT NEURON Efferent nerve *q.v.*

EFFICACY The extent to which an intervention can be shown to be beneficial under optimal conditions.

EFFICIENCY 1. The proportion of total costs that can be related to benefits achieved in practice. The relationship between the quantity of input or resources used in the production of medical services and the quantity of output produced.

EFFLEURAGE The circular stroking movement used in massage of the abdomen during labor in the Lamaze method *q.v.*

EFFUSION 1. The leakage of fluid from the tissue into a cavity, such as fluid in the pleural cavity *q.v.* 2. The escape of fluid from blood vessels or lymphatics into the tissues or a body cavity.

EFP An acronym for effective filtration pressure.

EGALITARIAN PRINCIPLE 1. Curriculum planning in which the learner is administered to in accordance to his or her needs. 2. Equality in education.

EGALITARIANISM Equalitarianism *q.v.*

EGEST To cast out as an indigestible food matter.

EGG 1. Ovum *q.v.* 2. A germ cell produced by a female organism. 3. Egg cell *q.v.*

EGG CELL 1. Ovum *q.v.* 2. Egg *q.v.*

EGO 1. The rational conscious aspect of a person's personality *q.v.* that regulates impulses enabling him or her to maintain self-esteem *q.v.* 2. The controller of personality. ~ allows for the expression of instincts in ways that are acceptable to society. It acts as the mediator between the id *q.v.* and the outside world. 3. In Freudian psychology, the component of personality concerned with responding to reality. 4. The conscious egocentric *q.v.* contact with reality. The self-assertive and self-preserving tendencies of a person. 5. The self. 6. The integrating core of the personality that mediates between needs and reality. ct: superego.

EGO ANALYSIS 1. An important set of modifications of classical psychoanalysis based on a conception of the human being as having a stronger, more autonomous ego *q.v.* with gratifications independent of id *q.v.* satisfactions. 2. Ego psychology.

EGO BOUNDARY The outer limits of what is familiar to a person. ~ expands as a person grows and acquires experience.

EGO DEFENSE MECHANISM 1. A type of reaction designed to maintain a person's feelings of adequacy and worth rather than to cope directly with the stress *q.v.* situation, usually unconscious and reality distorting. 2. Defense mechanism *q.v.*

EGO GAMES A deprecative term used by LSD *q.v.* users to social conformity and to normal activities, occupations, and responsibilities of the majority of people.

EGO IDEAL 1. A part of the superego *q.v.* that represents those things that are good and rewards the ego *q.v.* 2. The person or self that one thinks he or she could and should be.

EGO INVOLVEMENT The perception of a situation in terms of its potential effect on the person.

EGO ORIENTATION Instructions designed to produce personal involvement in a task. ct: task orientation.

EGO STATES A system of feelings that motivates *q.v.* a related set of behavior patterns.

EGO STRUCTURE The attitudes *q.v.*, defense reactions, and other aspects of the ego *q.v.* or self that form the integrating core of the personality *q.v.*

EGO-ALIEN Foreign to the self, e.g., compulsion *q.v.*

EGOCENTRIC 1. Limited to concern for oneself. 2. Selfish. 3. Self-centered. 4. Unable to take into account the views of others. 5. A person who is preoccupied with his or her own concerns and relatively insensitive to the concerns of others.

EGOCENTRIC THINKING 1. The assumption that other people view things the same way that you do. 2. The inability to imagine another person's viewpoint.

EGOCENTRISM 1. A defense mechanism *q.v.* 2. A reaction in which a person becomes preoccupied with his or her own concerns while being insensitive to those of others.

EGO-DYSTONIC HOMOSEXUALITY A disorder of people who are persistently dissatisfied with their homosexuality *q.v.* and who wish instead to be attracted to members of the opposite sex.

EGOISTIC SUICIDE 1. Self-destruction stemming from the lack of close relationships and meaningful social interaction. 2. As defined by Durkheim, self-annihilation committed because the person feels extreme alienation from others and from society.

EIDETIC MEMORY A sort of memory characterized by relatively long-lasting and detailed images of an event that can be recalled almost as though it were presently taking place.

EIO Exploratory, insight-oriented therapy *q.v.*

EJACULATION 1. A sexual response of the male occurring during the orgasmic phase *q.v.* of sexual arousal. 2. The forceful expulsion of the seminal fluid *q.v.* during orgasm *q.v.* cf: female ejaculation.

EJACULATION PRAECOX Premature ejaculation *q.v.*

EJACULATORY ANHEDONIA 1. Ejaculation *q.v.* not accompanied by orgasm. 2. Ejaculation with little pleasure or sensation. ~ is a difficulty usually of psychological *q.v.* origin.

EJACULATORY DUCT The short passage at the end of the vas deferens *q.v.* that empties into the urethra *q.v.*

EJACULATORY INCOMPETENCE Also referred to as retarded ejaculation, absence of ejaculation *q.v.*, ejaculatory impotence, and inhibited ejaculation. ~ is the inability to ejaculate even after sustained sexual stimulation through coitus *q.v.* Primary ejaculatory incompetence refers to never having ejaculated inside a woman's vagina *q.v.* Secondary ejaculatory incompetence involves having been able to ejaculate into a woman's vagina in the past, but not at the present time.

EJACULATORY INEVITABILITY The first stage of orgasm *q.v.* in men, a feeling of having passed the point where ejaculation *q.v.* cannot be controlled as the vas deferens *q.v.*, seminal vesicles *q.v.*, and prostate *q.v.* start contracting.

EJECTA Waste material excreted from the body.

EJUSDEM GENERIS 1. In law, of the same kind, class, or nature. In statutory construction, the ~ rule is that, where general words follow an enumeration of words of a particular and specific meaning, the general words are not interpreted in their broader sense but as applying to persons or things of the same general kind or class as those specifically mentioned. 2. The rule that if specific words are followed by general words, the specific words govern the character of the matter included in the general words.

ELABORATIVE ENCODING The enhancement of the organization and meaningfulness of information.

ELABORATIVE REHEARSAL 1. The process that facilitates transfer of information from the short-term to the long-term memory. 2. Rehearsal in which material is actively reorganized and elaborated while being held in short-term memory. ct: maintenance rehearsal.

ELASTIC TISSUE A specialized tissue lying in the lung and the great vessels and large arteries capable of stretching and recoiling.

ELATERS In botany, elongated cells with spirally thickened walls, associated with spores *q.v.* in the capsules of liverworts and mosses.

ELAVIL Brand name for amitriptyline *q.v.*

ELDER 1. Generally referring to persons over 60 years. 2. Elderly. cf: frail elderly; functional dependent elderly.

ELDERLY Elder *q.v.*

ELECTIVE MUTISM 1. A pattern of continually refusing to speak in almost all social situations, including school, even though the child understands spoken language and is able to speak. 2. A disorder of childhood where the child has speaking abilities but chooses not to use them.

ELECTIVE OFFICE A governmental or voluntary position which is filled through an election by the organization's constituents.

ELECTRA COMPLEX 1. Excessive emotional attachment of a daughter to her father. 2. According to Freudian psychology *q.v.*, a girl at about 4 years of age recognizes she has no penis *q.v.* and blames this lack on her mother. ct: Oedipus complex.

ELECTROCARDIOGRAM (ECG; EKG) 1. A tracing representing the heart's electrical action that is traced by amplifying the minutely small electrical impulses generated by the heart. 2. A tracing of the electrical potential produced by contractions of the heart.

ELECTROCARDIOGRAPH A device for recording the electrical activity that occurs during the heartbeat. cf: electrocardiogram.

ELECTROCARDIOGRAPH TECHNICIAN A person trained in the use of the electrocardiograph *q.v.*

ELECTROCOAGULATION 1. A treatment for killing cancerous tissue by the use of heat and electric current. 2. Electrodessication *q.v.*

ELECTROCONVULSIVE SHOCK THERAPY (ECT) 1. The passage of a controlled electrical current through the brain to promote a convulsion *q.v.* as a means of treating depression *q.v.* 2. The use of electrical shock to alter the neurotransmitter *q.v.* activity within the brain. cf: insulin shock treatment.

ELECTROCUTION Death caused by electricity.

ELECTRODESSICATION Electrocoagulation *q.v.*

ELECTROENCEPHALOGRAM (EEG) 1. A measure of brain function. 2. A recording of the electrical activity of the brain. 3. A record of brain waves. 4. A graphic recording of electrical activity of the brain, usually that of the cerebral cortex *q.v.*, but sometimes the electrical activity of lower areas of the brain. cf: electroencephalograph.

ELECTROENCEPHALOGRAPH (EEG) An instrument that measures the electrical activity of the brain, which is developed in the cerebral cortex *q.v.* as a result of brain functioning. Electrodes are attached to the scalp to record impulses, and these impulses are registered on graph paper as a brain wave pattern. An EEG is used to identify brain damage, tumors, or neurological disorders such as epilepsy *q.v.* cf: electroencephalogram.

ELECTROLYTE 1. A substance that, in solution, is capable of conducting an electric current. ~s are important in the prevention of heat cramps, heat exhaustion *q.v.*, and heat stroke *q.v.* 2. A substance that dissociates into ions *q.v.* when in solution and is capable of conducting electricity. Most common salts are ~s.

ELECTROLYTE BALANCE The proper concentration of various minerals within the blood and body fluids.

ELECTROMYOGRAM (EMG) A record of the electrical properties of skeletal muscles *q.v.*

ELECTRON 1. A negatively charged particle that revolves about the nucleus *q.v.* of an atom *q.v.* Its mass is negligible but its negative charge balances the single positive charge of one proton *q.v.* 2. Negative charge component of the neural atom; essential subatomic component that, by virtue of its quantitized energy state in a particular atom, permits the formation of chemical bonds between atoms.

ELECTRONIC DATA PROCESSING (EDP) Any systematic procedure for the handling or manipulating of information through the use of high-speed electronic devices.

ELECTRONIC FETAL MONITORING The observation of fetal *q.v.* heart rate and maternal uterine *q.v.* contractions through an internal or external monitoring device.

ELECTROPHORESIS The movement of charged particles suspended in a liquid on various media under the influence of an applied electric field. The migration of suspended particles in an electric field.

ELECTROSHOCK THERAPY Electroconvulsive shock therapy *q.v.*

ELECTROSURGERY The use of electricity to destroy surface lesions *q.v.*

ELEMENT A substance consisting of only one kind of atom *q.v.*

ELEMENTARY BODY A virus *q.v.* particle in an animal cell.

ELEMENTARY SCHOOL 1. Usually refers to kindergarten through the 6th grade. 2. Grades 1 through 6 or grades K through 6. cf: middle school; grammar school.

ELEPHANTIASIS A disease ordinarily found in tropical regions that involves a marked growth in subcutaneous *q.v.* tissues and the epidermis *q.v.* producing an enlargement varying from slight to monstrous. ~ may be caused by congenital *q.v.* circumstances, metastatic invasion *q.v.* of the lymph nodes *q.v.*, or infection by filariasis *q.v.* (*Wuchereria bancrofti*).

ELICIT To bring forth or cause to be revealed.

ELIMINATION Expulsion of wastes from the body.

ELISA 1. The enzyme-linked immunoabsorbent assay *q.v.*, a rapid screening test used to detect antibody to human immunodeficiency virus (HIV) *q.v.* 2. A blood test that indicates the presence of antibodies to a given antigen *q.v.* Various ~ tests are used to detect a variety of infections. The HIV ~ test does not detect AIDS *q.v.* but only indicates whether viral infection has occurred.

ELIXIR A sweetened liquid containing alcohol *q.v.* that is used to dissolve active ingredients in a drug or medicine.

EMACIATION 1. Excessive leanness. 2. A wasted condition of the body.

EMANCIPATION OF A CHILD Surrender of the right to care, custody, and earnings of a child by its parents who at the same time renounce parental duties.

EMASCULATE 1. To castrate *q.v.* 2. To deprive one of manliness or masculinity.

EMBALM The process of removing the blood from the corpse and replacing it with a preserving fluid.

EMBDEN–MEYERHOF PATHWAY 1. Glycolysis *q.v.* 2. The anaerobic *q.v.* pathway.

EMBEDDEDNESS To fix into a surrounding.

EMBOLISM Blockage of a blood vessel by a blot clot that is transported from some other area of the body.

EMBOLUS A blood clot or other substance inside a blood vessel that is carried in the bloodstream to a smaller blood vessel where it becomes an obstruction to circulation.

EMBRYO 1. The fertilized egg from the moment of conception through the 8th week of prenatal *q.v.* development, which is the period during which primary tissues differentiate and organs develop. 2. The developing creature in the uterus *q.v.* during the first trimester of pregnancy *q.v.* Embryonic tissue is more susceptible to teratogenic *q.v.* effects than is fetal *q.v.* tissue. 3. The period when basic structures form; it is the period of the most concentration of differentiation of cells. 4. In botany, the rudimentary plant formed in a seed or within the archegonium *q.v.* of lower plants.

EMBRYO SAC 1. In botany, a large thin-walled space within the ovule *q.v.* of the seed plant in which the egg and, after fertilization *q.v.*, the embryo develops. 2. The mature female gametophyte *q.v.* in higher plants. 3. The female gametophyte of angiosperms *q.v.*, consisting typically at maturity *q.v.* of the egg and two synergids *q.v.*, two polar nuclei *q.v.*, and three antipodal cells *q.v.*

EMBRYOLOGY The science that is concerned with the development of the embryo *q.v.*

EMBRYONIC PERIOD 1. The first 2 months of prenatal *q.v.* development. 2. Embryonic stage *q.v.*

EMBRYONIC STAGE 1. The stage of human development from the time of conception *q.v.* until the 8th week of gestation *q.v.* 2. Embryonic period. ct: fetal stage.

EMEGS An acronym for Environmental Medical Evaluation Guides *q.v.*

EMERGENCE OF COMMON MAN Coincides with the Age of Reason and emphasizes the rights of the common people for a better life, politically, economically, socially, and educationally. Rousseau was a leader of this movement.

EMERGENCY CERTIFICATE A substandard certificate for teachers who have not met all the requirements for certification.

EMERGENCY CLAUSE In politics, a phrase added to a bill to make it effective immediately after passage and signed by the governor or the president.

EMERGENCY MEDICAL RESPONSE PROTOCOLS A series of emergency medical response patient management protocols to be developed for the purpose of informing and guiding physicians on how to handle patients accidentally exposed to hazardous materials.

EMERGENCY MEDICAL TECHNICIAN (EMT) 1. A person trained in all aspects of first aid and emergency treatment and situations. 2. A paraprofessional emergency specialist who is trained to provide life-sustaining care and transportation of the injured and ill outside of a hospital or clinic setting.

EMERGENCY RESPONSE 1. The coordinated discharge of hormones *q.v.* and activity of the autonomic nervous system *q.v.* to prepare the body for flight or fight in a threatening situation. 2. The fight or flight response *q.v.*

EMERGENCY RESPONSE AND PREPAREDNESS DEMONSTRATION PROGRAM An ATSDR *q.v.*-supported demonstration program to facilitate development of emergency response and preparedness activities within the infrastructure of the public health community. These programs provide an opportunity for response and preparedness personnel to become oriented in health concepts and specific components of an integrated emergency response plan for chemical releases.

EMERITUS STAFF 1. In medicine, a retired physician *q.v.* who maintains a staff position within the hospital. 2. Retired faculty at universities. ct: active staff.

EMESIS Vomiting *q.v.* cf: emetic.

EMETIC A substance that causes vomiting *q.v.*

EMG An acronym for electromyogram *q.v.*

EMICBACK An acronym for Environmental Mutagen Information Center Backfile *q.v.*

EMISSARY 1. One of the channels of communication between the venous sinuses *q.v.* of the dura mater *q.v.* and the veins of the diploe *q.v.* and the scalp. 2. An outlet. 3. Providing an outlet.

EMISSION Discharge of semen *q.v.* from the penis *q.v.*, especially involuntary, as during sleep. cf: nocturnal emission.

EMMETROPIA Normal vision.

EMMETROPIC Normal vision as regards to accommodation *q.v.* and refraction *q.v.*

EMOLLIENT A substance that softens the skin.

EMOTION 1. An intense feeling that results in characteristic changes and the psychological *q.v.* need to act. Examples are love, hate, fear, anger, jealousy, guilt, envy, and others. There are three characteristics of ~ (a) they are conscious experiences, (b) they provoke physical response, and (c) they motivate *q.v.* behavior. 2. Emotive force *q.v.* 3. A stirred up state. 4. A felt tendency toward something assessed as favorable or away from something assessed as unfavorable. 5. ~s are either primary, those considered to be universal and basic, or secondary, those derived from some combination of these primary ~s.

EMOTIONAL CENTERS (OF THE BRAIN) 1. Center of emotions. 2. The limbic system *q.v.*

EMOTIONAL CONCEALMENT 1. Conscious or unconscious attempts to hide feelings interpreted as emotions *q.v.* 2. Conscious attempts are suppression *q.v.* while unconscious attempts are repression *q.v.*

EMOTIONAL CONTAGION An emotion *q.v.* that spreads to others as in a mob.

EMOTIONAL CONTROL The harnessing of emotions *q.v.* and using them for benefit or constructive results.

EMOTIONAL DISTRESS Feelings of frustration *q.v.*, fear, anxiety *q.v.*, or depression *q.v.* that occur when emotional needs *q.v.* are not being met.

EMOTIONAL DISTURBANCE 1. A condition characterized by the inability to learn, relate to others, or overcome depression *q.v.* 2. Behavior disorder *q.v.*

EMOTIONAL DIVORCE The state of a marriage in which the partners have ceased to have meaningful verbal or other interactions.

EMOTIONAL EXPRESSION 1. The means by which a person releases emotions *q.v.* or strong feelings. 2. Emotional behavior. cf: emotional control; emotional concealment.

EMOTIONAL EXPRESSIVENESS RESERVE A central orientation characterized by how much effort or feeling children typically express and by how important interactions with other people are to them. cf: central orientation; placidity explosiveness.

EMOTIONAL HEALTH 1. Mental health *q.v.* 2. Psychological health *q.v.* 3. A state in which a person is not troubled by ongoing conflicts among emotions *q.v.* to the extent that emotions do not interfere with everyday activities.

EMOTIONAL IMMATURITY The failure to develop normal adult degrees of independence and self-reliance with consequent use of immature *q.v.* adjustive patterns and the inability to maintain equilibrium under stress *q.v.* that most people can meet satisfactorily.

EMOTIONAL INSTABILITY REACTION An immature *q.v.* reaction to minor stress *q.v.* characterized by excitability and ineffectiveness.

EMOTIONAL INSULATION An ego *q.v.* defense mechanism *q.v.* in which the person reduces the tensions of need *q.v.* and anxiety *q.v.* by withdrawing into a shell of passivity.

EMOTIONAL INTIMACY A closeness between two or more people that includes a mutual awareness and influence of feelings.

EMOTIONAL ISOLATION 1. Lacking intimate relationships. 2. Having no emotional support system.

EMOTIONAL LAW OF EFFECT The fact that rewards tend to increase the probability of occurrence of rewarded responses and that punishments tend to decrease it.

EMOTIONAL MATURITY The extent to which a person manifests behavior appropriate to his or her age and intelligence *q.v.* levels.

EMOTIONAL NEEDS Psychological needs *q.v.*

EMOTIONAL REINFORCEMENT The reinforcement of adjustive patterns via the mobilized energy and drives of various emotional reactions *q.v.*

EMOTIONAL SYMPTOMS 1. Catatonia *q.v.*, mania *q.v.*, or depression *q.v.* 2. Psychotic symptoms *q.v.*

EMOTIONAL WELL-BEING Feeling good about self and others; being able to successfully resolve problems and to cope with the stresses *q.v.* and crises of life in socially acceptable ways. ~ reflects a person's subjective emotional, body image, and self-identity *q.v.*

EMOTIONALLY DISTURBED Behavior disordered *q.v.*

EMOTIONALLY UNSTABLE PERSONALITY 1. Characterized by excitability and ineffectiveness in the face of minor stress *q.v.* 2. Fluctuating emotional attitudes *q.v.* that upset interpersonal relations and impair judgment. 3. Difficulty in controlling hostility *q.v.*, guilt, and anxiety *q.v.*

EMOTIVE FORCE Emotion *q.v.*

EMOTIVE IDEOLOGY A life view that asserts the priority of emotions *q.v.* in the decision making of humans.

EMOTIVE IMAGERY A psychotherapeutic *q.v.* technique in which a child acquires anxiety-inhibiting *q.v.* responses by imagining an alter ego *q.v.* or favorite hero conquering his or her fears.

EMPATHY 1. The capacity to imagine oneself in the place of another person. 2. The ability to experience the feelings of another person. cf: primary empathy; advanced accurate empathy.

EMPHYSEMA 1. A condition in which the alveoli *q.v.* of the lungs become distended and/or ruptured and unable to hold or accept normal quantities of oxygen. 2. Swelling and inflammation *q.v.* of lung tissue resulting in tearing of the alveoli and decreased lung efficiency. 3. Loss of elasticity of the air sacs of the lungs. 4. A chronic disease in which the ability to move air in and out of the lungs is impaired. 5. A group of lung diseases that result in great difficulty in breathing and thus in poorly oxygenated blood. 6. Dilation of the pulmonary air vesicles, usually through atrophy *q.v.* of the septa between the alveoli.

EMPIRICAL That which is derived from observation or experimentation.

EMPIRICAL KEYING In research, the answer scored is determined by the answers given by some criterion group and discriminate that group from others.

EMPIRICISM In research, a philosophical orientation that contends that all reality can be observed and is quantifiable.

EMPLOYEE INFORMATION SYSTEM A system that provides information regarding the numbers, characteristics, skills, effectiveness, and promotion potential of existing employees.

EMPLOYEE SERVICES Programs, facilities, activities, and opportunities supplied by or through employers that are useful or beneficial to employees.

EMPLOYMENT Includes activities of civilian, noninstitutionalized persons such as (a) paid work during any part of a survey week; work at their own business, professional, or farm; or unpaid work for 15 h or more in a family-owned enterprise; or (b) temporary absence due to illness, bad weather, vacation, labor–management dispute, or personal reasons, whether or not another job is being sought.

EMPLOYMENT SECURITY COMMISSION A commission responsible for two major programs: (a) employment service, which provides unemployed persons with employment information; (b) administration of unemployment insurance that is given to qualified unemployed persons until they find work.

EMPTY CALORIES 1. Foods containing only calories *q.v.* but no significant amounts of other nutrients *q.v.* 2. Sugar foods. 3. Refined carbohydrates *q.v.*

EMPTY-CHAIR TECHNIQUE A Gestalt therapy *q.v.* procedure for helping the client become more aware of denied feelings. The client talks to important people or to feelings as though they were present and seated in a nearby vacant chair.

EMPTYSIS Expectoration *q.v.* of blood.

EMPYEMA 1. The accumulation of pus in a body cavity, especially the chest. 2. The presence of pus in any body cavity. 3. An accumulation of pus in the pleural cavity *q.v.*

EMT Emergency medical technician *q.v.*

EMULSIFICATION Any process by which a water-soluble substance is made more soluble. An emulsifier contains both water- and fat-soluble groups. It thus acts as a bridge between two substances that would not otherwise mix. cf: emulsion.

EMULSION A mixture of two immiscible liquids in which one is dispersed in very small globules throughout the other. cf: emulsification.

EN BANC 1. In law, the full court, all the judges sitting. 2. By all judges of the court.

EN BLOC VOTING In politics, to consider in a mass or as a whole, to adopt or reject a series of amendments with a single vote.

ENABLING ACT In politics, a statute that makes it lawful to do something that otherwise would be illegal. In some states, the legislature enacts a law that becomes operative only on the adoption by the people of an amendment to the constitution.

ENABLING FACTOR Any characteristic of the environment that facilitates health behavior and any skill or resource required to attain the behavior. cf: enabling goal.

ENABLING GOAL 1. The achievements necessary for the learner to achieve the terminal goal *q.v.* or objective *q.v.* 2. A goal that, when achieved, contributes to the achievement of the overall mission *q.v.* Sometimes called the enabling objective or simply objective *q.v.*

ENABLING OBJECTIVE The same as enabling goal *q.v.* May be written in more specific terms than a goal.

ENACTIVE REPRESENTATION The earliest form of symbolization in which infants represent their worlds in terms of interaction with the environment.

ENAMEL In dentistry, the outer covering of the crown of the tooth, which is an extremely hard tissue.

ENCEPHALITIS 1. Inflammation *q.v.* of the brain. 2. A general term for inflammation of the brain usually caused by a virus, but may also be caused by bacteria *q.v.* or chemicals.

ENCEPHALITIS LETHARGICA 1. Sleeping sickness. 2. A form of encephalitis *q.v.* that occurred in the early part of the twentieth century and was characterized by lethargy *q.v.* and prolonged periods of sleeping.

ENCEPHALIZATION The concept that, with increasing levels of phylogenic development, the cerebral cortex *q.v.* becomes increasingly important in the control of behavior.

ENCEPHALOGRAPHY An examination of the brain and mapping the result.

ENCEPHALON The brain.

ENCEPHALOPATHIES Neurologic disorders. Examples include (a) delirium tremens, (b) alcoholic hallucinosis, and (c) wet brain.

ENCODING 1. The conversion of information from its transmitted form to a form that can be interpreted. In information theory *q.v.*, the encoded message is the thought or idea converted into speech or language. 2. A component of information theory distinguished as the symbol of communication.

ENCODING SPECIFICITY PRINCIPLE The hypothesis *q.v.* that retrieval of information is most likely if the context at the time of recall approximates that during the original encoding *q.v.*

ENCOPRESIS 1. A disorder in which, through faulty control of the sphincters *q.v.*, a person repeatedly defecates *q.v.* in his or her clothing after an age at which continence *q.v.* is expected. 2. Lack of bowel control.

ENCOUNTER GROUP 1. A group of people that is organized for the purpose of learning about self and others. The usual focus of group discussion is on the concerns of the group participants, 2. Sensitivity group *q.v.*

ENCYST To surround with a protective coat.

END BULB 1. Presynaptic terminal *q.v.* 2. Part of the axon *q.v.* of the neuron *q.v.* where neurotransmitters *q.v.* are released.

END GOALS The ultimate goals a person sets for himself or herself.

ENDEMIC 1. A large number of cases of a disease that is usually found in a given population. 2. Pertaining to or prevalent in a particular geographic region or district. 3. Pertaining to a disease that has low incidence but is constantly present in a given geographic area. ct: pandemic; epidemic.

ENDEMIC DRUG USE Continuing presence of drug use/abuse behavior in a particular population or locality. cf: endemic.

ENDEMIC PREJUDICE Prejudice *q.v.* attitudes *q.v.* that are widely held and mostly taken for granted within some cultural groups and that children learn and may also unlearn. ct: pathological prejudice.

ENDEP A brand name of amitriptyline *q.v.*

ENDERGONIC A descriptive term for any reaction in which energy is absorbed.

ENDOCARDITIS Inflammation *q.v.* of the endocardium *q.v.*, usually associated with acute rheumatic fever *q.v.* or some other infectious agent *q.v.*

ENDOCARDIUM The inner layer of the heart.

ENDOCERVICAL CANAL A tubelike connection between the mouth of the cervix *q.v.* and the uterine *q.v.* cavity containing numerous secretory glands that produce mucus *q.v.*

ENDOCERVICAL CULTURES Laboratory tests in which secretions from the lining of the cervix *q.v.* are grown in a culture medium.

ENDOCHONDRAL Formed or occurring within a cartilage *q.v.*

ENDOCRINE GLANDS 1. Glands that secrete hormones *q.v.* into the blood stream or lymphatic system *q.v.* 2. Ductless glands. 3. Glands of internal secretion. 4. Organs that regulate body functions, such as energy supply and availability, sexual arousal, and physical growth, by secreting hormones into the blood and lymph system. cf: endocrine system.

ENDOCRINE SYSTEM 1. The group of glands that manufacture and secrete hormones *q.v.* directly into the bloodstream. 2. The system of ductless glands. 3. The glands of internal secretion. 4. One of the two major control systems of the body for homeostasis *q.v.* Endocrine glands *q.v.* secrete biochemical *q.v.* messengers, hormones, into the bloodstream or cerebrospinal fluid *q.v.*, which, when they reach their target tissue, adjust the tissue's activity.

ENDOCRINE THEORY OF ALCOHOLISM 1. This theory suggests that alcoholism *q.v.* may be caused by a dysfunction of the endocrine system *q.v.* However, some authorities believe that an endocrine dysfunction may be the result of alcoholism rather than its cause. 2. A physiological theory of causation. cf: hormone therapy.

ENDOCRINOLOGIST A medical practitioner who specializes in the diagnosis and treatment of diseases of the endocrine system *q.v.*

ENDOCRINOLOGY 1. The study of hormones *q.v.* secreted by the endocrine glands *q.v.* 2. The medical study of the structure, function, and diseases of the endocrine system *q.v.*

ENDODERM 1. The innermost layer of differentiated cells in the embryo *q.v.* from which the respiratory and digestive systems develop. 2. The innermost layer of the three primitive or primary germ layers of the embryo from which the digestive and respiratory systems of the body develop. 3. The innermost germ layers of the gastrula *q.v.* in subsequent stages, forming the lining of the essential parts of the digestive tract, and its derivatives.

ENDODONTIST A dentist *q.v.* who specializes in dental pulp and root canal therapy.

ENDOGENOUS DEPRESSION 1. Primary depression *q.v.* 2. A form of depression *q.v.* caused by the chemical makeup of the person. 3. A depression resulting from a genetically *q.v.* based abnormal production of neurotransmitter *q.v.* chemicals. 4. A profound sadness assumed to be caused by a biochemical *q.v.* malfunction in contrast to an environmental event, more recently regarded descriptively as having a more severe set of symptoms *q.v.* cf: melancholia.

ENDOGENOUS MICROORGANISMS Microscopic organisms that normally live within the human body, usually causing the body no harm and often contributing to its welfare, but sometimes causing disease.

ENDOGENOUS PIECE OR MATERIAL In genetics, some form of genetic *q.v.* material in a cell, but not part of the cell's normal complement.

ENDOGENOUS 1. Factors originating or produced within the person. 2. Intrinsic *q.v.* 3. Produced within or caused by factors within the organism. 4. Originating from within normal inhabitants of a region of the body. ct: exogenous.

ENDOGENOUS BETA ENDORPHINS Opiate-like substances within the central nervous system *q.v.* Endorphins *q.v.* are thought to produce euphoria *q.v.* 200 times more powerful than an equivalent amount of morphine *q.v.*

ENDOMETRIAL ASPIRATION The removal of the uterine *q.v.* lining through the use of a suction instrument (aspirator). ~ is sometimes used for menstrual extraction *q.v.*

ENDOMETRIAL CANCER Uterine cancer *q.v.*

ENDOMETRIOSIS 1. The aberrant presence of endometrial *q.v.* tissue in other parts of the female pelvic cavity, such as the fallopian tubes *q.v.*, ovaries *q.v.*, bladder, or intestines. 2. A condition in which the endometrium grows on other surfaces. 3. Pain during sexual intercourse *q.v.*, bowel elimination, and menstruation *q.v.* may be present. Endometriosis may be congenital *q.v.* or the result of surgery or pelvic infection. It may cause infertility.

ENDOMETRIUM 1. Tissues lining the uterus *q.v.* 2. The innermost layer of the uterus upon which the fertilized *q.v.* egg attaches and is nourished and develops prior to birth. The ~ is partly discharged during menstruation *q.v.* when pregnancy *q.v.* does not occur.

ENDOMITOSIS In genetics, duplication of chromosomes *q.v.* without division of the nucleus *q.v.* resulting in increased chromosome numbers within cells or endopolyploidy *q.v.* Chromosome strands separate but the cells do not divide.

ENDOMORPH One with endomorphy *q.v.* traits.

ENDOMORPHY One of the three body types identified by Sheldon as indicative of one's temperament: characterized by a person who is short and fat in the extreme and whose temperament is viscerotonia *q.v.*, that is, apprehensive, insecure, worried, amiable, and conforms to social conventions. cf: ectomorphy; mesomorphy.

ENDOPEPTIDASE One of a group of enzymes *q.v.* that hydrolyze *q.v.* dietary proteins *q.v.* by breaking peptide *q.v.* bonds.

ENDOPLASM The innermost portion of the cytoplasm *q.v.* of the microzoan *q.v.* cell, consisting of the fluid plasmasol *q.v.* with granules, vacuoles *q.v.*, and the nucleus *q.v.* ct: ectoplasm.

ENDOPLASMIC RETICULUM 1. An intracellular system of membranous channels that transport materials throughout the cell. Smooth ~ has no ribosomes *q.v.* attached to it, while rough ~ does. 2. A network of membrane-lined structures, a part of the submicroscopic structure of protoplasm *q.v.* 3. A double-membrane network that is filled with fluid and is found throughout the cytoplasm of many cells continuous with the plasma *q.v.* and nuclear membranes.

ENDORPHINS 1. A narcotic-like substance produced by the body that may relieve pain and produce euphoria *q.v.* 2. A type of neurotransmitter *q.v.*, sometimes found in the nerve cell, that prevents the transmission of electrochemical signals, especially of pain. 3. A collective term pertaining to any natural, internal body substance that has opioid-like activity. 4. A class of peptides *q.v.* from the pituitary gland *q.v.* and nervous tissue with action similar to morphine *q.v.* 5. Enkephalin *q.v.* 6. Opiates *q.v.* produced within the body, which may have an important role in the processes by which the body builds tolerance *q.v.* to drugs and is distressed by their withdrawal. cf: endogenous beta endorphins.

ENDOSCOPE 1. A small tube containing mirrors and lights that is inserted into the body. 2. An instrument for the examination of the interior of a canal or hollow viscus *q.v.*

ENDOSMOSIS Osmotic diffusion toward the inside of a cell or vessel.

ENDOSPORE A modified resistant bacterial cell.

ENDOSTEUM The internal lining of a bone.

ENDOTHELIAL INJURY–PLATELET AGGREGATION HYPOTHESIS Damage to inner blood vessel walls (endothelium) from a variety of sources causes platelet *q.v.* aggregation, vessel wall changes, and eventual atherosclerosis *q.v.*

ENDOTHELIUM A layer of flat cells lining blood and lymphatic *q.v.* vessels. ~ corresponds to the mesothelium *q.v.* of the serous cavities *q.v.*

ENDOTHRIX Infection of the hair in which the fungus mycelium *q.v.* penetrates the hair, forming spores *q.v.*, inside the hair shaft.

ENDOTOXINS 1. Toxins *q.v.* retained within a bacterial cell until freed by the disruption of the cell. 2. Toxins released from cells upon autolysis *q.v.*

ENDOTRACHIAL TUBE A tube that can be inserted into the trachea *q.v.* through the nose or mouth as an artificial airway.

ENDOWMENT The portion of an institution's income derived from donations. cf: endowment funds.

ENDOWMENT FUNDS Funds received from a donor with the restriction that the principle is not expendable. cf: endowment.

ENDURANCE 1. The ability of a muscle to remain contracted or to contract and relax many times. 2. The ability to carry out moderate to heavy physical activity over an extended period of time. The primary energy source is the aerobic system *q.v.* cf: muscular endurance.

ENEMA 1. Flushing the lower large intestine *q.v.* with a fluid. 2. The injection of a fluid into the rectum *q.v.*

ENERGETICS Human energetics *q.v.*

ENERGIZE To make an electrical circuit alive by applying voltage to allow current to flow through.

ENERGIZER 1. In medicine, a drug that has a stimulating effect on the central nervous system *q.v.* or other body organs or systems. 2. A stimulant *q.v.*

ENERGY 1. Measured in kilocalories *q.v.* or kilojoules *q.v.* One calorie equals 4184 joules. 2. The capacity to do work. 3. Among the various forms of ~ are radiant, heat, electrical, chemical, and kinetic.

ENERGY BALANCE The state that exists when caloric *q.v.* intake equals caloric expenditure.

ENFORCEABLE CONTRACT In law, any contract not void or voidable because of being defective.

ENFORCEMENT TECHNIQUES In drug law enforcement, methods used by local, state, and federal law enforcement agents to prevent illicit drug use, such as the use of informants, surveillance, undercover operations, drug raids, interdiction, and intelligence gathering.

ENGAGEMENT 1. A commitment to become married. 2. In pregnancy and childbirth, movement of the fetus *q.v.* into a lower position in the abdominal cavity prior to labor *q.v.*

ENGAGING 1. The settling of the fetal *q.v.* head into position against the pelvic bones for birth. ~ usually occurs during the last few weeks of pregnancy *q.v.* in women having their first child and during labor *q.v.* with subsequent pregnancies. 2. Dropping. 3. Lightening.

ENGLISH AS A SECOND LANGUAGE (ESL) A component of virtually all bilingual education programs in the United States that is designed to help instruct students whose primary language is not English.

ENGLISH GRAMMAR SCHOOL The model of elementary education in Colonial America.

ENGORGED 1. To become filled with blood or other fluid. 2. A swelling or filling with blood. cf: engorgement.

ENGORGEMENT Vascular congestion.

ENGRAM A pattern or trace that is theoretically left in the brain after a mental process takes place.

ENGROSSING In politics, a procedure for incorporating any amendments and checking the accuracy of a printed bill.

ENHANCER 1. A substance or object that increases a chemical activity or physiological *q.v.* process. 2. In genetic *q.v.*, a major or modifier gene *q.v.* that increases a physiological process.

ENJOIN 1. In law, to require a person, by writ of injunction from a court of equity, to perform, or to abstain or desist from, some act. 2. Command to maintain the status quo either by doing or refraining from doing a specific act. The writ is called an injunction.

ENKEPHALINS 1. The first internal body substance, extracted from the brain and the pituitary gland *q.v.* identified as having a narcotic *q.v.* effect within the body. 2. Endogenous *q.v.* peptides *q.v.* that bind to the same brain receptor *q.v.* sites as morphine *q.v.* and other opiates *q.v.* 3. A substance secreted in the brain and thought to produce a runner's high or euphoric *q.v.* feeling. 4. Hormones *q.v.* similar to endorphins *q.v.* with similar tranquilizing *q.v.* properties; the level of both drugs in the blood rises during strenuous exercise.

ENLIGHTENMENT EFFECT The change in a person's attitudes due to a knowledge of theoretical predictions about his or her behavior. Such effects may threaten accurate predictions of behavior.

ENLIGHTENMENT PERIOD The period in Europe during the eighteenth century.

ENRICHED The process of returning foods of some nutritional *q.v.* elements removed during processing. cf: enrichment.

ENRICHMENT 1. The addition of nutrients *q.v.* to foods according to standards established by the Food and Drug Administration *q.v.* ~ usually refers to the addition of nutrients to cereal products. 2. In education, experiences for gifted students that enhance their thinking and extend their knowledge of various areas or disciplines. cf: enriched.

ENROLLMENT 1. In education, the total number of entering students in a given school unit. 2. In health, the number of people being paid members of a particular health insurance plan.

ENT An acronym for otorhinolaryngology *q.v.*

ENTAMOEBA HISTOLYTICA The organism that causes amoebic dysentery *q.v.*

ENTELECHY In Aristotelian philosophy, true existence or the actualization of potentials. cf: actuality.

ENTERAL Pertaining to drugs that are taken orally.

ENTERIC Pertaining to digestion *q.v.*

ENTERIC INFECTION Infection *q.v.* of the intestine.

ENTERIC-COATED A medicinal preparation that is specially coated to allow it to pass through the stomach and to disintegrate in the intestine.

ENTERITIS 1. Inflammation *q.v.* of the alimentary canal *q.v.* usually characterized by severe diarrhea *q.v.* 2. Inflammation of the intestine. ~ is chiefly used to describe inflammation of the small intestine.

ENTEROHEPATIC CIRCULATION The return of the bile *q.v.* to the circulation and to the liver from the intestine.

ENTERON Intestine.

ENTEROSTOMY The surgical construction of an artificial outlet for the intestine.

ENTEROTOXIN Toxins *q.v.* excreted by the cells into the gastrointestinal tract *q.v.* of animals.

ENTITY Being or existence.

ENTODERM Endoderm *q.v.*

ENTOMOLOGY The science concerned with the study of insects.

ENTOZOIC Living with an animal.

ENTRAPMENT 1. In social psychology, when one invests in a given outcome, and over time, the investment becomes more costly while the outcome becomes less probable. 2. In law, the commission of a crime based on law enforcement's setting a trap or situation whereby the crime was imminent.

ENTRY LEVEL For health educators, the point at which an individual is capable of performing the specifications of the role identified. Skills and knowledge necessary to perform the role can be obtained through successful completion of a bachelor's degree program at an accredited university or college with major emphasis on health education.

ENURESIS 1. The involuntary discharge of urine after the age of 3. 2. Bed wetting. 3. A disorder in which, through faulty control of the urinary bladder, the person repeatedly wets during the night or during the day after an age at which continence *q.v.* is expected. 4. Nocturnal enuresis. 5. Lack of bladder control.

ENVELOPE PROTEINS Proteins *q.v.* that comprise the envelope or surface of a virus *q.v.*

ENVENOMATION The act of depositing toxins *q.v.*

ENVIRONMENT 1. The physical, social, emotional, effective, and noneffective influences of human functioning and behavior. 2. One's surroundings, animate and inanimate. 3. External and internal surroundings that have some influence upon the health and behavior of a person. 4. ~ is classified as (a) biological, (b) physical, (c) psychological, (d) social, (e) external, (f) internal, (g) effective, and (h) noneffective. 5. The complex of all factors that act upon an organism or an ecological *q.v.* community and ultimately determines its form. 6. One sector or element of the public health model of drug abuse prevention specifically related to the setting or context in which drug abuse occurs, and the group or community customs, mores, or folkways that influence drug takers.

ENVIRONMENTAL BIAS A subjective point of view based on the environment.

ENVIRONMENTAL CHARACTERIZATION DATA Information provided in site-specific reports on environmental contamination *q.v.* and environmental pathways.

ENVIRONMENTAL EDUCATION The study and analysis of the conditions and causes of pollution, overpopulation, and waste of natural resources and of the ways to preserve the planet's intricate environmental balance.

ENVIRONMENTAL HANDICAP In regards to differences in intelligence, the concept that low levels of intelligence scores on IQ *q.v.* tests result from environmental inadequacies.

ENVIRONMENTAL HEALTH The effect of external forces acting upon human, animal, insect, and plant life within the greater surroundings.

ENVIRONMENTAL MEDIA EVALUATION GUIDE (EMEG) Media-specific screening values that are used to select contaminants of potential health concern at hazardous waste sites. An ~ is expressed as the concentration of a specific chemical substance in a specific environmental medium such as water, air, and soil.

ENVIRONMENTAL MEDICINE A branch of medical practice that is concerned with the study of environmental causes of disease. cf: clinical ecologist.

ENVIRONMENTAL MUTAGEN INFORMATION CENTER BACKFILE (EMICBACK) A bibliographic database on chemical, biological, and physical agents that have been tested for genotoxic *q.v.* activity.

ENVIRONMENTAL PROTECTION AGENCY (EPA) The federal agency charged with the protection of natural resources and the quality of the environment.

ENVIRONMENTAL PSYCHOLOGY A recent community-oriented psychology *q.v.* that assumes that people's feelings and behavior are an important function of their physical setting.

ENVIRONMENTAL SCIENCES A specialized area of community health concerned with the identification and control of factors in the environment *q.v.* that affect health.

ENVIRONMENTAL TERATOLOGY INFORMATION CENTER BACKFILE (ETICBACK) A bibliographic database covering literature on teratology *q.v.* and developmental and reproductive toxicology.

ENZYMATIC Pertaining to an enzyme *q.v.*

ENVIRONMENTALITY The proportion of the variance in a trait that is attributable to the differences in the environments *q.v.* in which people develop.

ENZYMATIC ADAPTATION Adaptive nature of inducible bacteria.

ENZYME 1. Chemicals that are essential for such processes as digestion (catabolism *q.v.*) and protein synthesis *q.v.* in cells. 2. Substances that are capable of bringing about chemical changes in the body. 3. Protein substances that catalyze chemical reactions within the body. 4. A proteinaceous catalytic agent that increases the rate of a particular transformation of materials in plants and animals. At the end of the reaction, the ~ itself is unchanged. 5. A biological chemical, protein in nature, which is produced by living cells and which can influence the rate of body processes. ~s can act independently of the cells that produce them. 6. Biological catalysts, protein in nature, that have highly specific attachment and reaction sites for the reactants and products in a specific chemical reaction. As specific biocatalysts, they permit rapid reaction rates for complex chemical reactions at biological compatible temperatures.

ENZYME INDUCTION 1. An increase in the metabolic *q.v.* capacity of an enzyme system *q.v.* to detoxify *q.v.*, or metabolize, substances and clear them from the body. 2. Biotransformation *q.v.*

ENZYME SYSTEM A group of enzymes *q.v.* that act at consecutive steps in a metabolic *q.v.* pathway.

ENZYME-LINKED IMMUNOABSORBANT ASSAY (ELISA) A method in which an antibody *q.v.* or an antigen *q.v.*

can be coupled to an enzyme *q.v.* Some bacterial antigens and antibodies, along with certain hormones *q.v.*, can be detected by this assay method.

EOSINOPHILS 1. Granulocytes *q.v.* that constitute one of the two main types of leukocytes *q.v.* in the blood. 2. Acidophil *q.v.* 3. White blood cells readily stained by eosin *q.v.* (eosin is a dye derived from the action of bromine on fluorescein. It is a dye used frequently for staining microscopic specimens.)

EPA An acronym for Environmental Protection Agency *q.v.*

EPHEDRINE 1. A sympathomimetic *q.v.* drug used in treating asthma *q.v.* 2. A drug derived from the Chinese medicinal herb, *ma huang*, and used to relieve breathing difficulties in asthma victims. 3. A sympathomimetic from which amphetamine *q.v.* was derived.

EPICONDYLES The round articular processes on the ends of the long bones at the joint.

EPICRITIC Pertaining to a set of sensory nerve fibers supplying the skin by means of which one is able to appreciate the finer degrees of the sensations of touch, pain, and temperature.

EPIDEMIC 1. An unusual number of cases of a disease in a given population. 2. The rapid spread of a disease among people within a given area or population. 3. Widely diffused and rapid spreading of a disease. 4. When the incidence of a disease surpasses the expected rate in any well-defined geographic area. cf: epidemic disease.

EPIDEMIC CEREBROSPINAL MENINGITIS Inflammation *q.v.* of the meninges *q.v.* of the brain and spinal cord.

EPIDEMIC DISEASE A disease *q.v.* affecting a large number of people in a locality at the same time. cf: epidemic.

EPIDEMIC ENCEPHALITIS A disease of the brain caused by a virus *q.v.*

EPIDEMIOLOGIC ANALYSIS A type of analysis *q.v.* based on a statistical association between a characteristic and a disease *q.v.*

EPIDEMIOLOGIC MODEL 1. Consists of a susceptible host, agent, and suitable environment. 2. The relationship of the multicausal factors that exist in most disease states. cf: epidemiology.

EPIDEMIOLOGIC STUDIES Studies concerned with the relationship of various determining the frequency and distribution of certain diseases. cf: epidemiologic model; epidemiology.

EPIDEMIOLOGICAL Pertaining to the study of epidemics *q.v.* and how to control them. cf: epidemiology.

EPIDEMIOLOGICAL DATA Facts, figures, or information related to the causes, nature, distribution, and occurrence of diseases.

EPIDEMIOLOGICAL DIAGNOSIS The delineation of the extent, distribution, and causes of a health problem in a defined population.

EPIDEMIOLOGICAL EVIDENCE Facts based on the occurrence and distribution of a factor or factors associated with a particular health phenomenon in a given population.

EPIDEMIOLOGICAL METHOD A scientific approach to the study of situations that influence the health and well-being of the population. Also, epidemiologic method.

EPIDEMIOLOGIST A public health specialist concerned with the occurrence of disease by time, place, and persons involved. cf: epidemiology.

EPIDEMIOLOGY 1. The science that is concerned with the nature of disease among groups of people. 2. The science that uses the epidemiologic model *q.v.* to discover ways in which diseases can be prevented or controlled to raise the level of the health of populations. 3. ~ uses three areas of concentration: (a) descriptive ~, (b) analytic, ~ and (c) experimental ~. 4. ~ is a body of knowledge and a science or method of study. 5. The study of the frequency of illness in a population. Related terms are as follows: (a) endemic, found in a particular geographic area or among a particular group of people; (b) epidemic, spreading rapidly among many persons in an area, especially a contagious disease; and (c) pandemic, occurring over a large geographic area. 6. An investigation designed to ascertain and evaluate any causal relationship between exposure to a hazardous substance and the desired outcome in a defined population by testing scientific hypotheses. 7. The study of the factors that impact on the spread of disease in an area.

EPIDERMAL The outer, nonsensitive layer of the skin.

EPIDERMIS 1. In botany, the outermost layer of cells of the leaf and of young stems and roots. 2. In anatomy, the outermost layer of skin varying in thickness from 1/200th to 1/20th of an inch and containing cornified *q.v.*, external protecting cells.

EPIDERMOID CANCER A rapidly spreading type of skin cancer *q.v.* that may arise from aberrant epidermal cells *q.v.*

EPIDERMOPHYTOSIS Infection *q.v.* of the skin by a specific fungus *q.v.*

EPIDIDYMIS 1. An oblong-shaped body attached to each testicle *q.v.* in which sperm *q.v.* cells mature and are stored. 2. The network of tiny tubes in the male that connects the testicles with the sperm duct *q.v.* 3. The organ in which sperm are stored in the testes *q.v.* and where nutrients *q.v.* are provided to help the sperm mature.

4. A coiled tube about 18–20 ft long in the testes in which sperm mature after leaving the seminiferous tubules *q.v.* and before entering the vas deferens *q.v.*

EPIDIDYMITIS Inflammation *q.v.* of the epididymis *q.v.*, a common disorder affecting the male.

EPIDURAL External to the dura mater *q.v.*

EPIDURAL HEMATOMA A collection of blood clots or a clot *q.v.* caused by a laceration *q.v.* or rupture of a meningeal *q.v.* vessel lying external to the dura mater.

EPIDURAL INJECTION A procedure that may be used in labor to anesthetize *q.v.* the mother's lower body.

EPIGENERIC PROCESS A process of development that builds one stage of growth, maturity and development, upon another. cf: epigenetic principle; developmental tasks.

EPIGENESIS 1. The concept that the embryo *q.v.* develops anew from undifferentiated material in each generation. This is in contrast to preformation *q.v.* 2. The view that development is characterized by the emergence of new properties that are neither predestined nor predetermined. 3. In biology, ~ is in contrast to the view that knowledge of either nature or nurture alone is sufficient to predict developmental outcomes. 4. The theory that states that development involves a gradual diversification and differentiation of an initially undifferentiated entity. 5. The doctrine that development of an organism proceeds from a relatively simple germinal substance, with complexity arising through the interaction of the protoplasm *q.v.* and the environment.

EPIGENESIST A person who views embryological *q.v.* development as a progressive process from a relatively undifferentiated zygote *q.v.* to a complex adult.

EPIGENETIC PRINCIPLE The assumption that each body part develops at a particular time but all parts eventually merge into a functional whole. cf: epigeneric process.

EPIGLOTTIS A trapdoor-like valve that prevents food from entering the windpipe. 2. Covering of the glottis *q.v.* during swallowing.

EPILATION Pulling hair out by the roots.

EPILEPSY 1. A disease that affects the functioning of the cerebrum *q.v.* 2. A chronic *q.v.* disorder characterized by recurrent attacks or seizures whose onset is sudden and of short duration. There are four general characteristic seizures: (a) grand mal, (b) petit mal, (c) psychomotor attacks, and (d) epileptic equivalents. 3. A brain disorder accompanied by transient loss of consciousness or convulsions. 4. A disorder of the nervous system in which recurring periods of abnormal electrical activity in the brain produce temporary malfunctioning. There may or may not be a loss of consciousness or convulsive motor movements.

EPILEPTIC 1. A person suffering from epilepsy *q.v.* 2. A person with a disturbance characterized by generalized convulsions *q.v.*

EPILEPTIC EQUIVALENTS Associated with epilepsy *q.v.* and characterized by abdominal pain and mental confusion.

EPILEPTIC FUROR Psychomotor epilepsy *q.v.*

EPILEPTIC PATIENT A person suffering from a chronic *q.v.* nervous disorder characterized by attacks of unconsciousness or convulsions or both. cf: epileptic.

EPINEPHRINE 1. A hormone *q.v.* produced by the adrenal glands *q.v.* Under stress *q.v.*, ~ stimulates the autonomic nervous system *q.v.* and glycogenolysis *q.v.* 2. Adrenalin *q.v.* 3. A hormone produced by the medulla *q.v.* of the adrenal glands. ~ helps to regulate the sympathetic *q.v.* branch of the autonomic nervous system. 4. A monoamine *q.v.* hormone secreted by the adrenal medulla. The most powerful vasopressor *q.v.* known. ~ is used medicinally as a sympathomimetic *q.v.* 5. A powerful adrenal hormone whose presence in the bloodstream prepares the body for maximal energy production and skeletal muscle response.

EPIPHYSEAL INJURY An injury that results in a break of a bone at the cartilaginous *q.v.* epiphysis *q.v.*, or growth centers at the ends of the long bones. The most common site for ~ is the distal radial epiphysis *q.v.*

EPIPHYSEAL PLATE The disc of cartilage *q.v.* between the shaft and the epiphysis *q.v.* of a long bone during its growth.

EPIPHYSIS 1. Growth plate of the long bones. 2. Epiphyseal plate *q.v.* 3. A part of a long bone developed from a center of ossification *q.v.* distinct from that of the shaft and separated at first from the shaft by a layer of cartilage. 4. End of a long bone.

EPISIOTOMY 1. A surgical incision made at the entrance to the vagina *q.v.* extending toward the anal sphincter *q.v.* during birth to prevent undue tearing of the vaginal tissues and to assist in the expulsion of the fetus *q.v.* 2. A minor surgical procedure in which the perineum *q.v.* is cut to avoid the possibility of tearing the vaginal opening during childbirth.

EPISODIC MEMORY 1. Memory of particular events in a person's life. 2. Memories that have a personal reference for significance, usually to time and place. cf: generic memory.

EPISOME 1. A genetic *q.v.* element that may be present or absent in different cells, associated with a chromosome *q.v.* or independent in the cytoplasm *q.v.* 2. A bacterial replicon capable of attaching to the bacterial chromosome or existing in the cytoplasm and replicating there independently on the bacterial chromosome.

EPISPADIA A congenital *q.v.* defect in males in which the opening of the urethra *q.v.* is on the upper surface of the penis *q.v.* instead of at its tip. cf: hypospadia.

EPISTASIS The suppression of the action of a gene *q.v.* or genes by a gene or genes not allelomorphic *q.v.* to those suppresses. Those suppressed are said to be hypostatic *q.v.* This is distinguished from dominance *q.v.*, which refers to members of one allelomorphic pair.

EPISTAXIS 1. Nosebleed. 2. Hemorrhage *q.v.* from the nose.

EPISTEMOLOGY That branch of philosophy *q.v.* that focuses on the nature of knowledge.

EPISTROPHEUS The second cervical vertebra *q.v.*

EPITAPH An inscription on a grave marker or monument.

EPITESTOSTERONE A metabolic *q.v.* by-product of testosterone *q.v.*

EPITHECA Outer larger valve of the diatom thallus *q.v.*

EPITHELIAL CELLS 1. Cells that line or cover the body's surfaces. 2. The skin cells. 3. Cells lining the airways into the lungs and cells that line the surfaces of body organs. cf: epithelium.

EPITHELIAL TISSUE Tissue that forms the skin, glands, and the linings of the respiratory, gastrointestinal, urinary, and genital systems.

EPITHELIUM 1. The covering of both internal and external surfaces of the body. 2. The skin. 3. The outer layer of skin cells. cf: epithelial cells.

EPITHELIZATION Healing over a wound by the growing of epithelial cells *q.v.* of the skin.

EPITOPES Characteristic shapes of antigens *q.v.* found on an organism *q.v.*

EPSILON ALCOHOLISM 1. A form of alcoholism *q.v.* characterized chiefly by periods of excessive drinking of alcohol *q.v.* alternating with long periods of abstinence. 2. Dipsomania *q.v.*

EPSP An acronym for excitatory postsynaptic potential *q.v.*

EPSTEIN–BARR VIRUS (EBV) 1. The organism *q.v.* that causes the most common form of infectious mononucleosis *q.v.* 2. The virus that is the cause of infectious mononucleosis. It also has been linked with the development of Burkitt's lymphoma *q.v.* in Africa and nasopharyngeal carcinoma *q.v.* in China. 3. ~ is spread by saliva. EBV lies dormant in lymph glands *q.v.* and has been associated with cancer of the lymph tissue (Burkitt's lymphoma).

EPT An acronym for early pregnancy test.

EPULIS A type of tumor *q.v.* of the gums or jaw.

EQUAL EDUCATIONAL OPPORTUNITY Giving every student the educational opportunity to fully develop whatever talents, interests, and abilities he or she may have without regard to race, color, national origin, sex, handicap, or economic status. cf: equal employment opportunity.

EQUAL EMPLOYMENT OPPORTUNITY The Civil Rights Act of 1964 prohibits employers and labor unions from discriminating against a person because of race, color, religion, sex, or national origin. cf: equal educational opportunity.

EQUAL EMPLOYMENT OPPORTUNITY COMMISSION (EEOC) An agency established to enforce the laws that regulate recruiting and other managerial practices. cf: equal employment opportunity.

EQUAL PROTECTION OF THE LAW A guarantee that no person or class of persons shall be denied the same protection of the laws that is enjoyed by other persons or classes in similar circumstances. Denial of this right is prohibited by the Fourteenth Amendment to the United States Constitution.

EQUALIBRATION 1. The tendency for children to seek cognitive *q.v.* coherence and stability. 2. A self-regulatory process in intellectual growth, which encounters with new or discrepant information resulting in adaptation of intellectual structures so that they can handle the new information. 3. In dentistry, to equalize the stress of occlusal forces of the supporting tissues of the teeth. cf: adaptation.

EQUALITARIANISM 1. A doctrine asserting the similar worth of all groups of people. 2. Egalitarianism. cf: egalitarian principle.

EQUALITY RULE 1. A principle of social exchange in which each participant perceives that rewards and costs are equal for all. ~ considers each participant's abilities or needs. 2. Equity rule *q.v.*

EQUANIL 1. A minor tranquilizer *q.v.* 2. A commercial preparation of meprobramate *q.v.*

EQUATIONAL 1. A homotypic division of a cell. 2. Mitotic division which is usually the second division in the meiotic sequence. 3. Somatic mitosis *q.v.* and the nonreductional division of meiosis *q.v.*

EQUATORIAL PLATE The figure formed by the chromosomes *q.v.* in the center of the spindle in mitosis *q.v.*

EQUILIBRIUM Balance.

EQUIPOTENTIALITY The concept that all parts of the brain are capable of serving a variety of functions and taking over should the part that normally performs a certain function becomes destroyed.

EQUITABLE RELIEF In law, a decree of a court of equity *q.v.*

EQUITY RULE 1. Equality rule *q.v.* 2. A principle of social exchange in which each participant perceives that the relative rewards and costs are equal. ~ takes into account each participant's productivity.

EQUITY THEORY 1. A theory that specifies the way in which costs and rewards are to be distributed in society. 2. The idea that in some human relationships people's exchanges, although unequal, may over time, be deemed equitable.

EQUITY 1. In personal relationships, a perceived balance between the benefits the relationship provides and the personal investments it requires. 2. In law, the field of jurisprudence differing in origin, theory, and methods from the common law. 3. In labor relations, fair relationships between the rates of pay for workers and job classification.

EQUITY LAW A particular branch of law that differs from law. Primarily concerned with providing justice and fair treatment, ~ addresses issues the common law is unable to consider.

EQUIVALENCE RELIABILITY In research, evidence that a test measures consistently across different equivalent forms.

ER 1. In anatomy, an acronym for endoplasmic reticulum *q.v.* 2. In medical care, an acronym for emergency room.

ERECTILE In anatomy, tissues that are capable of erection *q.v.* cf: erectile tissue. ct: erectile dysfunction.

ERECTILE DYSFUNCTION (ED) 1. Impotence *q.v.* 2. Pertains to the inability of the male to achieve and maintain an erection *q.v.* sufficient for coitus *q.v.* to take place. ~ may be primary, in which the man has never been able to have sexual intercourse *q.v.*; secondary, in which the man has experienced coitus but at the present is unable to achieve an effective erection; or transient due to fatigue, alcohol, distraction, emotional stress, etc. 3. Erectile inhibition *q.v.*

ERECTILE INHIBITION 1. Impotence *q.v.* 2. The inability to achieve an erection *q.v.* ~ may be primary, in which case it is long lasting and has physical causes, or secondary, which is temporary and usually has emotional causes. 3. Erectile dysfunction *q.v.* ct: erectile.

ERECTILE TISSUE Tissue containing large vascular *q.v.* spaces that fill with blood upon stimulation. cf: erectile.

ERECTION 1. The condition of becoming rigid and elevated as in an ~ of the penis *q.v.* 2. The stiffening and enlargement of the penis or clitoris *q.v.* often as a result of sexual excitement. 3. The enlargement of erectile tissue *q.v.* with blood. cf: spontaneous erection.

EREPSIN A protein splitting enzyme *q.v.* of the intestine.

ERGOGENIC AGENT A drug used for purposes of artificially improving athletic performance. ~s include stimulants, narcotics, analgesics, and steroids.

ERGOMANIA 1. Compulsive worker. 2. A person who compulsively works at his or her occupation at the exclusion of other living activities. 3. Erroneously referred to as a "workaholic." Alcohol has no connection with ~. cf: mania.

ERGOMETER 1. An exercise device. 2. A stationary bicycle.

ERGONOMICS How the workplace, job practices, and equipment design interact to affect the well-being of the workers.

ERGOSTEROL 1. Provitamin D *q.v.* 2. A sterol *q.v.* found chiefly in plant tissues. Upon exposure to ultraviolet radiation, it becomes vitamin D *q.v.*

ERGOT 1. The substance from which LSD *q.v.* is synthesized. 2. Ergot fungus *q.v.*

ERGOT FUNGUS The sclerotium of the fungus *Claviceps purpurea*, which grows as a parasite *q.v.* on the rye plant and from which LSD *q.v.* is synthesized.

ERGOTISM 1. A condition caused by vasoconstrictive *q.v.* action of the chemical in ergot fungus *q.v.* related to LSD *q.v.*, which can cause delirium, hallucinations, convulsions, and gangrene. 2. St. Anthony's fire *q.v.* 3. A disease caused by eating grain infected with the ergot fungus. There are both psychological and physiological manifestations of the disease.

ERGOTROPIC 1. That which incites to activity. 2. That which can result in a state of hyperarousal. cf: trophotropic.

EROGENOUS 1. Exciting sexual desire. 2. Producing sexual arousal. 3. Capable of giving sexual pleasure when stimulated.

EROGENOUS ZONES 1. Areas of the body that are particularly sensitive to sexual stimulation. They include the genitals and surrounding areas. In males, the penis and the glans penis; in females, the clitoris and the vulva. General areas in both sexes are the breasts, armpits, small of the back, shoulders, neck, earlobes, scalp, eyelids, mouth, tongue, nose, and anus. 2. In psychoanalytic theory *q.v.*, the mouth, anus, and genitals. 3. Pleasure associated with the ~ are sexual in nature. 4. Those parts of the body that, when stimulated, give rise to sexual feelings.

EROS 1. The unconscious urge toward life and love. 2. In Freudian psychology *q.v.*, the powerful life force. 3. Self-integrating instinct *q.v.* or force of the id *q.v.*, sometimes equated with the sexual drive. 4. The Greek form of love most similar to romantic love.

EROSION 1. In ecology, the removal of soil and other materials by natural agencies, primarily water and wind. In pathology, ulceration or the eating away of a structure.

EROSIVE DISEASES The three minor venereal diseases *q.v.*: chancroid *q.v.*, lymphogranuloma venereum *q.v.*, and granuloma inguinale *q.v.*

EROTIC 1. Sexually stimulating. 2. Sexually arousing. 3. Pertaining to sexual love or sensation.

EROTIC DREAMS Dreams or fantasies whose nature elicits a sexual response.

EROTIC SENSATIONS Those sensory perceptions that are sexually gratifying.

EROTICA 1. Material aimed primarily at sexually arousing a consumer. ~ has a more positive connotation than pornography *q.v.* 2. There are two classes of ~: (a) hard-core, which explicitly displays the genitals in states of sexual excitation and the behaviors accompanying such states, and (b) soft core, which may display genitals but not in states of sexual excitement and often only simulations of sexual behaviors. 3. The graphic depiction of nudes in a manner that is a mutually pleasurable expression among people and not a debasing of the person.

EROTICAPHORES People who are highly offended by erotica *q.v.*

EROTOPHILIA A set of attitudes and behaviors that characterize a sexually liberal person. ct: erotophobia.

EROTOPHOBIA 1. A set of attitudes and behaviors that characterize a sexually conservative person. 2. Negative emotional response to sexual feelings and experiences. ct: erotophilia.

ERRORS OF METABOLISM 1. Inborn errors of metabolism *q.v.* 2. Genetic defects *q.v.* affecting the body's ability to metabolize *q.v.* certain substances. 3. The inability of the body to convert certain chemicals into other chemicals.

ERRORS OF REFRACTION Conditions in which the image does not fall clearly in the retina *q.v.* of the eye and causes sight to be distorted. There are three chief conditions: (a) hyperopia *q.v.*, (b) myopia *q.v.*, and (c) astigmatism *q.v.*

ERT Estrogen replacement therapy *q.v.*

ERUCTATION 1. The oral elimination of gas. 2. Belching.

ERV Expiratory reserve volume.

ERYSIPELAS An acute *q.v.* infectious disease *q.v.* of the skin caused by *streptococci q.v.*

ERYTHEMA A redness of the skin due to congestion of the capillaries *q.v.* or sunburn.

ERYTHROBLASTOSIS FETALIS 1. Destruction of red blood cells of the fetus *q.v.* or neonate *q.v.* usually resulting from Rh *q.v.* incompatibility. 2. A type of anemia *q.v.* caused by transmission of Rh antibodies *q.v.* from the mother to the child through the placenta *q.v.* 3. Associated with the Rh factor in the blood. A genetic *q.v.* defect in the blood characterized by an enlarged liver and spleen, which may result in stillbirth *q.v.* or death of the infant shortly after birth. When the infant is born alive, blood transfusion *q.v.* is essential to eliminate the high levels of bilirubin *q.v.* in the blood.

ERYTHROCYTE SEDIMENTATION RATE (ESR) The rate at which erythrocytes *q.v.* settle out of unclotted blood. Inflammation *q.v.* processes cause an aggregation of the red blood cells, which make them heavier and more likely to settle.

ERYTHROCYTES The red blood cells. ct: leukocytes.

ERYTHROMELAGIA A condition, esp. of the feet, characterized by intermittent feelings of burning and throbbing.

ERYTHROPOIESIS The formation of erythrocytes *q.v.* cf: erythropoietin.

ERYTHROPOIETIN A hormone *q.v.* produced by the kidneys that controls red blood cell production.

ERYTHROXYLON COCA The plant from which cocaine *q.v.* is derived.

ESCAPE LEARNING Instrumental learning *q.v.* in which reinforcement consists of the reduction of an aversion stimulus *q.v.*

ESCAPE MECHANISM 1. A defense mechanism *q.v.* characterized by a withdrawal from a frustrating situation. 2. Flight reaction *q.v.*

ESCAPE TRAINING Training that requires a person to escape from a noxious stimulus. cf: avoidance training; reward training.

ESCAPE-AVOIDANCE DRUG USE Drug-taking behavior motivated by the desire for relief from unpleasant sensations, tensions, disturbed interpersonal relationships, fears, and anxieties.

ESCHAR 1. The dead slough covering a severe burn wound. 2. Scab.

ESCHERICHIA COLI A bacterium *q.v.* normally found in the colon of humans.

ESKALITH A commercial preparation of lithium carbonate *q.v.*

ESL An acronym for English as a second language *q.v.*

ESOPHAGEAL CANCER A malignancy *q.v.* of the esophagus *q.v.*

ESOPHAGUS The muscular tube through which food and liquids pass from the mouth to the stomach.

ESR An acronym for erythrocyte sedimentation rate *q.v.*

ESSAY QUESTION In education, an evaluation item characterized by stimulating free thought and expression within the examinee.

ESSENCE That without which the thing being described would not exist. Its intrinsic and indispensable properties.

ESSENTIAL In nutrition, a substance that the body requires for growth and maintenance and cannot synthesize in sufficient amounts.

ESSENTIAL AMINO ACIDS 1. These include those amino acids *q.v.* that must be supplied to the body by the food a person eats. This is true because the body cannot manufacture them. These amino acids are isoleucine, leucine, lysine, methionine, phenylalanine, threonine, tryptophan, and valine. However, cystine, arginine, and histidine (nonessential amino acids in adults) are essential amino acids in infants. 2. The eight amino acids the body cannot synthesize.

ESSENTIAL ELEMENTS In botany, elements *q.v.* of the soil and air required by plants for normal growth and development.

ESSENTIAL FATS 1. The temporary reserve of fat for daily use. 2. Fat that is necessary for the body's normal physiological *q.v.* functioning in the storage and usage of nutrients *q.v.* cf: storage fat.

ESSENTIAL HYPERTENSION 1. High blood pressure that is of an emotional or psychological *q.v.* origin and not a secondary consequence of an identifiable physical disorder. 2. High blood pressure for which there is no apparent medically known cause. 3. A psychophysiological *q.v.* disorder characterized by high blood pressure that cannot be traced to an organic *q.v.* cause. Over a period of time ~ causes enlargement and degeneration of small arteries, enlargement of the heart, and kidney damage.

ESSENTIAL NUTRIENTS Specific nutrients *q.v.* that cannot be synthesized by the body and must be obtained through food.

ESSENTIALISM 1. An area of philosophy *q.v.* that believes a common core of knowledge and ideals should be the focus of the school curriculum *q.v.* 2. The doctrine that there is an indispensible, common core of culture (knowledge, skills, attitudes, ideals, etc.) that should be taught systematically to all, with rigorous standards of achievement. 3. Emphasis on physical sciences as used by authorities, with the assumption that there are no absolute truths and that success is based on absorption of knowledge about the physical world.

ESTEEM NEEDS According to Maslow, the fourth set of human needs that include the human desire for self-respect and respect form others.

ESTER A compound resulting from the combination of an alcohol *q.v.* and an acid *q.v.* Lipids *q.v.* are ~s formed from alcohols and fatty acids *q.v.*

ESTERIFICATION The process of forming an ester *q.v.* from an alcohol *q.v.* and an acid *q.v.*

ESTIMATED PREGNANCY RATE The sum of births plus abortions plus miscarriages *q.v.* Miscarriages are estimated as 20% of all births added to 10% of all abortions.

ESTIMATING 1. Making an educated guess. 2. Making a determination based on available data. cf: estimation.

ESTIMATION In research, the process in statistical inference whereby a confidence interval is constructed around an observed value within which the population value is presumed to lie with a confidence expressed by odds. cf: estimating.

ESTIVATION In biology, a state of sluggishness induced by the heat and dryness of summer.

ESTOP To prevent. cf: estoppel.

ESTOPPEL In law, a bar raised by the law, which prevents a person from alleging or denying a certain fact because of his or her previous statements or conduct.

ESTRADIOL 1. The major natural estrogen *q.v.* secreted by the ovaries *q.v.*, testes *q.v.*, and placenta *q.v.* 2. The most powerful of the estrogens, which are steroid hormones *q.v.*

ESTROGEN 1. A female hormone *q.v.* that is responsible for the development of the breast, nipple, areolae, and milk ducts. 2. A class of chemical compounds, some of which are synthetic and taken orally, that are similar to ovarian estradiol *q.v.* ~ is used in oral contraceptives *q.v.* 3. A female hormone produced primarily by the ovaries *q.v.* that stimulates the development of cervical *q.v.* mucus *q.v.* and ovulation *q.v.* and helps to prepare the uterine *q.v.* lining for implantation *q.v.* of the fertilized ovum *q.v.* 4. A hormone that stimulates the development of secondary sex characteristics *q.v.* in the female and the maintenance of menstruation *q.v.* Birth control pills contain ~ and are sometimes prescribed to control menopausal *q.v.* or postmenopausal symptoms.

ESTROGEN RECEPTOR ASSAY A diagnostic test to determine whether a cancer's *q.v.* growth is dependent upon estrogen *q.v.*

ESTROGEN REPLACEMENT THERAPY (ERT) A treatment sometimes recommended for women in the climacteric *q.v.* who experience severe symptoms. ~ reduces or completely alleviates hot flashes. However, there is some evidence that ~ may increase the risk of uterine cancer *q.v.*

ESTRUS 1. A recurrent period of sexual receptivity in female animals marked by an intense sexual urge. Slang: in heat. 2. The period in the cycle when the female is sexually receptive. 3. Nonprimate female animal's period of sexual readiness.

ET AL And others. Indicates that unnamed parties are involved in the proceedings.

ETHANOL Ethyl alcohol.

ETHER 1. A central nervous system *q.v.* depressant *q.v.* used as a general anesthetic *q.v.* until relatively recently. Now replaced by other more reliable, safer drugs. 2. Diethyl ether, used as an anesthetic with a chemical formula of $C_4H_{10}O$.

ETHICAL CODE The moral guideposts that direct a person, group, or profession in its decisions and behaviors; the philosophy that studies ethics *q.v.*

ETHICAL DRUGS 1. Drugs that are listed in the *United States Pharmacopeia* and found to be safe when used as directed or prescribed. 2. In pharmacy, medicines dispensed only by prescription. ct: over-the-counter drugs; patent medicines.

ETHICAL STANDARDS Rules that set limits on what can be done in good faith in a study; one of the three constraints on research.

ETHICS 1. The moral codes that guide a person, group, or profession in its decisions and behaviors. 2. The rationale behind decisions. 3. Philosophy *q.v.* that studies values. 4. A branch of philosophy that attempts to discover whether conduct is good or bad, right or wrong. An ethic is a value, a standard. Professions establish a code of ~ in order to govern conduct among its members.

ETHMOID 1. One of the nasal sinuses *q.v.* located behind the nose in the ethmoid bone *q.v.* 2. Specifically, sievelike.

ETHMOID BONE One of the nasal bones.

ETHNIC GROUP 1. A group of people who are treated as distinctive in terms of cultural patterns. 2. A group that is socially defined on the basis of its cultural characteristics.

ETHNIC MINORITY A minority group with certain observable cultural differences from the parent group.

ETHNOBIOLOGY 1. The study of biology *q.v.* in context; studying life forms in their natural environments.

ETHNOCENTRISM 1. The belief that a person's own group is superior to all other groups. The result of this belief is the rejection of all out-groups. 2. Pride in membership of a group, race, or religion.

ETHNOGRAPHER A person who studies a society and describes it for others. Usually the society is a nonindustrialized society and is not native to that of the ~. Cultural anthropologists *q.v.* are ~s.

ETHNOGRAPHIC MAP Used by anthropologists *q.v.* to plot the habits, conventions, and other pertinent data of cultures in a geographic area.

ETHNOGRAPHIC STUDIES Anthropologists' *q.v.* data on the habits and conventions within other cultures. cf: ethnographic map.

ETHNOMETHODOLOGY The study of the means by which people reach agreements about the nature of the world.

ETHOLOGY 1. A branch of biology *q.v.* that studies animal behavior under natural conditions.. 2. A branch of psychology that is dedicated to the naturalistic study of animal behavior and to the interpretation of animal behavior in terms of its evolutionary *q.v.* significance.

ETHYL ALCOHOL 1. Ethanol *q.v.* 2. Beverage alcohol *q.v.* 3. Liquid made from the fermentation *q.v.* of fruit or grains that is used in wine, whiskey, gin, beer, rum, etc., with the chemical formula C_2H_5OH. 4. A substance that produces intoxication *q.v.*

ETICBACK An acronym for Environmental Teratology Information Center Backfile *q.v.*

ETIOLATION The condition characterizing plants grown in the dark or in light of very low intensity.

ETIOLOGIC AGENT The organism that causes a disease.

ETIOLOGIC FACTORS 1. Things that cause disease. 2. Factors of disease causation.

ETIOLOGIC FRACTION In epidemiology, population attributable risk percentage *q.v.*

ETIOLOGIC HYPOTHESES Theories used to explain the cause or causes of a particular disease.

ETIOLOGICAL VALIDITY Validity *q.v.*

ETIOLOGY 1. The causation of disease. 2. The systematic study of the causes of disorders.

ETV An acronym for educational television.

EUBACTERIA True bacteria *q.v.*

EUCHROMATIN Parts of chromosomes *q.v.* that are genetically active and have characteristic staining properties. cf: heterochromatin.

EUGENICS 1. The science that seeks to improve future generations through the control of hereditary *q.v.* factors. 2. The science that deals with all influences that improve the unborn. 3. The science that is concerned with the influences that improve inborn qualities in a series of generations of a race or breed. cf: dysgenic; genetic.

EUKARYOTIC 1. Organisms showing mitosis *q.v.* with membrane-bound nuclei *q.v.* and other organelles *q.v.* 2. Description of cells with the hereditary *q.v.* information organized into chromosomes *q.v.* that are contained within the nucleus and are not in contact with the cytoplasm *q.v.* except at the time of cell division.

EULOGY A composition or speech that praises someone who has died. Usually delivered at a funeral or memorial service.

EUNUCH A castrated *q.v.* male.

EUNUCHOID A castrated male or one who is similar in appearance to a eunuch *q.v.*

EUPHORIA 1. An elevated positive mood. 2. A positive sign of phenothiazine *q.v.* drug response when it appears after a test dose of the drug. ct: dysphoria.

EUPLOID An organism or cell having a chromosome *q.v.* number that is an exact multiple of the monoploid *q.v.* or haploid *q.v.* number. cf: heteroploid.

EUPNEA Normal respiration.

EURHYTHMICS Aerobic *q.v.* dancing.

EUSTACHIAN TUBE The air tube extending from the middle ear to the throat that maintains the pressure equilibrium on the eardrum and drains the middle ear.

EUSTRESS 1. A tension appropriate for preparing the body for maximum functioning. 2. Stress *q.v.* that adds a positive, enhancing dimension to the quality of life. 3. Hans Selye's term for stressors. ct: distress.

EUTHANASIA 1. The process of bringing about the painless death of a person. 2. Mercy killing. 3. Assisting in or allowing a person to die for reasons of mercy.

EUTHENICS The science that is concerned with the betterment of living conditions to establish more efficient human beings.

EUTROPHICATION 1. The process by which oxygen is removed from water by the excessive growth of algae *q.v.* 2. Enrichment of a body of water with nutrients *q.v.*, which allows for overabundance of plant growth. 3. Aging of a large body of water.

EVAGINATION 1. A protrusion of some part of the body or of an organ. 2. The outfolding of a layer of cells from a cavity.

EVALUATION 1. An appraisal, assessment, or measurement in the broadest and most complete sense. 2. An estimation, calculation, determination, approximation, worth, or opinion. 3. A complex process of measurement and judgment, which includes gathering, organizing, and interpreting information. 4. Assessing the quality and effectiveness of programs for individuals and groups. 5. The comparison of an object of interest against a standard of acceptability. 6. A systematic approach used to determine the extent to which target goals have been achieved and whether program inputs are causally related to outputs. 7. An examination to determine how activities are carried out to achieve goals. 8. The process of determining the value or degree of success in achieving a predetermined objective. This may include formulation of objectives, identification of the criteria to be used in measuring success, and determination and explanation of the degree of success. 9. A means of making informed decisions about the quality of a product or a performance. ~ may be ongoing or formative as a means of assessing progress or summative as a means of determining total growth or change as a total outcome of some specified treatment or program, includes but is not limited to quantitative measurement.

EVALUATION APPREHENSION A person's concern with the possibility that other people will react to the quality of his or her performance.

EVALUATION DEVICES Instruments, procedures, and techniques available for assessing the elements of the school or community health program. ~ include the following: (a) observation, (b) interviews, (c) individual and group conferences, (d) self-appraisal checklists, (e) questionnaires (f) surveys, (g) general checklists, (h) records, (i) reports, (j) achievement tests, and (k) simulations.

EVALUATION PROGRAM The planned methods and procedures for measuring the extent to which the education program has achieved its objectives. cf: evaluation.

EVALUATION RESEARCH Programs of research that attempt to rigorously measure the results of implemented social programs. Such research can form the basis of changes in social policy.

EVANESCENT Tending to disappear early.

EVAPORATION A change in a compound from a liquid state to a vapor form. ct: condensation reaction.

EVENTS In the PERT *q.v.* network, events are the completions of major product tasks.

EVERSEARCHERS Swingers *q.v.* who wish to supplement routine marital sex.

EVERSION A turning outward or inside out, particularly of the eyelid lining.

EVERTED 1. Turned outward. 2. To turn a part outward.

EVIDENCE Facts, information, or data that support or refute a hypothesis *q.v.*

EVISCERATION 1. Disemboweling. 2. The protrusion of viscera *q.v.* from any body cavity or through an open wound.

EVOCATIVE Serving to call forth a response.

EVOKED POTENTIAL 1. An electrical discharge in a neutral center produced by stimulation elsewhere. 2. A specific, event-related response that can be detected in the brain using an electroencephalograph *q.v.*

EVOLUTION 1. Changes in the characteristics of living things as a result of an interruption in the genetic *q.v.* equilibrium of the species. Forces of evolution are chiefly gene mutation *q.v.*, natural selection *q.v.*, and genetic drift *q.v.* 2. The study of the development of humanity based on scientific data that proposes human beings developed from lower life forms. 3. The history of the development of a race, species, or larger group of organisms that, following modifications in successive generations, has acquired characteristics that distinguish it from other groups.

EVOLUTIONISM A concern for understanding the origins and development of natural phenomena.

EX OFFICIO 1. In politics, holding two offices, one of which is held by virtue or because of the first. 2. A nonvoting member of an organization.

EX POST FACTO 1. After the fact. 2. In law and politics, an ~ law is one passed after an act which retrospectively changes the legal consequences of that act. The United States Constitution prohibits the passage of ~ criminal laws. cf: bill of attainder.

EX POST FACTO ANALYSIS In correlational research *q.v.*, an attempt to reduce the third-variable *q.v.* problem by selecting subjects who are matched on characteristics that may be confounding *q.v.*

EX POST FACTO DESIGNS A procedure used in correlational studies *q.v.* to reduce the third-variable *q.v.* problem. Groups of subjects are carefully matched to eliminate variables likely to confound *q.v.* research results.

EX POST FACTO EXPERIMENT In research, an investigational procedure in which the independent variable *q.v.* is identified and related to behavior after the experiment *q.v.* is complete.

EX POST FACTO STUDIES After-the-fact natural experiments *q.v.*

EX REL 1. Ex relations. 2. On relation or information. 3. An action taken by an attorney general at the instigation of an individual with private interest. 4. On information supplied.

EXACERBATION 1. An increase in the severity of disease symptoms. 2. A flare up or worsening.

EXALTOLIDE A musky pheromone *q.v.* that is highly concentrated in the urine of adult males.

EXANTHEM Any contagious *q.v.* disease characterized by skin eruption.

EXCEPTION In civil procedure, a formal objection to the action of the court when it refuses a request or overrules an objection, implying that the party excepting does not acquiesce in the court's ruling and may base an appeal thereon.

EXCEPTIONAL In education, refers to any learner whose physical, mental, or behavioral performance deviates so substantially from the average that additional services are necessary to meet the learner's needs.

EXCEPTIONAL CHILDREN Learners with disabilities or talents that require specialized educational programs. cf: exceptional learner.

EXCEPTIONAL LEARNER One who deviates from the normal, intellectually, physically, socially, or emotionally in growth and development so markedly that he or she cannot receive the maximum educational benefits from a regular program.

EXCHANGE DIET A diet *q.v.* constructed around the interchanging of foods based on their nutrient composition. An important aspect is the management of Type 1 diabetes *q.v.*

EXCHANGE THEORY 1. A theory of interpersonal behavior that is based on four major assumptions: (a) human behavior is motivated primarily by pleasure and pain, (b) the actions of other people are primary sources of pleasure and pain, (c) a person's actions may be used to secure pleasure-giving actions from others, and (d) people attempt to gain maximum pleasure at minimum cost. 2. The concept that marriage or other serious romantic relationships are exchanges of resources. 3. An explanatory schema concerning human behavior that emphasizes the individual balancing of computed rewards and costs in making decisions.

EXCISION 1. Female circumcision *q.v.*, which varies in extent from the nicking of the clitoral hood *q.v.* to the removal of all external genitalia *q.v.* 2. The cutting out of a part or growth.

EXCISIONAL BIOPSY Total surgical removal of tissue to be examined.

EXCITATION In physiology, the process whereby activity is elicited in a nerve.

EXCITATION TRANSFER A process in which arousal that was generated by one stimulus can intensify unrelated activity.

EXCITATORY POSTSYNAPTIC POTENTIAL The potential change that takes place in a neuron *q.v.* when a nerve impulse is approaching it from a synapse *q.v.* This action is not subject to the all-or-none law *q.v.*

EXCITEMENT A generalized, usually pleasant, emotional state.

EXCITEMENT PHASE 1. The sexual response phase of arousal. 2. The initial stage of the human sexual response cycle *q.v.* that follows effective sexual stimulation. 3. The first of four stages of the sexual response cycle, vaginal lubrication and penile erection are the primary responses of females and males, respectively.

EXCLUSIONS Specific conditions listed in an insurance policy for which the insurance company will not pay.

EXCORIATION 1. Irritation of the superficial layers of the skin. 2. Pertaining to scratching. 3. A scratch mark or linear break in the skin surface usually covered with blood or serous crusts.

EXCRETE 1. To eliminate. 2. To separate from the blood and tissues and eliminate from the body. cf: excretory system. ct: secrete.

EXCRETION The elimination of waste products from the body.

EXCRETORY SYSTEM 1. The urinary system *q.v.* 2. Essentially the kidneys and connecting organs. 3. The kidneys, urinary bladder, ureters, and urethra.

EXECUTED CONTRACT A completed contract as opposed to one which is executory *q.v.*

EXECUTIVE A person having the authority to make policy decisions in an organization.

EXECUTIVE COMMITTEE ACTION The formal recommendation of a standing committee on any proposal referred to such committee for consideration.

EXECUTIVE FUNCTIONING The cognitive *q.v.* capacity to plan how to do a task, how to devise strategies, and how to monitor one's performance.

EXECUTIVE MBA A master's degree in business programs exclusively for executives who attend classes off-hours, such as on weekends, and progress through a program as part of an integrated group.

EXECUTIVE SESSION In politics, a session excluding from the chamber all persons other than members and essential staff personnel.

EXECUTOR In law, a person or institution authorized by the maker of a will to manage and distribute the property of a person who has died in accordance with the provisions of the will.

EXECUTORY CONTRACT In law, an incompletely performed contract. A contract to be completed sometime in the future.

EXEMPT In labor relations, employees whose rate of pay or position in the organization exempts them from the provisions of the Fair Labor Standards Act.

EXEMPT NARCOTIC A drug preparation containing a small amount of a narcotic *q.v.* substance that can be purchased legally in some states without a physician's written prescription.

EXERCISE Activities designed toward muscular development and/or cardiovascular fitness.

EXERCISE PHYSIOLOGY The study of the body's systems and processes during exercise *q.v.*

EXERCISE PRESCRIPTION A three-phase individualized exercise *q.v.* program. cf: training; conditioning.

EXERCISE TOLERANCE The maximum level of exercise *q.v.* to which the body responds favorably.

EXERGONIC Pertaining to any reaction in which energy is released.

EXFOLIATION 1. In botany, the falling off of superficial layers of growth or of leaves. 2. In anatomy, physiology, and medicine, the falling off of the outer layers of skin.

EXHAUSTION METHOD A method of habit breaking in which the undesirable response is allowed to occur without reinforcement until it disappears. cf: extinction; toleration method.

EXHAUSTIVE CATEGORIES In epidemiology, all subjects are classified in some category of the classification scheme for the variable.

EXHIBITIONISM 1. A sexual variance *q.v.* in which the person suffers from a compulsion to expose genitals publicly. 2. Sexual gratification from exposing one's genitals. Found most frequently among males. Slang: flasher. 3. Public display or exposure of genitals for the conscious or unconscious purpose of sexual excitement and pleasure.

EXHILARATION A feeling of gladness or extreme excitement.

EXISTENTIAL ANALYSIS 1. Humanistic–existential therapy *q.v.* 2. Existential therapy *q.v.*

EXISTENTIAL ANXIETY Anxiety *q.v.* concerning a person's ability to find a satisfying and fulfilling way of life.

EXISTENTIAL NEUROSIS A disorder in which the person feels alienation, considers life meaningless, and finds no activity worth selecting and pursuing. cf: premorbid personality.

EXISTENTIAL THERAPY 1. A form of therapy concerned with occurrences as they exist. The therapist helps the person to take responsibility for what happens and to seek success in self-actualization *q.v.* The person has control over the choices of behavior and the therapist attempts to find the original choices the person has made that resulted in maladjustment. 2. Therapy based on existential *q.v.* concepts emphasizing the development of a sense of self-direction and meaning in one's existence. 3. Intervention that encourages exploration of subjective experience as a means of reintegrating the self and emphasizes the potential for self-determination.

EXISTENTIALISM 1. A view of humans that emphasizes a person's responsibility for self and for becoming the kind of person he or she should be. 2. The philosophy *q.v.* that emphasizes individuals and individual decision making *q.v.* 3. A philosophy that emphasizes the ability of an individual to determine the course of his or her own life. 4. Emphasis on problem solving about highly controversial and emotional issues in any subject matter area. The assumption that learners define themselves and their relationships by their choices.

EXISTENTIALIST A person trained in existential therapy *q.v.*

EXOCRINE Secreting into a duct *q.v.* ct: endocrine glands.

EXOGENOTE A fragment of a bacterial chromosome *q.v.* of exogenous *q.v.* origin.

EXOGENOUS 1. Factors originating or produced by the social or physical environments. 2. Extrinsic *q.v.* 3. Originating outside or caused by factors outside the body. ct: endogenous.

EXOGENOUS DEPRESSION 1. A form of depression *q.v.* that results from factors outside the person. 2. Secondary depression *q.v.* 3. A profound sadness assumed to be caused by an environmental event.

EXOGENOUS MICROORGANISMS Microscopic organisms that are not normally found in the human body, many of which can cause disease when they enter the body.

EXOPHTHALMIC GOITER 1. Grave's disease *q.v.* 2. A disorder of the thyroid *q.v.* characterized by enlargement of this gland, protrusion of the eyelids, and several mental symptoms.

EXOPHTHALMOS Exaggerated protrusion of the eyelids. cf: hyperthyroidism; exophthalmic goiter.

EXORCISM A variety of techniques practiced since ancient times for casting out evil spirits that supposedly cause mental illness and organic diseases. ~ is based on the concept that illness is caused by the invasion of the body by demons and evil spirits.

EXOSMOSIS Osmotic diffusion *q.v.* toward the outside of a cell or vessel.

EXOSTOSIS An outgrowth of a bone.

EXOTOXINS 1. Soluble toxins *q.v.* that diffuse out of a living cell into the environment. 2. Toxins that are produced and excreted from cells during growth.

EXPECTANCE In research, a belief or subjective probability that a given act will result in a given outcome.

EXPECTANCY An aspect of cognitive theory *q.v.* relative to the acquisition of knowledge of what leads to what.

EXPECTED VALUE A measurement of the anticipated value of some event. ~ is determined by multiplying the income an event would produce by its probability of making that income.

EXPECTORANT 1. A drug that stimulates the flow of respiratory secretions. 2. A substance that stimulates fluid production in the throat to break up congestion. 3. Drugs that help bring mucus and phlegm up from the respiratory pathways.

EXPEDITED ARBITRATION In labor relations, arbitrators from a preselected list are instantly available to hear grievances and render quick decisions.

EXPERIENCE RATING A system of collecting insurance premiums on the basis of actual or anticipated use.

EXPERIENTIAL TEACHING 1. The provision of activities that are realistic, involve multiple senses, and require the learner to participate fully, effectively, physically, and cognitively. 2. Hands on learning. The learner does by doing. cf: experientially based learning.

EXPERIENTIALLY BASED LEARNING Changes in a person's knowledge, values, and skills resulting from participation in a variety of learning experiences. cf: experiential teaching.

EXPERIMENT 1. A study in which researchers manipulate one or more variables to determine its effect upon the subject's response. 2. The most powerful research technique for determining causal relationships, requiring the manipulation of an independent variable *q.v.*, the measurement of a dependent variable *q.v.*, and the random assignment *q.v.* of subjects to the several different conditions being investigated. 3. A procedure for making causal inferences from observations of the relationships that exist among variables.

EXPERIMENTAL BIAS 1. The distortions in the outcome of a study that are produced when the investigator communicates subtly and perhaps unconsciously how a subject should behave. 2. Subtly and unintended transmission of an experimenter's expectations. cf: demand characteristic.

EXPERIMENTAL EPIDEMIOLOGY 1. That phase of epidemiology *q.v.* that analyses prospective studies *q.v.* and retrospective studies *q.v.* 2. The historical analysis of two groups of people. 3. Used to evaluate *q.v.* the efficacy of some intervention procedure. cf: analytic epidemiology; descriptive epidemiology.

EXPERIMENTAL EVIDENCE Evidence derived from controlled research designed to test the validity *q.v.* of a hypothesis *q.v.* cf: descriptive evidence; epidemiological evidence.

EXPERIMENTAL GROUP 1. The group in an experiment *q.v.* whose behavior or condition is affected by the variable being tested. 2. The subjects who are exposed to the stimulus under study. cf: experimental method. ct: control group.

EXPERIMENTAL HYPOTHESIS What the investigator assumes will happen in a scientific investigation if certain conditions are met or particular variables are manipulated.

EXPERIMENTAL METHOD 1. An experiment in which something is done in one situation that is not done in another situation. The former is called the experimental group *q.v.*, while the latter is called the control group *q.v.* 2. A method of investigation in which one or more independent variables *q.v.* are manipulated, extraneous variables are controlled, and one or more dependent variables are observed. 3. A research method in which investigators try to isolate biological or environmental factors that they think may determine a particular behavior and then test subjects to see whether their behavior changes when such factors are present. cf: clinical method; observational method.

EXPERIMENTAL MODEL A nonhuman system used in research. The most common ~ is with animals other than humans. cf: animal model.

EXPERIMENTAL NEUROSIS Emotional disturbance produced by establishing the conditions of conflict *q.v.*

EXPERIMENTAL SCHOOLS Schools in which new methods or materials are tried under controlled conditions.

EXPERIMENTAL STUDY A research method that manipulates an independent variable *q.v.* and measures changes in a dependent variable *q.v.* according to a procedure designed to eliminate alternative explanations.

EXPERT SYSTEMS Computer problem-solving programs with a very narrow scope dealing only with problems in a limited domain of knowledge.

EXPERTISE-ORIENTED EVALUATION In research, judgments by experts of the value or worth of something.

EXPIATION Atonement *q.v.*

EXPIATIVE PUNISHMENT Punishment *q.v.* that is designed not to rectify a wrong but to gain revenge on the guilty.

EXPIRATION The act of breathing out or of expelling air from the lungs.

EXPIRE 1. To breathe out. 2. To die.

EXPLANATION CREDIBILITY In research, the plausibility of the explanation advanced for a phenomenon.

EXPLANATION GENERALITY In research, the generality that is claimed, implied, or must be inferred from a study's problem statement.

EXPLANATION, RATIONALE, THEORY, POINT OF VIEW In research, a description of the relationship among variables *q.v.* that portrays the sequence of events and attributes causal and mode-rating roles to certain variables or events in that sequence or, where this is not yet possible, as much of such description as the current state of knowledge permits.

EXPLORATION In research, to examine phenomena that have not previously been studied in the same way; to try different things in a situation to determine what happens; and to examine previously examined situations from new points of view to see whether a difference is significant.

EXPLORATORY EDUCATION Education that emphasizes children's need to discover answers themselves.

EXPLORATORY, INSIGHT-ORIENTED THERAPY (EOI) A therapeutic *q.v.* approach based on the Freudian model *q.v.* that emphasizes the attainment of insight and understanding of one's past and present difficulties.

EXPOSURE REGISTRY An official roster of persons exposed to hazardous substances that evolved from the need for fundamental information concerning the potential impact on human health of long-term exposure to low and moderate levels of hazardous substances.

EXPRESS Directly set forth in words.

EXPRESSED EMOTION In regards to schizophrenia *q.v.*, the amount of hostility and criticism directed from other people to the patient, usually within a family.

EXPRESSIONISTIC SEXUALITY Complete expression of a person's personality-defined concept of sexuality *q.v.*

EXPRESSIVE LANGUAGE DISORDERS Difficulties in language production.

EXPRESSIVE MOVEMENTS 1. Movements of the face and body that seem to reflect emotions *q.v.* 2. Built-in social displays.

EXPRESSIVE OBJECTIVES 1. Objectives *q.v.* described in a meaningful encounter or task rather than some exact outcome. 2. Evocative, wherein the impact is more in the nature of engaging the interest and impressing learners in new ways both intellectually and emotionally *q.v.*

EXPRESSIVITY A degree of expression of a trait controlled by a gene *q.v.* A particular gene may produce varying degrees of expression in different individuals.

EXPULSION In education, permanent withdrawal of a student's privilege to attend a certain school or class.

EXPUNGE 1. Obliterate. 2. Physically remove from its location.

EXTENDED CARE 1. Health care of a long-term nature with a minimum of nursing and rehabilitative services. 2. Essentially, custodial care as opposed to skilled nursing care *q.v.*

EXTENDED CARE FACILITY 1. A special convalescent wing of a hospital or a nursing home staffed by registered nurses *q.v.* 2. An institution designed to provide long-term medical or custodial care for people who do not require hospitalization.

EXTENDED FAMILY 1. A family *q.v.* in which children, parents, and grandparents live under the same roof. 2. Relatives other than spouse and children. 3. Close relatives to a family who visit or interact with the family on a regular basis.

EXTENDED INJUNCTION In labor relations, a national emergency strike remedy whereby a cooling off period is continued by Congressional action for an additional 30 days.

EXTENDED RADICAL MASTECTOMY The surgical removal of the breast, skin, pectoral muscles, all auxiliary mammary lymph nodes, fat, and sometimes a section of rib.

EXTENSION 1. Movement of a body joint such that the angle about the center of rotation (the fulcrum) increases. 2. The act of straightening. 3. The movement by which the two ends of any jointed part are drawn away from each other. ct: flexion.

EXTENT OF PERFORMANCE 1. Criterion of performance *q.v.* 2. The level of mastery of proficiency by which terminal behavior *q.v.* is evaluated.

EXTENUATING CIRCUMSTANCES In law, circumstances that make an offense seem less serious.

EXTERNAL COMMITTEE A group made up of people outside the organization or agency. ct: internal committee.

EXTERNAL CUES Environmental sensations that provide a person with information. ct: internal cues.

EXTERNAL ENVIRONMENT One's surroundings outside of the body. ct: internal environment.

EXTERNAL EVALUATION Evaluation *q.v.* of an agency, organization, or program conducted by people who have no significant attachment to the organization being evaluated.

EXTERNAL FRUSTRATION Environmental obstacles to achieving goals and need gratification.

EXTERNAL GENITALIA The reproductive structures visible by an external examination. ct: internal genitalia.

EXTERNAL ORGANIZATIONAL DIAGNOSIS The process of examining all outside factors that relate to organizational effectiveness.

EXTERNAL QUALITIES Those forces of the social and physical environments that act on the individual.

EXTERNAL RADIATION The use of X-rays or other sources of radiation *q.v.* for the treatment of a disease, e.g., cancer. Used for curing or palliation *q.v.* ct: internal radiation.

EXTERNAL STIMULUS Any stimulus *q.v.* energy that is outside of the nervous system *q.v.*

EXTERNAL URETHRAL SPHINCTER A circular muscle near the base of the penis *q.v.* that opens during a normal ejaculation *q.v.* allowing semen *q.v.* to flow through the penis to the outside.

EXTERNAL VALIDITY The extent to which conclusions of a research study can be generalized to other populations and settings. cf: validity.

EXTERNALITY A tendency of obese *q.v.* persons to be highly sensitive to food-related stimuli *q.v.*

EXTERNALITY HYPOTHESIS The theory that some obese *q.v.* people are relatively unresponsive to their own hunger state but are more susceptible to cues from the external environment.

EXTINCTION 1. In psychology, terminating the reinforcement of a behavior, which results in the behavior eventually being eliminated or stopped. 2. The elimination of a classically conditioned *q.v.* response by the omission of the unconditioned stimulus *q.v.* In operant conditioning *q.v.*, the elimination of the conditioned response by the omission of reinforcement. 3. In biology, the complete elimination of a species of plant or animal life. cf: instrumental conditioning.

EXTIRPATION 1. The removal of brain tissue for experimental purposes. 2. The complete removal of a part, usually an internal organ.

EXTRA PROCREATIVE SEX Sexual relations without the desire for children.

EXTRACELLULAR From outside the cell wall or membrane. ct: intracellular.

EXTRACELLULAR COMPARTMENT The approximate 40% of total body water that is found outside of body cells. Consists of intravascular, interstitial, and transcellular fluids *q.v.* Extracellular fluid *q.v.*

EXTRACELLULAR FLUID 1. Fluid found outside the body cells. 2. Tissue fluid. 3. Extracellular compartment.

EXTRACHROMOSOMAL 1. Structures that are not a part of the chromosomes *q.v.* 2. DNA *q.v.* units that control cytoplasmic *q.v.* inheritance *q.v.*

EXTRACTION 1. To free or remove from a difficult situation or position. ~ is often used to signify recovery of a person from a car wreck or other place of entrapment. 2. The removal of a tooth.

EXTRACURRICULAR In education, activities of learners outside the formal structure of the classroom. Sometimes referred to as cocurricular.

EXTRADITION In law, the legal surrender of an alleged criminal to a jurisdiction of another state, county, or government for trial.

EXTRADURAL HEMATOMA Hemorrhage *q.v.* and swelling between the skull and dura mater *q.v.* when a meningeal *q.v.* artery is ruptured by a fractured bone of the skull.

EXTRAGENITAL 1. A body part other than the reproductive organs *q.v.* 2. Outside of the genitals *q.v.* 3. Originating outside of the genital organs.

EXTRAGENITAL RESPONSES The responses of the parts of the body other than the reproductive organs *q.v.* to sexual arousal.

EXTRAMARITAL 1. Sexual relations with someone other than one's spouse. 2. Outside of marriage. 3. Adulterous *q.v.* sexual intercourse *q.v.*

EXTRAMURAL RESEARCH An investigative study that is undertaken outside the prescribed research agenda for the purpose of obtaining additional insight into some field of knowledge.

EXTRANEOUS DISTURBANCE In information theory *q.v.*, noise.

EXTRAPOLATION In epidemiology *q.v.* making quantitative or numerical predictions based on past or current rates or qualities.

EXTRAPUNITIVE 1. A tendency to evaluate the source of frustration as external and to direct hostility outward. 2. Extrapunitive aggression *q.v.*

EXTRAPUNITIVE AGGRESSION Aggressive *q.v.* behavior directed toward other persons. cf: extrapunitive.

EXTRAPYRAMIDAL Pertaining to a motor control system in the central nervous system *q.v.* that is responsible for maintaining muscle tone and posture. Parkinson's disease *q.v.* causes damage to this system. Antipsychotic drugs *q.v.* also interfere with the ~ system, producing similar symptoms to those of Parkinson's disease.

EXTRASCHOOL 1. Activities or programs conducted outside of the school setting. 2. Committees formed whose members are not associated directly with the school.

EXTRASYSTOLE An extra heart beat. cf: systole.

EXTRAUTERINE Outside of the uterus *q.v.* ct: intrauterine.

EXTRAUTERINE PREGNANCY 1. A pregnancy that occurs outside the uterus *q.v.* 2. Ectopic pregnancy *q.v.*

EXTRAVASATION 1. The act of escaping from a vessel into the tissues as associated with blood, lymph, or serum. 2. The spreading out of blood or other fluids into the tissue spaces.

EXTRAVERSION (EXTROVERSION) 1. An energy trait directed toward one's outer world of objects or other people. 2. The tendency to seek out stimulation from the world of people and things, characterized by a preference for novelty and variety. 3. A high sense of sociability. cf: extraversion/introversion. ct: introversion.

EXTRAVERSION/INTROVERSION A trait that refers to a person's main energy direction; toward the outer world with people or toward the inner world of self. cf: introversion; extraversion.

EXTRAVERT (EXTROVERT) In type theory *q.v.* a person whose personality *q.v.* is oriented outward, requiring continual stimulation from the social environment. ct: introvert.

EXTRINSIC 1. Outside of the body. 2. Chiefly environmental. ct: intrinsic.

EXTRINSIC FACTORS 1. The environment outside of the person. 2. In epidemiology, the factors of disease outside of the host.

EXTRINSIC MOTIVATION 1. Extrinsic reward *q.v.* 2. Incentive. 3. Behavior stimulated by the expectation of some sort of reward or avoidance of punishment. ct: intrinsic motivation.

EXTRINSIC REWARDS 1. Reward that is received from an external source as the result of a person's behavior or action. 2. Rewards that are extraneous to the task accomplished. ct: intrinsic motivation.

EXTRUSION REFLEX The instinctive motion of the tongue by which infants push food out of their mouths.

EXUDATE 1. Fluids that leak out of the blood vessels into an inflamed area causing swelling or edema *q.v.* 2. Pus *q.v.* 3. To produce liquid in response to disease.

EXUMBILICATION Protrusion of the navel.

EYE The organ of vision.

EYE–NECK REFLEX A reflex *q.v.* jerking of the head in infancy in response to light.

EYEPIECE A second series of lenses that magnifies the primary image, producing the image that is projected to the retina *q.v.* of the eye and recorded by the optic nerve *q.v.*

EYESPOT 1. In biology, a pigmented area that is sensitive to light. 2. A small, pigmented structure in algae *q.v.* that may be sensitive to light.

F

F′ An F^+ episome *q.v.* that also carries a piece of the bacterial chromosome *q.v.*

F_1 1. In genetics, the first generation following a cross. F_2 and F_3 are the second and third generations, respectively. 2. The first filial generation. 3. The first generation of descent from a given mating.

F_2 The second filial generation, produced by crossing inter se or by self-pollinating the F_1. The inbred grandchildren of a given mating. The term is loosely used to indicate any second-generation progeny from a given mating, but in controlled genetic experimentation, inbreeding of the F_1 (or equivalent) is implied.

FAAHB An acronym for Fellow of the American Academy of Health Behavior.

FAAN An acronym for Fellow of the American Academy of Nursing.

FABRICATION 1. Pertaining to imaginary events as though they were true without intent to deceive. 2. Confabulation *q.v.*

FACD An acronym for Fellow of the American College of Dentists.

FACE MASK In medicine, a device for the administration of anesthetic *q.v.* gases or oxygen.

FACE VALIDITY 1. The instrument, in the judgment of experts, will evaluate what it is purported to. The test obviously will elicit certain kinds of data. 2. The appearance of validity *q.v.* produced by the fact that a test requires a performance very similar to the task for which is designed to make predictions. 3. A quality of test design based upon the fact that the items do match the subject matter of concern.

FACEWORK The use of facial expressions to manage social relations.

FACIES The expression or appearance of the face. ~ may be characteristic of various disease conditions.

FACILITATED DIFFUSION Carrier-mediated diffusion *q.v.*

FACILITATION A disease in a neuron's *q.v.* resting potential to a point above its threshold of stimulation.

FACILITY 1. In public health, a place where health care is provided. 2. A health site: hospital, nursing home, clinic, or ambulatory center.

FACOG An acronym for Fellow of the American College of Obstetricians and Gynecologists.

FACP An acronym for Fellow of the American College of Physicians.

FACS An acronym for Fellow of the American College of Surgeons.

FACSM An acronym for Fellow of the American College of Sports Medicine.

FACT FINDING In labor relations, actions to investigate, assemble, and report the facts in an employment dispute, sometimes with authority to make recommendations for settlement.

FACTITIOUS DISORDER A disorder in which the person's physical or psychological *q.v.* symptoms *q.v.* appear under voluntary control and are adopted merely to assume the role of a sick person. This condition is not voluntary and implies a severe disturbance. cf: malingering.

FACTOR 1. In genetics, a gene *q.v.* 2. A specific germinal cause of a hereditary *q.v.* character.

FACTOR ANALYSIS 1. A complex statistical method for studying the interrelationships among various tests to determine what the tests have in common and whether these can be ascribed to one or several factors that run through some or all of the tests. 2. A statistical technique, employing the methods of correlation *q.v.*, designed to detect the factors that contribute to a complex trait. 3. Clustering the variables most highly correlated with each other into homogeneous *q.v.* groups called "factors" and making inferences of the constructs measured by the factors from the size of the variables' correlations with them.

FACTOR COMPARISON In job evaluation, monetary value assigned to each job for each compensable factor.

FACTORIAL DESIGN In research, a study design in which the data on every combination of variables *q.v.* in the study are provided by a separate group from which their effects can be determined.

FAD DIETS Eating practices that are popular with exaggerated excitement.

FADDIST A person who supports a popular craze with exaggerated zeal.

FACTOR VIII A naturally occurring protein *q.v.* in the plasma *q.v.* that aids in the coagulation *q.v.* of blood. A congenital *q.v.* deficiency of ~ results in the bleeding disorder known as hemophilia A *q.v.* cf: factor VIII concentrate.

FACTOR VIII CONCENTRATE A concentrated preparation of factor VIII *q.v.* that is used in the treatment of individuals with hemophilia *q.v.*

FAHRENHEIT SCALE The temperature scale in which the freezing point of water is 32° and the boiling point of water at sea level is 212°. Zero indicates the lowest ~ temperature that can be obtained with a mixture of ice and salt. ct: centigrade scale.

FAIL-SAFE MEDICINE Medicine that supposedly works safely on all people at all times.

FAILURE MODE AND EFFECT In safety epidemiology, each component is evaluated as to how it will affect the overall system if it fails. cf: epidemiology.

FAILURE-TO-THRIVE SYNDROME 1. A childhood condition characterized by a severely retarded growth rate. The condition can occur as a result of parental neglect and emotional upset. 2. Deprivation dwarfism *q.v.*

FAINT A temporary loss of consciousness, usually of brief duration. cf: fainting.

FAINTING 1. Syncope *q.v.* 2. ~ may be caused by either psychological *q.v.* or physiological factors. Blood tends to pool in the blood vessels of the viscera *q.v.* depriving the brain of sufficient oxygen.

FAIR EMPLOYMENT PRACTICES In labor relations, codes regulating hiring and other employment practices that consider race, color, creed, sex, religion, national origin, or other features or characteristics.

FAITH A predisposition to apply one's concept of an ultimate environment to life's experiences. The purpose and meaning that underlie a person's hopes, dreams, and strivings.

FAITH HEALING 1. Belief that religious faith or faith in the healer will cure disease. 2. Belief that the mind has control over the body and can cure disease through divine help.

FALLING A common problem experienced among older people due to a number of underlying causes. Evaluating people who have falls involves assessing the injuries sustained in the fall and the cause of the fall. In older people, ~ frequently results in broken bones and other serious injuries that may lead to disability and sometimes death.

FALLOPIAN TUBE 1. An anatomical structure of the female, which connects the ovary *q.v.* with the uterus *q.v.* 2. The duct through which the egg from the ovary passes to the uterus. 3. The place where the sperm *q.v.* usually fertilizes *q.v.* the egg. 4. The oviduct *q.v.*

FALLOUT 1. The descent to earth of radioactive *q.v.* particles. 2. The descent to earth of any particulate matter created by industry or a natural phenomenon.

FALSE LABOR 1. Irregular contractions of the undilated uterus *q.v.* that mimic true labor. 2. Conditions that tend to resemble the start of true labor. They may include irregular uterine contractions, pressure, and discomfort in the lower abdomen.

FALSE MOTION 1. Movement of an extremity of a part of the body where ordinarily there should be none, indicative of a fracture *q.v.* 2. Motion of the two ends of a fractured bone against one another.

FALSE NEGATIVES 1. In epidemiology, in test of validity *q.v.*, labeling cases or the presence of the attribute for which the test is conducted incorrectly. 2. Categorizing cases as noncases or failing to identify the characteristic when it was present. 3. The result that indicates that a condition does not exist when in fact the condition exists. ct: false positives.

FALSE POSITIVES 1. In epidemiology, in tests of validity *q.v.*, labeling noncases or the absence of a characteristic incorrectly. 2. Categorizing noncases as cases or identifying a characteristic when it was not present. 3. A test result that indicates that a condition exists when in fact the condition does not exist. ct: false negatives.

FALSE PREGNANCY 1. Pseudopregnancy *q.v.* 2. Pseudocyesis *q.v.* 3. Symptoms of early pregnancy without the presence of an embryo *q.v.*

FALSE TRANSMITTER In pharmacology, a method by which a drug may affect the nervous system *q.v.* The drug is taken into a neuron *q.v.* and acted upon by enzymes *q.v.* to produce a substance resembling the natural neurotransmitter *q.v.* but differing from it functionally.

FALSIFIABILITY 1. Testability *q.v.* 2. In research, one of the criteria for evaluating the scientific merit of theories. A theory is falsifiable when it is stated in such a way that it can be disproved.

FAMILIAL 1. Pertaining to characteristics that tend to run in families and have a higher incidence *q.v.* in certain families than in the general population. 2. Familial pattern *q.v.*

FAMILIAL PATTERN The higher than average occurrence of a disease among members of a blood-related family.

FAMILIARITY EFFECT In psychology, increased exposure to a stimulus tends to make the stimulus more pleasurable.

FAMILISM A high regard for the family, ancestors, and family traditions.

FAMILY 1. In sociology, a group of two or more people related by blood, marriage, or adoption who live together. 2. In biology, a category of classification above a genus *q.v.* and below an order *q.v.*, composed of one or a number of genera *q.v.*

FAMILY CLIMATE The degree of cohesiveness and harmony among family members characteristic of any given family *q.v.*

FAMILY GROUP THERAPY In psychology, the treatment of the family *q.v.* as a group rather than merely the treatment of the member apart from his or her family setting.

FAMILY HOUSEHOLD In sociology, a household maintained by a family *q.v.* and any unrelated persons (unrelated family members, other individuals, or both) who may be residing there. The number of family households is equal to the number of families. The count of family household members differs from the count of family members; however, in that the family household members include all persons living in the household, family members include only the householder and his or her relatives.

FAMILY INSTITUTION The normative ways in which a small kinship group performs the key function of nurturant of the newborn.

FAMILY INTERACTION METHOD In sociological research, a procedure for studying family *q.v.* behavior by observing its interaction in a structured laboratory situation.

FAMILY METHOD A research strategy in behavior genetics *q.v.* in which the frequency of a trait *q.v.* or of abnormal behavior *q.v.* is determined in relatives who have varying percentages of shared genetic *q.v.* background.

FAMILY PLANNING 1. Methods used to anticipate children, when they shall be born and the number to be born. 2. A method of birth control *q.v.*

FAMILY PRACTICE 1. A specialty of medical practice that is concerned with the overall health of a person or his or her family. 2. An intensification of general practice *q.v.* The physician trained in ~ gives basic, comprehensive medical care to all members of the family *q.v.* on a continuing basis and serves as a "gatekeeper" for insurance coverage.

FAMILY RESEMBLANCE CRITERIA In genetics, the set of criteria *q.v.* used in determining whether an object or trait *q.v.* falls into a given category.

FAMILY RESEMBLANCE STRUCTURE In genetics and sociology, an overlap of features among members of a group in such a way that none of the members has all of the features, but all members possess some of the features.

FAMILY STRUCTURE How a family is composed.

FAMILY STUDIES 1. Studies that chronicle the rate of particular forms of abnormal behavior in many generations of a family *q.v.* to test theories of genetic *q.v.* transmission. 2. Studies that determine the extent to which family members resemble one another on a trait *q.v.* Family studies are conducted to determine whether a trait might be inheritable.

FAMILY THERAPY 1. A form of group therapy *q.v.* in which members of a family *q.v.* are helped to relate better to one another. 2. Treatment of the entire family that focuses on the relationships and communication among family members rather than on the pathology *q.v.* of one person.

FAMWICH MOM 1. Women who spend approximately 18 years bringing up their children and another 19 years taking care of their mothers in later years. 2. Women who are sandwiched between their child care and their mothers' care.

FANG The front teeth of poisonous snakes through which the venom *q.v.* is injected into the wound.

FANTASY (PHANTASY) 1. Imagined happenings. 2. The expression or working through some psychological *q.v.* problem in the imagination. 3. Daydreaming. 4. An ego defense mechanism *q.v.* by means of which the person escapes reality and gratifies his or her desires in make-believe achievements. 5. Defense mechanisms *q.v.* 6. The process of adjusting to threatening situations by dreaming of imaginary achievements or by thinking of things that might have been. 7. A more or less pleasant mental image unrestrained by the realities of the external world.

FANTASY PHONE MATE Persons who engage in sexually stimulating talk on the telephone to a customer for a fee.

FANTASY TYPOLOGIES In psychology, ways of categorizing sexual fantasies *q.v.*, such as fantasizer as recipient, or sexual object as recipient.

FAO An acronym for Food and Agriculture Organization of the United States.

FAOTA An acronym for Fellow of the American Occupation Therapy Association.

FAPHA An acronym for Fellow of the American Public Health Association *q.v.*

FARSIGHTEDNESS Hyperopia *q.v.*

FARTLEK In physical fitness training, a form of training also known as speed play, which alternates fast and slow running over terrain for 3 or 4 miles.

FAS An acronym for fetal alcohol syndrome *q.v.*

FASCIA 1. In anatomy, a sheet or band of fibrous tissue, which covers muscles and various organs of the body. 2. ~ lies deep under the skin and forms an outer layer for the muscles and some organs of the body. 3. A sheet of connective tissue *q.v.*

FASCICULUS In anatomy, little bundle.

FASHA An acronym for Fellow of the American School Health Association *q.v.*

FAST FOODS 1. Convenience of foods. 2. Foods features in a variety of restaurants that are prepared in advance or quickly after an order is placed. ~ are sometimes erroneously described as junk food.

FASTIGIUM In pathology, the climax of a disease.

FASTING Choosing not to eat anything or a particular food item for a specified period of time. Frequently associated with religious observances or political protests. Unsupervised fasting to reduce weight can result in death.

FAST-TWITCH FIBERS 1. A type of muscle cells especially suited for anaerobic *q.v.* activities. 2. A type of muscle fiber used for sudden, powerful bursts of activity.

FAT 1. A major class of energy-rich food. 2. Adipose tissue *q.v.*

FAT-FREE MASS Lean body mass *q.v.*

FATHER OF HYGIENE Roger of Salerno.

FATHER OF MEDICINE Hippocrates of Cos.

FATIGUE 1. The desire or need to rest. 2. A condition characterized by continuous discomfort and decreased work output due to overexertion.

FATIGUE FRACTURE A fracture *q.v.* in which the bone breaks because of repeated stress that can no longer be tolerated by that particular bone. ~ can involve bones of the foot or leg.

FAT MASS The quantity of body fat *q.v.*, usually expressed as a percentage of total body mass *q.v.*

FATS 1. Lipids *q.v.* of both plant and animal origin. ~ consist of fatty acids *q.v.* of varying carbon chain lengths. Fats are important in the diet as (a) a concentrated source of energy, containing about twice as many calories *q.v.* as carbohydrates *q.v.* or proteins *q.v.* per gram; (b) a vehicle for satiety value of foods; (c) a source of linoleic acid *q.v.*; and (d) a vehicle for the fat-soluble vitamins *q.v.* 2. Mixture of glycerides *q.v.*, esters *q.v.*, glycerol *q.v.*, and fatty acids. 3. Organic compounds containing carbon, hydrogen, and oxygen. The proportion of oxygen to carbon is considerably less in fats than it is in carbohydrates. Fats in the liquid state are called oils.

FAT-SOLUBLE VITAMINS The group of vitamins *q.v.* identified as A, D, E, and K and are soluble in animal fats *q.v.* cf: water-soluble vitamins.

FATTY ACIDS 1. Short- and long-chain carbon substances that make up fats *q.v.* Short-chain ~ are liquid at room temperature, whereas whole long-chain ~ are solid at room temperature. Solid ~ are called saturated ~ *q.v.* because their carbon atoms contain all of the hydrogen possible. Liquid ~ are called unsaturated ~ *q.v.* because their carbon atoms lack two or more hydrogen atoms. Generally, fats from animal sources are saturated and high in cholesterol *q.v.* while vegetable fats are generally unsaturated and cholesterol free. 2. Organic acids composed of carbon, hydrogen, and oxygen that combine with glycerol *q.v.* to form fat. 3. Any acid derived from fats by hydrolysis.

FATTY LIVER The result of the liver metabolizing alcohol *q.v.* instead of fat. When alcohol is oxidized by the liver, there is a release of excess amounts of hydrogen and the cells make use of this hydrogen instead of the fatty acids *q.v.* As the fat is not oxidized, it is deposited in the liver. Once excess amounts of alcohol are eliminated from the diet, the fatty liver disappears.

FAUCES The passageway between the mouth and the pharynx *q.v.*

FAULT TREE In safety epidemiology, used after an accident occurs. Traces back to find what was the initial cause or causes of an accident.

FAUNA In biology or zoology, the animal life in a given geographic area. cf: flora.

FAVUS A disease caused by infection of hair follicles with *Trichophyton schoenleini.*

FDA The United States Food and Drug Administration, a branch of the US Department of Health and Human Services assigned with the task of protecting consumers against the dangers of contaminated food, hazardous drugs, medical devices, and cosmetics.

FEAR 1. One of the most powerful emotions *q.v.* May follow or accompany feelings associated with the inability to cope or to overcome a threatening situation. Most fears are irrational. One's reaction may be either to fight or to flee. 2. The conditioned form of a pain reaction. Associated with anxiety *q.v.* 3. An emotional response to an external threat, consists of subjective apprehension and physiological *q.v.* changes, including increased pulse and respiration rate, which prepare the body for a fight or flight response.

FEAR DRIVE According to Mowrer and Miller, an unpleasant internal state that impels avoidance. The need to reduce a fear drive can form the basis for new learning.

FEAR OF SUCCESS The tendency for a person to worry about being more successful than others because it may jeopardize his or her interpersonal relations.

FEAR RESPONSE According to Mowrer and Miller, a response to a threatening or noxious situation that is covert and unobservable but which is assumed to function as a stimulus to produce measurable physiological *q.v.* changes in the body and observable overt behavior. cf: fear drive.

FEAR SURVEY SCHEDULE II (FSS II) Descriptions of 51 stressful situations to which respondents relate their emotional response.

FEASIBILITY A measure of the workability of a plan or proposal.

FEATURE DETECTORS Neurons *q.v.* that respond to specific aspects of a stimulus such as movement or color.

FEBRILE 1. Feverish. 2. Having a fever. 3. Relating to fever.

FECAL Pertaining to feces *q.v.*

FECAL–ORAL ROUTE Leaving one's body with the feces *q.v.* and later entering another person's body by way of the mouth as in contaminated water or food.

FECES 1. Solid human waste. 2. Body waste as excreted from the colon and rectum *q.v.*

FECHNER'S LAW The strength of a sensation is proportional to the logarithm *q.v.* of physical stimulus intensity.

FECUNDITY The ability to produce offspring especially in a rapid manner and in large numbers.

FEDERAL ROLE The role of the federal government in education, health, and other state and local programs.

FEDERAL TRADE COMMISSION A federal agency that has authority to prevent the dissemination of false or misleading advertising of foods, cosmetics, and other health products.

FEDERATION Pertaining to a loosely knit league of affiliated national and international unions or associations.

FEEBLE MINDEDNESS 1. Mental deficiency. 2. The condition of a person with an intelligence quotient *q.v.* of 70 or below.

FEEDBACK 1. Verbal or nonverbal responses of a learner that may be interpreted by the teacher and used to guide learning. ~ may also originate with the teacher in verbal or nonverbal form, providing the learner with knowledge of what the teacher is aware of and understands the learner's coded message. 2. Stimuli provided by behavior. 3. The final step in the communication process that involves determining whether the receiver has received the intended message and produced the intended response. 4. The interpersonal communication situation, the decoder/destination's reaction to a message. cf: feedback system.

FEEDBACK CONTROL Control that takes place after some unit of work has been completed.

FEEDBACK SYSTEM 1. A system in which some action produces a consequence affecting action. The ~ consists of either (a) negative feedback, which tends to stop or reverse action, or (b) positive feedback, which tends to strengthen action. 2. The return of some output, or substance, in the body to the place of its origin by the system that receives it. ct: feedback.

FEE-FOR-SERVICE Payment of health or medical services based on the service rendered rather than through a salary or capitation *q.v.* policy.

FEELING 1. A mild form of an emotion *q.v.* 2. The pleasure and pain dimension of emotion or bodily sensation or function.

FELLATIO 1. Oral stimulation of the male's genitals *q.v.* 2. The act of taking the penis *q.v.* into the mouth and sucking it for erotic purposes.

FELLOWSHIPS Grants in aid and trainee stipends to graduate students. Usually excludes funds for which services to the institution must be rendered, such as payments for teaching or student loans.

FELON 1. A severe infection of the soft tissue of the end of a finger. 2. Whitlow. 3 One who has been convicted of a felony.

FELONY In law, a crime that is serious, such as robbery, and may result in confinement upon conviction. cf: misdemeanor.

FELT NEEDS In psychology, interests and concerns arising from intense desires to know about something or how to solve some problem.

FEMA An acronym for Federal Emergency Management Agency.

FEMALE 1. A gender *q.v.* designation distinguished by its anatomical structures, biochemistry, and the ability to conceive and procreate *q.v.* 2. A woman or girl child. ct: male.

FEMALE ABOVE A coital *q.v.* position in which the female *q.v.* is positioned above the male *q.v.* partner.

FEMALE EJACULATION The emission of fluid described as "watered down fat-free milk" from Skene's glands *q.v.*

located just inside the urethral opening that occurs in about 10% of women. Conversely, ~ is thought to be primarily urine *q.v.* ct: Grafenberg spot.

FEMININITY 1. A person's self-concept *q.v.* about possessed sexuality *q.v.* 2. Usually possessed by a female. 3. ~ is biologically *q.v.* and culturally *q.v.* influenced. 4. Being a woman. 5. Behavioral expressions traditionally observed in females. 6. Ladylike appearance and behavior. ct: masculinity.

FEMINISM The doctrine that asserts that women deserve equal rights with men in all spheres.

FEMORAL ARTERY 1. The principal artery of the thigh. 2. A continuation of the external iliac artery *q.v.* The ~ supplies blood to the lower abdominal wall, the external genitalia *q.v.*, and the lower extremities.

FEMORAL CONDYLE The rounded articular surface at the extremity of the femur *q.v.*

FEMORAL NERVE A major peripheral nerve *q.v.* originating in the lumbosacral plexus *q.v.*

FEMORAL VEIN 1. A continuation of the popliteal vein *q.v.* that becomes the external iliac vein *q.v.* 2. The major vein draining the leg.

FEMUR 1. The bone of the thigh. The ~ is the largest bone of the body. 2. The bone that extends from the pelvis to the knee. 3. The thigh bone.

FENESTRUM An opening on the inner wall of the middle ear leading to the cochlea *q.v.*

FENFLURAMINE 1. An appetite suppressant. 2. Pondimin is a brand name.

FENTANYL 1. A potent synthetic analgesic *q.v.* 2. Sublimaze is a brand name.

FERMENTATION 1. The action of yeast on sugar resulting in the formation of alcohol *q.v.* and carbon dioxide. 2. The chemical process whereby plant products are converted into alcohol by the action of yeast cells on carbohydrates *q.v.* 3. The conversion of sugar to ethyl alcohol *q.v.* by the action of yeast. 4. A respiratory process in which hydrogen released in glycolysis *q.v.* is recombined with pyruvic acid *q.v.* to form alcohol, lactic acid, and other products. 5. A controlled process by which a chemical is transformed by means of metabolic *q.v.* action of a microorganism to a predominant end product. A restrictive definition is often applied that limits the process to that which occurs in the absence of oxygen, the anaerobic *q.v.* production of alcohol by yeast.

FERRITIN The form in which iron is stored in the body. ~ is an iron–protein complex made up of iron and the protein apoferritin *q.v.*

FERTILE Able to reproduce.

FERTILE PERIOD The period each month during which a woman's ovum *q.v.* has been released and can most readily be fertilized *q.v.* by a sperm *q.v.*

FERTILITY 1. The capacity to conceive *q.v.* or to induce conception. 2. The capacity to become pregnant *q.v.* as in the case of the female or to impregnate as in the case of the male. 3. The ability to produce offspring. 4. The ability to reproduce. 5. The ability to cause or become pregnant. ct: sterility.

FERTILITY AWARENESS Contraception methods *q.v.* that attempt to pinpoint the time of ovulation *q.v.* cf: rhythm method; basal body temperature method; mucous method.

FERTILITY RATE The number of births per year per 1000 women aged 15–44 years. ct: total fertility rate.

FERTILIZATION 1. Conception *q.v.* 2. The union of a sperm *q.v.* with an egg. 3. The fusion of a sperm cell and the ovum *q.v.* 4. The union of two gametes *q.v.* to form a zygote *q.v.*

FERTILIZED OVUM 1. Fertilized egg. 2. A cell formed by the union of a sperm *q.v.* and an ovum *q.v.* from which a new human (or other organism) eventually develops.

FERTILIZERS In agriculture, materials added to the soil to provide elements essential to plant growth or to bring about a balance in the ratio of nutrients in the soil.

FESTINATING GAIT Uncoordinated, hurried, and uncertain walk in paralysis agitans *q.v.*

FETAL ALCOHOL SYNDROME (FAS) 1. Abnormalities present in neonates *q.v.* resulting from the mother drinking alcohol *q.v.* during pregnancy *q.v.* 2. A common pattern of birth defects and mental retardation that occurs among some children born of alcoholic *q.v.* or alcohol-consuming mothers, and manifest by central nervous system *q.v.* dysfunction, growth deficiency, facial abnormalities, and other major and minor malformations. ct: teratogen.

FETAL CARBOXYHEMOGLOBIN Hemoglobin *q.v.* within the fetal *q.v.* circulation that is carrying carbon monoxide *q.v.*

FETAL DEATH CERTIFICATE The certificate required when a baby is born dead: a stillbirth. Most states in the United States regard stillbirths of less than 20 weeks of pregnancy *q.v.* as abortions *q.v.* and may or may not require registration of a birth.

FETAL HYDROPS A form of dropsy *q.v.* in the newborn caused by incompatibility between an Rh-negative *q.v.* mother and her Rh-positive *q.v.* fetus during pregnancy *q.v.*

FETAL MEMBRANES Two sacs of tissue, the inner amnion *q.v.* and the outer amnion *q.v.*, that encloses the developing fetus *q.v.* in the uterus *q.v.*

FETAL STAGE 1. The stage of human development from the end of the 8th week of gestation *q.v.* until the time of birth. 2. Also interpreted as from the 12th week of pregnancy *q.v.* to birth. 3. Beginning at the end of the first trimester *q.v.* cf: embryonic stage.

FETISH An inanimate object or objects upon which a person becomes fixated, and which becomes a necessary part of achieving sexual fulfillment.

FETISHISM 1. A condition in which sexual impulses become fixated on a symbol. The symbol may be used in conjunction with masturbation *q.v.* or interpersonal sexual activity. 2. Sexual arousal and gratification stimulated by an inanimate object or nonsexual body part. 3. A sexual variance *q.v.* in which sexual gratification is achieved by means of an object, such as an article of clothing, that bears sexual symbolism for the person. cf: partialism.

FETOSCOPY 1. A method used for the detection of fetal *q.v.* abnormalities in which the fetus can actually be seen. ~ consists of inserting a needle containing a fiber optic lens into the amniotic sac *q.v.* 2. The insertion of a viewing instrument into the uterus *q.v.* to observe the fetus.

FETUS 1. The fertilized egg from the end of the embryonic period *q.v.* through birth. 2. The human organism from 8 weeks after conception until birth. 3. The developing organism in the uterus during the second and third trimesters of pregnancy. 4. Prenatal stage of a viviparous animal between the embryonic stage and the time of birth. In humans, the final 7 months before birth. cf: neonate; embryo.

FEVER An elevation of body temperature above normal. Normal human body temperature is designated as 98.6° F or 37° C.

F FACTOR Sex factor in male bacteria; capable of being transmitted across a conjugation bridge.

F^+ FACTOR 1. Fertility *q.v.* 2. The sex factor in male bacteria that is transmitted to F^- bacteria during conjugation *q.v.*

FIBER (DIETARY) 1. Roughage. 2. The parts of plant foods that cannot be readily digested by the body. 3. Cellulose *q.v.* 4. A nonnutritive substance in food that combines with water to form stools and to aid in digestion. 5. In anatomy, a threadlike structure.

FIBRILLATION 1. Spontaneous contraction of individual muscle fibers *q.v.* no longer under control of a motor nerve *q.v.* 2. Highly irregular heart beat.

FIBRIN 1. A sticky substance that combines with blood cells to form a clot in the healing of a wound. 2. Insoluble protein *q.v.* in clotted blood.

FIBRINADINOMA A benign tumor *q.v.* that is firm, round, and somewhat movable.

FIBRINOGEN 1. The protein *q.v.* that enables the blood to clot. 2. Soluble blood protein that is converted to insoluble fibrin *q.v.* during blood clotting.

FIBRINOLYSIS The activity of the fibrinolysin system that removes small clots from tiny blood vessels throughout the body.

FIBRINOPEPTIDE A A protein *q.v.* High levels in the blood may indicate the presence of cancer.

FIBROBLASTS Connective tissue *q.v.* cells that synthesize interstitial *q.v.* fibers *q.v.* and gels.

FIBROCYSTS Old fibroblasts *q.v.*

FIBROCYSTIC BREAST DISEASE 1. A benign *q.v.* but painful disorder characterized by lumps in the breasts. Consumption of caffeine may be related to this condition. 2. Fibrocystic disease *q.v.* cf: fibrocysts.

FIBROCYSTIC DISEASE 1. A benign *q.v.* breast condition consisting of an overgrowth of fibrous tissue often combined with formation of cysts *q.v.* 2. Fibrocystic breast disease *q.v.*

FIBROMA A benign *q.v.* type of growth composed of fibrous tissue *q.v.*

FIBROSIS The formation of fibrous tissue *q.v.* or scar. ~ is usually a reparative or reactive process.

FIBROUS TISSUE A scar.

FIBULA 1. The smaller and less important of the two bones of the lower leg. 2. The ~ extends from just below the knee to form the lateral wall of the ankle joint. ct: tibia.

FICS An acronym for Fellow of the International College of Surgeons.

FIDUCIARY Person or persons responsible for administering a retirement plan.

FIEDLER'S LEADERSHIP THEORY A perspective that considers the interaction between a leader's personal style and the leadership situation. There are two kinds of leaders: (a) task-oriented leaders who are most effective when a situation clearly favors success or failure and (b) relationship-oriented leaders who are successful when a situation is moderately favorable.

FIELD CAPACITY Field percentage *q.v.*

FIELD EXPERIMENT The experimental method *q.v.* applied to the ongoing activities of people in their natural environment.

FIELDNOTES In research, the observer's records of what has been observed.

FIELD OF FORCES In psychology, the various forces that act upon a person at any particular time.

FIELD PERCENTAGE The normal upper limit of the available capillary water. cf: field capacity.

FIELD RESEARCH Scientific study in which attempts are made to understand events that occur naturally. ct: laboratory research.

FIELD-REVIEW METHOD 1. Performance appraisal. 2. Personnel specialists provide ratings of employees from discussion with supervisors.

FIELD STUDY 1. A form of observation in which a researcher studies people in natural situations. 2. Naturalistic studies. cf: observational study.

FIELD THEORY 1. Lewin's theory that the way in which people represent their world psychologically *q.v.* is the primary determinant of their actions, and that social behavior is a function of both intrapersonal factors and the environment. 2. Structured organisms–environment field theory of behavior *q.v.*

FIELD TRIP In education, may be used to broaden the learner's view of the community and the world in general. ~s should be planned by the teachers and learners together with an opportunity for students to share their experiences upon return to class. A ~ is basically a learner observational method *q.v.*

FIELDWORK EXPERIENCE In education, a learner-centered method *q.v.* in which students spend part of their day working in a health-related community agency. The experience should result in students developing an appreciation for the health occupation, increasing their knowledge of the health problems, and the ways they are handled by the agency. Most importantly, students provide a community service by contributing to the functions of the community health agency.

FIFRA An acronym for Federal Insecticide, Fungicide, and Rhodenticide Act of 1972.

FIGHT/FLIGHT REACTION Physiological *q.v.* responses in which hormones *q.v.* cause an increase in heart rate, breathing rate, blood pressure, and perspiration. cf: flight reaction; fight reaction.

FIGHT REACTION A classification of defense mechanisms *q.v.* manifest in aggressive behavior *q.v.* ct: flight reaction.

FIGURAL AFTEREFFECT An apparent distortion of a figure following prolonged inspection.

FIGURE–GROUND ORGANIZATION 1. The separation of the visual field into a part that stands out against the rest of the field. 2. Figure–ground relationship. 3. Figure discrimination.

FILARIASIS A chronic disease caused by a filariae, a nematode *q.v.*

FILIAL 1. In Mendelian inheritance, designating a generation or generations successive to the parental generation. 2. The F_1 and F_2 generations.

FILIAL PIETY An unusual love and honor for parents.

FILM (SCREEN) In health screening, a mammography *q.v.* or X-ray.

FILTH-BORNE DISEASE Disease spread by germs *q.v.* transmitted through excretions.

FILTRATION 1. Fluid pressure in the blood vessels generated by the pumping action of the heart. 2. Hydrostatic pressure *q.v.*

FIMBRIA 1. The fingerlike upper end of the fallopian *q.v.* tubes that pick up the egg expelled from the ovary *q.v.* 2. The fibers *q.v.* on the fallopian tubes that pick up the egg expelled from the ovary 3. The ovarian end of the fallopian tube. 4. Fringe. The fimbria wave ova *q.v.* from the ovaries into the fallopian tubes.

FIMBRIAL HOOD An experimental form of contraception *q.v.* that operates by covering the fimbriae *q.v.* of the fallopian tubes *q.v.* thereby preventing eggs from entering them.

FINAL COMMON PATH In reflex physiology *q.v.*, the motor pathway upon which many neural pathways converge.

FINAL OFFER ARBITRATION In labor relations, each party submits its final proposal or offer and the arbitrator *q.v.* selects one of them.

FINGER OSCILLATION TEST A neuropsychological *q.v.* test used to assess possible impairment to the right or left side of the brain.

FIREMAN'S DRAG Drag *q.v.*

FIRST AID The immediate and temporary care given to the victim of an accident or sudden illness until qualified medical help is available.

FIRST-ORDER CHANGE In sociology, change from one behavior to another that occurs from within a group.

FIRST PROFESSIONAL CERTIFICATE An award that requires completion of an organized program of study designed for individuals who had completed the first professional degree. This usually involves 4 years of undergraduate college work.

FIRST-RANK SYMPTOM In schizophrenia *q.v.*, specific delusions *q.v.* and hallucinations *q.v.* as particularly for its more exact diagnosis *q.v.*

FIRST READING In politics, to read for the first time of three times, the bill or its title for consideration by the legislature.

FISCAL NOTE In politics, a note that states the estimated amount of increase or decrease in revenue or expenditures and the present and future fiscal implications of pending legislation.

FISCAL YEAR In politics, an accounting period of 1 year. Also used with most large businesses and industries.

FISHBEIN BEHAVIOR INTERACTION THEORY In psychology, attempts to bring cognitive *q.v.* theory and connectionist theory *q.v.* into focus. According to this theory, a person's behavior results from beliefs, values, attitudes, and desires. A person's beliefs determine attitude, which, in turn, determine behavior. People acquire beliefs from the many experiences they encounter incidentally, directly, or through observation of others (modeling). ~ has essentially four patterns: (a) information establishes beliefs, (b) those beliefs establish attitudes, (c) those attitudes establish intention to behave, and (d) that intention to behave results ultimately in the specific behavior. cf: Fishbein model.

FISHBEIN MODEL A model of attitude activation enabling one to make increasingly accurate predictions of behavior. cf: Fishbein behavior interaction theory.

FISH SCALE ANALOGY In research, knowing judgments made by each person in sequence extending from the researcher to laypersons. Each, being less expert than the previous person, looks at the evidence presented by previous judges and determines whether to accept their judgment.

FISSION 1. In physics, disintegration or splitting of an atom. 2. In biology, the form of reproduction found in lower plants and animals, e.g., bacteria *q.v.* 3. The division of a unicellular organism into two equal daughter cells. ct: fusion.

FISSURE 1. A major groove in the surface of the brain, teeth, or other organ. 2. Groove.

FISTULA An abnormal passage from an abscess *q.v.*, cavity, or organ to another.

FITNESS 1. A level of total health that makes it possible for a person to function effectively and efficiently. 2. The degree of adaptation of an organism of some specified genotype *q.v.* 3. In genetics, the number of offspring left by an individual as compared with the average of the population or compared to individuals of a different genotype. 4. A measure of a person's success in transmitting genes *q.v.* to the next generation. 5. Reproductive success.

FIVE DIMENSIONS OF HEALTH The major areas of health in which specific strengths or limitations are found: physical, emotional, social, intellectual, and spiritual. ct: three dimensions of health; dimensions of health.

FIVE TO SEVEN TRANSITION The shift from associative to cognitive *q.v.* responding assumed to take place for many children at about 5–7 years, in conjunction with the emergence of a generalized capacity for inhibition *q.v.*

FIXATED To become stationary.

FIXATION 1. Stereotyped response developed as a consequence of conflict *q.v.* 2. In psychoanalytic theory, an attachment of the libido *q.v.* to some particular stage of psychosocial *q.v.* development. 3. The arrest of psychosexual *q.v.* development at a particular stage through too much or too little gratification at that stage. 4. A defense mechanism *q.v.* 5. An exaggerated attachment to some person or the arresting of emotional development at a childhood or adolescent level. 6. Diffusion *q.v.* 7. Emotional immaturity *q.v.*

FIXATION OF COMPLEMENT TEST The entering of a complement into combination with an antigen/antibody *q.v.* aggregate so that it is fixed and not available for subsequent reaction. ~ is the basis of the Wassermann *q.v.*, Reiter protein *q.v.*, and other serologic *q.v.* tests.

FIXED-ACTION PATTERNS In ethology, a term used to describe stereotyped, species-specific behaviors set into motion by genetically *q.v.* preprogrammed releasing stimuli *q.v.*

FIXED ASSETS TURNOVER In management, an activity ratio that indicates the appropriateness of the amount of funds invested in plant and equipment relative to the level of sales.

$$\text{FAT} = \frac{\text{sales}}{\text{fixed assets}}$$

FIXED COSTS In management, expenses incurred by an organization regardless of the number of products produced.

FIXED INTERVAL SCHEDULE In psychology, reinforcement administered in accordance with a definite interval of time. cf: fixed-ratio schedule.

FIXED MODEL In research, a form of analysis of variance in which the treatments used are exactly those to which the researcher expects to generalize rather than being representative of them.

FIXED POSITION LAYOUT In industry, a layout pattern that, because of the weight and bulk of the product being produced, has workers, tools, and materials rotating around a stationary product.

FIXED-RATIO COMBINATION PRODUCT In pharmacology, a drug preparation containing a combination of two or more drug ingredients intended to relieve multiple symptoms.

FIXED-RATIO SCHEDULE The process of applying reinforcement after a fixed number of responses. cf: fixed interval schedule; schedule of reinforcement.

FLACCID 1. Nonerect. 2. The state of erectile *q.v.* tissue when vasocongestion *q.v.* is not occurring. 3. The unerected state of the penis *q.v.* 4. A state of limpness. 5. Soft, limp.

FLAGELLUM 1. A whiplike organ produced by some cells that makes motion possible. 2. An organelle *q.v.* of locomotion in certain cells. 3. Locomotor structures in flagellate protozoa.

FLAIL CHEST A condition of the chest wall following an injury characterized by a free segment that moves paradoxically when the person breathes. ~ is caused by fractures *q.v.* of several ribs in two or more places each.

FLAIL SEGMENT That portion of the chest wall in a flail chest *q.v.* injury lying between the rib fractures *q.v.* and moving paradoxically with respiration.

FLASH A short, intense, generalized sensation of total well-being experienced soon after intravenous injection of cocaine *q.v.* or methamphetamine *q.v.*, the so-called rush reaction.

FLASHBACK 1. The unpredictable phenomenon of undergoing again the effects of LSD *q.v.* weeks or even months after the last use of the drug. 2. Undesirable recurrence of a drug's effects with no recent consumption of drugs to explain changes in consciousness and experience of illusions *q.v.* and hallucinations *q.v.* 3. The unexpected return, without having taken the drug, of the subjective sensations from a hallucinogenic *q.v.* drug experience.

FLASHER 1. Slang for exhibitionist *q.v.* 2. A person who achieves sexual pleasure from exposing his or her genitals *q.v.* The term is usually associated with male exhibitionists.

FLAT EFFECT In psychology, a deviation in emotional response wherein virtually no emotion is expressed whatever the stimuli. Emotional expressiveness is blunted, or a lack of expression and muscle tone is noted in the face.

FLAT ORGANIZATIONAL CHART An organizational chart that is characterized by few levels and relatively large spans of management.

FLAT SCHEDULE In insurance policies, everyone in a group is insured for the same benefits regardless of salary or position.

FLATULENCE Excessive gassiness in the gastrointestinal tract *q.v.*

FLATUS Flatulence *q.v.*

FLAVOR ENHANCERS Artificial substances that are added to food to change one's perception of its flavor.

FLEABAGS 1. Slang for elderly bar girls. 2. Anything old, e.g., fleabag hotel.

FLEXIBILITY 1. The range through which a joint can move. 2. The ability of joints to function through their intended range of motion. 3. A willingness to change one's mind. 4. The ability to compromise.

FLEXIBLE HOURS In management, a practice whereby workers arrange their starting and stopping times to suit their personal requirements provided that they work a core time each day.

FLEXIBLE RETIREMENT An employment option allowing a person to retire at an age of his or her choice. cf: retirement; mandatory retirement.

FLEXIBLE SPLINT Rigid splint *q.v.*

FLEXION The movement of a body joint such that the angle about the center of rotation or fulcrum decreases. ct: extension.

FLEXITIME (FLEXTIME) Flexible hours arrangement where employees have several options for starting and stopping time. cf: flexible hours.

FLEXNER REPORT An in-depth study of medical education in the United States and Canada, directed by Abraham Flexner and funded by the Carnegie Foundation. Published in 1910.

FLIGHT INTO ILLNESS Escaping from some unpleasant situation or problem by simulating the symptoms of some organic condition and being convinced of one's illness.

FLIGHT OF IDEAS 1. The rapid succession of ideas without logical association or continuity. 2. A symptom of mania *q.v.* that involves a rapid shift from one subject to another in conversation with only superficial associative connections.

FLIGHT REACTION A classification of defense mechanisms *q.v.* manifest in withdrawal or passive behavior. ct: fight reaction.

FLIMMER In biology, fine projections from the side of the tinsel, fibrillose, or flimmer-geisel flagellum *q.v.*

FLOCCULATION The coagulation of finely divided particles or colloidal particles into larger particles that precipitate.

FLOODING 1. In psychology, experiencing something so often that a person is no longer aroused by it. ~ is a technique used to help a person to become more comfortable with sexual terminology. 2. A form of behavior therapy *q.v.* based on classical conditioning *q.v.*, used to extinguish a fear. cf: flooding therapy.

FLOODING THERAPY A behavior therapy *q.v.* procedure in which a fearful person exposes himself or herself to what is frightening, in reality or in the imagination, for extended periods of time without opportunity for escape. cf: flooding.

FLOOR In politics, that portion of the assembly chamber reserved for members and officers of the legislature and other persons granted the privilege of the ~.

FLORA In biology or botany, the plant life in any given geographic area. ct: fauna.

FLOW CYTOMETRY In medicine, the standard immunological laboratory tests to examine lymphocytes *q.v.* and measure cell-type ratios.

FLOWMETER A device to measure the rate of flow of any agent introduced into a person, such as oxygen or intravenous fluid.

FLOWRATE The rate at which oxygen flows from a cylinder. The ~ can be adjusted by a ~ control.

FLU Influenza *q.v.*

FLUCTUATION TEST A test designed to measure the frequency of spontaneous mutations *q.v.*

FLUENCY DISABILITIES Speech problems such as repetition, prolongation of sound, hesitations, and impediments in speech flow.

FLUID INTELLIGENCE The ability to deal with essentially new problems. cf: crystallized intelligence.

FLUORIDATION The addition of the chemical fluoride to water or other oral preparations for the purpose of preventing tooth decay. Usually, 1 part of fluoride to 1 million parts of water is used.

FLUOROCARBON 1. A gaseous chemical compound that contains fluorine *q.v.* 2. A group of gases that, when emitted into the atmosphere, may destroy the ozone layer *q.v.*

FLUOROSCOPE An instrument similar to an X-ray machine that is used to observe directly various structures of the body without taking a picture on film. cf: fluoroscopy.

FLUOROSCOPY The act of examining by means of a fluorescent screen. The use of a fluoroscope *q.v.*

FLUOROSIS (DENTAL) A mottled discoloration of the enamel of the teeth resulting from chronic ingestion (or exposure to) of excessive quantities of fluorine *q.v.*

FLUPHENAZINE 1. An antipsychotic drug *q.v.* 2. Permitil and Prolixin are commercial preparations.

FLURAZEPAM A nonbarbiturate *q.v.* sedative-hypnotic *q.v.* and a minor tranquilizer *q.v.* prescribed under the brand name of Dalmane. The only benzodiazepine *q.v.* promoted as a hypnotic *q.v.*

FLY AGARIC MUSHROOM Amanita muscaria *q.v.*, a hallucinogen *q.v.* mushroom that is also considered toxic *q.v.*

FLY ASH Particulates *q.v.* of soot and dust in the air.

FOAMS 1. Contraceptive foams. 2. Spermicidal *q.v.* chemicals.

FOCAL LESION A lesion *q.v.* in a particular area of the body.

FOCAL MOTOR SEIZURE A seizure *q.v.* that emanates from a particular area of the brain that governs or controls various motor functions. cf: focal seizures.

FOCAL SEIZURES Seizures *q.v.* that affect specific motor, sensory, and psychomotor functions. cf: focal motor seizures.

FOCUSED INTERVIEW Interview in which the respondent is allowed to set the initial course but increasingly focuses on the researcher's agenda as the interview progresses.

FOCUS GROUP In research, a panel, selected to be representative of a population, interviewed on a topic of interest. Probes determine the popularity of various comments and points of view and the depth of feeling toward them. There may also be trials of material to determine how the panel's reactions could be changed.

FOLACIN 1. A member of the vitamin B complex group *q.v.* ~ is necessary for cell growth and reproduction. A deficiency can result in megaloblastic anemia *q.v.* ~ is a water-soluble vitamin *q.v.* 2. Folic acid is used in the treatment of nutritional anemia *q.v.*

FOLIC ACID Folacin *q.v.*

FOLIE A` DUEX A psychotic *q.v.* interpersonal relationship involving two people who become psychotic with similar symptomatology *q.v.*

FOLK MEDICINE Treatment of disease traditionally practiced by lay persons within a cultural or subcultural context.

FOLLICLE 1. In anatomy, a small sac or vesicle *q.v.* 2. The structure in the ovary *q.v.* that nurtures the ripening ovum *q.v.* and from which the ovum is released into the oviduct *q.v.* 3. In botany, a dry fruit derived from a pistil *q.v.* and opening along only one side. 4. A structure produced by the ovaries that surrounds a mature ovum and when ripened releases the ovum from the ovary for fertilization *q.v.* 5. A deep, narrow pit containing the root of the hair ~. 6. A small sac or gland.

FOLLICLE-STIMULATING HORMONE 1. A hormone *q.v.* secreted by the anterior lobe of the pituitary gland *q.v.* ~ stimulates the primary graafian follicles *q.v.* to develop to the point of ovulation *q.v.* It also stimulates the development of the seminiferous tubules *q.v.* and maintains the process of spermatogenesis *q.v.* 2. In women, the hormone that stimulates a graafian follicle to mature into an ovum; in men, the hormone that stimulates the seminiferous tubules to produce sperm.

FOLLICULAR PHASE 1. Preovulatory phase *q.v.* 2. Proliferative phase. 3. That part of the menstrual cycle *q.v.* when hormonal signals prepare an ovum to ripen and the endometrium *q.v.* to receive it.

FOLLOW-THROUGH PROCEDURES Processes used to check on the outcome of a referral of a person for further diagnosis or treatment of a health problem or condition.

FOLLOW-UP STUDY A research procedure whereby individuals observed in an earlier investigation are contacted at a later time for further observation.

FOMENTATIONS Hot, wet dressings.

FOMITE 1. A contaminated *q.v.* object. 2. A nonliving carrier of disease.

FONTANELLE 1. A space between bones of the fetal *q.v.* or young skull covered with a membrane *q.v.* The ~ shows a rhythmic pulsation produced by the flow of blood in the vessels of the brain. 2. An infant's cranial soft spots. 3. Also fontanels. The openings between the bones of the skull in infants before the bones fuse together as the child matures. 4. Unossified areas in the infant's skull.

FOOD 1. Any substance that, when ingested, provides nutrients *q.v.* for the body. 2. Animal and vegetable products that are fit to eat. 3. A collection of nutrients in a form that is eaten, digested, and metabolized *q.v.* to provide energy, and chemicals that build and maintain the structure and regulates functions of the body. 4. An organic compound that can be respired to yield energy and that can be used in assimilation *q.v.*

FOOD ADDITIVE Any substance added intentionally or accidentally to foods that become an integral part of the food. cf: Food Additive Amendments.

FOOD ADDITIVE AMENDMENTS A series of amendments to the Pure Food and Drug Act designed to ensure safety of food additives.

FOOD AND AGRICULTURE ORGANIZATION OF THE UNITED NATIONS Established in 1945, the main purpose of ~ is to raise the levels of nutrition and the standards of living of the people of the United Nations' member states. Periodic estimates are made of the food available to each member nation in an attempt to improve food production and distribution. ~ is headquartered in Rome, Italy.

FOOD AND DRUG ADMINISTRATION (FDA) 1. The first consumer protection agency in the United States, established in 1931. It prevents some products from ever being sold; requires products to be redesigned, reformulated, relabeled, or packaged in a safer manner; initiates removal of products from the marketplace whenever new scientific data reveal risks that are unacceptable; enforces product standards and takes action against false and misleading labeling; and takes court action to seize illegal products, enjoins violative manufacturers, or prosecutes the manufacturer, packer, or shipper of adulterated or mislabeled products. 2. A branch of the United States Public Health Service. 3. The federal regulatory agency within the United States Department of Health and Human Services, with counterparts on the State level, responsible for assuring safety and effectiveness of drugs, protecting consumers against contaminants in food and against falsely represented, worthless, and dangerous drugs, medical devices, and cosmetics.

FOOD AND NUTRITION BOARD A member of the National Academy of Sciences, National Research Council. Established in 1940, this board serves as an advisory body to the federal government relative to food and nutrition. The ~ reviews and revises periodically the table of Recommended Daily/Dietary Allowances (RDAs) for specific nutrients *q.v.* essential for the maintenance of health for Americans.

FOOD CHAIN 1. A scheme or sequence of feeding relationships that link members of species of a biological *q.v.* community. 2. A group of plants or animals linked together by their food relationships.

FOOD–DRUG INTERACTION Interaction between certain foods eaten and drugs being taken, resulting in a speeding up or slowing down of drug effects, preventing effects, adversely affecting the body's use of food, and life-threatening conditions.

FOOD INTOXICATION Food poisoning *q.v.* cf: intoxication.

FOOD IRRADIATION The application of ionizing radiation, e.g., X-rays, or beta rays *q.v.*, to foods to kill organisms, inhibit growth, or delay ripening.

FOOD LABELING All food labels must contain the name of the product, the net contents or net weight, the name and place of business of the manufacturer, packer, or distributor. In addition, ingredients must be listed according to the largest amount by weight being listed first following in descending order of weight by the other ingredients. All additives must be listed on the label.

FOOD POISONING 1. A general term that encompasses foods that act as carriers of pathogenic *q.v.* organisms and substances that are inherently poisonous in humans. Obviously, food that are poisonous are not foods. Therefore, food poisoning is a term applied only to foods, in technical terms, that carry pathogens. 2. Food intoxication *q.v.*

FOOD PYRAMID Established by the US Department of Agriculture in 1993, the pyramid replaces the traditional reliance on the four food groups *q.v.* concept long advocated by nutritionists. It emphasizes a lowered intake of saturated fats and simple carbohydrates *q.v.* and an increased intake of vegetables and unsaturated fats and proteins.

FOOD SUPPLEMENTS 1. Commercially prepared nutrients *q.v.* for the purpose of adding nutrients to a person's diet. ~ consist mainly of vitamins *q.v.* and minerals *q.v.* 2. Chemical compounds that are taken in addition to those obtained through the diet, e.g., powdered protein, vitamins, and minerals.

FOODWAY 1. A stylized food habit that has evolved as an adaptation *q.v.* to the physical and social environments.

FOOT 1. In botany, in liverworts, mosses, and many vascular plants, the part of the embryo *q.v.* that remains in contact with gametophytic *q.v.* tissue, absorbing food from it and serving as an organ of attachment. 2. In anatomy, the lower end of the leg.

FOOTCANDLE 1. The amount of light on a surface that can be seen at a distance of one foot from a lightened standard candle. 2. A unit of light measurement.

FOOT-IN-THE-DOOR TECHNIQUE A technique of social influence in which a small favor is requested first in order to increase later compliance with a more extreme request.

FOOTLAMBERT The brightness of a surface resulting from illumination and reflection of the surface.

FOOTPRINT AREA The area of a tire that is in contact with the surface of the road.

FORAMEN 1. An opening. 2. A small perforation.

FORAMEN OVALE The opening between the atria *q.v.* of the fetal heart that normally closes shortly after birth.

FORCED-CHOICE ITEMS A format of a person inventory *q.v.* in which the response alternatives for each item are equated for social desirability *q.v.* cf: forced-choice method.

FORCED-CHOICE METHOD (PERFORMANCE APPRAISAL) Appraisers must choose the most descriptive statement for each category of performance rating. cf: forced-choice item.

FORCED COMPLIANCE EFFORT When a person is forced to speak publicly in a manner contrary to his or her own beliefs and there is a change in his or her views on a subject in the direction of the public action.

FORCED DISTRIBUTION (PERFORMANCE APPRAISAL) Allocation of employees' performance on the basis of their contribution on a scale of best to worst.

FORCIBLE RAPE Sexual intercourse achieved or attempted without the victim's consent and with the use of force or threat of harm. cf: rape.

FOREARM That part of the upper limb of the body between the elbow and the wrist.

FOREBRAIN 1. The bulk of the brain. 2. The foremost region of the brain, which includes the cerebral hemispheres *q.v.*; the rear portion of the brain, which includes the thalamus *q.v.* and the hypothalamus *q.v.*

FORECASTING A planning tool used to predict future environmental happenings that will influence the operation of an organization.

FORECASTS Giving a statement of what is likely to happen in the future based on considered judgment and analysis of data.

FORECLOSURE TYPE An adolescent who has unquestioningly endorsed the goals and values of his or her parents.

FORENSIC MEDICINE That branch of medical practice dealing with the legal questions surrounding death.

FORENSIC PSYCHIATRY (PSYCHOLOGY) That branch of psychiatry (or psychology) that deals with the legal questions raised by disordered behavior.

FOREPLAY In sexology, the preliminary stages of sexual arousal and intercourse in which partners usually stimulate each other in preparation for coitus *q.v.*

FORESKIN 1. A piece of skin that covers the head of the penis *q.v.* 2. Prepuce *q.v.* 3. The skin covering the tip of the penis or clitoris *q.v.*

FORGETTING A failure to recall materials previously learned. ct: retention.

FORMAL DISCIPLINE The theory (now discredited) that practice at learning strengthens the mind just as physical activity strengthens the muscles.

FORMAL EDUCATION Education *q.v.* received in schools separate from other aspects of learner's daily lives, by teachers trained for that purpose, with emphasis on verbal analysis and comprehension. ct: informal education.

FORMAL GROUP A group that exists within an organization by virtue of management decree to perform tasks that enhance the attainment of organizational objectives. cf: formal organization.

FORMAL OPERATIONS PERIOD 1. The developmental stage from 11 years onward characterized by the capacity to engage in abstract thinking. A point in development when egocentrism *q.v.* has been overcome. 2. Piaget's fourth major period of intellectual growth when children become capable of applying operational thinking to problems presented formally or propositionally. 3. Also, formal operation period, from about 11 or 12 years to late adolescence during which children develop the ability to think and reason about abstractions. As part of this process, they become capable of propositional logic, propositional reasoning, isolation of variables, and combinational reasoning. ct: concrete operational period.

FORMAL ORGANIZATION A group of people working together in some type of concerted or coordinated effort to attain objectives. cf: formal group.

FORMAL ORGANIZATIONAL COMMUNICATION Organizational communication that follows the lines of an organizational chart.

FORMAL STANDARD Within a particular culture *q.v.*, an idealization of how people should act sexually. cf: informal standard.

FORMAL STRUCTURE Relationships between organizational resources as outlined by management.

FORMAL THOUGHT DISORDER Disturbance in the normal thinking process in which the person shifts from one idea to other, unrelated ones, unaware of his or her own incoherence.

FORMATIVE EVALUATION 1. The use of tests to monitor progress or to facilitate remedial instruction. 2. Evaluation intended to provide information that can be used during the development of a project to guide progress toward its goals. cf: diagnostic evaluation. ct: summative evaluation.

FORM FETISH Sexual response to the shape and function of objects.

FORMICATION 1. Hallucination *q.v.* associated with stimulant-induced psychosis *q.v.* in which a person perceives imaginary ants, insects, or snakes crawling under the skin. 2. Cocaine bugs: a sensation of insects crawling underneath the skin, caused by stimulants *q.v.* such as cocaine *q.v.* or amphetamine *q.v.*

FORMULA GRANTS Educational funding based on the number of children eligible for various programs.

FORNICATION 1. Sexual intercourse between consenting unmarried adults. 2. Extramarital sexual relations. 3. Engaging in unlawful sexual intercourse. cf: adultery.

FORNICES Any anatomical structure with vault-like or arched shapes.

FORTIFICATION The addition of one or more nutrients *q.v.* to a food product in amounts so that the total amount will be larger than that contained in the natural food of its class. The FDA *q.v.* has established standards for ~ of food products.

FORTIFIED WINE Fermented *q.v.* fruits that have been strengthened by the addition of alcohol *q.v.* to bring the alcohol content to about 21%. ct: table wine.

FORWARD PAIRING A classical conditioning *q.v.* procedure in which the conditioned stimulus *q.v.* precedes the unconditioned stimulus *q.v.*

FOSSA In anatomy, a cavity or hollow.

FOSSIL A natural object preserved in the earth's crust that supplies information about a plant or animal of past geologic ages.

FOSSIL FUELS 1. Fuels derived from the remains of organic matter: coal, oil, and natural gas. 2. Fuels formed over millions of years of pressure of vegetation and other living things.

FOSTER CARE The temporary placement of children in private homes.

FOUNDATION An organization established by philanthropists to distribute financial resources to those who meet its specific eligibility requirements.

FOUNDATIONAL PERIOD In psychology, a period during ontogenesis *q.v.* when certain experiences must occur to provide developmental foundation for later experiences. Should the initial experiences not occur at their customary time, the developmental loss can be corrected by having the person go back to make up for the missed experience.

FOUNDATION PROGRAMS State funding programs that determine the dollar value of the basic educational opportunities that are desired in a state and referred to as the foundation level. These programs specify a minimum standard of local effort and determine an equitable way of distributing money to school districts based on local wealth.

FOUR BASIC FOOD GROUPS The traditional grouping of foods by category, formerly accepted by nutritionists as necessary for maintaining good health. These groups are (a) dairy products including eggs, (b) meat or meat substitutes, (c) cereals and grains, and (d) fruits and vegetables. cf: food pyramid.

FOURCHETTE In anatomy, the fold or mucous membrane *q.v.* at the posterior junction of labia majora *q.v.* in the female.

FOUR DIMENSIONS OF HEALTH Dimensions of health *q.v.*

FOUR-MAN ROLL 1. The back injury roll. 2. A method of placing a victim of injury on a carrying device, usually a long board or a flat litter, by rolling him or her on his or her side, then back onto the carrying device.

FOVEA 1. The region in the retina *q.v.* that is closely packed with cones *q.v.* 2. The region of the retina stimulated by the image at which a person is looking directly. 3. Small pit or depression. 4. A cup-shaped depression.

FOVEA CENTRALIS A small, rodless area of the retina *q.v.* that allows for acute vision.

FRACTURE Any break in the integrity of a bone. Specifically, ~s are identified as (a) simple, no external wound; (b) compound, an external wound; (c) complicated, injury to some internal organ; (d) comminuted, splintered; (e) impacted, one end of the bone is wedged into the interior of the other end; (f) incomplete, the ~ does not include the whole bone; (g) greenstick, the bone is bent and partially broken; (h) separation of an epiphysis, between the shaft of the bone and its growing end; and (i) depressed; a piece of the skull is driven inward (Table F-1).

FRAIL ELDERLY Elderly *q.v.* persons whose physical and emotional abilities or social support system is so reduced that maintaining a household or social contacts is difficult and sometimes impossible, without regular assistance from others. Healthy *q.v.* persons are usually not in this group until 75 years, and even then, many are not frail until they reach very late years.

FRAME OF REFERENCE The background or experience against which a person's judgments are made. cf: adaptation level.

FRAMING OF QUESTIONS In research and evaluation, stating a question in such a way that the respondent understands and reacts to the question exactly as intended. cf: validity; reliability.

FRATERNAL TWINS 1. Two offspring developed from two separate ova *q.v.* usually fertilized *q.v.* at the same time by two different sperm *q.v.* cells. ~ are no more genetically *q.v.* similar than ordinary siblings. 2. Dizygotic twins. ct: identical twins.

FRAUDULENT 1. Something that is not truthful. 2. A falsehood or deceptive practice.

FRC An acronym for functional respiratory capacity.

FRCP An acronym for Fellow of the Royal College of Physicians.

FRCS An acronym for Fellow of the Royal College of Surgeons.

FRECKLE A dense pigmented area of the skin.

FREE ANSWER TEST A test in which the learner uses his or her own words to respond to a relatively small number of questions.

TABLE F-1 SPECIFIC TYPES OF FRACTURES

Basal skull ~. Involves the base of the cranium.

Closed ~. A ~ in which there is no laceration in the overlaying skin.

Colles' ~. A ~ of the distal end of the radius.

Comminuted ~. A ~ in which the bone ends are broken into many fragments.

Compound ~. Open ~. One in which there is an open wound of the skin and soft parts leading down to the seat of the ~.

Depressed ~. A skull ~ with impaction, depression, or sinking in of the fragments of the bone.

Fatigue ~. A ~ in which the bone breaks as a result of repeated stress.

~ dislocation. A ~ near an articulation with a concomitant dislocation at the joint.

~ of the hip. A ~ that occurs at the upper end of the femur close to the hip joint.

Greenstick ~. An incomplete ~ causing partial disruption and bending of a bone, usually occurs in a child.

Linear ~. A ~ running parallel to the long axis of the bone.

Linear skull ~. A skull ~ in a straight line.

Muscle avulsion ~. A tearing away of a part of a bone, usually by a tendon, ligament, or capsule.

Oblique ~. A ~ that runs obliquely to the axis of the bone.

Open ~. Open dislocation. A ~ or dislocation having a direct communication with the outside of the skin. There may be a small wound over the ~ or dislocation or the ends of the bone may be protruding through the skin.

Pathological ~. A ~ in which a specific weakness or destruction of bone is caused by some disease process.

Simple ~. An uncomplicated ~.

Spiral ~. One in which the line of the break runs obliquely up one side of the bone.

Supracondylar ~. A ~ of the distal end of the humerus.

Transverse ~. A ~ whose line forms a right angle with the axis of the bone.

FREE ASSOCIATION 1. Consists of a person relating to a therapist any thoughts that come to mind. A method used in psychoanalytic therapy *q.v.* 2. Uninhibited expression of ideas as they enter consciousness during therapy. 3. A technique in psychoanalytic therapy in which the client is urged to talk about whatever comes to mind without censoring or interpreting those thoughts in order to reveal repressed ideas or memories for analysis. The assumption is that, over time, hitherto repressed *q.v.* material will come forth for examination by the analysand *q.v.* and analyst.

FREEBASE 1. The most potent part of cocaine *q.v.*, obtained by heating the drug with ether. 2. In general, when a chemical salt is separated into its basic and acidic components, the basic component is referred to as the ~. Most psychoactive *q.v.* drugs are bases that normally exist in salt form. Specifically, the salt, cocaine hydrochloride, can be chemically extracted to form the cocaine freebase, which is volatile and may, therefore, be smoked. cf: freebasing.

FREEBASING 1. A chemical process of changing common, white cocaine *q.v.* powder into a purer, more potent, smokable form of cocaine base, which the user then smokes in a glass water pipe that is heated by a butane lighter or small blowtorch. 2. Conversion of the stable salt form of an alkaloid into the less chemically stable but more biologically potent based form freed of ionic *q.v.* salt. Using a drug in this form. cf: freebase.

FREEDOM FROM COERCION In research, an ethical principle that requires that potential volunteers be free to participate or to decline participation in research without threat or punishment.

FREE FATTY ACID A fatty acid *q.v.* released from adipose *q.v.* tissue by hydrolysis *q.v.* of a triglyceride *q.v.*

FREE FLOATING ANGER A generalized displacement of anger to objects or persons that are neutral or that are unrelated to the true source of frustration. cf: displacement of anger.

FREE FLOATING ANXIETY 1. Anxiety *q.v.* not referable to any specific situation or cause. 2. Generalized anxiety disorder *q.v.*

FREEMARTIN A sexually underdeveloped female calf born twined with a male.

FREE RECALL A test of memory consisting of recalling as many items in a list as possible without regard to order.

FREE RUDER A group member who fails to contribute maximally to the group but benefits from others' efforts to do so.

FREE-WRITTEN RATING 1. Performance appraisal. 2. An overall appraisal that leaves raters complete flexibility on the form of rating.

FRENCH CULTURE In regard to sexual activity, oral stimulation of the genitals *q.v.*

FRENCH KISSING 1. A style of kissing in which the partner's tongues caress each other's. 2. Deep kissing. 3. Soul kissing. 4. Tongue kissing.

FRENULUM A delicate thin fold of skin that connects the foreskin *q.v.* with the undersurface of the glans penis *q.v.* Also, frenum.

FRENUM Frenulum *q.v.*

FREQUENCY 1. In physics, the rate at which a sound source vibrates, measured in cycles per second. 2. The number of cycles, repetitions, or oscillations of a periodic process completed during a given unit of time. 3. In physical training, the number of times per week a person should exercise to achieve a training effect *q.v.* 4. One of the chief variables of exercise prescription *q.v.*

FREQUENCY DISTRIBUTION 1. In statistics and epidemiology, an efficient method of presenting large numbers of data by grouping them into several categories. 2. Arranging scores according to frequency in which they occur. 3. A graphic presentation of the number of measures of each value or class of values.

FREQUENCY POLYGON A frequency distribution *q.v.* in which the *x*-axis *q.v.* is the measure or score, and the *y*-axis *q.v.* is the number of measures. ct: bar graph.

FREQUENCY THEORY An auditory theory *q.v.* according to which the basilar membrane *q.v.* responds with a frequency equal to that of the auditory *q.v.* stimulus *q.v.*

FREUDIANISM A set of beliefs derived from the ideas of Sigmund Freud, basic among them are the importance of the unconscious, the stages of psychosexual development, and the efficacy of helping persons resolve problems by exploring their earlier experiences.

FREUDIAN PSYCHOANALYSIS Analysis that aims at laying bare the complexes that have been repressed as a result of painful feelings associated with them.

FREUD'S THEORY OF DREAMS The aspect of Freudian psychology that at the root of all dreams there is an attempt to fulfill a wish. A dream consists of the latent aspect, which represents the hidden desire, and the manifest aspect, which is part of the dream that is remembered upon awakening.

FRIENDSHIP GROUPS Informal groups that form in organizations because of the personal affiliation members have for one another.

FRIGIDITY 1. Orgasmic dysfunction in the female. 2. A female dysfunction characterized by sexual coldness, indifference, or insensitivity to sexual intercourse or stimulation. 3. The inability to experience sexual pleasure. ct: impotence.

FRINGE BENEFITS In labor relations, any number of benefits provided to employees in addition to salary.

FROHLICH'S SYNDROME A disease of the anterior lobe of the pituitary gland *q.v.* occurring during adolescence *q.v.*, resulting in obesity *q.v.* and arrested development of the sex glands.

FRONTAL Pertaining to the region of the forehead.

FRONTAL LOBE 1. That part of the cerebral hemisphere *q.v.* forward of the central groove. 2. A lobe in each cerebral hemisphere that includes the motor area. 3. That portion of the brain that is active in reasoning and other higher thought processes. 4. The forward or upper half of each cerebral hemisphere in front of the central sulcus *q.v.* that is active in reasoning and other higher mental processes.

FRONTAL LOBOTOMY See lobotomy.

FRONTAL PLANE The anatomical plane of the body that divides the body in front and back, ventral and dorsal parts.

FROSTBITE 1. Destruction of tissue by freezing. 2. A deeper destruction than frost nip *q.v.*

FROST NIP Superficial local tissue destruction caused by freezing. ~ is limited in scope and does not destroy the full thickness of the skin. ct: frostbite.

FROTTAGE 1. The act of obtaining sexual gratification from rubbing against or pressing against the desired person, often while in a crowded place. A frotteur is a person who derives sexual pleasure from rubbing against a stranger. 2. A sexual variance *q.v.*

FRUCTOSE 1. A monosaccharide *q.v.* It is found in many fruits. It is also known as levulose or fruit sugar. It is a ready source of food energy. 2. A simple sugar. 3. A chemical substance that is responsible for making sperm *q.v.* mobile.

FRUIT A ripened ovary *q.v.* (or group of ovaries) containing seeds, together with any adjacent parts that may be found with it at maturity.

FRUSTRATION 1. Any situation that prevents a person from obtaining a desired goal. 2. Thwarting of a need or desire.

FRUSTRATION–AGGRESSION HYPOTHESIS Dollard's proposal that frustration *q.v.* always leads to some kind of aggression and that aggression is always the result of frustration.

FRUSTRATION TOLERANCE 1. The amount of frustration *q.v.* that a person can undergo without a disintegration of behavior *q.v.* 2. Stress tolerance *q.v.*

F-SCALE A method of measuring personality in which a questionnaire is used to assess the tendency to be subservient to authority. F stands for Fascist. cf: authoritarianism.

FSH Follicle-stimulating hormone *q.v.*

FTC Federal Trade Commission, a branch of the US Department of Commerce assigned the task of protecting the public against unfair methods of competition in interstate commerce.

FTE Full-time equivalency *q.v.*

FT FIBERS Fast-twitch fibers *q.v.*

FUGUE 1. A memory loss characterized by an actual physical departure from the stress-producing situation. The person may wander aimlessly and may manifest symptoms of amnesia *q.v.* 2. A neurosis *q.v.* 3. A dissociative reaction *q.v.* in which the person leaves his or her present life situation and establishes a somewhat different lifestyle in a new environment *q.v.* 4. Psychogenic fugue *q.v.*

FULGURATION In medicine, the burning away of a growth by means of a cautery *q.v.*

FULL POTENTIAL The talents, skills, and abilities an individual can acquire and/or develop if provided with the proper learning experiences and environments.

FULL-RANGE MOVEMENT In physiology, movement that starts from a fully extended, prestretched position and continues to a fully contracted position.

FULL-TERM INFANT 1. From conception *q.v.* to within 3 weeks of 280 days gestation *q.v.* 2. An infant born at 37 weeks or more of gestation.

FULL-TIME EQUIVALENCY (FTE) A funding model used at many universities where programs are funded based on the number of full-time students enrolled.

FULL-TIME STAFF People who are on the payroll of an institution and classified by the institution as full-time.

FULMINANT 1. In medicine, severe. 2. Flashes of pain. cf: fulminating anoxia.

FULMINATING ANOXIA In medicine, a sudden, intense, and severe anoxia *q.v.*

FUNCTIONAL 1. A dysfunction with no apparent alteration in tissues of the body as in functional disorder. 2. In sociology and social psychology, a part of the social system that tends to support another part of that system. ct: organic. cf: functional disease.

FUNCTIONAL AGE 1. An assessment of age based on physical or mental performance rather than on the number of years since birth. 2. A person's level of ability to perform various tasks relative to the average age of other who can perform the tasks. cf: chronological age.

FUNCTIONAL ANALYSIS OF BEHAVIOR A process used in naturalistic observations to record the person's behavior as well as the situational events surrounding it.

FUNCTIONAL AUTHORITY The right to give orders within a segment of the management system in which the right is normally nonexistent.

FUNCTIONAL AUTONOMY The hypothesis *q.v.* that sometimes habits become drives *q.v.* or ends in themselves, free of their original motivational origin.

FUNCTIONAL DEFECTS 1. Genetic defects *q.v.* affecting the body's ability to perform certain normal tasks. 2. Functional disorder: a form of psychopathological *q.v.* reaction without any known physiological *q.v.* basis.

FUNCTIONAL DEPENDENT (ELDERLY) Persons whose illnesses, disabilities, or social problems have reduced their ability to perform self-care and household tasks in an independent manner. cf: frail elderly.

FUNCTIONAL DISEASE 1. A condition lacking any physical or observable causes. 2. A disease *q.v.* that does not manifest any tissue change. 3. A disease with no organic *q.v.* basis. cf: functional. ct: organic disease.

FUNCTIONAL FIXEDNESS In psychology, a set *q.v.* to think of objects in terms of their normal function.

FUNCTIONAL GROUP In chemistry, an atom or group of atoms that determine or influence the chemical behavior of the molecule *q.v.* to which it is attached.

FUNCTIONAL HEALTH Homeostasis *q.v.*

FUNCTIONAL HEART DISEASE The presence of heart disease *q.v.* but without any known organic *q.v.* breakdown. cf: functional disease.

FUNCTIONAL HOMEOSTASIS 1. The internal mechanism that enables a person to retain and maintain biological, psychological, and sociological identity. 2. Adaptation *q.v.* cf: homeostasis.

FUNCTIONALLY EQUIVALENT GROUPS In research, groups that function as though they were identical to each other in every way that is relevant to the experiment.

FUNCTIONAL PSYCHOSIS 1. A psychotic *q.v.* reaction that is a functional disorder or defect *q.v.* 2. Severe disturbance of thought, emotion, and behavior without detectable brain pathology *q.v.* ct: organic psychosis.

FUNCTIONALS Homosexuals who live alone and have large numbers of sexual partners.

FUNCTIONAL SIMILARITY In management, a method of dividing job activities within the organization.

FUNCTIONAL SKILL The ability to apply appropriately the concepts *q.v.* of planning, organizing, influencing, and controlling the operation of a management system.

FUNDAMENTAL ATTRIBUTION ERROR In research, the tendency to disregard the effects that situations have on people's actions and to focus instead on people's personal disposition.

FUNDAMENTALIST A person who adheres to a very strict and literal interpretation of a particular set of religious beliefs.

FUNDAMENTAL TONE In the science of sound, the lowest tone in a complex tone. ct: overtone.

FUNDUS 1. In anatomy, the bottom or base of an organ. 2. The muscular top of the uterus *q.v.*

FUNGICIDE 1. A toxic *q.v.* substance causing destruction or inhibition of growth of fungi *q.v.* 2. An agent that destroys fungi.

FUNGUS A filamentous plant that lacks chlorophyll *q.v.* 2. A parasitic (parasite) *q.v.* plant that may cause disease *q.v.* 3. A group of plants, of which several microscopic *q.v.* varieties are pathogenic *q.v.* 4. Members of a class of relatively primitive organisms *q.v.* Fungi include mushrooms, yeasts, rusts, molds, and smuts.

FUROR In psychology, behavior characterized by transitory outbursts of excitement or anger during which the person may be dangerous.

FURUNCLE A form of small skin abscess *q.v.* involving a sebaceous gland *q.v.* cf: furunculosis.

FURUNCULOSIS 1. Boil caused by a coccus bacterium *q.v.* 2. A bacterial infection *q.v.* of the ear canal characterized by feelings of fullness in the ear and pain upon chewing. cf: boil; carbuncle.

FUSE In anatomy, to unite or join together. cf: fused joint; fusion.

FUSED CURRICULUM In education, the attempt to organize curriculum *q.v.* around a smaller number of subjects. It merges similar subjects into larger units of learning.

FUSED JOINT A joint that forms a solid, immobile, bony structure.

FUSIFORM ANEURYSM An aneurysm *q.v.* characterized by a bulging on both sides of a blood vessel. cf: aneurysm. ct: sacculated aneurysm.

FUSION 1. In physics, the putting together of atoms. 2. In medicine, joining together as in spinal fusion.

FUTURE-ORIENTED MANAGERS Managers who attempt to create their own future whenever possible, and adapt to this future, when necessary, through a continuous process of research about the future, long-range planning, and setting objectives.

FUTURE SHOCK A term coined by Alvin Toffler that refers to the accelerated pace of change and to the disorientation of people who are unable to adapt to altered norms, institutions, and values.

FUTURISM 1. The study of the future, including global concerns and more regional or local matters. 2. Focuses not only on predicting future developments but also on formulating techniques and procedures needed for preparing for such developments.

FY An acronym for fiscal year *q.v.*

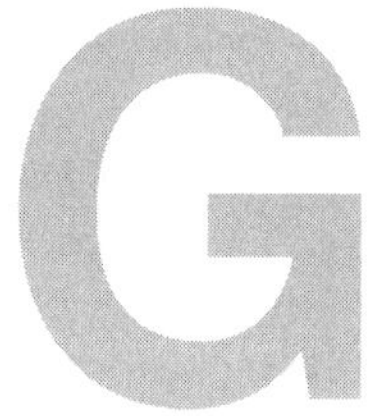

G An aeronautical unit of measure used to express the force of gravity.

GABA An acronym for gamma aminobutyrate *q.v.*

GAIT A person's pattern of walking.

GALACTOLINASE An enzyme *q.v.* essential for the metabolism *q.v.* of the sugar galactose *q.v.* cf: galactosemia.

GALACTORRHEA 1. A continued discharge of milk from the breasts in the intervals between nursing or after the child has been weaned. 2. Excessive or spontaneous flow of milk when not physiologically *q.v.* appropriate, and may be a side effect of drug use.

GALACTOSE 1. A monosaccharide *q.v.* 2. The major component of lactose *q.v.* 3. A simple sugar.

GALACTOSEMIA 1. A genetic defect *q.v.* characterized by the inability to metabolize *q.v.* the sugar, galactose *q.v.* 2. An inborn error of metabolism. The enzyme galactolinase *q.v.* is lacking in those persons with ~ and as a result, galactose builds up in the lens of the eye causing genetic cataract *q.v.* The toxicity *q.v.* may also cause damage to the liver and the brain. 3. The accumulation of galactose in the blood due to a lack of the enzyme galactose-1-phosphate uridyle transferase, which is necessary for the conversion of galactose into glucose. ~ is characterized by vomiting *q.v.* and diarrhea *q.v.*, abdominal distention, enlargement of the liver, and mental retardation *q.v.* 4. A type of mental retardation due to a metabolic deficiency.

GALEA APONEUROTICA 1. The fibrous aponeurosis *q.v.* connecting the occipitalis *q.v.* muscle posteriorly and the frontalis *q.v.* anteriorly and covering the skull. The tissue underlying the scalp.

GALL 1. Bile. 2. A secretion of the liver. cf: gallbladder.

GALLBLADDER 1. The sac located just beneath the liver which stores bile *q.v.* until needed. 2. A pear-shaped membranous sac on the underface of the liver. cf: gall; gallstone.

GALLERY In politics, balconies over chamber from which visitors may view proceedings of the legislature.

GALLSTONE Hard, calcium compounds formed in the gallbladder *q.v.* or bile duct *q.v.* cf: gall.

GALVANIC SKIN RESPONSE (GSR) 1. The electrical resistance of the skin in response to changes in a person's emotional state. 2. The electrical resistance of the skin in response to emotions *q.v.* 3. A drop in the electrical resistance of the skin often used as an index of autonomic *q.v.* reaction. 4. An index of sweat gland activity typically measured from the palm or surface by electrodes attached to the hand and connected to a polygraph *q.v.*; used to measure anxiety *q.v.*

GAMBLERS ANONYMOUS A voluntary organization made up of ex-gamblers whose purpose is to assist its members to resist the urge to gamble.

GAMEINSCHAFT In sociology, the close, personal relationships within the primary social group or within a primary community *q.v.*

GAMES (SIMULATION) In psychology, conditions are simulated and trainees make decisions that produce various outcomes that create new situations requiring further decisions.

GAMETANGIUM A general term applied to any cell or organ in which gametes *q.v.* are formed. ~ is usually restricted to reproductive bodies of lower plants in which the sex organs are alike.

GAMETE 1. Sperm or egg (ovum) *q.v.* 2. The mature reproductive cell of either sex. 3. Male or female germ cell, containing half the number of chromosomes *q.v.* as are in other cells of the body.

GAMETE TRANSFER A procedure in which a mature egg is placed in a woman's fallopian tube *q.v.* together with a sperm sample for fertilization *q.v.*

GAMETIC MUTATION A mutation *q.v.* of a germ cell.

GAMETOCYTE In biology, presexual stage in plasmodia, formed in definitive host's bloodstream.

GAMETOGENSIS The formation of gametes *q.v.*

GAMETOPHYTE That phase of the plant life cycle that bears the gametes *q.v.* Cells have *n* chromosomes *q.v.*

GAMETOPHYTE GENERATION The haploid (*n*) phase *q.v.* of the life cycle.

GAMETRICS 1. The application of biological and mathematical theory to gamete *q.v.* separation. The procedure involves identification, selection, and separation of y and x sperm *q.v.* which are artificially inseminated *q.v.* in the female to produce a baby of the desired sex or gender *q.v.* 2. The science that deals with controlling the sex of an embryo *q.v.* by sperm selection.

GAMMA One-thousandth of a milligram.

GAMMA ALCOHOLISM A form of alcoholism *q.v.* characterized by excessive drinking of alcohol *q.v.*, development of tolerance *q.v.*, withdrawal syndrome *q.v.*, craving, and inability to stop drinking once it has begun. The stereotyped alcoholic *q.v.*

GAMMA AMINOBUTYRATE (GABA) An amino acid *q.v.* that acts as a major inhibitory neurotransmitter *q.v.* in the central nervous system *q.v.*

GAMMAGLOBULIN 1. That part of the blood serum *q.v.* with which most of the immune antibodies *q.v.* are associated. 2. Certain blood proteins that contain antibodies. 3. The antibody component of the blood serum.

GAMMA RAYS 1. Radiation similar to X-rays but higher in energy output. 2. Electromagnetic waves emitted from radioactive *q.v.* material that have great penetrating power.

GANCICLOVIR (DHPG) An experimental antiviral drug used in the treatment of cytomegalovirus (CMV) retinitis. cf: cytomegalovirus.

GANGLIA 1. Groups of nerve cells outside the central nervous system *q.v.*, such as along the spinal cord. 2. A mass of nerve tissue containing nerve cells. 3. A nerve center.

GANGLION 1. A mass of nerve cells that serves as a center of nervous influence. 2. A small, hard tumor *q.v.* in a tender sheath. 3. A small swelling in the covering of a joint.

GANGPLANK A communication channel extending from one organizational division to another. This channel is not shown on the lines of communication outline on an organizational chart.

GANG RAPE A rape *q.v.*, usually performed by three or more assailants.

GANGRENE 1. Death of tissues in a localized area resulting from the loss of blood. 2. Necrosis *q.v.*

GANJA 1. West Indian name for marijuana *q.v.* 2. A preparation of *Cannabis* (marijuana) in which the most potent parts of the plant are used. It is more potent than Bhang *q.v.*

GANSER SYNDROME In psychology, the simulation of confusion, disorientation, or other supposed psychotic *q.v.* behavior. The ~ may involve malingering *q.v.*, neurotic *q.v.* behavior, or a combination of both.

GANTT CHART A scheduling tool essentially comprised of a bar chart with time on the horizontal axis and the resource to be scheduled on the vertical axis.

GARDNERELLA VAGINITIS A bacterial infection *q.v.* producing a thin odorous discharge in the genitalia *q.v.*

GARNISHES Condiments added to foods. A food added to main dishes for decorative purposes or as an added source of nutrients *q.v.*

GAS An acronym for general adaptation syndrome *q.v.*

GASEOUS PHASE That portion of tobacco smoke containing carbon monoxide *q.v.* and several other physiologically *q.v.* active gases. cf: particulate phase.

GAS GANGRENE A disease originating in a wound infected *q.v.* with *Clostridium perfringens q.v.*, resulting in rapid local tissue destruction and death of the person.

GASSERIAN Pertains to the ~ arteries. Named for Gasser, a sixteenth century Austrian surgeon.

GASTRIC Pertains to the stomach. cf: gastric digestion.

GASTRIC ASPIRATION A technique used to determine the contents of the stomach. cf: gastric.

GASTRIC DIGESTION That part of the digestive *q.v.* process that takes place in the stomach. cf: gastric.

GASTRIC JUICE 1. A mixture of hydrochloric acid and digestive enzymes *q.v.* secreted by the glands in the lining of the stomach. 2. The digestive fluid secreted by the glands of the stomach. 3. A thin, colorless liquid of acid reaction containing chiefly hydrochloric acid, pepsin, and mucus.

GASTRITIS 1. Inflammation *q.v.* of the stomach, causing damage to the blood vessels and erosion of stomach tissue. 2. Heartburn or upset stomach caused by an injury to, or the reaction of, the protective lining of the stomach and intestines.

GASTROCNEMIUS The large muscle that forms the calf of the leg.

GASTROENTERITIS A generalized infection *q.v.* of the gastrointestinal tract *q.v.*

GASTROENTEROLOGIST A physician who specializes in the diagnosis and treatment of problems of the stomach and intestines. cf: gastroenterology.

GASTROENTEROLOGY The medical specialty concerned with the health and disease of the stomach and intestines.

GASTROINTESTINAL DRUG A drug used to control or treat various disorders and diseases of the stomach and intestinal tract *q.v.*

GASTROINTESTINAL TRACT 1. The digestive pathway, including the esophagus, stomach, small intestine, and large intestine. 2. The stomach and intestines. 3. The digestive system. Also referred to as the GI *q.v.*

GASTROPLASTY A surgical alteration of the stomach, frequently for losing weight.

GASTRULA 1. The embryonic *q.v.* stage of development in which the cells form a double-layered hollow sphere. 2. An early animal embryo consisting of two layers of cells, an embryological stage following the blastula *q.v.*

GAVAGE Feeding by stomach tube.

GAW An acronym for guaranteed annual wage *q.v.*

GAY 1. Slang for homosexual *q.v.* 2. A colloquial term for homosexual, now often adopted by homosexuals who have openly announced their sexual orientation. 3. A male or female who engages in homosexual acts.

GAY COMMUNITY A colloquial term pertaining to homosexuals *q.v.* collectively.

GAY LIBERATION A movement, sometimes militant, seeking to achieve civil rights for homosexuals *q.v.* and recognition of the normality of homosexuality.

GEIGER COUNTER An instrument consisting of a Geiger–Muller tube and the electronic equipment used in conjunction with it to record the momentary current pulsations in the tube gas produced by the passage of radioactive particles.

GEL A jellylike colloid.

GELATIN A jellylike material obtained from boiling animal skin, ligaments, and bones.

GELATINIZATION Conversion to gelatin *q.v.*

GENDER 1. A person's genetic *q.v.* sex, biologically *q.v.* determined at the moment of conception *q.v.* by the pairing of the sex determining chromosomes *q.v.* 2. Male or female. 3. A cultural construct applied to the newborn usually according to their genital *q.v.* appearance. Some cultures have more than just the male and female gender, and allow for change of gender.

GENDER ADOPTION The lengthy process of learning the behaviors that are traditional for one's sex. cf: gender identity.

GENDER CONSTANCY 1. Recognition that a person's gender *q.v.* does not change as one grows older. 2. The belief that gender is a constant, inalterable attribute of people that persists no matter how they might change their appearance or behavior. cf: gender adoption.

GENDER DIFFERENCE A difference in physique, ability, attitude, or behavior found among groups of males and females.

GENDER DYSPHORIA 1. An uncomfortable feeling about one's gender identity *q.v.* ~ may range from a slight doubt about one's true sex to transsexuality *q.v.* 2. The feeling that one is definitely of the other sex.

GENDER IDENTIFICATION The achievement of a personally satisfying interpretation of one's masculinity *q.v.* or femininity *q.v.* cf: gender identity; gender adoption.

GENDER IDENTITY 1. How a person views himself or herself as a male or female. 2. Masculine *q.v.* or feminine self-concept *q.v.* 3. An environmentally, psychologically, or culturally determined feature. 4. Sexual orientation *q.v.* cf: sexual identity; gender identity disorder; gender role identification; gender adoption.

GENDER IDENTITY DISORDER 1. The expression of distaste and disgust for one's own genetic sex and a preference for and strong identification with the other sex. 2. Psychosexual *q.v.* disorientation in which a person lacks clear identification with his or her biological sex. 4. Disorders in which there is a deeply felt incongruence between anatomic *q.v.* sex and the sensed gender: transsexualism and gender identity of childhood are examples.

GENDER PREFERENCE The emotional and intellectual acceptance of the sex that a person is. cf: gender adoption; gender identity; gender role.

GENDER RATIO The proportion of one sex to the other in any particular societal subgroup.

GENDER ROLE 1. The socially accepted characteristics and behaviors typically associated with a person's gender identity *q.v.* 2. The set of external behavior patterns a culture deems appropriate for each sex. 3. The pattern of behavior considered usual for one's sex and the public expression of one's maleness or femaleness. 4. The set of rights and duties given by a particular society to those occupying the specific gender categories in that society. Such rights and duties apply to behavior and attitudes in all the major life areas of that society. cf: gender role identification.

GENDER ROLE IDENTIFICATION The process by which persons incorporate behaviors and characteristics of a culturally defined gender *q.v.* role into their own personalities.

GENDER ROLE SOCIALIZATION The training of children by parents and other caretakers to behave in ways considered socially appropriate for their gender *q.v.* cf: gender role identification.

GENDER SCHEMA The mental image of the cognitive *q.v.*, affective *q.v.*, and performance characteristics appropriate to a particular sex. A mental image of being a man or being a woman. cf: gender.

GENDER SCRIPT Script (sexual) *q.v.*

GENDER STABILITY The belief that gender *q.v.* is a stable attribute of people but that it can nonetheless change if people choose to dress or behave like a member of the opposite sex.

GENDER STEREOTYPE Behavior conforming to the norms that society has declared for its males and females.

GENE 1. A determiner of a hereditary *q.v.* trait. Genes together make up the chromosomes *q.v.* 2. Hereditary units that occupy a specific location on a chromosome. 3. The biological unit of heredity, self-reproducing and located at a definite position on a particular chromosome. 4. Chemical units, arranged linearly on chromosomes, that carry instructions for reproducing cells. Genes are the physical units that one generation inherits from another. 5. The basic unit of heredity, an ordered sequence of nucleotides *q.v.* A ~ contains the information for the synthesis of one polypeptide chain (protein).

GENEALOGICAL Refers to a record or account of a person's family and ancestry.

GENE EXPRESSION The production of RNA *q.v.* and cellular proteins.

GENE FREQUENCY The proportion of one allele *q.v.* as represented in a breeding population.

GENE INTERACTION The condition in which the usual expression of one gene is modified by the presence of other genes.

GENE MUTATION The appearance of new alleles *q.v.* through spontaneous change. It is an error that is made during cell division when DNA *q.v.* is being duplicated. These errors may be due to either internal or external forces such as radiation and the presence of some chemicals. An alteration in a gene *q.v.* affecting hereditary *q.v.* potential.

GENE POOL 1. The sum total of genetic *q.v.* material associated with large populations. 2. The sum total of all genes in a breeding population. cf: genetic pool.

GENERAL ADAPTATION SYNDROME (GAS) 1. The body's reaction to stress. The syndrome consists of (a) the alarm reaction, (b) the stage of resistance, and (c) the stage of exhaustion. 2. Sequenced physiological response to the presence of a stressor. 3. A three-staged physiological reaction to stress characterized by alarm, resistance, and finally exhaustion.

GENERAL ANESTHETIC A drug administered for the purpose of anesthetizing the entire body. ct: local anesthetic.

GENERAL CURRICULUM In education, basic curriculum *q.v.* required of all students.

GENERAL EDUCATION A broad area of the school program that attempts to develop common learning that is essential for success in society.

GENERAL EDUCATIONAL DEVELOPMENT (GED) PROGRAM Academic instruction to prepare persons to take the high school equivalency examination.

GENERAL ENVIRONMENT The secondary organizational environment that contains such variables as social norms, economic conditions, and government regulations.

GENERAL FACTOR In research, a factor that factor analysis *q.v.* suggests is involved in all tests for a particular trait.

GENERALITY In research, the ability to generalize to subjects, situations, treatments, measures, study designs, and procedures other than those used in a given study.

GENERALIZABILITY In research, the extent to which the results of a study with a particular sample *q.v.* represents the population from which the sample was taken.

GENERALIZATION 1. The automatic transfer of a response *q.v.* conditioned to a particular stimulus *q.v.* to all similar stimuli. 2. Stimulus generalization *q.v.* ct: generalization decrement.

GENERALIZATION DECREMENT The loss of response *q.v.* strength that occurs when a response is elicited by a stimulus *q.v.* other than the original stimulus. ct: generalization.

GENERALIZE 1. The extent or to go beyond. 2. To respond similarly to stimuli *q.v.* that resemble one another.

GENERALIZED ANXIETY DISORDER 1. A mental disorder *q.v.* whose primary characteristic is an all-pervasive, free-floating anxiety. Formerly called anxiety neurosis *q.v.* (reaction). 2. A state of hyperarousal typified by free-floating generalized anxiety and apprehension caused by a perceived omnipresent, unspecific threat. 3. One of the anxiety disorders *q.v.* where anxiety is so chronic *q.v.*, persistent, and pervasive that it seems free floating. The person is jittery and strained, distractible, and apprehensive that something bad is about to happen. A pounding heart, fast pulse rate and breathing, sweating, flushing, muscle aches, a lump in the throat, and an upset gastrointestinal tract *q.v.* are some of the bodily indicators of this form of extreme anxiety.

GENERALIZED CAPACITY FOR INHIBITION The ability to flexibly inhibit *q.v.* responses in a variety of circumstances assumed to emerge as part of the five to seven transition *q.v.*

GENERALIZED GRADIENT The curve that shows the relationship between the tendency to respond to a new stimulus *q.v.* and its similarity to the original conditioned stimulus *q.v.*

GENERALIZED OTHER A person's abstracted concept of other people.

GENERAL OBJECTIVES In education, 1. broad, abstract statements expressing educational goals *q.v.* for several years. ~ serve as guidelines for the more specific objectives *q.v.* of a given course of study *q.v.* 2. Goals. cf: mission.

GENERAL PARESIS 1. An organic *q.v.* mental illness characterized by destruction to parts of the brain *q.v.* as a result of the disease syphilis *q.v.* ~ manifests in progressive decline in cognitive *q.v.* and motor function culminating in death. 2. Neurosyphilis *q.v.*

GENERAL PRACTITIONER (GP) A physician who has a general or family practice. ct: medical specialist.

GENERAL SEXUAL DYSFUNCTION 1. Sexual unresponsiveness *q.v.* 2. A sexual problem in which the female arouses little, if at all, when sexually stimulated.

GENERATIONAL EPIDEMIC 1. Generational cycle *q.v.* 2. Health issues and problems that are perpetuated from parents to offspring. For example, child abusers are, generally, victims of child abuse.

GENERATIVE THEORY A theory *q.v.* that challenges the beliefs or assumptions that are common to a culture and in doing so develops alternatives to the status quo and furnishes a choice in the place of dogmatic belief.

GENERATIVITY A capacity shared by all languages for creating novel messages from a number of reusable linguistic units.

GENE RECOMBINATION Crossing over *q.v.*

GENERIC 1. Referring to a drug's basic chemical composition. 2. A drug that is sold under its chemical name rather than a trade name. 3. A drug product given an official or nonproprietary name, one that is not patented, trademarked, or owned by a private individual or company. The ~ name is often a contraction of the drug's more complex chemical name. 4. ~ drugs have the same active chemical ingredients as brand name drugs. Most ~ drugs are less expensive than brand name products, yet are as effective. cf: generic name.

GENERIC COMPETENCIES 1. Common competencies. 2. Basic skills and knowledge associated with a profession.

GENERIC MEMORY The ability to recall knowledge independent of the occasion when it was learned.

GENERIC NAME 1. The common or nonproprietary name of a drug. 2. For drugs, a name which specifies a particular chemical without being chemically descriptive. As an example, the chemical name sodium chloride is associated with the generic name table salt, of which there are several brand names. cf: generic.

GENETIC 1. Pertaining to, concerned with, or determined by the genesis of anything or its mode of reproduction or development. 2. Characteristics controlled by genes *q.v.* 3. Hereditary. 4. Pertaining to reproduction, or to birth, or origin. Inherited *q.v.*

GENETIC CAUSATION Something thought to be due to, or caused by, inherited *q.v.* factors.

GENETIC CLONING Cloning *q.v.* cf: genetic code.

GENETIC CODE 1. The hereditary *q.v.* characteristics contained within the germ cells *q.v.* of both sexes. 2. All of the genes *q.v.* contained within the gamete *q.v.* 3. The means by which DNA *q.v.* controls the sequence and structure of proteins manufactured within each cell and makes exact duplicates of itself. 4. The sequence of DNA nucleotides *q.v.*, providing information for sequence of amino acids *q.v.* in polypeptides *q.v.*

GENETIC COUNSELING A specialty of genetic *q.v.* medicine. Its goal is to present the occurrence of genetic defects *q.v.* The counselor determines the risks potential parents face in having a defective child. This is done through genetic screening *q.v.* and the establishment of family histories or pedigrees *q.v.* The genetic counselor determines the cause of a genetic defect in a family, whether it is due to a defective gene, chromosome *q.v.*, environmental factors, or a combination of these. The potential parents are then advised on the probability of passing a defect to their future offspring. cf: genetic counselor.

GENETIC COUNSELOR A person trained in genetic science and who counsels others in the probability of their passing genetic traits to the next generation.

GENETIC DAMAGE Damage to genes *q.v.* such as that produced by exposure to radioactivity *q.v.* cf: genetic defects.

GENETIC DEFECTS Defects and diseases *q.v.* caused by heredity *q.v.* or those classed as congenital *q.v.* ~ may result from defective genes, chromosomes *q.v.*, prenatal environment, or a combination of these factors, called multifactorial inheritance *q.v.* cf: genetic disease.

GENETIC DISEASE 1. Genetic defect *q.v.* 2. An abnormality determined at the moment of conception *q.v.* 3. Genetic disorder *q.v.*

GENETIC DISORDERS Genetic defects *q.v.* ct: genetic health.

GENETIC DISTURBANCE Genetic defect *q.v.*

GENETIC DRIFT 1. Random fluctuations in the frequencies of certain alleles *q.v.* occurring in small populations. 2. Drift *q.v.* 3. Random genetic drift *q.v.*

GENETIC ENGINEERING 1. The science that studies ways—surgical, physical, chemical, radiation—to alter the molecular *q.v.* structure of genetic *q.v.* material. 2. Molecular engineering *q.v.* cf: genetic medicine.

GENETIC EPISTEMOLOGY Piaget's name for the branch of cognitive science that concerns itself with the ontogenetic *q.v.* origins and development of the human ability to know and to reason.

GENETIC EQUILIBRIUM Condition in a group of interbreeding organisms in which particular gene *q.v.* frequencies remain constant through succeeding generations.

GENETIC HEALTH 1. The potential level of functioning ability as determined by genetic *q.v.* makeup. 2. The quality of functioning as determined by inherited *q.v.* potentials. ct: genetic disease; genetic defects.

GENETIC MEDICINE The study of cell biology and biomedical genetics. It includes a clinical discipline that concentrates its efforts on detecting, diagnosing, preventing, and treating genetic diseases and disorders *q.v.* cf: genetic engineering.

GENETIC MUTATION The alteration by chemicals or radiation of some portion of the DNA *q.v.* within the genes *q.v.*

GENETIC POOL The total genotype *q.v.* of a person or population. cf: gene pool.

GENETIC POTENTIALS A person's genotype *q.v.* cf: genetic predisposition.

GENETIC PREDISPOSITION An inherited tendency to develop a condition when certain environmental factors exist. cf: genetic potentials.

GENETIC SCREENING 1. Consists of examining (usually high risk populations) to determine whether certain persons are carriers of a specific genetic anomaly *q.v.* or whether there are familial risks related to certain genetic defects *q.v.* 2. A search in a population for persons possessing certain genotypes *q.v.* that are (a) already associated with disease or predisposed to disease, (b) may lead to disease in their descendents, or (c) produce other variations not known to be associated with disease.

GENETIC SEXUALITY A sexuality *q.v.* label that reflects either the XX or XY chromosome *q.v.* pattern.

GENETICS, SCIENCE OF 1. The science that strives to discover the truth about the development of life, its perpetuation and alterations as directed by the mechanisms contained within the genes *q.v.* 2. The science of heredity *q.v.* 3. The study of heredity and variation.

GENETIC THEORY OF ALCOHOLISM The cause of alcoholism *q.v.* is inherited. This theory suggests that as alcoholism seems to run in families, some people inherit a predisposition or susceptibility to the adverse effects of ingested alcohol *q.v.* cf: genetrophic theory of alcoholism.

GENETROPHIC THEORY OF ALCOHOLISM The causation of alcoholism *q.v.* is the interaction of a genetic *q.v.* trait and a nutritional deficiency *q.v.* A person inherits *q.v.* an abnormal need for some vitamins *q.v.* resulting in an abnormal craving for alcohol *q.v.* cf: genetic theory of alcoholism.

GENITAL 1. Pertaining to the organs of reproduction. 2. The sexual organs. 3. Genitalia *q.v.*

GENITAL APPOSITION A form of petting in which the partners rub their genitals *q.v.* together while lying close together with or without their clothes on and without coitus *q.v.*

GENITAL HERPES 1. Herpes simplex type 2 *q.v.* 2. A sexually transmitted *q.v.* viral *q.v.* infection *q.v.* that affects the genitals *q.v.* of either sex. 3. A sexually transmitted disease (STD) characterized by tiny fluid-filled blisters that appear on the genitals and in the genital tract. 4. An STD generally caused by herpes virus hominis type 2.

GENITALIA 1. The organs of reproduction, especially the external organs. 2. Genitals *q.v.*

GENITAL RESPONSE The responses of the reproductive organs *q.v.* to sexual arousal.

GENITAL SEXUALITY 1. Sexuality *q.v.* that is centered in the recreational use of the reproductive structures. 2. The sexuality that encompasses sexual performance and eroticism *q.v.* 3. The adult behavior that comes with the hormonal *q.v.* changes of puberty *q.v.*, according to Freud.

GENITAL STAGE 1. In Freudian psychology, the final stage of psychosexual *q.v.* development in which sexual pleasure shifts from self-pleasure through masturbation *q.v.* to interpersonal *q.v.* sexual pleasure. 2. The final stage in Freud's theory of psychosexual development in which heterosexual *q.v.* interests predominate (adulthood). ct: anal stage; oral stage.

GENITAL STIMULATION Fondling of the sex organs *q.v.* cf: masturbation.

GENITAL SYSTEM The system of the body including all the organs concerned with reproduction.

GENITAL TUBERCLE 1. Undifferentiated tissue within the embryo *q.v.* from which the penis *q.v.* or clitoris *q.v.* develops. 2. Part of the rudimentary genitals *q.v.* common to the male and female human embryos that will develop into either the penis or the clitoris. The other parts of the urogenital slit, urethral fold, and labio-scrotal swellings. The presence or absence of the hormone androgen *q.v.* will determine whether the genitals develop into, respectively, male or female form.

GENITAL WARTS 1. Sexually *q.v.* transmitted lesions *q.v.* that may appear in the cervix *q.v.*, vulva *q.v.*, urethra *q.v.*, or rectum *q.v.* 2. A viral disease characterized by wart-like lesions on the genitals *q.v.*

GENITOURINARY Pertaining to the reproductive and urinary organs, especially in males. cf: genitourinary tract.

GENITOURINARY TRACT 1. The anatomical structures of the male that are related to urinary excretion and sexual reproduction. 2. Pertaining to the urinary and reproductive structures; sometimes called the GU tract or system.

GENIUS 1. Very high intelligence *q.v.* 2. A person who possesses high intelligence or who has extraordinary achievements, either generally or specifically. 3. A person who has an intelligence quotient (IQ) *q.v.* of 145 or higher.

GENOCIDE The extermination of an entire ethnic *q.v.* group.

GENOID DNA *q.v.* carrying cytoplasmic particle *q.v.*

GENOME A complete set of chromosomes (hence of genes) inherited as a unit from one parent. 2. The genetic *q.v.* endowment of an organism.

GENOTOXIC A substance that has the ability to produce DNA *q.v.* damage.

GENOTYPE 1. The combination of genes *q.v.* that determines the genetic *q.v.* potentials. 2. One's actual gene combinations as determined at the moment of conception *q.v.* 3. The genetic combination, latent or expressed, of an organism. 4. The sum total of all the genes present in a person. 5. A person's total genetic makeup as represented by the sum of the genetic information in all the chromosomes *q.v.* or some particular aspect of this genetic makeup, such as the genotype for baldness or the genotype for albinism. ct: phenotype.

GENTLE BIRTH As advocated by French obstetrician, LeBoyer, childbirth in which the alert and responsive infant is born into a dimly lit, quiet room, allowed to lie on its mother's abdomen until the umbilical cord *q.v.* stops pulsing, and then is bathed calmly in a warm bath. ~ is thought to make neonates *q.v.* calmer and more alert than traditional childbirth.

GENUS 1. In biology, a group of closely related species clearly marked off from other groups. 2. A biological classification ranking between family and species. 3. A group of structurally or phylogenically related species.

GEO-ATMOSPHERE Atmosphere *q.v.* of the soil.

GEOGRAPHIC CONTIGUITY The degree to which subordinates are physically separated.

GEOPOLITICS 1. Political status of all countries of the world.

GEOTROPISM 1. A growth movement in response to the influence of gravity. Reactions of living organisms *q.v.* to gravity.

GERIATRICIAN A physician *q.v.* with special training in geriatric medicine *q.v.* In previous times, this training was self-taught through the special attention physicians gave their older patients. Presently, 1–3 years training programs that follow the regular medical curriculum are established in many of the teaching medical centers.

GERIATRIC MEDICINE 1. Geriatrics *q.v.* 2. The medical knowledge of physical disabilities in older persons, including the diagnosis *q.v.* treatment and prevention of disorders. ~ recognizes aging *q.v.* as a normal process, not a disease *q.v.* state.

GERIATRIC PSYCHIATRY 1. The medical specialty concerned with psychiatric *q.v.* conditions of older persons. cf: geriopsychiatry; psychiatrist.

GERIATRICS 1. The specialized branch of medicine concerned with treating the health conditions associated with senescence *q.v.* and senility *q.v.* 2. ~ is concerned with applying scientific findings to alleviating the diseases resulting from senescence. 3. The science of diseases and their treatment of the aged. 4. ~ was originally coined in 1909 by the American physician, Ingnaz L. Nasher when he recognized a similarity between the areas of aging and pediatrics *q.v.* Nasher is the founder of modern geriatrics in the United States. ct: gerontology. cf: geriatrician; geriatric medicine.

GERIOPSYCHIATRY Geriatric psychiatry *q.v.*

GERM 1. In biology, a small mass of living substance capable of developing into an animal or plant or into an organ part. 2. Any microorganism *q.v.* 3. The earliest stage of the embryo *q.v.* cf: germs.

GERMAN MEASLES 1. Rubella *q.v.* 2. Three-day measles.

GERM CELL 1. The sperm *q.v.* or ovum *q.v.* 2. A reproductive cell capable of being fertilized *q.v.* and reproducing an entire organism *q.v.* when mature.

GERMICIDE 1. A disinfectant *q.v.* 2. A substance that kills microorganisms *q.v.*

GERMINAL STAGE In embryology *q.v.*, the first 2 weeks after fertilization *q.v.*

GERMINATION Resumption of growth of an embryo *q.v.* or spore *q.v.*

GERM PLASM 1. In genetics, the germinal material or physical basis of heredity *q.v.* 2. The sum total of the genes *q.v.* 3. Idioplasm *q.v.*

GERMS 1. Infectious agents *q.v.* 2. Disease-producing microorganisms *q.v.*

GERM THEORY OF DISEASE 1. The concept that diseases *q.v.* are caused by microorganisms *q.v.* Discoveries by Louis Pasteur *q.v.* and Robert Koch *q.v.* established that several diseases are caused by bacteria *q.v.* and that putrification *q.v.* is also caused by microorganisms. These discoveries led to the establishment of the science of immunology *q.v.* and bacteriology *q.v.* 2. ~ states "that there is a single cause or pathological *q.v.* agent for each specific disease." 3. According to the ~, "the characters of a disease are determined more by response of the organism as a whole than by the characteristics of the causative agent."

GERONTOLOGIST A physician or other professionally trained person who examines the clinical, biological, psychosocial, and historical aspects of aging. cf: geriatrics; gerontology.

GERONTOLOGY 1. The specialized branch of medicine concerned with the scientific study of the aging process, clinical, biological, and social, and the problems that aging reveals. 2. The study of senescence *q.v.* 3. The interdisciplinary study of aging from the broadest perspective. Gerontologists *q.v.* examine not only the clinical and biological aspects of aging but also the psychosocial, economic, and historical conditions. Elie Metchnikoff, of the Pasteur Institute in Paris, France, first used the term in 1903 to describe the biological study of senescence.

GERONTOLOGY RESEARCH CENTER A branch of the National Institute on Aging *q.v.* Conducts research into behavior changes that take place with age, the aging process, age-related deterioration, and the inability of organisms to maintain their physiological control system and genetic *q.v.* information transfer system. cf: gerontology.

GERONTOSEXUALITY A sexual variance in which a young person gains sexual gratification from having sexual relations with a person who is much older.

GESELL DEVELOPMENTAL SCHEDULES One of the earliest instruments for assessing individual differences in the behavioral development of infants.

GESTALT A structure or configuration of physical, biological, or psychological phenomena so integrated as to constitute a functional unit with characteristics not derivable from its parts in summation. cf: gestaltism.

GESTALT FIELD THEORY The process of learning in which learning is defined as gaining new insight, outlooks, or thought processes. Gestalt theorists view individuals, their environments, and interactions with their environments as occurring simultaneously and define this as the field. cf: Gestalt therapy.

GESTALTISM The theory in psychology *q.v.* that the objects of the mind come as wholes which cannot be split into parts and which are unanalyzable. 2. Gestalt psychology *q.v.*

GESTALT PSYCHOLOGY 1. The hypothetical approach that emphasizes the role of wholes (gestaltism *q.v.*) in perception and other psychological processes. 2. An area of psychology *q.v.* that emphasizes the way in which a person's internal processes impose form on the external world. 3. The school of psychology that emphasizes patterns rather than elements or connections, taking the view that the whole is more than the sum of its parts. cf: Gestalt therapy; gestaltism.

GESTALT THERAPY A humanistic–existential *q.v.* insight therapy approach developed by Fritz Perls to integrate dissociated *q.v.* thought, feelings, and actions into a whole, well-functioning self; focuses on nonverbal clues to unacknowledged needs, which the therapist encourages the patient to confront. cf: Gestalt psychology.

GESTATE To carry a pregnancy to full term. cf: gestation.

GESTATION 1. The period of pregnancy. 2. The time of conception to the birth of a child. 3. The period of prenatal *q.v.* development. 4. The period from fertilization *q.v.* or conception *q.v.* to birth. 5. Ideal time of 280 days beginning with conception. 6. Average ~ period of 267 days or from 274 to 280 days from the beginning of the last menses *q.v.*

G FACTOR OF INTELLIGENCE 1. Generalized intelligence *q.v.* 2. Spearman's theory of general intelligence. 3. A general or unitary factor of intelligence that pervades all types of intellectual activity.

GH An acronym for growth hormone *q.v.*

GIARDIASIS 1. An infection *q.v.* of the intestines caused by a protozoan *q.v.* possessing flagella. 2. An infection of the intestinal tract with Giardia lamblia which may cause intermittent diarrhea *q.v.* of lengthy duration.

GIFTED LEARNER 1. Gifted *q.v.* 2. The term most frequently applied to those learners with exceptional intellectual ability, but may also refer to learners with outstanding ability in athletics, leadership, music, creativity, and the like.

GIFTED (TALENTED) 1. Children whose abilities are above those of most children of their age. These children, as students, require specialized educational programs. 2. Pertaining to those with extraordinary cognitive abilities and capable of superior performance in learning. cf: gifted learner.

GIGANTISM 1. An inherited *q.v.* condition that results in extremely large stature. It is caused by inheritance of genes *q.v.* for height and abnormal endocrine *q.v.* secretions resulting in the lack of closure of the epiphysis *q.v.* of long bones, and the eosinophil cells *q.v.* of the anterior pituitary gland *q.v.* secrete an excess of the principal growth hormone. 2. An abnormally tall stature resulting from hyperfunctioning of the pituitary gland.

GIGOLO A male prostitute *q.v.* who services women.

GINGIVA In dental anatomy, the gums, fibrous tissue covered by mucous membrane *q.v.* that covers the tooth and socket of the upper and lower jaws and surrounding the neck of the tooth. cf: gingivitis.

GINGIVITIS In dentistry, an inflammation *q.v.* of the gingivae *q.v.* due to infection *q.v.*, impaction of food, and faulty fillings.

GI TRACT An acronym for gastrointestinal tract *q.v.* The stomach and intestines.

GLAND 1. An organ made up of cells whose main function is to produce chemicals for secretion. 2. Examples of ~s are endocrine ~; exocrine ~ *q.v.* 3. A secreting structure of the body.

GLANDERS DISEASE 1. A vector-borne *q.v.* disease. 2. A contagious *q.v.* infection caused by *Pseudomonas mallei* in horses, donkeys, and mules. ~ is communicable *q.v.* to humans. It is characterized by fever, inflammation of the skin and mucous membranes.

GLANDS OF BARTHOLIN Two small glands *q.v.* located on each side of the vaginal orifice *q.v.* that provide a lubricating fluid during sexual arousal.

GLANS 1. A gland *q.v.* 2. Goiter *q.v.* 3. A nut. cf: glans clitoris; glans penis.

GLANS CLITORIS The head of the clitoris *q.v.* cf: glans penis.

GLANS PENIS The head of the penis *q.v.* The highly sensitive part of the penis. ct: glans clitoris.

GLARE Dazzling light.

GLAUCOMA 1. A disease in which pressure inside the eye increases. ~ can cause blindness if left untreated. 2. Increased pressure within the eye which can cause damage to the optic nerve *q.v.* 3. A disease of the eye in which the eyeball hardens, generally impairing sight and often leading to blindness when untreated. 4. A disease in which pressure builds up within the eye and causes internal damage, generally destroying vision. Often hereditary *q.v.* ~ usually affects persons after age 40 years. Symptoms may be blurred vision, difficulty in focusing, loss of peripheral vision, or slow adaptation to darkness. Often there are no symptoms until severe, irreversible loss of vision has occurred. While no method for preventing ~ exists, early diagnosis can prevent further damage.

GLENOHUMERAL JOINT 1. The shoulder joint. 2. The joint between the upper end of the humerus *q.v.* and the scapula *q.v.*

GLENOID FOSSA The hollow in the head of the scapula *q.v.* that receives the head of the humerus *q.v.* to make the shoulder joint. cf: glenohumeral joint.

GLIA CELL Neuroglia *q.v.* cf: glial cell.

GLIAL CELL 1. Cells that surround the neurons *q.v.* in the brain and that help form the blood–brain barrier; astrocytes (a star-shaped neurological cell with many branching processes). 2. Nonneuronal cells in the brain and spinal cord that provide structural and functional support for the neurons of the central nervous system *q.v.*

GLIOMA 1. Tumor *q.v.* 2. Specifically, cancer of nerve tissue.

GLOBAL TRENDS Forecasted developments that have an impact on the entire world, such as geopolitics, hunger, and population.

GLOBULIN 1. That portion of blood serum *q.v.* that contains the antibodies *q.v.* 2. Common proteins found in the blood that are insoluble in water and soluble in salt solutions. Alpha, beta, and gamma ~s can be distinguished in human blood serum. Gamma ~s are important in developing immunity *q.v.* to disease.

GLOBUS HYSTERICA A choking sensation in the throat; at one time, a common complaint in hysterical or conversion reactions *q.v.*

GLOMERULONEPHRITIS A type of kidney disease. The chronic *q.v.* form of ~ leads to impaired kidney function and eventual need for dialysis *q.v.* or transplantation *q.v.*

GLOMERULUS 1. A group of tiny blood vessels within the nephron *q.v.* of the kidney *q.v.* 2. A compact cluster. 3. A ball-like coil of capillaries *q.v.* at the enlarged end of each nephric tubule *q.v.* in the kidneys.

GLOSSAL Pertaining to the tongue.

GLOSSITIS Inflammation *q.v.* of the tongue.

GLOTTIS The vocal apparatus of the larynx *q.v.* consisting of the true vocal cords and the opening between them. cf: epiglottis.

GLOVE ANESTHESIA Loss of sensation in the hand but retaining full sensation in the arm above the wrist. Often seen in conversion disorders *q.v.*

GLUCAGON 1. A pancreatic *q.v.* hormone *q.v.* that triggers the breakdown of glycogen *q.v.* and is stored in the liver and some other tissues. 2. A compound *q.v.*

secreted by alpha cell *q.v.* of the islets of Langerhans *q.v.* that is hyperglycemic *q.v.*, glycogenolytic *q.v.*, and gluconeogenerin *q.v.*

GLUCOCORTICOIDS Hormones *q.v.* that influence food metabolism *q.v.* and secreted by the adrenal cortex *q.v.*

GLUCOGENIC Sugar producing.

GLUCOKINASE An enzyme *q.v.* that catalyzes *q.v.* conversion of glucose *q.v.* to glucose-6-phosphate.

GLUCONEOGENESIS The formation of glucose *q.v.* from noncarbohydrate *q.v.* sources, chiefly, certain amino acids *q.v.* and the glycerol *q.v.* portion of the fat molecule *q.v.* cf: glyconeogenesis.

GLUCOSE 1. A monosaccharide *q.v.* (dextrose, corn sugar). Found in sweet fruits and some vegetables. 2. A simple sugar that is the basic form of food energy. 3. Grape sugar, or dextrose, a 6-carbon sugar. 4. Free ~ occurs in the blood in a concentration of 60–120 mg per 100 ml of blood. In diabetes mellitus *q.v.*, it appears in the urine. cf: dextrose.

GLUCOSE TOLERANCE TEST A test indicating the efficiency of the body in its use of glucose *q.v.* Changes are noted in the concentration of glucose in the blood at determined intervals after ingestion of a standard amount of sugar. Recent research indicates that some increase occurs in blood glucose levels as people age.

GLUTEAL Of or near the buttocks *q.v.*

GLYCEMIA The presence of sugar in the blood.

GLYCERIDE 1. A compound (ester *q.v.*) formed by the combination of glycerol *q.v.* and fatty acids *q.v.* and the loss of water (the ester linkage). According to the number of ester linkages, the compound is a mono-, di-, or triglyceride *q.v.* 2. A glycerol ester formed from glycerol and a fatty acid. The mono-, di-, and triglycerides contain one, two, or three fatty acids, respectively. Glycerides constitute a major class of lipids *q.v.*

GLYCERIN 1. Glycerol *q.v.* 2. A product of fat digestion *q.v.*

GLYCEROL 1. Glycerin *q.v.* 2. The 3-carbon atom *q.v.* alcohol *q.v.* derived from the hydrolysis *q.v.* of fat. 3. A clear, colorless, and syrupy liquid made up of fats and oils. 4. An alcohol component that is a common constituent of dietary fats *q.v.*

GLYCOGEN 1. A polysaccharide *q.v.* of animal origin. It is synthesized *q.v.* during glucose *q.v.* metabolism *q.v.* ~ is the storage form of the body's energy supply; composed of a network of glucose *q.v.* molecules. 2. An animal starch *q.v.* which is stored in the animal body for future conversion into sugar (glucose *q.v.*) and for subsequent use as a source of energy.

GLYCOGENESIS 1. The formation of glycogen *q.v.* from glucose *q.v.* or from other monosaccharides *q.v.*, e.g., fructose *q.v.* or galactose *q.v.* 2. The production of glycogen in the body. Glycogen is the storage form of carbohydrate *q.v.* in animals.

GLYCOGENOLYSIS Hydrolysis *q.v.* of glycogen *q.v.* to glucose-6-phosphate or to glucose *q.v.* cf: glycogenolytic.

GLYCOGENOLYTIC A substance that hydrolyzes *q.v.* glycogen *q.v.* to glucose *q.v.* cf: glycogenolysis *q.v.*

GLYCOLYSIS 1. The production of energy from the anaerobic *q.v.* breakdown of glucose *q.v.* 2. Anaerobic pathway *q.v.* 3. Respiratory process in which sugar is changed anaerobically to pyruvic acid *q.v.* with the liberation of a small amount of useful energy. 4. A process of breakdown conversion of simple and complex carbohydrates *q.v.* to metabolic *q.v.* end products that are at a lower energy level than the original materials. 5. The conversion of glucose to lactic acid *q.v.* in body tissues, especially muscle tissue. As molecular *q.v.* oxygen *q.v.* is not consumed in the process, ~ is referred to as anaerobic glycolysis *q.v.*

GLYCOLYSIS ANAEROBIC 1. Anaerobic *q.v.* glycolysis *q.v.* 2. The metabolic *q.v.* pathway in muscles that breaks down sugars very rapidly into lactic acid *q.v.*, thereby liberating the large amounts of energy needed for speed and power activities.

GLYCONEOGENESIS The formation of glycogen from protein *q.v.* or frat compounds. cf: gluconeogenesis.

GLYCOPROTEINS Proteins *q.v.* with carbohydrate *q.v.* groups attached at specific locations.

GLYCOSIDE A plant product consisting of an organic molecule *q.v.* combined with sugar. Some very important drugs are ~s, e.g., cardiac ~s.

GLYCOSURIA Sugar in the urine typical of diabetes mellitus *q.v.*

GLYCOSYLATION The attachment of a carbohydrate *q.v.* molecule *q.v.* to another molecule such as a protein *q.v.*

GNP An acronym for gross national product *q.v.*

GOAL 1. In psychology, a commodity or condition capable of reducing or eliminating a drive *q.v.* 2. An incentive. 3. In education, the end toward which the learner strives. 4. The intermediary guidepost between the mission *q.v.* and objective *q.v.* 5. A broad, general statement of intent that gives direction to a plan, such as an educational process. 6. A long-range target indicating the ultimate outcome of some endeavor. 7. A desired end result target that provides general direction for a long-term program. 8. A quantified statement of a desired future state or condition.

GOAL-ATTAINMENT MODEL OF EVALUATION One of two major approaches to evaluation *q.v.* which views evaluation as a measure of the degree of success or failure encountered by a program. ~ uses program goals *q.v.* to measure outcomes. cf: goal-based evaluation.

GOAL-BASED EVALUATION The use of goals *q.v.* of the project as a basis for evaluation *q.v.* and for determining whether they have been met. ct: goal-free evaluation.

GOAL-FREE EVALUATION Inferring the goals *q.v.* of a project from observations and measures of what has occurred as a result of the project. These goals, and the success with which they have been achieved, are compared with the intended goals.

GOAL INTEGRATION Compatibility between individual and organizational objectives *q.v.*

GOAL-ORIENTED APPRAISAL 1. MBO appraisal *q.v.* 2. Actual accomplishments are measured against quantitative objectives *q.v.* jointly established by employees and their supervisors.

GOAL-SEEKING 1. Behavior directed toward the achievement of a particular goal *q.v.* or objective *q.v.* 2. Goal-seeking activity.

GOAL-SETTING A form of behavior that is directed toward the achievement of a particular goal *q.v.* cf: goal seeking.

GOBLET CELLS Cells within the epithelial *q.v.* lining of the airways that produce the mucus *q.v.* required for cleaning these passages.

GO-FAST A slang term referring to methamphetamine *q.v.*

GOING IN DRAG Dressing in female attire, usually with extensive makeup, by a male. These males may be homosexual *q.v.*

GOING RATE In business, the amount being paid in an area or industry for similar work.

GOING STEADY A loosely bound commitment between two people that they agree to date, socialize, and otherwise associate on a love relationship level only with each other. It is a preliminary stage that may be followed by an engagement period *q.v.*

GOITER A condition characterized by an enlargement of the thyroid gland *q.v.* ~s are often caused by an iodine deficiency.

GOITRIN The antithyroid or goitrogenic compound obtained from turnips and the seeds of cruciferous plants.

GOLGI BODY The cell organelle *q.v.* that functions in the packaging and storage of chemical substances before they are secreted.

GONAD 1. The testes *q.v.* in the males and the ovaries *q.v.* in the female. 2. The reproductive glands. 3. The ~ produces gonadotropin *q.v.* hormones *q.v.* that are responsible for the development of secondary sex characteristics *q.v.*

GONADAL HORMONES Hormones *q.v.* secreted by the gonads *q.v.* cf: gonadotropins.

GONADAL SEXUALITY A sexuality *q.v.* label that reflects the existence of either testicles *q.v.* or ovaries *q.v.*

GONADECTOMY The surgical removal of all or part of the gonads *q.v.*

GONADOTROPIN-RELEASING FACTOR (GRF) A hormone *q.v.*-like substance produced by the hypothalamus *q.v.* that controls the formation and release of the pituitary hormones *q.v.* concerned with sexual maturity and reproduction. cf: gonadotropin-releasing hormone.

GONADOTROPIN-RELEASING HORMONE (GnRH) A substance produced by the hypothalamus *q.v.* that controls the production and release of luteinizing hormone *q.v.* and follicle-stimulating hormone (FSH) *q.v.* cf: gonadotropin-releasing factor (GRF).

GONADOTROPINS 1. Male reproductive hormone *q.v.*: (a) follicle-stimulating hormone (FSH) *q.v.*, secreted by the anterior pituitary gland *q.v.* which stimulates the seminiferous tubules *q.v.* of the testes *q.v.* to produce sperm *q.v.* and also stimulates the ovary *q.v.* in the female; (b) interstitial-cell-stimulating hormone (ICSH) *q.v.*, secreted by the anterior pituitary gland which stimulates interstitial cells around the seminiferous tubules to produce testosterone *q.v.*

GONADS Reproductive glands: in males, the testes, and in females, the ovaries. cf: gonadal hormones; gonad.

GONOCOCCAL Pertaining to the bacterium that causes gonorrhea *q.v.*

GONOCOCCAL ARTHRITIS Inflammation *q.v.* of the joints of the body resulting from gonorrheal *q.v.* infection *q.v.*

GONOCOCCAL DERMATITIS Skin inflammation *q.v.* resulting from gonorrheal *q.v.* infection *q.v.*

GONOCOCCAL ENDOCARDITIS Inflammation *q.v.* of the heart valve resulting from gonorrheal *q.v.* infection *q.v.*

GONOCOCCAL PHARYNGITIS Inflammation *q.v.* of the throat caused by gonorrheal *q.v.* infection *q.v.*

GONOCOCCUS The specific etiologic *q.v.* agent of gonorrhea *q.v.* discovered by Neisser and named Neisseria gonorrhea.

GONOPHORE A gonad-bearing structure.

GONORRHEA 1. A sexually transmitted disease (STD) *q.v.* that is characterized by symptoms *q.v.* that explicitly manifest in the male, but may be asymptomatic *q.v.* in the female. The first symptoms to appear in the male are a slight milky discharge from the urethra *q.v.* and a burning sensation during urination *q.v.* Later symptoms include redness and swelling at the meatus *q.v.* of the penis *q.v.*

and an increase in the discharge, sometimes containing blood. ~ is caused by a gram-negative diplococcus bacterium, the Neisseria gonorrhea *q.v.* 2. Slang expressions include clap, whites, and morning drop.

GONORRHEAL Pertaining to gonorrhea *q.v.*

GOOD CONTINUATION A factor in visual grouping where contours tend to be perceived with little change in their direction.

GOOD SAMARITAN LAW Pertains to state laws that protect a person from liability lawsuits who assist a victim of an accident or sudden illness.

GOSSYPOL 1. A cotton seed derivative that blocks spermatogenesis *q.v.* 2. An experimental contraceptive for men that inhibits sperm production.

GOUT 1. A metabolic *q.v.* disease resulting in deposit of urates *q.v.* in the joints. 2. A form of arthritis *q.v.* 3. An inherited *q.v.* condition, ~ usually develops in men between the ages of 40 and 60. The condition results from an excess of uric acid *q.v.* in the blood that accumulates in the joints to produce severe inflammation *q.v.* Years ago, chronic pain and deformity were common characteristics of ~, but now medical treatment almost always controls the disease.

GOVERNMENTAL HEALTH AGENCY An organization concerned with some aspect of health that is tax supported and controlled by local, state, or federal government. ct: voluntary health agency.

GOVERNMENTAL IMMUNITY In law, immunity from tort *q.v.* actions enjoyed by governmental units in common-law states. cf: sovereign immunity.

GOVERNOR'S PROCLAMATION In politics, a means by which the governor may call an extra or special session of the legislature.

GP An acronym for general practitioner of medicine. cf: family doctor.

G PULL The force of the pull of gravity on the human body.

GRAAFIAN FOLLICLES Small sacs in the ovaries *q.v.* in which the egg matures and from which it is discharged at the time of ovulation *q.v.* When the ~ mature, an egg is discharged and the corpus luteum *q.v.* develops in the place from which the egg was released. Named after Graaf, a seventeenth century Dutch anatomist *q.v.*

GRADED SCHOOLS Schools organized using a step system whereby students are usually grouped related to chronological age rather than abilities.

GRADED SCHOOL SYSTEM A division of schools into groups of students according to the curriculum *q.v.* or the ages of pupils as in the six elementary grades. cf: graded schools.

GRADE EQUIVALENT SCORE A score on a standardized test *q.v.* that indicates the level of performance with reference to average performance at various grade levels.

GRADIENT A progressive change in a physical quantity over a period of time. cf: gradient of reinforcement.

GRADIENT OF REINFORCEMENT The curve that describes the declining effectiveness of reinforcement with increasing delay between the response and the reinforcer.

GRADUATED RECIPROCATION IN TENSION REDUCTION (GRIT) A proposal for the de-escalation of patterns of mutual exploitation in social change.

GRADUATE STUDENT A student who holds a bachelor's degree or first professional degree, or equivalent, and is taking courses at the post-baccalaureate level, generally working toward the master's or doctorate degree.

GRADUATION REQUIREMENTS Courses required of all students for graduation.

GRAE An acronym for generally recognized as effective, a term defined by the FDA *q.v.* with reference to the ingredients found in OTC *q.v.* drugs. cf: GRAS.

GRAFENBERG SPOT 1. G spot *q.v.* 2. An extremely sensitive area on the front wall of the vagina *q.v.* about 1 in into the opening. There is some controversy about the existence of the ~ as it cannot be located in all women.

GRAFT In medicine, the repair of a tissue defect by placement of a similar tissue from elsewhere in the body.

GRAHL An acronym for generally recognized as honestly labeled. cf: GRAE; GRAS.

GRAICUNAS' FORMULA In business management, a formula that makes the span of management point as the number of a manager's subordinates increases arithmetically, the number of possible relationships between the manager and those subordinates increases geometrically.

GRAIN 1. In botany, the fruit of the grass family; a small, dry, one-seeded fruit that does not open at maturity and in which the seed coat is fused with the pericarp *q.v.* 2. A measurement of weight formerly used in pharmacy, where one grain is equal to 65 mg.

GRAIN ALCOHOL Alcohol *q.v.* made from the fermentation *q.v.* of a cereal grain. Often used in reference to an alcohol product that is virtually pure ethyl alcohol *q.v.* cf: absolute alcohol.

GRAIN NEUTRAL SPIRITS Ethyl alcohol *q.v.* distilled to the purity of 190 proof or 95% alcohol *q.v.*

GRAM A basic unit of mass in the metric system of measurement.

GRAMMAR A structural characteristic of all languages; the ~s of human languages include phonological, morphological, syntactic, and semantic rules.

GRAMMAR SCHOOL Generally considered to be elementary school (grades K-6).

GRANDEUR (DELUSION) In psychology, a condition characterized by a person falsely believing that he or she is a person of great renown. cf: delusion.

GRANDFATHER CLAUSE In law and politics, laws providing new or additional professional qualifications often contain a ~ exempting persons presently practicing the affected profession from having to comply.

GRANDIOSITY 1. An inflated appraisal of one's own worth, power, knowledge, importance, or identity. 2. Delusion *q.v.* of exaggerated importance or power.

GRAND MAL EPILEPSY 1. A severe form of epilepsy *q.v.* involving periodic loss of consciousness and violent generalized convulsions. 2. Grand mal seizures *q.v.*

GRAND MAL SEIZURES 1. The most dramatic form of epilepsy *q.v.* characterized by visual or olfactory hallucinations *q.v.* called the aura *q.v.*, muscular movements of the mouth, numbness, tingling, or twitching of muscles. The person may fall, cry, lose consciousness, and have uncontrolled contractions of the muscles of the extremities. Seizures usually last up to 5 min. 2. Convulsions characterized by loss of consciousness and tonic spasm of the musculature, usually followed by repetitive clonic jerking.

GRANDMA'S RULE Premack principle *q.v.*

GRANOLA A commonly used term to describe the various mixtures of oats, wheat, and other grains, fruits, seeds, and nuts.

GRANT An award of money or direct assistance to perform activities or programs in which the outcome is seen as less certain than that from a contract, with expected results described in general terms. Application can be submitted without having been solicited or through a program announcement (request for application, RFA). Most federal grants fall into nine categories as follows: (a) entitlement, which is a noncompetitive award and given automatically on the basis of legally defined formula to all agencies that qualify; (b) competitive, which is awarded for specific types of research, demonstration, training, and the like (only nonprofit organizations are usually eligible); (c) block grants, in which the federal government merely stipulates in broad terms how the state and local governments should spend the aid. The purpose of these grants is to decentralize the federal government. (d) Categorical grants are more restrictive of the block grants as they spell out in detail the specific categories in which the money must be spent; (e) demonstration grants, where funds are used to underwrite a feasibility study; (f) formula grants are awarded by federal agencies on the basis of a set formula—chief recipients being state governments; (g) matching grants are the same as matching funds *q.v.*; (h) project grants include an overall term for the wide variety of grants that support specific projects; and (i) research grants provide funds to carry out specific investigations and clinical trials.

GRANULATION TISSUE 1. A growth of young capillaries *q.v.* and fibrous tissue *q.v.* cells which is the basis for healing in some wounds. 2. Proud flesh *q.v.*

GRANULOCYTES Phagocytic *q.v.* white blood cells filled with granules containing potent chemicals that allow the cells to digest microorganisms *q.v.* Neutrophils *q.v.*, eosinophils *q.v.*, basophils *q.v.*, and mast cells are examples of ~.

GRANULOMA 1. Infiltration of tissue phagocytes *q.v.*, producing a granular matrix in the area of the invading parasite *q.v.* 2. Any one of a large group of distinctive focal lesions *q.v.* that is granule-like or nodular *q.v.* and is formed as a result of inflammatory *q.v.* reactions, and ordinarily persists in the tissue as a slowly smoldering inflammation *q.v.*

GRANULOMA CELLS The cells lining the ovarian follicle *q.v.* that enlarge and form the corpus luteum *q.v.*

GRANULOMA INGUINALE 1. A sexually transmitted disease (STD) *q.v.* 2. An STD *q.v.* caused by the bacterium *Donovania granulomatis* *q.v.* It involves the skin and lymphatics *q.v.* Symptoms are the appearance of a painless vesicle or papule *q.v.* spreading to involve the abdomen, buttocks, and thighs. Eventually, the person becomes anemic *q.v.*, weak, and finally dies. It is curable by the use of antibiotics *q.v.*

GRAPEVINE In business and industry, a network of informal organizational communication *q.v.* The ~ may spread gossip, secrets, and other forms of information not publically available.

GRAPHIC SCALE 1. In business and industry, a performance appraisal. 2. An employee evaluation method that consists of descriptive phrases arranged on a scale, with ratings indicated by checking appropriate phrases.

GRAS 1. An acronym for generally recognized as safe. 2. A list of food additives exempted from the FDA's *q.v.* requirements for toxicological *q.v.* tests because they had been used in foods for many years without problems before the requirement for testing went into effect. cf: GRAE.

GRATIFICATION In psychology, a source of pleasure or satisfaction.

GRAVE'S DISEASE 1. Exophthalmic goiter *q.v.* 2. Hyperthyroidism *q.v.* 3. A disorder caused by overproduction of the hormone *q.v.*, thyroxin *q.v.*, marked by extreme weight loss, tremors, excessive anxiety, increased sweating, and psychomotor *q.v.* agitation.

GRAVID Pregnant *q.v.*

GRAVIDITY Pertains to the number of pregnancies *q.v.* a woman has had. cf: gravid.

GRAVITATIONAL WATER Water that the soil is unable to retain against the force of gravity.

GRAY LOBBY The advocacy movement whose members are concerned with the needs of the elderly. These persons come from the general public, organizations of older people, and health and welfare professionals.

GRAY MATTER The neural *q.v.* tissue made up largely of nerve cell bodies that constitutes the cortex *q.v.* covering the cerebral hemisphere *q.v.*, the nuclei *q.v.* in lower brain areas, columns of the spinal cord, and the ganglia *q.v.* of the autonomic nervous system *q.v.*

GRAY PANTHERS A political organization whose chief purpose is to combat ageism *q.v.* and old-age stereotyping.

GREATER TROCHANTER A large, bony prominence developed from an independent center near the extremity of the femur *q.v.* cf: trochanter.

GREAT FAMILY In sociology, the large, extended family *q.v.* as seen in the traditional Chinese family system.

GREEK CULTURE In regard to sexual activity, anal intercourse.

GREENHOUSE EFFECT The warming of the earth's surface that is produced when solar heat becomes trapped by layers of carbon dioxide and other gases.

GREEN MANURE In agriculture, a fresh green crop that is plowed under to increase the organic matter and nitrogen content of the soil.

GREENSTICK FRACTURE An incomplete fracture causing partial disruption and bending of the bone. cf: fracture.

GRF An acronym for gonadotropin-releasing factor *q.v.*

GRID ORGANIZATIONAL DEVELOPMENT (Grid OD) In business and industry, a commonly used organizational development technique based on a theoretical model called the managerial grid.

GRIEF 1. A powerful emotion *q.v.* Symptoms *q.v.* may include emotional debilitation, interference with mental, emotional, and physiological functioning. ~ can be mild, severe, momentary, or prolonged. Its stages are characterized by numbness, depression, and recovery. 2. Distress caused by bereavement *q.v.* ~ is usually self-limited and subsides after a reasonable length of time. On occasion, however, it can transform into depression *q.v.* ~ is associated with an important personal loss, e.g., death of a loved one.

GRIEVANCE PROCEDURE In business and industry, a procedure for the consideration and orderly resolution of disputes between management and employees.

GRIMACE A distorted facial expression, sometimes a symptom *q.v.* of schizophrenia *q.v.*

GRIT STRATEGY An acronym for graduated reciprocation in tension reduction *q.v.*

GROCER'S ITCH Eczema *q.v.* of the hands resulting from the handling of flour and sugar.

GROIN 1. The inguinal *q.v.* region of the body. 2. The junction of the abdomen *q.v.* with the thigh. 3. The topographical area of the abdomen related to the inguinal canal, lateral to the pubic region *q.v.*

GROSS NATIONAL PRODUCT (GNP) All the goods and services produced in a year in the United States changed to a dollar value.

GROUNDWATER Water in the water table below the earth's surface.

GROUP 1. In social psychology, two or more people who interact or communicate, perceive themselves as forming a unity, and typically share at least one common goal. 2. A unit of interacting personalities *q.v.* 3. A number of people who have common norms and patterned relationships with each other. 4. Any number of people who interact with one another, are psychologically aware of one another, and perceive themselves to be group. cf: group cohesiveness.

GROUP COHESIVENESS The attraction group *q.v.* members feel for one another in terms of desires to remain a member of the group and resist leaving it.

GROUP DYNAMICS The process of interaction of a person and the group *q.v.* ~ is concerned with the effect of a group on a person's readiness to change or to maintain certain standards or norms. 2. A group communication skill. Together they define the person and environment in mutual group-factor theory of intelligence. A factor-analysis *q.v.* approach to intelligence *q.v.* test performance which contends that intelligence is the composite of separate abilities without a sovereign capacity that enters into each. cf: Spearman's theory of general intelligence.

GROUPING PRACTICES In education, a set of criteria used to cluster students into different categories aimed at more efficient instructional delivery.

GROUP INVESTIGATION In education, a process of learning together in a cooperative manner. cf: cooperative learning.

GROUP MARRIAGE 1. Involves two marriages, two couples and an additional person, or one couple and an additional person. One of the most noteworthy experiments occurred through the establishment of the Oneida Community in upstate New York in 1884 by John Humphrey Noyes. The experiment ended in the 1880s when the community splintered and Noyes retreated to Canada. 2. A marriage in which there are multiple mates of more than one gender *q.v.*—a form of polygamy *q.v.*

GROUP MIND McDougalls' early concept for the shared beliefs or conceptions in a group *q.v.* said not to be reducible to individuals' mental processes.

GROUP NORMS Appropriate or standard behavior *q.v.* that is required of informal group *q.v.* members.

GROUP PLAN Representing the majority of health insurance policies; they are usually sold through one's employment. Such plans tend to be less expensive and broader in coverage than individual plans *q.v.*

GROUP PRACTICE In medicine, a medical practice in which two or more physicians share office space, nurses, and sometimes patients.

GROUP PROCESS In health education, the application of educational and communication principles in group situations, designed to facilitate problem solving and decision making through mutual stimulation of creative and critical thinking or to increase the credibility and attractiveness of recommended health practices.

GROUP-SUMMARY APPRAISAL In business and industry, managers reach a consensus of assessment of subordinates' performance.

GROUP TEST A test that can be administered to several people at the same time. ct: individual test.

GROUP THEORY A group *q.v.*: number, objects, concepts, or events. ~ explains change from within and change from outside.

GROUP THERAPY 1. A social interaction as a means for understanding and dealing with mental and emotional problems. ~ tends to help the persons in the group *q.v.* to clarify their values *q.v.* and establish new and more effective value systems. 2. Psychotherapy *q.v.* of several persons at one time. 3. A form of therapy in which one or two therapists meet with 6 to 10 clients and attempt to resolve emotional problems by analyzing intragroup relationships.

GROUPTHINK 1. The mode of thinking that people engage in when seeking agreement becomes so dominant in a group *q.v.* that it tends to override the realistic appraisal of alternative problems solutions. 2. A set of behavior patterns (including the delimiting of alternatives, the reduction of critical examination, and the stifling of expert opinion) that often undermines the decision-making process in group situations.

GROWTH 1. Changes in structure and function of cells, tissues, and organs. Cells grow in three ways: (a) increase in size, (b) increase in numbers, and (c) increase in intercellular material. 2. The process whereby the body increases in size. 3. Irreversible increases in number and size of cells due to division and enlargement, usually accompanied by cell differentiation. cf: development.

GROWTH AND DEVELOPMENT The changes in structure and function of cells, tissues, and organs. An increase in size and numbers of cells and improved functioning. A basis for motivation *q.v.* cf: growth.

GROWTH HORMONE A hormone *q.v.* that regulates growth *q.v.*

GROWTH MEDIUM In bacteriology, a substance containing appropriate nutrients for growing bacteria *q.v.*

GROWTH MOTIVATION In psychology, behavior designed to overcome weaknesses.

GROWTH NEEDS Self-actualization needs *q.v.*

GROWTH SUBSTANCE A synthetic *q.v.* chemical that affects growth *q.v.*

G SPOT 1. An abbreviation for Grafenberg spot *q.v.* 2. A spot on the anterior vaginal *q.v.* wall of some women that increases in size during sexual arousal. In some women, stimulation of the spot has been reported to lead to orgasm *q.v.* accompanied by ejaculation *q.v.*

GSR An acronym for galvanic skin response *q.v.*

G SUIT An inflatable coverall that can be used to exert general body compression. Originally designed for astronauts so that they could safely endure the force of sufficient acceleration to leave the gravitational pull of the Earth.

GUAIAC TEST A test to detect microscopic *q.v.* presence of blood in the feces *q.v.* that may be an early sign of colon cancer *q.v.*

GUANINE A purine base found in DNA *q.v.* and RNA *q.v.*

GUARANTEED ANNUAL WAGE (GAW) An agreement whereby an employer guarantees a certain number of weeks of employment.

GUARANTEED RENEWABLE A health insurance policy that states that the insured has the right to continue the policy in force by the payment of premiums to a specific age, during which period the insurance company has no right, on its own, to alter the provisions of the policy.

GUARDIANSHIP A legal process whereby another person assumes responsibility for managing an incompetent person's affairs.

GUEVODOCES In Spanish, literally means "penis at twelve." A group of 46, XY individuals in the Dominican Republic who, because of an inherited *q.v.* disorder in the production of androgen *q.v.*, are born with female-looking external genitals *q.v.* but become masculinized at puberty.

GUIDE CHART-PROFILE METHOD (JOB EVALUATION) Compensable factors used to evaluate positions. A method used in business and industry.

GUIDED DISCOVERY In education, a method of teaching in which the student is free to explore with directions from the teacher.

GUIDED EXPERIENCE In business and industry, a variety of approaches to individual development, especially job-rotation assignment. 2. In education, guided discovery *q.v.*

GUIDED IMAGERY In psychology, the process of visualizing oneself responding in a positive and controlled way to a stressor *q.v.*

GUIDELINE METHOD (JOB EVALUATION) In business and industry, salaries are established to reflect the current market prices of positions.

GUILLAIN–BARRE SYNDROME An uncommon, often temporary paralysis *q.v.* that results from exposure to certain influenza *q.v.* viruses *q.v.* or vaccinations *q.v.*

GUILT 1. A powerful emotion *q.v.* Results from remorse over events that have already occurred. 2. Anxiety reactions *q.v.* conditioned to aspects of one's own behavior *q.v.* 3. An unpleasant feeling of sinfulness arising from behavior or desires contrary to a person's ethical *q.v.* principles. ~ involves self-devaluation and apprehension growing out of fears of punishment.

GULLET 1. The esophagus *q.v.* 2. The passage leading from the pharynx *q.v.* to the stomach comprising a muscular tube lined with squamous epithelium *q.v.*

GUMBOIL 1. In dentistry, an infection related to a decayed tooth or irritation from a denture. Characterized by red and swollen gum tissue and may contain pus. 2. An abscess *q.v.* on the gum of the oral structures.

GUMMA 1. A lesion *q.v.* formed during the late stages of syphilis *q.v.* 2. A large, fast growing syphilis tumor *q.v.*

GUMS In dentistry, the dense, fibrous tissue, covered by mucous membrane *q.v.* that envelops the alveolar *q.v.* processes of the upper and lower jaws and surrounds the necks of the teeth.

GUNGEON Marijuana *q.v.* originating in Africa or Jamaica.

GUSTATORY Pertaining to taste.

GUTHRIE BLOOD TEST A test given to infants to detect the presence of phenylketonuria *q.v.* Routinely given to all new born infants.

GYANDROMORPH An individual in which one part of the body is female and another part is male. A sex mosaic.

GYNECOLOGIST A physician specializing in the treatment of the health problems of the female sexual and reproductive organs. cf: gynecology.

GYNECOLOGY 1. Usually, obstetrics and gynecology. Concerned with the health of the female, especially diagnosis and treatment of diseases of the reproductive organs, and care of pregnant women, delivery of the baby, and postnatal care. 2. The branch of medicine concerned with the health and disorders of the female reproductive system.

GYNECOMASTIA 1. The development of the breasts when physiologically inappropriate. 2. Female-like development of the male breasts. cf: galactorrhea.

GYRUS A ridge or convolution of the cerebral cortex *q.v.* A convoluted ridge.

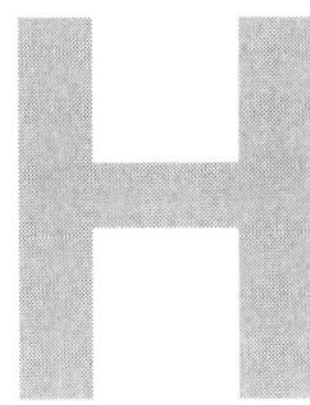

HABILITATION The process of making fit, often referring to training.

HABIT 1. Characteristic to behave in a particular way. 2. Characteristic form or bodily appearance of an organism *q.v.* 3. A learned act that is repeated when certain environmental cues are present. 4. Addiction *q.v.* to a drug. 5. Habituation *q.v.* 6. Any product of learning *q.v.* cf: health habit.

HABITAT The natural environment of a living organism *q.v.*; the place where it is usually found.

HABIT-FAMILY HIERARCHY An expression referring to the fact that any stimulus *q.v.* tends to elicit a group of responses *q.v.* that vary in strength.

HABITUATION 1. In psychology, a decline in the tendency to respond to stimuli *q.v.* that have become familiar because of repeated exposure. 2. Characterized by a psychological *q.v.* craving for a drug *q.v.* with an absence of the withdrawal syndrome *q.v.* A condition resulting from the repeated consumption of a drug which includes (a) a desire (but not a compulsion) to continue taking the drug for the sense of improved well-being that it engenders, (b) little or no tendency to increase the dose, (c) some degree of psychic dependence on the effect of the drug, but an absence of physical dependence *q.v.*, and (d) a detrimental effect, if any, primarily on the individual. 3. The process of allowing a person to become accustomed to a particular situation. 4. In physiology *q.v.*, a process whereby an organism's response to the same stimulus temporarily decreases with repeated presentation.

HABITUATION METHOD 1. A procedure that is widely used in infant research to investigate the discriminatory and memory abilities of infants. 2. Habituation procedure *q.v.*

HABITUATION PROCEDURE 1. A method used in the study of infant perception *q.v.* 2. Continuous exposure to a visual stimulus *q.v.* resulting in the infant ignoring it. 3. Habituation method *q.v.*

HAEC VERBA Pertains to the same words (identical).

HAIR FOLLICLE A small sac that extends from the epidermis *q.v.* into the subcutaneous *q.v.* tissue and which contains the individual hair root.

HAIR IMPLANTATION A surgical procedure of grafting hair-producing tissue from one part of the body to another part.

HALATION A blurring of vision resulting from light from the wrong direction.

HALCION A commercial preparation of triazolam *q.v.*

HALDOL A commercial preparation of haloperidol *q.v.*

HALF-LIFE 1. The time in which radioactivity originally associated with an isotope *q.v.* will be reduced by one-half through radioactive decay. 2. In pharmacology, the time required by the body tissue or organ to metabolize *q.v.* or inactivate half the amount of a substance taken. cf: biological half-life.

HALF-RING SPLINT A traction splint with a hinged half-ring at the upper end that allows the splint to be used on either the right or the left leg.

HALFWAY HOUSE 1. A treatment center for alcoholics *q.v.* or other drug addicts *q.v.* where they can receive support and are provided with a retreat to withdraw from addiction *q.v.* 2. In psychiatry, a treatment facility to assist in transition from a mental hospital to the community, usually of an inpatient type. 3. A homelike residence for people who are considered too disturbed to remain in their accustomed surroundings but do not require the total care of a mental institution. 4. Living arrangements in which formerly institutionalized patients prepare to readjust to reenter society. ct: day hospital; night hospital.

HALISTERESIS The lack of calcium in bones.

HALITOSIS Bad breath; a symptom of oral, digestive, or pulmonary disorder.

HALLUCINATION 1. A sensory perception that has no environmental stimulus to bring it about. The most common is auditory *q.v.* Psychotic *q.v.* persons may experience taste or small ~s. Visual ~s are very rare except in organic psychosis *q.v.* 2. A sensory experience which does not exist outside the mind of an individual and is a false perception of the real conditions. ct: illusion.

HALLUCINOGEN 1. Chemicals capable of inducing bizarre alterations in perceptions *q.v.* and states of consciousness. 2. Psychoactive *q.v.* chemicals that produce psychedelic effects *q.v.* 3. Any of several drugs or chemicals popularly called psychedelics, which produce sensations, such as distortion of time, space, color, sound, and other bizarre effects. While they are pharmacologically *q.v.* non-narcotic, some of these drugs, e.g., marijuana *q.v.*, are regulated under state or federal narcotic laws.

HALLUCINOGENIC 1. A chemical capable of producing distortions of the senses. 2. Causing or producing hallucinations *q.v.*

HALLUX (HALLUS) The great toe.

HALLUX VALGUS A bunion *q.v.*

HALO EFFECT 1. The tendency to assume that persons who possess one positive characteristic, also possess other positive characteristics. 2. In making judgments, the tendency to rate a person high or low on all traits because of the knowledge that he or she is high or low on one or a few traits.

HALOGENS Very active nonmetallic elements such as fluorine, chlorine, bromine, and iodine.

HALOPERIDOL 1. An antipsychotic *q.v.* drug. 2. Haldol *q.v.* is a brand name.

HALOPHILIC 1. Salt-tolerant. 2. Osmophilic *q.v.*

HALSTEAD–REITAN NEUROPSYCHOLOGY BATTERY A neuropsychology *q.v.* test for adults and children that measures functions such as concept formation, concentration, memory, motor coordination, and sensory awareness in order to assess the possibility of organic *q.v.* brain damage.

HALSTED RADICAL MASTECTOMY Surgical removal of the breast, skin, pectoral muscles, all auxiliary lymph nodes, and fat.

HAMILTON DEPRESSION SCALE A test used by psychologists or psychiatrists to assess the severity of depression *q.v.* of the patient.

HAND That part of the upper limb distal to the forearm *q.v.* consisting of the carpus *q.v.*, metacarpus *q.v.*, and fingers.

HANDICAP Pertains to persons who possess musculoskeletal disorders, neural disorders, cardiac disorders, hearing disorders, emotional disorders, and intellectual disorders. This term, however, has recently been replaced by the term handicapable *q.v.*

HANDICAPABLE 1. Handicapped *q.v.* 2. Refers to persons who possess a handicapping condition.

HANDICAPPED A person who has one or more of the exceptionalities: educable mentally retarded, trainable mental retarded, hard of hearing, deaf; speech-impaired, visually handicapped, seriously emotionally disturbed, orthopedically impaired, health impaired, specific learning disabled, deaf-blind, and multihandicapped.

HANDICAPPED CHILDREN Children who deviate from the norm due to physical, emotional, or mental disabilities. cf: handicapped.

HANDICAPPED LEARNER One who is mentally retarded, hard of hearing, deaf, speech impaired, visually handicapped, seriously disturbed, emotionally crippled, or health impaired. cf: handicapped.

HANDICAPPING CONDITION 1. A person possessing one or more conditions that limits capability. 2. Handicapable *q.v.* 3. Any condition that limits a person's mobility, strength, or well-being to the extent that special teaching may be required. cf: handicapped.

HANDLEBAR PALSY A condition characterized by a loss of sensation in the hands and an inability to coordinate finger movements due to ulnar nerve irritation. The condition results from excessive pressure being placed on the hands while riding a bicycle.

HANGNAIL A sliver of cuticle *q.v.* that is loose from around the edge of the finger nail.

HANGOVER 1. A disturbance in the body resulting from excessive use of alcohol *q.v.* Symptoms *q.v.* vary from person to person and even at different occasions for the same person. Symptoms may include headache, upset stomach, vomiting, thirst, and general weakness. 2. Temporary, acute *q.v.* physical and psychological distress following excessive consumption of alcoholic beverages.

HAPLOID 1. The reduced, or *n*, chromosome *q.v.* number, characteristic of the gametophyte *q.v.* generation. 2. Nuclear state of an organism in which cells have only one of each type of chromosome. 3. Monoploid. 4. An organism or cell having only one complete set (*n*) of chromosomes or one genome *q.v.* 5. Having the basic chromosome number for the species.

HAPLOPIA Single vision.

HAPTEN 1. A substance that does not stimulate *q.v.* antibody formation but that will combine with a carrier antigen to stimulate antibody formation. 2. An incomplete antigen *q.v.* incapable of producing antibodies *q.v.* until united with protein *q.v.*

HAPTIC Refers to touch sensation and information transmitted through body movement and/or position.

HAPTOGLOBIN A serum protein *q.v.*, alpha globulin *q.v.* in the blood.

HARD-CORE EROTICA Erotica that explicitly depicts genitals and sexual acts. cf: hard-core pornography.

HARD-CORE PORNOGRAPHY Materials aimed at sexually arousing a consumer, depicting sexual acts including penetration in close focus. cf: hard-core erotica. ct: soft-core pornography.

HARDENING OF THE ARTERIES Arteriosclerosis *q.v.*

HARDINESS A constellation of personality *q.v.* characteristics—commitment, control, and challenge—that has been linked to resistance to stress *q.v.*

HARD NARCOTICS Habit forming *q.v.* or addicting *q.v.* drugs derived from opium or identified as narcotics *q.v.* under federal law.

HARD-OF-HEARING A term used to categorize individuals with a sense of hearing that is defective but somewhat functional. cf: handicapped.

HARDWARE Mechanical and electronic devices that aid in classroom instruction, e.g., computers.

HARD WATER Water that contains a relatively large amount of minerals such as iron or calcium. ct: soft water.

HARELIP A congenital *q.v.* failure of the upper lip to fuse in the middle during embryonic *q.v.* development.

HARTMAN AND FITHIAN SEX THERAPY METHOD An approach to sexual dysfunction that combines procedures developed by Masters and Johnson with those of William Hartman and Marilyn Fithian that aims to help persons to learn more positive sexual behaviors. (Developed at the Center for Marital and Sexual Studies at Long Beach, California).

HAS An acronym for high-amplitude sucking method *q.v.*

HASHISH 1. A powered and sifted form of the unadulterated resin exuded from the flowering tops of the female hemp plant, *Cannabis sativa q.v.* or *Cannabis indica q.v.* 2. The dried resin of the cannabis plant, stronger in its effects than the dried leaves and stems which constitute marijuana *q.v.* cf: hashish oil.

HASHISH OIL 1. The dark, viscous liquid produced by repeated extraction of cannabis *q.v.* plant materials with a THC *q.v.* concentration greater than that of hashish *q.v.* 2. Hash oil. 3. A slang term for oil of cannabis, a liquid extract from the marijuana *q.v.* plant.

HAUSTORIA In biology, modified hyphal *q.v.* elements found in parasitic *q.v.* species that penetrate into the host for absorption. cf: haustorium.

HAUSTORIUM 1. In parasitic *q.v.* vascular plants, a specialized outgrowth from the stem or root that penetrates the living host tissues and absorbs foods or other materials. 2. A specialized fungus *q.v.* hypha *q.v.* that invades a host cell.

HAVERSIAN CANAL 1. A minute vascular *q.v.* canal located in osseous *q.v.* tissue. Named for Havers, an English anatomist of the late seventeenth century. 2. Small canals in bone to conduct blood and other fluids.

HAWTHORNE EFFECT 1. The tendency for subjects in a study to respond to almost any change as an indicator of appreciation that someone has taken the trouble to alter conditions. 2. Change in a subject's behavior caused by awareness of being in an experiment. 3. A change in performance that is attributable to the attention paid to subjects in an experiment.

HAY FEVER Allergic rhinitis *q.v.*

HAZARD ANALYSIS Identification of health or safety hazards before an accident or illness occurs. cf: hazardous.

HAZARDOUS A substance, situation, or behavior that is likely to result in injury or disease.

HAZARDOUS MATERIAL RESPONSE TEAM Emergency personnel who are trained in the identification, containment, and cleanup of hazardous *q.v.* materials.

HAZARDOUS SUBSTANCE DATA BANK (HSDB) A factual nonbibliographic data bank focusing on the toxicology *q.v.* of potentially hazardous *q.v.* chemicals. The data bank is enhanced with information from such related areas as emergency handling procedures, environmental fate, human exposure, detection methods, and regulatory requirements. Data are derived from a core set of standard texts and monographs, government documents, technical reports, and primary journal literature.

HAZARDOUS SUBSTANCE DATA MANAGEMENT SYSTEM (HAZDAT) The scientific database developed by ATSDR *q.v.* to manage data collection, retrieval analysis, and use through the more sophisticated technologies provided by computerization. ~ will allow agencies to locate information on the release of hazardous substances into the environment and ascertain the effects of hazardous *q.v.* substances on health with improved uniformity, efficiency, and precision.

HAZARDOUS SUBSTANCE LISTING A listing of 250 priority hazardous *q.v.* substances compiled by using an algorithm *q.v.* to weight the three basic criteria of toxicity *q.v.*, frequency of occurrence at superfund sites, and potential for human exposure.

HAZARDOUS WASTE WORKER SURVEILLANCE Activities that evaluate exposure or trends in adverse health effects over a specified period of time at the workplace. Because hazardous *q.v.* waste workers are potentially exposed to higher concentrations of contaminants, researchers can use information gathered from this population to evaluate a range of exposures.

HAZARD RANKING SYSTEM (HRS) EPA's system for ranking priority of sites designated for cleanup.

HAZDAT An acronym for Hazardous Substance Data Management System *q.v.*

HB An acronym for hemoglobin *q.v.*

HbO_2 An acronym for oxyhemoglobin *q.v.*

HCG An acronym for human chorionic gonadotropin *q.v.*

HDL An acronym for high-density lipoprotein *q.v.*

HEAD 1. In botany, inflorescence of sensile or nearly sensile flowers on a very short or flattened floral branch. 2. In human anatomy, that part of the upper extremity of the body containing the brain and the organs of sight, hearing, taste, and smell.

HEAD BAND In first aid and paramedics, a band used to fasten a victim's head to a spineboard *q.v.*

HEAD COLD Coryza *q.v.*

HEAD LOUSE 1. Infestation *q.v.* with the louse, Pediculosis humanis capitus *q.v.* 2. Pediculosis *q.v.*

HEAD START PROGRAMS Federally funded programs at the pre-elementary school level designed to provide learning opportunities for those children who have not had access to environments and experiences conducive to academic achievement. This program was spearheaded by Urie Bronfenbrenner at Cornell University.

HEAD-TILT MANEUVER In first aid and emergency care, the procedure for opening the airway to relieve obstruction caused by the tongue. With one hand beneath the victim's neck and one hand on the victim's forehead, the neck is lifted and the head tilted backward as far as possible. Note: The recommended method is now the chin-lift *q.v.*

HEAF TEST A tuberculin test in which the test material is pushed into the skin by six tiny needles.

HEALTH 1. A sense of physical, mental, and social well-being; effective functioning, both within the person and by the person in his or her environment *q.v.* 2. A state of complete physical, mental, and social well-being, not merely the absence of disease or infirmity (WHO). 3. A quality of life involving dynamic interaction and independence among the person's physical well-being, mental and emotional reactions, and the social complex in which he or she exists. 4. An integrated method of functioning that is oriented toward optimal functioning. 5. The quality of physical, psychological, and sociological functioning that enables a person to deal adequately with self and others in a variety of situations. ~ is related to self-sufficiency *q.v.* and effectiveness in living. 6. A dynamic and relative state of functioning. 7. Human effectiveness; the qualifying factor for living. 8. A quality of life. 9. The quality of the individual that makes it possible to function effectively. 10. A quality of life involving dynamic interaction and interdependence of the physical, social, mental, and emotional dimensions of a person's well-being. 11. An elusive term which usually encompasses the option of individual and collective well-being with physical, social, and psychological dimensions.

HEALTH ADVISING A process of informing and assisting individuals or groups in making decisions and solving problems related to health *q.v.* cf: health counseling.

HEALTH ADVISOR A competent professionally prepared person, associated with appropriate professional associations, who is skilled to counsel and/or treat a person.

HEALTH AFFAIRS The social issues that are related to health *q.v.* cf: health problems.

HEALTH AND MEDICAL SERVICES A component of the health program *q.v.* comprised of medical, dental, and psychological services. It provides for the treatment and intervention programs as well as educational functions within the health education program *q.v.* cf: health services; school health services.

HEALTH ASSESSMENT A written evaluation of available data and information on the release of hazardous substances into the environment in a specific geographic area. The evaluation is used to assess any pertinent current or future impact on public health *q.v.*

HEALTH ATTITUDES 1. The predisposition to behave in a particular way regarding health matters. They are characterized by health beliefs *q.v.* or feelings. 2. Relatively lasting clusters of feelings, beliefs, and behavior tendencies directed toward specific objects, persons, or situations related to health *q.v.* cf: attitude; health behavior.

HEALTH BEHAVIOR 1. Actions and reactions one makes to promote personal and social health *q.v.*, maintain health *q.v.*, or restore health. ~ may be either health-related or health-directed *q.v.* 2. ~ can be viewed in terms of human plasticity *q.v.* and human energetics *q.v.* 3. That which is related to the prevention of disease or injury. 4. Actions customarily taken by a person that have an impact on personal and community well-being. ct: illness behavior; sick-role behavior.

HEALTH BELIEF A health-related *q.v.* statement or sense, declared or implied intellectually or emotionally, and accepted as being true by a person or group, sometimes referred to as the conventional wisdom. cf: health belief model.

HEALTH BELIEF MODEL 1. Concerned with the development of a theory and a science of health behavior *q.v.* change. There are three phases that lead to a health action: (a) individual perception, (b) modifying factors, and (c) the likelihood of action. *Individual perception*:

an element or phase of the ~ which includes the person's subjective risk of contracting a disease. Perception includes (a) personal susceptibility to the disease and (b) the severity of the disease which are interacting and necessary for modifying behavior. *Modifying factors:* an element or phase of the ~ which includes (a) demographic variables, (c) sociopsychological variables, and (d) structural variables combined with a perceived threat of the disease and reinforced by cues to act. *Likelihood of action*: an element or phase of the ~ influenced by a person's perceived benefits of preventive actions minus his or her barriers to preventive action directly influenced by certain modifying factors. 2. A composite of theories that predicts or explains a given person's willingness to accept a procedure used to detect or prevent disease. 3. A psychosocial formulation that explains health-related behavior *q.v.* at the level of personal decision making. 4. As originally developed, a composite of theories that predicts or explains a given person's willingness to accept a procedure used to detect or prevent disease.

HEALTH CARE The planned process which includes procedures and techniques for the maintenance of health *q.v.* cf: health care dilemma.

HEALTH CARE DILEMMA The confusion and inconsistencies associated with a haphazard health care system.

HEALTH CARE SYSTEM 1. All of the facilities, people, and functions directed toward promoting, maintaining, and restoring health *q.v.* 2. An organized system of health care *q.v.* services, personnel, equipment, and facilities, in which persons, families, groups, and communities receive services to prevent, diagnose, and treat diseases and to promote general health and well-being. cf: health care dilemma.

HEALTH CONCEPTS Organized ideas of health *q.v.* facts demonstrating significance, relationships, and application. cf: health facts.

HEALTH CONSULTATION A written or verbal response from ATSOR *q.v.* to a specific request for information about health risks related to a specific site, chemical release, or hazardous material.

HEALTH CONSUMER Any person who purchases health services and/or products.

HEALTH CONSUMERISM Consumer health *q.v.*

HEALTH COUNSELING Procedures by which teachers, nurses, and physicians interpret a health problem to learners and their parents as a means of helping them find a solution. cf: health guidance.

HEALTH CRITERIA 1. Indicators of a person's levels of health *q.v.* 2. Standards to establish a level of health or of health status *q.v.* Criteria that have been suggested are as follows: (a) How well do you function in a variety of normal situations? (b) Can you function better in a particular situation? (c) Do you have significant handicaps? (d) Are you expending energy needlessly to accomplish tasks? (e) Are you accomplishing tasks efficiently? (f) Do you possess a sense of self-worth? (g) Do you have a sense of social sensitivity? (h) Are you free from diseases that interfere with your functioning ability? (i) Do you make judgments and choices based upon knowledge rather than feelings or emotions? (j) Do you avoid self-destructive forms of behavior? (k) Is your overall lifestyle both health-related *q.v.* and health-directed *q.v.* as conditions dictate?

HEALTH DIARY A record of behavior *q.v.* and circumstances interpreted as health-related, kept on a daily or, at least, frequent basis.

HEALTH-DIRECTED BEHAVIOR 1. The actions one takes to promote health *q.v.*, prevent the onset of disease or disability, maintain present health status *q.v.*, restore health that failed, or solve a specific health problem. 2. A conscious effort to behave healthfully. 3. Activities specifically designed to maintain health through the use of technologies, e.g., immunization *q.v.* cf: health maintenance. ct: health-related behavior.

HEALTH DISORDERS Conditions or diseases that interfere with an individual's functioning but not necessarily or initially have an impact on his or her ability to move about independently in various settings.

HEALTH EDUCATED PERSON A person who has acquired sufficient knowledge about health matters or issues to be able to make decisions that result in health promotion and health maintenance. cf: health belief model.

HEALTH EDUCATION 1. In community health, a specialized area of community health practice concerned with the process of influencing health-related *q.v.* social and behavioral change in human populations by predisposing, enabling, and reinforcing voluntary decisions conducive to health *q.v.* 2. All of the experiences—planned or unplanned, direct or indirect—that influence the way learners think, feel, and act in regard to their own health as well as that of the community *q.v.* in which they live. 3. ~ is a process affecting intellectual, psychological, and social dimensions that increase our capacity to make informed health decisions affecting self, family, and community well-being. It is one of several processes for improving human effectiveness. 4. The sum of all experiences which favorably influence habits, attitudes, and knowledge relating to individual, community, and social health. 5. The process of providing learning experiences for the purpose of influencing knowledge, attitudes, or conduct related to individual, community, and world health. 6. The aim of ~ is to help people achieve health by their own actions and efforts. ~ begins, therefore, with the interests of people in improving their conditions of living—in developing a sense of responsibility for their own health betterment and for the health of their families and government. 7. A process that bridges the gap between health information and health practices. ~ motivates the person to take information and do something with it, to keep himself or herself healthier by avoiding actions that are harmful and by forming habits that are beneficial. 8. A process with intellectual, psychological, and social dimensions relating to activities which increase the abilities of people to make informed decisions affecting their personal, family, and community well-being. This process, based on scientific principles, facilitates learning and behavioral change in both health personnel and consumers including children and youth. 9. Systematically organized activities designed to aid learners in acquiring the knowledge, skills, understandings, attitudes, and behavior patterns necessary for living healthfully. 10. The process by which individuals, organizations, communities, and societies learn to make informed decisions about issues related to health and disease. This process may be either planned or unplanned. The planned process includes a variety of scheduled activities to assist target populations in making decisions. 11. Any designed combination of methods to facilitate voluntary adaptation of behavior conducive to health. 12. ~ may be defined on two levels: (a) *operational*: a deliberately planned, structured learning opportunity about health that occurs in a given setting at a given point in time and involves an interaction between a health educator *q.v.* and a learner; (b) *process*: a change in health-related behavior in individuals or groups that leads to an improvement in health status *q.v.* for those individuals or groups.

HEALTH EDUCATION ADMINISTRATOR 1. An individual trained in health education and administration whose direction, supervision, and coordination is such that programmatic goals are achieved with a maximum amount of efficiency and a minimum expenditure of human energy. Functioning categories include planning, structuring, administering, communicating, and evaluating. 2. A professional health educator who has the authority and responsibility for management and coordination of all health education policies, activities, and resources within a particular setting. cf: health education coordinator.

HEALTH EDUCATION CENTER A focal point for the health education efforts of a geographic region comprised of five components: (a) research and evaluation, (b) personnel development, (c) community service, (d) communication and media development, and (e) program development.

HEALTH EDUCATION COORDINATOR A professional educator who is responsible for the management and coordination of all health education policies, activities, and resources within a particular setting. cf: health education administrator.

HEALTH EDUCATION CURRICULUM All of the planned and unplanned learning experiences that affect health learning. Usually, it is a term used to describe the planned health education program *q.v.* within the school. cf: health education curriculum guide.

HEALTH EDUCATION CURRICULUM GUIDE The culminating document of evaluation and planning related to the health education *q.v.* needs of the learner. A tool to help teachers and learners to systematically achieve health goals *q.v.* through predetermined processes. cf: curriculum guide.

HEALTH EDUCATION FIELD That multidisciplinary practice that is concerned with designing, implementing, and evaluating educational programs that enable individuals, families, groups, organizations, and communities to plan active roles in achieving, protecting, and sustaining health *q.v.*

HEALTH EDUCATION GOALS Long-range plans specified as the desired overall outcome of health instruction/education. cf: goals.

HEALTH EDUCATION METHODOLOGY The science and art of altering the environment *q.v.* for maximum learning to result. It consists of approaches that include teaching/learning techniques and strategies *q.v.*

HEALTH EDUCATION MOVEMENT 1. The events that have contributed to the progress of health education *q.v.* 2. The historical foundations of health education.

HEALTH EDUCATION OF THE PUBLIC 1. Community health education. *q.v.* 2. Public health education. 3. A process designed for improvement and maintenance of health, directed toward the general population as contrasted with health education *q.v.* for the preparation of a health professional *q.v.*

HEALTH EDUCATION PRACTICES 1. Professional procedures that affect health knowledge, attitudes, and behavior *q.v.* and, ultimately, health status *q.v.* 2. The application of theory to health learning *q.v.* The areas of ~ are classified as (a) professional preparation, (b) organization and administration, (c) theory and application of program development, (d) educational methodology and communication, and their application to health learning, and (e) evaluation.

HEALTH EDUCATION PROCESS That continuum of learning that enables people as individuals and as members of social structures to voluntarily make decision, modify behaviors, and change social conditions in ways that are health enhancing.

HEALTH EDUCATION PROFESSION The educational specialty concerned with health issues, health problems, and health affairs and composed of persons trained in educational processes related to these health matters. cf: professionalism.

HEALTH EDUCATION PROGRAM 1. A planned and organized series of health education *q.v.* activities and procedures implemented with (a) an educational specialist assigned primary responsibility, (b) a budget, (c) an integrated set of goals and objectives sufficiently detailed to allow for evaluation, and (d) administrative support. 2. A planned combination of activities developed with the involvement of specific populations and based on a needs assessment, sound principles of education, and periodic evaluation using a clear set of goals and objectives.

HEALTH EDUCATION PROGRAM AND CURRICULUM COMMITTEE Consists of representatives from health educators, elementary school teachers, school administrators, medical, dental, and psychological services, and students. This committee establishes the basis for curriculum development in health education.

HEALTH EDUCATION RESOURCES 1. The materials such as videos, printed materials, posters, computers, etc., and the people that contribute to the health learning of people. 2. All the assets, human and material, that may be enlisted in the school organization or community to enrich the health education *q.v.* experiences of individuals or groups. cf: health resources.

HEALTH EDUCATOR 1. A highly trained individual who attempts to improve the health of others through the use of the educational process. The ~ may function within the school, community, industrial, and/or clinical settings. 2. An individual prepared to assist individuals, acting separately or collectively, to make informed decisions regarding matters affecting their personal health and that of others. 3. A practitioner who is professionally prepared in the field of health education, who demonstrates competence in both theory and practice, and who accepts responsibility to advance the aims of the health education profession. A ~ may practice his or her profession in a number of settings including schools, communities, medical care facilities, voluntary health agencies, business and industry, rehabilitation centers, professional and private agencies, and governmental agencies.

HEALTH ENVIRONMENT The state of the environment *q.v.*

HEALTH EXAMINATION 1. A medical checkup. 2. A positive evaluation by a physician of the health status *q.v.* of a person. Generally, applicable to the physical examination.

HEALTH FACTS 1. Health information *q.v.* 2. Scientific knowledge related to the health of people.

HEALTH FOODS A misnomer since certain nutrients *q.v.* in quality and quantity are essential for maintaining health. No food is necessarily more healthful than another except in terms of its nutritional value, and whether or not it has been contaminated.

HEALTHFUL 1. Conditions that are conducive to the maintenance and/or promotion of one's health *q.v.* or well-being. 2. That which provides or gives health. ct: healthy.

HEALTHFUL LIFESTYLE A set of health-enhancing behaviors, shaped by internally consistent values *q.v.*, attitudes *q.v.*, beliefs, and external social and cultural forces.

HEALTHFUL LIVING Lifestyles *q.v.* conducive to health *q.v.* maintenance and promotion.

HEALTHFUL SCHOOL ENVIRONMENT 1. A division of the school health program *q.v.* 2. Procedures implemented by a school to provide for (a) healthful *q.v.* physical environment, (b) a mentally healthful environment, and (c) a socially healthful environment. 3. An element of the school health program that focuses on numerous responsibilities: (a) school administration, (b) board of education, (c) school plant architecture, (d) teachers, (e) pupils, (f) custodians, and (g) cafeteria staff. 4. The promotion, maintenance, and use of safe and wholesome surroundings, including physical settings, organization of day-to-day experiences, and planned learning procedures to influence favorably emotional, physical, and social health. 5. The quality of the physical, social, and emotional dimensions of a school, provided through procedures to maintain a safe and sanitary environment that promotes the health of students and school personnel.

HEALTH GOAL 1. Goal *q.v.* 2. General objective *q.v.* cf: health education goal; mission; health mission.

HEALTH GUIDANCE 1. A broad term that implies a variety of counseling techniques used to provide individuals or groups with insight into personal health problems.

2. Individual and/or group counseling regarding all aspects of personal and social health: promotion, prevention, control, improvement, appraisal, remedial, and referral. Emphasis is placed on health issues most significant to those being counseled. cf: health counseling.

HEALTH HABIT A health practice that has become a routine activity or behavior. cf: health-related behavior; habit.

HEALTH HISTORY A record of the health history of a person. Generally, conducted in a school setting, but private physicians also obtain the ~ of their patients.

HEALTH HUCKSTER Also health hawker, peddler. A person who sells health or medical products and services for commercial profit, frequently falsifying or distorting scientific truth about the product or service.

HEALTH INFORMATION 1. Facts related to the quality of individual and societal physical, psychological, and sociological effectiveness. 2. Communication of facts about health designed to develop a person's cognitive *q.v.* base for health action. 3. Facts about health. 4. Health knowledge *q.v.* 5. Scientific health or medical facts. ct: health fallacies; health misconceptions.

HEALTH INSTRUCTION 1. An obsolete term used in the past to describe direct and indirect health learning. Essentially, health teaching. More recently, health professionals have replaced this term with the broader one of health education *q.v.* which implies a focus on learning rather than on teaching. Instruction implies indoctrination. 2. The process of providing a sequence of planned and spontaneously originated learning opportunities comprising the organized aspects of health education in school or community.

HEALTH INSURANCE Probably more appropriately called disease insurance since most policies rarely cover "health." They tend to protect against the cost of illness, disability, etc. There are several modes of payment and forms of insurance: (a) direct payment, (b) copayment, (c) third-party payment, and others. Insurance may take the form of (a) governmental, (b) voluntary, (c) group, (d) individual, and (e) family.

HEALTH ISSUES Matters pertaining to individual and/or societal health. cf: health problems.

HEALTH KNOWLEDGE 1. The acquisition of health information *q.v.* which is assimilated *q.v.* and accommodated *q.v.* by the individual. ~ is health facts that become meaningful and a functional and integral part of the individual in making health decisions. 2. Authoritative concepts, generalizations, and supporting factual data deemed representative of the discipline of health education *q.v.*

HEALTH LEARNING Any of a variety of experiences which change the way a person feels and responds to health-related *q.v.* aspects of the environment. ~ can be either health-related or health-directed *q.v.*

HEALTH LEGISLATION Laws passed at the local, state, and federal levels to affect some aspect of societal health. They may be sanitary codes or public health laws, education laws, and others.

HEALTH LITERACY The capacity of an individual to obtain, interpret, and understand basic health information *q.v.* and services and the competence to use such information and services in ways that are health enhancing.

HEALTH MAINTENANCE 1. The actions one takes to preclude the onset of disease, disability, or premature death, including health-related *q.v.* and health-directed *q.v.* behavior. 2. Actions that direct a person to adapt to changes in the environment. 3. Those measures one takes to ensure that an optimal level of health continues. cf: interpretive level of health; biological level of health.

HEALTH MAINTENANCE ORGANIZATION (HMO) 1. An organizational health plan of total health care. 2. A health care system consisting of (a) an organized system for providing health care in a designated geographic area accepting responsibility for providing the essential health services, (b) an agreed upon set of basic and supplemental health maintenance and treatment services, (c) a voluntary, enrolled group of persons, and (d) the HMO is reimbursed through predetermined, fixed, periodic prepayments made by or on behalf of each enrolled person or family without regard to the amount of actual services provided. 3. A prepaid health insurance plan in which patients receive health care from designated health and medical providers.

HEALTH MISCONCEPTIONS Distorted or false ideas about health matters.

HEALTH MODELS 1. Illustrations and explanations of the various factors contributing to health and disease. 2. A comparison of health status *q.v.* to established or recognized standards or criteria. There are three major models: (a) medical or clinical, (b) statistical, and (c) holistic.

HEALTH MYTHS Health misconceptions *q.v.*

HEALTH NEEDS Basic needs *q.v.*

HEALTH OBJECTIVE A defined outcome of health learning. May be an enabling or a terminal objective.

HEALTH OUTCOME DATA A major source of data for health assessments. The identification, review, and evaluation of health outcome *q.v.* parameters is an interactive process involving the health assessors, data source generators, and the local community. Health outcome data should be community-specific and may be derived from databases at the local, state, and nations levels, as well as data collected by private health care organizations and professional institutions and associations. Databases to be considered include morbidity and mortality data, birth statistics, medical records, tumor and disease registries, surveillance data, and previously conducted health studies. Relevant health outcome data play an important role in assessing the public's health and in determining which follow-up activities are needed.

HEALTH OUTCOMES Any medically or epidemiologically defined characteristic of a patient or health problem in a population that results from health promotion or care provided or required as measured at one point in time. cf: health goal; health objective.

HEALTH PRACTITIONER One whose profession is one or more of the health professions *q.v.* They may be medical, nonmedical, or paramedical *q.v.*

HEALTH PROBLEM Health *q.v.* concerns that meet certain criteria to be classed as a problem. The criteria used revolve around (a) death rate *q.v.*, (b) family disruption, (c) extent of disability, (d) economic implications, (e) age of onset, (f) threat to large numbers of people, (g) relation to other health concerns, (h) preventability, (i) treatability, and (j) societal classes affected.

HEALTH PROFESSIONAL A person trained and qualified in one or more of the health professions. cf: health practitioner.

HEALTH PROFESSIONS Numerous occupations that are concerned with one or more aspects of human health. cf: health professional.

HEALTH PROGRAM 1. All of the activities within a school, community, or agency setting that are related to health, medical, dental, and psychological services; education and environment; and that are directed toward the improvement of personal and societal health. 2. A planned and organized series of health education *q.v.* activities or procedures implemented with (a) an educational specialist-assigned primary responsibility, (b) a budget, (c) an integral set of goals and objectives, (d) activities designed to achieve these goals and objectives, and (e) evaluation procedures to allow for determining success and needed revisions of the program.

HEALTH PROMOTION 1. A complex process of providing an environment conducive to optimal development of the individual and/or providing the necessary individual qualities for one to overcome obstacles standing in the way of growth and development. Specific intervention strategies that occur at the primary levels of prevention *q.v.* designed to make the host stronger or more resistant to infection, decrease the effect of the agent on the host, and create a barrier in the environment that prevents the agent from reaching the host. 2. Any combination of health education *q.v.* and related organizational, political, and economic interventions designed to facilitate behavioral and environmental adaptations to improve or protect health.

HEALTH PROMOTION AND DISEASE PREVENTION The aggregate of all purposeful activities designed to improve personal and public health through a combination of strategies, including the competent implementation of behavioral change strategies, health education, risk factor detection, health enhancement, and health maintenance.

HEALTH PROMOTION AND DISEASE PREVENTION A report by the U.S. Surgeon General in 1979 that presented five major goals of health for the United States: (a) to continue to improve infant health, and by 1990, to reduce infant mortality by at least 35% to fewer than nine deaths per 1000 live births; (b) to improve child health, foster optimum childhood development, and by 1990, reduce deaths among children 1–14 years by at least 20% to fewer than 34 per 100,000; (c) to improve the health and health habits of adolescents and young adults, and by 1990, to reduce deaths among people aged 15–24 years by at least 20% to fewer than 93 per 100,000; (d) to improve the health of adults, and by 1990, to reduce deaths among people aged 25–64 years by at least 25% to fewer than 400 per 100,000; (e) to improve the health and quality of life for older adults, and by 1990, to reduce the average annual number of days of restricted activity due to acute and chronic conditions by 20% to fewer than 30 days per year for people aged 65 years and older. Now called healthy people, the goals are updated in 10-year cycles.

HEALTH PROMOTIVE Something that promotes health *q.v.*

HEALTH QUACKERY Quackery *q.v.*

HEALTH-RELATED BEHAVIOR 1. All behavior, since all behavior is influenced by health, and health influences all behavior. 2. Any behavior that can affect one's health. 3. Those behaviors that are thought to be health maintenance *q.v.* activities. ct: health-directed behavior.

HEALTH RESOURCES People, facilities, materials, and products that are available for preventing disease and disability, promoting health, and treating diseases and disabilities, and restoring health and habilitating or rehabilitating the handicapped. ct: health education resources.

HEALTH RESOURCES ADMINISTRATION A branch of the United States Public Health Service (USPHS).

HEALTH RESTORATION The actions one takes to overcome a disease or disability.

HEALTH RISK APPRAISAL (HRA) An appraisal technique used to determine a person's probability of developing specific diseases.

HEALTH SCIENCE EDUCATION This refers basically to the acquisition of health facts, their relation to each other, and how these relationships can establish health principles or laws.

HEALTH SCIENCE EDUCATOR 1. Health educator *q.v.* 2. Pertains to instructors or teachers who teach life sciences, medicine, or allied professions that prepare health professionals *q.v.*

HEALTH SCIENCES Any number of sciences that directs its efforts toward solving and understanding health issues *q.v.*, e.g., epidemiology; medicine.

HEALTH SCREENING 1. The application of tests or other procedures that are easily administered, usually, to a high risk group, to determine the possible existence of a health problem *q.v.* Procedures include (a) multiphasic screening, (b) case finding, and (c) selective screening *q.v.* Data gathered during a ~ procedure should be evaluated in terms of validity *q.v.*, reliability *q.v.*, yield, cost, acceptance, and follow-up procedures. 2. Preliminary appraisal techniques used to identify people who appear to need diagnostic tests carried out by medical specialists.

HEALTH SERVICES 1. The medical and health-related functions found within the school and community which direct attention toward promotion of health, prevention of disease, disability, and premature death, and restoration of health. 2. Numerous health, medical, dental, and psychological professions concerned with the promotion, maintenance, and restoration of health. 3. In education, all the efforts of the school to conserve, protect, and improve the health of the school population. cf: school health services.

HEALTH SERVICES ADMINISTRATION A specialized area of community health that is concerned with the application and skills in resource management to accomplish the effective and efficient delivery of health services *q.v.*

HEALTH SERVICES ADMINISTRATION A branch of the United States Public Health Service (USPHS).

HEALTH SERVICES RESEARCH Research concerned with the organization, financing, administration efforts, or other aspects of health services *q.v.* ct: biomedical research.

HEALTH STATUS 1. The measurable level of functioning of the individual at any given moment in time. Also applicable to groups of people. 2. The general level of one's health at any given time under specific circumstances.

HEALTH STIMULI Stimuli *q.v.* that affect health responses or behavior.

HEALTH STUDY An investigation of exposed individuals designed to assist in identifying exposure or effects to public health. Health studies also define those health problems *q.v.* that require further inquiry through, for example, a health surveillance *q.v.* or epidemiological *q.v.* study.

HEALTH SURVEILLANCE The ongoing and systematic collection, analysis, and interpretation of health data while monitoring a health event.

HEALTH SYSTEMS AGENCIES (HSAs) Begun in the late 1970s and terminated during the early to the mid-1980s, a health management structure under federal law, controlled by consumers, for the planning of health priorities, activities, and funding on a regional basis.

HEALTH THREATENING A situation or condition that when present under certain circumstances may negatively influence health status *q.v.*

HEALTHY 1. An optimal state or quality of life. 2. Having health *q.v.* ct: healthful.

HEALTHY PEOPLE A series of publications that have set health goals for the nation in 10-year increments. There have been *Healthy People 1990*, *Healthy People 2000*, and *Healthy People 2010*.

HEARING 1. In politics, a session of a legislative committee at which witnesses present testimony on bills under consideration. 2. In anatomy and physiology, pertaining to the sense of hearing, the ability to perceive sound. 3. In law, judicial examination of factual or legal issues.

HEARING DISORDER Pertaining to the loss of hearing, the term includes both persons who are hard of hearing and persons who are deaf.

HEARING ON THE MERITS In law, trial on the substance of a case as opposed to consideration of procedure only.

HEARING SCREENING Procedures to detect hearing loss. The use of the pure tone audiometer by an audiometrician *q.v.* cf: health screening.

HEARSAY EVIDENCE In law, testimony given by any witness who relates what others have told him or her or what he or she has heard said by others, rather than what he or she knows personally.

HEART A four-chambered, muscular organ in humans that continuously pumps blood through the circulatory system *q.v.*

HEART ATTACK 1. Obstruction of the coronary arteries *q.v.* depriving the heart of blood and oxygen. 2. Death of heart muscle due to an occlusion or to an obstruction of blood supply that fails to meet the oxygen needs of the heart muscle. 3. Myocardial infarction *q.v.* 4. Damage to an area of the heart muscle due to an insufficient supply of blood. Various symptoms can indicate a heart attack is about to occur: chest pain, sweating, nausea, vomiting, shortness of breath, weakness. In older persons, there may be no symptoms. cf: coronary thrombosis.

HEART BLOCK 1. An interference with the conduction of the electrical impulses of the heart. Blockage can be either partial or complete. 2. Atrioventricular block *q.v.*

HEARTBURN A burning sensation in the esophagus *q.v.* that may be an indication of indigestion *q.v.*

HEART FAILURE A condition characterized by the inability of the heart to perform its proper pumping action.

HEART-LUNG MACHINE A device that oxygenates *q.v.* and circulates blood in the body during a coronary bypass or other appropriate surgical procedure.

HEART MURMUR The sound caused when a stream of blood rushes through a heart valve which has been scarred during an inflammation *q.v.* of the heart and its valves.

HEART MUSCLE Cardiac muscle *q.v.*

HEART RATE The number of times per minute that the heart fills with blood and then pumps the blood into the vascular system *q.v.*

HEAT COLLAPSE Heat exhaustion *q.v.*

HEAT CRAMPS A painful condition resulting in involuntary muscle contractions due to loss of body fluids and electrolytes during heavy exercise.

HEAT EXHAUSTION 1. A significant drop in sodium level in the body resulting in the withdrawal of water from the cells causing dehydration *q.v.* 2. A mild form of shock *q.v.* caused by a reduction in blood flow to the major organs of the body resulting from a loss of body fluids during strenuous exercise. 3. Heat prostration.

HEAT STROKE 1. Sunstroke *q.v.* 2. Failure of the body to regulate heat after exposure to high temperatures. 3. A condition that results from prolonged exposure to high temperatures characterized by cessation of sweating, extremely high body temperature, and collapse. ~ is extremely serious and may be fatal.

HEAVY METALS Metals, such as mercury, arsenic, lead, nickel, and zinc, that may enter the human food chain from industrial pollution. ~ slowly accumulate in the body and adversely affect the nervous system *q.v.*

HEBEPHRENIA Disorganized schizophrenia *q.v.* cf: hebephrenic reaction.

HEBEPHRENIC REACTION 1. A type of schizophrenia *q.v.* characterized by marked shallowness and distortion of affect *q.v.* and silly, inappropriate behavior. Hebephrenic schizophrenia *q.v.*

HEBEPHRENIC SCHIZOPHRENIA 1. A type of schizophrenia *q.v.* characterized by bizarre ideas and silliness. A term rarely used today by psychiatrists and psychologists. 2. Hebephrenic reaction *q.v.*

HEBIATRICS That branch of medicine that deals mainly with the diagnosis and treatment of disorders of adolescents.

HEDIR A listserv/discussion group, established in 1990, that encourages health educators from each area of practice to share ideas, seek advice, promote programs and conferences, etc.

HEDONISM 1. The doctrine that pleasure or happiness is the highest good. 2. In psychology, the theory that people's actions are driven by the search for pleasure and the avoidance of pain. 3. The philosophy that asserts that all people pursue pleasure and seek to avoid pain. This view goes back to Greek philosophers such as Epicurus but was popularized in the eighteenth and nineteenth centuries by British utilitarian philosophers such as Jeremy Bentham and John Stuart Mill. Mill added to the pursuit of pleasure a concern for producing the greatest amount of good by people's actions.

HEDONISTIC ETHIC A system of values maximizing pleasure and minimizing pain to all are the highest goods. cf: absolutist ethic; relativistic ethic.

HEEL COUNTERS Fitted heel cups inside shoes.

HEES An acronym for Health and Environment Electronic Seminars.

HEGAR'S SIGN Softness on a part of the uterus *q.v.* that is found in pregnant women.

HEIMLICH MANEUVER A technique for expelling foreign matter that has become lodged in a person's windpipe and who is choking.

HELIOTHERAPY The use of the sun's rays in treating a person.

HELIOTROPISM Response of organisms to light, especially the sun's rays.

HELIX Any structure with a spiral shape. The Watson and Crick model of DNA *q.v.* is in the form of a double ~.

HELMINTH A parasitic worm, example is a pinworm *q.v.* 2. A class of worms, many of which are parasitic *q.v.* to humans, e.g., the flatworms. These many-celled animal forms producing disease were formerly called metazoa *q.v.* cf: helminthiasis.

HELMINTHIASIS Infestation *q.v.* of the intestinal tract with worms. cf: helminth.

HELONA A corn *q.v.*

HELPER-SUPPRESSOR T-CELL RATIO Ration of the number of helper T cells to the number of suppressor T cells. The normal ration of 2:1 is reversed in people suffering from AIDS *q.v.*

HELPLESSNESS A construct *q.v.* referring to the sense of having no control over important events, considered by many theorists to play a central role in anxiety *q.v.* and depression *q.v.* cf: learned helplessness.

HEMAGGLUTINATION A process by which mammalian red blood cells are caused to clump or agglutinate as a result of the interaction of antigen *q.v.*, antibody *q.v.*, and complement, or directly by cells such as viruses *q.v.*

HEMANGIOMA A tumor composed of blood vessels or large spaces containing blood.

HEMARTHOSIS An accumulation of blood in a joint.

HEMATEMESIS Vomiting of blood.

HEMATIN The acid radical which unites with the protein globin *q.v.* to form hemoglobin *q.v.*

HEMATINIC Any drug that increases the hemoglobin *q.v.* and red blood cell count.

HEMATOCHEZIA The passage of grossly bloody stools or bright red blood from the rectum *q.v.*

HEMATOCRIT 1. The portion of whole-blood volume after centrifugation. 2. The solid component of blood which constitutes about 40% of the whole blood. 3. The volume percentage of erythrocytes *q.v.* in whole blood. It is determined by centrifuging a blood sample to separate the cellular elements from the plasma *q.v.* The results of the test indicate the ratio of cell volume to plasma volume.

HEMATOLOGY The study of the function and diseases of the blood.

HEMATOMA 1. The localized collection of blood in the tissues as a result of injury. 2. A bruise *q.v.* 3. A broken blood vessel.

HEMATOPOIESIS The production of various types of blood cells and platelets *q.v.* cf: hemopoiesis.

HEMATURIA Blood in the urine.

HEME 1. The iron-containing complex of the hemoglobin *q.v.* molecule *q.v.* 2. The nonprotein, insoluble pigment portion of the hemoglobin molecule. 3. The prosthetic group *q.v.* of the hemoglobin molecule. cf: heme iron.

HEME IRON The most biologically active form of iron available to the body. cf: heme.

HEMIANOPSIS The absence of vision in one-half of the visual field in one or both eyes.

HEMICELLULOSE Polysaccharides *q.v.* resembling cellulose *q.v.* but more soluble and less complex. Found particularly in cell walls.

HEMIC HYPOXIA A condition of insufficient oxygen in the blood related to a diminished capacity of the red blood cells to carry oxygen.

HEMIPLEGIA Paralysis of one-half of the body caused by damage to the opposite side of the brain. ~ is sometimes caused by a blood clot or hemorrhage *q.v.* in a blood vessel in the brain. cf: stroke.

HEMISPHERE DOMINANCE Refers to one hemisphere *q.v.* of the brain leading or having major control in certain behaviors.

HEMISPHERIC LATERALIZATION Differences in function between the right and left hemispheres of the brain.

HEMITHORAX One side of the chest.

HEMIZYGOUS 1. The condition in which only one allele *q.v.* of a pair is present, as in deletion or sex linkage *q.v.* 2. Pertaining to the alleles of the X chromosome in male cells.

HEMOCOEL A special part of the coelom *q.v.* for transporting blood.

HEMOCYTOMETER An instrument used in counting the blood corpuscles in a sample of blood.

HEMODIALYSIS A kidney machine that purifies a person's blood when the kidneys fail.

HEMODILUTION An increase in the fluid content of the blood resulting in diminution of the proportion of formed elements, red and white blood cells and platelets *q.v.*

HEMODYNAMIC 1. Related to the circulation or to the cardiovascular system *q.v.* 2. The movement of blood through the vast tubular network of the body.

HEMOGLOBIN 1. The oxygen-carrying portion of red blood cells which gives them a red color. 2. The red pigment (iron) of the erythrocytes *q.v.* that combines with oxygen. 3. The red protein of blood cells that transports oxygen and carbon dioxide. 4. A conjugated protein compound containing iron, located in the erythrocytes of vertebrates *q.v.*, important in the transportation of oxygen to the cells of the body. cf: heme.

HEMOGLOBINURIA The presence of hemoglobin *q.v.* in the urine, as in blackwater fever *q.v.*

HEMOLYMPH The mixture of blood and other fluids in the body cavity of an invertebrate *q.v.*

HEMOLYSIS 1. The liberation of the hemoglobin *q.v.* from the erythrocytes *q.v.* 2. The destruction of erythrocytes with the release of hemoglobin into the blood plasma *q.v.*

HEMOLYTIC Capable of dissolving red blood cells.

HEMOLYTIC STREPTOCOCCUS An organism that destroys red blood cells and allows hemoglobin *q.v.* to escape. cf: hemolytic.

HEMOPHILIA 1. A genetic *q.v.* disease almost exclusively of males, which interferes with blood coagulation *q.v.*, resulting in the person bleeding excessively when injured. 2. A hereditary *q.v.* bleeding disorder caused by a deficiency in the ability to synthesize *q.v.* one or more of the blood coagulation proteins, e.g., Factor VIII (hemophilia A) or Factor IX (hemophilia B). cf: hemophiliac.

HEMOPHILIAC A person who has hemophilia *q.v.*

HEMOPHILUS DUCREYI The infectious agent *q.v.* that causes chancroid *q.v.*

HEMOPNEUMOTHORAX Accumulation of air and blood in the pleural cavity *q.v.*

HEMOPOIESIS Blood cell formation. cf: hematopoiesis.

HEMOPTYSIS Coughing up blood from the lungs.

HEMORRHAGE 1. The escape of large volumes of blood from a blood vessel. May be external bleeding or internal bleeding. 2. To bleed. 3. Profuse bleeding.

HEMORRHAGIC SHOCK Shock *q.v.* resulting from hemorrhage *q.v.* sufficient to reduce blood volume markedly.

HEMORRHOIDECTOMY The surgical removal of hemorrhoids *q.v.*

HEMORRHOIDS 1. Swelling of the veins in the membranes *q.v.* of the anal canal *q.v.* and rectum *q.v.* 2. Varicose veins *q.v.* of the rectum. 3. Piles.

HEMOSTASIS Stopping hemorrhage *q.v.*

HEMOSTAT 1. Any agent that arrests, chemically or mechanically, the flow of blood from an open vessel. 2. An instrument for arresting hemorrhage *q.v.* by compression of the blood vessel.

HEMOTHORAX Blood in the pleural *q.v.* or thoracic *q.v.* cavity.

HEMP PLANT Leafy plant grown in temperate and tropical areas throughout the world; source of marijuana and other cannabis *q.v.* preparations. cf: *Cannabis indica*; *Cannabis sativa*.

HENBANE A poisonous anticholinergic *q.v.* plant that is sometimes used for its hallucinogenic *q.v.* properties, *Hyoscyamus niger*.

HEPAR Pertaining to the liver.

HEPARIN A substance obtained from the liver that inhibits blood clotting.

HEPATIC Pertaining to the liver.

HEPATIC FAILURE Failure of the liver to function properly.

HEPATIC NECROSIS Death of liver tissue.

HEPATIC PORTAL The circulatory pathway between the small intestine and the liver.

HEPATITIS 1. Inflammation *q.v.* of the liver due to many causes including viruses, several of which are transmissible through blood transfusions and sexual activity. 2. Inflammation of the liver usually from a viral infection. Type A may be transmitted by fecal–oral route and type B by injection of infected blood or use of contaminated needles. Types C, D, etc. are mainly transmitted through contaminated transplanted tissue or other clinical means.

HEPATOMEGALY Enlargement of the liver.

HEPATOSPLENOMEGALY Enlargement of the liver and spleen.

HERB In botany, a nonwoody plant—annual, biennial, or perennial—whose aerial portion is relatively short lived (in the temperate zone, only a single growing season).

HERBACEOUS Referring to any nonwoody plant. cf: herb.

HERBAL MEDICINE The use of plants and other natural substances in the treatment of diseases. ct: pharmacology. cf: pharmacognosy.

HERBALS Early botanical works of the sixteenth and seventeenth centuries. They described many of the plants known at the time, with special attention to their medicinal and other uses. Some contained attempts at classification.

HERBARTIAN MOVEMENT The development and extension of Herbart's psychology and educational methodology. Herbartianism exerted an influence on educational theory and practice nearly as great as that of Pestalozzi. cf: Herbartian teaching method.

HERBARTIAN TEACHING METHOD An organized method based on the principles of teaching of Pestalozzi that stresses learning by association and consists of five steps: (a) preparation, (b) presentation, (c) association, (d) generalization, and (e) application. cf: Herbartian movement.

HERBICIDE 1. A toxic chemical that kills unwanted plants. 2. A chemical compound used to destroy or kill vegetation.

HERBIVORE An animal that eats plants exclusively. cf: carnivore.

HERBIVOROUS An animal that feeds upon plants, as opposed to carnivorous *q.v.*

HERD IMMUNITY The point at which a disease can no longer spread through a population because of the lack of nonimmune hosts.

HEREDITARY POTENTIAL A person's genetic *q.v.* potentialities for physical and mental development.

HEREDITARY SYPHILIS Congenital syphilis *q.v.*

HEREDITY 1. Refers to factors or traits passed from one generation to another through the genes *q.v.* 2. Transmission of similar traits or features from parent to offspring. cf: heritability.

HERITABILITY 1. The degree to which a given trait is controlled by inheritance *q.v.* 2. The proportion of the variance in a trait that is attributable to the genetic *q.v.* differences that exist among individuals. cf: environmentality.

HERMAPHRODITE 1. One who possesses the sex organs of both sexes. 2. A person who, because of a rare congenital *q.v.* condition, cannot be clearly identified as either male or female. cf: bisexual; dysgenic.

HERMAPHRODITE, DYSGENIC A person who fails to develop completely the gonads *q.v.* of either sex. cf: hermaphrodite.

HERMAPHRODITE, FEMALE A person who possesses gonads *q.v.* that are ovaries *q.v.* but whose external genitalia *q.v.* are either ambiguous or male in appearance. cf: hermaphrodite, male.

HERMAPHRODITE, MALE A person who possesses gonads *q.v.* that are testes *q.v.* but whose external genitalia *q.v.* are either ambiguous or female in appearance. cf: hermaphrodite, female.

HERMAPHRODITE, TRUE A person who possesses both male and female gonads *q.v.* cf: hermaphrodite, female; hermaphrodite, male.

HERNIA 1. The protrusion of part of an organ through a portion of the abdominal wall. 2. Rupture. 3. Protrusion of a loop of an organ through an abdominal opening.

HERNIATED DISK A protrusion of an intervertebral disk *q.v.* from its normal position between adjoining vertebrae *q.v.*

HEROIN 1. A semisynthetic opiate *q.v.*, synthesized by Bayer Laboratories in 1874. 2. An addicting *q.v.* drug about three times more potent than morphine *q.v.* 3. An analgesic *q.v.* 4. A narcotic *q.v.* 5. Diacetylmorphine hydrochloride. 6. A narcotic in the form of a white crystalline powder. 7. An alkaloid prepared from morphine by acetylation, formerly used for relief of cough. Because of the danger of addiction *q.v.* and its growing popularity, its manufacture and importation into the United States has been prohibited by law since 1924.

HEROIN DEPENDENCY An addiction to heroin *q.v.*

HEROIN WITHDRAWAL SYNDROME The reaction upon sudden and prolonged abstinence from heroin after a dependency has developed. Symptoms include (a) drowsiness for several hours, (b) restlessness, yawning, profuse sweating, running nose and eyes, feelings of anxiety, insomnia *q.v.*, and muscular aches, (c) after 24 h, gooseflesh, uncontrolled muscular twitching, vomiting, diarrhea, muscular aches, a rise in body temperature, dehydration *q.v.*, and an increase in systolic blood pressure. These symptoms then gradually subside within 72 h.

HERPES A virus infection *q.v.* There are two types of herpes simplex: 1. Herpes simplex type 1 produces commonly known cold sores and fever blisters *q.v.* 2. Herpes simplex type 2, characterized by painful blisters on the genitals *q.v.*, thighs, and buttocks. It can cause central nervous system *q.v.* infection in infants born to mothers infected with the virus. Once infected with the virus, it remains in the body for life and symptoms may develop from time to time. It has been linked to the development of cervical cancer *q.v.* 3. Shingles and chicken pox are caused by the herpes zoster virus.

HERPES GENITALIS 1. A sexually transmitted disease *q.v.* caused by the herpes simplex virus *q.v.* 2. A virus-caused sexually transmitted disease manifested by multiple fluid containing blisters. 3. Genital herpes *q.v.* 4. A virus-caused sexually transmitted disease characterized by painful blister-like sores on or around the genital *q.v.* area.

HERPES SIMPLEX VIRUS 1 (HSV-1) A virus that results in cold sores or fever blisters, most often on the mouth or around the eyes. Like all herpes viruses, it may lie dormant for months or years in nerve tissue and flare up in times of stress, trauma, infection, or immunosuppression. There is no cure for any of the herpes viruses.

HERPES SIMPLEX VIRUS II (HSV-II) 1. Causes painful sores on the genitals or anus. It is one of the most common sexually transmitted diseases in the United States. 2. Also, herpes simplex type 2. 3. Genital herpes *q.v.* cf: herpes.

HERPES VARICELLA ZOSTER VIRUS (HVZ) The varicella virus causes chicken pox mainly in children, and may reappear in adulthood as herpes zoster. Herpes zoster, also called shingles, is characterized by small, painful blisters on the skin along nerve pathways.

HERPESVIRUS GROUP A group of viruses including herpes simplex virus *q.v.*, vericella zoster virus *q.v.*, cytomegalovirus *q.v.*, and Epstein–Barr virus *q.v.*

HERPES ZOSTER Shingles *q.v.* The infectious agent is the varicella zoster virus.

HERTZ (HZ) A unit used to measure the frequency of sound in terms of the number of cycles that vibrating molecules *q.v.* complete per second.

HETAIRAE A special class of Greek prostitutes who were sought by men because of their beauty and education.

HETEROCARYON A fungus hypha *q.v.* with two nuclei of different genotypes *q.v.* The nuclei do not fuse but divide independently and simultaneously as new cells are formed.

HETEROCATALYTICAL FUNCTION A molecule directing or catalyzing a molecule *q.v.* of a different structure.

HETEROCHROMATIN Chromatin *q.v.* staining differently and functioning differently than euchromatin *q.v.* which contains most of the genes *q.v.* In Drosophila salivary preparations, the heterochromatin is mostly in the chromocenter.

HETEROCHRONY A change in the normal temporal sequence for the development of tissues, organs, and other animal parts. Such changes are thought to have played a role in the origins of some species.

HETEROCYCLIC Pertaining to ring compounds that contain other atoms in addition to carbon atoms as part of the ring.

HETEROCYSTS 1. In botany, large, functionless cells in the filaments of certain algae. 2. A specialized schizophyte cell *q.v.* formed from vegetative cells by the development of a new cell wall, nonfunctional in many organisms, often serving as the site where breakage occurs when hormogonia *q.v.* develop.

HETEROFERMENTATION A fermentation *q.v.* in which the end products are varied.

HETEROGAMETIC SEX In genetics, producing unlike gametes *q.v.* particularly with regard to the sex chromosomes *q.v.* In species in which the male is "XY", the male is ~; the female (XX), homogametic.

HETEROGAMY 1. A condition in which gametes *q.v.* are morphologically distinguishable as male or female. 2. The union of unlike gametes.

HETEROGENEOUS Consisting of dissimilar elements. ct: homogeneous.

HETEROGENEOUS GROUPING In education, a group or class consisting of students who show normal variation in ability or performance. ct: homogeneous grouping.

HETERONOMOUS MORALITY The developmental precursor to autonomous morality; it is characterized by the belief in moral realism, expiative punishment, objective responsibility, and obedience to authority.

HETEROPLOID 1. Aneuploid *q.v.* 2. An organism characterized by a chromosome number other than the true haploid *q.v.* (monoploid) or diploid *q.v.* number. cf: euploid.

HETEROPYKNOSIS. (ADJ. HETEROPYKNOTIC) Property of certain chromosomes *q.v.* or their parts to remain more dense and stain more intensely than other chromosomes or parts during the nuclear cycle *q.v.*

HETEROSEXUAL 1. A person whose sexual preference is for persons of the opposite sex. 2. Involving both sexes. 3. Cross-gender *q.v.* sexual thoughts, feelings, or behavior. ct: homosexual.

HETEROSIS Hybrid vigor *q.v.*

HETEROSOME Sex chromosome *q.v.* ct: autosomes.

HETEROSPOROUS In botany, having spores *q.v.* of two kinds, usually designated as microspores and megaspores.

HETEROSTYLY In botany, the existence of long and short styles *q.v.* in different flowers of the same species.

HETEROTHALLIC In genetics, condition in which either male or female gametes *q.v.* develop on a single thallus *q.v.*

HETEROTHALLISM The condition in which two unisexual *q.v.* strains of a species are necessary for sexual reproduction. ct: homothallism.

HETEROTROPH 1. An organism that must obtain food from organic molecules *q.v.* 2. Heterotrophic *q.v.*

HETEROTROPHIC Organisms that must obtain some or all of their food from external sources. In general, applied to animals and nonphotosynthetic *q.v.* plants. cf: heterotroph.

HETEROZYGOTE (ADJ. HETEROZYGOUS) In genetics *q.v.*, an organism with unlike members of any given pair of series of alleles *q.v.* which consequently produces unlike gametes *q.v.*

HETEROZYGOUS 1. A genetic *q.v.* characteristic containing a dominant and recessive gene *q.v.* 2. The condition that exists when the genes for a given character on the homologous chromosomes *q.v.* are unlike. 3. Condition in a diploid *q.v.* cell when the genes for a trait are different alleles. ct: homozygous.

HETEROZYGOUS ALLELE An allele *q.v.* that contains one dominant gene *q.v.* and one recessive gene *q.v.*

HEURISTICS 1. In computer problem solving, a procedure that has often worked in the past and is likely to work again. 2. Methods or techniques of problem solving. ct: algorithm.

HEURISTIC VALUE One of the criteria for evaluating the scientific merit of theories. A theory has ~ if it proves to be useful either as a stimulus for new scientific discoveries or as a guide for practical applications.

HEW An acronym for the Department of Health, Education, and Welfare (now obsolete).

HEX A Hexosaminidase A *q.v.*

HEXOSAMINIDASE A (Hex A) An enzyme *q.v.* necessary for the body to properly use lipids *q.v.*

HEXOSE 1. A monosaccharide *q.v.* that contains six carbon atoms. 2. A six-carbon sugar, such as glucose or fructose *q.v.*

HFCS An acronym for high-fructose corn syrup *q.v.*

HFR 1. An acronym for high-frequency recombination. 2. Strains of male bacteria that readily transfer chromosomal *q.v.* genes to receptor strains.

Hg The chemical symbol for mercury.

HGH An acronym for human growth hormone.

HHS An acronym for the Department of Health and Human Services *q.v.*

HIATUS Any opening in the normal anatomical structures through which other structures pass.

HIBERNATE Passing the winter in a quiescent and torpid condition.

HIDDEN OBSERVER In hypnosis, the part of the self that is aware of things outside conscious awareness.

HIERARCHICAL ORGANIZATION An organization in which narrower categories are subsumed under broader ones which, in turn, are subsumed in still broader ones.

HIERARCHY The ranking of group members according to status and/or ability to control or influence events. More generally, a group of persons or things arranged in order of rank, grade, and so on.

HIERARCHY OF LEARNING In health education, the three levels of progressive learning: 1. the acquisition of health facts, 2. the development of positive health attitudes, and 3. the development of health values.

HIERARCHY OF NEEDS In psychology, the concept that needs *q.v.* arrange themselves in order of importance from the most basic biological needs *q.v.* to those psychological needs *q.v.* concerned with self-actualization *q.v.*

HIERARCHY OF OBJECTIVES 1. In business, the entire overall and related sub-objectives assigned to various segments of the organization. 2. In education, the arrangement of objectives to be achieved according to basic understandings to more complex understandings leading to a final achievement of the goals or mission established.

HIGH-AMPLITUDE SUCKING METHOD (HAS) In child development, a procedure for investigating infant cognition that takes advantage of infants' willingness to work to make interesting spectacles last. Infants are able to maintain a stimulus at an optimal level of intensity by sucking on a nipple that is electronically connected to an apparatus such as a video camera or voice recorder.

HIGH-DENSITY LIPOPROTEIN (HDL) 1. Protein-like structures that transport fats to the liver and lower the risk of cholesterol buildup in the arteries, thus lowering the risk of coronary heart disease. 2. The part of serum cholesterol *q.v.* responsible for transporting fats out of the bloodstream. The level of HDL increases with exercise. ct: low-density lipoprotein (LDL).

HIGH-ENERGY BONDS Energy-rich bonds. The pyrophosphate bonds on hydrolysis *q.v.* yield a standard free energy near 8000 kcal per molecule, whereas simple phosphate bonds on hydrolysis yield only 1000–4000 kcal of standard free energy.

HIGHER-ORDER CONDITIONING 1. In classical conditioning *q.v.*, a procedure by which a new stimulus comes to elicit the conditioned response *q.v.* by virtue of being paired with an effective conditioned stimulus *q.v.* 2. Classical conditioning in which the unconditioned stimulus *q.v.* is the conditioned stimulus from a previous experiment.

HIGH-FREQUENCY RECOMBINATION Hfr *q.v.*

HIGH-FRUCTOSE CORN SYRUP (HFCS) Corn syrup *q.v.* that has been industrially treated to break it down into glucose *q.v.* units, which are then converted into fructose *q.v.*

HIGH NICOTINE-LOW TAR CIGARETTE A cigarette whose high nicotine *q.v.* content could satisfy the user's dependency *q.v.* on nicotine while reducing the health risks associated with exposure to high levels of tar *q.v.*

HIGH PROBABILITY APPROACH An approach to planning that is based on the philosophy that there should be a high probability that the organization will be at least somewhat successful.

HIGH-RISK BEHAVIOR In epidemiology, a term used to describe certain activities that increase the risk of disease exposure. cf: high-risk groups.

HIGH-RISK GROUPS Those groups that show a behavior risk for exposure to a disease or condition. cf: high-risk behavior.

HIGH-RISK METHOD In research, a technique used in the study of schizophrenia *q.v.* involving the intensive examination of people who have a high probability of later becoming abnormal.

HIGH SCHOOL 1. A level of school organizational structure that generally includes grades 9–12. When grade 9 is organized as a part of a junior high school, ~ is grades 10–12.

HIGH SCHOOL DIPLOMA 1. A recognized equivalent. 2. A document certifying the successful completion of a prescribed secondary school program of studies or the attainment of satisfactory scores on the tests of general educational development (GED) *q.v.* or other state-specified examination.

HIGH TOLERANCE The ability for a person to adapt *q.v.* to excessive quantities of alcohol or other drugs without the usual affects. ct: loss of tolerance.

HILUM 1. In botany, the central part in a starch grain, surrounded by layers of starch. 2. The scar on the seed left by a stalk that attached the seed to the placenta. 3. In human anatomy, a depression where vessels enter an organ. 4. Hilus *q.v.*

HILUS Hilum *q.v.*

HINDBRAIN The most primitive part of the brain containing the medulla *q.v.* and the cerebellum *q.v.*

HINGE JOINT A joint *q.v.* in which a convexity on one bone fits into a corresponding concavity on another bone allowing motion in one plane only.

HIP 1. The lateral prominence of the pelvis from the waist to the thigh. 2. The hip joint *q.v.*

HIP JOINT The ball-and-socket joint *q.v.* between the head of the femur *q.v.* and the acetabular fossa *q.v.*

HIPPOCAMPAL GYRUS A portion of the temporal lobe *q.v.* of the cerebrum *q.v.*

HIPPOCAMPUS Phylogenetically older cortical *q.v.* tissues that are buried in the center of the cerebral hemispheres *q.v.*

HIPPOCRATES' BODY HUMOR THEORY One of the earliest body type theories, developed by Hippocrates *q.v.* The theory stated that a person's character could be determined through the identification of the balance of the four body humors: 1. blood, sanguine (hopeful, cheerful); 2. black bile, melancholic (sad, depressed); 3. yellow bile, choleric (irritable, irascible); and 4. phlegm, phlegmatic (apathetic, lethargic).

HIPPOCRATIC OATH The physician's oath attributed to Hippocrates. It is

> I swear by Apollo, the physician, by Aesculapius, by Hygeia, Panacea, and the gods and goddesses, that according to my ability and judgment I will keep this oath and stipulation. I will look upon him who shall have taught me this art even as one of my parents. I will share my substance with him, and I will supply his necessities, it he be in need. I will regard his offspring even as my own brethren, and I will teach them this art, if they would learn it, without fee or covenant. I will impart this art by precept, by lecture, and by every mode of teaching, not only to my own sons but to the sons of him who has taught me, and to disciples bound by covenant and oath, according to the law of medicine. The regimen I adopt shall be for the benefit of my patients according to my ability and judgment, and not for their hurt or for any wrong. I will give no deadly drug to any, though it be asked for me, nor will I counsel such, and especially I will not aid a woman to procure abortion. With purity and holiness will I pass my life and practice my art. I will not cut a person who is suffering with stone, but will leave this to be done by those who are practitioners of such work. Whatsoever house I enter, there I will go for the benefit of the sick, refraining from all wrongdoing or corruption, and especially from any act of seduction, of male or female, of bond or free. Whatsoever thing I see or hear concerning the life of men, in my attendance on the sick or apart therefrom, which ought not to be raised abroad, I will keep this oath inviolate, may it be granted to me to enjoy life and the practice of my art, respecting always all men; but should I break or violate this oath, may the reverse be my lot.

HIP POINTER An injury to the iliac crest (hip).

HIRSUTISM Abnormal hairiness, especially in women. cf: hypertrichosis.

HISTAMINE 1. A chemical normally present in all body tissues that, upon release, causes dilation of the capillaries *q.v.* and is associated with some allergic reactions *q.v.* 2. Biochemical substances (in the amino class) stored in mast cells and released by tissue injury, including allergic reactions; no known functional role, but may be a neurotransmitter *q.v.* 3. A substance released during allergic reactions which can result in localized redness, swelling, edema *q.v.*, mucous production, and increased gastric secretion.

HISTOCOMPATABILITY The degree of similarity between tissues from different persons as determined by the classes of antigens *q.v.* on cell surfaces. ~ is greatest between tissues of identical twins. Matching ~ is essential in organ and tissue transplants and in the transfusion of blood.

HISTOGENESIS Tissue formation and development.

HISTOGRAM A graphic presentation of a frequency distribution *q.v.* that reflects the distribution by a series of contiguous rectangles.

HISTOLOGICAL 1. Pertaining to the cellular makeup of a particular tissue. 2. Pertaining to microscopic structure. cf: histology.

HISTOLOGY The science that studies microscopic *q.v.* structures of living things. cf: histological.

HISTOPLASMOSIS A disease caused by a fungal infection that can affect all the organs of the body. Symptoms usually include fever, shortness of breath, cough, weight loss, and physical exhaustion.

HISTORICAL (ARCHIVAL) METHOD A technique for researching behavior in times past. cf: historical cohort study.

HISTORICAL COHORT STUDY 1. In epidemiology, a cohort study *q.v.* defined in the past. 2. Historical method. 3. Archival method. cf: cohort study.

HISTORICAL SOCIAL PSYCHOLOGY The study of social patterns as they change over time.

HISTORY OF EDUCATION Historical study of education.

HISTRIONIC PERSONALITY A person who is overly dramatic and given to emotional excess, impatient with minor annoyances, immature, dependent on others, and often sexually seductive, without taking responsibility for flirtations. Formerly called hysterical personality. cf: histrionic personality disorder.

HISTRIONIC PERSONALITY DISORDER A disorder marked by attention-seeking behavior such as excitability or self-dramatization; in spite of these emotional displays, the individual is perceived as shallow and lacking in genuineness. cf: histrionic personality.

HIV An acronym for human immunodeficiency virus. ~ causes AIDS *q.v.* by attacking the body's immune system *q.v.* making infected people vulnerable to fatal infections *q.v.*, cancer *q.v.*, and neurological disorders *q.v.* The target of ~ is the T4 subset of T lymphocytes, which regulate the immune system.

HIVES 1. An acute, itchy, rash-like outbreak of the skin as a result of sensitivity to a protein *q.v.* 2. An allergic reaction *q.v.* 3. Nettle rash. 4. Uticaria *q.v.* 5. A transient skin condition characterized by slightly raised, itching patches, often considered a psychophysiological disorder *q.v.*

HIV-POSITIVE Presence of the human immunodeficiency virus in the body.

HLA An acronym for human leukocyte antigens *q.v.*

HLA ANTIGENS Substances on the surface of white blood cells *q.v.* that are used to measure how similar tissues are between individuals. cf: histocompatability.

HMO An acronym for health maintenance organization *q.v.*

HOAX 1. An attempt to deceive. 2. A practical joke.

HOBBY An activity, voluntarily selected, that permits self-expression with a recreative purpose.

HODGKIN'S DISEASE A lymphoma *q.v.* Occurs mainly in people between 20 and 45 years. It is characterized by painless swelling of the lymph glands *q.v.* located in the neck, armpits, and groin. The cause is unclear; however, biopsy *q.v.* indicates malignancy of the reticular cells and the Reed–Sternberg cells *q.v.*

HOLANDRIC GENE In genetics, a gene carried on the Y chromosome *q.v.* and therefore transmitted from father to son. ct: hologynic.

HOLDFAST 1. In biology, flattened disc-like tip of a tendril *q.v.* used in attachment. 2. Basal part of an algal thallus *q.v.* that attaches it to a solid object, may be unicellular *q.v.* or composed of a mass of tissue.

HOLISTIC 1. Recognizing that health is influenced by an interaction of the three dimensions of health: psychological, physical, and social. 2. The ~ view of health is predicated upon the concept that all people are an integrated whole. 3. The ~ view of health recognizes our psychobiological *q.v.* integration and unity. 4. The functional interrelationship of all parts of the person: physical, psychological, and social. 5. Denoting the balanced state between mind, body, and spirit that allows for great vitality and excellence. 6. A systematic approach to science involving the study of the whole or total configuration: the view of humans as unified psychobiological organisms inextricably immersed in a physical and sociocultural environment.

HOLISTIC APPROACH 1. The simultaneous attention to the many factors that affect health. 2. Encompassing view of the nature of health. cf: holistic.

HOLISTIC HEALTH 1. The school of thought that views health in terms of its physical, emotional, social, intellectual, and spiritual makeup. 2. An approach to health that recognizes the interrelationships of physical, mental, emotional, spiritual, social, and environmental factors in the attainment of health. 3. The state of being in which a person's body, mind, and spirit are in balance, functioning with utmost capacity, or potential, and in tune with the natural and social environments. cf: holistic; holistic medicine.

HOLISTIC INDUCTIVE REASONING A method of reasoning used chiefly in the social sciences involving a process of thinking that moves from the specific to the general, from the part to the whole.

HOLISTIC MEDICINE 1. Medical treatment of all aspects of the person: physically and psychologically. This term is also used as a camouflage used by pseudoscientists to promote their unscientific treatment methods. 2. An approach to medical therapy that considers the life situation of the unwell person and not merely the elimination of specific symptoms *q.v.* Interacting variables considered are a person's physiology, nutrition, environment, emotional state, and lifestyle. ~ relies on the person becoming educated about his or her own medical care and taking responsibility to maintain health. cf: holistic health.

HOLISTIC MODEL OF HEALTH Based upon the concept that all persons are an integrated whole, with their biological, psychological, and sociological dimensions of health *q.v.* being in constant interaction. Factors affecting one dimension of health affect the other two and hence lowers one's health status *q.v.* cf: medical model; statistical model of health.

HOLMES GROUP Stands for a series of reforms posed by college deans. Reforms call for rigorous standards and moving teacher education to the graduate level.

HOLMES–RAHE SCALE (SOCIAL READJUSTMENT RATING SCALE) An instrument for assessing the stress on an individual by quantifying major life changes according to the difficulty people typically have readjusting to them.

HOLOGRAPHIC PHOTOGRAPHY Photography using lasers and mirrors to create a three-dimensional picture.

HOLOGRAPHIC WILL A will that is handwritten, dated, and signed by the maker of the will.

HOLOGYNIC In genetics, inheritance through females only. ct: holandric.

HOLOPHRASE A one-word utterance, which is to say, an utterance in which a single word carries the meaning of an entire sentence.

HOLOPHYTIC Pertains to plants that manufacture their own foods.

HOLOZOLIC 1. Ingestion of particulate food: typical animal-like nutrition. 2. Securing food after the manner of animals, involving ingestion and digestion of organic materials.

HOLTZMAN INKBLOT TECHNIQUE In psychology, a projective test containing two sets of 45 inkblots, similar to the Rorschach *q.v.*, but featuring better standardized administration, scoring, and interpretation.

HOME An acronym for home observation for measurement of the environment *q.v.*

HOME HEALTH AIDE Homemaker *q.v.*

HOME HEALTH CARE Health services provided in the home of the elderly, disabled, sick, or convalescent. The types of services provided include nursing care, social services, home health aide and homemaker services, and various rehabilitation services.

HOMEMAKER 1. Home health aide *q.v.* 2. A person who is paid to help in the home with personal care, light housekeeping, meal preparation, and shopping. Some states and agencies make a distinction between homemaking and personal care services.

HOME OBSERVATION FOR MEASUREMENT OF THE ENVIRONMENT (HOME) A process of assessment of the home environment in which family members and the actual setting are directly observed by the examiner.

HOMEOPATHY 1. A pseudoscience based upon the belief that medicines that are greatly diluted can possess powerful therapeutic benefits to the body. 2. Literally, same disease, a system of healing that involves the use of drugs to produce the same symptoms as the disease. 3. A type of therapy that emphasizes stimulation of the body's defenses by administration of a substance that can stimulate the symptoms of the disease.

HOMEOSTASIS 1. The tendency of an organism to maintain physiological equilibrium *q.v.* 2. It is also used to describe the tendency to maintain emotional and social equilibrium. 3. A tendency toward adaptation *q.v.* 4. The chemical equilibrium of the body. Psychological balance. 6. A dynamic equilibrium (changing balance) of an internal environment; in the body, this balance keeps the environment of the cells within the physical and chemical limits that support life. 7. The set of physiological mechanisms that maintains the internal environment *q.v.* as constant. 8. Maintenance of a stable biochemical environment within the body's cells and the fluid bathing the cells, in response to constant internal and external fluctuations, such as variations in nutrient supply and demands on organs, e.g., the liver, kidney, to metabolize and excrete natural and foreign substances. cf: homeostatic mechanism.

HOMEOSTATIC BALANCE The presence of physiological equilibrium in which body functions and conditions are within an acceptable and safe range. cf: homeostasis.

HOMEOSTATIC MECHANISM 1. A complex biological mechanism that attempts to moderate processes within the body so that a balance or equilibrium is maintained. 2. Responses developed by the body to achieve a stable state either for the whole organism or between different but interdependent body systems. cf: homeostasis.

HOMEOSTATIC RESERVE The ability of an organ, an organ system, or a person to maintain normal body functions. ~ is lowered by illness as well as the course of normal aging; illness causes far greater loss in reserve. cf: homeostasis.

HOMEOTHERMAL (ALSO, HOMOTHERMAL) Warm-blooded animals.

HOME SCHOOLING An educational model in which children are educated at home rather than attending school. Often, the parents are required to provide the children with minimum content established by the school district or the state, but the children may concentrate on subjects that are of interest to them.

HOME SIGN An idiosyncratic sign language spontaneously invented by deaf children who have not had the opportunity to learn a conventional sign language.

HOME STUDY A method of instruction designed for students who live at a distance from the teaching institution. Instructional materials are provided to the student, through various media, with structured units of information, assigned exercises, and examinations to measure achievement, which in turn are submitted to the teaching institution for evaluation.

HOMICIDE 1. Murder. 2. Taking the life of another.

HOMINID A human-like creature either prehistoric or extinct.

HOMOFERMENTATION A fermentation *q.v.* resulting in a high yield of a common end product.

HOMOGAMETIC SEX Producing like gametes *q.v.* ct: heterogametic sex.

HOMOGAMY 1. The existence of similar or shared traits among members of a group. 2. The tendency of like to marry like.

HOMOGENEITY OF VARIANCE In research, a circumstance wherein the variance of groups differs by no more than would be expected as a result of random sampling and chance error.

HOMOGENEOUS Of like characteristics. ct: heterogeneous.

HOMOGENEOUS GROUPING In education, the classification of pupils for the purpose of forming educational groups having a relatively high degree of similarity in regard to certain factors that affect learning.

HOMOGENIZE To break up the fat globules in milk to such an extent that no visible cream separation occurs.

HOMOIOTHERMOPHYTIC A warm blooded animal.

HOMOLOGOUS 1. Body organs in different sexed individuals that arise from the same embryological *q.v.* tissue. 2. Corresponding in position, structure, or origin to another anatomical *q.v.* entity.

HOMOLOGOUS CHROMOSOMES 1. Chromosomes *q.v.* which occur in pairs and are generally similar in size and shape, one having come form the male and one from the female parent. 2. Chromosomes that associate in pairs in the first stage of meiosis *q.v.*; each member of the pair is derived from a different parent. 3. A pair of chromosomes, one from each parent, which has a relatively similar value and structure. cf: homologous genes.

HOMOLOGOUS GENES Genes *q.v.* similarly situated in homologous chromosomes *q.v.* contributing to the same expression or different expression of a character.

HOMOLOGOUS ORGANS Structures in males and females that develop prenatally from similar tissue. For example, the penis and clitoris and scrotum and labia majora are homologous organs.

HOMOLOGUE 1. One pair of morphologically *q.v.* and genetically *q.v.* identical chromosomes *q.v.* 2. The two chromosomes of a pair.

HOMOLOGY 1. Similarity due to common origin. 2. Similarity that derives from having a common structure and evolutionary *q.v.* origin. cf: analogy.

HOMOPHILE 1. Preferences for the same sex. 2. Homosexual *q.v.*

HOMOPHILIC PERIOD A stage of maturation *q.v.* between 12 and 15 years wherein there is a preference for the same sex. It is also called the gang period.

HOMOPHOBIA 1. Fear of being homosexual *q.v.* 2. Intense irrational dislike of homosexual people and practices. 3. Negative bias toward or fear of individuals who are homosexual.

HOMO SAPIENS Humans.

HOMOSEXUAL 1. A person whose sexual preference is for persons of the same sex. 2. Involving the same sex, particularly in sexual preference. 3. Same-gender *q.v.* sexual thoughts, feelings, or behavior. cf: lesbian. ct: heterosexual.

HOMOSEXUAL ACT Erotic practice or feeling directed toward a member of the same sex. cf: homosexual identity.

HOMOSEXUAL IDENTITY Incorporation into one's self-definition the acceptance or an erotic or romantic attraction to a person of one's sex. cf: gender identity; homosexual act.

HOMOSOCIALITY Voluntary social segregation that occurs in late childhood, a period in which a person's social and personal activities are centered around members of the same gender *q.v.*

HOMOSPOROUS In botany, having but one kind of spore *q.v.*

HOMOTHALLIC 1. A condition in which both male and female sexual structures can develop on the same thallus *q.v.* 2. In bacteriology, the mating of cells from the same strain.

HOMOTHALLISM The condition in which the thallus *q.v.* is self-fertile, or bisexual *q.v.* Single individuals can form fertile zygotes *q.v.* cf: heterothallism.

HOMOTHERMAL 1. Provided with a mechanism that maintains the body at a particular and constant temperature, usually higher than that of the environment.

HOMOTYPIC DIVISION 1. Equatorial division *q.v.* 2. Pertaining to the same form or type.

HOMOVANILLIC ACID A major metabolite *q.v.* of dopamine *q.v.*

HOMOZYGOTE (ADJ. HOMOZYGOUS) An organism whose chromosomes *q.v.* carry identical members of any given pair of genes *q.v.* The gametes *q.v.* are, therefore, all alike with respect to this locus and the individual will breed true.

HOMOZYGOUS 1. A genetic *q.v.* characteristic containing either two dominant or two recessive genes *q.v.* 2. The condition that exists when the genes for a given character on homologous chromosomes *q.v.* are alike. An organism may be homozygous for one or several genes or, rarely, for all genes. 3. The condition in a diploid cell when both genes for a trait are the same allelic *q.v.* form. ct: heterozygous.

HOMOZYGOUS ALLELE An allele *q.v.* that contains two identical dominant genes *q.v.* or two recessive genes *q.v.*

HOMUNCULUS A miniature individual imagined by early biologists to be present in the head of the sperm cell *q.v.*

HOODED CLITORIS Clitoral foreskin adhesions. The condition in which the foreskin *q.v.* of the clitoris *q.v.* covers the glans clitoris *q.v.* to the extent that it interferes with adequate sexual stimulation. cf: clitoral hood.

HOOKWORM A tiny parasite *q.v.* that imbeds in the intestinal wall causing anemia *q.v.* and lack of energy. ~ is caused by the worm *Necator americanus.*

HOPE 1. According to Mowrer's theory, the emotion elicited by a stimulus *q.v.* that has been paired with a positive reinforcer *q.v.* 2. Positive anticipation.

HOPS The dried flowers of the *Humulus lupulus* vine that gives a bitter taste to beer.

HORDEOLUM A sty *q.v.*

HORIZONTAL CURRICULUM FORMAT In education, a design for a written curriculum *q.v.* guide where all information is presented across (horizontally) a page. More simplistic, flexible, and usable than the vertical format *q.v.* Provides teachers with suggestions for student learning, information, and methodology.

HORIZONTAL DECALAGE Within a given period of intellectual growth, the lag time as children apply the same intellectual structures to different content areas. ct: vertical decalage.

HORIZONTAL ENRICHMENT In education, the method whereby the teacher instructs students, who complete their work faster than classmates, to do more of the same type of assignment. ct: vertical enrichment.

HORMOGONIUM A subunit of the schizophyte thallus *q.v.* formed by fragmentation, and functioning is asexual *q.v.* propagation analogous to the trichome *q.v.* in other forms.

HORMONES 1. Chemicals that are manufactured and secreted by the endocrine glands *q.v.* that are essential for regulating specific body functions. 2. A specialized chemical secreted into the blood by a ductless *q.v.* gland and which has a specific effect on specific cells or tissues at some distance from the secreting gland. 3. A chemical product of an organ when secreted into body fluids has a specific effect on other organs. 4. A specific organic substance produced in one part of the organism and moving to and affecting reactions in other parts; in plants, frequently a growth substance or auxin *q.v.*

HORMONE THERAPY 1. Treatment by alteration of hormonal balance designed to adversely influence a tumor whose viability is dependent upon the presence or absence of particular hormones *q.v.* This may be accomplished by either surgery, radiation, or hormonal medication. 2. Treatment of people who have insufficient hormone production with synthetic *q.v.* hormone supplements.

HORNBOOK A single printed page containing the alphabet, syllable, a prayer, and other simple words and which was used in colonial times as the beginner's first book or pre-primer. ~s were attached to a wooden paddle for ease in carrying and were covered with a thin sheet of transparent horn for protection.

HOSPICE 1. Literal definition is an inn for travelers. 2. A facility for some terminally ill persons that provides the opportunity to die with appropriate medical care and in the presence of relatives. 3. The original ~ is St. Christopher's Hospice founded in 1948. cf: hospice care.

HOSPICE CARE An approach to caring for terminally ill people that maximizes their quality of life and allows death with dignity. cf: hospice.

HOSPITAL A facility equipped to deal with a variety of illnesses and injuries. ~s vary considerably in the types and quality of care provided and the types and quality of staffing. In addition, there are ~s that are publically operated, privately operated, and a combination of financial arrangements. Costs for services provided also have a various range. Essentially, ~s room and board, with medical, nursing, custodial, dietary, laboratory, and other services. cf: nursing home; day hospital; night hospital.

HOSPITAL INSURANCE Basically, a room and board coverage during a stay in hospital *q.v.* There are usually a variety of restrictions relative to coverage: limitations, copayments, deductibles, and others.

HOSPITAL OF St. BONIFACE Located in Florence, Italy, the insane asylum where Vincento Chiarugi introduced the moral treatment movement of the mentally ill.

HOST 1. In bacteriology and epidemiology, one sector or element of the public health model of drug abuse prevention, specifically relating to individuals and their knowledge about psychoactive drugs *q.v.*, the personal attitudes that influence drug use and patterns of abuse, and drug-taking behavior itself. 2. The individual or population with a disease *q.v.*

HOSTILE AGGRESSION In psychology, aggression *q.v.* that is designed to harm or injure. ct: instrumental aggression.

HOSTILITY 1. In psychology, anger *q.v.* 2. An emotion that has a basic release tendency toward destruction. 3. An emotional reaction or drive toward damage of an object interpreted as a source of frustration or threat.

HOST NEGLIGENCE The blame placed on a host who directly or indirectly contributes to the injury or death of a guest who consumes alcohol or other intoxicating *q.v.* drugs *q.v.*

HOT FLASHES 1. The temporary feelings of warmth experienced by women during and following menopause *q.v.* which is caused by blood vessel dilation *q.v.* May be caused by decreased production of estrogen *q.v.* 2. Flushes. 3. A transitory sensation of heat similar to blushing but often involving the whole body. ~ occur as blood vessels readjust to diminished amounts of estrogen being produced by the body.

HOUSE In government, the federal legislative body commonly known as the House of Representatives; the lower house. ct: senate.

HOUSEHOLD Consists of all the people who occupy a housing unit. A house, an apartment, or other group of rooms or a single room is regarded as a housing unit when it is occupied or intended for occupancy as separate living quarters, that is, when the occupants do not live with any other person in the structure and there is direct access from the outside or through a common hall. A household includes the related family members and all the unrelated persons, if any, such as lodgers, foster children, wards, or employees who share the housing unit. A person living alone in a housing unit, or a group of unrelated persons sharing a unit as partners, is also considered a household.

HOUSEHOLDER The person in whose name the housing unit is owned or rented or, if there is no such person, any adult member, excluding roomers, boarders, or paid employees. If the house is owned or rented jointly by a married couple, the householder may be either the husband or wife. The person designated as the householder is the "reference person" to whom the relations of all other household members, if any, are recorded. Before 1980, the husband was always considered the householder in married-couple households.

HOUSEHOLD SURVEY In nutritional studies, a method of dietary evaluation in which a trained interviewer visits the home to obtain information about family use of foods. Such a survey may also be done for other behavioral patterns, such as driving habits, the use of medications, etc.

HOUSE OF ORIGIN In politics, the chamber in which a measure is first introduced. A bill is filed either with the Clerk of the House or the Secretary of the Senate, is numbered, and is assigned to a committee.

HOUSE PROSTITUTES Brothel prostitutes *q.v.*

HOUSE STAFF Pertains to intern and residents within a particular hospital.

HP An acronym for hydrostatic pressure *q.v.*

HPL An acronym for human placental lactogen *q.v.*

HRA An acronym for health risk appraisal *q.v.*

HRAF An acronym for human relations area files.

HRD An acronym for human resources development *q.v.*

HRS An acronym for Hazard Ranking System *q.v.*

HRSA An acronym for Health Resources and Services Administration *q.v.*

HRSD An acronym for Hazard Ranking System Database *q.v.*

HS An acronym for house surgeon.

HSA An acronym for human serum albumin. Also, Health Systems Agency *q.v.*

HSDB An acronym for Hazardous Substance Data Bank *q.v.*

HTLV-I An acronym for human T-cell lymphotropic virus, type I. cf: HTLV-II; HTLV-III.

HTLV-II Human T-cell lymphotropic virus, type II. cf: HTLV-I; HTLV-III.

HTLV-III The human T-cell lymphotropic virus type III, the name once given by the National Cancer Institute *q.v.* to the virus now known as human immunodeficiency virus *q.v.*

HUE 1. A perceived *q.v.* color dimension of visual stimuli *q.v.* 2. Chromatin *q.v.* light stimulus. ct: brightness; saturation.

HUMAN ASSET ACCOUNTING A control tool based on the process of establishing the dollar value of human resources within an organization.

HUMAN CHORIONIC GONADOTROPIN (HCG) 1. A hormone *q.v.* produced by the placenta *q.v.* that can be detected in a woman's urine. 2. Chorionic gonadotropin hormone *q.v.* that maintains the ovaries' production of progesterone *q.v.* 3. A hormone produced during the early stages of pregnancy *q.v.* and used as the basis of pregnancy tests.

HUMAN DEVELOPMENT The study of the development of humans from infancy through adulthood.

HUMAN ECOLOGY 1. The study of the relations between humans and their environment. 2. The science concerned with the whole person in his or her reciprocal dynamic relationships with the total environment. cf: ecology.

HUMAN EFFECTIVENESS Generally, how well people perform in achieving predetermined goals. Factors that influence ~ are 1. hereditary makeup, 2. personal qualities that are developed, 3. the quality of the social and physical environments *q.v.*, and 4. the quality of the health care system *q.v.* ~ is variable since a person may be effective *q.v.* in one setting and ineffective in another setting. cf: levels of health.

HUMAN ENERGETICS Associated with motivation *q.v.* that influences the intensity of a person's response to internal and/or external stimuli *q.v.* When an external motivator is related to some internal need *q.v.*, it activates the energy *q.v.* necessary for appropriate action to take place. The intensity of motivation determines the amount of energy necessary for the endurance to achieve the goal or to satisfy the need.

HUMAN ETHOLOGY The application to human behavior *q.v.* of the research orientation based on the assumption that innate *q.v.* behavioral predispositions contribute to behavior development in important ways.

HUMAN FACTORS ENGINEERING Designed and constructed machines and controls to increase comfort, ease, and simplicity for users.

HUMAN GENOME PROJECT A multinational research effort begun in 1987 to map the entire sequence of the human genome. It was originally believed to be a project that would possibly take decades to complete. However, with the various technological advances that occurred, scientists completed the mapping in 2002. The medical/health benefits of the mapping are yet to be determined.

HUMAN IMMUNODEFICIENCY VIRUS (HIV) The retrovirus (RNA virus) that causes AIDS *q.v.* and AIDS-related complex (ARC). cf: HTLV-III.

HUMANISTIC EDUCATION 1. Humanistic therapies *q.v.* 2. An approach to instruction that stresses attitudes, values, personal fulfillment, and relationships with others.

HUMANISTIC–EXISTENTIAL THERAPY Insight psychotherapy that emphasizes the individual's subjective experiences, free will, and ever-present ability to decide on a new life course.

HUMANISTIC MEDICINE Medical practice and culture that respects and incorporates the concepts that the person is more than his or her disease and the professional is more than a scientifically trained mind using technical skills. People are more than their bodies. They are unique, interdependent relationships of body, mind, emotions, culture, and spirit.

HUMANISTIC PSYCHOTHERAPY Humanistic therapies *q.v.*

HUMANISTIC TEACHER EDUCATION An approach to teacher education that is concerned not only with teacher candidates' cognitive development but with their emotional and attitudinal development as well.

HUMANISTIC THERAPIES 1. Methods of treatment that are directed toward personal growth and self-fulfillment. 2. Nondirective techniques *q.v.* to help persons achieve the capacity for making personal choices. 3. Client-centered therapy *q.v.*

HUMANISTS Researchers who explain a particular effect in terms of the occurrence of a certain set of events. They seek the most powerful images and models that foster human understanding.

HUMAN LEUKOCYTE ANTIGENS (HLA) Protein *q.v.* markers of self used in histocompatibility testing. Some ~ types are also correlated with certain autoimmune *q.v.* diseases.

HUMAN MUTANT CELL REPOSITORY The Institute for Medical Research *q.v.* located in Camden, NJ. A branch of the National Institute of General Medical Sciences *q.v.* established in 1972.

HUMAN NEEDS 1. Urgencies essential for biological *q.v.* life and for mental, emotional, and social life *q.v.* 2. Basic needs *q.v.* 3. Biological needs *q.v.* and psychological needs *q.v.*

HUMAN PLACENTAL LACTOGEN (HPL) A hormone *q.v.* that stimulates *q.v.* breast growth during pregnancy *q.v.*

HUMAN PLASTICITY A learned phenomenon that is associated with the ability to change, adapt, or modify oneself or one's environment *q.v.*

HUMAN RELATIONS AREA FILES (HRAF) The original cross-cultural files started by George Peter Murdock in the late 1930s. Topics of interest on cultures were indexed on cards covering the information on that topic for all available cultures. Out of this endeavor came the Ethnographic Atlas *q.v.* and then the standard sample *q.v.*

HUMAN RESOURCE ACCOUNTING A proposed approach to accounting that involves an attempt to place a value on an organization's personnel.

HUMAN RESOURCE DEVELOPMENT (HRD) A continuous process of teaching and educating employees to improve their effectiveness in present and future jobs.

HUMAN RESOURCE PLANNING 1. Manpower planning. 2. The process by which an organization ensures that it has the right number of people and the right kind of people, at the right places, at the right time, doing the things for which they are economically most useful.

HUMAN RESOURCE PROGRAMMING The process of applying employee data and forecasts in the planning of programs to meet future human resource needs.

HUMAN RESOURCES 1. People in an organization. 2. People who possess certain productive skills in an organization.

HUMAN RESOURCES INVENTORY 1. An accumulation of information concerning the characteristics of organization members; this information focuses on the past performances of organization members as well as how they might be trained and best used in the future. 2. People resources *q.v.* 3. Provides employees' past experience with a company, job interests, capabilities, promotion potential, development needs, and other relevant personnel information.

HUMAN SERVICES Community services designed to meet the needs of its people. ~ include mental health, social health, educational, emergency, and safety services.

HUMAN SEXUALITY The broad concept that encompasses people's relationships, anatomy *q.v.*, behaviors *q.v.*, thoughts, and feelings, values, and variabilities regarding sex, and all of its ramifications. It is the state of being human.

HUMAN SEXUAL RESPONSE CYCLE As described by Masters and Johnson, the four phases of the sexual response are 1. excitement, 2. plateau, 3. orgasmic, and 4. resolution. These phases hold true for both men and women, although there are some gender differences in duration of time each stage lasts and there is a refractory period in the male after orgasm during which further stimulation will not result in further response.

HUMAN SKILLS The ability to build cooperation within the people being led.

HUMERAL EPICONDYLE A projection from the humerus *q.v.* near the articular extremity above or upon the condyle *q.v.*

HUMERUS The bone of the upper arm that extends from the shoulder to the elbow.

HUMIDIFICATION The process of adding water to a gas making it humid or moist. cf. humidifier.

HUMIDIFIER A device used with an oxygen supply to moisten the oxygen and prevent its drying effect on the nose and throat. cf: humidification.

HUMIDITY 1. Dampness. 2. Relative humidity is the water vapor content of air as a percentage of the saturation content at the same temperature.

HUMORAL Body fluids or the substances contained in them.

HUMORAL IMMUNITY 1. The presence of antibodies *q.v.* in the blood. 2. A form of acquired immunity *q.v.* that uses antibodies to counter specific antigens *q.v.* that enter the body. 3. The production of antibodies for defense against infection *q.v.* or disease *q.v.* 4. A defense mechanism involving production of antibodies in body fluids, such as serum *q.v.* and lymph *q.v.*, which are directed against bacteria *q.v.*, viruses *q.v.*, and other antigens.

HUMORS Proposed by Hippocrates, that the body contains four humors: blood, black bile, yellow bile, and phlegm. Proper balance of these humors was indicative of health, an imbalance indicative of illness. cf: Hippocrates' body humor theory.

HUMUS 1. In botany, a complex of incomplete decomposed organic materials in the soil. 2. Partially decayed plant material, constituting part of the organic matter of soils.

HUNCHBACK Kyphosis *q.v.*

HUNGER A sensation produced by a physiological *q.v.* need for food.

HUNGER CENTER In anatomy and physiology, the lateral hypothalamus *q.v.* cf: ventromedial region of the hypothalamus.

HUNTINGTON'S CHOREA 1. A rare and fatal hereditary *q.v.* disorder characterized by severe and progressive mental deterioration, muscular spasms, and psychotic behavior. 2. Huntington's disease *q.v.* 3. A fatal presenile *q.v.* dementia, passed on by a single dominant gene *q.v.*

HUNTINGTON'S DISEASE 1. An autosomal *q.v.* dominant genetic disease. 2. A late appearing genetic disease. 3. A genetic disease resulting in degeneration of nerve tissue usually appearing in midlife. 4. Huntington's chorea *q.v.* 5. An incurable disease, presumably of genetic origin that is manifest in jerking, twisting movements, and mental deterioration.

HURRY SICKNESS 1. An excessive time dependency *q.v.* 2. A condition seen in persons whose lives are geared to rigid schedules and high achievement aspirations.

HUSTLER A slang expression for a male prostitute *q.v.* who serves other males who are seeking homosexual *q.v.* relations.

HUSTLING THEORY The theory stating that the rituals and activities associated with the use of drugs reinforce addiction *q.v.* and abuse.

HUTCHINSON'S TEETH In dentistry, notched or peg-shaped teeth typically found in persons with congenital syphilis *q.v.*

HVZ An acronym for herpes varicella zoster virus *q.v.*

HYALINE 1. Clear or transparent. 2. Transparent, with a straw-colored tint.

HYALOPLASM The ground substance of living protoplasm *q.v.*

HYALURONIDASE An enzyme *q.v.* that helps sperm *q.v.* to penetrate ova *q.v.*

H-Y ANTIGEN 1. The substance that controls the transformation of the primitive gonads *q.v.* into testes *q.v.* in the embryo *q.v.* When ~ is not present, the primitive gonads develop into ovaries *q.v.* 2. A gene product triggered by a gene on the Y chromosome *q.v.* that causes undifferentiated gonads to develop into testes.

HYBRID 1. In genetics, the result of a cross between two species or incipient species. 2. The progeny of a cross between two individuals differing in one or more genes *q.v.* cf: hybridization.

HYBRIDIZATION 1. In genetics, the process of crossing individuals of unlike genetic *q.v.* constitution. 2. Interbreeding of species, races, varieties, etc., among plants and animals. 3. A process of forming a hybrid *q.v.* by cross pollination of plants or by mating animals of different types.

HYBRIDOMA A hybrid *q.v.* cell created by fusing a B lymphocyte *q.v.* with a long-lived neoplastic *q.v.* plasma cell *q.v.*, or a T lymphocyte *q.v.* with a lymphoma cell *q.v.* A B-cell hybridoma secretes a single specific antibody *q.v.*

HYBRID VIGOR 1. In genetics, the increased vigor that frequently is demonstrated by the progeny *q.v.* of a cross between inbred lines or between unrelated forms, varieties, or species. 2. Heterosis. 3. Unusual growth, strength, and health of hybrids *q.v.* from two less vigorous parents.

HYDRATED Technically, to indicate that a person is in a satisfactory state of water balance.

HYDRATION The process of returning the body fluid levels to normal. ct: dehydration.

HYDRAULIC-POWER UNIT A hand-operated hydraulic device used with attachments for the forceful raising, pushing apart, or pulling of vehicles or material useful in reaching and extricating trapped victims.

HYDROCARBON An organic compound that contains the elements of hydrogen and carbon.

HYDROCARBON SOLVENTS Fumes of hydrocarbons *q.v.* These compounds depress the central nervous system *q.v.*

HYDROCELE An accumulation of fluid in the scrotum *q.v.*

HYDROCEPHALUS 1. An abnormal increase in the amount of cerebral *q.v.* fluid resulting in an enlargement of the head and other symptoms. 2. A condition in which an excess of cerebrospinal fluid *q.v.* accumulates in the skull and results in potentially damaging pressure on the cerebral tissue. cf: hydrocephaly.

HYDROCEPHALY 1. A condition produced by an accumulation of cerebrospinal fluid *q.v.* in the cranial cavity. 2. Literally, water head. 3. Also, hydrocephalus *q.v.*, an enlargement of the cranium resulting from pressure of spinal fluid. 4. A blockage of an outlet of the ventricles *q.v.* of the brain which interferes with the drainage of the cerebrospinal fluid.

HYDROCHLORIC ACID The acid *q.v.* of gastric juices *q.v.* ~ gas and concentrated solution are strong irritants.

HYDROCODONE 1. Dihydrocodeinone *q.v.* 2. A synthetic derivative of morphine *q.v.* 3. A narcotic *q.v.* analgesic *q.v.*

HYDROCORTISONE 1. Cortisol *q.v.* 2. Compound F. 3. A hormone *q.v.* secreted by the adrenal cortex *q.v.*

HYDROGEN Chemical symbol is H. A gaseous element that combines with oxygen to form water (H_2O) and with carbon to form hydrocarbons *q.v.*

HYDROGENATION 1. The process of adding hydrogen to polyunsaturated *q.v.* oils to solidify them. 2. The process of changing a liquid fat to a solid fat by bubbling hydrogen *q.v.* through it.

HYDROGEN BOND A weak bond between a hydrogen *q.v.* atom attached to one oxygen *q.v.* or nitrogen *q.v.* atom and another oxygen or nitrogen atom. Important in water, proteins, and chromosomes *q.v.* cf: hydrogen bonding.

HYDROGEN BONDING Chemical bonds within compounds occurring at the points at which hydrogen *q.v.* atoms are found. cf: hydrogen bond.

HYDROGEN CYANIDE A gaseous compound of smoke that can damage the lining of the respiratory system *q.v.* when inhaled.

HYDROLOGIC CONDITION The location of underground water sources.

HYDROLYSIS 1. A chemical process whereby a compound is broken down into simpler units with the uptake of water. 2. A process in which a complex compound is digested into one or more simpler compounds through a reaction with water.

HYDROMORPHONE 1. Dihydromorphone *q.v.* 2. A semi-synthetic derivative of morphine *q.v.* 3. Dilaudid is a brand name.

HYDROPHOBIA 1. Rabies *q.v.* 2. Literally, fear of water. 3. See also Table P-1.

HYDROPHYTE In botany, a plant that grows wholly or partly submerged in water.

HYDROPLANING 1. Moving over the surface of water. 2. The action of a vehicle skimming over a wet pavement with the tires void of direct contact with the road surface because they are on a film of water.

HYDROPONICS The growth of plants in solutions containing essential elements.

HYDROSTATIC PRESSURE (HP) Filtration.

HYDROTHERAPY 1. A form of treatment in which water is used as the therapeutic agent. Used in the practice of physical therapy *q.v.* 2. The use of hot and/or cold baths, and/or ice packs for treatment.

HYDROTROPISM 1. Response of organisms, or parts of organisms, to moisture or water. 2. In botany, the bending of roots toward moist soil.

HYDROXYLATION The chemical change of a compound containing the hydrogen *q.v.* atom to acquisition of the hydroxyl radical *q.v.* A change from H to OH in the chemical structure of a compound.

HYGIENE 1. The science of preserving one's health and that of the community. 2. Personal health care, especially techniques and standards of grooming and cleanliness.

HYGIENE (MAINTENANCE) FACTORS 1. Items that influence the degree of job dissatisfaction. 2. Healthful or unhealthful environmental conditions.

HYMEN 1. The membranous fold that may partially or completely close the opening of the vagina *q.v.* 2. The maidenhead. cf: annular hymen; cribiform hymen.

HYMENIUM A fertile layer in a fructification *q.v.*

HYOID BONE 1. A bone in the throat just above the larynx *q.v.* at the base of the tongue. 2. A bone shaped like the letter U.

HYPERACIDITY Excessive acid *q.v.* condition.

HYPERACTIVE 1. In psychology, refers to a disorder characterized by short attention span and a high level of motor activity. 2. Excessively or pathologically *q.v.* active.

HYPERACTIVE CHILD SYNDROME An attention deficit disorder *q.v.* characterized by the inability to maintain concentration, overactivity, restlessness, etc. cf: hyperkinesis; hyperactivity.

HYPERACTIVITY 1. Above normal physical movement. Often accompanied by an inability to concentrate well on a specific task. 2. Hyperkinesis *q.v.* 3. Unusual activity, particularly for an individual of a given age in a given setting. Usually denotes disruptive activity.

HYPERAGGRESSIVE A person who is overly aggressive *q.v.*

HYPERALGESIA Excessive sensitivity to pain.

HYPERBULIA An occasional symptom of schizophrenia *q.v.* consisting of great reaction resulting from pressures (stress) from within oneself.

HYPERCALCEMIA An abnormally high concentration of calcium *q.v.* in the blood. ct: hypocalcemia.

HYPERCAPNEA Abnormally high blood carbon dioxide (CO_2) concentration.

HYPERCELLULARITY An abnormal increase in the usual number of cells. cf: hypercellular obesity.

HYPERCELLULAR OBESITY A form of obesity *q.v.* seen in people who possess an abnormally large number of fat cells. ct: hypertrophic obesity.

HYPERCHOLESTEROLEMIA A condition in which the person has excessively high levels of serum cholesterol *q.v.*

HYPEREMESIS GRAVIDUM 1. Excessive vomiting. 2. Severe nausea *q.v.* and vomiting in pregnancy *q.v.* that often leads to dehydration *q.v.* and loss of electrolytes *q.v.*

HYPEREMIA An increased amount of blood that expands or distends the blood vessels.

HYPEREPHROMA A malignant *q.v.* growth of the kidney.

HYPERESTHESIA Increased touch sensitivity. ct: hypoesthesia

HYPEREXTENSION 1. Extreme extension or overextension of a joint of the body. 2. Movement of a body joint such that the angle about the center of rotation, the fulcrum *q.v.*, increases beyond 0°. 3. Extension of a limb or part beyond its normal limit. ct: hyperflexion.

HYPERFLEXION Flexion *q.v.* of a limb or part beyond its normal limit. ct: hyperextension.

HYPERGLYCEMIA 1. A condition in which there is a high than normal concentration of glucose *q.v.* in the blood. 2. High blood sugar level characteristic of a person with diabetes mellitus (Type 1 diabetes) *q.v.*

HYPERIDROSIS Excessive sweating.

HYPERINSULINISM Too much insulin *q.v.* in the blood which lowers the blood sugar level and produces insulin shock *q.v.*

HYPERKALEMIA Higher than normal concentration of potassium *q.v.* in the blood.

HYPERKERATOSIS 1. An overdevelopment of the hard, horny layer of the skin. 2. A disease of the cornea *q.v.* of the eye.

HYPERKINESIS 1. Hyperactivity *q.v.*, a behavioral disorder in which the person, usually a child, is abnormally and uncontrollably active. 2. Excessive or exaggerated muscular activity. 3. Hyperkinetic *q.v.*

HYPERKINETIC 1. One who typically exhibits hyperactivity *q.v.* 2. Pertains to an excess of behavior in inappropriate circumstances. cf: hyperkinetic disorder.

HYPERKINETIC DISORDER A brain disorder characterized by extreme motor restlessness, poor attention span, and impulsive and sometimes disorderly behavior that, in children, is treated by prescribed amphetamines *q.v.*

HYPERLIPIDEMIA Generally, excessive levels of saturated fats *q.v.* in the blood.

HYPERMATREMIA A higher than normal concentration of sodium in the blood.

HYPERMNESIA An unusual retention of memory or clarity of memory images.

HYPEROPIA Farsightedness. The image theoretically falls behind the retina *q.v.* of the eye, either because the eyeball axis is too short or because the refraction of light rays entering the eye is too weak. cf: myopia.

HYPERPARATHYROIDISM A condition reflecting the overactive production of parathyroid hormone *q.v.* by the parathyroid gland *q.v.*

HYPERPERISTALSIS Increased activity of the musculature of hollow tube, especially of the intestine.

HYPERPHAGIA Chronic overeating brought about by lesion *q.v.* of the ventromedial region of the hypothalamus *q.v.* cf: bulimia.

HYPERPHOSPHATEMIA An abnormally high concentration of phosphates in the blood.

HYPERPITUITARISM A disease due to overactivity of the pituitary gland *q.v.* which produces a gigantic person with deformed bones.

HYPERPLASIA 1. Precancerous change in the lungs characterized by an increase in the number of layers of basal cells *q.v.* that underlie the inner surface of the bronchial tubes *q.v.* 2. The abnormal multiplication or increase in the number of cells in a tissue. 3. An increase in the number of fat or other cells, a cause of one form of obesity *q.v.* 4. New fat cell formation. cf: hypertrophy.

HYPERPNEA An increase in the rate and amplitude of respiration.

HYPERPYREXIA Abnormally elevated body temperature, as from a fever or activation of the sympathetic nervous system *q.v.* due to a drug, e.g., amphetamine *q.v.*

HYPERSENSITIVITY 1. Allergy *q.v.* 2. A tendency to be unusually sensitive to a particular drug or other agent. 3. Oversensitivity.

HYPERSEXUAL 1. Having an extraordinary high sex drive. 2. Oversexed. 3. Nymphomania *q.v.* in females; satyriasis *q.v.* in males.

HYPERTENSION 1. High blood pressure *q.v.* 2. Average blood pressure is about 120/70 mmHg, but can vary considerably. Generally, the lower the reading the better, unless shock symptoms are present. 3. Abnormally high arterial blood pressure, with or without known cause. cf: essential hypertension; organic hypertension.

HYPERTHERMIA 1. A treatment method in which the body's or a part of the body's temperature is raised. 2. An excess production of body heat. 3. Abnormally elevated core body temperature. 4. A condition in which the body temperature is so far above normal (104°F or 40°C) that irreversible damage or even death may result. ~ sometimes appears as heat stroke *q.v.* or heat exhaustion *q.v.* 5. Unusually high fever.

HYPERTHYROIDISM The overproduction of thyroxin *q.v.* from the thyroid gland *q.v.* which results in weight loss, restlessness, over-energetic activity, impulsive, and alert. ct: hypothyroidism.

HYPERTONIC A solution with a higher osmotic *q.v.* pressure (greater solute concentration) than a standard solution, usually water or physiological *q.v.* saline. ct: hypotonic.

HYPERTONIC SALINE SOLUTION A salt solution *q.v.* with a concentration higher than that found in human fluids. cf: saline solution.

HYPERTRICHOSIS Hair growth in excess of normal. cf: hirsutism.

HYPERTROPHIC OBESITY A form of obesity *q.v.* in which fat cells are enlarged. ct: hypercellular obesity.

HYPERTROPHY 1. An enlargement or outgrowth of a bodily part or organ because of enlargement of its constituent elements. 2. An enlargement of a tissue or organ due to exercise. cf: hyperplasia.

HYPERVENTILATION 1. Excessive rapid and deep breathing. May be brought on by excitement. 2. Very rapid and deep breathing associated with high levels of anxiety that causes levels of carbon dioxide *q.v.* in the blood to be lowered with possible loss of consciousness. 3. Increased pulmonary ventilation beyond that needed to maintain blood gases within the normal ranges. The expiration of excessive amounts of carbon dioxide causes a variety of symptoms such as dizziness or unconsciousness.

HYPERVITAMINOSIS 1. Symptoms of ill health resulting from the ingestion of large amounts of a vitamin *q.v.* 2. Vitamin poisoning. 3. An excessive accumulation of vitamins within the body associated with the fat-soluble vitamins *q.v.*

HYPERVOLEMIA Larger than normal volume of blood. ct: hypovolemia.

HYPESTHESIA Decreased sensitivity, especially to touch. ct: hyperesthesia.

HYPHA 1. In botany, a branched filament of a fungus *q.v.* 2. Basic unit of the fungus thallus *q.v.* cf: hyphae.

HYPHAE In botany, threadlike structures that compose the plant body of a fungus *q.v.*

HYPNOANALYSIS Analytic psychotherapy *q.v.* carried out under hypnosis *q.v.*

HYPNOANESTHESIA Insensitivity to pain and discomfort as a result of hypnosis *q.v.*

HYPNOGOGIC 1. A state between waking and sleep characterized by vivid and colorful images and thoughts; this state often includes a feeling of flying. 2. Drowsiness or sleeplike or trancelike state.

HYPNOSEDATIVES A group of drugs that have both sedative *q.v.* and hypnotic *q.v.* effects.

HYPNOSIS 1. An induced state susceptibility. Two aspects: 1. posthypnotic suggestion *q.v.* and 2. hypnotic regression *q.v.* 2. A state of focused mental attention in which the mind is particularly open to suggestion. 3. A trancelike state or behavior resembling sleep, characterized primarily by increased suggestibility and induced by suggestion.

HYPNOTHERAPY 1. The medical use of hypnosis *q.v.* for treating physical and emotional disturbances. 2. The use of hypnosis in psychotherapy *q.v.*

HYPNOTIC 1. A drug used to induce sleep. 2. A drug that induces sleep, such as barbiturate *q.v.*, flurazepam *q.v.*, methyl prylon *q.v.*, glutethimide *q.v.*, and chloral hydrate *q.v.*

HYPNOTIC REGRESSION The hypnotized person is returned to earlier years and allowed to relive some of the experiences that may be associated with emotional problems.

HYPNOTICS Drugs that induce sleep. They are generally slowly eliminated from the body and, therefore, make poor anesthetics *q.v.* cf: hypnotic.

HYPOACTIVE SEXUAL DESIRE A condition in which people who once cared about sex have lost sexual appetites. cf: desire; hypoactive sexual drive.

HYPOACTIVE SEXUAL DRIVE The lack of interest in sexual expression. cf: hypoactive sexual desire.

HYPOACTIVITY Lethargy. ct: hyperactivity.

HYPOAROUSAL A state in which the body is less aroused than normal.

HYPOCALCEMIA An abnormally low concentration of calcium in the blood. ct: hypercalcemia.

HYPOCHONDRIAC 1. A person with hypochondriasis *q.v.* 2. A person who is preoccupied with illnesses and their symptoms *q.v.* and who applies them to self. 3. A neurosis *q.v.*

HYPOCHONDRIAL A persistent concern with one's health, usually accompanied by real or imagined symptoms *q.v.* of a disease or illness. In elderly persons, ~ is frequently a sign of depression *q.v.* cf: hypochondriasis.

HYPOCHONDRIASIS 1. A condition characterized by preoccupation with illnesses, diseases, and morbid *q.v.* states. 2. A preoccupation with one's body, aches and pains, and presumed disease. 3. A neurotic *q.v.* conviction that a person is ill or afflicted with a particular disease or several diseases. 4. A neurotic condition characterized by excessive concern about one's health in the absence of related organic *q.v.* pathology *q.v.* 5. A somatoform *q.v.* disorder in which the person misinterprets rather ordinary physical sensations, is preoccupied with fears of having a serious disease, and is not dissuaded by medical opinion. Difficult to distinguish from somatization *q.v.* disorder.

HYPOCHONDRIUM The abdominal region or cavity.

HYPOCRITICAL 1. Pretending to be something that the person is not. 2. Hypocrisy *q.v.*

HYPODERMIC Under, or inserted under, the skin, as in hypodermic injection.

HYPODERMIC SYRINGE A device to which a hollow needle can be attached so that solutions can be injected through the skin. cf: hypodermic.

HYPODERMOCLYSIS The subcutaneous injection of a large quantity of saline solution.

HYPOGLYCEMIA 1. Low blood sugar. Physiological ~ is normal, which helps to make a person hungry. Pathological ~ is a rare condition in which severe symptoms *q.v.* occur when the blood sugar drops very low. 2. A condition characterized by a lower than normal level of glucose *q.v.* in the blood which results in irritability, confusion, depression, lethargy, and weakness. ~ is sometimes caused by the overuse of an antidiabetic *q.v.* drug such as insulin *q.v.* cf: reactive hypoglycemia. ct: hyperglycemia.

HYPOGONADISM Hormonal *q.v.* deprivation resulting in reduction or loss of sexual vigor and occurrence of certain negative emotional reactions, e.g., depression.

HYPOKALEMIA Lower than normal concentration of potassium in the blood.

HYPOKINESIS 1. Insufficient movement. 2. Krauss–Raab effect *q.v.* 3. Decreased motor activity. cf: hypokinetic.

HYPOKINETIC One who is typically hypoactive *q.v.*

HYPOKINETIC DISEASE A disease that relates to or is caused by the lack of regular physical activity.

HYPOMAGMESEMIA An abnormally low magnesium content of the blood plasma *q.v.*

HYPOMANIA 1. A mild form of manic *q.v.* excitement manifested in manic-depressive *q.v.* reactions. 2. An above normal elevation of mood, but not as extreme as mania. 3. A milder form of mania in which an individual is still able to function socially and professionally. ~ can be marked by slight psychomotor *q.v.* overactivity, pressured speech, elation, and irritability.

HYPONATREMIA Lower than normal concentration of sodium in the blood.

HYPOPARATHYROIDISM A condition due to a decrease or absence of parathyroid hormones *q.v.* usually resulting in hypocalcemia *q.v.* and severe muscle spasms.

HYPOPHALLUS A markedly small penis *q.v.* cf: congenital microphallus.

HYPOPHYSECTOMY Surgical removal of the hypophysis *q.v.* or pituitary gland.

HYPOPHYSIS 1. The pituitary gland *q.v.* 2. Greek for undergrowth, hence the pituitary gland which grows out from the undersurface of the brain.

HYPOPITUITARISM Inactivity of the pituitary gland *q.v.* characterized by the persistence of childlike features and excessive fat.

HYPOPLASIA The incomplete development of an organ or tissue.

HYPOSPADIA A congenital defect *q.v.* in males in which the opening of the urethra *q.v.* is on the underside of the penis *q.v.* instead of at the tip. cf: epispadia.

HYPOSTASIS Epistasis *q.v.*

HYPOSTOME The region around or under the mouth.

HYPOTENSION 1. Low blood pressure. 2. A blood pressure below the normal range. 3. An acute drop in blood pressure. 4. A blood pressure reading below 90 systolic and 50 diastolic.

HYPOTHALAMUS 1. A portion of the brain lying beneath the thalamus *q.v.* at the base of the cerebrum *q.v.* and forming the floor and part of the walls of the third ventricle *q.v.* 2. The ~ contains centers for temperature regulation of the body, appetite control, and other functions. 3. The ~ controls many of the body's metabolic *q.v.* activities and regulates physical body functions according to the person's emotional state at a given moment. 4. An area in the lower part of the brain that controls the pituitary gland's *q.v.* sexual functions. 5. The portion of the brain that is a prime site of action of many psychoactive drugs *q.v.*, which maintains homeostasis *q.v.* by regulating activities of the body cavity, emotions, and behavior. 6. Controls the reactions of the autonomic nervous system *q.v.* and is sensitive to internal changes (need states) in the body. 7. The region of the forebrain below the thalamus that is the major central control of the autonomic nervous system and is important in the regulation of body temperature, metabolism, and the endocrine system *q.v.*

HYPOTHECA Smaller inner valve of the diatom thallus *q.v.*

HYPOTHELICO Deductive reasoning *q.v.* A method of reasoning, used largely by natural scientists, that involves the use of assumptions in order to test ideas logically or empirically.

HYPOTHERMIA 1. A drop in body temperature below 95°F (35° C). 2. A condition in which a person's body temperature drops affecting the breathing centers of the central nervous system *q.v.* which may result in respiratory arrest and may cause death. Anyone exposed to severe cold can develop accidental ~; however, those at greater risk are older persons who have chronic illnesses, suffer from temperature regulation defects, or cannot afford heating fuel.

HYPOTHESIS 1. In scientific research, a prediction of the results of an experiment. The experiment is designed to test the validity *q.v.* of the ~. 2. A theoretical proposition used to predict behavior that is yet to be observed. 3. A tentative proposition to be confirmed or rejected by research. 4. A proposed relationship between two or more events or qualities. 5. A statement of a specific relationship between two or more variables *q.v.*

HYPOTHESIS GUESSING In research, subjects guessing what the researcher has in mind and reacting accordingly.

HYPOTHESIS TESTING In research, the process of statistical inference whereby the likelihood that an observed value, such as the difference between means, is typical of what might be expected as a result of random sampling variation and chance error or is atypically larger and, therefore, the result of some other influence.

HYPOTHYROIDISM The underproduction of thyroxin *q.v.* from the thyroid gland *q.v.* which results in listlessness, slow reactions, easily fatigued, and sluggishness. ct: hyperthyroidism.

HYPOTONIC A solution with a lower osmotic *q.v.* pressure (lesser salt concentration) than a standard solution, usually water or physiological saline *q.v.* ct: hypertonic.

HYPOVOLEMIA Abnormally decreased volume of circulating blood in the body.

HYPOVOLEMIC SHOCK Shock *q.v.* caused by a reduction in blood volume. ~ results from hemorrhage or from relaxation of blood vessel walls.

HYPOXIA 1. Low oxygen level. 2. Low oxygen content in the blood. 3. Deficiency of oxygen in inspired air.

HYPOXIC HYPOXIA A condition resulting from decreased oxygen reaching the blood in the lungs.

HYSTERECTOMY A surgical procedure to remove the uterus *q.v.*, either through the abdominal wall or through the vagina *q.v.* Total ~ is the removal of the uterus and both ovaries *q.v.*

HYSTERIA 1. A defense mechanism *q.v.* 2. A reaction to stress in which psychological *q.v.* turmoil is converted into physical disturbances with no organic cause. 3. Conversion reaction *q.v.* 4. Dissociative disorder *q.v.* ~ is no longer used as a diagnostic category since it erroneously implies that it is more prevalent in females than in males. ~ stems from the Greek *hystera* which means womb. 5. An early term for physical dysfunction (blindness, deafness, paralysis, and others) not caused by any known medical condition, also known as conversion hysteria.

HYSTERICAL NEUROSIS The DSM-IV category for dissociative and somatoform disorders *q.v.* 2. The conversion of mental conflict into extreme physical symptoms, e.g., blindness.

HYSTERICAL PERSONALITY A personality trait *q.v.* characterized by the attempt to control relations with others by simulation of sickness.

HYSTEROSALPINGOGRAM The use of a dye to determine whether the fallopian tubes *q.v.* are obstructed.

HYSTEROTOMY A form of abortion *q.v.* resembling a caesarian section *q.v.* An incision is made through the abdominal wall and the fetus *q.v.* and other products of pregnancy *q.v.* are removed. This method is used between the 13th and 19th weeks of pregnancy. cf: vacuum aspiration; dilation and curettage; menstrual extraction; saline induction.

Hz An acronym for Hertz *q.v.*

IAA An acronym for indoleacetic acid *q.v.*, an important growth hormone.

IAG An acronym for interagency agreement.

IATREION In ancient Greece, a physician's shop or office.

IATROGENIC 1. An adverse condition produced as a result of a diagnostic or treatment procedure. 2. Autosuggestion resulting from a clinician's discussion or examination. 3. A disorder caused by the treatment process. cf: iatrogenic disease.

IATROGENIC DISEASE 1. An illness caused by improper medication or medical care. 2. Iatrogenic illness. The illness may be caused by the effects of a physician or the efforts of a nurse or other health care practitioner. It can also be caused by the move of an older person's move to an unfamiliar setting such as a nursing home. cf: iatrogenic.

IC An acronym for inspiratory capacity.

ICD An acronym for International Classification of Diseases.

ICE A slang, or street term, for crystal-rock methamphetamine *q.v.* cf: crank; go-fast.

ICF An acronym for intracellular fluid *q.v.*

ICHTHYOSIS 1. Dry skin. 2. An inherited or systemic disorder characterized by mild to severe, disfiguring flaking, dry skin.

ICN An acronym of International Council of Nurses.

ICONIC REPRESENTATION Representation of the world through mental imagery.

ICS An acronym for International College of Surgeons.

ICSH An acronym for interstitial cell-stimulating hormone *q.v.*

ICT 1. Insulin coma therapy. 2. Insulin shock treatment *q.v.*

ICTERUS 1. Jaundice *q.v.* 2. The yellow appearance of the skin and other tissues due to an excessive accumulation of bile pigments.

ICU An acronym for intensive care unit.

ID 1. The primitive aspects of the psyche *q.v.* All psychic energy runs through the ~ from which all instincts *q.v.* or drives *q.v.* emanate. 2. In Freudian psychology *q.v.*, the component of personality concerned with need *q.v.* gratification. 3. The unconscious pleasure drive. 4. In psychoanalytic theory *q.v.*, that part of the personality present at birth. It is composed of all the energy of the psyche and expressed as biological urges that continuously seek gratification. 5. In Freud's theory, the component of the personality that is directed by biological cravings.

IDAV An acronym for immune deficiency-associated virus.

IDEAL HEALTH The state in which a person's maximum potentialities in the physical, mental, and social spheres are realized.

IDEALISM 1. The philosophy that holds that all knowledge is derived from ideas, emphasizing moral and spiritual reality. 2. A philosophy that emphasizes global ideas related to moral teachings.

IDEAL SELF A set of beliefs a person has concerning how he or she should behave and what he or she would like to be.

IDEAL WEIGHT Typically assumed to be the weight a person achieves at the age of 22–25.

IDEAS OF REFERENCE 1. A characteristic of some mental disorders *q.v.* in which the person thinks that external events are specifically related to them on a personal basis. 2. Delusional *q.v.* thinking in which the person believes that insignificant events and activities of others are extremely significant to them. Symptoms of the prodromal *q.v.* phase of schizophrenia *q.v.*

IDENTICAL TWINS 1. Two offspring developed from one ovum *q.v.* 2. Twins that originate from a single fertilized egg that splits into two exact replicas possessing identical genotypes *q.v.* 3. Monozygotic *q.v.* twins developed from a single fertilized egg. ct: fraternal twins.

IDENTIFICATION 1. Introjection *q.v.* 2. A defense mechanism *q.v.* that functions by a person assuming the identity of someone else. 3. In reference to gender role, the child takes on the demeanor and personality of the parent of the same sex. 4. In psychoanalytic psychology *q.v.*, a mechanism whereby a child models itself on the same-sexed parent in an unconscious *q.v.* effort to be like that parent. 5. In social psychology, the tendency to yield to group pressures because the group has attractive qualities. The process by which people pattern themselves on others and thus learn social roles.

IDENTITY 1. A person's concept of self. 2. The knowledge of who society says you are, combined with who you say you are. 3. A sense of psychological well-being produced by one's acceptance of one's appearance, goals, and recognition from others.

IDENTITY ACHIEVEMENT TYPE An adolescent *q.v.* who has made satisfying, self-chosen commitments relative to sex roles and occupational choice. ct: identity diffusion type.

IDENTITY CONFUSION Identity crisis *q.v.*

IDENTITY CRISIS 1. Identity confusion *q.v.* 2. A delay in structuring a mature identity *q.v.*, resulting in psychological distress.

IDENTITY DIFFUSION TYPE An adolescent who avoids thinking about goals, roles, and values. cf: identity achievement type.

IDENTITY DISSOLUTION A progressive, continuing loss of the immediate sense of self—a symptom of the prodromal stage of schizophrenia *q.v.*

IDEOGRAM A diagrammatic representation of the chromosomes of an individual illustrating their relative sizes and appearance.

IDEOGRAPHIC 1. The qualities possessed by individuals that make them different from others. 2. An approach to personality *q.v.* that emphasizes the unique aspects of the individual personality. 3. In psychology, relating to investigative procedures that consider the unique characteristics of a single person. ct: nomothetic.

IDEOGRAPHIC APPROACH An approach to the study of personality *q.v.* that emphasizes the unique aspects of the individual's personality.

IDEOGRAPHIC LAW Lawfulness within the behavior *q.v.* of a person. ct: nomothetic.

IDEOLOGY The fundamental beliefs of an individual or group concerning human nature. Specific ideologies relate to the level of agreement of the individual's personal beliefs with those of the culture.

IDIOPATHIC 1. Of unknown causation. 2. Inherent in the constitutional makeup of the person.

IDIOSYNCRASY A peculiar susceptibility to some foreign substance or physical agent.

IDIOSYNCRATIC A characteristic, habit, or mannerism unique to an individual.

IDIOSYNCRATIC RESPONSE Special sensitivity or unanticipated adverse reaction to a specific chemical substance. cf: allergy; hypersensitivity.

IDIOT 1. The term ~ is rarely used today to describe people possessing extremely low intelligence *q.v.* 2. A feebleminded *q.v.* person with an intelligence quotient *q.v.* of 25 or lower. 3. Mental retardation *q.v.*

IDIOT SAVANT An individual with a rare form of mental retardation *q.v.* but being extremely talented in one or several limited areas of intellectual achievement.

IDIOTYPES The unique parts and characteristics of an antibody's *q.v.* variable region. They may also serve as antigens *q.v.*

IEP An acronym for individualized education program *q.v.*

IF 1. Interstitial fluid *q.v.* 2. Intercellular fluid *q.v.*

IFIF An acronym for International Federation for Internal Freedom *q.v.*

IHS An acronym for Indian Health Services *q.v.*

IL-2 Interleukin-2 *q.v.*

ILEITIS An infection of the portion of the small intestine near the cecum *q.v.*

ILEOCECAL VALVE The portion of the terminal ileum *q.v.* into the large intestine at the ileocolic junction. The ~ protects the terminal ileum from feces *q.v.* being forced back from the cecum *q.v.*

ILEOCOLOSTOMY A short-circuiting surgical procedure that establishes a connection between the ileum *q.v.* and some part of the colon *q.v.*

ILEUM 1. The distal part of the small intestine opening into the cecum *q.v.* 2. The third and largest part of the small intestine, about 12 ft long and located between the jejunum *q.v.* and the colon.

ILEUS An intestinal obstruction resulting from paralysis *q.v.* of bowel motility caused by peritonitis *q.v.* or other inflammatory processes.

ILIAC CREST The large bony prominence at the top of each side of the hips.

ILLEGITIMATE Born to parents who are not married to each other.

ILLICIT DRUG 1. A drug that is not used in a legal way, even when it is not an illegal drug. 2. An illegal drug. 3. A legal drug used illegally.

ILLITERATE 1. The inability to read and/or write at a functional level. 2. Ignorant.

ILLITERATE E A visual acuity test using the letter E with the arms placed randomly facing in various directions. Generally used with very young children or those who are unable to read. cf: STYCAR; Snellen eye test.

ILLNESS 1. A condition that may or may not involve clinical signs and symptoms that form a known disease entity. 2. Symptoms or ill feelings experienced by an unwell person. 3. Ill health. 4. Disease *q.v.* 5. A negative state of health. cf: disease.

ILLNESS BEHAVIOR 1. Any activity undertaken by persons who feel ill to discover what is wrong and what can be done about it. 2. A component of the health belief model *q.v.* 3. According to SOPHE *q.v.*, that which occurs following the diagnosis of disease. cf: sick role behavior. ct: health behavior.

ILLNESS STAGE 1. One of the stages of disease characterized by the appearance of specific signs and symptoms *q.v.* 2. Acute stage.

ILLOCUTIONARY FORCE The effect of a spoken or written phrase, the meaning of which is different than its grammatical function. For example, the phrase, "What's up?" is not necessarily meant to be a question but rather a statement of greeting.

ILLUSINOGENS Psychedelic *q.v.* chemicals.

ILLUSION 1. The result when one erroneously organizes, then misinterprets, and misperceives stimuli *q.v.* from the physical environment as something contrary to reality. 2. A distorted perception. 3. Misinterpretation of sensory data. 4. False perception *q.v.* ct: hallucination.

ILLUSORY CORRELATION The tendency to seek information that supports and to avoid that which contradicts a particular belief.

ILP An acronym for individualized language plan *q.v.*

IM An acronym for intramuscular injection *q.v.*

IMA An acronym for Industrial Medical Association.

IMAGERY 1. The ability to see, hear, smell, taste, and feel through the mind's eye. 2. The ability to fantasize or daydream.

IMAGING The enhancement of memory through mentally picturing information.

IMBECILE 1. A rarely used term to describe people possessing extremely low intelligence *q.v.* 2. A feebleminded person with an intelligence quotient *q.v.* of 25–50. 3. A form of mental retardation *q.v.* ct: idiot; moron.

IMBIBITION The absorption of water and the swelling of colloidal material because of the absorption of water onto the internal surfaces of the materials.

IMC An acronym for Instructional Materials Center *q.v.*

I-MESSAGE The process whereby a teacher explains how he or she feels about an unsatisfactory situation.

IMIPRAMINE 1. An antidepressant *q.v.* drug. 2. One of the tricyclic *q.v.* group. 3. Tofranil is a brand name.

IMITATION (ON FOOD LABELS) Not the real thing and nutritionally inferior than the food it is imitating. cf: substitute.

IMITATION FOOD A term used in food labeling that designates according to government regulations that a food is nutritionally inferior to a food it is substituting.

IMMANENT JUSTICE The concept that no bad deed goes unpunished. Bad acts are inextricably tied to punishments.

IMMATURITY REACTION A mental disorder characterized by persons who are emotionally immature and are, therefore, unable to maintain their equilibrium and independence under stress *q.v.*

IMMEDIATE EFFECT Legislative action to render a law effective immediately upon being signed by the executive. Often, the phrase "takes effect upon passage" is written into the bill.

IMMERSION FOOT A disorder of the feet following prolonged immersion in water characterized by swelling, coldness of the feet, a waxy white appearance, cyanotic *q.v.* areas, and a loss of feeling. Later, the feet become red and hot, and swelling increases.

IMMOBILIZATION Holding a part of the body firmly in place.

IMMOBILIZE To make incapable of movement.

IMMUNE COMPLEX A cluster of interlocking antigens *q.v.* and antibodies *q.v.*

IMMUNE RESPONSE 1. The development by the body of antibodies *q.v.* specific for a particular disease. 2. The production of antibodies, B lymphocytes, in response to an antigen *q.v.* Direct attack on antigens by T lymphocytes. 3. The reaction of the immune system to foreign substances. cf: immunization.

IMMUNE STATUS The condition of the body's natural defenses to disease. ~ is influenced by a person's heredity, age, history of illness, diet, and physical and mental health. Included are the production of antibodies and their mechanism of action.

IMMUNE SURVEILLANCE HYPOTHESIS The proposal that specific cells of the immune system *q.v.* are able to detect and destroy cancer cells as they arise in the body.

IMMUNE SYSTEM 1. The body's ability to develop antibodies *q.v.* that resist disease-producing agents. The system of biochemical *q.v.* and cellular elements that protect the body from invading pathogens *q.v.* and foreign material. 2. The body's major mechanism for resisting disease-causing organisms, consisting of specialized cells and proteins in the blood and other body fluids. cf: immune response.

IMMUNITY 1. The power that a person may acquire to resist an infection *q.v.* to which most other people are susceptible *q.v.* 2. Safe from reinfection. 3. Resistance to disease. 4. Freedom from infection because of resistance. 5. The state of being resistant or not susceptible to a disease. Some immunities are natural; most immunities are produced by the body in the form of specific antibodies *q.v.* or by certain blood cells after exposure to antigens *q.v.*

IMMUNIZATION 1. Naturally or artificially induced resistance to disease. 2. Laboratory prepared pathogens that are introduced into the body for the purpose of stimulating the body's immune system *q.v.* cf: artificial immunity; natural immunity; immune response.

IMMUNIZE 1. To be vaccinated *q.v.* 2. To become immune *q.v.* to a disease. 3. To induce resistance to a parasite or foreign substance.

IMMUNOASSAY 1. A process for measuring an organic chemical by inducing an animal to develop an antibody to it. 2. The use of antibodies to identify and quantify substances. The antibody is often linked to a marker such as a fluorescent molecule or radioactive molecule or an enzyme.

IMMUNOASSAY PREGNANCY TEST A pregnancy *q.v.* test that uses an antigen–antibody response to determine the presence of HCG *q.v.* in a urine sample.

IMMUNOBLOT Western blot technique *q.v.*

IMMUNOCOMPETENT Capable of developing an immune response.

IMMUNODEFICIENT Having an impaired or nonfunctioning immune system.

IMMUNOGLOBULIN Serum globulin *q.v.* having antibody *q.v.* activity. Most of the antibody activity appears to be in the gamma *q.v.* fraction of globulin.

IMMUNOLOGICAL Treating an object or living thing as a foreign body, thus rejecting it.

IMMUNOLOGIC TOLERANCE A condition in which the body fails to reject a foreign object or pathogen *q.v.*

IMMUNOLOGY 1. The science that studies the body's immune system *q.v.* and methods for stimulating it to build antibodies *q.v.* to render a person resistant to a particular disease. 2. The study of the structure and function of the body's immune system.

IMMUNOSTIMULANT Any agent that will trigger an immune response *q.v.*

IMMUNOSUPPRESSANT A drug that decreases the body's defensive response to foreign substances. Used to prevent the body's rejection of transplanted organs and to treat autoimmune diseases.

IMMUNOSUPPRESSED Abnormal function of the immune system. Often the result of drugs used to treat certain illnesses.

IMMUNOSUPPRESSION A condition in which the immune system *q.v.* is not functioning normally. ~ may result from illness, certain drugs, or other environmental effects.

IMMUNOSUPPRESSIVE DRUGS Drugs that suppress the body's immune system *q.v.* and thus prevent the autoimmune *q.v.* destruction of normal body tissues. cf: immunosuppressive effect.

IMMUNOSUPPRESSIVE EFFECT Decreased effectiveness of the body's immune system resulting in the inability to provide protection from bacteria, molds, viruses, and toxins. cf: immunosuppressive drugs.

IMMUNOTHERAPY 1. Treatment technique using the body's immune system *q.v.* to combat a particular disease, e.g., cancer. 2. The use of highly complex vaccines *q.v.* and antibodies *q.v.* to stimulate the body's disease–defense mechanism.

IMPACTED 1. Wedged in a tissue. 2. Stuck within something, as an ~ wisdom tooth.

IMPACT EVALUATION A type of evaluation that measures the cumulative effect of educational programs on a community as a whole.

IMPAIRMENT A physical deviation or defect that reduces a person's ability to function effectively. An ~ may be acquired, genetically based, or congenital *q.v.*

IMPALED Pierced with a pointed object.

IMPERFORATE HYMEN 1. The presence of a hymen *q.v.* with no openings. Surgical incision at the time of first menstruation *q.v.* is indicated. 2. Unopened. 3. Unpierced. cf: cribriform hymen; annular hymen.

IMPETIGO Gym itch. A bacterial skin infection caused by either the *streptococci* or *staphylococcus* bacteria *q.v.* It is transmitted from the skin lesions, either directly or indirectly, from the infected person. Characterized by pink lesions filled with fluid that becomes pus-filled and finally crusty.

IMPLANT Transplanted or inserted material, e.g., artificial joints used in reconstructive surgery. cf: prosthetic device.

IMPLANTATION 1. The embedding of the embryo *q.v.* within the uterine wall. 2. The process of a fertilized egg fusing with the uterine lining to begin the gestational *q.v.* process. 3. Embedding of the blastocyst *q.v.* in the mucous membrane or endometrium *q.v.* lining the uterus *q.v.*

IMPLICIT KNOWLEDGE Understanding the nature of things through intuition and the drawing of conclusions as a result of experiences not necessarily directly related to the situation at hand.

IMPLICIT PERSONALITY THEORY The drawing of conclusions about a person's personality through relating certain characteristics in a seemingly logical way.

IMPLICIT TRIAL AND ERROR Trial and error *q.v.* behavior *q.v.* carried on covertly or at the level of thought rather than action.

IMPLOSIVE THERAPY 1. Based on the assumption that extinction of an unwanted response will occur as a person imagines the frightening stimuli that cause the fear or anxiety. 2. A form of behavior therapy *q.v.* in which the person is encouraged to imagine the worst or most frightening situations related to the fears being confronted. They can then be dealt with in more rational ways. cf: systematic desensitization; operant conditioning.

IMPOTENCE 1. Specifically, the lack of power. 2. The incapacity to perform sexually. 3. The inability to achieve erection *q.v.* ~ may be caused by physical or emotional disturbances. 4. The inability to achieve or maintain an erection. cf: erectile inhibition; erectile dysfunction.

IMPOTENCE—PRIMARY A condition in which a man has never been able to achieve or maintain an erection *q.v.* in either heterosexual *q.v.* or homosexual *q.v.* encounters.

IMPOTENCE—SECONDARY A condition in which a man has had at least one successful sexual encounter, but now has lost the ability to achieve or maintain an erection *q.v.* Its cause may be either physical or psychological *q.v.* This condition is now referred to as inhibited sexual excitement *q.v.*

IMPREGNATE To make pregnant *q.v.*

IMPREGNATION 1. Conception *q.v.* 2. The act of fertilization *q.v.* or fecundation *q.v.* 3. Making pregnant.

IMPRESSION FORMATION 1. In social psychology, the process of forming opinions of people. 2. Interpersonal perception *q.v.* 3. Person perception *q.v.*

IMPRESSION MANAGEMENT The process by which a person shapes other people's impressions of him or herself. cf: self-monitoring.

IMPRINTING 1. The development in the young of a filial attachment to the first large moving object they see. 2. A form of learning in very young animals that determines the exact course an instinctive behavior pattern will take.

IMPULSE 1. A spontaneous tendency to act upon a stimulus *q.v.* 2. A chemical–electrical wave along a nerve *q.v.*

IMPULSIVENESS A tendency to act without thinking about its consequences.

IMPUNITIVE The tendency toward a conciliatory attitude rather than blaming either the self or others.

IN ABSENTIA Literally, in one's absence. The person may be either physically or mentally absent from a proceeding for an action ~ to occur.

INADEQUATE PERSONALITY A personality pattern of disturbance *q.v.* characterized by one who is unable to adapt to varying situations, possesses poor judgment, is generally inept, lacks physical and emotional stamina, is socially incompatible, and does not appropriately respond to intellectual, social, emotional, and physical demands.

INANITION The result of starvation.

INAPPROPRIATE AFFECT Emotional reactions that are out of context with the particular environment. For example, laughing at a funeral, and having no emotion upon receiving bad news.

INBORN ERRORS OF METABOLISM See errors of metabolism.

INBREEDING 1. The breeding of close relatives in both plants and animals. 2. Continued inbreeding for several generations will lead to an increase in homozygosity in the offspring, which can, if continued, virtually eliminate genetic variability.

INCAP An acronym for Institute of Nutrition of Central America and Panama.

INCARCERATION The imprisonment of a tissue by surrounding bonds or adhesions *q.v.*

INCENTIVE 1. A commodity or condition capable of reducing or eliminating a drive or goal. It is an extrinsic *q.v.* motivational device and may take the form of reward or punishment. 2. An external reward or punishment that brings about motivation *q.v.*

INCENTIVE MOTIVATION Motivation generated by external stimuli *q.v.* rather than internal drives.

INCEST 1. Sexual intercourse between members of the same family. 2. Sexual intercourse between two people who are close genetic *q.v.* relatives.

INCEST TABOO Reflective of strong social norms or standards against sexual activities among members of the same family or blood relatives.

INCESTUOUS MOLESTER According to McGaghy, a person who has sexual contact with a child to whom he or she is closely related.

INCIDENCE 1. The number of new cases of a disease during a given period of time. 2. How frequently a disease occurs. 3. The rate of new cases occurring in a population *q.v.* during a given period of time. ct: prevalence.

INCIDENCE DENSITY (RATE) In epidemiology *q.v.*, a rate in which the number of new cases is divided by the number of people at risk. Usually stated as the number of new cases per 100,000.

INCIDENCE RATE 1. The amount or occurrence of disease, injury, or death in a given period of time. 2. In industry, a measure of illnesses and injuries combined, relative to total hours worked. cf: morbidity, mortality, incidence; ct: prevalence.

INCIDENCE STUDY Cohort study *q.v.*

INCIDENTAL ADDITIVE A substance that inadvertently enters food by migrating from packaging materials or contact with surfaces or as a result of processing aids.

INCIDENTAL HEALTH EXPERIENCE Health learning that is unplanned and indirect and that results from daily activities.

INCIDENTAL HEALTH LEARNING 1. Learning without trying to learn. 2. The acquisition of knowledge without a deliberate attempt to seek or acquire that knowledge. Learning of information incidental to, or not important for, the task at hand. ct: intentional learning. cf: individual health learning.

INCIDENT CONTROL METHOD In epidemiology *q.v.*, a case–control study *q.v.* where only new cases are investigated or studied.

INCIDENT PROCESS A problem-solving training method whereby trainees seek out pertinent details in order to make a decision.

INCINERATION The controlled burning of combustible waste at high temperatures.

INCISION A wound made with a sharp instrument.

INCISIONAL BIOPSY The surgical removal of a portion of tissue to be examined.

INCISORS The front teeth used to cut food, located between the left and right cuspids *q.v.*

INCLUSIONS Any foreign or heterogeneous *q.v.* substance contained in a cell or in any tissue or organ that was not introduced as a result of trauma *q.v.*

INCLUSIVE EDUCATION In education, the inclusion of the physically and mentally challenged students in regular classes, done largely as a result of federal law. cf: Public Law 94-142.

INCLUSIVE FITNESS A measure of the total contribution of genes *q.v.* to the next generation by oneself and those with whom one shares genes.

INCOHERENCE In schizophrenia, an aspect of thought disorder wherein verbal expression is marked by fragmented thoughts, disjointed sentences, garbled words and phrases, etc.

INCOMPATIBLE RESPONSE METHOD A method of breaking habits *q.v.* in which a new response *q.v.* is deliberately practiced in the situations that evoke the undesirable response.

INCOMPETENT A legal term designating a person as incapable of managing his or her affairs with ordinary prudence because of mental illness or mental deficiency.

INCOMPLETE DOMINANCE 1. In genetics, the result when two different alleles *q.v.* together produce an effect intermediate between the effects of these same genes in the homozygous *q.v.* condition. 2. An expression of heterozygous alleles different from those of the parents. 3. A condition when a heterozygote for a given trait is phenotypically *q.v.* different from either homozygote *q.v.*

INCOMPLETE PROTEIN 1. Dietary protein *q.v.* that contains fewer than the optimal number or amounts of the essential amino acids *q.v.* 2. Foods that lack one or more of the essential amino acids.

INCONTINENCE Lacking voluntary control over the bladder and bowel. In most people, ∼ can be treated and controlled, if not cured. Specific changes in body function, often resulting from disease or use of medications or other drugs, are the cause of ∼.

INCREASED AWARENESS A condition of stimulation allowing for changes in thought processes, ideas, and behaviors.

INCREASING SPECIFICITY OF DISCRIMINATION The ability of older children to discriminate and respond to as different stimuli *q.v.* that younger children respond to as the same.

INCUBATION 1. Incubation period *q.v.* 2. The development of an infection from the time the organism enters the body until the appearance of signs or symptoms *q.v.* of a disease *q.v.*

INCUBATION PERIOD 1. In the process of a communicable disease, the time from exposure to the infective agent *q.v.* to the onset of symptoms of the characteristic disease. 2. The time between the actual entry of an infectious agent into the body and the onset of disease symptoms. 3. The time it takes from the moment of entry into the body of a disease-producing agent until the signs and symptoms *q.v.* of the disease appear. 4. Incubation stage *q.v.*

INCUBATION STAGE Incubation period *q.v.*

INCUBATOR 1. A device that provides protection and temperature control for a newborn infant. 2. A device for culturing microorganisms *q.v.*

INCUS 1. One of the bones of the middle ear. 2. The anvil bone of the middle ear. ct: malleus; stapes.

IND Investigational New Drug number *q.v.*

INDEMNITY PAYMENT A system of paying insurance benefits by way of a flat amount for each day of care provided.

INDEPENDENT ASSOCIATION In epidemiology *q.v.*, a relationship between two variables that hold constant when controlling or changing for other variables.

INDEPENDENT ASSORTMENT 1. The segregation of two or more pairs of genes *q.v.* and their distribution into the gametes *q.v.* independent of one another. 2. Mendel's second law—random distribution of nonallelic genes during gamete formation.

INDEPENDENT COMBINATIONS 1. Independent assortment *q.v.* 2. The random behavior of genes *q.v.* in different chromosomes *q.v.* The distribution of one pair of genes is not controlled by other genes on nonhomologous chromosomes.

INDEPENDENT SCHOOL A nonpublic school not affiliated with any religion or other public or private agency.

INDEPENDENT VARIABLE 1. In epidemiology *q.v.*, a characteristic being considered or tested for its relationship to a health condition. 2. Any variable *q.v.* that serves as a basis for making a prediction. 3. A variable that researchers systematically vary in order to determine its possible effects on a dependent variable *q.v.* 4. In psychology, the factor or treatment that is under the control of the researcher and that is expected to have an effect on the subjects as determined by changes in the dependent variable. 5. The factor whose effects are being evaluated. In health education, the independent variable is the method, technique, or strategy. cf: experiment. ct: dependent variable.

INDEX CASE The person, who in a genetic investigation, bears the diagnosis *q.v.* or trait *q.v.* that the researcher is interested in. cf: proband.

INDIAN HEALTH SERVICES (IHS) A federal bureau focused on the delivery of health and medical services to Native Americans, particularly those residing on Indian reservations.

INDIAN HEMP An inaccurate term popularly used to describe all forms of cannabis *q.v.*

INDIFFERENT GONADS The potential sex organs of both sexes in prenatal development. This occurs during the 5th week of prenatal development. The gonad precursors consist of outer cells (the cortex) that can develop into ovaries *q.v.* and inner cells (the medulla) that can develop into testes *q.v.*

INDIGESTION An inability or difficulty in digesting food.

INDIRECT ASSOCIATION 1. In epidemiology *q.v.*, a dependent relationship between two variables that appears to exist because of the confounding influence of a third variable and disappears when the third variable is controlled. 2. A secondary association *q.v.*

INDIRECT CALORIMETER The measurement of the amount of oxygen consumed.

INDIRECT CONTACT A means of transmitting a communicable disease *q.v.* indirectly by contact with contaminated objects. ct: direct contact.

INDIRECT EUTHANASIA Passive euthanasia *q.v.* The process of allowing a person to die by discontinuing life-support systems or withholding life-saving techniques.

INDIRECT METHOD OF AGE ADJUSTMENT In epidemiology *q.v.*, standard rates are applied to the population being studied so as to calculate the expected number of events that is then compared with the observed number of events.

INDIRECT TRANSMISSION The transmission of a disease to a susceptible host by means of vectors, fomites *qq.v.*, or through the air.

INDIVIDUAL EDUCATION PROGRAM (IEP) A specially planned instruction program and evaluation designed for a particular handicapped learner. This program is required by Public Law 94-142 *q.v.*

INDIVIDUAL FINANCING In health care and health services, the financing of health costs without the benefit of any prepayment or insurance plan.

INDIVIDUAL HEALTH LEARNING See individualized learning.

INDIVIDUALIZED INSTRUCTION Educational activities that are tailored to the needs and interests of individual learners. Each student receives his or her own learning plan, associated activities, and evaluation mechanisms. cf: individualized learning.

INDIVIDUALIZED LANGUAGE PLAN (ILP) A language learning program designed to fit each student's language skills and background. Similar to an IEP *q.v.*, students who are challenged in the area of language are targeted by such a plan.

INDIVIDUALIZED LEARNING A means of arranging the learning environment so that all learners have the opportunity to satisfy their health needs and interests according to their personal capabilities, at times and in ways best suited to their motivation and speed of learning. It is the use of methods, techniques, or strategies that influence the learning of each individual most effectively. cf: individualized instruction.

INDIVIDUALLY GUIDED EDUCATION (IGE) An individualized educational plan in which the teacher and students plan the learning objectives and how best to achieve them.

INDIVIDUALLY PRESCRIBED INSTRUCTION (IPI) An individualized learning *q.v.* program that follows a formalized structure that leads to the achievement of behavioral objectives.

INDIVIDUAL OBJECTIVES Personal objectives formulated by each member of an organization that outline how he or she could improve the functioning of the organization.

INDIVIDUAL PERCEPTION See perception.

INDIVIDUAL PLAN An insurance plan sold to a person rather than to a group. Such plans tend to be more expensive and narrower in coverage than a group plan *q.v.*

INDIVIDUAL RELATIVITY Internal relativity *v.*

INDIVIDUAL SPORTS Physical activities that require only one participant, e.g., jogging, golf.

INDIVIDUAL TEST A test that is designed to be administered to one person only at a given time. ct: group test.

INDIVIDUAL THEORY 1. The premise that a person is inherently social with social urges, values, and interests. 2. A person is constantly striving for self-actualization and fulfillment.

INDIVIDUATION 1. A pattern of development from the general to the specific. 2. A characteristic of human maturation *q.v.*

INDIVIDUATIVE-REFLECTIVE STAGE 1. The state of faith development generally associated with the young adult. 2. The stage in which a person translates symbols into personally meaningful concepts. Living within one's own structure of faith.

INDIVISIBLE CONTRACT A contract in which the performance of any one part of the contract binds the party to the fulfillment of the whole contract, in contrast to a divisible contract in which each part stands alone and binds the party only as far as it goes.

INDOLE A type of chemical structure. The neurotransmitter *q.v.* serotonin *q.v.* and the hallucinogen LSD *q.v.* both contain an indole nucleus.

INDOLEACETIC ACID (IAA) An important growth hormone *q.v.*

INDOLEAMINES Monoamine *q.v.* compounds (NH_2) each containing an indole *q.v.* portion (C_8H_7N) believed to act in neurotransmission and serotonin *q.v.* and tryptamine *q.v.*

INDOLENT 1. Indisposed to action. 2. Sluggish. 3. Slow in healing.

INDUCED ABORTION Purposeful termination of a pregnancy *q.v.*

INDUCED LABOR 1. Labor *q.v.* started artificially, usually by infusing oxytocin *q.v.* into a vein. 2. A method of induced abortion *q.v.* in which salt water is injected through the abdominal wall into the uterus *q.v.* to bring about the onset of labor, from which the dead fetus *q.v.* and placenta *q.v.* are expelled.

INDUCED MOVEMENT Perceived movement of an objectively stationary stimulus *q.v.* that is enclosed within a moving framework.

INDUCED MUTATION Mutation *q.v.* caused by the presence of a mutagenic *q.v.* agent.

INDUCER SUBSTANCE A chemical substance produced by the male embryo *q.v.* that helps support the development of the male internal reproductive structures.

INDUCIBLE BACTERIA Bacteria *q.v.* that produce specific enzymes *q.v.* only in the presence of their substrate.

INDUCTION 1. In reflex *q.v.* psychology, an increase in the strength of a reflex that follows a period of inhibition *q.v.* 2. In parental control, techniques of discipline *q.v.* in which parents attempt to control children by giving explanations or reasons why the child's behavior is good or bad. 3. In embryology *q.v.*, the process by which the development of undifferentiated cells or tissues is determined through the release of chemicals from neighboring cells and tissues. cf: power assertion; love withdrawal.

INDUCTION PROGRAMS Programs designed to help teachers during their first few years on the job. cf: mentoring programs.

INDUCTIVE DISCOVERY LEARNING Educational programs designed to present learning experiences that are clustered into generalizations.

INDUCTIVE LEARNING A methodology that begins with a health problem or issue followed by an accumulation of empirical evidence. This method tends to expose new health issues, resulting in broadened learning. Inductive reasoning is essentially the scientific method *q.v.* cf: problem-solving method. ct: deductive learning.

INDUCTIVE REASONING 1. The observation of a number of particular instances with an attempt to determine the general rule that pertains to them all. 2. A methodology that begins with a health problem or issues followed by an accumulation of empirical evidence. It is related to the scientific method *q.v.* cf: inductive learning.

INDULGENCE A strong emotional desire to engage in a particular behavior solely for one's own enjoyment or benefit.

INDURATION Hardening or firming of a tissue as the result of cellular infiltration due to infection, inflammation, or trauma.

INDURISM An epidural outgrowth covering the sorus in ferns.

INDUSTRIAL HYGIENE Those aspects of health and medicine that apply to the workplace environment and how they affect the well-being, health, and safety of the workers.

INDUSTRIAL SECURITY Measures taken to protect the safety and security of a workplace against criminal or malicious activities that may adversely affect productivity and the health and well-being of the workers.

INDUSTRY VERSUS INFERIORITY Erickson's fourth stage of psychosocial development *q.v.* during which predominantly positive interactions with others result in a sense of industry, competency, interest in doing things, whereas predominantly negative interaction with others results in a sense of inferiority.

INEXACT LABELING A form of cognitive *q.v.* distortion in which the individual overreacts to a situation by mislabeling it, then responds to the label rather than the event itself.

INFANTICIDE The murder of infants *q.v.* or young children.

INFANTILE AUTISM A childhood disorder characterized by profound isolation, inhibited speech, and intolerance of variance in routine or surroundings. cf: autism; idiot savant.

INFANTILE ENTERITIS Diarrhea *q.v.* occurring in children under 2 years.

INFANTILE IMMUNITY Natural passive immunity *q.v.* of the infant during the first 3–6 months after birth that is acquired from the mother during gestation *q.v.*

INFANTILE PARALYSIS Poliomyelitis *q.v.*

INFANTILE PERSEVERATION Speech immaturity that is characterized largely to sound omissions and substitutions, where the person uses speech as a major mechanism of communication, but it is like that of a much younger person.

INFANTILE SPASMS Muscular spasms that infants, 3 months to 2 years of age, experience, characterized by flexor spasms of the arms, legs, and head. Also known as jackknife seizures.

INFANTILISM Persistence of infantile emotional attitudes and behavior patterns into adulthood.

INFANT MORTALITY RATE The number of deaths under 1 year per 1000 live births in a given year.

INFANT–MOTHER ATTACHMENT The special affectionate relationship between a mother and child, providing the infant *q.v.* with security and comfort necessary for healthful development.

INFARCT 1. The death of tissue as a result of oxygen deprivation. 2. The area of tissue that is damaged as a result of receiving too little blood. cf: myocardial infarction.

INFECT 1. To enter, invade, or inhibit another organism, causing infection *q.v.* or contamination *q.v.*

INFECTED PARTNER In regards to AIDS *q.v.*, a person in a sexual relationship who is carrying the AIDS virus (HIV) *q.v.* in his or her body.

INFECTION 1. The introduction of a foreign organism into the body that can result in damage to cells, organs, or tissues. 2. An illness caused by an organism, such as a virus *q.v.*, bacterium *q.v.*, or fungus *q.v.* cf: inflammation.

INFECTIOUS 1. A disease that is caused by a microorganism. It may be communicable *q.v.* 2. An organism that can be transmitted from host *q.v.* to host. 3. Capable of being transmitted by infection, with or without actual contact.

INFECTIOUS AGENT A disease-causing agent, such as bacteria *q.v.* or virus *q.v.*

INFECTIOUS DISEASE 1. An illness caused by a microorganism, such as a virus or bacterium, that upon entering the body attacks a specific organ or organ system. 2. An infection *q.v.* in the body that may be either communicable *q.v.* or noncommunicable *q.v.*

INFECTIOUS DISEASE CLASSIFICATION Generally, classified according to mode of transmission: 1. respiratory diseases *q.v.*, 2. alvine discharge diseases *q.v.*, 3. vector-borne diseases *q.v.*, and 4. open lesion diseases *q.v.*

INFECTIOUS HEPATITIS An acute infection *q.v.* of the liver caused by a virus *q.v.* Transmitted from feces *q.v.* to hands to oral portal of entry. Characterized by fever, headaches, nausea, loss of appetite, tenderness, and pain in the region of the liver. Sometimes jaundice *q.v.* is present. cf: serum hepatitis.

INFECTIOUS MONONUCLEOSIS A system disease *q.v.* caused by the Epstein–Barr virus *q.v.* Symptoms include fever, fatigue, swollen lymph glands, and sore throat. Recovery may be slow, taking several weeks or months.

INFECTIVITY The ability of microbes to lodge and multiply in a human host.

INFERENTIAL STATISTICS 1. Estimations, generalizations, or predictions about a particular group. 2. Comparisons of differences between groups to test the probability that the differences could be reliably replicated. cf: descriptive statistics.

INFERIOR Lower or toward the lower end. Used frequently to indicate an anatomical position.

INFERIORITY COMPLEX Strong feelings of inadequacy and insecurity that influence a person's adjustive efforts.

INFERIOR VENA CAVA The large vein that returns blood from the lower body regions to the right atrium *q.v.* of the heart.

INFERTILITY 1. The inability to conceive a child as in reproduction. 2. The inability to reproduce. 3. The inability of a heterosexual *q.v.* couple to conceive *q.v.* a pregnancy *q.v.* after 1 year of regular, unprotected coitus *q.v.* 4. ~ may result from conditions in both sexes, many of which are curable. cf: sterility.

INFIBULATION A custom consisting of the surgical removal of the clitoris and part of the labia and sewing of the remaining labia so as to render coitus extremely difficult if not impossible.

INFILTRATION A stage of cancer in which cancer cells extend into surrounding tissues. cf: metastasis.

INFIRMITY Debilitative illness.

INFLAMMATION 1. A reddening of tissues resulting from irritation. Irritation may originate from infection *q.v.*, chemicals, mechanical trauma *q.v.*, or radiation. 2. Local reaction characterized by pain, swelling, and warmth. 3. The condition into which tissues enter as a reaction to injury or infection. Symptoms include pain, heat, redness, and swelling. cf: infection. 4. A morbid series of reactions produced in the tissues by an irritant characterized by an influx of blood with exudation *q.v.* of plasma *q.v.* and leukocytes *q.v.*

INFLAMMATORY RESPONSE 1. Redness, warmth, and swelling as a result of infection *q.v.* This reaction results from increased blood flow and a gathering of immune cells *q.v.* and secretions. 2. A general defense mechanism *q.v.* in the blood and tissues aimed at warding off any irritant or foreign body. 3. An allergic *q.v.* reaction in which blood flows to the site of a cell injury and massive amounts of plasma *q.v.* escape from the blood vessels producing swelling, redness, and a fever.

INFLECTION A morpheme *q.v.* placed at the end of a word that alters its meaning or interpretation.

INFLORESCENCE 1. A flower cluster. 2. The arrangement of flowers on the floral axis.

INFLUENCE In social psychology, a resulting personal change of attitude *q.v.* or opinion as a result of the suggestion of others.

INFLUENCING The process of guiding an individual or a group of people toward a desired goal.

INFLUENCING SUBSYSTEM A part of the overall system of management of an organization. The purpose of the ~ is desirable organization member behavior. The ~ performs four major management activities: 1. leading, 2. motivating, 3. considering groups, and 4. communicating.

INFLUENZA (FLU) 1. An infectious *q.v.* respiratory disease caused by a virus and characterized by headache, fever, chills, gastrointestinal disturbances, and muscular aches and pains. 2. ~ may also result from infection with *Hemophilus influenza* bacillus *q.v.*

INFORMAL EDUCATION Learning experiences encountered in the course of daily life out of school, often with tutoring from others not explicitly trained to do so.

INFORMAL GROUPS Groups that naturally develop in organizations as people interact.

INFORMAL ORGANIZATION A loosely structured and loosely defined interaction pattern that tends to develop in formal organizations.

INFORMAL ORGANIZATIONAL COMMUNICATION Organizational communication that does not follow the lines of communication set forth on the organizational chart.

INFORMAL STANDARD Within a particular culture, the expectations of most of the people as to how to behave without it being mandated in law or religion or by some other controlling body.

INFORMATION 1. Conclusions derived from data analysis. 2. Data *q.v.* 3. In law, an accusation against a person.

INFORMATION AGE A view of society that recognizes the increasing role of technology and resultant ease of communication and the sharing of information.

INFORMATIONAL APPROACH A method of teaching concerned with the acquisition of health knowledge and its comprehension and with its application to the issues being explored.

INFORMATIONAL APPROACH TO CURRICULUM DEVELOPMENT Concerned with the acquisition of health knowledge and its comprehension and with application to the health issues being explored. This approach places emphasis on the acquisition of health facts.

INFORMATIONAL CONTENT The content areas related to health topics or issues. cf: content areas.

INFORMATION APPROPRIATENESS The degree to which information is relevant to the decision-making process.

INFORMATION-EXCHANGE INTERVIEW The acquisition or exchange of information or ideas.

INFORMATION PROCESSING 1. The process whereby crude and new materials are refashioned into items of knowledge. The process includes perceptual organization, relationships, and significances. 2. The storing and using of information within a system. 3. An approach to understanding and thinking as a complex of different intellectual processes engaged in by people having particular processing capabilities and limitations.

INFORMATION PROCESSING THEORY A study of the ways that sensory input is transformed, stored, recovered, and used.

INFORMATION QUALITY The degree to which information represents reality and is correctly perceived.

INFORMATION THEORY The field of study of communications systems which is concerned with the principles governing understanding, control, and predictability in communications.

INFORMATION TIMELINESS A measurement of the timing and significance of the information received as it relates to the benefit of an organization or individual.

INFORMED CONSENT 1. Agreement based on full knowledge. 2. Extending permission to perform based on an understanding of the circumstances surrounding said performance. 3. The permission of a person to serve as a subject in a research study or to enter therapy after being told of the possible risks or other outcomes.

INFRACLAVICULAR NODES Lymph nodes *q.v.* located beneath the clavicle *q.v.* (collar bone).

INFRADIAN RHYTHM 1. A relatively long biological *q.v.* cycle. 2. A physiological *q.v.* cycle, e.g., the menstrual cycle.

INFRARED 1. Beyond the red end of the spectrum. 2. A section of the electromagnetic spectrum invisible to the eye and characterized by waves of increasing length.

INFRINGEMENT An encroachment or invasion of one's rights.

INFUNDIBULUM 1. A funnel-like outgrowth from the ventral wall of the diencephalon *q.v.* 2. The funnel-shaped end of the fallopian tube *q.v.* cf: fimbria.

INFUSION 1. The liquid produced by soaking a substance in water and extracting the soluble parts. 2. The injection of a fluid into a vein. 3. The administration intravenously by gravity of any of a number of cell-free fluids.

INFUSION CAVERNOSOGRAPHY Used in diagnosing the cause of erectile dysfunction *q.v.* in men, the injection of the genitals *q.v.* with radioactive substances to monitor blood flow.

INGESTION 1. The swallowing of food. 2. The act of taking food or other substances into the body by mouth.

INGRATIATION STRATEGY Manipulating another person by making oneself seem likable.

IN-GROUP A social group with which a person identifies and to which a person feels close. ct: out-group.

INGUINAL 1. That region of the body located between the abdomen and thigh. 2. Groin. 3. Pertaining to or situated in the groin.

INGUINAL CANAL The passageway from the abdominal cavity to the scrotum *q.v.* in the male through which the testicles *q.v.* descend shortly before birth or just after birth.

INGUINAL HERNIA A condition in which the inguinal canal *q.v.* has not closed completely after the testes *q.v.* have descended through it. Portions of intestine may enter the canal and the scrotum *q.v.* Strenuous exercise may produce symptoms of pain. ~ is often treated surgically.

INHALANTS 1. Volatile chemicals that evaporate easily, that when inhaled *q.v.* produce psychoactive *q.v.* effects. 2. Psychoactive drugs that enter the body through inhalation.

INHALATION 1. The process of breathing in. 2. The absorption of volatile chemicals into the blood by passing through the lungs. 3. The drawing of air and other substances into the lungs. 4. Inspiration.

INHERENT INSUSCEPTIBILITY A physiological state that renders some people, with or without antibodies *q.v.*, immune *q.v.* to certain infections *q.v.*

INHERITED A condition or trait that is passed from parents to offspring by way of the genes *q.v.* or chromosomes *q.v.*

INHIBIN A protein that may be a hormone *q.v.* and that may inhibit secretion of the follicle-stimulating hormone (FSH) *q.v.*

INHIBITED FEMALE ORGASM A delay in or inability to achieve orgasm *q.v.* during sexual activity, with or without accompanying sexual arousal. cf: inhibited sexual excitement. ct: inhibited male orgasm.

INHIBITED MALE ORGASM 1. A delay in or inability to achieve orgasm *q.v.* after arousal. 2. A condition in which the male can become aroused and achieve and maintain an erection *q.v.*, but is not able to achieve orgasm during sexual intercourse *q.v.* cf: inhibited sexual excitement. ct: inhibited female orgasm.

INHIBITED SEXUAL DESIRE (ISD) 1. Sexual apathy. 2. The condition in which a person lacks the desire for sexual activity. 3. A person who never initiates sexual activity and is rarely receptive to another person who does initiate the activity. Two forms are noted: 1. primary, in which the person has never been interested in sex, and 2. secondary, in which the person was at one time interested in sex but is no longer interested. ct: inhibited male orgasm. cf: inhibitions of sexual desire; inhibited sexual excitement.

INHIBITED SEXUAL EXCITEMENT A term replacing the terms of impotence in men and frigidity in women. Characterized by a persistent lack of sexual arousal during sexual activity. cf: inhibited female orgasm; inhibited sexual desire; inhibited male orgasm.

INHIBITION 1. The inner controls that prevent a person from engaging in certain types of behavior. 2. Any temporary interference with a response *q.v.* 3. In motor learning, the suppressive effect of massed practice *q.v.* 4. In personality theory, an interference with the expression of some tendency or with the recall of some event. 5. In Pavlovian theory, the ~ developed during extinction *q.v.* and with respect to the nonreinforced stimulus *q.v.* in discrimination *q.v.* learning (internal inhibition). 6. Conscious restrain of impulse or desire. 7. In physiology, interference with, or slowing down of, some body activity. 8. An increase in a neuron's resting potential above its usual level.

INHIBITIONS OF SEXUAL DESIRE (ISD) A category of sexual dysfunction in which sexual desire for another person is missing or adversely affected. cf: inhibited sexual desire.

INHIBITOR 1. Any chemical or substance that retards or inhibits a chemical reaction. 2. A genetic cause of interference with a particular reaction or process. 3. The inhibition of postsynaptic potential.

INJECTION 1. Introduction of a drug or other substance into the bloodstream through the use of a syringe. 2. Administering a drug or other substance intravenously *q.v.*, intramuscularly *q.v.*, or subcutaneously *q.v.* 3. The act of forcing a liquid into a part of the body, as into the subcutaneous tissues *q.v.*, the blood, or an organ through a needle or tube introduced through the skin.

INJUNCTION 1. To enjoin. 2. A writ issued by a court forbidding the defendant from doing an act(s) that is or may be injurious to the plaintiff and cannot adequately be redressed by other legal means.

INJUNCTION, TEMPORARY An act of the court to prohibit certain acts relating to the case being litigated and which may be reversed depending on the outcome of the case.

INJURY Damage to a part of the body. It may be accidental *q.v.* or intentional. Caused by chemicals, physical objects, or trauma. *q.v.*

INJURY CONTROL A relatively new term being used by some public health educators to replace accident prevention.

IN-KIND CONTRIBUTIONS Donations of goods or services in lieu of funds.

IN LOCO PARENTIS 1. In place of or acting on behalf of the parent. 2. A term used to describe the implied power of schools to act in place of and the best interests of the student.

INN An acronym for *International Nonproprietary Names*, published by the World Health Organization.

INNATE 1. Inborn. 2. Genetically determined.

INNATE IMMUNITY Inborn or hereditary immunity.

INNATE RELEASING MECHANISM In ethology *q.v.*, the mechanism that releases instinctive *q.v.* behavior *q.v.* in the presence of appropriate stimuli *q.v.* cf: action-specific energy.

INNER CONTROLS Reality, value, and possibility assumptions that serve to inhibit *q.v.* dangerous or undesirable behavior. May be applied to conditioned avoidance reactions.

INNER DIRECTED A person who has an inner set of principles that guide his or her behavior. ct: outer directed.

INNER LANGUAGE Language of thought, possibly developed before other language that can be verbalized.

INNER LIPS Labia minora *q.v.*

INNERVATIONS The nerve or group of nerves that controls the activity of a muscle or other organ.

INNOCUOUS 1. Not harmful. 2. Not poisonous or toxic. 3. Harmless.

INNOMINATE 1. Pertaining to certain structures formed by the fusion *q.v.* of other separate structures. 2. Not named, anonymous, e.g., innominate bone.

INNOMINATE ARTERY The brachiocephalic artery *q.v.* giving rise to the right subclavian *q.v.* and right common carotid *q.v.* arteries.

INNOMINATE BONE The bone forming one half of the pelvic girdle *q.v.* and arising from a fusion of the ilium *q.v.*, the ischium *q.v.*, and the pubis.

INOCULATION An injection of any biological *q.v.* substance intended to confer protection against disease.

INOCULATION STRATEGY A strategy for the prevention of drug abuse through education, the promotion of healthful behaviors, appropriate decision-making skills, and placing limits on drug intake.

INORGANIC Compounds that do not contain carbon. Compounds not living or have never lived. ct: organic.

INOSITOL 1. A sugar-like substance included in the B-complex vitamins *q.v.* that is an important growth factor for certain yeasts. 2. A B-complex vitamin often found as an adulterant in street cocaine *q.v.*

IN PARI MATERIA On the same subject matter.

INPATIENT A person being treated in a hospital or other facility as a resident. ct: outpatient.

INPUT FUNCTION A computer function that enters the data to be analyzed and the type of analysis to be performed.

INPUT MEASURE A measure of the quality of service based on the number, type, and resources used in the production of the services being measured. Health services are often evaluated by measuring the education and experience of the health provider *q.v.*, the reputation and accreditation of the institution, the number of health personnel involved, and the amount of money spent for services, administration, and supplies.

INPUT OVERLOAD 1. Pertains to an excess of stimuli *q.v.* 2. Overstimulation that interferes with the ability to respond.

INPUT PLANNING The development of strategies that will provide sufficient resources, both financial and administrative, for reaching the organizational objectives.

INQUIRY 1. A process of asking questions. 2. Questioning the learner not only to determine what he or she has learned but what the needs of the learner are and how best to satisfy them.

IN RE 1. In the matter of. 2. Entitling a judicial proceeding in which there are no adversaries but issues requiring judicial action.

INSANITY 1. A legal term describing a person who may not be convicted of a crime *q.v.* when it is shown that he or she is not legally responsible for the criminal behavior *q.v.* Legal definitions are within (a) the Currens formula, (b) the Durham decision, or (c) the McNaghten decision. Some states also allow an insanity decision based on a psychotic condition called an irresistible impulse *q.v.* 2. A legal term for a mental disorder implying a lack of responsibility and inability to manage one's affairs.

INSANITY DEFENSE The legal argument that a person accused of a crime should not be held responsible for his or her actions because of his or her inability to distinguish between right and wrong.

INSECTICIDE A toxic chemical that kills unwanted insects.

INSEMINATION 1. The deposit of semen *q.v.* within the vagina *q.v.* 2. The impregnation, either by natural or artificial means, of sperm *q.v.* into the uterine *q.v.* cavity.

INSENSIBLE PERSPIRATION Perspiration that evaporates before it appears as fluid on the skin.

INSERTION OF MUSCLE The place of attachment of a muscle to the bone that it moves.

IN-SERVICE EDUCATION Continuing education of teachers, health care professional, or others to maintain their professional qualifications and/or certifications.

IN-SERVICE TRAINING Educational programs directed toward advanced training or review training of persons in the profession and on the job.

INSIDIOUS DISEASE A disease that is especially treacherous in that there are no previous warning signs and symptoms.

INSIDIOUS ONSET In psychology, the gradual appearance of a psychotic disorder.

INSIGHT 1. A sudden grasp or understanding of the significance and relationships of factors. 2. Understanding. 3. Clinically, a person's understanding of his or her illness or of the motivations underlying the behavior. 4. In general psychology, the sudden grasp or understanding of meaningful relationships. 5. In education, learning that occurs when a learner perceives new relationships.

INSIGHTFUL LEARNING Learning that is characterized by understanding the relationships and significances between and among components of a problem. cf: trial and error learning.

INSIGHT THERAPY The general term for psychotherapy *q.v.* that is designed to enhance a patient's insight into what motivates his or her behavior, thereby facilitating the resolution of conflicts that have caused problems for the patient.

IN SITU Localized, confined to the site of origin.

IN SITU CANCER Cancer *q.v.* confined to the site of origin. No metastasis *q.v.* has yet occurred.

INSOMNIA The inability to sleep. ~ in the elderly is frequently a manifestation of depression. Often, ~ is treated with hypnotic *q.v.* drugs.

INSPECTION A process used to detect physical abnormalities by using the sense of sight.

INSPECTIONALISM Scoptophilia *q.v.*

INSPIRATION 1. The act of breathing in or drawing air into the lungs. 2. Inhalation *q.v.*

INSPIRE To breathe in.

INSPISSATED Thickened by evaporation or absorption of fluid.

IN-STATE STUDENT A legal resident of a state for the purposes of calculating tuition at a school or college.

IN STATU QUO In the situation that existed previously.

INSTIGATION 1. That which sets the occasion for behavior *q.v.* 2. A combination of appropriate stimuli *q.v.* and motivation *q.v.*

INSTILLATION 1. An abortion *q.v.* technique in which a foreign substance is injected into the uterus *q.v.* to induce labor *q.v.* 2. Intraamniotic infusion *q.v.* 3. Putting drops of medication in the eye or any body cavity.

INSTINCT 1. A behavior pattern whose underlying biological pattern is produced by maturation *q.v.* rather than learning and which appears full-blown upon the first occasion that an adequate stimulus *q.v.* is presented, without the organism having previous opportunity to learn. Common in lower animals but rare in humans. 2. An unlearned biologically based form of behavior *q.v.* 3. In ethology *q.v.*, a rigidly stereotyped complex bit of behavior that is specific to a species. 4. A subconscious, fixed reflex *q.v.* act due to a definite arrangement of inherited *q.v.* patterns of nerve cells and tissues. cf: primary drive.

INSTITUTE OF SOCIETY, ETHICS AND LIFE SCIENCES Founded in 1969 and consists of leading authorities in biology, medicine, philosophy, law, and the social and behavioral sciences.

INSTITUTION 1. An organization that has a special mandate, certain prescribed procedures for processing people or services, and serves a well-defined population. 2. One of the more durable social systems focused around meeting basic social needs. 3. An organized set of groups or organizations with prescribed norms and values, having a defined purpose, and meeting social needs.

INSTITUTIONAL CARE Medical care provided by hospitals, rehabilitation facilities, and nursing homes.

INSTITUTIONALISM 1. A patient's gradual acceptance to the authority of the institution to a point where apathy and unquestioned acceptance exists. 2. The routine, bureaucratic structure that exists in many large institutions, leading to a stifling of creativity on the part of employees.

INSTITUTIONALIZATION Admission of a person to an institution, such as a nursing home, where he or she will reside for an extended period of time or indefinitely. cf: institutionalized.

INSTITUTIONALIZED 1. Incorporated into the regular operations of a larger organization. 2. The result of a person being admitted to an institution, especially against his or her will.

INSTITUTIONAL MARRIAGE A marriage *q.v.* that conforms to society's expectations and standards.

INSTITUTIONAL PRACTICES Those practices that are implemented by an institution to serve its purposes and to enhance its structure and power.

INSTITUTIONS OF HIGHER EDUCATION Postsecondary institutions providing course work leading to a degree, usually at the associate or bachelor level and often at the graduate level.

INSTRUCTION 1. Teaching. 2. Often equated with training and not with the complex process of education. 3. That which is done by a teacher to engage his or her students in the learning process.

INSTRUCTIONAL FACULTY Staff employed full or part time whose regular assignment is instruction.

INSTRUCTIONAL OBJECTIVES Statements of what learners are supposed to know and under what conditions they are to know the curricular material to have successfully completed the lesson, unit, or program.

INSTRUCTIONAL TECHNOLOGY Typically refers to electronic hardware and software used by students and faculty to enhance the curriculum being offered by an educational institution.

INSTRUCTIONAL TELEVISION (ITV) Educational programs telecast for educational institutions, frequently on a closed-circuit basis, to enhance student learning and to enable the educational institution to offer courses to students living or working at long distances from the school or college. cf: educational television.

INSTRUCTION EXPENDITURES Funds spent to support the instructional efforts of an educational institution.

INSTRUCTION MATERIALS CENTER (IMC) An area where students may use books, journals, computer software, recordings, etc., to enhance their learning experiences.

INSTRUMENTAL AGGRESSION Aggressive acts that are designed to achieve a goal other than that of hurting another person.

INSTRUMENTAL BEHAVIOR Behavior *q.v.* that leads to the attainment of a goal.

INSTRUMENTAL COMPETENCE An overarching ability to function effectively, characterized by social responsibility, independence or self-sufficiency, and an achievement orientation.

INSTRUMENTAL CONDITIONING 1. Operant conditioning. 2. A form of learning in which a reinforcer is provided only when the person performs the intended response. 3. A type of conditioning in which the subject learns to make a predetermined response in order to obtain a reward. ct: classical conditioning.

INSTRUMENTAL LEARNING 1. A learning theory that asserts that learning consists of the strengthening or weakening of particular responses. 2. Learning that occurs because a response is instrumental in producing a reinforcement. cf: instrumental conditioning. ct: cognitive theory.

INSUFFICIENCY A condition that results when a heart valve cannot close fully, thus allowing blood to return to the chamber from which it just left.

INSUFFLATION The blowing of a medical powder into any body cavity.

INSULATION A nonconducting substance that offers a barrier to the passage of heat or electricity.

INSULIN 1. A pancreatic hormone *q.v.* that plays a crucial role in regulating glucose metabolism *q.v.* Interference with ~ production in the islet cells of Langerhans *q.v.* will produce symptoms of diabetes mellitus *q.v.* 2. A hormone secreted by the beta cells of the islets of Langerhans.

~ facilitates glucose oxidation *q.v.* as well as the synthesis *q.v.* of glycogen, fat, and protein. 3. An antidiabetic drug that helps maintain the diabetic's blood sugar at near-normal levels and keeps the urine free of sugar. 4. A hormone that promotes glucose use, protein synthesis, and storage of neutral lipids *q.v.*

INSULIN DEPENDENCE A condition in diabetes *q.v.* in which the pancreas produces insufficient quantities of insulin *q.v.*, requiring the person to obtain a supply through injections.

INSULIN REACTION 1. A condition that occurs when the blood sugar level becomes too low. 2. Hypoglycemia *q.v.*

INSULIN REBOUND Reactive hypoglycemia *q.v.*

INSULIN SHOCK Characterized by trembling, faintness, palpitations, excessive perspiration, and hunger. Present on occasion with people who suffer from diabetes mellitus *q.v.* The symptoms will disappear when the person drinks orange juice or eats some form of carbohydrate.

INSULIN SHOCK TREATMENT (THERAPY) 1. Insulin coma therapy. 2. Injection of insulin *q.v.* in large enough doses to produce profound hypoglycemia *q.v.* resulting in coma. Formerly used primarily in the treatment of schizophrenia *q.v.* Rarely used today in the United States since the development of tranquilizers *q.v.* and other antipsychotic drugs *q.v.* 3. A form of convulsive therapy *q.v.* in which the agent is insulin.

INSURANCE Financial protection against injury, death, illness, or any of a variety of other losses.

INSURANCE CLAUSE The statement in a health insurance policy or contract that indicates the parties involved and that states what is covered by the policy or contract.

INTEGRATED HEALTH EXPERIENCES Health learning that is a component of another curricular discipline. ct: integrated health experiences.

INTEGRATED RISK INFORMATION SYSTEM (IRIS) An online database built on the Environmental Protection Agency (EPA) *q.v.*, which contains EPA carcinogenic *q.v.* and noncarcinogenic health risk and regulatory information on some 400 chemicals.

INTEGRATION 1. The organization of parts, psychological and biological functions, to make a functional whole. 2. The coordination of specific responses with unified patterns. 3. The process of assigning students to schools to achieve a racial mix reflective of the society as a whole.

INTEGRATION IN CURRICULUM Methods used to introduce a subject area in a particular educational situation so that subject areas are not treated separately, but logically as they relate to a broad unit of study. cf: integrated health experiences.

INTEGRITY The acceptance of the self and the living up to one's moral values.

INTEGUMENT 1. In botany, one or sometimes two outer layers of the ovule *q.v.*, which develop into the seed coat. 2. In anatomy, the skin or a covering or investment.

INTELLECTUAL DEVELOPMENT The development or maturation *q.v.* of the intellect.

INTELLECTUAL HEALTH 1. Rational behavior. 2. Accepting intellectual challenges. 3. Intellectual maturity *q.v.* 4. Rational behavior rather than impulsive or emotional behavior.

INTELLECTUAL QUOTIENT See intelligence quotient.

INTELLECTUALIZATION 1. A defense mechanism *q.v.* 2. A compromise *q.v.* reaction in which problems and frustrations are dealt with by the intellect through rationalization *q.v.* or other means of reality distortion. 3. An ego defense mechanism *q.v.* by which a person achieves some measure of insulation from emotional pain by cutting off or distorting the emotional charge that normally accompanies painful situations. 4. A justification of behavior by assigning intellectual justification for it rather than by responding through emotion.

INTELLIGENCE 1. The capacity to learn and the capacity to use appropriately that which is learned. 2. The term that refers to intellectual ability. An ability or pattern of abilities influencing intellectual functioning. ~ is related to learning, memorizing, reasoning, comprehending, conceptualizing, wisdom, and problem solving. 3. The capacities that are essential to success and are measured by intelligence tests.

INTELLIGENCE QUOTIENT (IQ) A ratio measure to indicate whether a person's mental age (MA) *q.v.* is ahead of or behind the chronological age (CA) *q.v.* The formula for determining ~ is as follows: $IQ = MA \times CA \times 100$. cf: deviation IQ.

INTELLIGENCE TEST A standardized test of assessing a person's mental ability. cf: Stanford–Binet test; Wechsler Adult Intelligence Scale.

INTENSION MOVEMENTS In ethology, ~ pertain to displays that represent anticipations of an impending response.

INTENSITY 1. The strength or loudness of a particular sound, measured in decibels *q.v.* 2. The level of effort a person puts into an activity. 3. The degree of vigor of any phase of an exercise prescription *q.v.* ct: frequency.

INTENTIONAL LEARNING 1. A deliberate attempt to acquire knowledge for a purpose. 2. Learning when the learner is informed that there will be an evaluation of knowledge following the learning period. ct: incidental learning.

INTERACTION 1. A statistical term pertaining to the fact that the influence of a particular variable *q.v.* depends upon the value of other variables. 2. In sociology, the ways in which two or more persons in contact influence the behavior of each other. 3. In chemistry, the way two or more elements or compounds combine chemically to form new substances. 4. In nutrition, a serious illness may be produced in a poorly nourished person that may produce few, if any, symptoms in a well-nourished person. There is an ~ between disease severity and nutrition *q.v.* 5. The relationships between or among variables in a particular situation.

INTERACTIVE LEARNING A process whereby students are active participants in the learning situation.

INTERACTIVE TEACHING A teaching method in which the teacher and students interact with each other.

INTER ALIA Among other things.

INTERCELLULAR Between the cells.

INTERCOURSE An interaction between two or more people in any social interaction.

INTERCOURSE, ANAL A form of sexual intercourse *q.v.* in which the penis is inserted into the partner's anus *q.v.* cf: sodomy.

INTERCOURSE, INTERFEMORAL Nonvaginal method of coitus *q.v.* that uses the space between the thighs to hold the penis *q.v.*

INTERCOURSE, SEXUAL 1. Traditionally, a sexual union between a male and a female in which the penis *q.v.* is inserted into the vagina *q.v.* 2. Coitus *q.v.*

INTERCURRENT INFECTION An infection *q.v.* that occurs in an already ill person during the course of some other disease state.

INTERDICTION The prevention of, or interruption of, the smuggling of illegal drugs into the United States at boarder crossings, at sea, and through air surveillance and interception.

INTEREST CENTERS Areas within a classroom that focus on a particular subject area. Particularly geared toward an open classroom *q.v.* setup where students can move from one area to another with minimal restriction.

INTEREST GROUPS Usually focused upon a particular target area, e.g., the environment, politics, education, etc., where members informally coalesce to discuss the issue at hand and to advocate for particular action to promote their cause.

INTEREST INVENTORIES Questionnaires designed to measure a person's various areas of interest to assist in determining a particular academic area of study or area of vocational interest.

INTERFERENCE In genetics, studies of three or more linked genes have revealed that a crossover *q.v.* at one point reduced the likelihood of another crossover in adjacent regions.

INTERFERENCE OF FORGETTING The assertion that items are forgotten because they are somehow interfered with by other items learned before or after.

INTERFERON 1. A protein substance produced in minute quantities by the body's immune system *q.v.*, which aids the body in combating viral infections. In the experimental stage, there is evidence that ~ may be useful in combating some forms of cancer. 2. One of a group of proteins *q.v.* released from virus-infected cells preventing viral *q.v.* replication in healthy cells. 3. A chemical produced by the body in response to viral infections. Injections of ~ have been shown to reduce the risk of contracting certain diseases. 4. A class of glycoproteins *q.v.* thought to inhibit viral infection.

INTERINDIVIDUAL A term used to describe a person's performance in comparison to that of others.

INTERJUDGE RELIABILITY The extent of agreement by trained observers of the evaluation of a particular event or phenomenon.

INTERLEUKIN-2 1. An anticancer drug researched in 1987, ~ appears to stimulate the body's immune system *q.v.* to destroy cancer cells. 2. Chemical messengers that travel from leukocytes to other white blood cells. Some promote cell development while others promote rapid cell division.

INTERMEDIATE CARE FACILITY Provides health-related care and services to persons who do not require the degree of care or treatment normally provided by a hospital or skilled treatment facility *q.v.* but who do require health-related institutional care beyond the level of room and board. Eligible for Medicaid *q.v.* reimbursement. cf: domiciliary care facility.

INTERMEDIATE GRADES The grades in elementary school normally including grades 4, 5, and 6.

INTERMEDIATE HOST A mode of disease transmission where the infectious agents must spend a part of their life cycle in a host between the infected person (source of the agent) and the new host (to become infected). For example, the malaria plasmodium *q.v.* must spend a part of its life cycle in the body of the anopheles mosquito to mature sufficiently to infect the new host.

INTERMEDIATE INHERITANCE An alternative to dominance *q.v.* in which the heterozygotes *q.v.* are different from both homozygotes *q.v.*

INTERMEDIATE LEVEL 1. Middle school *q.v.* 2. Generally grades 4–6. 3. One of two divisions of elementary school organization. ct: primary level.

INTERMEDIATE LEVEL OF HEALTH Health status *q.v.* measured in terms of temporary, curable conditions. Persons falling within this level of health have contracted or developed a disease condition that interferes with functioning ability, but with proper treatment will return to the primary level of health *q.v.* cf: secondary level of health.

INTERMEDIATE OBJECTIVES Targets to be achieved within 1–5 years.

INTERMEDIATE SCHOOL A synonym for middle school *q.v.*

INTERMEDIATE UNIT 1. A division of elementary school comprised of grades 4–6. 2. A level of school organization, usually on a county-wide or multicounty basis, between the state and local school districts.

INTERMITTENT DUTY As applied to emergency situations, communications equipment that is not operational continuously. ct: continuous duty.

INTERMITTENT EXERCISE Activities performed with alternate periods of intense physical activity interspersed with varying periods of rest.

INTERMODAL ORGANIZATION In perception, the concentration of more than one sensory modality to the production of unified experience.

INTERNAL COMMITTEE A committee completely made up of people within the organization.

INTERNAL CUES Sensations from within the body that provide information. ct: external cues.

INTERNAL ENVIRONMENT 1. Consists of the body's processes that tend to maintain a state of homeostasis *q.v.* 2. The set of conditions, processes, and substances found inside an organism. ct: external environment.

INTERNAL EVALUATION Evaluation *q.v.* by people within the organization.

INTERNAL FRUSTRATION Barriers to goal achievement and need *q.v.* satisfaction arising from personal limitations or attitudes *q.v.*

INTERNAL GENITALIA The reproductive structures that are not visible by external examination. ct: external genitalia.

INTERNAL INHIBITION Inhibition *q.v.*

INTERNALIZATION 1. The process whereby moral codes are adopted by the person so that they control his or her behavior even when there are no external rewards or punishments. 2. The incorporation into things that are learned into one's own system of values. 3. Yielding to the beliefs of a group because of the belief that the group is correct.

INTERNAL LOCUS OF CONTROL A person's belief that he or she, not outside forces or other people, is largely responsible for what happens to him or her in life.

INTERNAL MEDICINE A medical specialty concerned with the diagnosis and treatment (including surgery) of diseases of the internal organs, e.g., liver, lungs, and heart. Internists are diagnosticians, personal physicians for adult medical care, health counselors, and consultants to other physicians. Many subspecialize in such areas as cardiology, hematology, allergy, and rheumatology.

INTERNAL ORGANIZATIONAL DIAGNOSIS The process of examining all factors within an organization that relate to its effectiveness in carrying out its mission.

INTERNAL QUALITIES The qualities of a person that stem from within or from the internal environment.

INTERNAL RADIATION The implantation of a radioactive substance into the body for treating a disease, e.g., cancer.

INTERNAL RELATIVITY Labeling that occurs when an individual imposes a label on him or herself.

INTERNAL RELIABILITY Similarity or consistency between the results of one part of a measurement and those of other parts or the whole of that being observed.

INTERNAL STIMULUS 1. A stimulus *q.v.* arising from inside the body. 2. Motivation *q.v.*

INTERNAL VALIDITY The extent to which a particular variable being manipulated can be assigned the responsibility of the effect observed.

INTERNATIONAL EDUCATION The study of the educational, economic, political, and other social forces that affect international relations. ~ also includes programs to foster the development of nations.

INTERNATIONAL FEDERATION FOR INTERNAL FREEDOM An organization established by Dr. Timothy Leary for the purpose of studying the psychedelic *q.v.* effects of certain hallucinogenic drugs *q.v.*, chiefly LSD *q.v.* and psilocybin *q.v.* The organization was short lived because of lack of support.

INTERNATIONAL MANAGEMENT Conducting management activities across national borders.

INTERNATIONAL UNIT (IU) 1. An international standard of the biological effects of a particular amount of a substance, e.g., vitamin. 2. A standard unit of measurement representing the biological activity of a nutrient *q.v.*

INTERNEURONS 1. Neurons *q.v.* that receive impulses and transmit them to other neurons. 2. Internuncial neurons. 3. Intercalated neurons. 4. Neurons that lie entirely within the central nervous system *q.v.* and that conduct impulses from sensory *q.v.* to motor *q.v.* neurons.

INTERNEUROSENSORY That which involves more that one system of the brain. ct: intraneurosensory.

INTERNIST 1. One who practices internal medicine. 2. One who practices a specialty of medicine directed toward treatment through the use of medicines, a general practitioner of medicine.

INTERNSHIP (MEDICAL) A period of study for medical students that provides for the practice of medicine within a hospital setting under the supervision of a resident physician.

INTERNUNCIAL NEURON Any neuron *q.v.* in a chain of neurons that is situated between the primary afferent neuron *q.v.* and the final motor, or efferent, neuron *q.v.*

INTEROBSERVER RELIABILITY In epidemiology, the degree to which two or more observers classify consistently among themselves the same observation on a group of subjects being studied.

INTEROCEPTIVE CONDITIONING Classical conditioning *q.v.* in which some important component is inside the body.

INTERPERSONAL AWARENESS A dimension of recognition of the attributes of persons and social interactions assumed to be reflected in developing ideas about friendship, role-taking, peer interactions, and other social processes.

INTERPERSONAL FACTORS Any event, element, individual, or group that influences positively or negatively the quality of relationships between individuals or groups.

INTERPERSONAL PERCEPTION Impression formation *q.v.*

INTERPERSONAL PSYCHOTHERAPY (IPT) A short-term therapy designed to address interpersonal relationships and their improvement rather than attempting to treat maladaptive cognitive issues. Primarily used to help depressed people function effectively. cf: interpersonal therapy.

INTERPERSONAL RELATIONSHIP 1. Social intercourse. 2. The quality of one's own actions while in the presence of other people. 3. Social interactions. cf: intrapersonal relationship.

INTERPERSONAL SEXUALITY Mutual emotional and physical sexual relationships between people. ct: intrapersonal sexuality.

INTERPERSONAL THERAPY Treatment that concentrates upon a person's marital and family problems that may contribute to the emotional or other mental health problems. Used frequently to treat alcoholism *q.v.* cf: interpersonal psychotherapy.

INTERPHASE 1. The stage between the time one mitosis takes place and the beginning of the next mitotic division. 2. The stage when the cell is not dividing.

INTERPOSITION A secondary cue to depth *q.v.* in which an object whose outline interrupts that of a second object is seen as nearer than the latter object.

INTERPRETATION The act by the therapist of reforming the views of the client so that they may be looked at by the client in a new way, thus gaining insight into the causes of the mental health issue.

INTERPRETIVE LEVEL OF HEALTH 1. Characterized by a person's need to establish feelings of self-worth, to interact socially, and to behave in ways that result in personal satisfaction, growth, and actualization *q.v.* 2. A level of health maintenance *q.v.* cf: biological level of health.

INTERSENSORY KNOWLEDGE The ability to predict how one sense will interpret an object or event after experiencing it with another sense. For example, if we smell a new food, we can predict whether or not we will like its taste.

INTERSEX An organism that displays phenotypic characteristics more-or-less intermediate between male and female.

INTERSTIMULUS INTERVAL In classical conditioning *q.v.*, the interval separating the conditioned stimulus *q.v.* and the unconditioned *q.v.* stimulus.

INTERSTITIAL 1. Spaces in a structure of the body, e.g., tissue. 2. Situated within a tissue. 3. Intercellular *q.v.*

INTERSTITIAL CELLS 1. Specialized cells in the testicles *q.v.* that produce the male sex hormone *q.v.*, testosterone *q.v.* 2. The cells between the seminiferous tubules *q.v.* cf: Leydig's cells.

INTERSTITIAL CELL-STIMULATING HORMONE (ICSH) 1. Associated with development of the testicles *q.v.* and the secretion of testosterone *q.v.* 2. A hormone *q.v.* secreted by the pituitary gland that stimulates the maturation of the sperm cells *q.v.*

INTERSTITIAL FLUID Together with transcellular fluid *q.v.* accounts for 80% of all extracellular *q.v.* fluid in the body. ~ consists of body fluids that bathe all body cells.

INTERSTITIAL PNEUMONITIS 1. An acute *q.v.* inflammation of the lungs. 2. An inflammation of the lungs which, if it persists for more than 2 months, is indicative of AIDS *q.v.* in children unless another cause is diagnosed.

INTERTRIGO An eruption of the skin due to chafing.

INTERTROCHANTERIC AREA The area between the two trochanters *q.v.* of the femur *q.v.*

INTERVAL SCALE A scale in which equal differences between the scores can be treated as equal so that the scores can be added or subtracted. cf: categorical scale; ordinal scale; ratio scale.

INTERVAL TRAINING 1. Alternate periods of rigorous activity and reduced activity. 2. A training routine consisting of four elements: (a) intensity, (b) duration, (c) repetitions, and (d) rest intervals. 3. Repeated bouts of exercise performed at an intensity above the anaerobic *q.v.* threshold, culminated with periods of rest or light exercise.

INTERVENING VARIABLE 1. A hypothetical concept. 2. A construct.

INTERVENTION 1. An active advocacy for change. 2. Sometimes done to alcoholics *q.v.* or other drug abusers *q.v.*, a planned encounter of the drug user's close friends and relatives to convince him or her to seek rehabilitation services. 3. An effort to change abnormal behaviors.

INTERVENTRICULAR SEPTUM The tissue that separates the right and left side of the heart.

INTERVERTEBRAL CARTILAGE Intervertebral disc *q.v.*

INTERVERTEBRAL DISC 1. The connective tissue *q.v.* formed between each vertebra *q.v.* in the spinal column. 2. Intervertebral cartilage *q.v.* 3. Layers of fibrocartilage between the bodies of adjacent vertebrae.

INTERVIEW 1. A research technique in which an investigator or his or her representative seeks one-on-one information from the subject with respect to the issue being studied. 2. The exchange of information from one person to another.

INTESTATE A person who dies without leaving a valid will.

INTESTINAL LIPASE An enzyme *q.v.* that hydrolyzes *q.v.* medium- and short-chain triglycerides *q.v.* to glycerol *q.v.* plus short- and medium-chain fatty acids *q.v.*

INTESTINE 1. Tubular structures at the lower end of the alimentary canal. There are two kinds of ~: (a) Large ~, the terminal portion of the intestinal tract that runs in an inverted V shape from the right lower abdomen up across and down to the rectum *q.v.* totaling about 5 ft in length and 3 inches in breadth. The ~ consists of the ascending colon, transverse colon, descending colon, sigmoid colon. (b) Small ~, that portion of the digestive tube leading from the stomach to the ascending colon, averaging about 22 ft in length and 2 inches in diameter. 2. That portion of the alimentary canal *q.v.* extending from the pyloric *q.v.* opening of the stomach to the anus *q.v.* The ~s are the (a) small ~, which is that portion of the digestive tube between the stomach and the cecum *q.v.* consisting of the duodenum *q.v.*, jejunum *q.v.*, and the ileum *q.v.* Also called the small bowel. (b) The large ~, which is that portion of the digestive tube extending from the ileocecal valve *q.v.* to the anus and consists of the cecum *q.v.*, colon, and rectum. Also called the large bowel.

INTIMA 1. The lining of an artery. 2. The innermost coat of a structure.

INTIMACY 1. A state of warm friendship and the sharing of innermost feelings and emotions. ~ develops through long association with another person. 2. A feeling of emotional closeness to another person. ~ may or may not involve sexual activity.

INTIMACY NEEDS Needs *q.v.* for companionship, love, and mutual respect.

INTIMATE Characterized by sharing innermost thoughts and feelings.

INTOLERANCE An allergy or sensitivity to a subject.

INTOXICATE To excite or stupefy by alcohol *q.v.* or a narcotic *q.v.* to the point where physical and mental control are markedly diminished.

INTOXICATION 1. Drunkenness as a result of the chemical action of alcohol on the central nervous system *q.v.* 2. The process of depressing the activities of the central nervous system by the chemical action of alcohol and some other drugs or chemicals. 3. The temporary reduction of mental and physical control or the stupefaction of normal functions because of the effects of drugs or chemicals. 4. Under the influence of a drug.

INTOXIFICATION COMA A deep state of unconsciousness caused by a drug from which the person cannot be aroused.

INTRAAMNIOTIC INFUSION 1. The injection of a substance into the amniotic sac *q.v.* to induce premature labor. 2. Instillation. 3. The replacement of amniotic fluid *q.v.* either with prostaglandins *q.v.* or with a salt solution causing circulatory arrest of the fetus *q.v.* Used in second trimester *q.v.* abortions *q.v.*

INTRACELLULAR Within a cell or cells.

INTRACELLULAR COMPARTMENT The approximately 60% of body water that is contained within body cells. ct: extracellular compartment.

INTRACELLULAR FLUID Fluid found within the cell wall or membrane.

INTRACEREBRAL Within the cerebrum *q.v.*

INTRACEREBRAL HEMATOMA Extravasation of blood within the brain substance.

INTRACRANIAL Within the skull.

INTRACUTANEOUS Within the skin.

INTRAINDIVIDUAL Comparisons of an individual's levels of performance in different area, e.g., motor skills versus musical skills.

INTRAMUSCULAR Within a muscle.

INTRAMUSCULAR INJECTION (IM) Hypodermic injection of drugs or fluids into a muscle.

INTRANEUROSENSORY A neural function that involves only one system in the brain. ct: interneurosensory.

INTRAOCULAR Between the cornea and the lens of the eye.

INTRAOCULAR LENS A lens made of plastic or other synthetic material used to replace an abnormal eye lens, as in the removal of a cataract *q.v.*

INTRAOCULAR TENSION The pressure of the vitreous humor *q.v.* within the eyeball.

INTRAPERSONAL RELATIONSHIP 1. How a person views the self. 2. Self-concept. 3. Self-esteem. cf: mental health; ct: interpersonal relationship.

INTRAPERSONAL SEXUALITY The sex drive within each person as manifested in sexual fantasies and masturbation *q.v.* ct: interpersonal sexuality.

INTRAPSYCHIC FACTORS Any factor, physical, psychological, or social, that influences a person's ability to function mentally and emotionally.

INTRAPSYCHIC METHODS (THERAPY) Techniques used to treat behavioral problems, such as alcoholism, that include role-playing, psychodrama, and group therapy. These methods are based on the somewhat controversial assumption that behavioral problems stem from emotional or unconsciously motivated factors.

INTRAPSYCHOTIC CONFLICT 1. Inner conflict. 2. Conflict between personal values.

INTRASCHOOL Within the confines of the school. ct: extraschool.

INTRAUTERINE Within the uterus *q.v.* Inside of the uterus. ct: extrauterine.

INTRAUTERINE DEVICE (IUD) 1. A method of birth control *q.v.* 2. An object inserted directly into the uterus *q.v.* that prevents the implantation of a fertilized egg *q.v.* They are of two types: (a) inert, a plastic device that inhibits implantation of the fertilized egg as a result of its presence in the uterus, and (b) active, a device wound with copper wire that releases ions *q.v.* that inhibits implantation of the fertilized egg. 3. A small plastic or metal object that prevents the zygote *q.v.* from implantation in the uterine wall.

INTRAVASCULAR FLUID The liquid part of the blood. ~ constitutes 20% of the intracellular *q.v.* fluid in the body.

INTRAVENOUS Within a vein.

INTRAVENOUS AGENTS Substances, drugs, fluids, or blood products introduced into a person by way of a vein *q.v.* for the purpose of hydration *q.v.* to increase the volume of the circulating blood or to provide faster action of a drug.

INTRAVENOUS DRUGS Drugs that are administered through a needle and syringe and injected directly into a vein and thus into the bloodstream.

INTRAVENOUS INJECTION (IV) 1. To administer into a vein. 2. An injection directly into the bloodstream. ct: intramuscular injection; subcutaneous injection.

INTRINSIC Within the individual arising inside the mind or the body. ct: extrinsic.

INTRINSIC FACTOR A transferase *q.v.* microprotein *q.v.* secreted by the mucosal cells of the stomach, which is required for the absorption of vitamin B_{12} *q.v.* through the intestinal wall. A lack of ~ will produce pernicious anemia *q.v.*

INTRINSIC MOTIVATION 1. Displayed when a person engages in action or behavior for its own sake or reward. 2. Personal reward that arises from an action. 3. Internal satisfaction. ct: extrinsic motivation; incentive.

INTRODUCER In politics, one who presents a bill or resolution for consideration. Cointroducers are those who signed onto the bill or resolution before its enactment.

INTRODUCTION In politics, the formal presentation or submission of a bill for consideration by the legislative body.

INTROITUS 1. The opening of the vagina *q.v.* 2. Any aperture of the body.

INTROJECTION 1. A defense mechanism *q.v.* 2. A process in which a person incorporates into his or her personality *q.v.* structure those characteristics of others who are threatening or, positively, those characteristics that are admired. 3. The acceptance of the values of another person into the self.

INTROMISSION The insertion of the penis *q.v.* into the vagina *q.v.* cf: sexual intercourse.

INTROPUNITIVE Responding to frustration *q.v.* by tending to blame oneself.

INTROPUNITIVE AGGRESSION Aggression *q.v.* directed against oneself. cf: extrapunitive aggression.

INTROSPECTION 1. The process of examining one's own thoughts and feelings. 2. In research, a process in which trained observers record their own subjective sensations as stimuli are changed.

INTROSPECTIVE METHOD Systematically begun in early twentieth century psychology, a process whereby trained subjects record their conscious experiences, thus giving a broader understanding of psychological processes.

INTROVERSION 1. An energy trait directed toward one's own inner world of thoughts and feelings. 2. The tendency to reject or resist the influence of others or of the external environment. cf: extraversion/introversion; ct: extraversion.

INTROVERSION/EXTRAVERSION TYPOLOGY 1. The theory *q.v.* that persons may be divided into two types of personality *q.v.*: (a) introverts *q.v.* and (b) extraverts *q.v.* 2. According to Eysenck's theory, ~ refers mainly to a person's susceptibility to conditioning. An extrovert is likely to be conditioned slowly and loses the responses rapidly, whereas the introvert is the opposite.

INTROVERT 1. A person who shows a strong tendency to find satisfaction in an inner life of thought and fantasy *q.v.* 2. A personality *q.v.* type characterized by the direction of interest toward oneself and one's inner world of experiences. ct: extravert.

INTRUSION ERROR In verbal learning *q.v.*, an error of commission in which a correct item as a response *q.v.* elsewhere in the list occurs as a mistake.

INTUBATION The act of inserting a tube into the larynx to relieve a respiratory obstacle.

INTUITION Direct perception of truth, fact, etc., independent of any rational, logical process.

INTUSSUCEPTION 1. The invagination of a segment of the intestine *q.v.* into itself, most common in children. 2. Telescoping of a segment of the intestine into the next most distal *q.v.* one. 3. The infolding of one segment of the intestine within another segment. 4. The deposition of new particles of formative material among those already embodied in a tissue or structure, as in the growth of living organisms.

IN UTERO In the uterus *q.v.*

INVAGINATE To fold in.

INVAGINATION The pushing of the wall of a cavity into the cavity.

INVALID 1. In law, not binding, lacking in authority. 2. In health, a person whose physical or mental health is compromised, necessitating the care of others.

INVARIABLE BEHAVIOR Determined by innate potentials, such as reflex actions. cf: automatic behavior. ct: variable behavior; adaptive behavior.

INVARIANT Some aspect of the proximal stimulus *q.v.* pattern that remains unchanged despite various transformations of the stimulus.

INVASIVE CANCER A cancer that infiltrates and destroys surrounding tissue.

INVASIVE CERVICAL CANCER 1. Cancer *q.v.* that has invaded a wide area of cervical tissue. 2. A malignancy *q.v.* that has spread through the cervix *q.v.*

INVERSION 1. A turning inward, as of the eyelid or the foot. 2. In genetics *q.v.*, a rearrangement of a group of genes *q.v.* in a chromosome *q.v.* in such a way that their order in the chromosome is reversed. 3. In ecology, a reversal of the atmospheric temperature gradient in which a layer of warm air traps a layer of cooler air beneath and keeps it from rising. ~ causes air pollution, smog *q.v.*, and related environmental health problems in industrial areas.

INVERT 1. In sexual psychology, a homosexual *q.v.* 2. A person who is sexually attracted to persons of the same sex.

INVERTASE Sucrase *q.v.*

INVERTED APPRAISAL Evaluation of superiors by their employees.

INVERTED NIPPLES 1. A congenital condition in which the nipples are not protuberant *q.v.* 2. A normal condition in which the nipple turns inward rather than outward from the areola *q.v.*

INVERT SUGAR Chemically treated sucrose *q.v.* ~ is sold as a liquid form of a mixture of glucose and fructose and primarily used to sweeten baked goods.

INVESTIGATIONAL NEW DRUG NUMBER (IND) An FDA *q.v.*-assigned code number used during human clinical trials of a new drug prior to the granting of permission to market it.

INVESTOR-OWNED HOSPITALS 1. Proprietary hospitals. 2. Hospitals that are operated as profit-making institutions.

IN VITRO 1. On (in) glass. 2. Experiments performed outside the living organism, within the laboratory. 3. Test tube experiments. 4. Outside the body in an artificial environment. ct: in vivo. cf: in vitro fertilization.

IN VITRO FERTILIZATION 1. "In glass" fertilization *q.v.* 2. A procedure in which the human ovum *q.v.* is fertilized in a laboratory dish and then reintroduced into the mother's uterus *q.v.* for gestational *q.v.* development. cf: in vitro; ct: in vivo.

IN VIVO 1. A reaction within a living organism. 2. In psychology *q.v.*, a real-life situation. ct: in vitro.

INVOLUNTARY ACTION 1. Any action performed independent of the will. 2. Not voluntary.

INVOLUNTARY MUSCLE 1. Muscles that make up the blood vessels and other organs such as the stomach. 2. Muscles not under the control of the will. ~ is smooth with the exception of the heart. 3. Nonstriated muscle tissue. ct: voluntary muscle.

INVOLUNTARY SMOKING With reference to tobacco smoke, passive smoking from "side stream" or second-hand smoke that is inhaled as a result of being in close proximity to one who is smoking.

INVOLUTION 1. An inward curvature. 2. A shrinking or return to a former size, as the uterus *q.v.* after child-birth. 3. The regressive alterations in the body or its parts characteristic of the aging process.

INVOLUTIONAL MELANCHOLIA 1. An outdated term referring to a depressive psychotic *q.v.* reaction characterized by depression, agitation, and apprehension. 2. Involutional psychotic reaction. Involutional psychosis *q.v.*

INVOLUTIONAL PSYCHOTIC REACTION 1. Involutional melancholia *q.v.* 2. Involutional psychosis *q.v.*

IOM An acronym for Institute of Medicine.

ION 1. Any atom that has lost one or more electrons or that has gained one or more electrons. 2. An electrically charged atom that is positive or negative depending upon whether or not it has gained or lost electrons. 3. A charged subatomic particle.

IONIZATION 1. Dissociation into ions *q.v.* 2. A process that occurs when a salt or similar substance composed of negatively and positively charged ions is dissolved in water and the two ions separate.

IONIZATION CHAMBER A chamber for detecting the ionization *q.v.* of an enclosed gas. The ~ is used for determining the intensity of ionization radiation *q.v.*

IONIZE 1. To separate into ions *q.v.* 2. To dissociate atoms or molecules into electrically charged atoms or radicals.

IONIZING RADIATION 1. A form of radiation *q.v.* capable of releasing electrons from atoms *q.v.* 2. Electromagnetic radiation *q.v.* (X-rays and gamma rays) and atomic particles that are energetic enough to knock electrons from elements and produce ions *q.v.* 3. A form of radiation often used in the treatment of cancer and is a major cause of gene *q.v.* mutation *q.v.* 4. Radiation that results when a stable, neutral atom is disrupted, releasing individual ions *q.v.* that bear either positive or negative charges.

IPCS An acronym for International Program on Chemical Safety, WHO *q.v.*

IPECAC 1. The dried root of *Uragoga ipecacuanha*, a shrub found chiefly in Brazil that can cause vomiting. 2. Syrup of ipecac.

IPRONIAZID An MAO *q.v.* antidepressant *q.v.* by elevating neurotransmitter levels by inhibiting their metabolism.

IPSATIVE STABILITY Stability that is achieved by maintaining the constancy of some trait or tendency. cf: normative stability.

IPSILATERAL On the same side. ct: contralateral.

IPSO FACTO 1. As a necessary consequence. 2. By the fact itself.

IPSP An acronym for inhibitory postsynaptic potential *q.v.*

IPT An acronym for interpersonal psychotherapy *q.v.*

IQ An acronym for intelligence quotient *q.v.*

IRIDOLOGY 1. A pseudoscience that is based on the belief that most abnormalities of the body cause abnormal markings in the eye. 2. The diagnosis of disease based on observations of the iris *q.v.* of the eye.

IRIS 1. The pigmented membrane *q.v.* in front of the lens of the eye that acts as a diaphragm to control the amount of light entering the eye through its central opening, the pupil *q.v.* 2. The circular pigmented membrane behind the cornea *q.v.* perforated by the pupil. The ~ is made up of circular muscle fibers and a thin layer of radial muscle fibers that dilate and constrict the pupil.

IRIS An acronym for Integrated Risk Information System *q.v.*

IRIS DIAPHRAGM A diaphragm that automatically adjusts to match the optical values of the objective.

IRITIS Inflammation of the iris *q.v.*

IRON A mineral element essential in forming red blood cells.

IRON DEFICIENCY ANEMIA Anemia *q.v.* resulting from a low hemoglobin *q.v.* level and a low hematocrit level *q.v.* Symptoms include irritability, fatigue, inability or difficulty in concentrating, and headaches.

IRRADIATION 1. Treatment by radiation *q.v.* 2. Used to irradiate foods to eliminate microorganism *q.v.* contamination. 3. In psychology, Pavlov's term for generalization *q.v.* that occurs because of a spread of excitation in the brain.

IRRATIONAL BELIEFS Beliefs that have no basis in reality, thought by rational-emotive psychologists *q.v.* to underlie psychological distress.

IRREGULAR 1. In botany, a term applied to a flower in which the floral whorls are unequal. 2. In physiology, unpredictable bowel movements. 3. Constipation *q.v.*

IRRESISTIBLE IMPULSE 1. An insanity *q.v.* plea following the commitment of a crime in some states. This is based on the concept that a person is not responsible for a crime committed when the act was precipitated by a psychotic condition that motivated the act and the person was unable to control his or her actions. 2. Based on a legal precedent in an 1834 Ohio court ruling in which it was decided that an insanity defense can be established by showing that the accused had an uncontrollable urge to commit the act. cf: Currens formula; McNaghten decision; Durham decision.

IRRITABILITY 1. In psychology, the ability to respond to stimuli. 2. The ability of protoplasm *q.v.* to respond to external stimuli.

IRV An acronym for inspiratory reserve volume.

IS An acronym for intercostal space.

ISCHEMIA 1. A narrowing of the coronary artery *q.v.* or arteries due to atherosclerotic plaque *q.v.* obstructing the flow of blood to the cardiac muscle *q.v.* resulting in coronary heart disease *q.v.* 2. Disruption or cutting off of the blood supply to a body part.

ISCHIAL TUBEROSITY A protuberance on the inferior surface of the ischium *q.v.* lateral to the anus *q.v.* and bearing weight when one is seated.

ISCHIOCAVERNOUS MUSCLE The muscle that extends from the hip bone to the penis *q.v.* or clitoris *q.v.*

ISCHIUM 1. One of the bones of the pelvis. 2. The inferior dorsal part of the hip bone. The ~ is a separate bone in early childhood. 3. The dorsal and posterior of the three principal bones composing either half of the pelvis.

ISCLT An acronym for International Society of Clinical Laboratory Technologists.

ISD An acronym for inhibited sexual desire *q.v.*

ISD An acronym for inhibitions of sexual desire *q.v.*

ISLANDS (ISLETS) OF LANGERHANS 1. Clusters of cells in the pancreas *q.v.* that produce insulin *q.v.* 2. Irregular microscopic *q.v.* structures scattered throughout the pancreas and comprising its endocrine *q.v.* portion.

ISO An acronym for International Standards Organization.

ISOAGGLUTINOGEN An antigen such as A or B blood-type factor that normally occurs without artificial stimulation in an individual.

ISOCALORIC Providing the same number of kilocalories *q.v.*

ISOCARBOSAZID 1. An MAO inhibitor *q.v.* used as an antidepressant. 2. Marplan is a brand name.

ISOELECTRIC POINT The pH level at which protein shows no net charge.

ISOGAMETE A gamete *q.v.* of a type not exhibiting sexual or other differentiations.

ISOGAMY 1. Sexual reproduction *q.v.* in algae and fungi in which the gametes are all alike in size. 2. A condition in which the gametes are structurally indistinguishable.

ISOIMMUNIZATION Incompatibility of blood type *q.v.* between the mother and her fetus *q.v.*

ISOKINETIC CONTRACTION 1. A muscular contraction performed against a controlled maximum resistance throughout the full range of motion. 2. A type of muscle contraction in which the speed of the contraction and the resistance encountered are unchanged during the entire range of motion. cf: isokinetic exercise.

ISOKINETIC EXERCISE Activity involving contraction of muscles throughout the full range of motion possible. cf: isometric exercise; isotonic exercise.

ISOLATE 1. Social isolate. 2. A child whose group status is characterized by low social impact as well as low social preference by other children.

ISOLATION 1. In epidemiology, a method of controlling the spread of a communicable *q.v.* disease by separating the infected person from those who are well. 2. In psychology, an ego defense mechanism *q.v.* by means of which contradictory attitudes or feelings that normally accompany particular attitudes are kept apart, thus preventing conflict or emotional pain. 3. A defense mechanism in which the individual inhibits emotions associated with unwanted desires.

ISOLATION OF VARIABLES A mental process that allows one to distinguish which variable is causally related to another and which is not.

ISOLEUCINE An essential amino acid *q.v.*

ISOMER One or two or more compounds that are identical in chemical composition but differ in atomic structure.

ISOMETRIC Same measure; exercise in which muscles contract but do not shorten. cf: isometric exercise.

ISOMETRIC CONTRACTION An system of exercise in which the muscle contracts but does not shorten when force is exerted on a stationary object. cf: isometric exercise.

ISOMETRIC EXERCISE Those activities characterized by pushing or pulling against an immovable object or against other muscles. ct: isotonic exercise; isokinetic exercise.

ISOMORPHISM The degree to which two things are seen as identical in form.

ISOTONIC A solution having the same osmotic pressure as physiological saline *q.v.*

ISOTONIC CONTRACTION A muscular contraction in which the length of the muscle shortens while overcoming resistance. 2. Dynamic contraction. cf: isotonic exercise. ct: isometric exercise.

ISOTONIC EXERCISE 1. Those activities that are characterized by placing resistance on a muscle or group of muscles but gradually allowing the muscle to move through its full range of motion. 2. Exercise in which muscles are allowed to contract and shorten. cf: isotonic contraction; ct: isometric exercise.

ISOTONIC SOLUTION A solution with an osmotic pressure equal to that of protoplasm *q.v.*

ISOTOPE An element *q.v.* of a chemical character identical with that of another element, occupying the same place in the periodic table *q.v.* but differing from it in other characteristics, as in radioactivity or in the mass of its atoms *q.v.*

ISSUE A matter or question disputed between two contending parties. Both issues are neither right or wrong; only the evidence used to support the contention is right or wrong. Issues are usually settled by the weight of the evidence.

ISTHMUS 1. The narrow connection between two larger bodies or parts of an organ. 2. The narrow end of the fallopian tubes *q.v.*

ITAI-ITAI A bone disease resulting from cadmium poisoning.

ITEM BANK In testing and evaluation, a collection of test items that are systematically stored and easily retrieved as needed by individual teachers so that they may devise and create tests for specific purposes by using previously designed and tested test items.

ITEM CARD Before computerized data storage, a card that used a standardized format for preparing, storing, and retrieving test items from the item bank *q.v.*

ITV An acronym for instructional television *q.v.*

IUD An acronym for intrauterine device *q.v.*

IV 1. Intravenous *q.v.* 2. Intravenously.

JACKSONIAN EPILEPSY 1. A form of epilepsy *q.v.* 2. Muscle spasms usually restricted to a small muscle group or to one-half of the body associated with an epileptic *q.v.* seizure *q.v.*

JAMES–LANGE THEORY OF EMOTIONS The hypothesis *q.v.* that the subjective experience of emotion *q.v.* is the awareness of one's own bodily reactions in the presence of certain arousing stimuli *q.v.*

JANIMINE A commercial preparation of imipramine *q.v.*

JAUNDICE 1. A yellowish pigment of the skin, eyes, and other tissues caused by an accumulation of bile pigments from the liver. The bile pigment, bilirubin *q.v.*, is diffused into the blood causing a yellowing of the tissues. 2. A symptom of an inflamed liver (hepatitis *q.v.*).

JAW THRUST MANEUVER A procedure for opening the airway. The jaw is lifted and pulled forward to keep the tongue from falling back into the airway. The lower lip is pulled down to force the mouth open.

JCAH An acronym for Joint Commission on Accreditation of Hospitals.

J-CURVE CONCEPT 1. Any system that grows by doubling is involved in geometric and exponential growth. 2. A frequency distribution *q.v.* in which the modal value is the most extreme measure, typically zero.

JEALOUSY 1. A powerful emotion *q.v.* in which the person experiences extreme fear that he or she might lose that which is loved to someone or something else. 2. A love–hate conflict. cf: sexual jealousy.

JEJUNUM 1. The second portion of the small intestine *q.v.* about 8 ft long. 2. That portion of the small intestine that extends from the duodenum *q.v.* to the ileum *q.v.*

JELLINEK THEORY OF ALCOHOLISM Named after its developer E. M. Jellinek (1890–1963), a theory claiming that alcoholics may present their patterns of alcohol use in a wide range of patterns. The theory is flawed and has little scientific validity, though its influence has been quite significant.

JND An acronym for just noticeable difference *q.v.*

JOB ANALYSIS 1. In the construction of aptitude tests, the analysis *q.v.* of the criterion performance *q.v.* into subskills. 2. A technique used to gain an understanding of what a task entails and the skills an individual must have to perform it.

JOB CLASS 1. The categorization of jobs based on skill and experience level linked to a particular salary scale. 2. Job classification.

JOB DESCRIPTION 1. Specific activities that a particular job entails and the desired qualifications of the person who holds the job. 2. Job specifications.

JOB DESIGN A specification of the responsibilities to be carried out by the person who holds the job and the methods needed to be used to fulfill the requirements for the job.

JOB ENLARGEMENT The addition of meaningless tasks to a job not expressed in the original job description.

JOB ENRICHMENT The addition of motivators or incentives to a particular job with the purpose of increasing productivity.

JOB EVALUATION An objective and systematic approach to evaluating the value of a particular job to an organization.

JOB ROTATION A formal process of moving employees from one job to another on a periodic basis in order to enhance the dynamism of the organization.

JOCK ITCH Tinea cruris *q.v.*

JOHN A slang expression for the customer of a prostitute *q.v.*

JOINT 1. The articulation *q.v.* or place of union or function between two or more bones of the skeleton *q.v.* 2. A slang term for a marijuana *q.v.* cigarette.

JOINT CAPSULE A fibrous sac with its synovial *q.v.* lining enclosing a joint *q.v.*

JOINT COMMISSION ON MENTAL ILLNESS AND HEALTH Established under the provisions of the Mental Health Study Act of 1955, conducted a comprehensive study of mental health programs and resources in the United States.

JOINT COMMITTEE ON CAREERS IN NURSING Founded in 1948 and consolidated with the National League for Nursing in 1952.

JOINT COMMITTEE ON HEALTH EDUCATION AND PROMOTION TERMINOLOGY (HEPT) Established in 2000, a continuance of the National Committee on Health Education Terminology of 1990. It refined the terminology included in the 1990 final document and added new content that has become more-or-less standardized as the professional language of health education.

JOINT COMMITTEE ON HEALTH EDUCATION TERMINOLOGY Established in 1990, a committee comprised of representatives of the various professional associations with a significant interest in health education, it developed a list of health education terms and phrases used by health educators. It was the first major attempt to standardize the definitions of key health education professional terminology.

JOINT COMMITTEE ON PRACTICAL NURSES AND AUXILIARY WORKERS IN NURSING SERVICE Founded in 1945 and consolidated with the National League for Nursing in 1952.

JOINT MOUSE Any loose calcareous deposit in a joint.

JOULE A unit of energy measurement in which 4.184 J equals 1 cal *q.v.*, or 4.184 kJ *q.v.* equals 1 kcal *q.v.* or 1 j equals 0.0002 kcal.

JOURNAL In politics, the official chronological record of the proceedings of the respective houses of the legislature.

JUDGMENT In law, a decision of the court, often involving the payment of damages.

JUDGMENT PROOF In law, a term applied to those against whom a judgment has been rendered and who do not have the ability or resources to pay damages.

JUGULAR Pertaining to the neck.

JUGULAR NOTCH The bony depression at the superior end of the manubrium *q.v.* sterni.

JUGULAR VEINS The main blood vessels collecting blood from the head and neck: (a) external bilateral ~ are the major veins draining the scalp and face and (b) internal bilateral ~ are the major veins draining the brain.

JUMP KIT A closed container fitted with necessary portable equipment and supplies to be used in the emergency care of victims away from the ambulance.

JUNIOR HIGH SCHOOL 1. A level of school organizational structure that generally includes grades 7 and 8 or grades 7, 8, and 9. 2. A level of adolescent education largely replaced by middle school *q.v.* ct: elementary school; high school.

JUNK FOODS 1. Foods very low in or lacking in essential nutrients. 2. Foods high in calories, salt, sugar, fat, and the like, but low in the micronutrients *q.v.* Erroneously compared with fast foods.

JURY OF EXECUTIVE OPINION METHOD The process of gaining input from the various executives of an organization in predicting future sales of products or future programmatic needs as they see it.

JUST CAUSE In law, what a person, given the conditions at the time and the standards of justice, would have done under similar circumstances.

JUST NOTICEABLE DIFFERENCE (JND) 1. Difference threshold *q.v.* 2. The smallest difference between two stimuli *q.v.* that can be detected reliably.

JUST-WORLD HYPOTHESIS The belief that people can get what they deserve from life, and thus deserve what they get.

JUVENILE DELINQUENCY 1. Behavior that is legally prohibited and manifest by persons who are under the legal age. 2. Criminal behavior committed by a minor.

JUVENILE ERA The first part of the school year when children first begin to interact with a diversity of adults besides their parents and to spend a large proportion of their time with their peers. cf: prepubescence.

JUVENILE ONSET DIABETES 1. Type I diabetes mellitus *q.v.* 2. Usually manifests itself in children or young adults. Treatment consists of daily injections of insulin *q.v.* as there is a total or substantial lack of it being secreted by the islet cells of Langerhans. Cardiovascular *q.v.* complications often result after several years. ct: maturity diabetes; adult onset diabetes.

JUVENILE PARESIS 1. General paresis *q.v.* in children who are usually of congenital *q.v.* origin. 2. Resulting from untreated syphilis *q.v.*, the onset of symptoms is usually at 12–14 years after a symptom-free childhood.

JUVENILE RHEUMATOID ARTHRITIS 1. A disease of the joints *q.v.* similar to adult rheumatoid arthritis *q.v.* except that it occurs in joints that are undergoing growth. 2. A childhood viral disease characterized by inflammation and swelling of the joints.

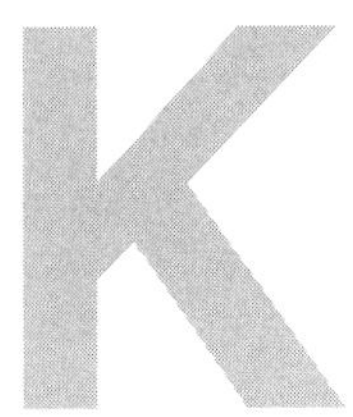

KALLMANN'S SYNDROME A disorder that occurs in males at puberty *q.v.* where the hypothalamus *q.v.* fails to signal for the release of male hormone, thus preventing the development of adult secondary sex characteristics.

KAMASUTRA An ancient manual originally developed in India, depicting sex techniques.

KAPLAN'S SEX THERAPY METHOD A blend of psychodynamic *q.v.* and behavioral techniques. Developed by Helen Kaplan at Cornell University Medical Center.

KAPOSI'S SARCOMA 1. A cancer *q.v.* of the blood and/or lymphatic *q.v.* vessel walls. It usually appears as blue–violet to brownish skin blotches or papules. A common result of AIDS *q.v.* 2. A spreading cancer of the connective tissue, principally involving the skin. Prior to 1978, ~ was largely confined to men over 50 years. Since the appearance of AIDS, however, it is a common affliction of men and women of all ages who have contracted AIDS.

KARYOLYMPH The ground substance of a cell nucleus *q.v.*

KARYOTYPE 1. In genetics, all of the characteristics of the chromosomes *q.v.* of a cell. 2. The arrangement of the chromosomes. 3. The appearance of the metaphase chromosomes of an individual or species. ~ is of comparative size, shape, and morphology *q.v.* of the different chromosomes.

kcal An abbreviation for kilocalorie *q.v.*

KEEP AMERICA BEAUTIFUL, INC. One of the chief voluntary organizations for the prevention of littering.

KEGEL EXERCISES 1. Repeated contractions *q.v.* of the pubococcygeal muscles *q.v.* designed to strengthen them. 2. An exercise for toning *q.v.* vaginal *q.v.* and perineal *q.v.* muscles. It is performed by repeatedly tightening the muscles that stop the flow of urine.

KELLER PLAN A teaching technique in which learners proceed at their own pace in mastering a series of units in some subject.

KELOID An overgrowth of fibrous tissue in a scar.

KELP A large, brown seaweed.

KERATIN 1. An insoluble substance that forms the basis of horns, nails, and hoofs. 2. A waterproofing protein *q.v.* for the skin. 3. A horny protein-like substance in the upper layers of the skin and which is the principal constituent of hair and nails.

KERATINIZED 1. Cells that have become toughened with an excess protein *q.v.* substance. 2. To become horny or cornified *q.v.*

KERATINOPHILIC Growing upon substances rich in keratin *q.v.*, such as hair, feathers, nails, and hoofs.

KERATITIS Inflammation *q.v.* of the cornea *q.v.* due to infection *q.v.* or injury.

KERATOCONJUNCTIVITIS Inflammation *q.v.* of both the cornea *q.v.* and the overlying conjunctiva *q.v.*, giving a diffuse inflamed appearance to the eye.

KERATOMALACIA An affliction of the cornea *q.v.* characterized by dryness with ulceration *q.v.* and perforation resulting from vitamin A deficiency *q.v.*

KERATOMETER An instrument measuring the curves of the cornea *q.v.*

KERATOSIS 1. A small skin thickening, swelling, or lump that may be a precursor to cancer *q.v.* 2. Any horny growth of skin.

KERATOTOMY A surgical procedure to correct nearsightedness *q.v.* by incising the cornea *q.v.* of the eye.

KETALAR A commercial preparation of ketamine *q.v.*

KETAMINE 1. A dissociative *q.v.* anesthetic *q.v.* 2. Ketalar is a brand name.

KETOACID A product of fats that is unused as a result of diabetes *q.v.* ~ destroys brain tissue and causes diabetic coma *q.v.*

KETOACIDOSIS Acidosis *q.v.* found in diabetics *q.v.* and associated with increased production of ketone bodies *q.v.* from incomplete metabolism *q.v.* of fats *q.v.*

KETOGENIC 1. That which is conducive to the formation of ketone *q.v.* bodies, e.g., a high-fat, low-carbohydrate *q.v.* diet. 2. Producing ketones *q.v.*

KETONE 1. A chemical compound that contains the carboxyl group *q.v.* 2. An acid produced during fat catabolism *q.v.*: acetoacetic, β-hydroxybutyric, and acetone.

KETONE BODIES Fatty acid *q.v.* derivatives that can function as energy sources in the body. ~ include β-oxybutyric acid, acetoacetic acid, and acetone.

KETOSIS 1. An excessive accumulation of ketone bodies *q.v.* caused by accelerated rate of tissue lipolysis *q.v.* 2. An abnormal metabolic condition caused by an incomplete breakdown of fatty acids *q.v.* into ketone bodies. ~ may result from a low-carbohydrate or starvation diet. The by-products of incomplete fat metabolism may result in an acidic blood condition.

KEYING Activating a transmitter as used in emergency vehicle and by dispatchers.

KEYWORD METHOD A mnemonic device used to learn a foreign language word by forming a visual image or link to an English word. Applicable in health education in regards to learning technical terminology.

kg An abbreviation for kilogram *q.v.*

kg m/min Kilograms times meters per minute. A kilogram meter (kg m) is a measure of work. A kilogram meter per minute is the rate of doing work.

KHAT (catha) A shrub of Africa and Arabia. People chew the leaves and twigs of the shrub, or brew it like tea. ~ causes a stimulating, euphoric effect.

KI A Japanese term for a form of energy that flows through the body.

KIDDIE PORN A slang term for child pornography *q.v.*

KIDNEY 1. Humans possess two ~s located posteriorly in the abdominal cavity. There are three main functions of the ~s: (a) to produce urine for excretion, (b) to produce a hormone *q.v.* called renin *q.v.*, (c) to produce a hormone called erythropoietin. 2. Either of the two retroperitoneal organs in the lumbar *q.v.* region that filter the blood, excreting the end products of metabolism as urine and regulating salt and water content in the body.

KIDNEY DISEASE 1. Any agent, biological, chemical, or physical that causes dysfunction of the kidneys or related structures. 2. A renal disorder *q.v.* cf: six warning signs of kidney disease.

KIDNEY STONES Concentrations of insoluble material ranging from a fraction of an inch to several inches in diameter that are formed in the urinary tract.

KIEF Arabic for marijuana *q.v.* in dried resin form. cf: kif.

KIF A Moroccan cannabis *q.v.* preparation. cf: kief.

KILO A kilogram, the equivalent of 2.2 pounds. The usual package of marijuana *q.v.* sold in Mexico.

KILOCALORIE (kcal) 1. The basic unit of energy in the body. 2. The amount of energy required to raise the temperature of 1 l of water from 15°C to 16°C. 3. A unit of heat measure equivalent to 1000 gram calories. cf: calorie.

KILOGRAM (kg) A metric unit of weight that is equivalent to 2.2 pounds or 1000 g.

KILOJOULE (kj) A metric unit of energy that is equivalent to 0.239 kcal *q.v.* cf: joule.

KINDERGARTEN A term coined by Froebel, who began the first schools for children aged 4–6.

KINESIOLOGY 1. The science that studies the mechanisms and anatomy of motion and movement. 2. The science that deals with the functions of muscles. cf: kinesthesia; ct: applied kinesiology.

KINESTHESIA 1. The sense through which the organism perceives muscle movement. 2. Muscle sense. 3. A sense of position and movement of body parts. cf: kinesiology.

KINESTHESIS Sensory information generated by receptors in the muscles, tendons, and joints that inform a person of skeletal movement. cf: kinesiology.

KINESTHETIC Pertaining to, and relating to, sensations derived from muscles or movement.

KINESTHETIC METHOD A technique for teaching the learning disabled pupil that makes use of several sense modalities.

KINESTHETIC SENSE 1. The sensation of body position and movement perceived through nerve end-organs in muscles, tendons, and joints. 2. The ability to perceive body part positions without actually visualizing their location.

KINETIC ENERGY 1. Energy *q.v.* that is producing work. 2. Energy due to movement of an object. ct: potential energy.

KINETOCHORE Centromere *q.v.*

KINETOSOME A granular body at the base of a cilium *q.v.* or flagellum *q.v.*

KININS Hormones *q.v.* involved in cell division and other processes.

KIN-SELECTION HYPOTHESIS A proposition that altruism *q.v.* has biological survival value because the altruist's beneficiaries tend to be closely related relatives who carry a high proportion of his or her own genes *q.v.* cf: reciprocal-altruism hypothesis.

KINSHIP A social bond based upon genetic relationship or by marriage or other partnership arrangement. In some societies, there are also ties, called fictive kin, where there is closeness by arrangement, such as godparents.

KLEBSIELLA PNEUMONIAE A bacterium *q.v.* that can cause pneumonia *q.v.*

KLEPTOMANIA 1. A neurosis *q.v.* characterized by compulsive stealing. 2. An obsessive-compulsive reaction *q.v.*

(neurosis). 3. An irresistible compulsion to steal, usually without regard to the use for the article stolen.

KLINEFELTER'S SYNDROME An abnormality affecting males in which the sex-determining chromosomes are XXY instead of the normal XY. One gamete *q.v.* somehow contributes an extra X chromosome at the time of fertilization. Symptoms include small testicles, sterility, and, frequently, feminine physical features.

KLISMAPHILIA 1. A sexual variance *q.v.* 2. A person who gains sexual gratification from giving or receiving enemas *q.v.*

KNEE A hinge joint *q.v.* between the femur *q.v.* and the tibia *q.v.*

KNEECAP Patella *q.v.*

KNOWLEDGE 1. Job-relevant information a person needs to perform activities. 2. Assimilation *q.v.* and accommodation *q.v.* of information. 3. An understanding of facts. A synthesis of facts. 4. Insight *q.v.* into the relationship and significance of factual information.

KNOWLEDGE BASE A term referring to the information upon which a profession or professional education program is built.

KNOWLEDGE NEEDS The need for cognitive *q.v.* development; the acquisition of knowledge, comprehension, and wisdom.

KNOWLEDGE TEST A test for evaluating *q.v.*, recall, recognition, and understanding. cf: knowledge.

KOANS Puzzles or dilemmas, usually with no definitive answer.

KOPLICK'S SPOTS Red and white pinpoint eruptions that occur on the lining of the cheeks when a person has rubeola *q.v.*

KORSAKOFF'S PSYCHOSIS Characterized by disorientation, failure of memory, and substituting imagined episodes for the loss of memory. It results from a combination of excessive alcohol intake and a deficiency of niacin *q.v.* Symptoms of neuropathy associated with ~ include impairment of reflexes, loss of sensation of pain, progressive muscular weakness, and difficulty in walking. ~ was first described and named ~ in 1887 by S. S. Korsakoff.

KORSAKOFF cf: Korsakoff/Wernicke's syndrome.

KORSAKOFF/WERNICKE'S SYNDROME See Korsakoff's psychosis; Wernicke's disease.

KRAUSE'S END BULB A sensory receptor *q.v.* thought to respond to cold.

KRAUSS–RAAB EFFECT The symptoms that accompany a lack of exercise, characterized by lethargy, stiffness, depression, and the like; hypokinetic disease *q.v.*

KREBIOZEN An unproven method of cancer *q.v.* treatment. cf: Laetrile.

KREBS CYCLE 1. The aerobic pathway *q.v.* for oxidation *q.v.* of carbohydrates *q.v.*, protein *q.v.*, and lipids *q.v.* to CO_2, H_2O, and energy. 2. A series of biochemical reactions by which carbon chains or sugars, fatty acids *q.v.*, and amino acids *q.v.* are metabolized *q.v.* to yield carbon dioxide, water, and energy.

KRETEK A clove cigarette.

KS An acronym for Kaposi's sarcoma *q.v.*

KUSSMAUL RESPIRATION Deep, rapid respiration characteristic of the air hunger found in diabetic acidosis *q.v.* or coma *q.v.*

KWASHIORKOR A protein deficiency disease of children characterized by edema *q.v.*, changes in the health of the hair and skin, growth failure, and apathy. cf: marasmus.

KYNURENINE A derivative of tryptophan *q.v.* metabolism, present in the urine of rabbits and occasionally other animals.

KYPHOLORDOSIS Round, hollow back.

KYPHOSIS 1. Forward head. 2. Humpback.

L

LAAM A synthetic *q.v.* narcotic *q.v.* that is chemically similar to methadone *q.v.* that has a duration of action that lasts 48–72 h.

LABELING In education, the classifying or categorizing of students based on their ability or aptitude *q.v.* for the purpose of placement.

LABELING THEORY OF MENTAL DISORDERS The assertion that the label "mental illness" acts as a self-fulfilling prophecy that perpetuates the condition once the label has been applied.

LABIA 1. The liplike structures of the female external genitalia *q.v.* 2. The genital lips of the female. 3. Lips. 4. The external female genitalia, including the outer lips, the labia majora *q.v.*, and the inner lips, the labia minora *q.v.*

LABIA MAJORA The outer and larger pair of lips of the female vulva *q.v.* ct: labia minora.

LABIA MINORA The inner or lesser lips of the female genitalia *q.v.* or vulva *q.v.* ct: labia majora.

LABILE Easily moved or changed, as in shifting from one emotion to another, or becoming quickly aroused.

LABILITY Instability, particularly with regard to affect *q.v.*

LABIOSCROTAL SWELLING 1. Undifferentiated tissue within the embryo *q.v.* that becomes either the scrotum *q.v.* in males or the labia majora *q.v.* in females. 2. Rudimentary genitals *q.v.* that develop into either the scrotum in males or the labia majora in females depending on the presence of androgen *q.v.* The presence of androgen will cause scrotal development, an absence will result in the development of the labia majora.

LABIUM (PL. LABIA) 1. A fleshy border or edge. 2. Lip. 3. A part of the vulva *q.v.* 4. The lips of the vagina *q.v.*

LABOR 1. The series of processes by which the fetus *q.v.* and other products of pregnancy *q.v.* are expelled from the uterus *q.v.* 2. Delivery, birth, and expulsion of the child and placenta *q.v.* as a result of uterine contractions. 3. The process by which the muscles of the uterus open the birth canal *q.v.* and push the baby down and through so that it can be born. cf: birth.

LABORATORY METHOD A type of experimental learning occurring within a community or group. New patterns of behavior are invented and tested in a climate supportive of behavior change.

LABORATORY RESEARCH Scientific study or experiment characterized by controlled experimentation. ct: field research.

LABORATORY SCHOOL A school under the control of, and often operated by, a college or university that has a teacher preparation program. A ~ provides a setting for student teaching experiences, the study of teaching methods, and the implementation of new curricula or school structuring. Also called a campus school.

LABOR FORCE Data reflecting the total number of people employed or unemployed, be they civilians or in the military. These data are usually gathered on a weekly basis.

LABOR FORCE PARTICIPATION RATE 1. The ratio of the labor force to the noninstitutionalized population (does not include those who are incarcerated or those institutionalized for medical reasons). 2. The percentage of eligible people who are working.

LABOR INTENSIVE Refers to the amount of high-intensity labor necessary for a particular production or other work process.

LABOR PNEUMONIA A disease caused by a specific type of bacterium *q.v.* and characterized by inflammation of one or more of the lobes of the lungs.

LABYRINTH 1. A structure containing many passageways. 2. The internal ear.

LACERATE To tear or cut roughly.

LACERATION 1. A wound made with a dull instrument. The wound may have jagged edges. 2. In neurology, a tearing of tissues by an object entering the skull.

LACHES In law, the failure to assert a right for an unreasonable and unexplained length of time, rendering the circumstances prejudicial to the opposing party.

LACRIMAL Pertaining to tears. cf: lacrimal system.

LACRIMAL GLANDS The tear glands. cf: lacrimal system.

LACRIMAL SYSTEM The system pertaining to the tears consisting of (a) lacrimal duct *q.v.* that is a short canal leading from each lower eyelid to the nose, conducting tears into the nares *q.v.*; (b) lacrimal gland *q.v.*, which is a small gland located in the upper outer angle of the orbit and that secretes tears; and (c) punctum lacrimale, which is the small mound as the inner angle of each lower eyelid containing the upper opening of the lacrimal duct.

LACRIMATION Secreting and discharging tears.

LACTASE An enzyme *q.v.* required for the digestion of lactose *q.v.* into glucose *q.v.* and galactose *q.v.*

LACTATING Breastfeeding. Nursing. cf: lactation.

LACTATION The production of milk in the breasts of the female shortly before and after the birth of a baby. cf: colostrum.

LACTATIONAL AMENORRHEA The tendency for women to be less fertile when they are lactating *q.v.* The operational term here is "less fertile," as breast feeding is not an effective birth control for most women.

LACTATOR A female who is producing breast milk. cf: lactating; lactation.

LACTEAL 1. One of the lymphatic vessels of the small intestine *q.v.* that conveys the chyle from the intestine through the mesenteric glands *q.v.* to the thoracic duct *q.v.* 2. Resembling milk.

LACTENIN Bacteriostatic *q.v.* substances innate to milk.

LACTIC ACID 1. A compound formed in the body during anaerobic *q.v.* glycolysis *q.v.* ~ is also produced in milk by the bacterial fermentation *q.v.* of lactose *q.v.* 2. A chemical by-product of anaerobic activity. 3. A chemical causing fatigue caused by an insufficient supply of oxygen during exercise and is capable of terminating muscular contraction if concentration is high enough.

LACTIFEROUS SINUS A vessel that transports milk from the milk-producing acini *q.v.* to the opening of the nipple.

LACTOBACILLI Bacteria in the vagina that aid in keeping it (the vagina) healthy. cf: *Doderlein's bacilli.*

LACTOBACILLUS ACIDOPHILUS A bacterium *q.v.* believed to be responsible for tooth decay (dental caries *q.v.*).

LACTOGENESIS The initiation of milk production after delivery of the baby. cf: lactogenic hormone.

LACTOGENIC HORMONE Prolactin *q.v.*

LACTOSE Milk sugar. A disaccharide *q.v.* produced from the condensation of glucose *q.v.* and galactose *q.v.*, a significant dietary carbohydrate *q.v.* from animal origin.

LACTO VEGETARIAN DIET A vegetarian diet *q.v.* that permits the use of dairy products.

LACUNA 1. The space in which cells are located. 2. A pit. 3. A space or a cavity. Lacunae in bone.

LAD An acronym for language acquisition device *q.v.*

LADDER SPLINT A flexible splint consisting of two stout parallel wires and five cross-wires that resemble a ladder.

LAETRILE An unproven method of cancer *q.v.* treatment. It is derived from apricot kernels and contains a chemical substance known as amygdaline, a poisonous compound that releases cyanide when acted upon by the body's enzymes *q.v.* ~ is forbidden in interstate commerce in the United States but is a legal drug in some states. To date, there is no scientific evidence that ~ has any effects upon the prevention or treatment of cancer.

LAISSEZ FAIRE 1. A doctrine that government should not interfere with business or personal activities. 2. Noninterference with the affairs of others.

LAMINARIA Plugs made of seaweed that, on exposure to moisture, expand and dilate *q.v.* the canal into which they have been placed.

LAMARCKISM A theory concerning the environmental origin of adaptive variation.

LAMAZE 1. A method of muscle relaxation by mothers in childbirth. 2. A so-called form of natural childbirth. 3. The ~ method was developed by Fernand Lamaze as a childbirth alternative characterized by the couple attending a series of instructional sessions to teach them about childbirth and to prepare them to participate as a couple in the childbirth experience.

LAMBERT'S TREATMENT Gradual reduction of the dosage of opium *q.v.* with increased dosage of codeine *q.v.* Codeine dosage is continued for 7–10 days following complete withdrawal form opium.

LAMELLA 1. The structure made of small plates, such as the bony concentric layers surrounding the Haversian canals *q.v.* 2. The unit of arrangement in bone. 3. Cells, together with the matrix, forming a sheet.

LAMELLAE 1. In botany, layers of protoplasmic membranes *q.v.* observed in the protoplast, particularly in and between the grana of the chloroplasts *q.v.* 2. A thin layer, as of bone.

LAMINA 1. A thin plate or flat layer. 2. The flattened portion of either side of a vertebral arch.

LAMINECTOMY The surgical removal of a portion of a vertebra.

LAMPBRUSH CHROMOSOMES Greatly enlarged chromosomes *q.v.* in the oocytes *q.v.* of amphibians. ~ have a main axis and side loops, which is how its name is derived.

LANCEOLATE Narrow, tapering to a point at the apex and sometimes at the base.

LAND GRANT COLLEGE A college established to carry out the intent of the Morrill Act of 1862, which provided public lands to states for the establishment of colleges focusing on the practical arts and agriculture, and mechanical arts.

LAND POLLUTION Pollution *q.v.* of the land with chemicals and other physical materials. ~ may result from erosion, agricultural manure, chemicals from industry and other sources, dumps, junk yards, septic systems, incineration residue, and radioactive waste.

LANGERHANS CELLS Dendritic cells *q.v.* in the skin that pick up antigens *q.v.* and transport them to the lymph nodes *q.v.*

LANGUAGE The systematic linkage of utterances that convey a message.

LANGUAGE ACQUISITION DEVICE (LAD) Chomsky's name for the innate knowledge that humans appear to have regarding the possible rules and meanings of language. This "device" enables anyone at a very early age to infer the grammar of whatever language is first spoken to him or her.

LANGUAGE ACQUISITION SUPPORT SYSTEM The features or characteristics of a child's linguistic environment that enables him or her to acquire language skills.

LANGUAGE DELAY The interruption of the normal developmental process of language acquisition, while retaining the typical sequence of development.

LANGUAGE DISORDER Refers to an irregularity of the normal sequence of language acquisition. This acquisition is not systematic and sequential as is normally the case.

LANUGO Fine hair that appears on the developing fetus during the fifth or sixth month of fetal *q.v.* development.

LAPAROSCOPE 1. A lighted tube used for examination and surgery in the abdomen. Used in female sterilization. 2. An instrument used to electrically sever the fallopian tubes *q.v.* 3. An instrument inserted into the abdominal cavity *q.v.* used to visualize its contents or to perform surgery. cf: laparoscopy.

LAPAROSCOPIC STERILIZATION Involves making two incisions through the abdominal wall, one just below the umbilicus *q.v.* and a second about 8 cm below the umbilicus. The abdomen is distended with an inert gas through the first incision, giving the surgeon a clear view of the fallopian tubes *q.v.* The tubes are tied off through the second incision. Also called the band aid operation.

LAPAROSCOPY Laparoscopic sterilization *q.v.*

LAPAROTOMY 1. A type of tubal ligation *q.v.* procedure. 2. A sterilization procedure involving a major abdominal incision through which the fallopian tubes *q.v.* are cut and tied. 3. A procedure, now largely replaced by laparoscopy, used to perform tubal ligations. 4. Any surgical procedure involving an incision through the abdominal wall.

LOPHOPHORA WILLIAMSII Peyote *q.v.*

LARGE INTESTINE See intestine.

LARYNGEAL Pertaining to the larynx *q.v.*

LARYNGECTOMY Surgical removal of all or part of the larynx *q.v.*

LARYNGITIS Inflammation of the larynx *q.v.*

LARYNGOSCOPE An instrument for directly visualizing the larynx *q.v.* and its related structures.

LARYNX 1. The structure in the neck that contains the vocal cords. 2. The Adam's apple. 3. The voice box. 4. Site of the vocal cords. 5. The musculocartilaginous structure lined with mucous membrane *q.v.*, situated superior to the trachea *q.v.* and inferior to the root of the tongue, guarding the entrance to the trachea and functioning secondarily as the organ of the voice.

LARYNXGOLOGY The study and treatment of the diseases of the throat.

LAS An acronym for lymphadenopathy syndrome *q.v.*

LASCIVIOUS Tending to stimulate lustful urges.

LASER 1. An instrument for producing an enormously intense and sharply directed beam of light. 2. *L*ight *a*mplification by *s*timulated *e*mission of *r*adiation. 3. A device that produces a beam of nonspreading, monochromatic, visible light. High energies are concentrated into a narrow beam, and laser treatment can be completed with so brief a flash that damaging surrounding areas by heat is precluded.

LASS An acronym for language acquisition support system *q.v.*

LASSITUDE A feeling of tiredness or weakness.

LATENCY 1. The period of time between the administration of a drug and the beginning of a response. 2. Generally, the interval before some reaction takes place. 3. In psychology, the time between the presentation of a stimulus *q.v.* and the occurrence of the response *q.v.* 4. A period of time during which a virus or other organism is inactive in the body. cf: latency period.

LATENCY PERIOD 1. In psychoanalytic psychology *q.v.*, a stage in psychosexual development *q.v.* in which sexuality *q.v.* lies essentially dormant—from ages 5 to 12. 2. The period of psychosexual development following the phallic stage *q.v.* during which psychodynamic conflicts are repressed and latent *q.v.* 3. The fourth stage of Freud's theory of psychosexual development; preadolescence.

LATENCY STAGE OF SYPHILIS Refers to a period in syphilitic *q.v.* infection when all symptoms disappear. It may last as long as 30 years. However, during this time, the disease is invading muscles and nerve tissues.

LATENT 1. Hidden. 2. Quiet. 3. Not active. 4. Inactive or dormant.

LATENT CONTENT In psychoanalytic theory *q.v.*, repressed wishes that are indirectly expressed in the manifest content *q.v.* of dreams.

LATENT DREAM The wish fulfillment during dreams that represents the person's hidden desires. cf: Freud's theory of dreams.

LATENT FUNCTION In sociology, the results or consequences neither expected nor intended by participants in a social system.

LATENT HOMOSEXUAL A person with hidden homosexual *q.v.* impulses.

LATENT LEARNING Learning that occurs without manifestation of any performance.

LATENT STAGE A period of a disease in which there are no signs or symptoms of the disease.

LATENT VIRAL INFECTION The period in which the virion *q.v.* becomes part of the host's cell's DNA *q.v.*

LATERAL 1. On one side of an organ. 2. To one side. 3. Away from the middle of the body. ct: medial; terminal.

LATERAL ASYMMETRY The difference in the functioning between the right and the left hemispheres of the brain.

LATERAL COLOR The spectrum of colors seen as a result of the spherical surface of the lens.

LATERAL HYPOTHALAMUS 1. A region of the hypothalamus *q.v.* that is said to be a hunger center and to be in an antagonistic relation to a supposed satiety center. 2. The ventromedial region of the hypothalamus.

LATERAL INHIBITION The tendency of adjacent neural elements of the visual system to inhibit each other; it underlies brightness contrast *q.v.* and accentuation of contours.

LATERALITY A sense of "sideness," including the tendency to use one hand for specific tasks.

LATERALIZATION An asymmetry of function of the two cerebral hemispheres *q.v.* In most people who are right handed, the left hemisphere is specialized for language, while the right hemisphere is better at visual and special tasks.

LATERAL MALLEOLUS The rounded projection on the lateral *q.v.* side of the ankle joint. ct: medial malleolus.

LATERAL MERISTEMS Secondary tissue, such as cambium and cork cambium, that are produced by ∼.

LATERAL ORGANIZATIONAL COMMUNICATION An organizational structure allowing for communication to flow horizontally to another part on the organizational chart.

LATERAL SULCUS A major horizontal fissure on each side of the cerebral hemisphere *q.v.*, separating the frontal and parietal lobes *q.v.* from the temporal lobe *q.v.*

LATEX A milky fluid found in certain plants, such as the opium poppy *q.v.*, dandelion, milkweed, and the Brazilian rubber tree.

LATIN GRAMMAR SCHOOL 1. A classical secondary school with a curriculum largely centered around Greek and Latin; its primary purpose being preparation for college. 2. The type of schools that proliferated from 50 B.C. to A.D. 200. The chief elements of the curriculum were Latin, grammar, literature, mathematics, music, and dialectics.

LATROGENIC An illness resulting from actions taken by the healer to treat a disease. cf: iatrogenic.

LAUDANUM 1. The earliest example of a patent medicine *q.v.* containing opium *q.v.* ∼ was first concocted by Paracelsus *q.v.* in the early part of the sixteenth century. Thomas Sydenham *q.v.* is also credited with its development, but it was somewhat different in its ingredients. A more powerful mixture was compounded by Thomas Dover *q.v.* in 1732, known as Dover's powder. 2. A tincture of 10% opium. A hydroalcoholic mixture.

LAV Lymphadenopathy-associated virus; the name given by French researchers to the human immunodeficiency virus (HIV) *q.v.*

LAVAGE A washing out of a hollow organ, such as the stomach.

LAW 1. A statute. 2. A bill that is passed by the legislature and signed by the executive. 3. In science, a basic principle that has been demonstrated to be true on innumerable occasions without variation in outcome.

LAW OF CLOSURE The tendency to perceptually close gaps in slightly incomplete figures. cf: Gestalt psychology.

LAW OF EFFECT 1. The premise that learning takes place when responses *q.v.* are rewarded. 2. Empirical law of effect *q.v.* 3. The proposition that reward is necessary for learning to take place. 4. The theory that asserts that the tendency of a stimulus *q.v.* to evoke a response is strengthened when the response is followed by reward and is weakened when the response is ignored. 5. In instrumental learning *q.v.*, as trials proceed, incorrect bonds will weaken, while the correct bonds will be strengthened.

LAW OF PROXIMITY The tendency to respond to stimuli *q.v.* that are arranged close to each other as groups rather than as separate entities.

LAW OF RECAPITULATION 1. Biogenetic law. 2. The theory that ontogeny *q.v.* recapitulates phylogeny *q.v.*; a belief that was widely held in the late nineteenth century.

LAXATIVE A drug *q.v.* whose purpose is to stimulate the large intestine *q.v.* to pass waste materials along to the rectum for excretion. Some may also act as waste product softeners to expedite passage along the large intestine. ~s are also used to treat constipation *q.v.*, but overuse may actually cause constipation as well as other bowel problems.

LAY MIDWIFE 1. A person who has received specialized training in midwifery *q.v.*, but who does not possess the academic credentials of the registered nurse midwife *q.v.* 2. A person without formal nursing or midwifery training who assists in childbirth. 3. An unlicensed midwife.

LAZY EYE Amblyopia *q.v.*

LCU 1. Life change units *q.v.* 2. Life change unit score *q.v.*

LD An acronym for lethal dose *q.v.*

LDL An acronym for low-density lipoprotein *q.v.*

L-DOPA Levodopa *q.v.*

LEA An acronym for local education agency *q.v.*

LEAD COLIC Intense abdominal pain associated with overexposure to lead. A form of lead poisoning.

LEAD COMPOUNDS Chemical air pollutants *q.v.* originating from the combustion of leaded automobile fuels.

LEADER NUTRIENTS Basic nutrients that must be listed on labels specifying nutritional content of the packaged food. ~ include protein, carbohydrates, fat, vitamins A and C, thiamin, riboflavin, niacin, calcium, and iron.

LEADERSHIP The process of directing the behavior of others toward the achievement of objectives.

LEADERSHIP EFFECTIVENESS The degree to which a leader is able to elicit the desired response from others.

LEADERSHIP STYLE The behavioral pattern of a leader that is used to elicit the desired response.

LEAGUE OF NATIONS HEALTH SECTION Established in 1923, dissolved with the creation of the World Health Organization.

LEAGUE OF SPIRITUAL DISCOVERY A quasi-religious organization founded in 1966 by Timothy Leary. ~ was based on the belief that psychedelic *q.v.* drugs can assist a person in finding religious revelation. The ~'s credo was, "Turn on, tune in, and drop put." LSD *q.v.* was the League's sacrament. The ~ folded shortly after its founding for lack of support.

LEAN BODY MASS 1. A measure of body composition. Fat-free body weight. 2. Lean body weight consisting of the bones, muscles, connective tissues, and vital organs.

LEARNED BEHAVIORAL TOLERANCE Apparently normal behavior in a person with a high blood alcohol content *q.v.*

LEARNED HELPLESSNESS 1. A condition created by exposure to inescapable aversive events. ~ retards or prevents learning in subsequent situations in which escape or avoidance is possible. 2. A learned condition that is produced when the environment has total control over a person. cf: learned helplessness theory of depression.

LEARNED HELPLESSNESS THEORY OF DEPRESSION 1. The hypothesis that depression is analogous to learned helplessness *q.v.* effects produced in the laboratory by exposing subjects to uncontrollable aversive events. 2. The perception of oneself as unable to surmount failure and associated with falling apart when failure is encountered. 3. Attribution of failure to uncontrollable factors.

LEARNER One who learns: pupil, student, or scholar.

LEARNER-CENTERED CURRICULUM GUIDE A written document describing what learners will be doing to achieve their objectives, rather than what teachers will be doing. ct: teacher-centered curriculum guide.

LEARNER-CENTERED METHODS Includes a variety of approaches based on the premise that learning is most effective when the learner is actively involved in all phases of the learning process: planning, selecting objectives, selecting the learning processes, and self-evaluation. These methods emphasize learning as opposed to teaching.

LEARNER-OBSERVATIONAL METHODS These include a wide variety of methods that provide the learner with the opportunity to observe others who are actively engaged in some sort of health activity. Essentially, a passive form of learning. The field trip and demonstration methods *q.v.* are examples.

LEARNER'S MODEL A subcategory of the pathology model *q.v.* that views mental disorders *q.v.* as the result of some form of faulty learning, and believes that these should be treated by behavior therapists *q.v.* according to the laws of classical and instrumental conditioning *q.v.*, or by cognitive therapists *q.v.* who try to affect faulty modes of thinking. cf: medical model; psychoanalytic model.

LEARNING 1. A change in behavior *q.v.* Potentiality that occurs as a result of reinforced practice. 2. A change in behavior resulting from experience. 3. The acquisition of knowledge, attitudes, skills, and experience resulting in behavior change. 4. A change in behavior resulting from an individual's participation in various experiences with the environment. Positive learning results in improved adaptation to the environment. 5. ~ is essentially an intellectual change that may be observed through changes in skills—artistic, musical, athletic, and others. 6. A relatively permanent change in behavior that occurs as the result of practice. cf: health learning; theories of learning.

LEARNING CURVE A curve in which some index of learning is plotted against trials or sessions.

LEARNING DISABILITIES 1. Problems in mastering language, reading, mathematics, or other subject area that are not caused by heredity, economic, or social status. Also called specific developmental disorders. 2. Significant discrepancies between the child's ability to develop language skills and those expected of children his or her age and development. 3. A disorder in one or more psychological processes in understanding or developing language skills.

LEARNING DISABILITY SYNDROME 1. An attention deficit disorder *q.v.* 2. A discrepancy between achievement and ability in one or more of several areas of performance. 3. Learning disability.

LEARNING DISORDERED A term used to describe those with significant deficiency in learning performance when compared with those of a comparable chronological age.

LEARNING METHODS Those procedures that the learner uses to acquire insight into a new or familiar situation. They may originate from the teacher, from other outside sources, or from the learner. ct: teaching methods.

LEARNING OPPORTUNITY A situation in which relevant knowledge and activities are provided to stimulate the learner to become actively involved in the development of knowledge and skills.

LEARNING PARADIGM In abnormal psychology, the premise that abnormal behavior is learned in the same ways as other types of behavior.

LEARNING RESOURCE CENTER A specifically designated area containing a wide variety of materials and equipment for the use of students individually or in small groups for independent study.

LEARNING RESOURCES Used as techniques or strategies to enhance learning. They may be either materials or people.

LEARNING RESOURCES AND EVALUATION COMMITTEE A committee that functions to review, evaluate, and make recommendations regarding the varieties of learning resources available; makes recommendations regarding policies for the selection and use of material and human resources; and assists in the development of the evaluation program.

LEARNING SET The increased ability to solve problems, especially in discriminative learning *q.v.*, as a result of previous experience with problems of a similar nature.

LEARNING STRATEGIES 1. The skills used by the learner to facilitate learning that are generally energized by the strategies used by the teacher. 2. An integrated system for improving a person's ability to learn *q.v.* ct: teaching strategies.

LEARNING THEORY OF ALCOHOLISM A proposition that suggests that alcoholism can be explained by the approach–avoidance reaction *q.v.* People are generally attracted to pleasant situations and repelled by unpleasant situations. Alcoholic beverages reduce tensions and anxiety associated with feelings of unpleasantness. Alcohol establishes a state of euphoria *q.v.* ~ is associated with reward and punishment.

LEARNING TO LEARN Improvement in learning *q.v.* that occurs as a result of previous learning.

LEAST RESTRICTIVE ALTERNATIVE 1. A concept supported by legal precedent that mandates that a mental patient must be treated in a setting that is least restrictive on his or her freedoms. 2. For special education students, learning experiences in a setting that most closely resembles a normal classroom.

LEAST RESTRICTIVE ENVIRONMENT (LRE) The most normal environment possible for learning, treatment, and/or living. cf: least restrictive alternative.

LE BELLE INDIFFERENCE 1. In hysteria *q.v.*, an expression of the fact that the person appears to enjoy illness and to be indifferent to the symptoms *q.v.* that are present. 2. A characteristic of people with a conversion disorder *q.v.* in which they have little concern toward their illness symptoms.

LEBOYER METHOD 1. A method of subdued conditions in the environment during childbirth. 2. A method of childbirth that emphasizes gently easing the neonate *q.v.* into the world. 3. A method of childbirth that attempts to lessen the shock of birth to the neonate by minimizing the differences between the uterine *q.v.* and external environments.

LECHERY Excessive indulgence of sexual desires.

LECITHIN 1. A lipid composed of chlorine, glycerol *q.v.*, phosphoric acid, and fatty acids *q.v.* 2. Any of a group of phospholipids *q.v.* An important emulsifier *q.v.* Phosphatidyl chlorine *q.v.*

LECTURE METHOD A traditional teacher-centered approach to learning. It is characterized by one-way communication resulting in very little learning. The ~ may be used to cover a large body of information in a short period of time. cf: lecture recitation.

LECTURE RECITATION A teacher-centered approach to education consisting of a presentation by the teacher, followed by student responses to questions asked by the teacher concerning the subject just presented. cf: lecture method.

LEFT ATRIUM The atrium *q.v.* situated on the left side of the heart.

LEFT VENTRICLE The ventricle *q.v.* situated on the left side of the heart.

LEG The lower extremity, generally. Specifically, that part of the lower limb extending from the knee *q.v.* to the ankle.

LEGAL DETERRENCE MODEL A concept used in some drug education curricula and in public education efforts of law enforcement officials that emphasizes the legal consequences of using illegal drugs in hopes that people will not use such drugs in order to avoid fines or imprisonment.

LEGAL DISABILITY A lack of legal capacity to perform a given act.

LEGALISM The adherence to a strict set of laws or codes of conduct as a guide to decision making.

LEGALIZATION The legislative act or administrative executive order authorizing a particular action. ct: decriminalization.

LEGAL POWER The legal authority to engage in some act.

LEGEND DRUG 1. A prescription drug. 2. A drug that bears on its label, "Caution: Federal Law Prohibits Dispensing Without a Prescription." ct: over-the-counter drug.

LEGIONNAIRE'S DISEASE An infection causing a form of bronchopneumonia *q.v.* First identified in 1976, after an outbreak at a Legionnaire's convention in Philadelphia. It is caused by a gram-negative microorganism, *Legionella pneumophila*.

LEGION OF DECENCY An organization established by the Roman Catholic Church in the 1930s to rate films on their violence and sexual content.

LEGISLATION Acts or bills passed by the legislative branches of local, state, and national governments that become laws.

LEGISLATIVE STUDY COMMITTEE Most frequently, an ad hoc committee established by the leadership of a legislative chamber to study a particular issue and to issue recommendations for legislation that will be acceptable to the legislature and to the executive.

LEGUMES 1. Peas and beans. 2. Plant sources high in the essential amino acids *q.v.*

LEMNISCUS (MEDIAL) A flat band of sensory *q.v.* fibers extending up from the medulla *q.v.* through the pons *q.v.* and midbrain *q.v.* to the thalamus *q.v.*

LENGTH OF ACTION The period of time that a drug is effective.

LENS The transparent body through which images are focused on the retina *q.v.*

LENTIVIRUSES Viruses *q.v.* that cause disease very slowly. HIV *q.v.* is thought to be this type of virus.

LEPROSY A chronic, contagious disease caused by a bacterial infection characterized by large nodules on the surface of the body, loss of sensation, paralysis, wasting of muscles, and body deformities.

LEPTONEMA A stage in meiosis *q.v.* immediately preceding synapsis *q.v.* in which the chromosomes *q.v.* appear to be single, threadlike structures.

LEPTOSOME A body type identified by Kretschmer *q.v.* whose temperament was supposed to be schizothymic *q.v.* cf: pyknic.

LEPTOSPIROSIS A rare bone disease whose causative agent is *Leptospira*, a genus of spirochetes *q.v.*

LESBIAN A female who is homosexual *q.v.*

LESBIANISM Homosexuality *q.v.* in women.

LESCH–NYHAN SYNDROME A relatively rare genetic disease characterized by mental retardation and compulsive self-mutilation accompanied by uremia *q.v.*

LESION 1. A break in the cellular integrity of a tissue or organ. Lesions may be caused by infections, chemicals, or trauma to the tissue. 2. An abnormal change in the structure of a tissue or organ such as cuts, burns, and tumors. 3. A wound or injury. 4. Any pathological or traumatic disruption of the integrity of normal tissue.

LESION, NEURAL Injury in a specific area of the brain or nervous system *q.v.*

LESSON PLAN 1. The functional culmination of all curriculum planning and development. It describes what will happen to the learner and how it shall take place on a day-to-day basis. 2. A tool used by the teacher that lists objectives, materials, and techniques to be used and how the material will be presented.

LESSONS AND UNITS Subcategories of a curriculum that center on specific themes or a central purpose. Each lesson or unit has a set of objectives that center on the theme of the lesson or unit.

LETDOWN A tingling sensation in the breasts when milk is forced out shortly after the baby begins to suckle.

LETHAL DOSE (LD) The dose of a drug that will cause death. For example, an LD_{50} signifies a dose that will kill 50% of the test subjects. ct: therapeutic index.

LETHAL FACTOR In genetics, a genetic factor that brings about the early death of the organism.

LETHAL GENE A gene that results in a cell that cannot replicate or the death of the organism.

LEUCINE An essential amino acid *q.v.*

LEUCOPLAST A colorless plastid *q.v.* commonly the center of starch formation.

LEUCORRHEA Excessive vaginal mucus discharge, but not a disease entity within itself. A condition caused by a chemical, physical irritation, dysfunction, or infection.

LEUCOTOMY A brain operation involving the severing of association pathways in the frontal lobes *q.v.* of the brain in which the surgical instruments are inserted transorbitally. cf: frontal lobotomy.

LEUKEMIA Cancer *q.v.* of the blood and lymphatic *q.v.* systems. There are two kinds of leukemias: 1. Acute leukemia *q.v.*, which is most common among children. 2. Chronic leukemia *q.v.*, which is most common in adults over 40 years. Death from leukemia usually results from increased susceptibility to infection *q.v.* and hemorrhage *q.v.* Causes range from exposure to radiation, certain chemicals, and viruses.

LEUKOCYTES 1. The white cells of the blood *q.v.* 2. White blood cells that combat infectious organisms and other foreign substances in the body. ct: erythrocytes.

LEUKOCYTOSIS An abnormally large number of white blood cells, often brought about by acute infections *q.v.*

LEUKODERMA A deficiency of pigmentation of the skin.

LEUKOPENIA An abnormally low number of white blood cells.

LEUKOPLAKIA A precancerous condition in which white patches occur or form on mucous membranes, such as the tongue, cheek, or female genitalia.

LEVATOR A muscle that serves to raise some part.

LEVATOR ANI 1. The muscle that draws the anus *q.v.* upward in defecation *q.v.* and aids in the support of the pelvic *q.v.* floor. 2. The major muscle affording fecal *q.v.* continence *q.v.*

LEVATOR PULPEBRAE The muscle that raises the upper eyelid.

LEVEL OF ASPIRATION The tendency of persons to set goals in an effort to succeed at the highest possible level while avoiding failure.

LEVEL OF CONFIDENCE The probability that the value of a statistic is equal to or exceeds its observed value.

LEVEL OF EFFORT An expression of the amount of time required to complete a project, often based on labor hours.

LEVEL OF INTIMACY Refers to Levinger's model of the progression of the development of deep relationships.

LEVELS OF COMMUNICATION There are four types of communication based on function and emotional needs, and which progress from giving information to disclosing emotions: (a) giving of information, (b) directive or argumentative, (c) exploratory, and (d) self-disclosing.

LEVELS OF DEFENSE Biological, psychological, or sociological adjustive reactions.

LEVELS OF HEALTH A person's health status *q.v.* as measured in terms of (a) primary level *q.v.*, (b) intermediate level *q.v.*, or (c) secondary level *q.v.*

LEVIRATE A custom that mandates that when an older brother dies, his younger brother should marry his widow.

LEVIRATE MARRIAGE An ancient custom whereby when a Jewish husband dies without heirs, his closest male relative is obliged to provide the widow with children.

LEVODOPA 1. L-Dopa. 2. A medication used for alleviating symptoms of Parkinson's disease *q.v.* by compensating for the loss of dopamine *q.v.* in the brain.

LEVULOSE 1. Fruit sugar. 2. Fructose *q.v.*

LEWD Intended to stimulate sexual excitement, particularly in an offensive manner.

LEXICAL ACCESS The process of recognizing and understanding a word, which is presumably achieved by making contact with the word in the mental lexicon.

LEXICON The vocabulary of a language.

LEYDIG'S CELLS The cells found in the seminiferous tubules *q.v.* that secrete the male sex hormone *q.v.*, testosterone *q.v.*

LGV An acronym for lymphogranuloma venereum *q.v.*

LH An acronym for luteinizing hormone *q.v.*

LHD An acronym for local health department.

LIABILITY 1. Legal responsibility. 2. Being responsible for a loss.

LIBERTINISM A disregard for authority or for convention in sexual or religious matters.

LIBIDO 1. The psychic energy of the id *q.v.* Viewed by Freudian psychologists as sexual in nature. 2. The sexual drive. 3. In psychoanalytic theory *q.v.*, the instinctual drives of the id. 4. The drive for sexual gratification. cf: eros.

LIBRARIAN An individual who has formal training in the theoretical and scientific aspects of library work.

LIBRARY An organized collection of books, electronic media, and other sources of information, located in one or more places, providing equipment and services to the public, students, and faculty.

LIBRIUM 1. Chlordiazepoxide hydrochloride *q.v.* 2. A commercial preparation of one of the minor tranquilizers *q.v.* 3. A benzodiazepine sedative *q.v.*

LICE Pediculosis *q.v.*

LICENSE An authorization to function in a particular skill or profession.

LICENSED CLINICAL SOCIAL WORKER A person with academic training in social work who specializes in emotional or psychological adjustment.

LICENSED PRACTICAL NURSE A trained professional in basic nursing skills who assists in providing the medical and other health needs of patients.

LICENSURE The process by which an agency or government grants permission for practicing a profession by certifying that those licensed have attained the minimal degree of competency necessary to ensure that the public health, safety, and welfare will be reasonably protected. In most instances, ~ also implies that those who are not licensed must not claim the title of a licensed profession.

LID Either of the two movable conjuctival–cutaneous folds that protect the anterior *q.v.* surface of the eyeball.

LIFE-ADJUSTMENT EDUCATION A program providing experiences for the learner in which the unique talents and resources of each individual are nurtured and developed.

LIFE CHANGE UNITS (LCU) 1. According to the Holmes and Rahe Scale, the measure of stress *q.v.* 2. The stress value assigned to various lifetime events as listed in the Holmes–Rahe Social Readjustment Rating Scale *q.v.* cf: life change unit score.

LIFE CHANGE UNIT SCORE A score determined by totaling the scores assigned to each stressful event a person has experienced in the recent past. The higher the score, the greater the likelihood of developing health problems. cf: life change units.

LIFE CYCLE 1. The artificial segments of the life span. Each segment represents a developmental period: birth, maturity, aging, and dying. 2. The entire course of a person's life from infancy through old age. Health, social roles and expectations, and socioeconomic status tend to change as a person moves from one phase of life to the next.

LIFE CYCLE THEORY OF LEADERSHIP A view of leadership styles that suggest successful leaders reflect the maturity level of the followers.

LIFE EXPECTANCY 1. A measure of how long a person can expect to live from birth. 2. A mathematical average based on death rates *q.v.* for various ages. 3. A statistical *q.v.* projection of the number of years a person is expected to live. ~ can be calculated from birth, or it can be calculated from some other point; e.g., the number of years left after reaching a given age. Persons of the same age can have different life expectancies depending on their race, sex, or socioeconomic status.

LIFE HISTORY METHOD A technique of psychological observation in which the development of particular forms of behavior are traced by means of records of the person's past or present behavior.

LIFE SPACE 1. A term coined by Lewin referring to the entire complex psychologic world; and it is the person's perception that determines what his or her actions will be. 2. In field theory, the psychological representation of the person and the environment. 3. Everything that a person needs to know about a person in order to understand behavior at a given moment.

LIFE SPAN 1. The time that a person actually lives. 2. The years a person would live if negative variables *q.v.*, e.g., disease or accidents, did not shorten their number. An ideal number, probably approaching 110 years. cf: life expectancy.

LIFE SPAN DEVELOPMENT ORIENTATION The orientation toward psychological development that maintains that development continues throughout a person's life rather than ending at some point.

LIFESTYLE 1. Activities that are a regular part of a person's daily pattern of living. 2. A person's pattern of behavior. 3. The general pattern of assumptions, motives, cognition, and coping techniques that characterizes the behavior of a person and gives it consistency. 4. Ways of behaving, referring to the sequence of physical, social, and psychological experiences that make up the existence of individuals or groups.

LIFE-SUPPORT TECHNOLOGY The use of artificial body parts and machines to maintain physiological (but not necessarily functional) life.

LIFE-TABLE ANALYSIS In epidemiology *q.v.*, a method of including subjects in a cohort study *q.v.* for different durations of time during the overall study period.

LIFE, THE (THE LIFE) Jargon for the lifestyle of a prostitute *q.v.*

LIGAMENT 1. A band or sheet of fibrous tissue connecting two or more bones, cartilages *q.v.*, or other structures, or serving as a support for muscles. 2. A tough band of tissue serving to connect the articular extremities of bones or to support or retain an organ in place.

LIGATION To cut.

LIGATURE 1. A thread or wire tied tightly around a blood vessel, the pedicle of a tumor, or other structure in order to constrict it. 2. A string made from any material, such as catgut, silk, or cotton, that is used for the purpose of controlling bleeding, to tie shut blood vessels, which have been cut.

LIGHTENING 1. A labor process in which the uterus sinks downward because the fetus's presenting part settles far down into the pelvic area. 2. Engaging *q.v.*

LIGHTNESS CONSTANCY The tendency to perceive the lightness of an object as more or less the same despite the fact that the light reflected from the object changes with the illumination that falls on it.

LIGHT SOURCE A source of illumination with filters and controlled color balance for use with a microscope.

LIKERT SCALE The use of scaled agree–disagree statements in attitude measurement.

LIMBIC SYSTEM 1. The center of emotions connecting the reptilian brain and the neocortex *q.v.* It is concerned with self-preservation and guides emotional feelings and behavior toward satisfaction of basic biological needs *q.v.* and away from threats. The neocortex responds to the external stimuli with trust while the limbic system responds to the repetition of inner stimuli. 2. A group of regions in the brain including the thalamus *q.v.*, amygdala *q.v.*, hippocampus *q.v.*, limbic cortex, and parts of the hypothalamus *q.v.* 3. Neurons in the hippocampus, amygdala, and other structures integrating the cerebral cortex and the hypothalamus. ~ is concerned with emotion and motivation. cf: neocortex.

LIMBRI LOBE Limbic system *q.v.*

LIMERENCE 1. Romantic love *q.v.* 2. A state of high arousal often experienced at the onset of romance. 3. Coined by Tennov to describe a blind, intense kind of love outside the person's rational control.

LIMITED-ENGLISH PROFICIENCY Students who have a limited ability to read, speak, or comprehend English and who have a primary language other than English spoken at home.

LINEAR FRACTURE A fracture *q.v.* running parallel to the long axis of a bone.

LINEAR PERSPECTIVE A secondary cue to depth *q.v.* or distance promoted by the fact that parallel lines appear to converge in the distance.

LINEAR PROGRAM An educational approach wherein a single sequence of frames is presented to all learners.

LINEAR RELATIONSHIP In epidemiology *q.v.*, when two variables are considered together, the first increases or decreases as the second variable increases or decreases so that, when plotted on a graph, a straight line results.

LINE AUTHORITY The authority and responsibility to make decisions and give directives to subordinates within an organization.

LINE BREEDING The mating of selected members of successive generations among themselves to strengthen the given genetic traits *q.v.*

LINEMAN'S GLOVES Rubber lined leather gloves, esp. designed to be nonconductive of electricity.

LINE OF BEST FIT A line drawn through points in a scatter diagram that yields the best prediction of one variable *q.v.* when given the value of the other variable.

LINGUISTICS The study of language.

LININ 1. A fine, threadlike structure associated with the chromatin *q.v.* of the nucleus of a cell. 2. The faintly staining substance composing the fine netlike threads in the nucleus of the cell bearing chromatin in the form of granules.

LINKAGE 1. In genetics *q.v.*, the inheritance of traits in groups because their genes *q.v.* are in the same chromosome *q.v.* 2. The tendency of two or more genes to be inherited together because they are present on the same chromosome. 3. Nonrandom assortment of genes on homologous *q.v.* chromosomes.

LINOLEIC ACID 1. An essential nutritional substance found in animal and vegetable fats and essential for growth. 2. The essential fatty acid *q.v.*, ~ , is unsaturated and occurs widely in plant glycerides *q.v.*

LIPASE An enzyme *q.v.* that converts fats to fatty acids *q.v.* and glycerine *q.v.*

LIPECTOMY The surgical removal of excess body fat.

LIPID INFILTRATION HYPOTHESIS The development of lipid *q.v.* material in the walls of arteries *q.v.* as a result of elevated serum *q.v.* lipid levels.

LIPIDS 1. Fat found in foods. Sources are both animal and vegetable products. 2. One of a major class of nutrients. Any one of a group of fats or fat-like substances. 3. Substances that are diverse in chemical nature but soluble in fat solvents. ~ include fats and oils, phospholipids *q.v.*, glycolipids *q.v.*, and lipoproteins *q.v.*, fatty acids *q.v.*, alcohols (glycerol, sterols, and carotenoids *q.v.*). 4. Cholesterol *q.v.* and triglycerides *q.v.*

LIPOGENESIS 1. The process by which lipids *q.v.* are synthesized *q.v.* in the body. 2. The formation of fat. 3. The process whereby the body develops adipose *q.v.* cells.

LIPOID Of a fatty nature.

LIPOLYSIS The breakdown of triglycerides *q.v.* to glycerol *q.v.* and fatty acids *q.v.*

LIPOMA Any tumor *q.v.* composed principally of fat.

LIPOPHILIC A drug *q.v.* or other chemical that is more soluble *q.v.* in fat than in water.

LIPOPROTEIN Molecular structures comprised of proteins *q.v.* and cholesterol *q.v.* There are two kinds: (a) high-density lipoprotein (HDL) and (b) low-density lipoprotein (LDL). LDL appears to be associated with atherosclerosis *q.v.* as it has a tendency to accumulate in the inner lining of arteries.

LIPOPROTEIN PROFILE An analysis of the relative amounts of high-density lipoproteins (HDL) *q.v.* to low-density lipoproteins (LDL) *q.v.* in the blood.

LIQUOR A distilled alcoholic beverage.

LISTENING A process that takes place when a person comprehends and/or responds to a verbal stimulus.

LITER A unit of volume in the metric system.

LITERACY The possession of the skills and cultural content to comprehend written, oral, and visual information.

LITERACY EVENTS Action sequences in a child's life in which the production and/or comprehension of print plays some part.

LITHANE A commercial preparation of lithium carbonate *q.v.*

LITHIASIS The presence of a stone in any organ or duct *q.v.*

LITHIUM 1. An element used for the treatment of gout *q.v.* and, more recently, for the treatment of mania *q.v.* It was approved for this latter use by the Food and Drug Administration in 1970. 2. Lithium carbonate *q.v.* 3. Lithium citrate. 4. An element used in the treatment of both mania and bipolar disorder *q.v.*

LITHIUM CARBONATE Lithium *q.v.*, used in the treatment of mania *q.v.* and bipolar disorders *q.v.*

LITHIUM CITRATE Lithium carbonate *q.v.*

LITHOBID A commercial preparation of lithium carbonate *q.v.*

LITHOTOMY POSITION A position in which a woman lies on her back with her feet in stirrups, often during a pelvic examination or in childbirth.

LITIGATION 1. A lawsuit. 2. The formal contesting of a dispute in court.

LITTER In first aid, a stretcher or device for carrying a victim of an accident or illness. In zoology, the multiple birth of some animals.

LIUNA An acronym for Laborers International Union of North America.

LIVE BIRTH CERTIFICATE A document that states that a live birth has occurred regardless of the length of pregnancy. This certificate is required in all states in the United States. The ~ is usually signed by the person attending the birth and who may not necessarily be a trained medical person.

LIVE PEEPS Slang for small booths in which customers watch a model pantomime sexual acts.

LIVER A large, vascular organ of the body that lies in the upper right section of the abdominal cavity directly beneath the diaphragm *q.v.* The ~ produces bile *q.v.*, glycogen *q.v.*, and antibodies *q.v.* It also interconverts proteins *q.v.*, carbohydrates *q.v.*, and fats; stores iron, copper, vitamins A and D *q.v.*; and detoxifies *q.v.* harmful substances.

LIVER INDUCTION Enzyme induction *q.v.*

LIVER MICROSOMAL ENZYME An enzyme in the liver that is essential in the metabolism of many drugs.

LIVID Suffused with blood to give a bright, congested appearance, usually applied to the face.

LIVING TOGETHER An arrangement in which two people live together without the formality of marriage. ~ implies intimacy. ~ does not constitute a common law marriage.

LIVING WILL A document in which the signer requests to be allowed to die rather than to be kept alive by artificial means in the event of becoming terminally ill.

LMP The first day of the last menstrual period *q.v.*

LNHSF An acronym for Laborers National Health and Safety Fund.

LOBBYIST In politics, a representative of a special interest who makes contact with members of the legislature to influence the passage or rejection of specific pieces of legislation.

LOBE Any anatomically well-defined part of a large organ separated from the rest of the organ by clefts, e.g., ear lobe, lobe of the lungs.

LOBECTOMY 1. Excision or removal of parts of the prefrontal lobes *q.v.* of the brain by surgical methods. ~ was formerly used in the treatment of certain types of mental illness. 2. A surgical removal of one part of an organ. cf: lobotomy.

LOBELINE A nicotine *q.v.* substitute sometimes used in stop smoking programs.

LOBOTOMY 1. A surgical procedure to sever the connections between two or more lobes of the brain. 2. Prefrontal lobotomy *q.v.* 3. The severing of the prefrontal from the frontal lobes of the brain to reduce severely disturbed behavior. ct: lobectomy.

LOCAL ANESTHETIC A drug administered for the purpose of anesthetizing a restricted area of the body. ct: general anesthetic.

LOCAL BASIC ADMINISTRATIVE UNIT 1. Local school district. 2. Local education agency (LEA) *q.v.*

LOCAL EDUCATION AGENCY (LEA) 1. Local school districts. 2. The basic educational unit in all states. 3. The board of education or other public authority that controls the administration of, and sets policy for, the functions of public elementary and secondary schools in a particular district.

LOCAL ILLNESS Pathological *q.v.* changes in a single group of cells that make up one of the body's organs or systems.

LOCALITY DEVELOPMENT One of the three major approaches used to create change at the community *q.v.* level. ~ emphasizes process goals *q.v.* designed to improve the capacity of the community to engage in cooperative problem solving *q.v.* The use of democratic methods is of central importance.

LOCALIZED CANCER 1. A cancer *q.v.* confined to the site of origin. 2. A cancer that has not yet metastasized *q.v.*

LOCAL STIMULUS THEORY OF DRIVE The hypothesis *q.v.* that motives *q.v.* are intense stimuli *q.v.* cf: drive-stimulus reduction theory.

LOCHIA The discharge from the uterus and vagina that takes place during the first few weeks following childbirth. cf: endometrium.

LOCI METHOD A mnemonic device that involves associating items to be learned with familiar locations or places.

LOCKJAW 1. Tetanus *q.v.* 2. ~ is caused by the *Clostridium tetani* microorganism.

LOCOMOTION Movement from one location to another by means of walking, crawling, running, etc.

LOCOMOTOR ATAXIA Muscular uncoordination usually resulting from syphilitic *q.v.* damage to the spinal cord pathways.

LOCULE A functional cavity or chamber.

LOCUS The position on a chromosome *q.v.* that is occupied by a gene *q.v.*

LOCUS OF CONTROL 1. The degree to which a person views outcomes as happening because of his or her own ability or because of chance, fate, or other. 2. A person's sense of control over his or her life, either through internal or external causes.

LOGAGNOSIA Aphasia *q.v.*

LOGARITHM The exponent that indicates the power to which a number must be raised to produce a given number.

LOGIC TIGHT COMPARTMENTS A form of intellectualization *q.v.* in which contradictory devices or attitudes *q.v.* are sealed off in separate areas of consciousness *q.v.*

LOGOGRAPHICS Writing systems in which picture symbols stand for words.

LOGOTHERAPY 1. A subtechnique of existential therapy *q.v.* 2. The school of existential analysis that focuses on the person's need to see meaning in life. 3. An existential therapy technique developed by Victor Frankl to help a patient identify meaning in life by placing the person's conflicts in a larger spiritual and philosophical context.

LOIN Part of the back between the ribs and hip bones.

LONELINESS An emotional state in which a person feels a lack of social relationships, or ones that produced little or no satisfaction.

LONELINESS ANXIETY The fear that one may be left alone or left out and thus have to spend one's life in solitude.

LONGEVITY The condition or quality of being long-lived.

LONGITUDINAL FISSION A split in the cytoplasm *q.v.*, the axis of which is parallel to the long axis of the cell.

LONGITUDINAL RESEARCH 1. Research that follows the same group of people and collects information from them repeatedly over a significant period of time. 2. Studies that examine one group of people over a long period of time as they grow, develop, and age. This is in contrast to cross-sectional research *q.v.* in which persons of different ages are compared with one another at one point in time. 3. A research design that measures age-related change in a single group over time. cf: longitudinal study.

LONGITUDINAL STUDY 1. A study that measures subjects on the dependent variables at many points in time. 2. Scientific research in which a group of subjects is studied over the course of many years. 3. Long-term studies. cf: longitudinal research.

LONG-RUN OBJECTIVES Targets to be achieved over an extended period of time. In management, this time span is usually set at 5–7 years.

LONG-TERM CARE The medical and social care given to persons who have severe, chronic impairments. ~ can consist of care in the home, by family members, assistance through voluntary or employed help, or care in institutions. Various types of ~ facilities exist throughout the United States that frequently differ in their available staff, reimbursements, and services. cf: domiciliary care facility; intermediate care facility; skilled nursing facility.

LONG-TERM MEMORY (LTM) 1. The storehouse of permanently recorded information in a person's memory. 2. Long-term memory store *q.v.* 3. A memory system that keeps memories for long periods, has a large capacity, and stores items in relatively processed form. cf: sensory registers. ct: short-term memory.

LONG-TERM MEMORY STORE 1. According to Atkinson and Shiffrin, a storage area that is distinct from the short-term memory store and retains an indefinite amount of information indefinitely. 2. Long-term memory *q.v.*

LOOK-ALIKES Drugs sold legally, often through the mail or over the Internet, that are made to look like prescription drugs or illegal drugs, e.g., caffeine *q.v.* tablets that are made to look like amphetamine *q.v.* tablets.

LOOKING GLASS The theory that a person's self-concept *q.v.* is reflected in the way a person perceives how others look at him or her.

LOOSE ASSOCIATION A thought disorder in which the person has difficulty sticking to one topic and drifts from one thought to another in a disjointed manner. A symptom of schizophrenia *q.v.*

LOPHOTRICHOUS An arrangement of flagella *q.v.* at one or both ends of a cell.

LORAZEPAM 1. A benzodiazepine *q.v.* 2. Ativan is a brand name.

LORDOSIS 1. Swayback. 2. Ventral curvature of the vertebral column. 3. Hollow back. ct: scoliosis; kyphosis.

LORDOTIC A position for sexual intercourse *q.v.*, common in primates, in which the female is bent over and the male enters her from the rear.

LORDOTIC CURVATURE A characteristic curve in the lower portion of the spinal column *q.v.* cf: lordosis.

LOSS EFFECT The deterioration of health and/or the quality of life as one mourns the loss of a loved one.

LOSS OF CONTROL With respect to drug use, the inability of one who is drug dependent *q.v.* to consistently predict the frequency of use or the amount consumed once use has begun.

LOSS OF INCOME (INSURANCE COVERAGE) An insurance policy that makes provision for payments directly to the policy holder to compensate for loss of income due to illness or injury.

LOSS OF TOLERANCE Especially with alcohol use; after several years of excessive use of alcohol, a person experiences intoxication *q.v.* with ingestion of relatively small amounts of alcohol. ct: high tolerance.

LOUDNESS 1. A dimension of auditory perception related to the intensity of the stimulus *q.v.* 2. The volume of sound.

LOVASTATIN A drug *q.v.* used to lower serum cholesterol *q.v.* levels.

LOVE 1. One of the most powerful emotions, characterized by an urgency to possess. 2. A strong emotional attachment, typically to another person, but also to objects, ideas, or gods.

LOVE WITHDRAWAL 1. Techniques of parental discipline *q.v.* based on direct, nonphysical expression of anger designed to arouse a child's feeling of guilt and shame. 2. Attempts to control children by expressing dislike for them. cf: power assertion; induction.

LOW ADAPTATION ENERGY Low constitutional energy; the ability to adjust to changing circumstances.

LOW CALORIE (ON FOOD LABELS) Forty calories or less per serving or no more than 0.4 calories per gram. Foods naturally low in calories cannot be labeled low calorie. ct: reduced calorie.

LOW CHOLESTEROL (ON FOOD LABELS) Twenty milligrams or less per serving. ct: reduced cholesterol.

LOW-DENSITY LIPOPROTEIN (LDL) The part of serum cholesterol *q.v.* that tends to accumulate in the walls of arteries, contributing to the development of atherosclerosis *q.v.* ct: high-density lipoprotein (HDL).

LOWEST COMMON DENOMINATOR EFFECT The tendency for an educational program writer to prepare and arrange frames for the least capable learners who will be requested to master them.

LOW FAT (ON FOOD LABELS) A listing in which dairy products must be between 0.5% and 2.0% milk fat to be labeled low fat; meat must be less than 10% fat to be labeled low fat.

LOW SODIUM (ON FOOD LABELS) One hundred forty milligrams or less per serving. cf: very low sodium; unsalted.

LOW-YIELD CIGARETTE A cigarette containing relatively low amounts of tar *q.v.* and nicotine *q.v.*, defined as yielding less than 15 mg of tar per cigarette.

LOXAPINE 1. An antipsychotic *q.v.* medication. 2. Loxitane is a brand name.

LOXITANE A commercial preparation of loxapine *q.v.*

LPN An acronym for licensed practical nurse *q.v.*

LRE An acronym for least restrictive environment *q.v.*

LSD 1. D-Lysergic acid diethylamide 25. 2. A semisynthetic derivative of lysergic acid, an alkaloid found in the fungus *Claviceps purpurea q.v.* 3. A psychoactive *q.v.* chemical that creates hallucinogenic reactions in people who use it. A popular drug of abuse in the 1960s and 1970s; it has recently regained some popularity. 4. A hallucinogen. 5. A drug synthesized in 1938 by Albert Hofmann. Its hallucinogenic properties were recognized in 1943.

LTM Long-term memory *q.v.*

LUDIOMIL A commercial preparation of maprotiline *q.v.*

LUES Syphilis *q.v.*

LUMBAGO Backache in the lumbar *q.v.* region.

LUMBAR 1. Of, or pertaining to, or near the loins. 2. Near the loins or just below the chest. 3. The region of the spine and surrounding trunk between the thorax and the brim of the pelvis.

LUMBAR KYPHOSIS Flat back.

LUMBAR PUNCTURE 1. A procedure for obtaining a sample of cerebrospinal *q.v.* fluid by inserting a hollow needle into the back between the vertebrae in the lumbar *q.v.* region. 2. Spinal tap.

LUMBAR REGION The lower back area.

LUMBAR SPINE That part of the spine consisting of the most inferior five individual vertebrae *q.v.* located just superior to the sacrum *q.v.*

LUMBOSACRAL PLEXUS 1. The network of nerves formed by the union of the anterior pituitary division of the lumbar *q.v.*, sacral *q.v.*, and coccygeal *q.v.* nerves. 2. A network of nerves containing the motor and sensory innervations of the leg. cf: plexus.

LUMEN 1. The cavity or channel within a blood vessel. 2. The passageway inside a tubular organ. The vascular lumen in the passageway inside a blood vessel.

LUMINAL 1. A barbiturate *q.v.* 2. A commercial preparation of barbituric acid *q.v.* first compounded in 1912. 3. A long-acting, slow-starting barbiturate. 4. Phenobarbital *q.v.*

LUMPECTOMY 1. Surgical removal of a lump—usually in the breast—and immediate tissues surrounding the lump. 2. Tylectomy. 3. Removal of a malignant mass. cf: mastectomy; radical mastectomy; modified mastectomy.

LUNACY A legal term that is synonymous with insanity *q.v.* ~ is derived from luna (Latin for moon). Historically, mental illness was associated with the moon as a presumed cause.

LUNAR MONTH Four weeks or 28 days.

LUNG 1. The organ that accommodates the exchange of oxygen and carbon dioxide between the blood and the external environment. 2. Either of the pair of organs that aerate *q.v.* the blood. The ~s occupy the lateral cavities of the chest separated from each other by the heart and mediastinal structures. cf: alveoli.

LUNG CANCER 1. A malignancy *q.v.* of the lung. 2. A bronchogenic carcinoma *q.v.* 3. Uncontrolled cellular growth in the lungs.

LUPUS Tuberculous *q.v.* infection of the skin.

LUPUS ERYTHEMATOSIS An autoimmune *q.v.* disease in which the body destroys its own tissues.

LURIA–NEBRASKA TEST A battery of neuropsychological *q.v.* tests that can detect impairments of different parts of the brain.

LUTEAL PHASE 1. The last 14 days of the ovulatory *q.v.* cycle in which the corpus luteum *q.v.* is formed and the uterus *q.v.* is prepared to nourish a fertilized *q.v.* egg. 2. That part of the ovulatory cycle, following ovulation *q.v.*, that the fertilized egg implants itself into the uterine lining. If fertilization does not occur or if the fertilized egg does not become implanted, the ~ gives way to menstruation.

LUTEINIZING HORMONE (LH) 1. A hormone *q.v.* that causes ovulation *q.v.* in women and is associated with the secretion of progesterone *q.v.* and estrogen *q.v.* 2. A hormone secreted by the pituitary gland *q.v.* that stimulates the formation of the corpus luteum *q.v.* in the female. In the male, the ~ stimulates testosterone *q.v.* production and the production of sperm *q.v.* 3. The female gonadotropic *q.v.* hormone required for fullest development of and release of ova *q.v.* cf: interstitial cell-stimulating hormone (ICSH).

LUTEOTROPIC HORMONE Prolactin *q.v.*

LUTEUM Golden yellow.

LYCANTHROPY The delusion *q.v.* of being a wolf.

LYE A solution of alkaline *q.v.* salts obtained by the leaching of wood ashes.

LYMPH 1. A fluid that circulates within the lymphatic vessels and is eventually added to the venous *q.v.* blood circulation. ~ arises from tissue fluid and from intestinal absorption of fatty acids *q.v.* ~ is colorless, odorless, slightly alkaline *q.v.*, and slightly opalescent. 2. A transparent, slightly yellow fluid that carries lymphocytes *q.v.*, bathes body tissues, and drains into the lymphatic vessels.

LYMPHADENITIS Inflammation of the lymph glands *q.v.*

LYMPHADENOPATHY Enlargement of the lymph glands *q.v.* cf: lymphadenopathy syndrome.

LYMPHADENOPATHY-ASSOCIATED VIRUS LAV *q.v.*

LYMPHADENOPATHY SYNDROME A generalized, persistent enlargement of the lymph nodes *q.v.*, sometimes accompanied with a mild fever and weight loss. ~ is associated with HIV *q.v.* infection. ~ is also known as generalized lymphadenopathy syndrome.

LYMPHATIC The tiny vessels that carry lymph *q.v.* from the tissues to the bloodstream or to the lymph glands *q.v.*

LYMPHATIC GLANDS 1. Lymph nodes *q.v.* 2. Glands scattered along a path of the lymphatics, especially in the neck region, armpits, and at the bend of the elbow and knee. They store and produce white blood cells and act as filters to remove harmful substances. cf: lymphatic system.

LYMPHATIC SYSTEM 1. All of the vessels and structures that carry lymph *q.v.* from the tissues to the blood.

2. A glandular system involved in the immune response *q.v.* 3. A circulatory network of lymph-carrying vessels, and the lymph nodes *q.v.*, spleen *q.v.*, and thymus *q.v.*, which produce and store infection-fighting cells.

LYMPHATIC TISSUES A three-dimensional network of reticular fibers *q.v.* and cells, the meshes of which are occupied in varying degrees of density by lymphocytes *q.v.*; there are nodular, diffuse, and loose ~.

LYMPH NODE 1. Lymph gland *q.v.* 2. One of numerous round- or oval-shaped bodies located along the course of lymphatic vessels *q.v.* They vary in size from 1 to 25 mm in diameter. They function in the defense mechanisms *q.v.* of the body and swell greatly when infected.

LYMPHOCYTE 1. White blood cells that can produce antibodies *q.v.* and interferon *q.v.* 2. A type of white blood cell that is produced in the bone marrow. Some of these cells migrate to the thymus *q.v.*, where they develop as T cells *q.v.* Other ~s that mature in the bone marrow or in organs other than the thymus are called B cells. The B cells produce antibodies, and the T cells regulate antibody production. In healthy people, about 60% of circulating ~s are helper T cells. With AIDS *q.v.*, only about 2% of the ~s are helper T cells. With fewer T cells, the body is unable to recognize and attack invading organisms.

LYMPHODEMA Chronic edema *q.v.* of the extremities as a result of an accumulation of fluid because of an obstruction or severance of the lymph nodes *q.v.*

LYMPHOGRANULOMA VENEREUM (LGV) A sexually transmitted disease that affects the lymph nodes *q.v.* ~ is a disease that is endemic *q.v.* in the southern United States. Caused by a filterable virus and is characterized by ulcerative lesions on the genitalia *q.v.*, spreading to the lymph channels *q.v.* and lymph nodes *q.v.* and becoming systemic *q.v.* ~ is self-limiting. Tetracycline *q.v.* is used to treat the disease.

LYMPHOID Pertaining to the lymphatic system *q.v.*

LYMPHOID ORGANS The organs where lymphocytes *q.v.* develop and congregate: bone marrow, thymus *q.v.*, lymph nodes *q.v.*, spleen *q.v.*, and other lymphoid tissues.

LYMPHOKINES Chemical messengers produced by T cells *q.v.* and B cells *q.v.*

LYMPHOMA 1. Cancer *q.v.* of the lymphatic system *q.v.* The chief forms are Hodgkin's disease *q.v.*, lymphosarcoma *q.v.*, and reticulum cell sarcoma *q.v.* 2. Leukemia *q.v.* 3. An unregulated proliferation of lymphocytes *q.v.*

LYMPHOMATOSIS The growth of lymphomas *q.v.* in several areas of the body.

LYMPHOSARCOMA A general term describing neoplastic disorders *q.v.* not including Hodgkin's disease.

LYMPH STAGNATION An accumulation of fluid in the tissues.

LYOSOME 1. A cell organelle *q.v.* 2. A membrane-bound vesicle *q.v.* containing digestive enzymes *q.v.* that break down intracellular products and debris.

LYSERGIC ACID DIETHYLAMIDE (LSD) 1. A semisynthetic hallucinogen derived from the fungus, ergot. 2. One of the most potent psychedelic *q.v.* chemicals known.

LYSIN 1. A substance that destroys cells or tissues. 2. Antibodies *q.v.* that function in antigen *q.v.* disruption or lysis *q.v.*

LYSINE An essential amino acid *q.v.*

LYSIS 1. The destruction of bacteria *q.v.* by a bacteriophage *q.v.* 2. The gradual fall in body temperature, improvement of a disease state, or the subsidence of an infection.

LYSOENZYME 1. An enzyme *q.v.* in tears capable of dissolving bacterial *q.v.* cell membranes. 2. In plants, an enzyme capable of disintegrating the constituents that constitute to plant cell wall.

LYSOGENIC BACTERIA Bacteria containing a bacteriophage *q.v.*

LYSOSOME 1. In botany, bodies in the protoplasm *q.v.* that lack a double membrane, and contain enzymes for the lysis *q.v.* of proteins and lipids. 2. In physiology, the membranous organelles *q.v.* containing various enzymes that can dissolve most cellular compounds. Also referred to as digestive bags or suicide bags.

LYTIC CYCLE The cycle of a virulent *q.v.* bacteriophage *q.v.* in which nearly all cells infected are lysed *q.v.*

LYTIC INFECTION After a virus *q.v.* invades a cell, new viruses are produced that break open the cell, releasing the viruses.

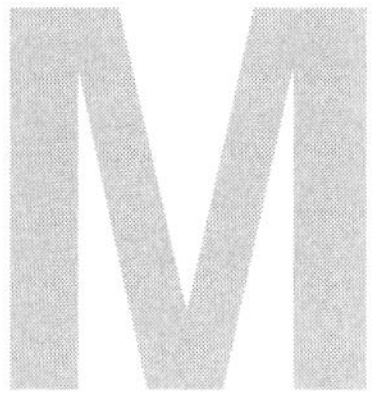

MA Mental age *q.v.*

MACHIAVELLIANISM A style of behavior *q.v.* in which a person manipulates others to achieve his or her own objectives *q.v.*

MACERATION Softening, reddening, and superficial ulceration *q.v.* of the skin due to prolonged exposure to moisture.

MACHISMO A male gender role characteristic in which the male displays physical aggression, risk-taking behavior, and has casual sexual relations with women. cf: macho.

MACHO Aggressively male. The adjective form of machismo *q.v.* that describes a complicated set of masculine *q.v.* attitudes *q.v.* and behaviors *q.v.*, originally from South America and Mediterranean cultures *q.v.*

MACRO In sociology *q.v.*, a level of analysis that searches for relationships among the larger segments of society, such as between the political and economic institutions. Sociologists also compare entire societies with each other. These sociologists are called comparative sociologists. Macrosociologists are closer to anthropology *q.v.* in their interests. ct: micro.

MACRO-APPROACH An all-inclusive drug abuse prevention strategy in which preventive efforts are on the entire environment in the promotion of a drug-abuse–free environment.

MACROBIOTIC DIET A restricted diet that is rich in whole grains and claimed by its advocates to improve health and prolong life.

MACROCEPHALY An enlarged head.

MACROCONIDIUM In microbiology, a large multicelled asexual fungus spore *q.v.*, especially in the dermatophytes *q.v.*

MACROCYTE The largest type of erythrocyte *q.v.*

MACROCYTIC ANEMIA 1. Chronic macrocytic anemia *q.v.* 2. A form of anemia in which large red blood cells *q.v.* predominate, but in which total red blood count is depressed.

MACROGAMY Conjugation or fusion of two adult cells or gametes *q.v.*

MACROMASTIA 1. The condition of having an abnormally large breast *q.v.* or breasts. 2. Mammary hyperplasia *q.v.*

MACROMOLECULE A large molecule *q.v.* ~ is a term used to identify large structures, such as ribosomes *q.v.*, in living cells.

MACRONUTRIENTS Carbohydrates *q.v.*, lipids *q.v.*, and proteins *q.v.* Their chief function is to provide the body with the energy necessary to carry on all of the activities of life. ct: micronutrients.

MACRO-OBJECTIVE 1. Goal *q.v.* 2. Terminal objective *q.v.*

MACROPAPULAR FLUSH Sex flush *q.v.*

MACROPHAGE 1. A large immune cell *q.v.* that destroys invading microorganisms *q.v.* 2. A white blood cell that destroys foreign particles. 3. Specialized phagocytic *q.v.* cells that ingest and destroy foreign substances and microorganisms.

MACROPSIA An abnormal condition in which objects are perceived as larger than they really are. ct: micropsia.

MACROSYSTEM A large, interrelated system, e.g., a state with its cities, counties, and villages, or a group of organizations having common alliances or purposes. ct: microsystem.

MACULA 1. A part of the retina *q.v.* 2. Any lesion of the skin that is not raised above the surface. 3. The area on the retina, near the optic nerve, that is the area of most sensitive vision.

MACULA LUTEA 1. The yellow spot of the retina *q.v.* where only cones *q.v.* are present. 2. The point on the retina of clearest vision.

MACULAR DEGENERATION Progressive, irreversible damage to the macula *q.v.* which results in a gradual loss of fine reading vision and, eventually, blindness. The use of lasers *q.v.* can, in some instances, halt the degenerative process.

MACULE A discolored spot or patch on the skin that is not raised above the skin's surface.

MACULOPAPULAR Spotted and raised or elevated.

MADAM Jargon for women who manage a brothel *q.v.*

MADNESS A nonscientific synonym for mental illness.

MAGICAL THINKING A delusional *q.v.* thought process characteristic of schizophrenia *q.v.* in which the individual believes that his or her actions will have a profound impact on the course of events defying the laws of cause and effect.

MAGNET SCHOOLS Schools, often offering a specialized curriculum *q.v.* that attract students from throughout the district. Admission is frequently done on a lottery basis.

MAHU Originating in Polynesian culture, a Mahu was a male transvestite *q.v.* who served as a sexual outlet for some of the heterosexual *q.v.* males in the village.

MA HUANG A Chinese herb containing ephedrine *q.v.*, a central nervous system stimulant *q.v.*, used for its stimulating qualities.

MAIDENHEAD The hymen *q.v.*

MAIN EFFECT A drug's primary effect. It may be positive or negative, depending upon the dose, its potency, and the purpose for which it is taken.

MAINLINING 1. A mode of drug administration in which the drug is injected directly into a vein. 2. Intravenous administration.

MAINSTREAMING 1. An educational process or organization that integrates handicapped *q.v.* pupils in the school's general curriculum and other activities. 2. A policy of placing handicapped learners in regular classes. 3. A plan by which special education students receive as much of their instruction as possible in the regular classroom.

MAINSTREAM SMOKE Tobacco *q.v.* smoke that is inhaled by the smoker.

MAINTENANCE OF HEALTH The avoidance of ill health.

MAINTENANCE OR DEVELOPMENTAL BILINGUAL EDUCATION An attempt to preserve and develop a student's first language while developing competence in a second language.

MAINTENANCE LOAD A measure of the amount of exercise required to maintain a given level of conditioning.

MAINTENANCE-MOTIVATION MODEL (HERZBERG) A theory of motivation that suggests that work-related factors can be lumped into two categories: (a) maintenance factors that will not produce motivation but can prevent it and (b) factors that can encourage motivation.

MAINTENANCE-OF-MEMBERSHIP AGREEMENT An agreement that provides for continued membership in a union for the duration of a contract.

MAINTENANCE REHEARSAL Rehearsal in which learned material is merely held in short-term memory *q.v.* for a while. ct: elaborative rehearsal.

MAJOR DEPRESSION 1. A condition in which a person experiences episodes of significant depression without periods of mania *q.v.* 2. Unipolar depression. ct: bipolar disorder; mania.

MAJOR HISTOCOMPATIBILITY COMPLEX (MHC) A term for a group of genes that controls several aspects of the immune response *q.v.*

MAJORITY LEADER A member of the legislative body chosen by members of the majority party *q.v.* as their leader. ct: minority leader.

MAJORITY OPINION 1. The formal statement issued by the majority of judges in a particular court decision. 2. The statement of reasons for the views of a majority of the court with respect to a decision, when some members of the court may have dissented.

MAJORITY PARTY The political party having the greatest number of members in the legislative body.

MAJORITY RULE A legal principle in which the previous opinions of the courts have prevailed as precedent. ct: minority rule.

MAJORITY WHIP A member of a legislative body appointed by the majority party to perform partisan political functions. Often the ~ is second in command to the majority leader.

MAJOR MEDICAL EXPENSE COVERAGE (INSURANCE) Usually a supplement to a general health insurance policy. It generally provides protection against a catastrophic illness or accident. It is typically designed to cover illness or injury costs beyond the basic policy coverage.

MAJOR MINERALS 1. Macrominerals. 2. Dietary minerals *q.v.* required in amounts of 100 mg or more each day. ct: trace elements.

MAJOR ROLE THERAPY (MRT) A counseling technique primarily used on mental patients who are preparing to reenter the general community that focuses on reestablishing productive relationships and assuming a positive social role.

MAJOR TRANQUILIZERS 1. Drugs used to treat some psychoses *q.v.*, such as schizophrenia *q.v.*, derived from phenothiazine *q.v.*, first synthesized in 1883. Commercial preparations include Thorazine, Vesprin, Prolixin, Compazine, Mellaril, Dartal, and Stelazine. 2. A pharmacological and chemical classification of the phenothiazine type. ct: minor tranquilizers.

MALACIA Softening of a part or of tissues. cf: osteomalacia.

MALADAPTIVE A characteristic of a response that makes it inappropriate in dealing with stress *q.v.*

MALADJUSTMENT 1. An enduring failure of adjustment *q.v.* 2. A lack of harmony with self or the environment.

MALADY Any disease afflicting the human body.

MALAISE 1. A general feeling of discomfort or fatigue. 2. A general feeling of illness, characterized by restlessness, lack of appetite, and decreased energy.

MALARIA A disease caused by infection of the red blood cells with one of several types of protozoan *q.v.* parasites *q.v.* of the genus *Plasmodium q.v.*

MALE A gender *q.v.* designation distinguished by the anatomical structures, biochemistry, and ability to cause procreation. ct: female.

MALE ABOVE The coital *q.v.* position in which the male is positioned above his female partner. The missionary position or male superior.

MALE CLIMACTERIC Male menopause *q.v.*

MALE MENOPAUSE The time during middle age when a male *q.v.* begins to respond to a lowered production of testosterone *q.v.* ct: menopause.

MALFEASANCE The commission of an unlawful act, typically applied to public officials or employees.

MALICE Intentionally committing an unlawful or wrongful act without proper motive or justification.

MALIGNANT 1. A neoplasm *q.v.* that is cancerous *q.v.* 2. Tending to become progressively worse and to result in death. 3. Having the properties of invasion and metastasis *q.v.*, said of cancerous tumors *q.v.* 4. Harmful, injurious.

MALIGNANT MELANOMA 1. A type of skin cancer *q.v.* arising from blue–black moles. 2. A type of skin cancer that metastasizes *q.v.* readily and is not typically as controllable as other types of skin cancers.

MALIGNANT TUMOR A tumor made up of cancerous *q.v.* cells. The cells of the tumor may either invade other tissues immediately surrounding the site of the tumor or break away and metastasize *q.v.* to other parts of the body.

MALINGERING 1. A faked illness. 2. A faked physical or psychological disorder in order to avoid responsibility or to gain an advantage over others. cf: conversion reaction; psychophysiologic disorder.

MALLEOLUS 1. The rounded projection on either side of the ankle joint. 2. Lateral ~ *q.v.* 3. Small hammer. 4. The projection at the distal *q.v.* ends of the tibia *q.v.* and fibula *q.v.*

MALLEUS 1. One of the three bones of the middle ear. 2. The hammer bone. 3. The first of the three bones or ossicles *q.v.* of the middle ear that is attached to the tympanic membrane *q.v.* ct: incus; stapes.

MALLEUS MALEFICARUM (THE WITCHES HAMMER) A document written by two Dominican monks in the fifteenth century to aid in the identification and trying of witches.

MALNUTRITION 1. An overall term for poor nourishment *q.v.* ~ may be due to an inadequate diet or to some defect in metabolism *q.v.* that prevents the body for utilizing nutrients properly. 2. Lacking one or more nutrients *q.v.* necessary for the maintenance of health.

MALOCCLUSION 1. A dental condition characterized by the irregularity of teeth and improper alignment of the biting surfaces of the teeth. 2. A marked overbite or underbite and poorly aligned teeth.

MALPRACTICE 1. The failure of a health care provider to provide appropriate health, medical or surgical treatment, or care. 2. Negligence through commission or omission of care.

MALPRESENTATION A condition in which a fetus *q.v.* does not move through the birth canal *q.v.* in a normal manner. A Caesarian section *q.v.* is indicated.

MALT A cereal grain that has been allowed to sprout and then is dried and ground.

MALTASE An enzyme *q.v.* that breaks down maltose *q.v.* into dextrose *q.v.*

MALTED Sprouted, as in a grain used in the brewing process.

MALTING The wetting of a grain to allow it to sprout to maximize its sugar content prior to fermentation *q.v.*

MALTOSE A disaccharide *q.v.* It is an intermediate product formed in the breakdown of starch during digestion *q.v.*

MALUM PROHIBITUM An act prohibited by law; but one that is not necessarily wrong or immoral.

MALUNION Improper healing or lack of healing of a fracture *q.v.*

MAMILLARY Like a nipple.

MAMMALIAN DIVING REFLEX A complex series of bodily responses that reduce oxygen requirements of the major body organs occurring when a person's face and head are submerged in cold water.

MAMMALS Animals that are warm-blooded who bear live young.

MAMMARY Pertaining to the breast. cf: mammary glands.

MAMMARY GLANDS Milk-producing glands located in the female breasts. cf: mammary.

MAMMARY HYPLASIA Macromastia *q.v.*

MAMMILLARY BODY Either of two small structures located in the hypothalamus *q.v.* and consisting of nuclei *q.v.*

MAMMOGRAM The X-ray image produced by a mammography *q.v.* that details the structure of the breast.

MAMMOGRAPHY 1. A diagnostic technique using radiation to detect breast cancer in its early developmental stages. 2. X-ray that is often capable of detecting cancer at a stage at which it may be successfully treated. 3. Eaton test *q.v.* cf: xeroradiography; thermography.

MAMMOPLASTY The surgical procedure for reshaping the breasts.

MANAGEMENT The process of organizing, coordinating, directing, evaluating, and utilizing human and financial resources to achieve the objectives of an organization. cf: leadership.

MANAGEMENT BY EXCEPTION A system of managerial control in which only significant deviations from the goals and objectives of the organization are brought to the manager's attention.

MANAGEMENT BY OBJECTIVES (MBO) A system of management based on the establishment of specific actions to be carried out or end results to be achieved. ~ includes information regarding the resources and time periods necessary to carry out the tasks as well as the identity of those responsible for implementation.

MANAGEMENT BY OBJECTIVES APPRAISAL MBO appraisal *q.v.*

MANAGEMENT COMPENSATION All salaries, incentives, and fringe benefits paid to managers in return for their services to the organization.

MANAGEMENT DEVELOPMENT The process of enhancing the qualifications of individuals on staff for current and future employment opportunities.

MANAGEMENT FUNCTIONS The planning, organizing, evaluating, and allocating resources within an organization. cf: management.

MANAGEMENT INFORMATION SYSTEM A network, be it electronic or person to person, within an organization designed to provide managers and other employees with information to enhance the functioning of an organization.

MANAGEMENT INVENTORY An accounting of the strengths and weaknesses of the employees of an organization, including titles, age, length of service, development needs, etc.

MANAGEMENT RESPONSIBILITY GUIDE A document available to all employees clarifying the role and responsibilities of the various managers within an organization.

MANAGEMENT-RIGHTS CLAUSE A section of the labor–management contract that gives management a list of specific rights or general freedom to act on matters not specifically excluded by the contract.

MANAGEMENT SCIENCE APPROACH TO MANAGEMENT The use of the scientific method *q.v.* and quantitative techniques to increase the level of attainment of organizational goals.

MANAGERIAL OBSOLESCENCE A case in which a manager is no longer considered to be up-to-date.

MANDAMUS 1. A court order compelling a person or an institution to perform a particular duty. 2. A writ ordering the execution of a nondiscretionary duty by the person changed with its responsibility.

MANDALA 1. A sight or geometric pattern which is focused upon during meditation. 2. An artistic, religious design used as an object of meditation. cf: mantra.

MANDATE 1. Something that is essential; required by statute or regulation. 2. A law that requires that certain actions be carried out in a prescribed manner. 3. A judicial command, order, or direction.

MANDATORY 1. A compulsory requirement. 2. A command that if ignored, disregarded, or violated is unlawful.

MANDATORY RETIREMENT A policy, now largely abandoned for legal reasons, of requiring a person to retire upon reaching a designated age. Some unique occupations may still legally impose age restrictions, but, in general, there is no longer a mandated *q.v.* retirement restriction based on age. cf: retirement; flexible retirement.

MANDIBLE 1. The jaw. 2. The bone of the lower jaw.

MANDRAKE 1. An herb whose root resembles the human form and was widely used for its aphrodisiac *q.v.* properties. 2. A plant with a branched root that contains an anticholinergic *q.v.* chemical that causes hallucinations *q.v.* when ingested.

MANIA 1. A highly emotional state characterized by excitement, elation, and restlessness, resulting in the expenditure of high levels of energy. Frequently used as a suffix. 2. Hyperactive *q.v.* state with marked impairment of judgment and usually accompanied by intense euphoria *q.v.*, irritability, and/or paranoia; also, mental and physical activity characterized by a lack of concentration, impulsiveness, inflated self-esteem, and hypersexuality.

MANIACAL A mental state in which the person is in a state of uncontrollable excitement. cf: mania.

MANIC-DEPRESSION 1. A type of mental illness characterized by extreme and sudden swings of mood. 2. A bipolar disorder *q.v.* cf: manic-depressive psychosis.

MANIC-DEPRESSIVE PSYCHOSIS 1. Extreme reactions of elation and deep depression. 2. A psychosis *q.v.* 3. A major affective *q.v.* disorder. There are three subgroups: (a) depressed type, consisting exclusively of depressive episodes; (b) circular type, consisting of at least one depressive episode and one manic episode; and (c) manic type, consisting exclusively of manic episodes. 4. Bipolar disorder *q.v.* 5. Manic-depressive reaction.

MANIFEST CONTENT In psychoanalytic theory *q.v.*, the apparent meaning of a dream that masks the latent content *q.v.* cf: manifest dream.

MANIFEST DREAM The portion of a dream that the person remembers upon awakening. cf: Freud's theory of dreams; ct: latent dream.

MANIPULATIVE THERAPY Manual adjustments of the spine to relieve ailments. cf: chiropractic.

MANOMETER An instrument used for measuring the pressure of fluids.

MANUBRIUM 1. Handle. 2. The upper part of the sternum *q.v.*

MANNERISM A recurring stereotyped gesture, posture, or movement.

MANNITOL 1. Mannite. 2. A white powderlike type of sugar frequently used as an adulterant in street cocaine *q.v.* and heroin *q.v.* 3. Hydrogenation *q.v.* of invert sugar syrup *q.v.* that is approximately three-fourths as sweet as sucrose *q.v.*

MANOMETER 1. An instrument for external measurement of arterial blood pressure. 2. Sphygmomanometer *q.v.*

MANTOUX TEST A tuberculin *q.v.* test in which the test material is injected under the skin.

MANTRA 1. A word or sound used in meditation to focus attention. 2. A phrase that is repeated in the mind to help to produce a meditative state. cf: mandala.

MANUAL STIMULATION A sexual activity in which the genitals *q.v.* of one partner are caressed, manipulated, and stimulated by the hands of the other partner. ct: masturbation.

MANUBRIUM 1. The main section of the sternum *q.v.* or breastbone. 2. Manubrium sterni *q.v.*

MANUBRIUM STERNI The cranial portion of the sternum *q.v.* that articulates *q.v.* with the clavicles *q.v.* and the first two pairs of ribs.

MAO INHIBITORS 1. Monoamine oxidase, a drug having a central nervous system *q.v.* stimulating effect. 2. ~ block a specific enzyme, resulting in an increase in neurotransmitter *q.v.* levels that results in elevated mood and a relief of depression *q.v.*

MAPROTILINE A heterocyclic antidepressant *q.v.* Ludiomil is the brand name.

MAP UNITS In genetics *q.v.*, 1% of crossing over *q.v.* represents one unit on a linkage map.

MARASMUS 1. A condition that results from a diet inadequate in both protein and calories. It results in extreme emaciation *q.v.* and growth failure. ~ is the result of starvation and characterized by abnormal growth rate, extreme thinness, wasted tissues, and apathy. 2. Extreme emaciation due to insufficient food. 3. Gradual withering of tissues. cf: kwashiorkor *q.v.*

MARATHON A race covering 26 miles, 385 yards.

MARATHON GROUP A session of a committee or other group run continuously for a day or more for such purposes as sensitivity training, or contract negotiations, so that fatigue will aid in the breakdown of defenses resulting in agreement or insight.

MARCHIAFAVA'S SYNDROME A disease associated with alcoholism *q.v.*, characterized by degeneration of the corpus collosum *q.v.* It probably has a nutritional deficiency basis associated with excessive alcohol intake over a long period of time. ~ was first described by Marchiafava *q.v.* and Bignami *q.v.* in 1897.

MARCH OF DIMES/BIRTH DEFECTS FOUNDATION Formerly the National Foundation for Infantile Paralysis, founded by President Franklin D. Roosevelt in 1938. In 1958, the agency changed its name to the National Foundation following the development of the Salk vaccine.

MARFAN'S SYNDROME 1. Athlete's heart. 2. A genetically based heart disease. 3. A form of cardiac arrest frequently observed in young, tall, slender, athletic persons.

MARGIN OF SAFETY The difference between the drug dosage required to produce the desired effect and the dosage that will cause death (lethal dose). cf: therapeutic index.

MARIANI'S WINE A beverage made from the coca leaf and introduced in the nineteenth century. Named after Angelo Mariani.

MARIJUANA A psychoactive drug, the active ingredient of which is delta 9-tetrahydrocannabinol (THC) *q.v.* THC was first synthesized in 1966. The marijuana plant is *Cannabis sativa* or *Cannabis indica*. It is metabolized in the liver and produces a feeling of stimulation, well-being, and tranquility. It may also produce feelings of hilarity or a desire for contemplative silence. ~ may be either smoked or eaten.

MARIJUANA HIGH The variety of effects that may be experienced from marijuana use, including a sense of well-being, relaxation, and a dreamlike state.

MARITAL AIDS Slang for devices and erotic materials, including dildos *q.v.*, vibrators, sexually oriented videos, etc.

MARITAL COMMUNICATIONS A basis for a stable marital relationship. According to Cox, there are three processes for positive ~: 1. commitment, 2. growth orientation, and 3. noncoercive atmosphere.

MARITAL INSTITUTION The concept that a man and a woman create a legitimate role for parenthood through marriage.

MARITAL INTERCOURSE Traditionally, coitus *q.v.* between a man and a woman who are legally married to each other.

MARITAL RAPE EXEMPTION A traditional legal precedent exempting a husband from being prosecuted for raping his wife.

MARITAL THERAPY Professional intervention which treats a couple for significant marital issues.

MARKER In genetics *q.v.*, a trait that is followed during its recombination *q.v.* among the progeny of a test cross *q.v.*

MARPLAN A commercial preparation of isocarboxazid *q.v.*

MARRIAGE 1. A legal bond between two people. 2. A commitment between two people bonding them to a life together. 3. A holy, spiritual, and legal bond between two people. 4. A legal, spiritual, religious, and personal bond between two or more people. 5. Marriages may be any one of five forms: (a) monogamy, (b) polygamy, (c) polygyny, (d) polyandry, or (e) group *qq.v.*

MARRIAGE CONTRACT An agreement prior to marriage outlining the rights and roles of each partner concerning issues of importance to them. cf: prenuptial agreement.

MARXISM The economic theory of Karl Marx, in which it is purported that economic institutions create and/or become exploitative ruling groups, resulting in oppression of the masses.

MASCULINITY 1. A person's self-concept about possessed sexuality. Usually possessed by a male. ~ is biologically and culturally influenced. 2. Being a man. 3. Behavioral expressions, traditionally observed in males. ct: femininity.

MASCULINIZATION The process by which tissues in the embryo that are sex-neutral become masculine in their structure and function.

MASKING In hearing, the obliteration of one tone by another tone.

MASLOW'S HOLISTIC-DYNAMIC THEORY OF MOTIVATION Developed by Abraham Maslow; also known as Maslow's hierarchy of needs. Maslow suggested there are the biological needs which are the most urgent and the emotional needs as the most complex. They are 1. basic needs, the physiological and emotional needs and 2. metaneeds, self-actualization, knowledge, and aesthetic needs.

MASOCHISM A sexual variance *q.v.* characterized by acts in which sexual pleasure and gratification are derived from being the object of physical or psychological punishment. This punishment is usually planned with a sadistic *q.v.* partner. It may be that for both sadism and masochism there is an attempt to punish or to be punished for feeling sexual pleasure, which may be perceived as "dirty". ct: sadism.

MASS ACTION Behavior *q.v.* involving the entire organism.

MASS ACTION DIFFERENTIATION SEQUENCE In psychological *q.v.* development, a progression from activity that involves the entire body to a more precise control over parts of the body.

MASS COMMUNICATION In health education, the transfer of health information to a large population, usually by means of direct mail, newspapers, the internet, magazines, and other electronic media.

MASS MADNESS 1. A group outbreak of conversion reaction *q.v.* 2. Hysteria *q.v.*

MASS PERSUASION The act of convincing large groups of people to behave in a certain way.

MASSED PRACTICE 1. Programming long study periods at frequent intervals. 2. A practice situation in which the trials are crowded closely together. 3. Practice schedules in which there is little time allowed between sessions of the activity being practiced. ct: spaced practice.

MASSEUR A male who practices massage. ct: masseuse.

MASSEUSE A female who practices massage. ct: masseur.

MAST An acronym for Military Assistance to Safety and Traffic *q.v.*

MASTALGIA Painful swelling of the breasts.

MAST CELL 1. A granulocyte *q.v.* found in tissue. The contents of ~s along with those of the basophils *q.v.* cause the symptoms of allergies *q.v.* 2. A cell that contains a toxic substance called histamine *q.v.* that, when released into the blood, causes an allergic reaction *q.v.*

MASTECTOMY Surgical removal of the breast. The types of ~ are 1. simple: removal of the breast; 2. modified radical: removal of the breast and some axillary *q.v.* lymph nodes *q.v.*; and 3. radical: removal of the breast axillary lymph nodes and pectoral muscles *q.v.*

MASTER PLAN 1. A written guide that describes elements that constitute the total health program *q.v.* 2. Describes the elements that constitute the total health program of the school. It is a statement of the school's philosophy of health education, the aim of health education, and the overall plans for program evaluation. It is characterized chiefly by its lack of detail. ct: curriculum guide.

MASTERS AND JOHNSON SEX THERAPY An approach to sexual dysfunction that revolves around exercises to help persons to learn new ways of sexually relating. Developed by William Masters and Virginia Johnson at the Masters and Johnson Institute located in St. Louis, MO.

MASTERY When applied to growth, ~ implies becoming more self-aware, independent, responsible, and socially interactive.

MASTERY LEARNING A technique of teaching whereby learners are given many opportunities to master a series of examinations, evaluated with reference to specified criteria.

MASTICATION Chewing.

MASTITIS A milk-borne disease characterized by inflammation of the breast and most common in women during lactation. The two types of ~ are (a) ~ interstitial, which is inflammation of the glandular substance of the breast and (b) ~ stagnation, characterized by caked breast.

MASTODYNIA A tight sensation in the breasts.

MASTOID The nipple-shaped bone protuberance of the temporal bone *q.v.* Mastoid cells or sinuses *q.v.* connect with the middle ear. The sinuses may become infected as the result of untreated middle ear infections; a condition known as mastoiditis *q.v.*

MASTOIDITIS An infection of the sinuses *q.v.* of the mastoid *q.v.* bone, usually resulting from untreated middle ear infection.

MASTOID PROCESS The nipple-like projection of the mastoid portion of the temporal bone *q.v.*

MAST PANTS Military antishock trousers *q.v.*

MASTURBATION 1. Sexual stimulation of the self. 2. Manual stimulation of the genitals *q.v.*, usually to orgasm *q.v.* cf: autoeroticism.

MASTER'S DEGREE A graduate studies degree, usually entailing 1–2 years of full-time academic study beyond the bachelor's degree.

MATCHING In epidemiology *q.v.*, a technique for controlling variables that are actual or confounding *q.v.*

MATCHING FUNDS Funds or in-kind contributions *q.v.* that must be provided by a third party in order for a grant or other type of funding to be approved. The prospective funding source often specifies the type of and the percentage of funding that must be matched.

MATCHING HYPOTHESIS The hypothesis that persons of a given level of physical attractiveness will seek out partners of a similar level. 2. Matching process *q.v.*

MATCHING PROCESS 1. The theory that a person will select a prospective romantic relationship from those who are approximately equivalent to himself or herself in terms of physical attractiveness. 2. Matching hypothesis *q.v.*

MATCHING TEST ITEM A two-column item wherein the learner is to match by some criteria items that are related.

MATCHING TO SAMPLE A procedure in which a person has to choose one of two alternative stimuli which is the same as a third sample stimulus *q.v.*

MATE EXCHANGE A situation in which spouses change partners for purposes of sexual intercourse.

MATERIAL RESOURCE An object that is used as an aid to learning, e.g., a textbook, CD-ROM.

MATERNAL DEPRIVATION A lack of adequate care and stimulation by the mother or mother surrogate.

MATERNAL INHERITANCE (MATERNAL EFFECT) Inherited traits from the mother to her offspring that is unaffected by the inheritance from the father.

MATERNAL MORTALITY 1. Maternal deaths. 2. Deaths of women associated with deliveries, complications of pregnancy, childbirth, and puerperalism *q.v.*

MATERNAL MORTALITY RATE The number of deaths of mother from childbirth per 10,000 live births in a given year.

$$\frac{\text{Number of deaths of mothers from childbirth}}{\text{Number of live births}} \times 10,000.$$

MATERNAL SUPPORTIVE TISSUES A general term referring to the development of the placenta *q.v.* and other tissues specifically associated with pregnancy *q.v.*

MATERIA ALBA A whitish food residue that adheres to the teeth near the gums.

MATERIA DENTICA That branch of dental studies that deals with medicinal substances used in the practice of dentistry.

MATERIALISM A system of values *q.v.* in which goods and their acquisition have special significance.

MATERIA MEDICA That branch of medical science concerned with the sources, preparation, properties, and uses of the drugs in preventing, diagnosing, treating, and controlling diseases. cf: toxicology; pharmacognosy.

MATE SWAPPING A sexual variance *q.v.* (also called swinging) that involves the sexual exchange of partners of two or more married couples. In most cases, all of those involved are aware of the swapping activities.

MATHEMATICAL MODELS Variables expressed quantitatively within functional relationships.

MATING GRADIENT A gradient referring to the practice of a young, attractive woman marrying a better educated, well-established less attractive male.

MATING TYPE A strain of organisms in which they cannot reproduce with themselves but are able to reproduce with others of different strains, but within the same species.

MATRIARCHY In sociology, the control of the family or other groups by the female. ct: patriarchy.

MATRILINEAL A kinship system in which family ties and succession are traced through the mother and her female ancestors. ct: patrilineal.

MATRILOCAL 1. A society in which young couples reside with or near the bride's mother's family. 2. Uxorilocal.

MATRIX The noncellular material in which bone and cartilage cells are embedded.

MATTER Anything that occupies space and has mass or weight.

MATURATION 1. The process of development to full effectiveness of cells, tissues, organs, and systems of the body or the person in general. Also applied to social, emotional, and intellectual development *q.v.* 2. A preprogrammed growth process based on changes in underlying neural structure that are relatively unaffected by environmental conditions. 3. Changes in behavior *q.v.* that occur as a result of physiological growth. 4. The biological changes taking place in the cells, tissues, organs, and systems of the body and the improvement in their functioning. ~ is influenced by such factors as genetic potentials *q.v.*, nutrition, rest, recreation, and the richness of the culture or other environmental stimuli that affect personality *q.v.*, emotional and social growth, and intellectual development.

MATURATIONAL READINESS A stage of development where the person is optimally prepared to acquire some particular kind of habit. cf: critical period.

MATURITY The degree of physical and psychological development demonstrated by an individual to function effectively in a particular environment.

MATURITY DIABETES 1. Type 2 diabetes. 2. Traditionally, ~ afflicted people primarily in their 50s or 60s. Now, it is increasingly common among young people as obesity *q.v.* rates have risen. Quite often, those with ~ do not require insulin *q.v.* injections so long as they maintain their diet. Long-term complications are common usually affecting the vascular system *q.v.* The risk of cardiovascular *q.v.* complications is increased if the diabetic patient also has high blood pressure *q.v.*, high blood cholesterol *q.v.*, and is a smoker. cf: juvenile onset diabetes; Type 1 diabetes.

MAUSOLEUM An above-ground structure into which caskets can be placed for later disposition. A ~ frequently resembles a small stone house. cf: crypt.

MAXILLA 1. The upper jaw. 2. The irregularly shaped bone that helps to form the upper jaw on either side of the face. The ~ contains the upper teeth and the orbit of the eye, the nasal cavity, and the palate *q.v.* The ~ is formed by the *q.v.* fusion of several smaller bones.

MAXILLARY ARTERY The artery *q.v.* on either side of the face that supplies blood to the face. The ~ is palpable *q.v.* in front of the angle of the mandible *q.v.*

MAXILLOFACIAL SURGERY A dental specialty (especially of oral surgery *q.v.*) concerned with surgery to correct malformations of the jaws and related facial structures.

MAXIMAL AEROBIC CAPACITY 1. Maximal oxygen consumption. 2. The maximal amount of oxygen that can be transported from the lungs *q.v.* to the working muscles in heavy or exhausting exercise. 3. Maximal aerobic power *q.v.* cf: oxygen transport.

MAXIMAL AEROBIC POWER 1. The point at which the heart and circulatory system *q.v.* cannot deliver more oxygen to the tissues without approaching exhaustion. 2. Maximal aerobic capacity *q.v.*

MAXIMUM OXYGEN UPTAKE The maximum amount of oxygen that can be utilized at the tissue level during vigorous exercise.

MAXIMIZING APPROACH A planning process in which the maximum level of production dictates the type of programs implemented.

MAXIMUM AUDITORY ACUITY The highest degree of clarity or sharpness at which a person can hear. cf: auditory acuity.

MAXIMUM CARRYING CAPACITY The upper limits of population that the available resources can carry or tolerate regardless of quality of life. ct: optimum carrying capacity.

MAXIMUM HEART RATE The highest number of times the heart can beat per minute, calculated as 220 minus age. cf: heart rate.

MAXIMUM JOINT PAYOFF In social exchange theory, the tendency to make choices that benefit each party either monetarily or in terms of pleasure. cf: accommodation process.

MAXIMUM LIFE SPAN The age beyond which no person can survive. cf: mean life span.

MAXIMUM OXYGEN CONSUMPTION (MOC) The maximum amount of oxygen that the body can burn during strenuous exercise.

MAXIMUM PULSE RATE The fastest rate at which the heart will beat.

MAXIMUM REPETITION (MR) The amount of weight with which an individual can perform a specific number of repetitions.

MAZANOR A commercial preparation of mazindol *q.v.*

MAZEWAY A term used to describe the unique path an individual follows as he or she interacts with the collective truth held by all humans.

MAZINDOL An appetite suppressant. Mazanor and Sanorex are brand names.

MBD An acronym for minimal brain dysfunction *q.v.*

MBO An acronym for management by objectives *q.v.*

MBO APPRAISAL A process in which actual performance is measured against established performance objectives.

MBRS An acronym for Minority Biomedical Research Support *q.v.*

MCNAGHTEN DECISION 1. An insanity *q.v.* plea following commitment of a crime *q.v.* This is based on the concept that a person committing a crime is not responsible for the crime while suffering from a defect of reason from a mental illness rendering him or her unable to know the nature of the act or, if he or she did, was unable to know that the act was wrong. 2. Based on a British court decision in 1843, an insanity defense can be established by showing that the defendant did not know his or her act was wrong or did not realize that it was wrong. cf: Durham decision; Currens formula.

MD An acronym for doctor of Medicine Degree.

MDA 1. A synthetic hallucinogen *q.v.* 2. Methylenedioxyamphetamine. First synthesized in 1910.

MDMA 1. A synthetic hallucinogen *q.v.*; methylenedioxymethamphetamine. 2. A catechol *q.v.* hallucinogen. Referred to as ecstasy in the drug culture.

MEAD See metheglin.

MEDIAN A measure of central tendency *q.v.* that occupies the middle position in the rank order of values.

MEALS-ON-WHEELS A program that delivers meals to the homebound.

MEAN (M) 1. In statistics, the average. 2. The most commonly used measure of central tendency *q.v.* ~ is calculated by the sum of the scores divided by the number of scores. ct: median.

MEAN GOAL The habits or characteristics which a person would like to acquire.

MEANING I 1. Operational meaning. 2. Meaning that a concept *q.v.* possesses as a result of translatability into publicly observable operations. cf: meaning II.

MEANING II 1. Significance. 2. The meaning that a concept possesses as a result of the valid relationship to dependent variables *q.v.* cf: meaning I.

MEAN LENGTH OF UTTERANCE (MLU) The average length of a child's utterances as measured in morphemes *q.v.*

MEAN LIFE SPAN The age by which half of the individuals in a population have died.

MEANS-ENDS ANALYSIS The process of evaluating the means by which various organizational objectives can be achieved.

MEAN TEST SCORE The score obtained by dividing the sum scores of all individuals in a group by the number of individuals in the group.

MEASLES 1. Rubella *q.v.* or rubeola *q.v.* 2. A communicable disease. 3. Also referred to as one of the childhood diseases. 4. A contagious viral disease characterized by a cough and raised red circular spots on the body.

MEASURABLE OBJECTIVES An objective *q.v.* whose achievement can be assessed by means of an evaluation *q.v.* procedure that exactly matches the objective's expressed intent cf: behavioral objective.

MEASUREMENT 1. Quantitative description of the learning process. 2. Status determination. 3. A term often used interchangeably with evaluation *q.v.* 4. The gathering of data.

MEASURE OF ATTENTION SPAN An auditory test in which a series of letters are read to a child, who then repeats them in their exact order.

MEATUS 1. A passage or channel. 2. The external opening of a canal. 3. The opening at the end of the urethra *q.v.* in the penis *q.v.* In the female, the external orifice *q.v.* of the urethra.

MEBARAL A commercial preparation of mephobarbital *q.v.*

MECHANISM 1. A view or theory that is in contrast to vitalism *q.v.* and states that life can be explained in terms of natural transformations of energy and matter, without the introduction of any immaterial or extranatural vital forces. 2. A device by which a person unconsciously attempts to protect his or her ego *q.v.* integrity. cf: defense mechanism.

MECHANISM OF DEFENSE 1. Some line of behavior designed to protect a person from uncomfortable anxiety *q.v.* 2. Defense mechanism *q.v.*

MECHANIZATION 1. In psychology *q.v.*, the lack of adequate material love. 2. Coldness in mother–infant or parent–child relationships.

MECONIUM The material in the intestinal tract of a newborn infant before true feces *q.v.* are formed.

MEDIA Any of several information sources, such as radio, television, print materials, the Internet.

MEDIA ADDICTION Spending excessive time with media to the exclusion of other activities and social interactions. May be an indication of personal maladjustment *q.v.*

MEDIA FETISH A sexual response to the texture of an object, e.g., silk, leather, rubber, or wax.

MEDIAL In or toward the middle or center. ct: lateral.

MEDIAL FOREBRAIN BUNDLE A group of nerve fibers connecting the forebrain, midbrain, and hypothalamus. It is the location of the pleasure center of the brain. Norepinephrine *q.v.* and dopamine *q.v.* are the active neurotransmitters in this area.

MEDIAL MALLEOLUS The rounded projection on the medial *q.v.* side of the ankle joint. ct: lateral malleolus.

MEDIAN 1. A measure of central tendency *q.v.* of a frequency distribution *q.v.* 2. ~ is the point that divides the distribution into two equal parts when all scores are arranged is ascending order. 3. The exact middle score. ct: mean.

MEDIAN AGE The age at which half of the group in question has experienced a particular behavior or event.

MEDIAN NERVE A nerve that arises by two roots from the medial *q.v.* and lateral *q.v.* cords of the brachial plexus *q.v.* The ~ controls sensation of the central palm, the thumb, and the first three fingers, as well as the ability to oppose the thumb to the fifth finger.

MEDIA RESOURCES These include any sensory stimuli *q.v.* that enhance learning when used in conjunction with other methods.

MEDIASTINUM 1. A cavity between two major portions of an organ, esp. in reference to the area of the thoracic cavity *q.v.* containing all of the structures except the lungs. 2. The space between the lungs containing the heart, great vessels, nerves, trachea, and esophagus. 3. The middle section of the thorax *q.v.*

MEDIATED GENERALIZATION Stimulus generalization *q.v.* that occurs because the new stimulus *q.v.* evokes a response *q.v.* which, in turn, evokes the conditioned response. cf: semantic generalization.

MEDIATION 1. An attempt to reconcile differences between two sides of an issue, particularly as it relates to labor relations. 2. In psychology, a process that serves to link a stimulus *q.v.* and a response *q.v.* cf: arbitration; mediated generalization.

MEDIATION DEFICIENCY An inability to use a strategy to improve learning *q.v.* and memory.

MEDIATION THEORY In psychology *q.v.*, the view that certain stimuli *q.v.* do not themselves evoke a response, but rather activate intervening processes that result in a response.

MEDIATOR 1. In psychology *q.v.*, a thought, drive, emotion, or belief. 2. A construct *q.v.*

MEDICAID 1. Federal and state government-financed health insurance for individuals and families whose financial status is below the poverty level. 2. Title XIX of the Social Security Act *q.v.* provides medical care for persons who are indigent; a noncontributory governmental health insurance for persons receiving other types of public assistance.

MEDICAL COMMUNITY The medical professions as a group or collectively.

MEDICAL DEATH Death as defined by the absence of spontaneous voluntary movement, brain controlled reflexes, and electrical energy in the brain.

MEDICAL DEVICE An appliance or equipment intended to help a person to maintain or improve health.

MEDICAL EXPENSE COVERAGE (INSURANCE) Health care coverage that may or may not be associated with hospital or surgical coverage *q.v.* Benefits may include physician's fees, diagnostic procedures, etc.

MEDICAL HISTORY An account of a person's past medical conditions, problems, treatments, and outcomes.

MEDICAL MODEL 1. In psychology, a means of explaining abnormal behavior in ways similar to those used in the study of physical diseases, in which the symptoms of the disorder are treated and/or their causes sought. 2. An assumption that abnormal behavior is a symptom resulting from a disease. cf: medical model of health.

MEDICAL MODEL OF HEALTH 1. Criteria of health status *q.v.* in terms of reactions to medical examinations, screenings, and results from laboratory tests. 2. Health is measured in terms of illness or disability that is diagnosed based on the presence of symptoms. 3. In psychology *q.v.*, a subcategory of the pathology model *q.v.* that holds that the underlying pathology is organic and that the treatment should be conducted by physicians. cf: statistical model; holistic model; psychoanalytic model; medical model.

MEDICAL PRACTITIONER A person who provides health services and who possesses a medical degree, e.g., MD and DO.

MEDICAL SPECIALIST A medical doctor who receives additional training and experience in a specific area of medical practice (Table M-1).

MEDICAL TECHNOLOGY The practice of medical laboratory procedures.

MEDICAL TREATMENT (FOR ALCOHOLISM) Includes intervention–emergency treatment and medical

TABLE M-1 MEDICAL SPECIALTIES

SPECIALTY	SPECIALIST	DESCRIPTION
Anesthesiology	Anesthesiologist	The study of anesthetics and anesthesia. A person who specializes in the administration of drugs necessary to produce anesthesia during surgery or for diagnosis of a health or medical condition
Allergy	Allergist	Concerned with the causes, diagnosis, and treatment of diseases resulting from sensitivity to certain substances
Cardiology	Cardiologist	The specialty concerned with the health of the heart and cardiovascular system
Dermatology	Dermatologist	Concerned with the diagnosis and treatment of diseases of the skin
Emergency medicine	Emergency medicine physician	Concerned with the treatment of diseases and injury on an emergency basis, often in an emergency room of a hospital or an emergency medical clinic
Gastroenterology	Gastroenterologist	Concerned with health and diseases of the stomach and intestines
General practice, including family practice	General practitioner or family practitioner	Concerned with all health matters and diseases of people, their diagnosis, and treatment
General surgery	Surgeon	Concerned with the surgical treatment of disease or disability
Internal medicine	Internist	Concerned with the diagnosis and treatment of diseases of the internal organs, often by the administration of drugs
Neurological surgery	Neurologist	Concerned with the diagnosis and operative treatment of the brain, spinal cord, and disorders of the nerves
Obstetrics and gynecology	Obstetrician and gynecologist	Concerned with the health of women, especially the diagnosis and treatment of diseases of the female reproductive organs and the care of pregnant women, delivery of the baby, and prenatal and postnatal care
Ophthalmology	Ophthalmologist	Concerned with the health of the eyes and the diagnosis, treatment (including surgery) of diseases of the eyes
Orthopedic surgery	Orthopedist	Concerned with the diagnosis and treatment (including surgery) of diseases, injuries, and deformities of the bones, joints, and related structures
Otolaryngology	Otolaryngologist	Concerned with the diagnosis and treatment of diseases of the ear
Otorhinolaryngology	Otorhinolaryngologist	Concerned with the totality of the ear, nose, and throat
Pathology	Pathologist	Concerned with the study of the changes in tissues, organs, and cells as a result of disease or other phenomena
Plastic surgery	Plastic surgeon	Concerned with the corrective or reparative surgery for restoring deformed or mutilated parts of the body or to improve features, esp. facial features
Pediatrics	Pediatrician	Concerned with the health of children (usually under the age of 13 years) and the prevention, diagnosis, and treatment of their diseases
Proctology	Proctologist	Concerned with the diagnosis and treatment of diseases of the colon and rectum
Psychiatry	Psychiatrist	Concerned with mental and emotional disorders and their diagnosis and treatment
Radiology	Radiologist	Concerned with the diagnosis and treatment of diseases through the use of radiation
Urology	Urologist	Concerned with the diagnosis and treatment of diseases and disorders of the kidneys, urinary bladder, and related structures, and the male reproductive organs

approaches based on the metabolism of alcohol *q.v.* and its pharmacological *q.v.* effects on the body. The intervention–emergency treatment consists of detoxification *q.v.* and the use of anticonvulsive *q.v.* drugs and sedatives *q.v.* to reduce mortality and morbidity rates from severe intoxication *q.v.* and past intoxication complications. These are associated with the withdrawal syndrome *q.v.* In addition, complications from prolonged, excessive alcohol intake such as gastritis, liver disease, and nutritional deficiencies are treated.

MEDICAL WASTE TRACKING ACT OF 1988 (MWTA) Legislation passed by the U.S. Congress to assist in developing a national policy on the management of medical waste.

MEDICARE Originally established in 1966, ~ is a federally financed health insurance program for persons 65 years of age and older and others who are in special categories. The basic plan, Part A (Title XVIII of the Social Security Act *q.v.*) provides for payment for hospitalization up to 90 days but the person must pay a deductible. Hospital costs are provided for another 60 days, but the person must pay a fixed amount for each of the 40 days of additional hospitalization. ~ pays the cost of home care up to 100 visits and posthospital care for 20 days, in addition to 80 days copayment. Part B provides medical care as well as various types of therapy. The insured must pay a premium for this coverage. cf: Medicaid.

MEDICINAL Having the power to heal.

MEDICINE 1. Drug *q.v.* 2. A drug substance used in the diagnosis, cure, treatment, and prevention of disease or in the relief of symptoms of illness.

MEDIEVAL PERIOD The period in Europe from A.D. 476 to 1300.

MEDIGAP INSURANCE 1. Supplementary health insurance. 2. An insurance policy for the purpose of supplementing Medicare *q.v.*

MEDITATION 1. A process of focusing attention. 2. A state of constant attention to one chosen object to maintain a thought-free state of mind. 3. A quiet, passive state in which the mind is alert and awake and yet calm and relaxed.

MEDIUM 1. The substance or material in which anything moves or acts. 2. A substance that supports the growth and multiplication of microorganisms *q.v.* 3. The nutrient substance used in a laboratory setting for growing bacteria *q.v.*

MEDROXYPROGESTERONE ACETATE (MPA) Depo-Provera *q.v.*

MEDULLA 1. The deep, inner substance or tissue of an organ or part, as of the kidney or of a hair. 2. In embryology *q.v.*, the central cells of the human embryo's *q.v.* undifferentiated gonad *q.v.* 3. Latin for marrow; the inner part of an organ. cf: medulla oblongata. ct: cortex.

MEDULLA OBLONGATA 1. The cone of the nervous tissue continuous above the pons *q.v.* and below the spinal cord *q.v.* Concerned with involuntary vital actions such as breathing. Many depressant drugs have secondary effects on the ~. 2. The structure that is a direct upward continuation of the spinal cord within the skull. 3. The medulla *q.v.* 4. An area of the brainstem through which nerve fibers ascend or descend from higher brain centers.

MEDULLARY PLATE (GROOVE AND TUBE) The three successive shapes in the embryonic *q.v.* development of the central nervous system *q.v.* of vertebrates.

MEDULLARY SHEATH The layer surrounding a medullated nerve fiber.

MEGABLAST A large, nucleated embryonic *q.v.* type of cell. A ~ is found in the blood in cases of pernicious anemia *q.v.*, vitamin B_{12} *q.v.* deficiency, and folacin *q.v.* deficiency.

MEGADOSE A large quantity of medication.

MEGALOMANIA A delusion of grandeur *q.v.* in which a person believes that he or she is an unusually great person or is carrying out spectacular plans and events.

MEGASPORANGIUM The structure containing megaspores *q.v.*

MEGASPORE 1. A large spore that germinates to form a female gametophyte *q.v.* 2. A spore that gives rise to an embryonic sac *q.v.* bearing only female gametes *q.v.* cf: megasporogenesis.

MEGASPOROGENESIS The process of production of megaspores *q.v.*

MEGASPOROPHYLL A leaflike organ that bears one or more megasporangia.

MEGASPORE-MOTHER-CELL 1. Megasporocyte. 2. The cell which undergoes two meiotic divisions to produce four megaspores *q.v.*

MEGATON The equivalent to a million tons. Often used to describe the explosive power of an atomic bomb, e.g., a 1 megaton bomb has the explosive power of one million tons of TNT.

MEGAVITAMIN Dosages of vitamins *q.v.* in amounts that far exceed the recommended daily allowances. cf: megavitamin therapy.

MEGAVITAMIN THERAPY Treatment of a disease with large dosages of vitamins *q.v.* The consumption or administration of vitamins in dosages exceeding the RDAs *q.v.* by a factor of 10 or more.

MEHP An acronym for Minority Environmental Health Program *q.v.*

MEIOSIS 1. A form of cell division that takes place in the germ cells *q.v.* resulting in daughter cells containing one-half the chromosomes *q.v.* of the mother cell. Also called reduction division. 2. The process by which the chromosome number of a reproductive cell becomes reduced to half the diploid *q.v.* or somatic *q.v.* 3. Cellular reduction division, as in spermatogenesis *q.v.* and oogenesis *q.v.*, in which the daughter cells are produced containing one-half the number of chromosomes as present in the mother cell. ct: mitosis.

MEIOSPORE A haploid cell *q.v.* formed in meiosis *q.v.*

MELANCHOLIA A mental disorder characterized by extreme depression *q.v.*

MELANCHOLY Sadness. Pensiveness.

MELANIN 1. A substance beneath the skin that causes the dark pigment color; freckles. 2. Brown or black pigment characteristic of animals. cf: melanocyte.

MELANOCYTE The cell that produces melanin *q.v.*

MELANOCYTE-STIMULATING HORMONE (MSH) The hormone *q.v.* that regulates skin pigmentation.

MELANOMA A skin tumor containing dark pigment.

MELANOPHORE A chromatophore *q.v.* containing black pigment.

MELENA The passage of dark stools stained with blood pigments and digested blood. Essentially, the stools are black and of a sticky, tarry consistency.

MELLARIL 1. A phenothiazine *q.v.* 2. One of the commercial preparations of major tranquilizers *q.v.*, thioridazine *q.v.*

MELTING POT THEORY The theory that people from all cultures can form a common culture over time.

MEMBERS ELECT Members of a legislative body who have been elected, but have not yet assumed office.

MEMBRANE A thin layer of tissue (skin) that covers a surface or divides a space or organ.

MEMORANDUM OF AGREEMENT A written agreement that is often informal but sets the parameters for further discussion. Also, MOU *q.v.*

MEMORIAL SERVICE A form of funeral service in which the body is not present.

MEMORY DRUM A mechanical device for presenting verbal materials for studies of rote material.

MEMORY SPAN 1. The number of items a person can recall after just one presentation or exposure. 2. The recall capability of a person with respect to his or her short-term memory.

MEMORY TRACE The change in the nervous system *q.v.* left by an experience that is the physical basis of its retention in memory.

MENARCHE 1. The first menstrual period *q.v.* Typically, ~ occurs between the ages of 11 and 14. 2. The onset of menstruation *q.v.* 3. The onset of menstruation in the human female occurring in late puberty *q.v.* and ushering in the growth period of adolescence *q.v.*

MENDELIAN POPULATION A naturally interbreeding unit of sexually reproducing plants or animals.

MENINGES 1. The three membranes *q.v.* that cover the brain and spinal cord. 2. The three layers of nonneural tissue the cover the brain and spinal cord: (a) the dura mater *q.v.*, (b) the arachnoid *q.v.*, and (c) the pia mater *q.v.*

MENINGITIS 1. An inflammation of the meninges *q.v.* of the brain. 2. An inflammation of the meninges through infection, usually caused by a bacterium or through irritation.

MENINGOCOCCUS MENINGITIS A meningococcal bacterial *q.v.* infection caused by *Neisseria meningitides*, transmitted by nose and throat discharges from an infected person, either directly or indirectly. It is characterized by an acute *q.v.* onset, headache, fever, nausea, stiff neck, and irritability. It is fatal in about 10% of those who contract it.

MENINGOMYELOCELE A congenital *q.v.* deformity.

MENISCUS A cartilage that acts as a cushion between the opposing surfaces of the knee joint.

MENOPAUSE 1. The period in life when the menstrual cycle *q.v.* ceases. 2. A permanent cessation of the menstrual cycle, usually between 40 and 55 years. 3. Change of life *q.v.* 4. Climacteric *q.v.*

MENORRHAGIA Prolonged menstruation *q.v.*

MENSES 1. The menstrual *q.v.* flow. 2. The products of menstruation *q.v.* 3. A periodic, physiologic, vaginal hemorrhage *q.v.*, occurring at approximately 4-week intervals and taking its source from the uterine *q.v.* mucous membrane *q.v.*, which is shed. Under normal circumstances, the bleeding is preceded by ovulation *q.v.*

MENSTRUAL CRAMPS Pain experienced by a woman before or during her menstrual period *q.v.* The problem may have a physical and/or psychological basis. cf: premenstrual syndrome.

MENSTRUAL CYCLE 1. The regularly recurring cycle of physiological events, including ovulation *q.v.* and menstruation *q.v.* 2. The lapse of time from the first day of one menstrual flow to the day before the next menstrual flow—usually between 24 and 32 days.

MENSTRUAL EXTRACTION A form of therapeutic abortion *q.v.* performed within 2 weeks after the first missed menstrual period *q.v.* It makes use of a suction technique by inserting a fine, flexible plastic tube into the uterus *q.v.* cf: vacuum aspiration; dilation and curettage; hysterotomy; saline induction.

MENSTRUAL FLOW 1. The regular monthly vaginal *q.v.* discharge consisting of blood and the shed endometrium *q.v.* 2. Menses *q.v.*

MENSTRUAL PERIOD The time of the menstrual flow *q.v.*, usually 3–7 days.

MENSTRUAL PHASE Menstruation *q.v.*

MENSTRUAL REGULATION (EXTRACTION) A vacuum aspiration *q.v.* of the uterus *q.v.*, performed up to 6 weeks after the beginning of the last menstrual period *q.v.*

MENSTRUATE To undergo cyclic buildup and destruction of the uterine *q.v.* wall. cf: menstruation.

MENSTRUAL SYNCHRONY The simultaneous occurrence of the menstrual cycles of women living in close proximity to one another. This is thought to evolve over the course of a few months through a gradual synchronization process.

MENSTRUATION 1. The cyclic uterine *q.v.* bleeding resulting from degeneration of the endometrium *q.v.* 2. The discharge of blood from the uterus through the vagina *q.v.* that normally recurs at about 4-week intervals in women beginning with menarche *q.v.* to menopause *q.v.* cf: menstrual cycle.

MENTAL ABILITY TEST A test measuring general learning ability. Used to measure potential for success in education or in career choice.

MENTAL AGE (MA) 1. A score devised by Binet to represent a person's test performance. 2. ~ represents the chronological age *q.v.* at which 50% of the people in that age group will perform. 3. A person's degree of mental development as measured against means. cf: intelligence quotient. ct: chronological age. 4. The numerical index of an individual's cognitive development as determined by standardized intelligence tests.

MENTAL ALERTNESS TEST A test that measures an individual's ability to comprehend and rapidly indentify verbal, mathematical, and visual symbols.

MENTAL ATTRIBUTES Hereditary *q.v.* intelligence.

MENTAL DEFICIENCY 1. Mental retardation. 2. An obsolete term pertaining to low intelligence. cf: idiot; imbecile; moron.

MENTAL DISEASE A mental disorder *q.v.* associated with an organic *q.v.* or functional *q.v.* disease *q.v.* of the nervous system.

MENTAL DISORDER 1. Mental illness *q.v.* 2. Psychopathology *q.v.*

MENTAL HEALTH 1. The quality of one's psychological dimension of health *q.v.* which makes it possible to function effectively with self and others. 2. A relative, rather than an absolute, state of functioning. 3. The quality of a person's usual or integrated intrapersonal and interpersonal relationships. Characteristics include (a) intrapersonal: (i) understanding feelings and emotions, (ii) understanding and accepting failures and successes, talents and shortcomings, (iii) possessing a sense of humor, (iv) possessing a positive self-concept *q.v.*, self-respect, sense of dignity, and worthwhileness, and (v) enjoying life, making plans, carrying them through and making the most of personal resources; (b) interpersonal: (i) giving and receiving love, (ii) being trusted and trusting others, (iii) making and keeping friends, (iv) projecting self-respect to others, (v) possessing a sense of belonging and contributing, (vi) accepting social responsibilities; (c) application of capabilities: (i) facing everyday problems, (ii) making appropriate decisions, (iii) seeking help when necessary, (iv) adjusting to existing environments, (v) working to improve the environment, (vi) feeling excitement about the future, (vii) planning for the future, (viii) working for the future, (ix) accepting the challenges of life, (x) expressing responsible and meaningful behavior, (xi) controlling behavior rationally, intellectually, and with wisdom, (xii) making effective use of innate and developed talents and skills. 4. Emotional and intellectual maturity *q.v.*

MENTAL ILLNESS 1. The inability for a person to cope adequately and appropriately with life. 2. Any number of psychological *q.v.* or behavioral disorders that impair a person's functioning. The causes may be social, psychological, genetic, or chemical. ~ is usually characterized either by a psychosis *q.v.* or a neurosis *q.v.* 3. Disorders of the nervous system *q.v.* 4. A term that implies acceptance of the medical model *q.v.* of mental disorders *q.v.*

MENTAL HYGIENE A scientific discipline primarily concerned with healthful personality development and the prevention of psychiatric *q.v.* disorders. cf: mental health.

MENTALLY HANDICAPPED STUDENT A student whose mental capacity lacks maturity or is so deficient as to hinder normal achievement.

MENTAL RETARDATION 1. Low intelligence *q.v.* that renders a person to some extent ineffective in dealing with his or her affairs. 2. A person whose intelligence quotient *q.v.* is 70 or below. 3. A condition that usually manifests itself during childhood, characterized by low intelligence and maladaptive behavior. cf: mental deficiency.

MENTAL WELL-BEING 1. Control over everyday life and successful adaptation *q.v.* to stress. 2. A manifestation of a sense of personal worth, feeling and drives, and a sense of meaning and purpose in life.

MENTOPLASTY The surgical procedure to change the shape of the chin.

MENTOR 1. A person who functions as a teacher, counselor, and role model for a younger person. 2. In education, a senior teacher who serves as a role model and makes constructive suggestions to a younger member of the faculty.

MENTORING PROGRAMS Programs utilizing mentors *q.v.* to improve the performance of students or faculty.

MEPERIDINE 1. A synthetic derivative of opium *q.v.* 2. An analgesic *q.v.* 3. A narcotic analgesic. 4. Demerol is a brand name.

MEPHOBARBITAL A barbiturate sedative/hypnotic *q.v.* Mebaral is a brand name.

MEPROBRAMATE 1. A minor tranquilizer *q.v.* 2. The first minor tranquilizer marketed as Miltown and Equanil. cf: chlordiazepoxide; diazepam.

MEQ Milliequivalent *q.v.*

MERE EXPOSURE HYPOTHESIS The belief that an increase in attraction to a person or an object is related to the frequency of observation of the person or object.

MERIT PAY A salary increase based on performance and not upon years of service.

MEROGENOTE A piece of chromosome *q.v.* that has entered a bacterium *q.v.* from the environment.

MEROZOITE The infective stage of *Plasmodium q.v.* that invades red blood cells *q.v.*

MEROZYGOTE 1. A partial zygote *q.v.* produced by a partial genetic exchange in bacteria *q.v.* 2. A partially diploid *q.v.* bacterium.

MESCAL Peyote *q.v.*

MESCALINE 1. The chief psychoactive *q.v.* chemical found in peyote *q.v.* 2. A poisonous oil extracted from peyote (*Lophophora williamsii*). ~ produces an intoxication with delusions of color and sound. 3. From the "buttons" of a small cactus, *L. williamsii*, that produces effects similar to those caused by LSD *q.v.*

MESENCEPHALON The midbrain. cf: cerebrum.

MESENTERY 1. A membrane to invest and suspend internal organs. 2. The tissue by which the intestines *q.v.* are attached to the back surface of the abdominal cavity *q.v.* which contains the blood vessels, lymphatics *q.v.*, and nerves supplying the intestines.

MESEROLE Marijuana *q.v.* from Central or South America.

MESIAL 1. Situated in the middle. 2. Median *q.v.*

MESMERISM Associated with theories of "animal magnetism" that were formulated by Anton Mesmer. cf: hypnosis.

MESMERIZE The first term referring to hypnosis, after Anton Mesmer.

MESODERM 1. The middle tissue developed in the gastrula *q.v.* stage of the embryo lying between the ectoderm *q.v.* and the endoderm *q.v.* 2. The middle layer of tissue in the embryo from which skeletal, muscular, circulatory, and reproductive systems develop.

MESOLIMBIC DOPAMINE SYSTEM A group of dopamine-containing neurons *q.v.* that have their cell bodies in the midbrain *q.v.* and their terminals in the forebrain *q.v.*; the ~ plays an important role in the effect of antipsychotic medications.

MESOMORPH A somatotype *q.v.* represented by the broad-shouldered, well-muscled person. cf: mesomorphy.

MESOMORPHY One of the three body types identified by Sheldon as indicative of one's temperament, characterized by a muscular body form and whose temperament is somatotonia *q.v.*, i.e., adventurous, likes strenuous exercise, and withstands pain easily. ct: endomorphy; ectomorphy.

MESON An unstable nuclear particle that has a mass between that of an electron and a proton.

MESONEPHRIC The duct system *q.v.* within the male embryo *q.v.* that gives rise to several internal reproductive structures.

MESOPHILIC Descriptive of organisms that grow at medium range temperatures, esp. microorganisms *q.v.*

MESOPHYLL Thin-walled parenchyma tissue containing chloroplasts *q.v.* that composes the bulk of the upper and lower epidermis *q.v.*

MESORIDAZINE 1. An antipsychotic drug. 2. Serentil is a commercial preparation.

MESSAGE Encoded information that the source–encoder intends to share with others.

MESSAGE FROM THE SENATE OR HOUSE Official communication from the opposite house read into the official record.

MESSAGE INTERFERENCE Stimuli that interfere with the message being communicated interrupting the attention of the message's destination.

MESSENGER RNA (MRNA) 1. RNA *q.v.* that serves as the template for protein synthesis *q.v.* It carries the information from the DNA *q.v.* to the protein synthesizing site to direct the process. 2. RNA produced in the nucleus *q.v.* and moves to the ribosomes *q.v.* where it determines the order of the amino acids *q.v.* in a polypeptide *q.v.* cf: ribonucleic acid.

MET An acronym for metabolic equivalent of resting oxygen uptake. It is expressed in millimeters per kilogram of body weight per minute.

METABOLIC ACTIVITY Chemical processes that involve the body's use of food to convert it into energy and to create new or repair old tissues. cf: metabolism.

METABOLIC ANTAGONIST A substance that reverses or inhibits the physical or chemical processes by which living organisms produce and maintain life.

METABOLIC CELL A cell that is not dividing.

METABOLIC DISTURBANCE A disruption of the normal processes of anabolism *q.v.* or catabolism *q.v.* cf: inborn errors of metabolism.

METABOLIC FUNCTIONS Activities related to metabolism *q.v.*

METABOLIC PATHWAYS The chemical changes that a substance undergoes in its passage through the body. cf: metabolism.

METABOLIC POOL The total amount of a specific substance in the body that is in a state of active turnover, e.g., the amino acid *q.v.* pool or vitamin D *q.v.* pool. Subtractions from and additions to the pool are constantly being made. cf: metabolism.

METABOLIC PSYCHOSES Psychotic *q.v.* reactions associated with metabolic disturbances *q.v.*

METABOLIC RATE The intensity at which the body produces energy.

METABOLIC SIZE The body weight raised to the three-fourths power ($W^{3/4}$). cf: metabolism.

METABOLIC THERAPY An unorthodox program of treatment that may include megadoses of vitamins *q.v.*, oral enzymes, pangamic acid, coffee enemas, and a low-protein diet.

METABOLIC WASTE The unusable end products of anabolic *q.v.* and catabolic *q.v.* processes that are excreted *q.v.* from the body.

METABOLISM 1. The sum of the chemical processes within the body necessary for building protoplasm *q.v.*, breaking down chemical substances, and providing energy for maintenance of the vital process. 2. Consists of anabolism *q.v.* and catabolism *q.v.* within the body. 3. Complex chemical changes that alter drugs and convert them to substances that can be eliminated from the body. 4. Biotransformation. 5. The process by which the body transforms a drug or other substance, preparing it for excretion. 6. The sum total of all chemical and energy transformation within a cell or organism that serve to maintain the health of the organism.

METABOLITE 1. Any compound produced during metabolism *q.v.* 2. Any substance that the body uses to promote cell growth and maintenance.

METABOLITE, ESSENTIAL A substance whose presence in very low concentration must be supplied from an external source in order that the organism may carry out its functions or that a specific biochemical reaction may be allowed to proceed.

METACARPAL BONES 1. The bones between the wrist and fingers. 2. The bones of the palm of the hand. 3. The five cylindrical bones of the hand extending from the carpus *q.v.* to the phalanges *q.v.*

METACARPUS 1. That part of the hand between the wrist and fingers. 2. After the wrist.

METACERCARIA An encysted cercaria. If present in fluke life history, it is ingested passively by the final host.

METACOGNITION 1. Knowledge about knowledge. 2. A person's knowledge about own and other's cognitions *q.v.* 3. Knowledge about persons as intelligent beings. cf: social cognition.

METACOGNITIVE EXPERIENCE Being or becoming aware or conscious of some metacognition *q.v.*

METACOGNITIVE KNOWLEDGE Everything a person knows about cognizing: (a) knowledge about persons as cognizers, (b) knowledge about tasks and their demands, and (c) knowledge about strategies for accomplishing cognitive ends.

METALLOENZYME An enzyme *q.v.* containing a metal (ion *q.v.*) as an integral part of its active structure.

METAMEMORY 1. Memory, as knowing about knowing. 2. A person's knowledge or awareness of his or her own memory and how it works.

METAMORPHOSIS A marked and more-or-less abrupt change in the form or structure of an animal during postembryonic *q.v.* development.

METANEEDS 1. According to Maslow, needs for self-actualization *q.v.*, knowledge *q.v.*, and aesthetics *q.v.* 2. Needs beyond the normal survivor needs. 3. The higher transcending needs.

METAPHASE 1. A period preceding the anaphase *q.v.* in mitosis *q.v.* 2. The mitotic stage in which the chromosomes *q.v.* are arranged as a spindle, midway between the two poles. 3. The stage in mitosis in which the chromosomes are arranged in an equatorial plate.

METAPHYSICS The branch of philosophy that studies the nature of reality.

METAPLASM The lifeless materials of living protoplasm *q.v.*

METASTASIS 1. A cancer *q.v.* that has spread through the various systems. 2. The process by which tumor *q.v.* cells are carried by the blood and lymph *q.v.* to diverse parts of the body to form new tumors. 2. The spread of disease from one part of the body to another.

METASTATIC GROWTH Metastasis *q.v.*

METATARSAL Any one of the fine bones forming an arch across the foot near the base of the toes.

METATARSUS 1. That part of the foot between the tarsal bones *q.v.* and the toes. 2. After the instep.

METAZOA A many-celled organism of higher organization, e.g., hookworm, louse, itch mite.

METER A measurement of the metric system, equal to about 39.5 in.

METHADONE 1. A synthetic opiate *q.v.* whose pharmacological properties resemble those of morphine *q.v.* but is slightly more potent *q.v.* 2. An addicting drug used in maintenance treatment of morphine or heroin *q.v.* addicts. ~ is prescribed in daily maintenance doses that supposedly make the addict more amenable to rehabilitation efforts. 3. A synthetic narcotic that resembles heroin and morphine in terms of its effect, having a duration of action of up to 24 h. ct: Cyclazocine.

METHADONE MAINTENANCE The chronic use of methadone, administered orally, in order to reduce the person's need for heroin or morphine and to eliminate the "rush" that occurs when heroin or morphine is injected.

METHAMPHETAMINE 1. A powerful stimulant of the amphetamine *q.v.* group. Used in the treatment of narcolepsy *q.v.* 2. The most common ~ abused in the United States is Methedrine *q.v.* 3. A synthetic amphetamine, known as "meth" or "speed" and abused by injection for the rapid, intense "flash" effect.

METHAPYRILENE An antihistamine *q.v.* removed from over-the-counter drugs in 1979.

METHAQUALONE 1. Used as a substitute for barbiturates *q.v.* as a drug of abuse in the early 1970s. It was referred to as the "intellectual heroin" because it was thought to be nonaddicting. It was introduced in 1966 under the trade name Quaalude by William H. Rorer Company as a substitute for barbiturates for people who could not tolerate the chemical action of the barbiturates. It was prescribed as a sleeping aid. It is addicting *q.v.* with a withdrawal syndrome *q.v.*, characterized by convulsions, gastrointestinal hemorrhaging, and possibly death. 2. A synthetic, nonbarbiturate sedative-hypnotic. Because of its high abuse popularity, it was removed from the market in 1983. 3. Sopor is a second brand name.

METHADRINE 1. An amphetamine *q.v.* 2. A powerful methamphetamine *q.v.*; the most commonly abused amphetamine in the United States.

METHEGLIN (MEAD) A fermented drink made from water, honey, malt, and yeast, and usually contains spices. Probably one of the first forms of alcoholic beverage used by humans.

METHIONINE A sulfur-containing essential amino acid *q.v.*

METHOD OF CONSTANT STIMULI A psychophysical method in which a difference threshold *q.v.* is obtained in which the subject attempts to detect the difference between a selected set of stimuli and a standard stimulus *q.v.* of fixed value.

METHOD OF ENTRY 1. Mode of entry. 2. The manner in which organisms enter the host's *q.v.* body. ct: method of escape.

METHOD OF ESCAPE 1. Mode of escape. 2. The manner in which organisms leave the host's body. ct: method of entry.

METHOD OF FRACTIONATION A psychophysical method in which a subject selects a stimulus *q.v.* which appears to be a certain fraction of a second stimulus.

METHOD OF MAGNITUDE ESTIMATION A psychophysical method in which a reference stimulus *q.v.* is assigned an arbitrary value and the subject is required to state the value of another stimulus. ct: method of magnitude production.

METHOD OF MAGNITUDE PRODUCTION A psychophysical method in which a reference stimulus *q.v.* is assigned an arbitrary value and the subject is required to set a variable stimulus to some stipulated value. ct: method of magnitude estimation.

METHOD OF RATIO ESTIMATION A psychophysical method in which the subject is required to estimate the ratio of two stimuli *q.v.* ct: method of ratio production.

METHOD OF RATIO PRODUCTION A psychophysical method in which the subject is required to adjust a variable stimulus *q.v.* to some stated ratio to another stimulus. ct: method of ratio estimation.

METHODS OF SYSTEMS SAFETY ANALYSIS Techniques that identify contributing factors in accident causation and identify major hazards before an accident occurs.

METHODOLOGY The techniques, strategies, and other procedures used to achieve goals and objectives. cf: health education methodology.

METHODS 1. In health education, communication techniques through the use of printed and electronic media, group interactions, group instruction, role playing, etc., that assist in the learning process. 2. Planned, organized techniques that are used to assist learners achieve certain objectives. 3. A way of learning and teaching. 4. A sequence of steps and procedures enabling a person to carry out a specific activity toward a specific goal with consistency. ct: technique; strategy.

METHYL ALCOHOL An alcohol *q.v.* used for industrial purposes. Not fit for human consumption. Its chemical formula is CH_3OH. ct: ethyl alcohol.

METHYLMORPHINE Codeine *q.v.*

METHYLPHENIDATE 1. A stimulant used in the treatment of ADHD *q.v.* 2. Ritalin is a brand name.

METRAZOL A commercial preparation of pentylenetetrazol *q.v.*

METRAZOL THERAPY 1. A form of shock therapy in which convulsions are produced by injections of metrazol. This treatment is rarely used today. 2. The administration of metrazol to produce epileptiform convulsions.

METRORRHAGIA Bleeding from the uterus *q.v.* between menstrual periods *q.v.*

MG An abbreviation for milligram *q.v.*

MHz Megahertz.

MHC An acronym for major histocompatibility complex *q.v.*

MI An acronym for myocardial infarction *q.v.*

MIASMA Historically, a term used to indicate a vapor or mist that was thought to cause illness. cf: miasmatic theory of disease.

MIASMATIC THEORY OF DISEASE The theory of the causation of disease that arose during the Middle Ages *q.v.* It proposed that mysterious poisons from decaying matter were carried in the atmosphere causing disease. ct: germ theory of disease.

MICELLE A specialized aggregate of monoglycerides *q.v.*, fatty acids *q.v.*, cholesterol *q.v.*, phospholipids *q.v.*, and bile *q.v.*

MICKEY FINN Slang for chloral hydrate mixed in alcohol.

MICRO In sociology, a level of analysis that searches for relationships within a single institution or within the smaller segments of society. ~ sociologists are chiefly concerned with the psychology of the situation rather than the anthropological aspects. ct: macro.

MICROAEROPHILIC Requiring a relatively low oxygen tension for growth. There may be a requirement for a higher carbon dioxide concentration.

MICROBE A microscopic organism, particularly bacteria, viruses, fungi, and protozoa.

MICROBIAL AGENT Pertaining to a microbe-caused disease.

MICROCROBIAL CLASSIFICATION The categories that pathogenic *q.v.* organisms are placed. There are two general classifications with several subclasses for each: 1. plants: (a) bacteria (bacillus, coccus, spirillum), (b) rickettsia, (c) virus, (d) fungus (molds and yeasts); 2. Animals: (a) protozoa (amoeba, plasmodium), (b) spirochete, (c) metazoa (roundworm, tapeworm, trichinella), (d) schistosomes *qq.v.*

MICROBIOLOGY The study of microbes and their interaction with the ecosystems *q.v.*

MICROCEPHALY 1. A condition often associated with feeblemindedness *q.v.* 2. Literally, small head. 3. Abnormal smallness of the head with associated mental retardation *q.v.*

MICROCOMPUTERS Generally, an outmoded term referring to computers that are manufactured for personal use to be used for testing, data storage and analysis, and computer-aided instruction.

MICROCONIDIA Small unicellular fungus spores.

MICROCYST Small, rounded, resistant cells with thick walls.

MICROFILARIA Infective larvae of some roundworms, usually produced in the host's bloodstream.

MICROGAMETE The male gamete *q.v.* of *Plasmodium q.v.* that develops in the mosquito.

MICROGLIA One type of connective tissue *q.v.* cell found in the brain and spinal cord.

MICROGRAM A metric unit that is equivalent to one-millionth of a gram *q.v.*

MICRON One thousandth of a millimeter or one twenty-five thousandth of an inch.

MICRONUTRIENTS Vitamins *q.v.* and minerals *q.v.* ~ are necessary for regulating body functions and for becoming integral components of various body structures and fluids. ct: macronutrients.

MICRO OBJECTIVE Enabling objective *q.v.*

MICROORGANISMS Microscopic *q.v.* plants or animals.

MICROPENIS A penis *q.v.* that is correctly formed, but that is less than 2 cm long.

MICROPHTHALMOS An abnormally small eyeball.

MICROPSIA The perception *q.v.* of objects as smaller than they actually are. ct: macropsia.

MICROPYLE 1. A small opening. 2. The opening in the integuments *q.v.* of the ovule *q.v.*

MICROSCOPE A laboratory instrument used to magnify objects. Many disease-producing organisms are so small that they can be observed only through the use of a ~. These organisms are said to be microscopic *q.v.*

MICROSCOPIC Pertaining to objects that can be observed only with the aid of a microscope. Invisible to the naked eye.

MICROSOMAL ENZYMES Enzymes located in the liver that break down substances into simpler compounds.

MICROSPORANGIUM A structure producing microspores *q.v.*

MICROSPORE 1. A small spore that germinates to form a male gametophyte *q.v.* 2. A spore giving rise to a gametophyte bearing only male gametes *q.v.*

MICROSPORE-MOTHER-CELL Pollen mother cell *q.v.*

MICROSPOROGENESIS The process of producing microspores *q.v.*

MICROSPOROPHYLL A leaflike organ bearing one or more microsporangia *q.v.*

MICROSYSTEM A small system, such as the organization, that exists within a community *q.v.* system. ct: macrosystem.

MICROTEACHING An experiential-based experience in which a prospective teacher practices a particular teaching method to a group of his or her peers. Often this session is recorded so that it can be examined and critiqued.

MICROVILLI Cylindrical outgrowth from villi *q.v.* and surrounding epithelial cells. They constitute the brush border *q.v.* and function in absorption of nutrients.

MICROZOA Any microscopic *q.v.* animal.

MICTURITION 1. Urination *q.v.* 2. Voiding.

MIDBRAIN 1. The middle of the three primitive enlargements of the developing brain in the embryo *q.v.*, connecting the pons *q.v.* and the cerebellum *q.v.* with the hemispheres of the cerebrum *q.v.* 2. A component of the brain between the brainstem and the forebrain. The ~ has tracts from the spinal cord and the medulla oblongata *q.v.* going to the cortical centers and has relays that control vision and hearing. 3. That part of the brain that includes some lower centers for sensorimotor integration and part of the cochlea *q.v.* 4. Part of the brain immediately above the pons. ct: forebrain; hindbrain.

MID-CLAVICULAR LINE A line dropped from the midpoint of either clavicle *q.v.*

MIDDLE EAR 1. An antechamber to the inner ear *q.v.* that amplifies sound vibrations of the eardrum *q.v.* and transmits them to the cochlea *q.v.* 2. The tympanic cavity with its ossicles *q.v.*

MIDDLE LAMELLA Intercellular layer *q.v.*

MIDDLE SCHOOL A school for the intermediate grades that has largely replaced the junior high school *q.v.* Most often, ~ includes grades 5–8 or 6–8. ct: elementary school; high school.

MIDLIFE The period of the life cycle *q.v.* between 45 and 65 years.

MIDLIFE CRISIS The period of emotional upheaval noted among some midlife *q.v.* persons as they struggle with the finality of death and the nature of their past and future accomplishments.

MIDWIFERY A process or art of assisting in childbirth. The person trained in ~ is a midwife.

MIGRAINE A psychosomatic *q.v.* disorder characterized by recurrent severe headaches, often accompanied by visual disturbances and nausea. cf: migraine headache.

MIGRAINE HEADACHE 1. A type of periodically recurring headache, often confined to one side of the head. 2. A headache caused by altered blood flow to the brain. 3. An extremely debilitating headache caused by sustained dilation of the extracranial arteries *q.v.*, the temporal artery in particular. The dilations trigger pain-sensitive nerve fibers in the scalp.

MIGRAVIDA A woman who is pregnant *q.v.* for the first time. ct: multigravida.

MILBANK MEMORIAL FUND Founded in 1905 for the purpose of improving the physical, mental, and moral condition of humanity and the advancement of charitable and benevolent projects.

MILD LEARNING AND BEHAVIOR DISORDERS A general classification for disorders that involve learning and/or social or interpersonal behavior disorders that generally are discovered in a school-based setting. Usually this classification is assigned to those who fall 1–2 standard deviations from the norm and can still be taught in a regular class setting for the majority of a day.

MILD MENTAL RETARDATION A limited intellectual development reflected in an IQ *q.v.* score between 50 and 70. Children in this range are considered to be educably mentally retarded.

MILIARIA 1. Heat rash. 2. A diffuse pimple-like eruption of the skin common in infants but may occur in adults as the result of excessive heat and the inability to perspire freely.

MILIARY TUBERCULOSIS The type of tuberculosis *q.v.* in which the tubercle bacilli *q.v.* spread into the circulatory system *q.v.* and are carried to other vital organs of the body.

MILIEU 1. The environment *q.v.* 2. The immediate environment, physical or social or both. ~ is sometimes used to include the internal state of an organism.

MILIEU THERAPY A treatment procedure in which the total environment of a treatment facility, the patients and the staff, are conducive to psychological improvement and that this improvement is expected through more normal behavior and responsibility.

MILITARY ANTISHOCK TROUSERS 1. MAST pants *q.v.* 2. Pressure pants for the control of severe hemorrhage *q.v.* Used to apply counter pressure over the entire lower half of the body in victims with extensive lacerations *q.v.* or fractures *q.v.* of the lower extremities, or fractures of the pelvis *q.v.* or hip joint.

MILITARY ASSISTANCE TO SAFETY AND TRAFFIC 1. MAST. 2. A program using military helicopters and medical corpsmen as a supplement to an existing local emergency medical service system for the purpose of providing emergency assistance to civilian victims.

MILITARY PSYCHOLOGY A subcategory of psychology *q.v.* that deals with psychological problems within the armed forces or military forces.

MILK DUCT The connections between the mammary glands *q.v.* and the nipple of the female breast *q.v.* cf: mammary glands.

MILL A tenth of a cent or one thousandth of a dollar. Used to assess the rate of property taxes.

MILLIEQUIVALENT (mEq) A measure of the chemical combining power of electrolytes *q.v.* in solution. One ~ has the chemical combining power of 1 mg *q.v.* of hydrogen *q.v.* and is usually expressed in terms of the number per liter. The formula for calculating is

$$\frac{\text{mEq}}{1} = \frac{\text{Mg\%} \times \text{valence} \times 10}{\text{atomic weight}}.$$

MILLIGRAM (mg) A metric unit of weight that is equivalent to 1/1000 g *q.v.* or 1000 μg *q.v.*

MILLILITER (ml) A metric unit of liquid measure that is equivalent to 1/1000 l.

MILLIMETER (mm) 1. A metric unit of length that is equivalent to 1/10 centimeter (cm). 2. 0.001 m. 3. About 1/25 of an inch.

MILLIMICRON A thousandth part of a micron or a millionth of a millimeter.

MILLIROENTGEN One thousandth of a roentgen *q.v.*

MILLIVOLT One thousandth of a volt.

MILTOWN 1. A commercial preparation of the first minor tranquilizer *q.v.* developed in 1952. 2. ~ has the generic name meprobramate. 3. Equanil is another trade name.

MIND 1. Pertaining to the brain. 2. The functional aspects of the brain. 3. Intellectual, emotional, perceptual functioning. 4. The thought processes emanating from the brain. 5. Freudian theory *q.v.* states there are three level of the mind: (a) conscious, (b) preconscious, and (c) subconscious.

MIND-EXPANSION A hallucinogenic or psychedelic state characterized by heightened awareness, an enhanced sense of clarity, and a general alteration of the conscious state.

MINERALS 1. Inorganic, crystalline chemicals that perform vital functions in the body including controlling water balance, regulating acid–base balance, acting as catalysts *q.v.* for a variety of body functions, and becoming integral components of body structures, such as bones, teeth, enzymes, hormones *q.v.*, and blood. Some ~ are needed in relatively large amounts and are called macrominerals; others are needed in small trace amounts and are called microminerals. 2. Components of various hormones, enzymes, and other substances that help regulate chemical reactions in cells. 3. Chemical elements that serve as structural elements within the body tissues or that participate in physiological processes. Included are calcium, phosphorus, iron, and zinc.

MINERAL ACID A strong acid such as sulfuric, nitric, or hydrochloric.

MINERALOCORTICOIDS Hormones *q.v.* that influence mineral *q.v.* salt metabolism *q.v.* Secreted by the adrenal cortex *q.v.*

MINICOURSE A short, usually narrowly focused, instructional experience.

MINIMAL AGE The youngest age at which a person can be married, whether or not parental consent is given.

MINIMAL BRAIN DAMAGE A term sometimes used to describe a hyperactive child reflecting the belief that at least some hyperactive children suffer from minor brain defects.

MINIMAL BRAIN DYSFUNCTION 1. A group of conditions characterized by attention dysfunction. 2. A condition characterized by hyperactivity, impulsiveness, distractibility, and short attention span. 3. A condition in which an individual exhibits behavioral and sensorineural problems. cf: attention deficit disorder.

MINIMAL RISK LEVEL (MRL) An estimate of the daily human exposure to a chemical that is likely to be without an appreciable risk of deleterious effects (noncancerous) over a specified duration of exposure.

MINIMAL MEDIUM A chemically defined medium that will support the growth of an organism.

MINIMAL SUFFICIENCY PRINCIPLE A principle that holds that appropriate behavior can be best achieved by deemphasizing the external factors that are contributing to the inappropriate behavior. In other words, minimal rewards and punishments should be used to enforce appropriate behavior.

MINIMATA DISEASE A disease, first made notable in Minimata, Japan, in 1956. Caused by mercury poisoning. The disease is characterized by delirium, paralysis, and brain damage.

MINIMAX STRATEGY (IN SOCIAL EXCHANGE) The attempt by individuals to minimize the cost of achieving their goals in order to maximize their pleasure when the goals are achieved.

MINIMUM COMPETENCY TESTING Exit level testing to determine whether students have achieved basic standards of performance in various academic areas.

MINIMUM FOUNDATION PROGRAM A funding model common in most states that attempts to guarantee a basic minimal education program for all children funded at an average minimal level.

MINIPILL A hormonal *q.v.* contraceptive *q.v.* The ~ was introduced in 1973 as an alternative to existing oral contraceptives. ~s contain only progestogen *q.v.* which inhibits the ability of a fertilized egg to become implanted in the uterine wall. ~s do not prevent ovulation *q.v.*

MINI-RESIDENCY Training designed to provide ample opportunity for trainees to acquire experience in the basic principles of environmental disease and to better understand how to assess the exposure of an individual patient to hazardous substances and any attendant health effects.

MINNESOTA MULTIPHASIC PERSONALITY INVENTORY (MMPI) 1. An inventory that uses several psychiatric criterion groups to its subscales. 2. A lengthy personality inventory through which an individual diagnosis is made as a result of responses to questions related to anxiety, depression, masculinity/femininity, and paranoia. 3. An inventory that is easily administered, covering a wide range of topics, while providing important diagnostic information.

MINORITIES Any group that has a relatively small representation in comparison to the whole population with respect to employment, school, voting eligibility, etc.

MINORITY ENVIRONMENTAL HEALTH PROGRAM (MEHP) A program initiated by the ATSDR *q.v.* to improve data acquisition, research, and health information dissemination and education programs regarding minorities, with specific emphasis in three main areas: 1. demographic analysis *q.v.*, 2. health perspectives, and 3. health communications.

MINORITY GROUP A small number of people within a society. Members of racial minority groups who are elderly bear a double burden of discrimination *q.v.* based on both race and age.

MINORITY LEADER In politics, a member of the minority party designated to be leader.

MINORITY PARTY The political party holding less than a majority of seats in a legislative body.

MINORITY OPINION A statement expressing the views of a justice who has voted in dissent of the majority opinion with respect to a particular case. There may be several minority opinions expressed from different members of the court.

MINORITY REPORT A report reflecting the views of the minority of members or a court or legislative body with respect to a particular matter.

MINORITY RULE A decision of the court that runs contrary to the opinions of the majority of courts on a particular matter. ct: majority rule.

MINORITY WHIP A member of the minority party in a legislative body who is second in command with respect to minority party leadership.

MINOR MOTOR SEIZURES Seizures *q.v.* that are (a) myoclonic—shock-like contractions of muscles or muscle groups, (b) akinetic—sudden loss of muscle tone, and (c) infantile spasms—"jackknife" seizures.

MINOR TRANQUILIZERS 1. Drugs used to treat anxiety, nervous tension, and some neuroses *q.v.* They are addicting *q.v.* and produce withdrawal syndrome *q.v.* 2. A pharmacological and chemical classification of tranquilizers *q.v.* 3. Antianxiety agents that function somewhat like a sedative-hypnotic *q.v.* including meprobramate *q.v.* and the benzodiazepines *q.v.* ct: major tranquilizers.

MINUTES An accurate record of the proceedings of a meeting.

MIOSIS Constriction of the pupils of the eyes. ct: mydriasis.

MIRROR-IMAGE Applied to antagonistic groups, each believing that they are right and their enemy was mistaken and threatening.

MIRRORING A technique used in psychodrama *q.v.* in which an individual attempts to see himself or herself as another person, thereby acquiring an understanding of how others view him or her.

MIS 1. An acronym for management information system *q.v.* 2. An acronym for Mullerian inhibiting substance *q.v.*

MISATTRIBUTION (MISLABELING) The erroneous interpretation of physical cues.

MISCARRIAGE 1. Spontaneous abortion *q.v.* 2. The spontaneous expulsion of the product of conception early in pregnancy. 3. The premature and spontaneous expulsion of the fetus *q.v.*, esp. between the 4th and 7th month of pregnancy.

MISCONCEPTION (HEALTH) 1. An erroneous conception. 2. The erroneous acquisition of health information. 3. An erroneous health attitude. 4. The erroneous acquisition of health information that may influence the development of erroneous health attitudes resulting in unhealthful behavior.

MISDEMEANOR 1. A criminal offense lower than a felony and usually punished by a fine, imprisonment, or both. 2. A minor crime *q.v.* such as disorderly conduct. ct: felony.

MISFEASANCE 1. The improper performance of an act for which one is responsible. 2. The improper performance of a lawful act.

MISSION The total and complete end result of all learning experiences. The achievement of the sum total of all goals and objectives.

MISSIONARY POSITION A front-to-front position in sexual intercourse with the male above the female. Introduced by missionaries to the "heathens."

MISTRESS A woman whose lifestyle as a sex partner is maintained by a man to whom she is not married and who does not provide her with other payment for sexual intercourse.

MITIGATING CIRCUMSTANCES Those circumstances that may exonerate a person charged with a crime or which may reduce the extent of the person's culpability in the commission of the crime.

MITOCHONDRIA 1. The largest organelles *q.v.* in the cytoplasm *q.v.* The cell ~ contain important enzymatic *q.v.*, oxidative *q.v.*, and respiratory systems. 2. Small bodies in the cytoplasm of most cells. 3. The site of cellular respiration. 4. Cytoplasmic organelles that contain enzymes of the Krebs cycle *q.v.* and of oxidative phosphorylation *q.v.*

MITOSIS 1. Cell division in which the daughter cells contain precisely the same gametic *q.v.* material as the mother cell. 2. The process by which the body grows and replaces cells. 3. Ordinary cell division involving nuclear *q.v.* and cytoplasmic *q.v.* fission *q.v.* and resulting in two new cells, each containing the full complement of 46 chromosomes.

MITRAL Shaped like a miter.

MITRAL VALVE 1. Bicuspid valve. 2. A two-cusp valve that regulates blood flow between the left atrium *q.v.* and the left ventricle *q.v.* of the heart.

MITRAL VALVE PROLAPSE (MVP) 1. A common but rarely dangerous heart valve dysfunction. The mitral valve, which separates the upper and lower chamber in the left side of the heart, may not close properly causing a click sound to the physician through a stethoscope and may be followed by a murmur. 2. A defect of the mitral heart valve; considered a predisposing factor for a panic disorder *q.v.*

MITTELSCHMERZ 1. Intermenstrual pain. Signals the moment of ovulation *q.v.* 2. German for "middle pain," the discomfort some women feel at the time of ovulation.

MIXED DESIGN A research strategy in which both experimental and classificatory variables are used. Assigning subjects from discrete populations to two experimental conditions is an example.

MIXED (CEREBRAL) DOMINANCE A term applied to certain learning disorders, particularly in terms of language, caused because neither hemisphere of the brain is dominant. cf: cerebral dominance.

MIXED HEARING LOSS A hearing impairment caused by both a conductive disorder and sensorineural problems.

ml An abbreviation for milliliter *q.v.*

ml O_2/min/kg 1. Milliliters of oxygen consumed per minute, divided by body mass in kilograms. 2. The measure of maximal oxygen consumption during exercise.

MLV An acronym for mean length of utterance *q.v.*

mm An abbreviation for millimeter *q.v.*

mmHg PRES Millimeter mercury pressure.

MMPI An acronym for Minnesota Multiphasic Personality Inventory *q.v.*

MMR An abbreviation for measles, mumps, and rubella vaccine.

MNC An acronym for multinational corporation.

MNEMONIC DEVICE A memory aid or system designed to improve a person's ability to recall. cf: mnemonics.

MNEMONICS Deliberate devices for helping memory. cf: mnemonic device.

MOBAN A commercial preparation of molindone *q.v.*

MOBILE 1. A radio, cell phone, or other device designed for installation in and operation from a vehicle. 2. Movable.

MOBILE INTENSIVE CARE UNIT A vehicle designed to provide specialized emergency care of serious conditions such as cardiac *q.v.* damage, or a severe trauma *q.v.*, and containing operating room facilities and other special emergency equipment.

MOBILITY 1. The movement of people from one position in a system or stratification to another. 2. Geographic mobility. 3. Social mobility.

MOCK-UP A simplified and clarified working model of part or all of a real device or situation.

MOC An acronym for maximum oxygen consumption *q.v.*

MODE 1. In statistics *q.v.*, any class occurring most frequently. 2. A measure of central tendency *q.v.*

MODEL 1. A composite of concepts delineated in a manner that illustrates the ways in which a program shall be implemented. 2. A concept, usually depicted in the form of a chart or diagram, around which a set of principles, relationships, and conclusions can be discussed. 3. A method of theorizing in which there is an attempt to understand the information of one field of study in terms of the formal structure of some other field of study, e.g., psychology and physiology.

MODELING 1. Learning through observation. 2. Observational learning *q.v.* as in social learning theory *q.v.*

3. Adoption by one individual, often a child, of another's practices or attitudes.

MODELING THEORY A theory of pornography's effects on the future behavior of those exposed to pornographic materials. cf: catharsis; null theory.

MODEL PSYCHOSIS Psychotic *q.v.*-like states produced by certain hallucinogenic *q.v.* chemicals or drugs.

MODELS OF HEALTH See health models.

MODERATE CONSUMPTION Infrequent and relatively light ingestion of foods, alcohol, and other substances. Applied chiefly to alcohol.

MODERATE LEARNING AND BEHAVIOR DISORDERS Individuals who exhibit learning and behavioral disorders that are 2–3 standard deviations below the norm. The causes for the deficits may or may not be known. These individuals require substantially altered environmental accommodations and patterns of treatment.

MODERATE MENTAL RETARDATION A description of an individual whose intelligence quotient *q.v.* is between 35 and 49. Children with this level of intelligence are often institutionalized, with their training focused on self-care.

MODIFIED MASTECTOMY Surgical removal of the breast and lymph nodes *q.v.* cf: mastectomy; radical mastectomy; lumpectomy.

MODIFIED RADICAL MASTECTOMY Surgical removal of the breast, some fat, and most of the axillary lymph nodes *q.v.*, leaving the chest muscles intact.

MODIFIED UNION SHOP Any modification from the standard union shop which requires that all employees join a union after they are hired.

MODIFIER (MODIFYING GENE) A gene *q.v.* that affects or influences the expression of another nonallelic *q.v.* gene.

MODULAR SCHEDULING In education, the scheduling of classes for varying lengths of time to allow for greater flexibility.

MODULAR UNIT A unit responds to a relatively narrow band of wavelengths. May be related to color vision. ct: dominator unit.

MODUS OPERANDI The manner or mode of behavior.

MOIST SNUFF A type of smokeless tobacco, which is finely ground and moist. A pinch is held behind the lower lip or between the cheek and gum with nicotine absorbed through the mucous membranes of the mouth.

MOLAR BEHAVIOR Behavior *q.v.* that is viewed in terms of large units. ct: molecular behavior.

MOLAR BONE The cheekbone.

MOLAR CONCENTRATION The number of grams *q.v.* solute *q.v.* per liter *q.v.* of solution *q.v.* divided by the solute's molecular weight.

MOLARS The teeth used to grind food located posterior to the bicuspids *q.v.* Also called first and second molars or 6-and 12-year molars. Wisdom teeth located in the far most posterior part of the mouth are the third molars.

MOLD A plant, some of which are pathogenic *q.v.* Examples of diseases caused by a mold are mycosis *q.v.* and ringworm (tinea) *q.v.*

MOLE 1. Molecular weight of a compound expressed in grams *q.v.* 2. Gram molecular weight.

MOLECULAR BEHAVIOR Behavior *q.v.* analyzed into its components.

MOLECULAR BIOLOGY Genetic medicine *q.v.*

MOLECULAR MEDICINE Genetic medicine *q.v.*

MOLECULAR WEIGHT The weight of a molecule *q.v.* of a chemical compound *q.v.* as compared with the weight of an atom of hydrogen *q.v.* ~ is equal to the sum of the weight of the constituent atoms.

MOLECULE 1. Matter *q.v.* consisting of two or more atoms *q.v.* The atoms may be the same, as in oxygen (O_2), or different, as in water (H_2O). 2. The smallest amount of a specific chemical substance that can exist alone. 3. In chemistry, a unit of matter, the smallest portion of an element or compound that retains chemical identity with the substance in mass. Usually consists of a union of two or more atoms.

MOLES Densely packed skin cells that are pigmented brown or black.

MOLESTATION An act of meddling or interfering. Often a result of abnormal sexual motivation or activity.

MOLINDONE An antipsychotic *q.v.* Moban is the brand name.

MOLT The shedding of an outer covering.

MONGOLISM 1. A type of mental retardation *q.v.* resulting from the presence of one extra chromosome *q.v.* in each body cell. 2. Down syndrome *q.v.* 3. A label for those with Down syndrome. No longer acceptable as a descriptor for this condition.

MONILLA 1. Candida *q.v.* 2. Moniliasis *q.v.*, a yeast infection resulting in itching and inflammation of the vagina *q.v.* 3. An infection of practically any tissue of the body with a mold known as *Candida albicans*.

MONISM A philosophy that holds that reality is a unified whole and that mental and physical attributes are one and the same. ct: dualism.

MONITOR 1. A person who receives, and often records, radio or other electronic messages without himself or herself transmitting. 2. To attend to, by person or device, the physiological activities of a person, usually a victim of an accident or one who is critically ill.

MONITORIAL SCHOOLS 1. Schools developed by Joseph Lancaster and Andrew Bell in which one teacher taught a number of bright students with monitors who, in turn, taught other groups of students. 2. Schools in which the brightest students were taught and in turn they taught other students.

MONOAMINE An organic compound containing nitrogen in one amino group (NH_2). Some of the neurotransmitters *q.v.* in the central nervous system *q.v.* are ~s.

MONOAMINE OXIDASE 1. A drug having a central nervous system *q.v.* stimulant effect and that blocks a specific enzyme *q.v.*, increasing a neurotransmitter *q.v.* that helps to elevate and relieve depression *q.v.* 2. An antidepressant drug *q.v.* 3. An enzyme that deactivates catecholamines *q.v.* and indoleamine *q.v.* within the presynaptic neuron *q.v.*

MONOAMINE OXIDASE INHIBITORS A group of antidepressant drugs that prevents the enzyme *q.v.* monoamine oxidase *q.v.* from deactivating neurotransmitters *q.v.* in the central nervous system *q.v.* With the resultant increase in norepinephrine *q.v.* and serotonin *q.v.* available in the synapse, the mood is elevated.

MONOCLONAL ANTIBODIES 1. Homogenous antibodies from clones of a single cell. ~ recognize only one chemical structure which make them highly specific in their action. 2. Antibodies *q.v.* produced by clones *q.v.* from one original antigen–antibody complex.

MONOCLONAL CELL PROLIFERATION THEORY A theory that holds that there is a proliferation of an atherosclerotic *q.v.* stem from one mutated *q.v.* cell.

MONOCULAR DEPTH CUES Various features of the visual stimulus that indicate depth, even when viewed with only one eye.

MONOCULAR MOVEMENT PARALLAX Apparent motion *q.v.* seen when the eye is fixed on a particular stimulus *q.v.* when the body is in motion.

MONOCYTE 1. A large phagocytic *q.v.* white blood cell which, when it enters a tissue, develops into a macrophage *q.v.* 2. A large white blood cell having a single nucleus *q.v.*

MONOGAMOUS A paired relationship with one partner. cf: monogamy.

MONOGAMY 1. A condition in which a man has one wife and a woman has one husband. 2. A man and a woman married to each other and to no one else. 3. A homosexual relationship in which two people maintain an exclusive relationship. ct: polygamy.

MONOGENETIC MODEL The theory that considers a disorder to be the result of a single gene.

MONOGENETIC TRAIT A trait that is controlled by a single gene.

MONOGLYCERIDE A glycerol *q.v.* ester *q.v.* containing one fatty acid *q.v.*

MONOHYBRID 1. A cross between two parents differing only in a single gene. 2. Monohybrid cross.

MONOKIINES Powerful chemical substances secreted by monocytes *q.v.* and macrophages *q.v.* that help direct the immune response *q.v.*

MONOMANIA A compulsive preoccupation with one idea or activity.

MONOMER A simple molecule *q.v.* of a compound of relatively low molecular weight.

MONONUCLEAR LEUKOCYTES Large white blood cells that have only one nucleus *q.v.*

MONOECIOUS 1. Having both male and female reproductive organs in the same individual. 2. Hermaphroditic.

MONONUCLEOSIS An acute infection caused by an unidentified virus. Most prevalent among children and adolescents. Transmitted by direct contact with an infected person. Characterized by fever, sore throat, headache, fatigue, chills, malaise *q.v.*, lymph node *q.v.* involvement, and an excess of agglutinins *q.v.* present in the blood.

MONOPHOSPHOESTERASE Milk enzyme.

MONOPLEGIA A paralysis in one arm or one leg. ct: paraplegia.

MONOPLOID 1. Haploid. 2. An individual having a single set of chromosomes *q.v.* or one genome *q.v.*

MONORCHISM The condition of having only one testicle *q.v.* in the scrotum *q.v.*

MONOSACCHARIDES 1. Simple sugars: glucose, fructose, and galactose *qq.v.* 2. Carbohydrate *q.v.* compounds of one saccharide unit. cf: disaccharides; polysaccharides.

MONOSODIUM GLUTAMATE (MSG) An artificial flavor enhancer commonly used in restaurants and in processed foods.

MONOSOMIC A diploid *q.v.* organism lacking one chromosome *q.v.* of its normal complement.

MONOTHEISM The acceptance of or belief in one god.

MONOTONIC RELATIONSHIP In research, any relationship in which steady increases or decreases of the dependent variable *q.v.* are associated with increases of the independent variable *q.v.*

MONOTRICHOUS A flagellar arrangement with a single flagellum arising at the end of the cell.

MONOSATURATED FATTY ACID 1. A fatty acid *q.v.* with one double bond, as in oleic acid *q.v.* 2. Fats *q.v.* made of compounds in which one hydrogen-bonding position remains to be filled. 3. ~ is semisolid at room temperature and derived chiefly from peanut and olive oils.

MONOXIDIL A drug used for the treatment of hypertension *q.v.* Side effects include an increase in body hair growth. The drug is used for the treatment of baldness.

MONOZYGOTIC TWINS 1. Identical twins *q.v.* 2. Two infants developed from one fertilized egg. ct: dizygotic twins.

MONS PUBIS The mound consisting the pubic hair in the female. Also called the mount of Venus. cf: mons veneris.

MONS VENERIS 1. The mount of Venus. 2. The rounded fleshy prominence over the symphysis pubis *q.v.* 3. A triangular shaped mound of fat at the symphysis pubis of a woman, just above the vulval area. cf: mons pubis.

MOOD 1. Moderate changes in emotions *q.v.* 2. An emotional state of relatively long duration, but usually less intense than an emotion.

MOOD MODIFICATION A change in thinking, feeling, and possible behavior. Frequently caused by the use of a psychoactive drug *q.v.*

MOONLIGHTING The process of accepting additional employment outside of a regular teaching position. Also descriptive of a physician who works at a different hospital or clinic in his or her off hours from regular employment.

MOONSHINING The illegal production of distilled spirits.

MOOT CASE In law, a case in which the facts do not support the proposed litigation, either because of legal precedent or because the facts of the case have changed.

MOR A GRIFA Marijuana *q.v.*

MORAL ANXIETY In psychoanalytic theory *q.v.*, fear of punishment based in the ego *q.v.* for failure to adhere to the superego's *q.v.* standards of proper conduct.

MORAL DEVELOPMENT Stages in the development of the concepts of right and wrong.

MORALITY OF CONSTRAINT 1. Moral thinking typical of children up to about the age of 10, characterized by sacred rules, no exceptions, no allowance for intentions. 2. Moral realism. ct: morality of cooperation.

MORALITY OF COOPERATION Moral thinking typical of children about 12 years and older characterized by flexible rules, mutual agreements, and allowance for intentions. ct: morality of constraint.

MORAL JUDGMENT The process through which a person decides that some action is good or bad.

MORAL MAJORITY Those persons who possess a conservative religiously oriented view of life.

MORAL MORON A person who fails to develop adequate moral *q.v.* values.

MORAL REALISM 1. Morality of constraint *q.v.* 2. A literal interpretation of rules. 3. Real values as opposed to idealistic assumptions. 4. The belief that rules governing human social behavior are as fixed and inalterable as the laws of physics. ct: moral relativism.

MORAL RELATIVISM 1. The concept of rules as changeable human conventions based on reciprocal agreement among those who use them. 2. The belief that rules governing social behavior as arbitrary conventions were adopted by society for the mutual benefit of members of a society. ct. moral realism.

MORALS Concrete decisions pertaining to right and wrong.

MORAL TREATMENT MOVEMENT 1. An innovative method of treating the mentally ill in "hospitals" during the late eighteenth century. Introduced by Philippe Pinel *q.v.* in 1792 and characterized by removal of the chains and shackles from the mentally ill patients at the Bicetre hospital *q.v.* See also Vincenzo Chuarugi *q.v.* 2. Characterized by treating the mentally ill more humanely—patients were given sufficient food, chains removed, and attempts at habilitation. 3. A method whereby patients were treated with compassion and dignity rather than with contempt and denigration. cf: milieu therapy.

MORAL VALUES Those values that relate to a person's behavior or conduct with and treatment of other people.

MORATORIUM TYPE An adolescent *q.v.* who is suffering an identity crisis because of confusion or indecision about sex role and/or occupational choice.

MORBID 1. Unhealthy. 2. Pathological *q.v.*

MORBIDITY 1. Illness, sickness, or disease. 2. ~ rates measure the level of illness in a given population. The case-specific formula is

$$\frac{\text{Number of cases of a specific disease}}{\text{Total population}} \times 1000.$$

3. The ratio of persons who are ill or disabled to the total number within a population *q.v.*

MORBIDITY RISK The probability that a person will develop a particular disease or disorder.

MORBIDITY STATISTICS The reported incidence *q.v.* of specified diseases and other health issues.

MORDANT Substances that provide the necessary prerequisites for dye absorption.

MORES Customs or conventions enforced by social pressure.

MORNING-AFTER CONTRACEPTIVE 1. A contraceptive that may be used after unprotected coitus *q.v.* has taken place. 2. An oral or injectable procedure used to prevent pregnancy if no other contraceptives have been used and if later abortion is not preferable, such as when a rape has occurred.

MORNING NAUSEA Morning sickness *q.v.*

MORNING SICKNESS A condition consisting of a group of symptoms including feelings of nauseousness and vomiting shortly after awakening in the morning and associated with early pregnancy *q.v.*

MORON A form of mental retardation *q.v.* in which the person has an intelligence quotient *q.v.* of 50–70. It is a term that is considered obsolete. ct: idiot; imbecile.

MORPHEME 1. The smallest significant unit of meaning in a language. 2. A word or part of a word that cannot be subdivided into other meaningful elements. cf: closed-class morphemes; open-class morphemes.

MORPHEUS The Greek god of dreams. Morphine *q.v.* derived its name from ~.

MORPHOGENESIS The origin and development of form and structure in an organism.

MORPHINE 1. An opiate *q.v.* 2. A narcotic *q.v.* drug. 3. Morphine sulfate crystallized by Frederick Serturner in 1803. 4. A highly effective pain killer and a treatment for dysentery *q.v.* 5. The standard by which all other analgesics are measured.

MORPHINE ADDICTION A dependency *q.v.* on morphine *q.v.* Psychological and physiological dependency with the withdrawal syndrome *q.v.* upon denial of the drug.

MORPHINE SULFATE 1. Crystallized from opium *q.v.* 2. Morphine *q.v.* 3. A narcotic *q.v.*

MORPHINISM An outdated term used to describe dependency *q.v.* on the use of morphine *q.v.*

MORPHOGENESIS The morphological *q.v.* and physiological *q.v.* events involved in the formation of an organism.

MORPHOLOGICAL RULES Those rules of grammar that deal with the combination of morphemes *q.v.* into words.

MORPHOLOGY 1. The study of the form and structure of organisms. 2. The form and structure of a person as a whole. 3. The study of the form, structure, and development of plants and animals. 4. The form and structure of words.

MORTALITY Death.

MORTALITY RATE 1. Death rate. 2. The number of deaths in relation to population, usually given per 100,000 population. 3. The ratio of persons who have died to the total number of persons in the population during a given period of time.

MORULA 1. A round mass of cells that develops from the original fertilized egg within a few days after fertilization *q.v.* 2. A cell mass formed by cleavage of the ovum *q.v.* shortly after fertilization and before the blastocyst *q.v.* stage and implantation *q.v.*

MOSAIC An organism, part of which is made up of tissue genetically different from the remaining part.

MOSAIC EGG A fertilized egg in which a high degree of development has already occurred at the time of fertilization *q.v.*

MOSAICISM 1. The presence of different chromosome *q.v.* numbers in different body cells. In humans, some contain 46 chromosomes, while others contain 47 chromosomes. 2. A form of Down syndrome *q.v.* 3. A type of Down syndrome in which the chromosomal abnormality occurs after fertilization *q.v.*

MOTHERESE The speech pattern that adults use (esp. mothers) when talking to infants.

MOTILE Capable of spontaneous movement.

MOTILITY 1. Pertaining to motion or movement. 2. The ability to move spontaneously. 3. Sperm *q.v.* motility.

MOTION In parliamentary procedure, a formal proposal offered by a member of a deliberative body.

MOTION PARALLAX A visual cue to depth created when images of distant objects are displaced less than the images of near objects when the object themselves or the observer moves.

MOTION SICKNESS A sensation induced by repetitive motion and characterized by nausea *q.v.* and light-headedness.

MOTION STUDY Finding the best way to accomplish a task by analyzing the movements necessary to perform the task.

MOTION TO RECONSIDER In parliamentary deliberations, a motion to place the question in the same status it was in prior to the vote on the question.

MOTIVATED PERCEPTION The tendency to view people or events in self-gratifying ways.

MOTIVATING FACTORS Items that influence the type of behavior to be performed and the degree of satisfaction received in performing the behavior.

MOTIVATION 1. An internal urge to behave. ~ may be automatic and intrinsic *q.v.*; extrinsic *q.v.* as from an environmental factor, or from conscious desires and aspirations. 2. An intervening variable *q.v.* that refers to the energizing of behavior *q.v.* 3. A cue to all motivation in education is the natural human desire for self-status through attention, achievement, advancement, improvement, superiority, praise, and recognition. 4. A drive or activation. 5. A person's behavior is partly determined in direction and strength by his or her own inner nature. 6. Arousal, selection, direction, and continuation of behavior. 7. An internal urge to behave. An individual's inner state that causes him or her to behave in a way that ensures the achievement of some predetermined goal. cf: motivational force; motive.

MOTIVATIONAL FORCE A stimulus *q.v.* or stimuli that results in behavior *q.v.* cf: motivation; motive.

MOTIVATIONAL SEQUENCE Need-goal-means-satisfaction sequence. cf: need-satisfaction sequence.

MOTIVATION STRENGTH An individual's level of desire to perform or engage in a behavior.

MOTIVE 1. An internal force that compels a person to behave in a particular way under particular circumstances. 2. An internal condition that directs a person's action toward some goal. 3. A drive and goal toward which action is directed.

MOTONEURON 1. Motor neurons *q.v.* 2. Efferent neurons *q.v.* 3 ~ transmits nerve impulses away from the brain or spinal cord.

MOTOR DEVELOPMENT The development of behaviors involving the skeletal muscles *q.v.* and the motor neurons *q.v.*

MOTOR DIVISION That part of the peripheral nervous system *q.v.* that transmits messages outward from the central nervous system *q.v.* to effectors *q.v.*

MOTORS NERVES 1. A bundle of nerves, conducting impulses independently, connecting the central nervous system *q.v.* to the effectors *q.v.* 2. Fibers of tissue that conduct impulses from the brain to muscle tissue. 3. An efferent nerve that stimulates a muscle contraction in response to a conscious, willed thought or reflex *q.v.*

MOTOR PROJECTION AREAS One aspect of projection areas *q.v.* ct: sensory projection areas.

MOTOR TENSION Physical signs of anxiety including shaking, jitters, restlessness, and the like.

MOTOR THEORY OF CONSCIOUSNESS The theory *q.v.* that mental experience results from stimulation arising from muscular activity.

MOU An acronym for memorandum of understanding.

MOUNT OF VENUS 1. The mons pubis. 2. The mons veneris.

MOURNING PROCESS The period of time and the emotional stages of grief *q.v.* from the time of a tragedy through recovery and acceptance.

MOURNING WORK According to Freud's theory of depression *q.v.*, the recall of memories of the lost one that assists in separating the individual from the deceased.

MOUTH GAG A device for protecting a victim's tongue during a convulsion and/or controlling the tongue during the insertion of an artificial airway.

MOUTH-TO-MOUTH RESUSCITATION The oral technique of resuscitation *q.v.* whereby the paramedic *q.v.* places his or her mouth over the mouth of the victim who is not breathing and blows air into the victim's lungs.

MOUTHWASH A chemical substance in liquid form used as an oral rinse.

MPA Medroxyprogesterone acetate *q.v.*

MPC An acronym for maximum permissible concentration of radiation.

MRI An acronym for magnetic resonance imaging.

MPN An acronym for most probable number.

MRL An acronym for minimal risk level *q.v.*

MRNA RNA molecule formed in the transcription process—messenger RNA *q.v.*

MRT An acronym for major role therapy *q.v.*

MSG An acronym for monosodium glutamate *q.v.*

MSH An acronym for melanocyte-stimulating hormone *q.v.*

M-space The term used by Pascual-Leone to label the storage capacity of short-term memory *q.v.*

MTF An acronym for medical treatment facility.

MUCIN 1. Secretions containing mucopolysaccharides *q.v.* 2. The chief constituent of mucus *q.v.*

MUCOID Resembling mucus *q.v.*

MUCOPOLYSACCHARIDE A complex of protein *q.v.* and polysaccharides *q.v.*

MUCOPROTEIN A complex of protein *q.v.* and oligosaccharides *q.v.*

MUCOSA 1. A mucous membrane *q.v.* 2. A thin tissue whose surface is kept moist by the secretion of mucus *q.v.*

MUCOUS 1. Pertaining to or resembling mucus *q.v.* 2. Secreting mucus. cf: mucous membrane.

MUCOUS MEMBRANE 1. Mucosa *q.v.* 2. The lining of body cavities and passages which communicate directly or indirectly with the exterior.

MUCOUS PATCHES White patches, usually found in the mouth, which may be highly infectious symptoms of secondary syphilis *q.v.*

MUCUS 1. A viscous secretion produced by the mucous membranes *q.v.* that moisten and protect the membranes. 2. A thick, slippery substance secreted by the mucosa *q.v.* ~ traps much of the suspended particulate *q.v.* matter present in tobacco smoke or other air contaminants.

MUCOUS METHOD A method of predicting the fertile period in a woman's cycle by means of the texture, color, and quantity of the cervical *q.v.* mucus *q.v.* cf: ovulation method.

MULLERIAN DUCTS 1. Ducts *q.v.* in the embryo *q.v.* that develop into the fallopian tubes *q.v.*, the uterus *q.v.*, and possibly the upper region of the vagina *q.v.* in females. 2. The primitive genital ducts that, under hormonal *q.v.* influence, evolve into the female genitalia *q.v.* cf: Wolffian ducts.

MULLERIAN DUCT SYSTEM The tissue in a fetus *q.v.* that develops into the internal female reproductive structures when the fetus is genetically female.

MULLERIAN INHIBITING HORMONE 1. A hormone *q.v.* produced by the testes *q.v.* that prevents the development of female internal genitalia *q.v.* 2. A hormone secreted by the fetal testes that inhibits the growth and development of the Mullerian duct system *q.v.* 3. Also called Mullerian inhibiting substance (MIS).

MULTIAXIAL In psychology, having several dimensions, each of which is used in determining diagnosis. cf: multiaxial diagnosis.

MULTIAXIAL DIAGNOSIS A diagnostic system for classifying behavior on several dimensional axes.

MULTICENTRIC Having many centers.

MULTICULTURALISM An environment with many cultures working together with mutual respect toward complementary goals.

MULTICULTURAL EDUCATION Education for cultural understanding and respect.

MULTIEJACULATORY Repeated orgasms *q.v.* and ejaculations *q.v.* without the male experiencing the typical refractory period *q.v.*

MULTIFACTORIAL Referring to many variables *q.v.* concurrently influencing the development, maintenance, or operation of a phenomenon.

MULTIFACTORIAL INHERITANCE Genetic *q.v.* traits caused by a combination of factors, genes, chromosomes, prenatal development. cf: genetic defects; genetic health.

MULTIFACTORIAL THEORIES Explanations of phenomena based on two or more interacting factors or causative influences.

MULTIGRAVIDA Having given birth earlier. Pertains to a woman who has been previously pregnant *q.v.* and who has given birth. ct: primigravida.

MULTIMODAL APPROACH 1. A combination of therapies, e.g., drug therapy, behavioral therapy, psychoanalysis, used to assist a patient with mental illness. 2. Multimodality therapeutic approach.

MULTIORGASMIC 1. Multiorgasmic capacity *q.v.* 2. The potential ability to experience a series of identifiable orgasmic responses without dropping below the plateau level *q.v.* of arousal.

MULTIORGASMIC CAPACITY 1. The potential to have several orgasms *q.v.* within a single period of sexual arousal and activity. 2. Multiorgasmic *q.v.*

MULTIPARA A woman who has given birth to two or more children.

MULTIPHASIC SCREENING A health screening *q.v.* procedure consisting of a battery of tests administered at one time.

MULTIPLE ALLELES Three or more alternative genes *q.v.* representing the same locus on a given pair of chromosomes *q.v.*

MULTIPLE-BASELINE DESIGN An experimental design in which two behaviors of a single subject are selected with one being treated. The behavior that is not treated is used as a baseline against which the treatment can be compared.

MULTIPLE BIRTH The birth of more than one baby at a time, twins, triplets, etc.

MULTIPLE CAUSATION The concept that a given disease *q.v.* has a number of different but interrelated causes. Three general categories exist: (a) host-related factors, (b) agent-related factors, and (c) environmental factors.

MULTIPLE CHOICE TEST ITEMS A test item consisting of a stem and several possible answers or responses, only one of which is correct.

MULTIPLE GENES Two or more independent pairs of genes *q.v.* whose functions complement each other to produce a cumulative effect upon the same trait.

MULTIPLE MYELOMA A form of bone cancer *q.v.* centering its growth in the bone marrow *q.v.*

MULTIPLE ORGASMS Multiorgasmic *q.v.*

MULTIPLE PERSONALITY 1. A rare neurosis *q.v.*, characterized by the person developing more than one distinct personality. The personalities are usually in traits. These are representative of competing motives *q.v.* of behavior and are perceived as two different people within the same physical or biological structure. 2. A dissociative reaction involving the expression by one individual of two or more distinct personalities that have varying degrees of awareness of each other.

MULTIPLE PREGNANCY A pregnancy in which there is more than one fetus *q.v.*

MULTIPLE REGRESSION A form of multivariate analysis used when three or more variables are examined. It allows the researcher to determine the net effect of each independent variable on the dependent variable.

MULTIPLE SCLEROSIS A group of diseases in which the myelin sheath *q.v.* of nerves is destroyed and replaced with scar tissue.

MULTIPLEXING Transmitting several messages simultaneously on the same radio circuit or channel.

MULTIPURPOSE HIGH SCHOOL Features comprehensive curricula in a variety of subject areas to meet the needs of all students regardless of their needs, interests, or aptitudes.

MULTISITE EPIDEMIOLOGIC STUDIES Studies that increase the sample sizes for statistical analysis by combining populations from several sites to draw more definitive conclusions between exposure and outcome.

MUMPS 1. Parotitis *q.v.* 2. A disease caused by an unidentified virus *q.v.* Transmitted by salivary droplets from an infected person directly or indirectly. Characterized by fever, tenderness, and swelling of the glands under the jaw and in front of the ears (one side or both), possible involvement of the ovaries or testes *qq.v.* in persons who are reproductively mature. ~ can be prevented by proper immunization *q.v.*

MURIFORM A multicelled conidia with cross walls at right angles to each other.

MURINE TYPHUS Typhus *q.v.* spread by the bite of a rat flea.

MURMUR 1. An abnormal heart sound-like fluid passing an obstruction. The sound is heard between the normal hearty beats. 2. An atypical heart sound that suggests a backwashing of blood into a chamber of the heart from which it has just left.

MUSCA DOMESTICA The housefly.

MUSCARINIC CHOLINOCEPTIVE SITE A postjunctional receptor for acetylcholine.

MUSCLE An organ which by contraction produces movement of an organism. There are three types: striated, cardiac, and smooth *qq.v.*

MUSCLE ACTION POTENTIAL An electrical discharge associated with the activity of muscles *q.v.*

MUSCLE AVULSION FRACTURE A tearing away of a part of bone, usually by a tendon *q.v.*, ligament *q.v.*, or capsule *q.v.*

MUSCLE FATIGUE The inability of muscle tissue to maintain a desired exercise intensity.

MUSCLE FIBER 1. The basic structural unit of muscle *q.v.* 2. The muscle cell.

MUSCLE-TENSION-RELAXATION EXERCISE An exercise that uses progressive tension-relaxation to reduce the effects of stress *q.v.*

MUSCLE TONE A tension or slight contraction of the muscle *q.v.*

MUSCULAR DYSTROPHY 1. A genetic defect *q.v.* affecting the muscles and nerves. 2. A group of inherited *q.v.* disorders characterized by a gradual wasting or weakening of skeletal muscles *q.v.*

MUSCULAR ENDURANCE 1. The ability of a muscle or muscle group to continue functioning. ~ depends upon well-developed respiratory and circulatory systems. 2. A muscle's ability to continue submaximal contractions against a resistance. cf: endurance; muscular strength.

MUSCULAR ENDURANCE EXERCISE Repetitive, submaximal muscular contractions measured by the time to fatigue and performed by the major muscle groups of the body.

MUSCULAR STRENGTH 1. The ability to contract skeletal muscles to engage in work. 2. The amount of force a muscle must exert for one repetition. cf: strength; muscular endurance.

MUSCLE TONE The firmness of a muscle group in a relaxed state.

MUSCULOSKELETAL SYSTEM 1. The structural and functional independence of the muscular and skeletal systems *q.v.* 2. All the bones, muscles, and tendons of the body collectively.

MUTABLE GENES 1. Those genes *q.v.* with an unusually high mutation rate. 2. Unstable genes.

MUTAGEN A chemical or physical agent that caused genetic *q.v.* mutations *q.v.*

MUTAGENESIS Damage to genes *q.v.*

MUTAGENIC Capable of promoting genetic *q.v.* alterations in cells. cf: mutagenic effect.

MUTAGENIC EFFECT A production of a sudden change in the parent's genes that appears in the offspring due to a chemical or physical force. cf: mutagenic.

MUTANT A cell or individual organism that shows changes brought about by alterations (mutations) in genes *q.v.*

MUTATION 1. In genetics *q.v.*, a permanent change in the genetic material, usually a single gene *q.v.* 2. A spontaneous alteration of genetic material. 3. A change from one allelic *q.v.* form to another. 4. A chemical or physical change in the structure of a gene. 5. To mutilate. 6. To destroy. 7. A stable, transmissible change in a DNA *q.v.*

pattern. 8. A term that is loosely used to describe either a point mutation involving a single gene or chromosomal changes.

MUTATION, DIRECTED, OR SPECIFIC A mutation with a specific environmental cause.

MUTATION PRESSURE A constant mutation rate that adds mutant genes to a population.

MUTATION RATE The chance of occurrence of a mutation in a given length of time.

MUTATOR GENES Genes *q.v.* that increase the frequency of mutations *q.v.* in other genes.

MUTISM A refusal or an inability to speak.

MUTON The smallest unit of DNA *q.v.* that can undergo change resulting in a mutation *q.v.*

MUTUALITY According to Levinger, the stage of a relationship in which a couple thinks of themselves as "we."

MUTUALISM The cohabitation of two or more organisms in an association that is mutually beneficial. cf: symbiosis.

MUTUALLY EXCLUSIVE CATEGORIES In epidemiology *q.v.*, a situation in which each subject appears in only one category.

MUTUAL MASTURBATION Masturbation *q.v.* as a couple activity in which each person sexually stimulates himself or herself while the partner does the same or observes the other.

mV An abbreviation for millivolt.

MVP An acronym for mitral valve prolapse *q.v.*

MW An acronym for molecular weight.

MWTA An acronym for Medical Waste Tracking Act of 1988 *q.v.*

MYALGIA Muscle pain.

MYASTHENIA GRAVIS A progressive, fatal disease of the muscles characterized by slow paralysis *q.v.* of various muscle groups.

MYCELIUM A collective term applied to a mass of hyphae *q.v.*

MYCOBACTERIUM AVIUM-INTRACELLULARE A rare form of bacteria, related to the bacteria that causes tuberculosis, that is common in AIDS, but uncommon in those with healthy immune systems.

MYCOLOGY 1. The study of fungi *q.v.* 2. The study of diseases caused by fungi. Symbiotic *q.v.* relationship.

MYCOSIS A disease caused by a fungus *q.v.*

MYDRIASIS Dilation of the pupils of the eyes. ct: miosis.

MYELIN 1. The white, fatty insulating material that surrounds the axons *q.v.* of many nerve cells. 2. Lipoid *q.v.* substance in the myelin sheath *q.v.*

MYELINIZATION The process of a nerve developing a myelin *q.v.* sheath, which serves to speed nerve impulses.

MYELIN SHEATH Myelin. cf: myelinization.

MYELITIS 1. Inflammation or infection of the nerves of the spinal cord *q.v.* 2. Inflammation of the bone marrow *q.v.*

MYOCARDIAL CONTUSION A bruise of the muscular tissue of the heart.

MYOCARDIAL INFARCTION 1. Heart attack. 2. The death of cardiac muscles due to a severe lack of oxygen to the cells. Caused when a coronary artery or one of its branches becomes blocked, eliminating or severely limiting blood flow to a specific area of the heart. Coronary arteries may be blocked by a blood clot *q.v.*, spasms of the muscles in the walls of the arteries, or a buildup of atherosclerotic plaque *q.v.* in the lining of the arteries. 3. Damage or death of an area of the heart muscle, the myocardium *q.v.*, resulting from a reduction in blood supply reaching the area of the heart.

MYOCARDITIS Inflammation of the heart muscle.

MYOCARDIUM 1. The middle layer of the heart, consisting of the cardiac muscle. 2. The heart muscle.

MYOCLONIC JERKS Sudden, involuntary muscle spasms that accompany the onset of sleep.

MYOCLONIC SEIZURES A seizure *q.v.* that is characterized by shock-like contractions involving a muscle or group of muscles.

MYOCLONUS A condition wherein the muscles jerk involuntarily.

MYOGLOBIN The oxygen transporting protein of muscles, resembling hemoglobin *q.v.* in function.

MYOGLOBINURIA The excretion of myoglobin *q.v.* in the urine *q.v.* caused by certain instances of crush syndrome *q.v.* or an advanced or protracted ischemia *q.v.* of muscles.

MYOMA 1. A tumor *q.v.* consisting of muscle tissue that grows in the wall of the uterus. 2. Fibroid tumor.

MYOMETRIUM 1. The smooth muscle layer of the uterine *q.v.* wall. 2. Uterine muscles that contract and aid in delivery during childbirth. 3. The middle layer of the uterus consisting of smooth muscle *q.v.*, thereby aiding in the pushing of the fetus through the cervix *q.v.* during labor *q.v.*

MYONEURAL 1. Relating to both muscle and nerve. 2. The nerve terminations in muscular tissue.

MYOPIA Nearsightedness. The image theoretically falls in front of the retina *q.v.* of the eye because the axis of the eye is too long or the refractive power of the lens of the eye is too strong. ct: hyperopia.

MYOSIN One of the chief proteins *q.v.* of muscle.

MYOSITIS Inflammation *q.v.* of a muscle.

MYOTONIA 1. Muscle tension; sometimes resulting in muscles contractions and spasms. ~ increases during sexual arousal. 2. The delayed relaxation of a muscle following a contraction. 3. Involuntary muscle contraction.

MYOTONIC RESPONSE The muscle contractions that accompany sexual arousal.

MYRINGOTOMY An incision of the eardrum to establish drainage in infection of the middle ear *q.v.*

MYSTIC A person who alleges to have powers to communicate directly with god or with the dead.

MYRISTICIN A compound found in nutmeg thought to be responsible for its hallucinogenic *q.v.* effect following ingestion of large amounts of nutmeg.

MYSTICAL EXPERIENCE An experience often linked with the use of psychedelic *q.v.* or other psychoactive *q.v.* drugs in which the person feels extreme joy and contentment and a loss of sense of self.

MYSTIFICATION A repeated parental denial of a child's feelings and perceptions that results in the child losing his or her self-concept and sense of reality, resulting in chronic feelings of fear and guilt.

MYXEDEMA 1. A disorder resulting from a thyroid *q.v.* deficiency in adulthood and characterized by mental dullness. 2. An endocrine disorder of adults produced by thyroid deficiency, where metabolic processes are slowed and the person becomes lethargic, slow-thinking, and depressed. 3. Hypothyroidism *q.v.*

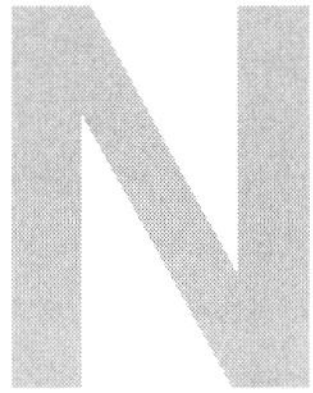

N 1. Newton *q.v.* 2. The chemical symbol for nitrogen.

Na The chemical symbol for sodium.

NABOTHIAN GLANDS Little glands *q.v.* at the neck of the cervix *q.v.* ~ may form cysts and require treatment.

NACHO An acronym for National Association for County Health Officials.

NaCl 1. Sodium chloride. 2. Table salt.

NAD 1. Nicotinamide adenine dinucleotide *q.v.*, frequently found as coenzymes *q.v.* in oxidation–reduction *q.v.* reactions. 2. ~ is also called DPN (diphosphopyridine nucleotide *q.v.*).

NADLE A third gender *q.v.* in the Navajo culture. Members of this gender are those who are dissatisfied or uncomfortable with the male and female gender roles as well as those born with ambiguous genitalia *q.v.*

NADP 1. Nicotinamide adenine dinucleotide phosphate *q.v.* 2. TPN, triphosphopyridine nucleotide *q.v.*

NAGELE'S RULE A method for determining the expected date of confinement *q.v.* relative to pregnancy *q.v.*, determined by adding 7 days to the first day of the last normal menstrual period *q.v.* and subtracting 3 months from this date.

NAILBED The area of the corium *q.v.* on which the toe or finger nail rests.

NALAXONE A drug *q.v.* that inhibits the effect of morphine *q.v.* and similar opiates *q.v.* and blocks the pain alleviation ascribed to endorphins *q.v.*

NALLINE 1. A semisynthetic derivative of morphine *q.v.* 2. Nalorphine hydrochloride *q.v.*

NALORPHINE HYDROCHLORIDE Nalline *q.v.*

NALOXONE 1. A narcotic antagonist *q.v.* 2. Narcan is a commercial preparation.

NALTREXONE 1. A narcotic antagonist *q.v.* 2. Trexan is a commercial preparation.

NAMH An acronym for National Association for Mental Health.

NARAPATHY A system of healing that asserts that disease originates in disturbed ligaments *q.v.* and connective tissue *q.v.*

NARCAN A commercial preparation of naloxone *q.v.*

NARCISSISM Excessive self-love. Sexual excitement through admiration of one's own body.

NARCISSISTIC PERSONALITY One who is extremely self-centered and selfish. The person who possesses this type of personality has a grandiose view of himself or herself and an insatiable craving for recognition and admiration from others. cf: narcissistic personality disorder.

NARCISSISTIC PERSONALITY DISORDER A disorder in which the person has a grandiose sense of self-importance, while having mood vacillations swinging from overidealization of self to extreme self-devaluation. cf: narcissistic personality.

NARCOANALYSIS 1. Narcotherapy *q.v.* 2. Narcosynthesis *q.v.*

NARCOLEPSY 1. A condition characterized by uncontrollable sleepiness. 2. A condition characterized by recurrent attacks of sleep, often induced by emotional stress. ~ has a neurological *q.v.* basis. 3. A sleep disorder characterized by muscle weakness and falling asleep involuntarily. Most commonly treated with stimulant drugs to maintain wakefulness. ct: neurasthenia.

NARCOSYNTHESIS 1. A psychotherapeutic procedure in which the person is under the influence of some hypnotic *q.v.* drug, e.g., sodium amytal *q.v.* 2. Narcoanalysis. 3. Narcotherapy *q.v.* 4. A psychiatric *q.v.* procedure originating during World War II in which drugs were employed to assist stressed soldiers in recalling their battle trauma.

NARCOTHERAPY 1. Narcosynthesis *q.v.* 2. Carrying on psychotherapy *q.v.* while the person is under the influence of a narcotic drug *q.v.*

NARCOTIC 1. A drug derived from opium *q.v.* or opium-like compounds that are analgesics, also producing significant alterations in mood and behavior. Addiction *q.v.* is possible, followed by a withdrawal syndrome *q.v.* upon the sudden, prolonged abstinence from the drug. 2. A group of drugs similar to morphine *q.v.* and used medicinally primarily for their analgesic effects.

NARCOTIC ANALGESICS A group of drugs that act on the central nervous system *q.v.* to eliminate or relieve pain without causing loss of consciousness.

NARCOTIC ANTAGONISTS 1. A group of drugs that act on the central nervous system *q.v.* to eliminate or relieve the effects of narcotics. They may block the euphoric effects of the narcotics being used or trigger a withdrawal syndrome *q.v.* Often used to treat overdose cases. 2. A drug or chemical that tends to neutralize the pharmacological *q.v.* effects of narcotic drugs *q.v.* 3. Drugs that tend to block or reverse the effects of narcotics.

NARCOTICS 1. Drugs that induce sedation *q.v.* in small amounts, coma and death in large amounts, insensitivity to pain, and feelings of euphoria. There are four legal classes: (1) class A ~, which include opium and its derivatives, coca leaves—their alkaloids and derivative—meperidine, methadone *q.v.*, and other synthetic opiates; (2) class B ~, which include drugs having relatively little addicting potential, including papaverine and codeine; (3) class M ~, which include those drugs that are especially exempt and may be prescribed by a physician, without filling out a narcotics order. Drugs in this class are considered nonaddicting. (4) Class X ~, which includes drugs containing a prescribed minimum amount of narcotic and are nonaddicting as prescribed. 2. Medically defined ~: any drug that induces sleep or stupor and relieves pain. 3. Legally defined as any drug regulated under the Harrison Narcotic Act *q.v.* and other federal narcotic laws. Some of these drugs are pharmacologically non-narcotics. 4. A drug that dulls the senses, reduces pain, and induces sleep. Large doses may result in stupor, coma, or convulsions. Heroin, morphine, and opium are narcotics.

NARCOTIZE To bring under the influence of a narcotic *q.v.*

NARDIL A commercial preparation of phenelzine *q.v.*

NARES Nostrils.

NAS An acronym for National Academy of Sciences.

NASAL Pertaining to the nose.

NASAL BONE Either of the two small oblong bones that together form the bridge of the nose.

NASAL CANNULA An apparatus for providing supplemental oxygen through a small tubular prong, which fits into the person's nostrils.

NAS/NRC An acronym for National Academy of Sciences, National Research Council *q.v.*

NASOLACRIMAL DUCT The passage leading downward from the lacrimal sac *q.v.* on each side of the inferior *q.v.* meatus *q.v.* of the nose through which tears are conducted into the nasal cavity.

NASOPHARYNGEAL Pertaining to the pharynx *q.v.* at the back of the nose.

NASOPHARYNX The internal portions of the nose and throat.

NASTIC MOVEMENTS A response to external stimuli *q.v.* in which the reaction to it is independent of the direction from which it comes.

NATAL Birth. cf: prenatal.

NATIONAL ACADEMY OF SCIENCES, NATIONAL RESEARCH COUNCIL (NAS/NRC) A scientific group founded over a century ago to serve science and the U.S. government. The ~ is composed of distinguished scholars in scientific and engineering research dedicated to the furtherance of science and its use for the general welfare. The ~ was chartered by the U.S. Congress on March 3, 1863, to serve as an official advisor upon request and without fee to the federal government.

NATIONAL ADVISORY COUNCIL FOR DRUG ABUSE PREVENTION Created in 1972 through authorization granted to the director of the Special Action Office for Drug Abuse Prevention.

NATIONAL ASSESSMENT A comprehensive, nationwide analysis of educational objectives and their achievement in 10 learning areas.

NATIONAL ASSOCIATION FOR THE PROTECTION OF THE INSANE AND PREVENTION OF INSANITY Founded in 1872. For the first time, the word "prevention" was used in the title of a professional association. The ~ was in existence until 1888.

NATIONAL BETTER BUSINESS BUREAU Provides the public with information relative to business and industry practices—some of which may involve fraudulent practices.

NATIONAL CENTER FOR CHILD ABUSE AND NEGLECT Established in 1974 under authority granted by the passage of the Child Abuse Prevention and Treatment Act. The ~ was organized as a part of the (then) Department of Health, Education, and Welfare. Its basic functions were to compile and analyze child abuse research, establish a clearinghouse for information, develop and publish documents to be used in training personnel, provide technical assistance to states and agencies, and conduct research.

NATIONAL CENTER FOR HEALTH EDUCATION Organized within the Centers for Disease Control [although the President's Committee on Health Education recommend it be established within the (then) Department of Health, Education, and Welfare].

NATIONAL COMMISSION FOR HEALTH EDUCATION CREDENTIALING (NCHEC), INC A national organization designed to ensure rigorous professional standards for health educators and to issue credentials to qualified individuals (CHES *q.v.*).

NATIONAL COMMISSION ON EXCELLENCE IN EDUCATION A study group formed in the early 1980s to investigate the status of public education in the United States.

NATIONAL COMMISSION ON MARIJUANA (SIC) AND DRUG ABUSE Chaired by Raymond P. Shafer, the commission was comprised of 13 prestigious persons who represented medicine, education, government, and law enforcement. The first of two reports was transmitted to President Nixon on March 22, 1972, and titled *Marijuana: A Signal of Misunderstanding.* The President rejected the entire report.

NATIONAL COMMITTEE FOR MENTAL HYGIENE Founded in 1909 and is considered the beginning of the mental health movement.

NATIONAL COMMITTEE FOR THE IMPROVEMENT OF NURSING SERVICES Founded in 1949 and consolidated with the National League for nursing in 1952.

NATIONAL COMMITTEE ON HEALTH EDUCATION Appointed by President Nixon in 1971, the Committee's mission was to 1. describe the state of the art of health education; 2. define the need for health education in the United States; 3. establish goals, priorities, and objectives for health education; and 4. determine the most appropriate structure, organization, and function for a national health education foundation. The Committee's report in 1973 led to the establishment of the Bureau of Health Education in 1974 within the structure of the U.S. Public Health Service. In 1975, the National Center for Health Education was established.

NATIONAL COUNCIL FOR THE ACCREDITATION OF TEACHER EDUCATION (NCATE) An accrediting agency that certifies the quality of teacher education programs nationwide.

NATIONAL COUNCIL ON HEALTH PLANNING AND DEVELOPMENT Authorized by the enactment of the National Health Planning and Resources Development Act of 1974. Focused on consumer-driven state and regional health planning efforts through the establishment of Health Systems Agencies.

NATIONAL DISEASE REGISTRY An ATSDR *q.v.*-proposed registry designed to ascertain the effects of waste sites on public health by examining existing health outcomes while using existing databases and information as much as possible.

NATIONAL DRUG ABUSE TRAINING CENTER Created in 1972 through authorization granted to the director of the Special Office for Drug Abuse Prevention.

NATIONAL EDUCATION ASSOCIATION (NEA) The largest teachers' professional organization in the United States.

NATIONAL EMERGENCY STRIKES Circumstances in which a curtailment of services and social order is likely to occur, which put the social order at risk and endanger the safety and lives of a substantial portion of the public.

NATIONAL EXPOSURE REGISTRY A listing of persons exposed to hazardous substances. This listing is composed of chemical-specific sub-registries. The primary purpose of the registry program is to create a large database of similarly exposed persons. This database is to be used to facilitate epidemiological research in ascertaining adverse health effects of persons exposed to low levels of chemicals over a period of time.

NATIONAL FORMULARY (NF) A standard directory of drugs and their formulas. cf: *United States Pharmacopeia.*

NATIONAL FOUNDATION FOR INFANTILE PARALYSIS, INC Following the development of a vaccine in 1957 to prevent polio, the ~ changed its name to the National Foundation/March of Dimes *q.v.*, focusing its attention on birth defects.

NATIONAL FOUNDATION/MARCH OF DIMES Formerly the National Foundation for Infantile Paralysis. Following the development of the Salk vaccine, the organization changed its name to the ~, focusing on birth defects.

NATIONAL HEALTH AND NUTRITION EXAMINATION SURVEY (NHANES II) A comprehensive population survey that included a detailed dietary questionnaire from which intakes were calculated in a sample of over 10,000 adults.

NATIONAL HEALTH COUNCIL A voluntary organization made up of representatives of various health organizations to coordinate efforts to deal with health issues affecting the country. Established in 1921.

NATIONAL HEALTH COVERAGE The concept of a comprehensive health insurance coverage provided by the federal government for all its citizens. cf: Medicare; Medicaid; National Health Insurance.

NATIONAL HEALTH INSURANCE 1. A proposed federally controlled health insurance that would be available to all U.S. citizens. 2. A system involving government subsidization of health care costs. cf: national health coverage.

NATIONAL HEART INSTITUTE One of the National Institutes of Health. Established through the passage of the National Heart Act of 1948.

NATIONAL HEART, LUNG, AND BLOOD INSTITUTE (NHLBI) Organized within the National Institutes of Health, the ~ is concerned with research and prevention activities related to the heart, blood, lungs, sleep disorders, and the Women's Health Initiative.

NATIONAL HIGHWAY TRAFFIC SAFETY ADMINISTRATION Organized within the Department of Transportation. It develops and enforces safety standards for certain parts of motor vehicles.

NATIONAL INSTITUTE FOR MENTAL HEALTH, THE Established in 1946 by passage of the National Mental Health Act.

NATIONAL INSTITUTE FOR OCCUPATIONAL SAFETY AND HEALTH (NIOSH) Responsible for identifying occupational health and safety hazards, determining methods to control them, and recommending exposure limits to hazardous substances.

NATIONAL INSTITUTE OF ALLERGY AND INFECTIOUS DISEASES A part of the National Institutes of Health, established in 1887 at the Marine Hospital on Staten Island, NY.

NATIONAL INSTITUTE OF CHILD HEALTH AND GENERAL MEDICAL SERVICES A part of the National Institutes of Health, established in 1962.

NATIONAL INSTITUTE OF DENTAL AND CRANIOFACIAL RESEARCH (NIDR) A part of the National Institutes of Health, established in 1948.

NATIONAL INSTITUTE OF MENTAL HEALTH A part of the National Institutes of Health. Focuses on the diagnosis, treatment, and cure of mental disorders.

NATIONAL INSTITUTE OF NEUROLOGICAL AND COMMUNICATIVE DISORDERS AND STROKE Established as a part of the National Institutes of Health in 1950, the institute sponsors biomedical research on issues related to the brain and nervous system.

NATIONAL INSTITUTE ON AGING (NIA) One of the National Institutes of Health, the ~ was established by Congress on May 31, 1974 (PL 93-296). As a federal agency, the ~ supports research on conditions that affect the aging process. The activities range from investigations on biological, social, and psychological issues to training personnel for related research.

NATIONAL INSTITUTE ON ALCOHOL ABUSE AND ALCOHOLISM (NIAAA) Established in 1970 as a branch of the National Institute of Mental Health.

NATIONAL INSTITUTE ON DRUG ABUSE (NIDA) Established within the National Institute of Mental Health by authority granted to the director of the Special Action Office for Drug Abuse Prevention. This authority was granted by a bill passed by Congress in 1972.

NATIONAL INSTITUTES OF HEALTH (NIH) A branch of the United States Public Health Service (USPHS) *q.v.*

NATIONAL INTERAGENCY COUNCIL ON SMOKING AND HEALTH As a result of the first Surgeon General's report on smoking, the ~ was established in 1964. It was the first national antismoking coalition.

NATIONAL LEAGUE FOR NURSING Founded in 1952 as a consolidation of the National League of Nursing Education, the National Organization for Public Health Nursing, the Association of Collegiate Schools of Nursing, the Joint Committee on Practical Nurses and Auxiliary Workers in Nursing Services, the Joint Committee on Careers in Nursing, the National Committee for the Improvement of Nursing Services, and the National Nursing Accrediting Service. ~ purpose is "that the nursing needs of the people may be met."

NATIONAL NURSING ACCREDITATION SERVICE Founded in 1949 and consolidated with the National League for Nursing *q.v.* in 1952.

NATIONAL PERIOD The period in American education from 1788 to the present.

NATIONAL PRIORITIES LIST (NPL) A listing of sites that have undergone preliminary assessment and inspection with respect to toxic chemical spills and other discharges to determine which locations pose immediate threats to persons living or working near the release. These sites are most in need of cleanup, promulgated by EPA *q.v.* under CERCLA *q.v.*

NATIONAL RESEARCH COUNCIL (NRC) Organized by the National Academy of Sciences *q.v.* in 1916 in the interest of national preparedness, it served the purpose of encouraging a broader participation by American scientists and engineers in the service of the Academy to the nation.

NATIONAL SAFETY COUNCIL A nonprofit, nongovernmental agency dedicated to promoting the safety of individuals and communities throughout the United States. The ~ was founded in 1913 and chartered by Congress in 1953.

NATIONAL TOXICOLOGY PROGRAM ~ conducts toxicology testing on those substances most frequently found at sites on the National Priorities List *q.v.* of the EPA *q.v.* and has the greatest potential for human exposure.

NATIONAL URBAN LEAGUE Founded in 1910. Its basic functions are the promotion of health through education and other health-related activities, as well as the advocacy of basic civil rights.

NATION AT RISK REPORT Issued in 1983 by the National Commission on Excellence in Education. It called for significant reform in public education as a matter of national security, because of the many major deficiencies in public education at the time.

NATIVE AMERICAN CHURCH A religious organization that blends traditional Indian beliefs with Christianity. The hallucinogenic drug mescaline *q.v.*, gotten from the peyote *q.v.*, is used as a part of the religious ceremonies.

NATIVISM The view that some important aspects of perception *q.v.* and of other cognitive *q.v.* processes are innate.

NATURAL ATTITUDE The common agreements and assumptions in a culture concerning human nature.

NATURAL CATEGORIES Basic concepts caused by the natural impact of the physical world on the senses.

NATURAL CHILDBIRTH 1. A method of childbirth that is directed toward minimizing labor *q.v.* pain through techniques of physical and psychological training prior to delivery, rather than a reliance on the use of drugs. A form of educated childbirth *q.v.* 2. Pertains to a variety of childbirth methods that emphasize the preparation of the couple for labor and delivery. cf: LeBoyer; Lamaze.

NATURAL EXPERIMENTS Naturally occurring situations that allow researchers to test the effects of one variable upon another.

NATURAL FAMILY PLANNING 1. The combined use of all three rhythm techniques *q.v.* of contraception. 2. The ovulation method *q.v.*

NATURAL FOOD Any food that is minimally processed and contains no artificial ingredients.

NATURAL "HIGH" Feeling elation or euphoria without the use of psychoactive drugs.

NATURAL HISTORY 1. The stages through which a disease passes. 2. The description of what happens following the development of disease, including complications, cure, death, symptom changes, remissions, etc., without medical intervention.

NATURAL IMMUNITY 1. A condition of immunity *q.v.* that results when a person has a disease, builds antibodies *q.v.* against the disease, and recovers from the disease. 2. A component of the immune system *q.v.* that uses chemicals produced by the body to destroy pathogens *q.v.*

NATURALISM A philosophy that contends that whatever occurs naturally is good.

NATURALISTIC OBSERVATION 1. Observation. 2. The observation of behavior *q.v.* under natural conditions of life. 3. A diagnostic procedure in which individuals are observed in their own natural settings, with minimal intrusion by the observer.

NATURALISTIC STUDIES 1. Noninvasive, nonexperimental studies conducted under natural conditions primarily through observation. 2. Field studies.

NATURAL KILLER (NK) CELLS A type of white blood cell *q.v.* that recognizes and kills certain tumor *q.v.* cells.

NATURAL MEDIUM An inanimate medium consisting of plant and/or animal components, occurring naturally in which other organisms can grow.

NATURAL SELECTION 1. Determined by environmental *q.v.* factors that favor the reproduction of certain alleles *q.v.* or gene *q.v.* combinations over others. Results from constant interplay between the organism and the environment. However, ~ does not produce new genes. 2. The explanatory principle that underlies Darwin's theory of evolution. Some organisms produce offspring that are able to survive and reproduce while others of the same species do not. 3. A process in which fertility is varied among competing organisms resulting in a change in the genetic composition of a particular species.

NATURE–NURTURE PROBLEM 1. The pervasive question of whether behavior *q.v.* is the result of heredity *q.v.* or environment *q.v.* 2. Nature–nurture controversy.

NATUROPATH A health practitioner who attributes disease to an imbalance of the natural forces within the body and treats disease by employing natural forces, such as air, light, heat, water, electricity, and diet.

NATUROPATHY 1. A pseudoscience that is based on the belief that the fundamental cause of diseases is the violation of nature's laws. 2. A system of healing that attempts to restore or maintain a balance of the body's mental and physiological functioning. 3. A system of disease treatment that employs natural means and rejects the use of drug therapy.

NAUSEA Sickish feelings in the stomach characterized by a feeling to vomit.

NAVAL 1. Bellybutton. 2. The spot where the umbilical cord *q.v.* is attached.

NAVANE A commercial preparation of thiothixene *q.v.*

NCATE An acronym for the National Council for the Accreditation of Teacher Education *q.v.*

NCHEC An acronym for National Commission for Health Education Credentialing, Inc. *q.v.*

NCI An acronym for National Cancer Institute; a part of NIH *q.v.*

NDA An acronym for new drug application, required of pharmaceutical companies by the FDA *q.v.* The ~ provides data from both human and animal studies demonstrating the safety and effectiveness of the drug in question.

NDPCAL Nondietary protein calories.

NE An acronym for norepinephrine *q.v.*

NEA An acronym for National Education Association *q.v.*

NEAR-GENIUS 1. A level of intelligence for above the average, but short of genius *q.v.* 2. A person who has an intelligence quotient *q.v.* of 130–145.

NEARSIGHTEDNESS Myopia *q.v.*

NEBULIZATION The process of breaking up a liquid solution into the form of a fine spray or vapor.

NEBULIZER An apparatus for distributing a liquid in the form of a spray or vapor.

NECATOR AMERICANUS The parasite *q.v.* that causes hookworm *q.v.* in humans.

NECK The supporting structure of the head, formed by the seven cervical vertebrae *q.v.* and lying between the head and the shoulders.

NECROPHILIA 1. A rare sexual variance *q.v.* in which sexual gratification is achieved by looking at or having intercourse with a corpse. In extreme cases, a necrophiliac may kill to provide himself with a corpse. This is considered by some authorities as the most deviant of all sexual variances. 2. Morbid sexual attraction to a corpse.

NECROPSY 1. Autopsy *q.v.* 2. Examination of a dead body by dissection.

NECROSIS 1. Dead. 2. Necrotic *q.v.* tissue. 3. Death of a cell or group of cells due to irreversible damage.

NECROTIC Dead.

NECROTIZING ULCERATIVE GINGIVITIS Vincent's disease *q.v.*

NEED 1. A variety of felt urgencies related to existence, continuation, maintenance of life, and enhancement of living. The biological *q.v.* and psychosocial needs *q.v.* are interrelated. 2. Urgencies whose satisfaction is essential for continuance of health and life. 3. A state of lack or excess that underlie a drive *q.v.* 4. A biological or psychological *q.v.* condition whose gratification is necessary for the maintenance of homeostasis *q.v.* or self-actualization *q.v.* 5. In health education, whatever is required for well-being or a requirement of an individual or group to be conscious of that which demands certain levels of comfort or wellness. 6. The degree to which the present condition of a person differs from some acceptable norm *q.v.* 7. The natural urge to maintain a balance between internal drives *q.v.* and external conditions. 8. Interpretive ~. 9. Felt ~. cf: basic need; metaneed.

NEED FOR ACHIEVEMENT A need that motivates a person to seek out opportunities in the environment and to take advantage of them.

NEEDLE ASPIRATION Removal of fluid from a tumor *q.v.* or cyst *q.v.* by a fine needle.

NEEDLE BIOPSY 1. The removal of a small sample of tissue from an area of the body using a wide-bore needle. 2. A minor surgical procedure in which a needle is inserted into an anesthetized portion of tissue and a sample of the tissue is removed for microscopic examination.

NEEDLES AND WORKS The devices used to prepare and inject drugs directly into the vein and, thus, into the bloodstream.

NEEDLE SHARING 1. One of the most common means for the transmission of the human immunodeficiency virus *q.v.* 2. Sharing needles for IV *q.v.* drug use without sterilizing the needles and syringes before each use.

NEED-REDUCTION THEORY The theory *q.v.* that associates reinforcement *q.v.* with the reduction of a need *q.v.*

NEEDS ASSESSMENT 1. The process by which both the perceived and unperceived needs of an individual or group are identified. 2. The process of identifying what is needed or desired for inclusion in a program or curriculum. 3. A process used by health educators to identify the health needs of a population. ~ includes working with the population to determine what needs should be met and exploring alternative ways or methods to bring about appropriate changes.

NEED-SATISFACTION SEQUENCES Behavior leading to the gratification of needs *q.v.* with accompanying pleasure or gratification. cf: motivational sequence.

NEEDS-GOAL MODEL A model of motivation that hypothesizes that felt needs cause behavior *q.v.*

NEEDS HIERARCHY Referring to Maslow's theory, indicative of the motivational force of one's own needs as they are perceived. cf: basic needs; hierarchy of needs.

NEGATED In pharmacology *q.v.*, the process in which one drug cancels or neutralizes the effects of another drug.

NEGATIVE ACCELERATION A curve of diminishing returns. Increases in the independent variable *q.v.* produce smaller increases in the value of the dependent variable *q.v.* ct: positive acceleration. cf: negative association.

NEGATIVE AFTERIMAGE A visual experience that follows stimulation. ~ takes the form of an image that is complementary in color to the original stimulus *q.v.*

NEGATIVE (INVERSE) ASSOCIATION In epidemiology *q.v.*, as the amount of the characteristics increases, the rate of the health state decreases. cf: negative acceleration. ct: positive association.

NEGATIVE CONSEQUENCES Events and situations that follow a behavior and are unpleasant, e.g., punishments.

NEGATIVE CORRELATION A relationship between two measures of behavior *q.v.* in which high values of one are associated with low values of the other. ct: positive correlation.

NEGATIVE DEPENDENCY BEHAVIOR Actions that create psychological dependence *q.v.* and harm structures and functions of the body.

NEGATIVE FEEDBACK An action that produces a consequence that stops or reverses the action. cf: feedback system. ct: positive feedback.

NEGATIVE IDENTITY The process of adopting forms of behavior opposite to those that are regarded as desirable by parents, most adults, and society in general.

NEGATIVE NORMS The dynamics and standards of a group that limit or inhibit productivity.

NEGATIVE REINFORCEMENT 1. Punishment designed to reduce the frequency of negative behavior. 2. Removal of an adverse stimulus when appropriate behavior is exhibited. 3. A reward that is the elimination of an undesirable consequence of behavior. 4. Increasing the frequency of a behavior by associating it with the removal of something aversive. ct: positive reinforcement. cf: aversion therapy.

NEGATIVE REINFORCER 1. A punishment. 2. An event that a person will learn to escape or avoid.

NEGATIVE RELATIONSHIP A relationship in which increases in the independent variable *q.v.* are associated with decreases in the dependent variable *q.v.* cf: negative correlation. ct: positive relationship.

NEGATIVE RESISTANCE The lowering phase of weight lifting.

NEGATIVE SYMPTOMS Behavioral deficits such as flat affect *q.v.* or apathy *q.v.*, esp. in schizophrenia *q.v.*

NEGATIVE TRANSFER Transfer in which practice in one task interferes with the learning *q.v.* of another task. ct: positive transfer.

NEGATIVE TRANSFERENCE See analysis of transference *q.v.*

NEGATIVISM 1. A defense mechanism *q.v.* 2. A form of aggressive withdrawal in which a person exhibits a tendency to want forbidden things and has an aversion to those things for which one is praised; it involves refusing to cooperate with commands or doing the opposite of what has been requested. 3. A tendency to behave in a manner opposite to that which is expected or appropriate. 4. Behavior in children who refuse to perform when expectations are exceeding their level of tolerance.

NEGLIGENCE 1. Failure to do something that a reasonable person would do, or doing something that a reasonable and prudent person would not do. 2. Failure to act responsibly.

NEGOTIATING In collective bargaining, a process of joint decision making involving representatives of the management of an organization and representatives of the workers in that organization. Decisions are made with respect to salary, working conditions, fringe benefits, and the like. Most often, such decisions require the ratification of those being represented.

NEHA An acronym for National Environmental Health Association.

NEI An acronym for National Eye Institute (part of the National Institutes of Health).

NEISSERIA GONORRHEA A gram-negative diplococcus bacterium *q.v.* that causes gonorrhea.

NEISSERIAN INFECTION Gonorrhea *q.v.*

NEMATODE A parasitic round worm.

NEMBUTAL A commercial preparation of a barbiturate *q.v.*

NEOBEHAVIORISM 1. The behaviorist orientation that advocates the relationship between environmental events and social behavior, but also recognizes the importance of internal properties of the individual in determining this relationship. 2. The general point of view that emphasizes the central position of response *q.v.* in psychology *q.v.* cf: behaviorist orientation.

NEOCORTEX 1. The highest center of intelligence in the brain. 2. The center of the brain that responds to external stimuli with trust. cf: limbic system.

NEO-DARWINISM The theory that adaptation is the result of natural selection of variations caused by spontaneous mutations and/or genetic recombinations.

NEOENDOTHRIX An infection of the hair in which the fungus mycelium develops both inside and outside the hair shaft.

NEO-FREUDIANS 1. Theorists who accept the psychoanalytic theory *q.v.* of unconscious *q.v.* conflict but who, in contrast, describe these conflicts in social terms rather than in terms of bodily pleasures or frustrations, and in maintaining that many of these conflicts arise from the specific cultural *q.v.* conditions rather than being biologically *q.v.* established. 2. Psychoanalysts who believe that therapy must be aimed at understanding the person's present situation as well as his or her childhood experiences and unconscious mental processes.

3. A person who has modified the practice of Freudian psychology.

NEOLOCAL RESIDENCE In sociology, a residence outside the homes of parents of either the husband or wife.

NEOLOGISM 1. A word coined by a patient who is in psychotherapy *q.v.* 2. A word made up by the speaker that is usually meaningless to a listener.

NEONATAL Pertaining to or related to the first month of life following birth.

NEONATAL SEIZURES Seizures evidenced by alternating contractions of various muscle groups in newborns.

NEONATE The newly born infant.

NEOPHOBIA In nutrition *q.v.*, the tendency for a person to refuse to eat new and unfamiliar foods.

NEOPLASM 1. Any new growth of tissue. 2. A tumor *q.v.* 3. Any abnormal formation or growth.

NEOPLASTIC CELLS 1. Referring to new, abnormal formation of tissue cells. 2. Cells formed that are larger and multiply more quickly than do normal cells.

NEOTENY The retention of juvenile features of ancestral species in the adult features of later species.

NEPHRECTOMY The surgical removal of a kidney.

NEPHRITIS 1. Inflammation of the kidney. A progressive degenerative lesion affecting the renal system *q.v.* 2. Inflammation of the glomeruli *q.v.* of the kidney causing impairment of the filtering process so that blood and albumin are excreted in the urine.

NEPHROLOGY The medical study of the structure, function, and diseases of the kidneys.

NEPHRON The functional unit of the kidney *q.v.* made up of the glomerulus *q.v.* Each kidney contains about one million ~s.

NEPHROSIS Any disease of the kidney, particularly the type that involves the tubules *q.v.*

NERVE A cord-like structure comprising a collection of fibers that convey impulses between a part of the central nervous system *q.v.* and some other region of the body and vice versa.

NERVE BLOCK 1. A method of analgesia *q.v.* in which a nerve-destroying agent is injected close to the affected nerve *q.v.* 2. The use of drugs to stop the flow of electrical impulses through the nerves.

NERVE GROWTH FACTOR A chemical substance that stimulates the growth of developing nerves as they establish connections with various parts of the body.

NERVE IMPULSE Action potential *q.v.*

NERVE ROOT One of two bundles of nerve *q.v.* fibers emerging from the spinal cord *q.v.* at each vertebra to join and form a spinal nerve.

NERVOUS BREAKDOWN 1. Pertaining to lowered integration and the inability to deal adequately with one's life situation. 2. A nonscientific term and somewhat of a misnomer that refers to an apparent, sudden onset of emotional and/or mental illness.

NERVOUSNESS A state of emotional *q.v.* tension, restlessness, and hypersensitivity *q.v.*

NERVOUS SYSTEM 1. A system of microscopic cells that specialize in the conduction of impulses and are located in the central nervous system *q.v.* and the peripheral nervous system *q.v.* 2. One of two major control systems that transmit impulses and interprets stimuli *q.v.* cf: autonomic nervous system; central nervous system.

NERVOUS TENSION 1. Stress *q.v.* 2. An emotional *q.v.* state.

NESTING 1. Frenetic housecleaning by a pregnant woman in the late stage of pregnancy. 2. The increased urge by some to make the home more comfortable, particularly when pregnant. cf: cacooning.

NET PROTEIN UTILIZATION (NPU) 1. Proportion of dietary nitrogen that is retained by the body. 2. An index of protein *q.v.* quality.

NET VENATION The patterns of veins in a leaf that form a network.

NETWORK (NET) In a communications system, an orderly arrangement of stations interconnected through communications channels that form a coordinated entity.

NEURAL Pertaining to any part of the nervous system *q.v.*

NEURALGIA 1. A painful inflammation *q.v.* of a nerve. 2. Sharp pain along the path followed by a nerve *q.v.*

NEURAL GROOVE A groove on the embryo *q.v.* formed by the unfolding of the outer layer of cells and destined to become the nervous system *q.v.* in humans.

NEURAL LESION Lesion, neural *q.v.*

NEURAL OBSERVATION SHEET 1. Neural watch sheet *q.v.* 2. A chart constructed to provide a convenient record of sequential observations of the neurological *q.v.* status of a person.

NEURAL TUBE The epithelial *q.v.* tube that develops from the neural plate to form the embryo's *q.v.* central nervous system *q.v.* and from which the brain *q.v.* and spinal cord *q.v.* develop.

NEURAL WATCH SHEET Neural observation sheet *q.v.*

NEURASTHENIA 1. A psychoneurosis *q.v.* (nervous exhaustion) characterized by abnormal fatigability. 2. Asthenic reaction *q.v.* 3. A neurotic *q.v.* reaction characterized by chronic mental and physical fatigue and listlessness. cf: narcolepsy.

NEURILEMMA Nerve sheath.

NEURITIS 1. Inflammation of the peripheral nerves *q.v.* that link the brain *q.v.* and the spinal cord *q.v.* with muscles, skin, organs, and other parts of the body. 2. The inflammation of a nerve characterized by pain, tenderness, paralysis, and loss of reflexes.

NEUROCHEMISTRY The study of the chemical interactions of the brain *q.v.* and nervous system *q.v.*

NEUROCYTE A nerve cell.

NEURODERMATITIS 1. A chronic psychophysiological *q.v.* disorder characterized by patches of skin becoming inflamed. 2. An itching eruption of the skin that is due to some nervous disorder.

NEUROENDOCRINE SYSTEM 1. The combined interaction of the nervous system *q.v.* and the endocrine system *q.v.* 2. Pertains to the nervous system and the endocrine system.

NEUROENDOCRINOLOGY The study of the ways in which the central nervous system *q.v.* and the endocrine system *q.v.* interact to promote normal body functioning.

NEUROFIBROMATOSIS (NF) A genetic (autosomal dominant) disorder characterized by skin lesions and cutaneous *q.v.* tumors. In some people, severe disfiguring may occur and skeletal abnormalities may also be present. There is no effective treatment at this time other than surgical correction.

NEUROGENIC SHOCK A state of shock *q.v.* as a result of generalized vasodilation *q.v.*, produced by action of the nervous system *q.v.*

NEUROGLIA 1. Connective tissue *q.v.* forming the supporting structure of the nerve cells of the cerebrospinal *q.v.* axis. 2. Glia cell. cf: astrocyte.

NEUROHORMONES 1. The hormones *q.v.* produced by the hypothalamus *q.v.* 2. Transmitter chemicals secreted by nerve endings that excite or inhibit the transmission of nerve impulses.

NEUROHYPOPHYSIS The posterior pituitary gland *q.v.*

NEUROLEPTIC 1. A psychoactive drug *q.v.* that reduces psychotic symptoms but produces some side effects resembling neurological diseases. 2. Antipsychotic *q.v.* 3. Major tranquilizers *q.v.*

NEUROLOGICAL 1. Pertaining to the diagnosis and treatment of diseases of the nervous system *q.v.* 2. Pertaining to the nervous system.

NEUROLOGIST A doctor of medicine who specializes in the diagnosis and treatment of diseases or injuries of the brain and branches of the nervous system *q.v.*

NEUROLOGY The medical specialty that is concerned with diagnosis, operative, and medical treatment of the brain, spinal cord, and disorders of the nerves.

NEUROMUSCULAR DISEASES 1. A group of muscle-destroying disorders that vary in hereditary pattern, age of onset, initial muscles attacked, and rate of progression. 2. Muscular dystrophy *q.v.* 3. A neurological disease that attacks the myelin sheath *q.v.* of nerve fibers in the brain *q.v.* and spinal cord *q.v.* 4. Multiple sclerosis *q.v.*

NEUROMUSCULAR EFFICIENCY Control of muscles by the motor nerve stimuli in the most frugal manner.

NEUROMUSCULAR MATURATION Maturation involving the muscles and the skeletal system, the nerves that innervate them, and the motor areas of the brain that control voluntary muscle movement.

NEUROMUSCULAR TENSION Buildup of energy in the nerves and muscles throughout the body sometimes caused by sexual arousal.

NEUROMUSCULAR TONUS The level of nervous tension within a muscle.

NEURON 1. A nerve cell. 2. The basic unit of the nervous system *q.v.* cf: axon; dendrite; end bulb; receptor; synapse.

NEUROPHRENIA A term used to describe the behavioral symptoms resulting from central nervous system *q.v.* impairment.

NEUROPHYSIOLOGICAL 1. Nervous system *q.v.* function. 2. The processes through which the body senses and responds to internal and external environments. cf: neurophysiology.

NEUROPHYSIOLOGY The physiology of the nervous system *q.v.* cf: neurophysiological.

NEUROPSYCHIATRY The scientific discipline concerned with the diagnosis, treatment, and prevention of all psychiatric *q.v.* disorders.

NEUROPSYCHOLOGICAL BATTERIES A series of psychological *q.v.* tests used to detect and understand behavioral disturbances that relate to organic *q.v.* brain dysfunction.

NEUROPSYCHOLOGY A psychological specialty concerned with the relationships among cognition *q.v.*, affect *q.v.*, and behavior and the functioning of the brain.

NEUROSCIENTIST A person who studies the anatomical *q.v.* and physiological *q.v.* relationships of the nervous system *q.v.*

NEUROSIS 1. A form of compulsive, ineffective behavior of which the person is aware but is unable to control. 2. Conditions characterized by behavior and feelings that are considered abnormal but that are not severe enough to prevent most kinds of normal functioning. 3. In psychoanalytic psychology *q.v.*, a broad term pertaining to mental disorders *q.v.* whose primary symptoms are anxiety and defenses against anxiety. 4. Psychoneurotic disorder *q.v.* 5. Neurotic disorder *q.v.* 6. Psychological difficulty created when significant conflict and its associated emotions are unresolved and repressed *q.v.* 7. One of a large group of nonpsychotic disorders characterized by unrealistic anxiety.

NEUROSYPHILIS 1. Syphilitic *q.v.* infection of the nervous system *q.v.* 2. General paresis *q.v.* 3. Infection of the central nervous system *q.v.* by the spirochete, *Treponema pallidum*, resulting in destruction of brain tissue affecting behavior or the senses depending on the area of the brain destroyed.

NEUROTIC ANXIETY 1. Unrealistic fear. 2. A general, undercurrent of anxiety that irrationally causes a fear of the consequences of performing normal activities.

NEUROTIC BEHAVIOR Psychogenic *q.v.* reactions or actions characteristic of those of a child: compulsive, ineffective, and inefficient.

NEUROTIC-DEPRESSIVE REACTION A psychoneurotic reaction *q.v.* characterized by marked, persistent dejection, and discouragement.

NEUROTICISM Emotional instability and maladjustment.

NEUROTIC NEEDS Needs *q.v.* that are unrealistic.

NEUROTIC PARADOX The use of temporary relief of tension and a tendency to repeat an ineffective behavior which in turn may increase frustration.

NEUROTOXIC Poisonous to the nervous system *q.v.*

NEUROTOXICOLOGY The science of poisons, their effects, and antidotes as they relate to nerves or the nervous system *q.v.*

NEUROTRANSMITTER 1. A chemical substance in the axon *q.v.* of a nerve that carries an impulse to the dendrites *q.v.* of another nerve cell. 2. An organic substance produced by nerve cells, necessary for the electrochemical functions of the neuron. 3. Biochemical substance released at the synapse that either excites the receiving neuron enhancing the impulse transmission or inhibits the receiving neuron to stop the transmission of an impulse.

NEUROVASCULAR THEORY A theory of thermal sensitivity that attributes the experience of warmth and cold to changes in the peripheral blood vessels.

NEUROVESICLES Microscopic *q.v.* sacs in axon *q.v.* terminals that contain a transmitter substance.

NEUTRALIZATION 1. In pathology *q.v.*, the binding of an antibody *q.v.* to an antigen *q.v.* in such a way that the antigen is no longer harmful. 2. In psychology, a therapeutic process by which the subject learns to reduce the frequency and intensity of irrational thoughts by reciting reasons why they are not valid.

NEUTRALIZE 1. To render neutral. 2. The chemical combination of hydrogen and hydroxyl ions *q.v.* to form water, thereby rendering each ion harmless.

NEUTRAL STEER Pertaining to the handling characteristics of a vehicle that has a center of gravity in the middle of the vehicle making it easy to handle.

NEUTRON An electrically neutral particle located in the nucleus of the atom *q.v.*

NEUTROPHIL A type of white blood cell. 2. A polymorphonuclear *q.v.* leukocyte *q.v.* that is important in combating infection. ~s stain readily with neutral dyes.

NEVOID AMENTIA A rare condition characterized by extensive blood vessel tumors, convulsions, hemiplegia *q.v.*, and severe mental deficiency resulting in a shortened life span.

NEVUS 1. A birth mark. 2. A congenital discoloration of a circumscribed area of the skin resulting from accumulation of pigment. 3. Pigmentation in a localized area of the skin present at birth.

NEW CORTEX 1. The outside layer of the brain that appeared late in human evolution and controls complex behavior and mental activity. 2. Cortex *q.v.* 3. Cerebral cortex *q.v.* ct: old cortex.

NEW ENGLAND PRIMER An early textbook used in colonial schools.

NEW HOST A previously uninfected person now infected with a disease agent *q.v.*

NEW RIGHT A term used to describe extremely conservative groups that attempt to influence politics or educational programs.

NEWTON (N) A unit of measure of force.

NEW YORK ACADEMY OF MEDICINE Conducted research into the problems associated with marijuana between 1940 and 1944 at the request of New York City Mayor Fiorella La Guardia. The ~ issued its report, "The Marijuana Problem In the City of New York," in 1944. Among many of its conclusions, the report stated the following: 1. marijuana does not cause a person to become violent or criminal, 2. marijuana does adversely affect a person's intellectual ability, 3. marijuana does not result in any basic changes in a person's personality, 4. marijuana does produce a sense of euphoria *q.v.* and well-being, 5. there is no evidence that marijuana use results in physical or mental deterioration, and 6. the use of marijuana does not lead to morphine, heroin, or cocaine addiction.

NF An acronym for National Formulary *q.v.*

NGA An acronym for National Governors Association.

NGO An acronym for nongovernmental organization. cf: voluntary health agency; private health agency.

NGU An acronym for nongonococcal urethritis *q.v.*

NHANES II An acronym for National Health and Nutrition Examination Survey *q.v.*

NHLBI An acronym for National Heart, Lung, and Blood Institute (part of NIH *q.v.*).

NIA An acronym for National Institute on Aging *q.v.*

NIAAA An acronym for National Institute on Alcohol Abuse and Alcoholism (part of NIH *q.v.*).

NIACIN 1. One of the B complex vitamins *q.v.* that was discovered in 1937. It aids in the release of energy during metabolism. A severe deficiency results in pellagra *q.v.* 2. A water-soluble vitamin *q.v.*

NIACINAMIDE An antidote *q.v.* for LSD *q.v.*, used to interrupt a bad LSD trip.

NIAID An acronym for National Institute for Allergy and Infectious Diseases (part of NIH *q.v.*).

NICOTIANA A genus *q.v.* of several types of tobacco plant, e.g., *Nicotiana tabacum*; *Nicotiana rustica*.

NICOTIANA TABACUM The botanical name of the tobacco plant named after Jean Nicot.

NICOTINAMIDE ADENINE DINUCLEOTIDE (NAD) 1. Diphosphopyridine nucleotide (DPN). Attached as a prosthetic group *q.v.* to a protein. ~ serves as a respiratory enzyme *q.v.*, i.e., part of an oxidative–reduction system, converting substrates to carbon dioxide (CO_2) and water (H_2O) and the transfer of electrons *q.v.* removed to oxygen (O_2). 2. A coenzyme *q.v.* that participates in oxidation–reduction processes. 3. Also called DPN, a hydrogen acceptor molecule *q.v.* in respiration *q.v.*

NICOTINAMIDE ADENINE DINUCLEOTIDE PHOSPHATE (NADP) Also called TPN (triphosphopyridine nucleotide), a hydrogen acceptor molecule in photosynthesis *q.v.*

NICOTINE 1. A chemical found in tobacco q.v., responsible for some of the physiological *q.v.* effects of smoking. 2. A physiologically active, dependence *q.v.*-producing drug found in tobacco. 3. A chemical constituent in tobacco that produces rapid pulse rate, increased alertness, and a variety of other physiological effects. 4. The most powerful pharmacological agent in tobacco smoke. It is an oily, alkaloid *q.v.* poison that is metabolized in the liver.

NICOTINE RECEPTORS Specialized cells within the central nervous system *q.v.* that are sensitive to the level of nicotine *q.v.* in body tissues.

NICOTINIC CHOLINOCEPTIVE SITE A postjunctional receptor for acetylcholine *q.v.* that is affected by nicotine.

NIDA An acronym for National Institute on Drug Abuse, part of PHS *q.v.*

NIDATION The implantation *q.v.* of the blastocyst *q.v.* in the lining of the uterus *q.v.* in pregnancy *q.v.*

NIDR An acronym for National Institute of Dental Research, part of NIH *q.v.*

NIEMANN–PICK DISEASE A genetic *q.v.* disorder of fat metabolism *q.v.* resulting in mental retardation *q.v.* and brings early death.

NIGHT BLINDNESS The inability to see in dim light.

NIGHT HOSPITAL 1. A treatment center providing night care for alcoholics *q.v.* or other addicts *q.v.* The persons using these facilities have a place to go during the day, such as a job, but need care during the night. 2. A mental hospital in which a person may receive treatment during all or part of the night while carrying on his or her usual occupation in the daytime. ct: day hospital.

NIGHTINGALE PLEDGE 1. A pledge often recited at graduation ceremonies for nurses. 2. Written in 1893, "I solemnly pledge myself before God and in the presence of this assembly, to pass my life in purity and to practice my profession faithfully. I will abstain from whatever is deleterious and mischievous, and I will not take or knowingly administer any harmful drug. I will do all in my power to maintain and elevate the standard of my profession, and will hold in confidence all personal matters committed to my keeping and all family affairs coming to my knowledge in the practice of my calling. With loyalty will I endeavor to aid the physician in this work, and devote myself to the welfare of those committed to my care."

NIGROSTRIATAL DOPAMINE SYSTEM A group of dopamine-containing neurons *q.v.* that have their cell bodies in the midbrain *q.v.* and their terminals in the basal ganglia *q.v.*, which is part of the extrapyramidal motor system. This pathway deteriorates in Parkinson's disease *q.v.* and on which antipsychotic drugs *q.v.* act to produce side effects resembling Parkinson's disease.

NIH An acronym for National Institutes of Health *q.v.*

NIHILISTIC DELUSION A fixed belief that everything is unreal, that nothing really exists.

NIMH An acronym for National Institute of Mental Health (part of NIH *q.v.*).

NINCDS An acronym for National Institute of Neurological and Communicative Disorders and Stroke (part of NIH *q.v.*).

NIOSH An acronym for National Institute for Occupational Safety and Health (part of NIH *q.v.*).

NIPPLE 1. A protuberance *q.v.* located at the tip of the breast consisting principally of smooth muscle fibers and a network of nerve endings and containing, in the female, the outlets of the milk ducts *q.v.* 2. The pigmented projection on the breast that is surrounded by, but does not include, the areola *q.v.* 3. The central area, made of smooth muscle, of the breasts in males and females.

NIPPLE BANKING A surgical method by which a nipple is grafted to another part of the body until the breast is reconstructed and then replaced onto the reconstructed breast.

NISSL'S GRANULES Discrete bodies present in the cytoplasm *q.v.* of a nerve cell associated with their activities.

NIT The egg of the louse that is responsible for pediculosis *q.v.* infestation.

NITRATE See sodium nitrate.

NITRIFICATION The conversion of ammonia nitrogen to nitrate nitrogen by two specific groups of bacteria *q.v.*, the nitrifying bacteria *q.v.*

NITRIFYING BACTERIA The bacteria that carry on nitrification *q.v.*

NITRITE 1. Sodium nitrate. 2. A food additive used to inhibit spoilage and to give color to cured meats.

NITROBACTERS Microorganisms that convert nitrites into nitrates in the nitrogen cycle *q.v.*

NITROGEN 1. Chemical symbol N. 2. A gaseous element that is a constituent of air and is found in all proteins *q.v.*

NITROGEN CYCLE The process of decomposing certain waste products by bacterial *q.v.* action. The ~ consists of the following: 1. Decomposition of animal protein *q.v.* by bacteria, converting it into its amino acids *q.v.* 2. The amino acids are further broken down into ammonia. 3. The ammonia combines with carbon dioxide *q.v.* to form ammonium carbonate, which is then connected to nitrites. 4. Nitrites combine with sodium and potassium, being converted into nitrates by nitrobacters *q.v.* 5. Nitrates that are dissolved in water diffuse into the root systems of plants, combining with carbon dioxide and water to form plant proteins. 6. The plant proteins are eaten by animals and converted into animal proteins.

NITROGEN-FIXING BACTERIA Bacteria, living in the soil or in the root systems of legumes, that convert atmospheric nitrogen into nitrogen compounds in their own bodies.

NITROGEN NARCOSIS 1. A drugged condition that can be created in a person when the nitrogen *q.v.* in the body is exposed to great pressure as in a deep dive. 2. Rapture of the deep.

NITROGEN OXIDE A gaseous compound of smoke that may be a cause of emphysema *q.v.*

NITROGEN TRICHLORIDE A toxic gas produced by mixing cleaning agents that contain chlorine and ammonia.

NITROGLYCERINE 1. A drug that dilates the arteries and is used to treat attacks of angina pectoris *q.v.* 2. A vasodilator *q.v.*

NITROSAMINES 1. End products of the combination of nitrites *q.v.* and nitrates *q.v.* with amines in meat. ~ have been shown to produce cancer in test animals. 2. Cancer-producing substances that are found in some foods and that can also be synthesized *q.v.* in the body. 3. At least four ~ have been found in tobacco, which may account for much of the cancer caused by tobacco use.

NITROSIFICATION Oxidation of ammonia to nitrite.

NITROUS OXIDE 1. An anesthetic *q.v.* gas sometimes used recreationally as an inhalant. 2. Laughing gas.

NK Natural killer cells *q.v.*

NLM An acronym for National Library of Medicine, NIH *q.v.*

NLRB An acronym for National Labor Relations Board.

NMR An acronym for nuclear magnetic resonance *q.v.*

NOCICEPTOR A sensory receptor *q.v.* that transmits a pain signal when stimulated.

NOCTURIA The necessity to get up at night to urinate.

NOCTURNAL EMISSION 1. The discharge of semen *q.v.* by males during sleep. This first occurs shortly after puberty *q.v.* 2. An involuntary male orgasm *q.v.* and ejaculation *q.v.* of semen during sleep. 3. Wet dream. cf: nocturnal orgasm.

NOCTURNAL ENURESIS Bedwetting at least once a month beyond the age of 3–4 years.

NOCTURNAL MYCLONUS Uncontrolled leg jerks during sleep.

NOCTURNAL ORGASM Female vaginal *q.v.* vascular *q.v.* engorgement during sleep while having an erotic dream. cf: nocturnal emission.

NOCTURNAL PENILE TUMESCENCE An erection during sleep.

NOD 1. Behaving in a lethargic manner, if not in a somnolent one, when under the influence of drugs. 2. A dozing state due to the effects of an opiate *q.v.*

NODE 1. In botany, the region of the stem where one or more leaves are attached. 2. In anatomy, the lymph node *q.v.*

NODULE 1. A small node *q.v.* that can be detected by touch, e.g., lymph nodes. 2. In botany, enlargements or swellings on the roots of legumes inhabited by nitrogen-fixing bacteria *q.v.*

NO-FAULT DIVORCE The granting of a divorce *q.v.* without either partner having to prove the other was the cause of the failure of the marriage.

NO-FURLOUGH POLICY A contractual agreement that employees will not be temporarily or permanently laid off because of insufficient work.

NOISE Extraneous disturbances in the learning environment that may interrupt or interfere with communication.

NOLENS VOLENS With or without consent.

NO LOSE METHOD 1. The process whereby the teacher (or other adult) and learners discuss a problem until they reach a mutual agreement about how to solve it. 2. A method of resolving parent–child conflict in which a solution acceptable to both parent and child is reached through discussion.

NOMADISM 1. A defense mechanism *q.v.* 2. A withdrawal reaction in which a person attempts to avoid frustration *q.v.* by continually moving from place to place or from job to job. 3. Wandering.

NOMENCLATURE A system or set of names or designations used in classifying or identifying subjects, e.g., species, mental illnesses, and geologic timeframes.

NOMINAL VARIABLE 1. In epidemiology *q.v.*, the data from variables that name things; they do not measure or quantify amounts. 2. Qualitative variables *q.v.*

NOMOGRAM A series of graphs that interpolate human data and predict degree of body fat, metabolic rate *q.v.*, and desirable caloric intake.

NOMOTHETIC 1. The characteristics possessed by individuals that make them similar. 2. The qualities that make all people more or less alike. ct: idiographic learning.

NONASSERTIVE Giving up one's basic rights so others may achieve theirs. ct: assertion; aggression.

NONCANCELABLE A health insurance policy that states that the insured has the right to continue in force the policy by payment of the designated premiums and that the insurance company cannot alter the provisions unilaterally.

NONCOMMUNICABLE Not transmittable. cf: noncommunicable disease.

NONCOMMUNICABLE DISEASE 1. A disease *q.v.* that cannot be transmitted from one person to another. 2. Usually, degenerative *q.v.* or chronic disease *q.v.* ct: communicable disease.

NONCONDUCTOR 1. Anything that does not transmit an electrical current or any other form of energy. 2. An insulator.

NONCONSCIOUS IDEOLOGIES Beliefs and attitudes *q.v.* about which a person has acquired such uniform messages in socialization that the person is not aware that he or she holds such beliefs and attitudes because no alternative is available.

NONCONTINUITY THEORY The theory *q.v.* that learning *q.v.* occurs in an all or none way.

NONDEBATABLE Subjects or motions that cannot be discussed or debated under strict rules of order.

NONDIRECTIVE TECHNIQUES (THERAPY) Methods for psychological treatment developed by Carl Rogers wherein the therapist refrains from offering advice or interpretations, but only tries to clarify the person's feelings by repeating or restating what is said. cf: client-centered therapy.

NONDISJUNCTION Failure of chromosomes *q.v.* to separate in cell division, with the result that both go to the same cell. Particularly, failure of maternal and paternal chromosomes to separate in the reduction division of meiosis.

NONEFFECTIVE ENVIRONMENT That part of the external environment *q.v.* to which a person is not responding at any given time. ct: effective environment.

NONEMISSIVE ERECTION A sexual dysfunction *q.v.* in which a man is able to achieve an erection *q.v.* but is not able to ejaculate *q.v.*

NONESSENTIAL AMINO ACIDS The amino acids *q.v.* needed for protein synthesis *q.v.* within the cell that can be formed by the body. Examples include alanine, arginine, histidine (see essential amino acids), tyrosine, and cystine.

NONEXEMPT EMPLOYEES Employees who are covered by the Fair Labor Standards Act.

NONFAMILY HOUSEHOLDER A person who lives alone or with nonrelatives only.

NONFASTING REACTIVE HYPOGLYCEMIA The most common form of hypoglycemia *q.v.* Symptoms appear 2–5 h after meals and are short-lived.

NONFEASANCE Failure to perform a required duty.

NONGONOCOCCAL URETHRITIS (NGU) Inflammation of the urinary tract *q.v.* usually by *Chlamydial trachomatis* or *Ureaplasma urealyticum*. Symptoms are similar to those of gonorrhea *q.v.*, but ordinarily it is not considered a sexually transmitted disease *q.v.*

NONGOVERNMENTAL ORGANIZATION (NGO) An organization not supported with public funds. cf: voluntary organization.

NONGRADED SCHOOL An organizational structure in which students are grouped as to their interests and abilities rather than being assigned to a particular grade based on chronological age *q.v.*

NONINSITUTIONAL POPULATION All those who are not residents of hospitals, nursing homes, mental institutions, orphanages, special schools, or correctional institutions.

NONMEDICAL PRACTITIONER A person who provides health services but does not possess the Doctor of Medicine (MD) degree. ct: medical practitioner.

NONNUTRIENTS Food components, e.g., fiber, that pass undigested through the intestinal tract *q.v.* but are important for digestion *q.v.*

NONOBSERVABLE HEALTH BEHAVIOR 1. Those instances in which an individual is functioning outside of the educational setting. 2. Those feelings and thoughts occurring within the individual. 3. Health attitudes *q.v.*, a form of nonobservable behavior, may be inferred from observable health behavior *q.v.*

NONPARAMETRIC STATISTICS In epidemiology *q.v.*, statistical techniques that can be used on nominal *q.v.* or ordinal *q.v.* data.

NONPROCREATIVE SEX Any sexual activity that does not result in pregnancy or the production of offspring.

NONPROFESSIONAL CAREERS A broad category of careers *q.v.* that usually does not require college training.

NONPROGRAMMED DECISIONS Decisions that are nonplanned with little structure.

NONPSYCHOTIC DISORDERS Mental disorders in which the person's functioning is seriously inhibited but in which thought processes are not as grossly distorted as in some of the psychotic *q.v.* disorders and the person recognizes the symptoms *q.v.*

NONREACTIVE MEASURES Techniques for conducting research, such as the study of archives and anonymous observation, that eliminate the problem of subjects' reactivity to the experiment.

NONREMEDIABLE HEALTH CONDITION A condition for which there is no effective treatment.

NONSALICYLATES Nonaspirin, over-the-counter analgesics.

NONSENSE SYLLABLE A combination of letters, usually consisting of two consonants with a vowel in between, that do not form a word in the language of the person using it. Used by Effinghaus *q.v.* in experiments investigating memory and rote learning *q.v.*

NONSMOKERS' RIGHTS The concept that people who do not smoke have the right to breathe air free from smoke, especially tobacco smoke *q.v.*

NONSPECIFIC EFFECTS The effects of a drug that are not directly associated with the chemical action of the drug. cf: placebo effect.

NONSPECIFIC IMMUNE MECHANISM A part of the body's immune system *q.v.* that is activated regardless of the nature of the invading foreign substance. ct: specific immune mechanism.

NONSPECIFIC PRESENTATION OF ILLNESS Symptoms appearing in a person that do not clearly indicate a single disease or single organ system disorder. Older persons more than those in other age groups come to the attention of health care providers due to nonspecific reasons.

NONSPECIFIC URETHRITIS (NSU) An inflammation *q.v.* of the urethra *q.v.* before a causative agent was known. Since 1974, ~ is referred to as nongonococcal urethritis *q.v.*

NONSPECIFIC VAGINITIS A classification used when all the symptoms of vaginitis *q.v.* are present but no specific cause can be found.

NONSUIT A judgment against a plaintiff *q.v.* when he or she is unable to prove a case or when the case is not pursued to trial.

NONTRADITIONAL STUDENTS An administrative term used by colleges and universities to describe students who are pursuing undergraduate degrees at an age other than that associated with traditional college years.

NONVERBAL COMMUNICATION 1. The sharing of meanings in a social setting without the use of words. 2. Relating information by means of physical gestures and mannerisms.

NONVERBAL FEEDBACK Nonverbal communication *q.v.*

NORADRENALINE 1. A hormone *q.v.* that maintains high blood pressure during periods of physical shock. 2. A neurotransmitter *q.v.* 3. Norepinephrine *q.v.*

NOREPINEPHRINE (NE) 1. A neurohormone *q.v.* that activates nervous impulses in the sympathetic nervous system *q.v.* ~ is normally stored in the nerve endings. 2. A hormone *q.v.* secreted by the adrenal medulla *q.v.* that possesses the excitatory actions of epinephrine, with minimal inhibitory effect. 3. A catecholamine *q.v.* that is the neurotransmitter *q.v.* by which the sympathetic fibers exert their effects on internal organs. ~ is the neurotransmitter of various arousing systems in the brain. 4. Disturbances in the tracts of ~ play a role in mania *q.v.* and depression *q.v.* In addition to its stimulant effects, it is also a powerful vasodilator *q.v.*

NORM 1. A widely shared pattern of behavior. 2. A pattern of cultural behavior adhered to by members of a group. 3. A social standard or rule. 4. The average score on a standardized test based on data obtained through its application to a population of persons of a specified developmental level or age.

NORMAL That which is socially accepted as the usual. cf: normal behavior.

NORMAL ANXIETY Anxiety *q.v.* as experienced by most people. ~ controls behavior *q.v.* without producing maladjustment. ct: pathological anxiety.

NORMAL BEHAVIOR Any form of behavior *q.v.* that results in effectiveness in responding to internal or external stimuli. Any behavior that is constructive, purposeful, and does not interfere with other social activities.

NORMAL CURVE 1. A symmetrical, bell-shaped curve that describes the probability of obtaining various combinations of chance events. The ~ describes the frequency distributions of many physical and psychological attributes of people. 2. Normal probability curve. 3. The bell-shaped curve. cf: normal distribution; frequency distribution.

NORMAL DEVIANCE According to Gagnon and Simon, widely practiced deviant *q.v.* behavior.

NORMAL DISTRIBUTION 1. A frequency distribution *q.v.* 2. The normal curve *q.v.* 3. Normal probability curve.

NORMALITY Inclusive of all characteristics, except those that would prevent a person from functioning in society.

NORMALIZATION 1. Making an individual's life and surroundings as close to normal as possible. 2. Creation of a lifestyle for mentally challenged individuals as close as possible to that of the mainstream society.

NORMAL SCHOOL The college training programs for the training of teachers.

NORMATIVE The process of being shaped by norms *q.v.*

NORMATIVE PRESSURE A social influence by which a group exerts influence on an individual by befriending that person.

NORMATIVE STABILITY A stability that is achieved when one maintains a constant ranking within a social group over an extended period of time.

NORMATIVE STANDARDS Statements of social expectations concerning behavioral conduct.

NORML An acronym for National Organization for the Reform of Marijuana Laws.

NORM OF REACTION The range of phenotypes *q.v.* that is possible as a result of changes in the environment for a given genotype *q.v.*

NORMOGLYCEMIA The condition of the body having normal levels of blood glucose *q.v.*

NORM-REFERENCED ASSESSMENT A measurement that compares an individual's performance to that of others.

NORM-REFERENCED DATA Data *q.v.* based on local, state, or national norms *q.v.*

NORM-REFERENCED GRADING A learner's performance is evaluated by comparing it to the performance of other learners in the same learning environment. cf: norm-referenced tests.

NORM-REFERENCED TESTS Tests that enable one to compare a student's scores to a "norm" group. cf: norm-referenced grading.

NORMS 1. A standard based on measurement of a large group of persons, used for comparing the scores of a person with those of others in a defined group. 2. Standards of behavior that are shared by the members of a group.

NORPRAMINE A commercial preparation of desipramine *q.v.*

NORTRIPYLINE 1. A heterocyclic antidepressant *q.v.* 2. Aventyl and Pamelor are commercial preparations.

NOSEBLEED Bleeding from the nose channel by a rupture of blood vessels in the nostril(s).

NOSE PAINTING Slang for reddening of the nose that sometimes occurs in alcoholics *q.v.* as a result of the bursting of capillaries *q.v.* in the nose. cf: sludging.

NOSOCOMIAL Pertains to illness or injury caused by contact with a hospital/medical institution, ranging from a fall from bed to an infection to a fatal surgical error.

NOSOLOGY The naming and classification of diseases.

NO-STRIKE CLAUSE An agreement by the union with management not to go on strike for the duration of the contract.

NOSTRUM 1. A device or drug that is ineffective as claimed by a quack *q.v.* to produce miraculous results. 2. A fraudulent device, drug, or routine. 3. Ineffective medications or devices sold or used by quacks.

NOTEC A commercial preparation of chloral hydrate *q.v.*

NOTOCHORD A longitudinal rod of cells in the embryo *q.v.* of a vertebrate *q.v.* that gives rise to the backbone of the adult.

NOVOCAIN 1. A drug used for local anesthesia *q.v.* 2. A commercial name of procaine hydrochloride *q.v.*

NOXIOUS Harmful.

NP An acronym for nurse practitioner *q.v.*

NPL An acronym for National Priorities List *q.v.*

NPU An acronym for net protein utilization *q.v.*

NRC An acronym for 1. National Research Council *q.v.* 2. Nuclear Regulatory Commission.

NSU An acronym for nonspecific urethritis *q.v.*

NTP An acronym for National Toxicology Program *q.v.*

NUCHAL Pertaining to the nape of the neck *q.v.*

NUCLEAR ENERGY 1. The energy *q.v.* contained within the atomic nucleus *q.v.* 2. Atomic energy.

NUCLEAR FALLOUT Radioactive debris that reaches the earth's surface following a nuclear explosion.

NUCLEAR FAMILY A family *q.v.* in which children and parents live together with only incidental contact with other relatives.

NUCLEAR MAGNETIC RESONANCE (NMR) A brain imaging technique that uses a magnetic field and radio waves to produce an image. Also known as magnetic resonance imaging (MRI).

NUCLEAR MEDICINE A branch of radiology that uses nuclear physics to diagnose and treat disease.

NUCLEAR MEMBRANE The outer bounding membrane of the nucleus *q.v.*

NUCLEIC ACID 1. Complex, high-molecular-weight molecules that contain phosphate, ribose, and four bases: (a) adenine, (b) guanine, (c) cytosine, and (d) thymine. 2. A nucleotide *q.v.* 3. DNA, deoxyribonucleic acid *q.v.*, and RNA, ribonucleic acid *q.v.*, found in the cell nucleus. 4. An acid composed of phosphoric acid, pentose sugar, and organic bases.

NUCLEIN Material from the cell nucleus containing nucleic acid *q.v.* and protein *q.v.*

NUCLEOLUS 1. One or more spherical, dark-staining bodies in the nucleus that are rich in RNA *q.v.* and protein *q.v.* 2. Structures within the nucleus of some metabolic cells.

NUCLEOPLASM The protoplasm *q.v.* composing the nucleus *q.v.* of a cell.

NUCLEOPROTEIN A complex of protein *q.v.* and nucleic acid *q.v.* making up the chromosomes *q.v.*

NUCLEOTIDE 1. A combination of purine *q.v.* and pyrimidine bases, 5-carbon atom sugar, and phosphoric acid *q.v.* 2. A hydrolytic *q.v.* product of nucleic acid *q.v.* 3. A constituent of the coenzymes *q.v.* NAD *q.v.* and NADP *q.v.* 4. Compounds composed of an organic phosphate, a pentose sugar, and a nitrogen base. They are the structural units of DNA *q.v.* and RNA *q.v.*

NUCLEUS 1. Typically, the largest structure within cells. The ~ contains DNA *q.v.*, RNA *q.v.*, and, usually, a distinct body called the nucleolus *q.v.* 2. In anatomy, a mass of nerve cell bodies (gray matter) within the brain and spinal cord. 3. A spherical body within a cell containing the chromosomes *q.v.* 4. The central part of an atom consisting of neutrons *q.v.* and positively charged protons *q.v.* (except for hydrogen, which contains only a proton).

NUCLEUS BASALIS A group of large cell bodies found just below the basal ganglia *q.v.* and containing acetylcholine *q.v.* These cells send impulses to the cerebral cortex *q.v.* A loss of these neurons *q.v.* and a subsequent reduction in the amount of acetylcholine is common in people with Alzheimer's disease *q.v.*

NUDISM The social practice of some people who prefer to be nude rather than clothed. Often erroneously linked with exhibitionism *q.v.* ~ is considered by some to be a sexual variance *q.v.*

NUISANCE A continuous disruption or misuse of property or social activity that prevents the normal function of a community.

NULL HYPOTHESIS 1. In epidemiology *q.v.*, a statement expressing no relationship between two or more variables. 2. No differences. 3. The true meaning difference is zero. 4. A tentative proposition that is being tested. cf: alternative hypothesis.

NULLIPARA A woman who has not yet had her first baby.

NULLIPAROUS Never having given birth to a child.

NULLISOMIC A diploid *q.v.* cell or organism lacking both members of a chromosome *q.v.* pair.

NULL THEORY A theory of pornography's effects that holds that pornography neither stimulates nor depresses sexual behavior. ct: catharsis theory; modeling theory.

NUMORPHAN A commercial preparation of oxymorphone *q.v.*

NUNC PRO TUNC Acts permitted to be performed after they should have been performed and given retroactive effect.

NUNCUPATIVE WILL An oral will.

NURSE 1. A paramedical profession requiring training in general aspects of nursing and requiring licensing or certification. 2. A person who performs a variety of services for the sick, injured, elderly, etc. These services include emergency care, routine care, administration of drugs as directed by a physician, social care, etc.

NURSE PRACTITIONER (NP) A registered nurse (RN) with advanced training in a particular medical specialty.

NURSERY SCHOOL A school that offers supervised educational experiences for prekindergarten children.

NURSING AIDE One who performs limited nursing services usually under the supervision of a registered nurse.

NURSING HOME A facility that provides secure, protective, custodial care of the sick, elderly, or disabled.

NURTURANCE 1. Comfort and support in the interest of personal growth. 2. Being concerned for and responsible to the needs of others.

NURTURE 1. Environmental *q.v.* influence and care of the young. 2. The giving of emotional support.

NUTATION 1. In botany, the movement of growing parts, such as stems, leaves, or flowers. 2. In physiology *q.v.* nodding, as of the head. 3. In birth, ~ of the sacrum to give greater space for passage of the fetus *q.v.*

NUTRIENT 1. The chemical substances in foods necessary for health and for maintenance of life: vitamins, minerals, carbohydrates, proteins, and fats *q.v.* Water is sometimes regarded as a nutrient. 2. Nutritional substances found in food. 3. Chemical substances that nourish. 4. The energy-yielding substances and building materials obtained from food. 5. Elements in foods that are required for the growth, repair, maintenance, and regulation of body tissues and processes.

NUTRIENT DENSITY The ratio of calories *q.v.* to other nutrients *q.v.* in food.

NUTRITION 1. Refers to the quality and quantities of nutrients *q.v.* taken into the body over a specified period of time. 2. The study of nutritional processes. 3. The overall process in which food is taken into the body and then transformed and used for proper functioning of the body. 4. A specialized area of community health that is concerned with the study of the interaction between nutrients, nutrition, and health and with the application of scientific nutritional principles and maintenance of health.

NUTRITIONAL ABUSES Refers to actions taken relative to foods, nutrients, and diets that are contrary to scientific evidence or are harmful to health.

NUTRITIONAL ANTHROPOLOGY A discipline or science that is concerned with patterns of food acquisition and consumption. cf: anthropology.

NUTRITIONAL DEFICIENCY Symptoms indicating a lack in the body of one or more of the essential nutrients *q.v.*

NUTRITION LABELING A listing of nutritive content of packaged foods on the product label as required by the Food and Drug Administration *q.v.*

NUTRITION QUACKERY Quackery *q.v.* in regards to foods. Food quackery is identifiable by the catch phrases frequently used by the nutrition quack: health food, organic foods, natural foods, miracle foods, and others. ~ is also found in regards to various miracle diets, none of which has been found scientifically to be effective over the long run.

NYMPHOMANIA 1. A rare phenomenon involving uncontrollable desire of a woman for sexual fulfillment. A true nymphomaniac *q.v.* will seek sexual gratification no matter what the consequences may be. 2. A sexual variance *q.v.* ct: Satyriasis.

NYMPHOMANIAC A woman who suffers from nymphomania *q.v.*

NYSTAGMUS 1. A rapid, uncontrollable oscillation of the eyeballs, usually side-to-side. 2. Uncontrollable eye movements in a to-and-fro motion due to disease of the internal ear or central nervous system *q.v.*

OASH An acronym for Office of Assistant Secretary for Health.

OBEDIENCE A change in belief or behavior as a result of pressure from an authority figure.

OBESE An excess of body weight as a result of the presence of surplus fat tissues.

OBESITY 1. A condition characterized by being 20% or more above one's ideal body weight *q.v.* 2. The accumulation of fat beyond the amount needed for health. 3. A condition of marked overweight produced by a variety of factors, e.g., metabolic *q.v.* disorders or overeating.

OBITUARY NOTICE A biographical sketch that appears in a newspaper or on the Internet shortly after a person's death.

OBJECT CHOICE In the psychology *q.v.* of sex, the type of person or thing selected as a focus for sexual activity.

OBJECT CONSTANCY The main achievement of the sensorimotor period *q.v.* when the infant realizes that objects exist independent of the infant's sensory and/or motor contact with them.

OBJECT FETISH A sexually arousing inanimate object.

OBJECTIVE 1. In education, a purpose or goal. 2. In science, a compound lens system that is nearest the specimen. The ~ is prepared with various magnifications, and the image produced is called the primary image. 3. A statement that describes the outcome of teaching or learning. Objectives may be classified as teacher, learner, or method. 4. Learner objectives are expressed in behavioral terms and fall within the cognitive *q.v.*, affective *q.v.*, or psychomotor domains *q.v.* 5. An ~ states precisely what the learner will be doing as a result of the learning experience, and ~s are quantitatively measurable. cf: behavioral objective.

OBJECTIVE ANXIETY In psychoanalytic theory *q.v.*, the ego's *q.v.* reaction to danger, the same as realistic fear.

OBJECTIVE MORAL REASONING In moral judgment *q.v.*, judging an act as good or bad on the basis of its consequences. ct: subjective moral reasoning.

OBJECTIVE RESPONSIBILITY A belief that the magnitude of an offense can be judged solely by the magnitude of its consequences regardless of the intensions of the offender.

OBJECTIVE SELF-AWARENESS A perception of self often accompanied by feelings of anxiety *q.v.* over meeting standards.

OBJECTIVE TEST A test yielding results that can be scored by anyone with like outcomes.

OBJECTIVE TEST INSTRUMENT 1. An evaluation instrument that is consistently scored in the same manner each time it is used. 2. An evaluation instrument that requires no judgment in scoring. ct: subjective test instrument.

OBJECTIVE TESTS OF PERSONALITY Tests that take the form of questionnaires or rating scales. ct: projective tests of personality.

OBJECTIVE THEORY One of three major systems of rules and principles that guides persons in making value judgments. ~ holds that one perfect set of values exists, which is binding to all persons in all places at all times and is not subject to change.

OBJECTIVITY One of the criteria for evaluating the scientific merit of observations. All subjective judgments are avoided and all descriptive statements are made in a manner that is objectively verifiable.

OBJECT PERMANENCE The conviction that an object remains perceptually constant over time and exists even when it is out of sight.

OBJECT RELATIONSHIP Refers to the parent–child relationship in which the parent functions as an object of admiration and a role model for the child.

OBLIQUE FRACTURE A fracture *q.v.* that runs obliquely to the axis *q.v.* of the bone.

OBSCENE 1. Disgusting, repulsive, filthy, shocking. 2. That which is abhorrent to accepted social standards or morality and decency.

OBSCENE TELEPHONE CALLING A variant sexual behavior in which there is anonymous telephone communication involving lewd language.

OBSCENITY 1. Something offensive to modesty or decency, often sexually related. 2. Pictures or writings that are disgusting to the senses, abhorrent to morality or virtue, and/or specifically designed to incite lust or depravity. In this definition, ~ is not constitutionally protected. 3. In law, a concept that the act or materials in question appeal to the prurient interest, violate community standards, and have no scientific or other value. cf: pornography.

OBSERVABLE HEALTH BEHAVIOR Behavior that can be evaluated during or immediately after the learning experience, or when the learner uses what is learned in a later life situation. ~ is the overt behavior of the individual toward various aspects of the environment that affect health.

OBSERVATIONAL LEARNING 1. Modeling *q.v.* as related to social learning theory *q.v.* 2. The acquisition of a new form of behavior as a result of observing another person benefit from using a particular form of behavior.

OBSERVATIONAL METHOD 1. A research technique in which people observe and describe subjects' behavior. 2. Participant observation. cf: clinical method; experimental method.

OBSERVATIONAL STUDY A study in which the investigator does not manipulate any of the variables but simply observes their relationships as they occur.

OBSERVATION TECHNIQUES In education, structured methods for observing various aspects of a particular class or the entire school.

OBSERVER DRIFT The tendency of two observers of an activity or a process to begin to agree with each other. This is regarded as a threat to reliable *q.v.* and valid *q.v.* behavior assessment.

OBSERVING EGO According to Selman's theory of self, the ~ represents a view of self that is characteristic of late childhood or early adolescence, when children tend to think that they have an inner self who is in charge of both their behavior and thoughts.

OBSESSION 1. A persistent impulse that cannot be relieved by logic. 2. The unintentional, repetition of thoughts. 3. A recurring thought or thought process that is intrusive and repetitive that the person believes is irrational. cf: obsessive; obsessive-compulsive reaction (disorder).

OBSESSIVE A person suffering from a neurosis *q.v.*, characterized by the persistent recurrence of some irrational thought or idea, or by an attachment to or fixation on a particular or individual or object. cf: obsessive-compulsive reaction (disorder).

OBSESSIVE-COMPULSIVE REACTION (DISORDER) 1. A neurosis *q.v.* 2. The chief characteristics of ~ are uncontrollable thoughts (obsessions) and actions (compulsions). 3. There are three main subdivisions of ~: 1. ambivalence *q.v.*, 2. isolation *q.v.*, and 3. undoing *q.v.* cf: generalized anxiety disorder; phobia.

OBSTETRICAL ANALGESIA A nondrug pain reliever used in childbirth, e.g., hypnosis *q.v.*

OBSTETRICIAN A physician specializing in the care of women during pregnancy, labor, and the period immediately following delivery of the child. cf: gynecologist.

OBSTETRICS 1. Gynecology *q.v.* 2. One of the medical specialties that deals with the scientific management of women during pregnancy, childbirth, and postpartum *q.v.*

OBSTRUCTION A blockage or clogging.

OCCIPITAL The region pertaining to the back part of the head. cf: occipital lobe; occipital bone.

OCCIPITAL BONE The posterior region of the cranium *q.v.* or skull.

OCCIPITAL LOBE 1. The most posterior lobe of the cerebral hemisphere *q.v.* 2. A lobe in each cerebral hemisphere that includes the visual projection area *q.v.*

OCCIPUT The back of the head.

OCCLUDE 1. To close off or stop up. 2. Obstruct *q.v.*

OCCLUSION 1. The contact of the teeth of both jaws when the mouth is closed or during the movements of the mandible *q.v.* in mastication *q.v.* 2. The closing and fitting together of dental structures.

OCCLUSIVE DRESSING A dressing or bandage that closes a wound and protects it from the air.

OCCULT 1. A philosophy of hidden matters that includes practices based on those theories and beliefs that are beyond human understanding. 2. Obscure, unknown, not obvious.

OCCULT BLOOD Blood in such minute quantities that it can be seen only by microscopic *q.v.* examination.

OCCULT TUMOR A tumor *q.v.* that is concealed or hidden.

OCCUPATIONAL CLUSTERS Several kinds of jobs that require similar skills and are grouped together.

OCCUPATIONAL DRINKING The excessive consumption of alcohol that is associated with some occupations, frequently on the job, e.g., bartending.

OCCUPATIONAL HEALTH EDUCATION 1. Corporate health education *q.v.* 2. Health education *q.v.* in the workplace.

OCCUPATIONAL HEALTH SERVICES Health services *q.v.* concerned with the physical, mental, and social well-being of people in relation to their work and working environment and with the adjustment of the people to their work and vice versa.

OCCUPATIONAL ILLNESS Any abnormal condition, other than those resulting from injury, caused by exposure to environmental factors in the workplace. cf: occupational injury.

OCCUPATIONAL INJURY Any injury that results from a work-related accident. cf: occupational illness.

OCCUPATIONAL PRESTIGE In sociology, the relative social status generally attributed to some occupations.

OCCUPATIONAL SAFETY AND HEALTH A specialized area of community health that is concerned with the identification of health and safety hazards related to work and the work environment and with their prevention and control.

OCCUPATIONAL SAFETY AND HEALTH ADMINISTRATION (OSHA) A federal agency that attempts to assure a safe and healthful environment in the workplace by setting and enforcing health and safety standards.

OCCUPATIONAL THERAPY 1. A form of psychological *q.v.* treatment that involves habilitating or rehabilitating a person in occupational activities. 2. Training a person to perform work-related activities necessary to make a living. 3. The use of occupational training in psychotherapy *q.v.*

OCEANIC KISS An ancient way of kissing in Polynesia that involves placing one's face to the cheek of the other person and smelling his or her skin.

OCKHAM'S RAZOR The principle that if one is confronted with more than one possible solution to a problem, one should choose the simplest. Named after a fourteenth century British Franciscan.

OCTOPLOID A cell or organism with eight genomes *q.v.* or monoploid *q.v.* sets of chromosomes.

OCULAR Pertaining to the eye.

OCULOMOTOR Moving the eyeball.

ODDS RATIO In epidemiology *q.v.*, a technique for estimating relative risk from case–control studies *q.v.* cf: relative odds.

ODONTALGIA A toothache.

ODONTOBLASTS One of the connective tissue *q.v.* cells that constitutes the outer surface of the dental pulp *q.v.* adjacent to the dentin *q.v.*

ODONTOLOGY 1. Dentistry *q.v.* 2. The scientific study of the teeth.

OEDIPAL CONFLICT 1. In Freud's theory of psychosexual development *q.v.*, the conflict of a boy between a desire for his mother and the fear of punishment by his father. 2. According to Freud, the key to resolving the basic conflict of sexual development involving hostility toward the same-sex parent for usurping the sexual love for the parent of the opposite sex. cf: Oedipus complex.

OEDIPUS COMPLEX 1. Excessive emotional attachment, involving conscious or unconscious incestuous *q.v.* desires, of a son in relation to his mother. 2. In Freudian theory *q.v.*, the emotional attachment of a boy to his mother. 3. Oedipal conflict. cf: Oedipal conflict. ct: Electra complex.

OFFICE OF CONSUMER AFFAIRS Organized within the Department of Health and Human Services *q.v.* and serves as a coordinating body for inquiries and complaints on such subjects as consumer prices, quality, and safety of products and services.

OFFICE OF DISEASE PREVENTION AND HEALTH PROMOTION Concerned with coordination and policy development in matters concerned with the promotion of health.

OFFICERS In politics, those of the legislative staff elected by the membership, e.g., speaker of the house, and majority and minority whips.

OFFICIAL HEALTH AGENCY A publicly supported governmental organization mandated by law and/or regulation for the protection and improvement of the health of the population. ct: voluntary health agency; NGO.

OGIVE A monotonic relationship *q.v.* in which a period of positive acceleration *q.v.* is followed by a period of negative acceleration *q.v.*

OHDS An acronym for Office of Human Development Services.

OHIHP An acronym for U.S. Office of Health Information, Health Promotion, and Physical Fitness and Sports Medicine *q.v.*

OIL In nutrition *q.v.*, a lipid *q.v.* that is liquid at room temperature.

OLD CORTEX A small, hidden part of the brain that governs the sense of smell. cf: new cortex.

OLDER AMERICANS ACT Enacted in 1965 (PL 89-73), the purpose of the ~ was to give elderly citizens more opportunity to participate in and receive the benefits of modern society: adequate housing, income, employment, nutrition, and health care.

OLECRANON 1. The back of the elbow, formed by the tip of the ulna *q.v.* which curves around the lower end of the humorous *q.v.* 2. ~ process.

OLECRANON PROCESS Olecranon *q.v.*

OLEIC ACID An 18-carbon fatty acid *q.v.* that contains one double bond. ~ is found in animal and vegetable fat.

OLFACTION 1. The sense of smell. Olfactory *q.v.*, pertaining to the organs of smell. cf: olfactory nerve.

OLFACTORY Pertaining to the sense of smell.

OLFACTORY NERVE The first cranial nerve *q.v.* associated with the sense of smell. cf: olfaction.

OLIGODENDROGLIA A type of connective tissue *q.v.* cell found in the brain and spinal cord *q.v.*

OLIGOGMENORRHEA Unpredictable, irregular menstrual *q.v.* periods.

OLIGOSACCHARIDE A carbohydrate *q.v.* consisting of 2–10 monosaccharide *q.v.* units.

OLIGOSPERMIA A condition wherein a man's sperm *q.v.* count is too low to ensure fertilization *q.v.*

OLIGURIA Too little output of urine.

OMB An acronym for Office of Management and Budget.

OMENTUM The apron of fatty tissue that hangs down from the stomach to cover most of the front surface of the abdominal region.

OMMOCHROME A product of tryptophan *q.v.* that gives rise to pigments, particularly of the eye in animals.

OMNIVORE An organism that eats both plant and animal products.

OMNIVOROUS The consumption of both plants and animals.

OMPHALITIS Inflammation *q.v.* or infection *q.v.* of the naval.

ONANISM 1. Withdrawal of the penis *q.v.* from the vagina *q.v.* before ejaculation *q.v.* 2. Coitus interruptus *q.v.* 3. Ejaculation outside of the vagina.

ONCHOCERCIASIS River blindness. Caused by a tiny worm transmitted to humans by the bite of infected flies. Most prevalent in Central America and Africa.

ONCOGENE 1. A hypothetical gene *q.v.* that is passed from parent to offspring that has the potential of developing cancer *q.v.* 2. Genes that are believed to activate the development of cancer.

ONCOGENE HYPOTHESIS The concept that mammalian cell chromosomes *q.v.* harbor unexpressed viral DNA *q.v.* and that virus *q.v.* growth can be initiated by ionizing radiation *q.v.* or by cocarcinogens *q.v.* causing the cells in which the viruses grow to become cancerous *q.v.*

ONCOGENESIS Refers to tumors *q.v.*, cancer *q.v.*, and other neoplasms *q.v.*

ONCOGENIC 1. Anything that may give rise to or cause cancer *q.v.* 2. Pertaining to the cancer-producing potential of a virus *q.v.*

ONCOLOGIST A physician who specializes in the study and treatment of malignancies *q.v.*

ONCOLOGY The science that studies tumors *q.v.*

ONDONTALGIA A toothache.

ONE GENE-ONE ENZYME HYPOTHESIS The belief that separate enzymatic steps in metabolic *q.v.* pathways are controlled by genes *q.v.*

ONE GENE-ONE FUNCTION HYPOTHESIS The hypothesis *q.v.* that a gene *q.v.* performs a single function in a cell.

ONE-PARENT FAMILY A nuclear family *q.v.* in which only one parent is living with the children. May be caused by death, divorce, separation, desertion, or children born out of wedlock.

ONE-ROOM SCHOOL A setting in which all grade levels are taught by a single teacher in a single room.

ONE-STEP PROCEDURE (ONE-STAGE) A type of surgery that involves biopsy *q.v.* and surgery in a single operation.

ON-THE-JOB TRAINING Skills learned at the place of employment.

ONTOGENESIS The development of a single member of a species. ct: phylogenesis.

ONTOGENY 1. The history of the development of an individual organism. 2. The life history of an individual. ct: phylogeny.

ONYCHECTOMY The surgical removal of a finger or toe nail.

ONYCHOMYCOSIS A fungal infection of the nails.

OOCYST A cyst formed from the zygote *q.v.* of plasmodium *q.v.*

OOCYTE 1. An ovum *q.v.* in an immature stage of development. 2. The egg-mother cell. The cell that undergoes two meiotic divisions to form the egg cell.

OOGAMY A kind of sexual reproduction in which one gamete *q.v.* (the egg) is large and nonmotile, and the other gamete (the sperm) is smaller and motile.

OOGENESIS The maturation of ova *q.v.* in the female.

OOGONIUM 1. A cell in the female prior to meiosis *q.v.* 2. In some thallophytes *q.v.*, a structure that contains one or several eggs. 3. A structure in which the female gametes *q.v.* develop.

OOPHORECTOMY 1. Ovariectomy *q.v.* 2. The surgical removal of an ovary *q.v.* or ovaries.

OP An acronym for osmotic pressure.

OPACITY Obscuring the normal transparency of the cornea *q.v.* or lens of the eye.

OPEN-CLASS MORPHEMES Consists of the nouns, adjectives, verbs, and adverbs of a language. cf: morphemes. ct: closed-class morphemes.

OPEN CLASSROOM An organizational structure in schools in which self-contained classrooms are replaced by an open plan where students have the freedom to move about the school for different educational experiences. ct: traditional classroom.

OPEN COUPLES Among homosexuals *q.v.* and heterosexuals, couples who live together but who engage in sexual relations with others. cf: open marriage.

OPEN DISLOCATION An open fracture *q.v.*

OPEN-DOOR POLICY An administrative policy in which employees are encouraged to express complaints, ask questions, make suggestions, without the threat of reprisal.

OPEN EDUCATION A form of teaching that stresses learner activity and interaction, learning centers, cooperative planning, and individualized learning activities. ct: traditional education.

OPEN-ENDED A question or statement that allows the subject freedom to respond in any way he or she wishes.

OPEN ENROLLMENT The practice of allowing students to attend the school of their choice within a particular school district.

OPEN FRACTURE A fracture *q.v.* or dislocation *q.v.* having a direct communication with the outside through the skin. There may be a small wound over the fracture or dislocation, or the ends of the bone may be protruding through the skin.

OPEN HEAD INJURY A trauma to the brain in which the skull is opened by the injury. ct: closed head injury.

OPEN INSTITUTION An organization that is subject to pressures from outside its domain.

OPEN LESION DISEASES A class of infectious diseases *q.v.* that are generally transmitted by direct contact with the lesions of an infected person.

OPEN MARRIAGE A relationship in which the couples are committed to each other but are free to engage in sexual activities with others.

OPEN PANEL A prepaid insurance plan or policy in which any health or medical provider may become the provider of the health and medical services needed.

OPEN SPACE SCHOOL A school building without interior walls.

OPEN SYSTEM A system that is influenced by and is in constant interaction with the environment.

OPEN WOUND A wound *q.v.* in which the affected tissues are exposed by an external opening.

OPERANT BEHAVIOR A response that is generated or modified through the expectation of a reward.

OPERANT GOALS The end result and the process for achieving this end. These goals are values clarification *q.v.*, decision making, and self-actualization *q.v.*

OPERANT (INSTRUMENTAL) CONDITIONING 1. The process adhered to be one subschool of the associationist school of thought, rewarding or punishing an organism's emitted behavior. 2. A form of behavior therapy *q.v.* 3. A form of learning in which the correct response is reinforced and becomes more likely to occur again. cf: systematic desensitization; implosive therapy. ct: classical conditioning theory.

OPERANT LEARNING Learning that occurs as a result of the consequences of a behavior. Positive consequences increase the frequency of the behavior, while negative consequences decrease the frequency of the behavior.

OPERANT PAIN Learned pain behavior that may respond to behavior modification *q.v.* cf: respondent pain.

OPERATION In educational psychology *q.v.*, a mental action that can be reversed. cf: organization; reversibility.

OPERATIONAL DEFINITION The definition of a variable *q.v.* in such a way that it can be measured.

OPERATIONAL OBJECTIVES Objectives that are stated in measurable or observable terms.

OPERATIONS In developmental psychology, those skills and thought processes that are experienced as one grows and develops. cf: concrete operational period.

OPERATIONISM A position in the philosophy of science that maintains that scientific concepts acquire their meaning in terms of publicly observable operations that can be measured.

OPERATIVE VALUES One's feelings of right or wrong that influence one's decisions.

OPERATOR GENE A gene that is part of an operon *q.v.* that controls the activity of one or more structural genes *q.v.*

OPERON In genetics *q.v.*, a group of genes *q.v.* that are linked and have regulatory elements that function as a unit.

OPHTHALMIA A generalized inflammation of the eye.

OPHTHALMIA NEONATORUM An infection of the eye by the gonococcal *q.v.* bacterium of a newborn infant.

OPHTHALMIC Pertaining to the eyes.

OPHTHALMOLOGIST 1. A physician who specializes in the diagnosis and treatment of diseases and disorders of the eyes. 2. ~s are Doctors of Medicine (MD) or Doctors of Osteopathy (DO) who perform all types of eye surgery as well as prescribe corrective lenses and medicines for the eye. ct: optometrist.

OPHTHALMOLOGY The medical study of the structure, function, and diseases of the eye.

OPIATES 1. Narcotics (with the exception of cocaine). 2. Drugs derived from the opium poppy: heroin, morphine, and codeine, and synthetic and semisynthetic derivatives.

OPIOID 1. A narcotic *q.v.* so named because its actions resemble those caused by opium q.v. 2. Synthetic narcotics that resemble opium in action but are not derivatives of opium.

OPISTHOTONUS A convulsive rigid arching of the back that is characteristically seen in severe meningitis *q.v.*

OPIUM 1. A milky exudate of the unripe seed pod of the opium poppy, *Papaver somniferum q.v.* 2. A naturally occurring narcotic that is considered to be the "mother drug" of nonsynthetic narcotics.

OPIUM ADDICTION Dependence *q.v.* upon opium *q.v.*

OPPONENT-PROCESS THEORY OF COLOR VISION The theory of color vision that asserts that there are three pairs of color antagonists: red-green, blue-yellow, and white-black. Stimulation of one member of a pair inhibits the other member of the pair.

OPPONENT-PROCESS THEORY OF MOTIVATION The theory that asserts that the nervous system *q.v.* has the tendency to counteract any deviation from the neutral point of the pain–pleasure dimension. When the original stimulus *q.v.* is maintained, there is an attenuation of the emotional state that a person is in. When the stimulus is withdrawn, the opponent process reveals itself and the emotional state swings in the opposite direction.

OPPORTUNISTIC INFECTION An infection *q.v.* caused by a microorganism that rarely causes disease in persons with a normal immune system *q.v.* ~ is a term generally used in connection with AIDS *q.v.*

OPPORTUNISTIC ORGANISMS Organisms in the body that are activated by other organisms or conditions to cause a disease.

OPSONIN A substance in the blood that aids phagocytes *q.v.* in destroying bacteria *q.v.*

OPTICAL ISOMERS Alternate forms of the same substance which differ only in terms of the arrangement of molecules.

OPTIC ATROPHY A disease that results from deteriorating nerve fibers *q.v.* connecting the retina *q.v.* to the brain.

OPTIC CHIASMA The crossing of the optic nerves *q.v.* on the ventral *q.v.* surface of the brain.

OPTIC DISC The entrance of optic nerves *q.v.* into the retina *q.v.*

OPTICIAN 1. A person who specializes in the preparation of corrective lenses. 2. One who fills prescriptions from an ophthalmologist *q.v.* or from an optometrist *q.v.* but who does not examine the eyes.

OPTIC NERVE 1. The nerve of sight that enables visual images to pass from the retina *q.v.* to that portion of the brain where they are interpreted. 2. Second cranial nerve *q.v.*

OPTIMAL HEALTH 1. The highest level of functioning of which a person is capable under the existing environmental constraints. 2. The highest possible level of health.

OPTIMAL INTELLIGENCE The intelligence *q.v.* that is most appropriate to a particular task. Not necessarily maximal intelligence.

OPTIMIZING ATTENTION The ability to direct attention toward relevant attributes and to obtain desired information from the environment *q.v.*

OPTIMUM CARRYING CAPACITY The level of population that allows all people to have a high quality of life. ct: maximum carrying capacity.

OPTOGRAM A picture (image) on the retina *q.v.*

OPTOMETRIST A person with specialized training in the diagnosis and correction of visual problems. An ~ cannot prescribe drugs or perform surgery; holds a degree of Doctor of Optometry (DO). cf: optometry. ct: ophthalmologist.

OPTOMETRY A nonmedical *q.v.* specialty concerned with examining a person's eyes for refractory problems and correcting them by fitting eye glasses. cf: optometrist; ophthalmology.

ORAL ADMINISTRATION The introduction of a drug into the body through the mouth.

ORAL CANCER Malignancy *q.v.* of the mouth or oral cavity *q.v.*

ORAL CAVITY Pertaining to the mouth.

ORAL CONTRACEPTIVES 1. Drugs taken through oral administration *q.v.* to prevent conception *q.v.* 2. Pills taken orally, composed of synthetic female hormones *q.v.* that prevent ovulation *q.v.* or implantation *q.v.* of a fertilized *q.v.* egg.

ORAL DISEASES Diseases of the oral cavity *q.v.* These diseases include tooth decay, pulpitis *q.v.*, periodontal diseases *q.v.*, and halitosis *q.v.*

ORAL EROTICISM 1. Oral gratification *q.v.* 2. Pleasurable sensations centered in the lips and mouth and is related to early pleasure arising from nursing during infancy.

ORAL FIXATION In Freudian psychology *q.v.*, gratification or stimulation of the mouth enhancing emotional security.

ORAL GRATIFICATION 1. Satisfaction or need fulfillment obtained through the use of the mouth or by placing something in the mouth. 2. Oral eroticism *q.v.*

ORAL PATHOLOGY 1. That specialty of dentistry *q.v.* that is concerned with the treatment of diseases of the mouth. 2. Dental pathology *q.v.* cf: pathology; oral diseases.

ORAL SEX Fellatio *q.v.* or cunnilingus *q.v.*

ORAL STAGE In Freudian psychology *q.v.*, the first of four psychosexual stages *q.v.* in which sexual pleasure is derived through stimulation of the lips and mouth and extends from birth to age two. ct: anal stage; genital stage; latency period.

ORAL SURGEON 1. A dentist *q.v.* specializing in surgery of the mouth or oral cavity *q.v.* 2. A dentist specializing in dental extractions and surgery on related structures. cf: maxillofacial surgery.

ORAL SURGERY 1. A dental specialty concerned with surgery of the oral cavity such as dental extractions and related structures. 2. The specialized branch of dentistry *q.v.* that treats conditions of the oral cavity *q.v.* by surgical methods.

ORCHIECTOMY The surgical removal of one or both testicles *q.v.*

ORCHITIS 1. A complication of mumps *q.v.* resulting in a swelling of the testicles *q.v.* and in severe cases sterility *q.v.* 2. Inflammation or infection of the testicles.

ORDER In the classification of living things, a category above the family and below the class.

ORDINAL SCALE A scale in which responses are ranked-ordered by relative magnitude but in which the intervals between successive ranks are not necessarily equal. cf: categorical scale; interval scale; ratio scale.

ORDINAL VARIABLE In epidemiology *q.v.*, a variable having values that can be meaningfully ordered or ranked.

ORGAN A part of the body consisting of two or more tissues organized to perform a specific function.

ORGAN DONOR A person who donates one or more of his or her organs to another person whose organ is diseased, injured, or lacking.

ORGANELLE A subcellular structure that performs a specialized function in the cell.

ORGANIC 1. A dysfunction caused by a change in tissues, as in organic disease *q.v.* 2. Compounds containing one or more carbon atoms. 3. Food that is grown without the use of pesticides. ct: functional; inorganic.

ORGANIC BRAIN SYNDROME 1. A disorder characterized by mental confusion, disorientation, and decreased intellectual function. Possibly caused by the prolonged use of psychoactive *q.v.* drugs. 2. Abnormal mental functioning brought about by degeneration or injury to brain tissue. 3. A mental disorder in which there is an impairment of intellectual and emotional functioning.

ORGANIC CHEMICAL A substance, such as an acid, alkali, salt, or synthetic compound obtained by a chemical process, prepared for use in chemical manufacture, or used for producing a chemical effect. ct: inorganic chemical.

ORGANIC COMPOUND 1. A carbon-containing compound *q.v.* There are four classes of major nutrients: (a) carbohydrates *q.v.*, (b) proteins *q.v.*, (c) lipids *q.v.*, and (d) vitamins *q.v.* 2. A compound containing carbon and often hydrogen that may also contain other elements.

ORGANIC DISEASE A disease *q.v.* condition characterized by an abnormal alteration of tissues.

ORGANIC EVOLUTION The theory that existing living forms have been derived by gradual modification from earlier and simpler forms.

ORGANIC FOODS Foods grown without chemical pesticides *q.v.* or chemical fertilizers.

ORGANIC HEART DISEASE The presence of symptoms of disease of the heart due to changes or breakdown of cardiac *q.v.* tissues. cf: functional heart disease.

ORGANIC HYPERTENSION Hypertension that develops as a result of a specific physical cause. cf: hypertension.

ORGANICITY Impairment of the central nervous system *q.v.*

ORGANIC MENTAL DISORDER A disorder that is caused by a physical change in brain tissue or brain functioning. Withdrawal syndrome from drugs or Alzheimer's disease are examples of ~s. cf: organic psychosis.

ORGANIC PSYCHOSIS 1. A psychosis *q.v.* with a known physiological or neuroanatomical basis or cause. 2. A psychosis associated with brain pathology *q.v.* 3. A severe mental disorder known to be caused by a physical disease or condition. cf: organic mental disorder. ct: functional psychosis.

ORGANIC VIEWPOINT The theory in psychology *q.v.* that all mental disorders have an organic *q.v.* basis.

ORGANISM Any living thing capable of performing all of life processes.

ORGANISMIC VARIABLE A physical or psychological factor that makes an organism or individual unique and is subject to evaluation through behavior assessment.

ORGANIZATION 1. A group of people working in concert to achieve common goals. 2. Pertaining to intellectual structures, a universal attribute of biological characteristics. 3. In the case of intelligence *q.v.*, ~ is manifested by recurrent, identifiable sequences of behavior. cf: scheme; operations.

ORGANIZATIONAL ANALYSIS A study of the organizational structure, work climate, functions, and relationships to determine training needs and other needs of the organization.

ORGANIZATIONAL DEVELOPMENT 1. A continuous effort to increase productivity and effectiveness of an organization. 2. Based on a systems perspective, a process of change in an organization's structure and personnel through the application of knowledge gained from the behavioral sciences.

ORGANIZATIONAL STRUCTURE The way in which an organization *q.v.* is structured or put together to efficiently achieve its goals.

ORGANIZATION ENVIRONMENT The environment *q.v.* within an organization—physical, cultural, and emotional climate.

ORGANIZATION OF BLOOD CLOT A blood clot in which connective tissue and blood vessels have formed.

ORGANIZED ELEMENTS The range of subject areas or health topics considered to constitute the body of knowledge of health education *q.v.*

ORGANIZER 1. An inductor. 2. A chemical substance in a living system that determines the development of cells or groups of cells.

ORGANIZING The process of establishing orderly processes for the utilization of all resources within an organization.

ORGANIZING EFFECTS Influences on the directions and forms that behavior takes. ct: activating effects.

ORGANIZING THREADS Continuing curriculum *q.v.* emphasis, health concepts, values, and problem-solving *q.v.* skills that provide the basis for continuity and integration.

ORGANOGENESIS The processes by which organs form and develop. Much of these processes occur during embryonic *q.v.* development and continue during the fetal *q.v.* period and after birth.

ORGANOTROPIC Having an attraction for certain organs or tissues of the body.

ORGASM 1. A series of involuntary muscular contractions accompanied by emotional and nervous system *q.v.* pleasurable sensations and usually accompanied by ejaculation *q.v.* in the male and vaginal *q.v.* and uterine *q.v.* contractions in the female. 2. One of the four basic phases of sexual arousal, the orgasmic phase *q.v.* 3. The peak or climax of sexual excitement in sexual activity.

ORGASM DISCLOSURE RATIO For a given time frame, the number of people who have witnessed a given person experience an orgasm divided by the number of people with whom the person is interacting.

ORGASMIC DYSFUNCTION The complete inability to achieve orgasm or the inability to achieve orgasm when desired.

ORGASMIC PHASE 1. One of the four phases of sexual arousal *q.v.* 2. Achieving orgasm *q.v.* 3. The third stage in the human sexual response cycle *q.v.* during which orgasm occurs.

ORGASMIC PLATFORM 1. The narrowed lower vaginal *q.v.* canal during sexual arousal. 2. The area comprising the outer third of the vagina *q.v.* and the labia minora *q.v.*, which displays marked vasocongestion *q.v.* in the plateau phase *q.v.* of the female sexual response cycle *q.v.*

ORGASMIC RECONDITIONING Orgasmic reorientation *q.v.*

ORGASMIC REORIENTATION 1. Orgasmic reconditioning. 2. An approach used to condition a person away from an undesirable or unsuitable stimulus to a more desirable one by rewarding the latter and/or making the former unattractive.

ORGASMIC STAGE Orgasmic phase *q.v.*

ORIENTATION The person's ability to comprehend the environment with reference to time, place, and person.

ORIENTING RESPONSE In classical conditioning *q.v.*, a person's initial reaction to a new stimulus *q.v.*

ORIFICE An opening.

ORIGINAL JURISDICTION The court that originally entertains a case from its inception, as opposed to appellate jurisdiction.

ORIGIN OF MUSCLE The place where a muscle *q.v.* is firmly attached to the skeleton, as distinguished from its insertion, which is where the muscle is attached to the bone that moves.

OROPHARYNGEAL AIRWAY A device that can be placed in the mouth to make it easier to breathe by lifting the tongue away from the palate *q.v.*

OROPHARYNX The central portion of the pharynx *q.v.* extending from the level of the palate *q.v.* to the vestibule *q.v.* of the larynx *q.v.*

ORPHAN DRUG A drug that typically is used for the treatment of a rare condition, making it exorbitantly expensive and/or difficult to obtain.

ORTHOBIOSIS The proper style of living that fulfills a person's health needs, promotes optimal well-being, and prolongs life. ~ is made up of positive and constructive behaviors.

ORTHODONTIA A dental specialty concerned with correcting malocclusion *q.v.*, proper alignment of the teeth. cf: orthodontics.

ORTHODONTICS Orthodontia *q.v.*

ORTHOGENESIS The development or evolution in a definite direction.

ORTHOMOLECULAR MEDICINE 1. Treatment based on the use of large amounts of naturally occurring substances, such as vitamins *q.v.* ~ is not an accepted medical practice. 2. Correction of mental disorders with nutrition *q.v.* 3. Treating a disease by determining whether it is caused by chemical imbalances and correcting them with nutrition. cf: orthomolecular nutrition.

ORTHOMOLECULAR NUTRITION Supplying a person with a chemically perfect diet for his or her individual nutritional *q.v.* needs. cf: orthomolecular medicine.

ORTHOMOLECULAR PSYCHIATRY Correcting mental disorders with nutrition *q.v.*

ORTHOMOLECULAR TREATMENT 1. An unorthodox method of treatment that claims that diseases should be treated by administering the right nutrient molecules at the right time. 2. Meganutrient therapy *q.v.*

ORTHOPEDICS 1. Refers to postural or structural condition. The person who has an orthopedic handicap may encounter problems associated with ambulation. 2. The medical knowledge, diagnosis, and treatment of the skeletal system *q.v.* 3. A medical specialty concerned with the diagnosis, treatment (including surgery) of diseases, injuries, and deformities of the bones, joints, and related structures.

ORTHOPSYCHIATRY The area of psychiatry *q.v.* that is primarily concerned with unhealthful personality trends and the maladjustments *q.v.* of children.

ORTHOPTICS 1. The science of treating visual defects of a mechanical nature. 2. The practice of correcting visual defects through the use of exercises of the muscles controlling the eyes.

ORTHOSTATIC ALBUMINURIA 1. Postural albuminuria *q.v.* 2. Albuminuria *q.v.* that disappears when a person lies down for a period of time.

ORTHOSTATIC HYPERTENSION A drop in blood pressure caused by standing up from a prone position, resulting in dizziness or fainting.

OS 1. A mouth or orifice *q.v.* 2. The opening of the vagina *q.v.* into the uterus *q.v.* 3. Latin for mouth or for bone.

OSCULUM An excurrent opening.

OS EXTERNUM UTERI The mouth or orifice *q.v.* to the uterus *q.v.*

OSHA An acronym for Occupational Safety and Health Administration *q.v.*

OSMOPHILIC 1. Salt loving. 2. Organisms that can tolerate high salt concentrations. 3. Halophilic.

OSMORECEPTORS Receptors *q.v.* that help to control water intake by responding to the concentrations of body fluids.

OSMOSIS 1. The movement of a liquid through a semipermeable membrane from a less dense to greater density medium. 2. The passage of a solvent through a membrane separating two solutions from the solution of lesser concentration to that of greater concentration.

OSMOTIC PRESSURE (OP) The pressure that develops or is present when two solutions of different concentrations are separated by a membrane that is permeable only to the solvent. cf: osmosis.

OSSCULAR CHAIN The three small bones of the middle ear (malleus, incus, and stapes) that transmit vibrations to the inner ear.

OSSICLE 1. One of the small bones of the tympanum *q.v.* of the ear, malleus *q.v.*, incus *q.v.*, or stapes *q.v.* 2. Any small bone.

OSSIFICATION The presence of bone formation.

OSTEITIS Inflammation of a bone.

OSTEOARTHRITIS 1. A chronic *q.v.* degenerative *q.v.* disease *q.v.* of the joints. 2. Arthritis *q.v.* resulting from a degeneration of the joint. 3. ~ usually produces stiffness or pain in the fingers or in weight-bearing joints. Inflammation *q.v.* is rare. While the cause of ~ is unknown, recent research indicates that the cartilage *q.v.* in persons with severe ~ symptoms is different from the cartilage in persons without symptoms. Wear and tear on joint surfaces appears to contribute to the condition. Most people over 60 years have this type of arthritis but only about 50% experience symptoms.

OSTEOARTHROPATHY Any disease involving the bones and joints.

OSTEOBLAST An immature bone-producing cell.

OSTEOCHONDRITIS An inflammatory process of bone and cartilage about a joint.

OSTEOCLAST A bone cell that helps to resorb bone.

OSTEOCYTE Bone cell.

OSTEOMALACIA 1. A condition characterized by resorption of calcium from bones and resulting from a deficiency of vitamin D *q.v.* in the diet. 2. Adult rickets *q.v.* A softening of the bones caused by a vitamin D deficiency in adults. cf: osteoporosis.

OSTEOMYELITIS 1. Infection of a bone. 2. An infectious inflammatory *q.v.* disease of the bone evidenced by localized death of the bone and separation of the tissue.

OSTEOPATHIC MEDICINE A field of medicine emphasizing diagnosing and treating structural problems through manipulating the musculoskeletal system *q.v.* Practitioners receive much the same training and perform similar functions as medical doctors.

OSTEOPATHIC PHYSICIAN 1. A practitioner who diagnoses and treats disease. 2. A person who possesses the Doctor of Osteopathy (DO) degree. In general, the ~ is licensed to practice medicine in the same manner as a medical doctor who possesses the MD degree.

OSTEOPATHY 1. That system of treating illnesses that are presumed to be caused by pressure of displaced bones upon nerves and are cured by manipulation. 2. A medical treatment involving the manipulation of the spine and other body parts. 3. A system of medical practice similar to allopathy *q.v.* cf: osteopathic physician.

OSTEOPOROSIS 1. A reduction in bone size resulting from a depletion of calcium levels in the body. Relatively common in postmenopausal *q.v.* women. 2. A reduction in the normal quantity of bone tissue. 3. A loss of calcium from the bones, characterized by brittle, fragile bones. Treated through exercise and dietary calcium supplements. 4. A decrease in the density of the bones causing structural weakness throughout the skeleton *q.v.* Fractures can result from even a minor injury or fall. Some bone loss is normal in older adults, but ~ develops most often in white women after menopause.

OSTIUM A small opening, especially one of entrance into a hollow organ or canal.

OTA An acronym for Office of Technology Assessment (part of the U.S. Congress).

OTITIS (ACUTE EXTERNAL) A bacterial infection of the ear canal *q.v.* Usually caused from swimming. Symptoms include inflammation of the ear canal.

OTITIS MEDIA Inflammation of the middle ear *q.v.*

OTOCEPHALY An abnormal development of the head of a fetus *q.v.*

OTOLARYNGOLOGICAL Pertaining to diseases of the ear and respiratory *q.v.* passages.

OTOLARYNGOLOGY A medical specialty concerned with the diagnosis and treatment of diseases of the ear, nose, and throat.

OTOLOGIST A physician specializing in the health of the ear.

OTOLOGY A medical specialty concerned with the diagnosis and treatment of diseases of the ear.

OTOMYOSIS A fungal *q.v.* infection of the external ear characterized by itching or pain.

OTOPLASTY The surgical procedure for restructuring the shape of the ear.

OTORHINOLARYNGOLOGY (ENT) A medical specialty concerned with the totality of the ear, nose, and throat.

OTORHINOLOGY The study of the diseases of the ear and nose.

OTOSCLEROSIS 1. A pathological *q.v.* change that occurs in the middle and inner ear, causing progressive impairment of hearing. 2. The formation of spongy bone about the stapes *q.v.* and fenestra nestibuli *q.v.* in the ear.

OTOSCOPE An instrument for inspecting the ear canal and ear drum.

OTOTOXIC DRUGS Drugs that can have an adverse effect on the eighth cranial nerve *q.v.* or on the organs of balance and hearing.

OUTBREEDING The mating of individuals who are not closely related.

OUTCOME EVALUATION 1. The level of evaluation that measures whether a program has met its own objectives. 2. A process of determining a student's accomplishment based on stated objectives.

OUTCOME MEASURE A measure of the quality or effectiveness of health education in which the standard of judgment is the attainment of a specified end result.

OUTCOME RESEARCH Research that is concerned with the effects of treatment or other procedures upon behavior *q.v.* ct: process research.

OUTDOOR EDUCATION Activity and study in an outdoor setting.

OUTER DIRECTED A person who seeks guidance from others in behavioral matters. ct: inner directed.

OUTER LIPS Labia majora *q.v.*

OUT-GROUP In sociology, groups with which a person does not identify or which a person is antagonistic towards. ct: in-group.

OUT OF ORDER Business that is not proper under parliamentary procedures.

OUT-OF-POCKET PAYMENTS Pertains to those medical expenses such as deductibles and coinsurance for which the insured person is responsible.

OUTPATIENT A person who is treated at a facility without residing there. ct: inpatient.

OVARIAN CANCER Malignancy *q.v.* of the ovary *q.v.*

OVARIAN FOLLICLE 1. The small sac or vesicle near the surface of the ovary *q.v.* in the female that contains a developing egg cell. 2. Follicle.

OVARIECTOMY 1. Oophorectomy *q.v.* 2. The surgical removal of the ovaries *q.v.*

OVARY 1. The anatomical structure in the female located one on either side of the uterus *q.v.* and whose function is to produce ova *q.v.* for fertilization *q.v.* and reproduction *q.v.* The ~ also produces sex hormones *q.v.* 2. The primary female sex gland that produces estrogen *q.v.* and progesterone *q.v.* Each ovary contains up to 200,000 immature ova at a female's birth. 3. In botany, the swollen part at the base of a pistil, containing the ovules or seeds.

OVATESTIS An organ that contains both ovarian and testicular tissue, found in some hermaphrodites *q.v.*

OVERACHIEVEMENT The act of performing above expectations based on measures of ability.

OVERCOMPENSATION A marked exaggeration of compensatory behavior *q.v.* in an effort to cover up weakness or inferiority. cf: compensation.

OVERCONTROLLED In reference to childhood disorders, a situation in which a child cannot adequately cope with stress and anxiety and may withdraw socially because of a very controlling environment.

OVEREXTENSION A child's tendency to use a rather specific term to refer to a wide class of referents.

OVERFAT A condition in which a person possesses more body fat than is normal for people of the same height and sex. cf: overweight; obesity.

OVERGENERALIZATION The tendency to draw an inappropriately general or illogical conclusion from very limited data or experience.

OVERLAPPING DISTRIBUTION A statistical term describing situations in which, although a difference exists between the overall values of a particular variable for two groups, the values of the variable for some individual members of the two groups are the same.

OVERLAPPING RESPONSIBILITY A situation in which several people may be responsible for the same activity.

OVERLEARNING Practice beyond the point of mastery in learning *q.v.* a set of material.

OVERLOAD 1. A training principle in which those being trained are required to work at a level beyond normal demands. 2. A work schedule in which a person is either forced or elects to assume more responsibility than is normally required.

OVERLOADING 1. Subjecting a person to excessive stress *q.v.* 2. Forcing a person to handle or process an excessive amount of information. cf: overload principle.

OVERLOAD PRINCIPLE Used in training programs to increase muscular strength. The concept whereby a person gradually increases the resistance load on muscles.

OVERPOPULATION A condition where the population exceeds the ability of the land to sustain it.

OVERPROTECTION Shielding a child to the extent that he or she becomes overly dependent upon the parent or other adult.

OVERRIDING AORTA A condition in which the aorta *q.v.* takes blood from the right ventricle *q.v.* as well as from the left ventricle *q.v.*

OVERSHADOWING An effect produced when two conditioned stimuli *q.v.* are both presented at the same time with the unconditioned stimulus *q.v.* When one conditioned stimulus is more intense than the other, it tends to overshadow the other and will prevent the formation of an association between the second and the unconditioned stimulus.

OVERSTEER Pertaining to the handling characteristics of a vehicle that has a center of gravity behind the center of the car, making it necessary to steer continuously during a turn as the rear tires must develop more drift angle than the front tires.

OVERT BEHAVIOR 1. Activities that can be observed by an outsider. 2. Observable behavior. 3. Behavior that can be observed, such as overt movement, gland secretions, muscular contractions, and the like.

OVER-THE-COUNTER DRUG (OTC) 1. Refers to patent medicines *q.v.* that can be sold directly to the consumer. 2. Nonprescription drugs.

OVERTONE In a complex tone, any of the tones of higher pitch *q.v.* The frequencies of the ~ are multiples of those of the fundamental tone *q.v.*

OVERTRAINING 1. Excessive hard training on a frequent basis. 2. Failure to alternate light and heavy workouts.

OVERWEIGHT A condition characterized by being 10% above one's ideal weight *q.v.* cf: obesity.

OVIDUCT 1. The tube that carries the ova *q.v.* from the ovary *q.v.* to the uterus *q.v.* 2. The fallopian tube *q.v.*

OVIST A preformationist *q.v.* who believed that the egg rather than the sperm carried the miniature but complete organism.

OVOLACTOVEGETARIANISM A diet that excludes the ingestion of all meats but that does allow for the consumption of eggs and dairy products.

OVO VEGETARIAN DIET A vegetarian diet *q.v.* that permits the use of eggs.

OVULATION 1. The process of the ovary *q.v.* expelling an ovum *q.v.* in preparation for fertilization *q.v.* ~ takes place approximately once every 28 days or once during the menstrual cycle *q.v.* during the reproductive years of the female. 2. The discharge of the mature ovum from the graafian follicle *q.v.* of the ovary.

OVULATION METHOD 1. A contraceptive method *q.v.* entailing the identification of the approach and occurrence of ovulation *q.v.* by interpreting the cervical mucous *q.v.* pattern. When ovulation is occurring, abstinence from coitus *q.v.* is advised. 2. Natural family planning.

OVUM 1. The egg. 2. The female reproductive cell. ct: spermatozoon.

OWN CHILDREN Family members who are the sons and daughters, including stepchildren and adopted children, of the householder *q.v.*

OWSLEY'S ACID Good quality LSD *q.v.* originally manufactured by Augustus Owsley Stanley III.

OXAZEPAM 1. A benzodiazepine *q.v.* sedative. Serax is the brand name.

OXIDANT Chemical substances having an oxygen molecule that is a by-product of photochemical smog *q.v.*

OXIDATION 1. The chemical combining of oxygen with other substances as during burning. 2. The increase of positive charges on an atom or loss of negative charges. ~ is one of the changes that takes place when fats become rancid *q.v.* 3. The chemical reaction that involves the addition of oxygen or the removal of hydrogen or of electrons. 4. The chemical conversion of alcohol by the liver into water, carbon dioxide, and heat energy (calories).

OXIDATIVE PHOSPHORYLATION Phosphorylation *q.v.*

OXYCODONE 1. Dihydrohydroxycodeinone *q.v.* 2. A semisynthetic derivative of morphine *q.v.* 3. Percodan is the commercial preparation. 4. A narcotic analgesic *q.v.*

OXYGEN 1. The chemical symbol is O. A gaseous element that combines with other elements to form oxides. 2. The gas that constitutes 20.93% of air at sea level. 3. An essential component of metabolism *q.v.*

OXYGEN CONSUMPTION The amount of oxygen *q.v.* utilized by the body, expressed in liters per minute. cf: oxygen uptake.

OXYGEN DEBT 1. A physical state that occurs when the body can no longer process and transport sufficient amounts of oxygen *q.v.* for continued muscle contraction. A result of vigorous exercise. 2. The difference between the ideal amount of oxygen needed for the performance of a task and the actual amount of oxygen taken in.

OXYGEN DRIVE The stimulus to breathe, provided by a low actual level of oxygen *q.v.* in the blood.

OXYGEN EXTRACTION The amount of oxygen that can be extracted from 100 ml of blood.

OXYGEN MASK A device that fits over a person's nose and mouth to permit the breathing of oxygen *q.v.* The ~ should be semiopen, valveless, and made of transparent plastic.

OXYGEN TOXICITY An unusual condition caused by an excessive concentration of oxygen *q.v.* in inspired air resulting in damage to lung tissue.

OXYGEN TRANSPORT IN EXERCISE The delivery of oxygen *q.v.* by the lungs *q.v.*, heart *q.v.*, and vascular system *q.v.* to the working muscles where large quantities are needed for the aerobic *q.v.* production of energy.

OXYGEN UPTAKE The volume of oxygen *q.v.* able to be extracted from inspired air, usually expressed as liters per minute.

OXYHEMOGLOBIN A compound formed by the union of oxygen *q.v.* with hemoglobin *q.v.*

OXYMORPHONE A narcotic analgesic *q.v.* Nuomorphan is the brand name.

OXYTETRACYCLINE A generic name for Terramycin, a commercial antibiotic *q.v.* preparation.

OXYTOCIC A drug that stimulates the uterus to contract. cf: oxytocin.

OXYTOCIN 1. A female hormone *q.v.* that causes contraction of cells around the milk-producing glands in the breast, which force milk into the ducts *q.v.* and out the nipple. 2. A hormone secreted by the pituitary gland *q.v.* that stimulates the muscles of the uterus *q.v.* to contract. cf: oxytocic.

OXYURIASIS An intestinal infestation with pinworms.

OZONE 1. A form of oxygen consisting of molecules *q.v.* of three oxygen atoms (O_3), as compared with atmospheric oxygen with two oxygen atoms (O_2). 2. An irritating gas found in photochemical smog *q.v.*

OZONE LAYER The layer of triatomic oxygen *q.v.* that surrounds the Earth and filters much of the sun's radiation before it can reach the earth's surface.

P

P In genetics *q.v.* and sociology *q.v.*, ~ symbolizes the parental generation or parents of a given individual.

PABA An acronym for *para*-aminobenzoic acid *q.v.*

PACCHIONIAN BODIES Small projections of the arachnoid *q.v.* tissue chiefly into the venous sinuses *q.v.* of the dura mater *q.v.*

PACEMAKER 1. A small group of specialized cells in the heart that produce electrical impulses to start heart contractions. 2. An artificial device used as a substitute for the heart's natural ~ and controls heartbeats through a series of electrical discharges. This device may be placed on the outside of the chest or implanted within the chest wall. 3. The sinoatrial node *q.v.*

PACHYNEMA A midprophase *q.v.* stage in meiosis *q.v.* In well-prepared microscope slides, the chromosomes *q.v.* are visible as long, paired threads.

PADOPHYLLIN A medication used in the treatment of genital warts *q.v.* ~ acts as an irritant to cause sloughing off of the area affected by the wart virus *q.v.*

PAGAN A person who is not Jewish, Christian, or Moslem.

PAGER A compact, pocket carried radio receiver for providing one-way communication that is used to locate or direct persons within a limited geographic area.

PAGET'S DISEASE 1. An inflammatory cancerous *q.v.* condition of the areola *q.v.* and nipple, usually associated with carcinoma *q.v.* or the milk ducts and other tissues of the breast. 2. A disease of the skeleton *q.v.* of the elderly with chronic *q.v.* inflammation of bones. 3. Osteitis deformans *q.v.*

PAH An acronym for *para*-aminohippuric acid *q.v.*

PAIN An extremely uncomfortable signal of possible damage to the body. Subclassified as visceral (nonskeletal), or somatic (skeletal muscle or bone), and sharp (carried by A-delta fibers), or dull (carried by C-fibers).

PAIN GATE A hypothetical system in the spinal cord *q.v.* thought to account for moderating the signals being sent to the brain. The "gate" can be closed by such techniques as acupuncture and hypnosis, by sending inhibitory signals back down the spinal cord, effectively "closing" the gate.

PAIN THRESHOLD That level of tolerance at which pain becomes uncomfortable. cf: pain tolerance.

PAIN TOLERANCE A threshold, influenced by psychological *q.v.* factors, at which a person indicates that he or she cannot tolerate any further stimulation.

PAIR BONDING The process by which two people form an extremely close attachment.

PAIRED ASSOCIATE LEARNING Learning *q.v.* pairs of terms. Subjects are required to respond with the second member of the pair of terms when presented with the first term of the pair.

PAIRED ASSOCIATE METHOD A procedure in which subjects learn to provide particular response terms to various stimulus *q.v.* items. cf: paired associate learning.

PAIRED ASSOCIATION LEARNING (PAL) A technique of studying memory involving the presentation of pairs of words, pictures, or phrases. cf: paired associate method.

PAL An acronym for paired association learning *q.v.*

PALATE 1. The roof of the mouth. 2. The bony and muscular partition between the oral and nasal cavities *q.v.*

PALEOBOTANY The study of plant life of the geologic past.

PALEONTOLOGY The science that deals with the life of past geological periods.

PALINOPIA A condition of experiencing prolonged visual afterimages.

PALLIATION 1. To reduce pain. 2. To cover or cloak without a cure. 3. A treatment that lessens symptoms but does not cure.

PALLIATIVE Inducing relief, but not cure.

PALLIATIVE REHABILITATION Rehabilitation designed to enhance and prolong functioning ability. Part of a broad palliative care program. cf: palliation.

PALLOR 1. A lack of color. 2. Paleness.

PALMATE Having lobes radiating from a common point.

PALMITIC ACID A saturated fatty acid *q.v.* with 16 carbon atoms. ~ is common in fats *q.v.* and oils *q.v.*

PALPABLE Perceptible by touch.

PALPATE To examine or feel by the hand.

PALPATION The act of feeling or touching with light finger pressure.

PALPEBRAE The eyelids.

PALPITATION 1. A noticeably forceful heartbeat. 2. A fluttering of the heart at an abnormal rate or rhythm that a person can feel.

PALSY Paralysis *q.v.*

PAMELOR A commercial preparation of nortriptyline *q.v.*

PAN An acronym for peroxyacetyl nitrate *q.v.*

PANACEA A cure-all. A chemical, drug, medicine, or treatment that is claimed to be effective for all diseases. Historically, derived from Panakeia, the Greek goddess of healing who searched for a universal cure-all.

PAN AMERICAN HEALTH ORGANIZATION (PAHO) Established in 1902 under the authority of the Second International Conference of the American States in 1901. Its name was changed to the Pan American Sanitary Bureau in 1911. It is now one of the regional offices of the World Health Organization *q.v.*

PANCREAS A large gland located behind the stomach, producing the enzymes *q.v.* insulin *q.v.* and glucagon *q.v.*

PANCREATIC CANCER A malignancy *q.v.* of the pancreas *q.v.*

PANCREATITIS Inflammation of the pancreas *q.v.* Most common in alcoholics *q.v.*

PANDEMIC 1. A widespread epidemic *q.v.* over a large geographic area. 2. An epidemic of disease occurring in worldwide proportions. cf: epidemic; endemic.

PANDERER A person who obtains customers for prostitutes *q.v.* cf: pimp.

PANEL A group of research subjects followed during a longitudinal study *q.v.*

PANGENESIS An unaccepted theory proposed by Darwin that all body cells give rise to minute particles called pangenes, which migrate to the germplasm and impress their characteristics upon the latter.

PANIC A severe personality *q.v.* disorganization involving intense anxiety *q.v.* and usually paralyzing immobility or blind flight. cf: panic disorder.

PANIC DISORDER 1. A psychological condition in which the person experiences a series of panic *q.v.* attacks, characterized by fear, anxiety *q.v.*, a loss of breath, pounding heart, etc., without their being an obvious threat to the person. 2. An anxiety disorder in which the person has sudden, inexplicable bouts with fear and anxiety.

PANOPHTHALMITIS A generalized severe inflammation of all the ocular structures.

PANSINUSITIS An infection of all the sinuses *q.v.*

PANTOTHENIC ACID A component of coenzyme A *q.v.* ~ is essential for the metabolism of carbohydrates, fats, and proteins to produce energy. It is plentiful in foods, and consequently deficiency symptoms have not been observed in humans.

PAPAIN An enzyme *q.v.* found in the latex of the fruit and leaves of the papaya plant.

PAPAVERINE A class B narcotic *q.v.*

PAPAVER SOMNIFERUM The botanical name for the opium poppy, from which raw opium is derived. cf: opium.

PAPILLA 1. In botany, a budlike structure associated with reproduction in certain algae. 2. In anatomy, a small vascular process at the root of a hair. 3. A small, nipple-shaped elevation.

PAPILLARY Pertaining to the pupil *q.v.*

PAPILLEDEMA A swelling of the head of the optic nerve *q.v.*, usually due to increased intracranial pressure.

PAPILLOMA Any wart-like growth of the skin or mucous membrane *q.v.*

PAPILLOMA VIRUSES A group of viruses *q.v.* that cause genital *q.v.* and other warts and are strongly linked to cervical cancer *q.v.*

PAP SMEAR Pap test *q.v.*

PAP TEST Developed by George Papanicolaou and consists of obtaining cells from the cervix *q.v.* of the uterus *q.v.* and examining them under the microscope for any abnormal conditions that could indicate the presence of a malignancy *q.v.* cf: pap smear.

PAPULE 1. A vesicle *q.v.* 2. A red, elevated area on the skin; solid and circumscribed, varying in size from a pinhead to that of a pea.

PAPYRUS EBERS Also Ebers Papyrus. Dates to 1550 B.C.; an Egyptian document containing descriptions of over 700 different drugs that were used at that time. Most of the descriptions were of drugs from botanical sources, but many were also of animal and mineral sources.

PAR An acronym for population at risk *q.v.*

PARACENTESIS Drainage of fluid from the peritoneal cavity *q.v.* by means of a large needle inserted through the abdominal wall *q.v.*

PARACENTRIC INVERSION An inversion that is entirely within one arm of a chromosome *q.v.*

PARACERVICAL ANESTHETIC 1. Paracervical block *q.v.* 2. An anesthetic *q.v.* injected into tissues surrounding the cervical opening *q.v.*

PARACERVICAL BLOCK 1. Paracervical anesthetic *q.v.* 2. A common procedure in labor *q.v.* in which the vagina *q.v.* and cervix *q.v.* are anesthetized.

PARACHLOROPHENYLALANINE (PCPA) A drug that blocks serotonin *q.v.* synthesis resulting in a deficiency of that neurotransmitter *q.v.*

PARADIGM 1. A way of viewing life. A world view or belief pattern that is overriding. 2. A set of basic assumptions that outline the universe of scientific inquiry. 3. Provided the context in which research is conducted and knowledge is accumulated.

PARADIGM CLASH The conflict that is created when one set of beliefs threatens to replace an established belief pattern.

PARADOXICAL EFFECTS Effects that conflict with expectations. In pharmacology *q.v.*, effects that are the opposite of what a drug usually produce.

PARADOXICAL MOVEMENT The motion of an injured segment of a flail chest *q.v.*, opposite to the normal motion of the chest wall.

PARALDEHYDE 1. A nonbarbiturate sedative-hypnotic *q.v.* drug whose action on the central nervous system *q.v.* resembles that of alcohol *q.v.* It was replaced by the barbiturates *q.v.* in medicinal use, and more recently with other sedative-hypnotic drugs. 2. A fast-acting nonbarbiturate sedative.

PARALINGUISTIC Relating to audible *q.v.* components of speech that communicate meaning beyond the actual content of the words.

PARALLEL PLAY Play that occurs alongside rather than with other children.

PARALYSIS 1. The inability to move. There are two general forms: (a) spastic ~, in which injury is located in the brain or spinal cord *q.v.* and (b) flaccid ~, in which injury is located in a nerve *q.v.* between the spinal cord and the affected muscle. 2. The loss or impairment of motor function in a part of the body.

PARALYSIS AGITANS Parkinson's disease *q.v.*

PARALYTIC ILEUS 1. The obstruction of the intestines due to paralysis *q.v.* 2. The loss of normal intestinal function due to paralysis.

PARALYTIC POLIO A form of polio *q.v.* in which large numbers of motor nerves *q.v.* are destroyed by the polio virus *q.v.*

PARAMEDICAL PRACTITIONER 1. A person who assists a physician *q.v.* in providing health services. 2. Emergency specialists who are trained to deliver advance life support in an emergency situation. Their emergency actions include endotracheal intubation *q.v.*, intravenous *q.v.* therapy, cardiac *q.v.* monitoring, injections of specified medications, and defibrillation *q.v.* 3. Having a medical aspect or a secondary relation to medicine.

PARAMESONEPHRIC The duct *q.v.* system within the female embryo *q.v.* that gives rise to several internal reproductive structures.

PARAMETER 1. In epidemiology *q.v.*, the true value of a population of health attributes. 2. Within the boundaries of a population. 3. A value or constant based on an entire population.

PARAMETERS OF CLASSIFICATION The basis used for classification.

PARAMETRIC STATISTICS In epidemiology *q.v.*, statistical techniques that can be used on quantitative data *q.v.*

PARAMNESIA A false memory in which the person recalls events that did not occur.

PARANASAL SINUS An air-filled hollow in the facial or cranial bones, communicating with the nasal cavity.

PARANOIA 1. A psychotic *q.v.* symptom. The paranoid psychotic possesses persistent delusions *q.v.* of persecution *q.v.* or grandeur *q.v.* A paranoid reaction may take one of two forms: (a) classic ~ *q.v.* or (b) paranoid state *q.v.* 2. A mental disorder in which the person has unsubstantiated fears that others are threatening him or her or are hostile. 3. Delusions of persecution. 4. Irrational suspiciousness and distrust of people.

PARANOIAC A person suffering from paranoia *q.v.*

PARANOID DISORDER A disorder in which a person has persistent delusions *q.v.* but has no thought disorder and does not hallucinate *q.v.*

PARANOID PERSONALITY A personality or character disorder characterized by an abortive paranoid reaction *q.v.* manifested by projection *q.v.*, suspiciousness, jealously, and stubbornness. 2. Paranoid personality disorder *q.v.*

PARANOID PERSONALITY DISORDER 1. A disorder characterized by long-standing, pervasive, suspiciousness of others, hypersensitivity, and aggressive behavior if a threat is felt. 2. Paranoid personality *q.v.*

PARANOID PSYCHOSIS Paranoia *q.v.*

PARANOID SCHIZOPHRENIA 1. A type of schizophrenia *q.v.* characterized by dissociation, particularly between the intellectual processes and the affective *q.v.* dimension, disorganization with auditory and visual hallucinations *q.v.*, and paranoid delusions *q.v.* 2. Schizophrenia in which the major symptom is delusions. 3. A psychotic disorder in which the person experiences delusions (particularly of reference *q.v.*) and hallucinations, accompanied by agitation, anger, and violence.

PARANOID STATE A psychotic *q.v.* condition characterized by the person responding inadequately to situations, the responses including affective *q.v.* reactions and progressive disorganized associations. The person attempts to maintain self-esteem *q.v.* by carrying these reactions to an extreme.

PARAPHERNALIA In the area of the drug culture, equipment used in the taking of drugs, including syringes, pipes, scales, and mirrors.

PARAPHILIA 1. A sexual variance *q.v.* 2. Aberrant sexual activity. 3. A heterosexual condition in which the person is dependent on an unusual or unacceptable stimulus for sexual excitement and orgasm *q.v.* 4. A class of deviant sexual activities including voyeurism, fetishism, transvestism, and pedophilia *qq.v.*

PARAPHRASE The relation between two sentences whose meanings are essentially the same but whose surface structures differ.

PARAPHRENIA A term referring to schizophrenia *q.v.* in an older adult.

PARAPLEGIA Paralysis of the legs and lower part of the body. cf: monoplegia. ct: quadriplegia.

PARAPROFESSIONAL In education, a person working in a school who is not fully trained and licensed as a teacher, but who performs educational duties, such as tutoring and monitoring study halls.

PARAQUAT 1. An herbicide or plant killer that has been used to eradicate marijuana *q.v.* plants. 2. A marijuana contaminant that is associated with temporary and permanent damage to various organ systems of the body. 3. A defoliant.

PARASITE A plant or animal that lives off the host *q.v.* but does not contribute anything to the welfare of the host. ct: symbiotic relationship.

PARASITIC WORMS Many-celled animals that live in humans causing illness, e.g., pinworms and flukes.

PARASYMPATHETIC DIVISION Parasympathetic nervous system *q.v.*

PARASYMPATHETIC NERVOUS SYSTEM 1. A part of the autonomic nervous system *q.v.* that tends to slow down actions of various organs. 2. A division of the autonomic nervous system that mediates functions that occur in a relaxed state. 3. A division of the autonomic nervous system that is stimulated by the emotional state of the person. The ~ acts to restore and conserve body energy. ct: sympathetic nervous system.

PARASYMPATHETIC OVERSHOOT A rebound effect in which the parasympathetic *q.v.* system responds above its normal level after the inhibition from its sympathetic *q.v.* antagonist *q.v.* is suddenly removed.

PARATAXIC DISTORTION According to Harry Stack Sullivan, a hypothesis consisting of an unconscious misrepresentation of reality in childhood interpersonal relationships that extends to all later relationships.

PARATHORMONE A hormone *q.v.* released by the parathyroid gland *q.v.* that causes the release of calcium from the bones and causes reabsorption of calcium by the kidneys *q.v.*

PARATHYROID GLAND One of two glands located on each side in or near the thyroid gland *q.v.* that mainly controls calcium metabolism *q.v.* and muscle tone *q.v.* Failure to function properly results in convulsions.

PARATYPHOID An infectious intestinal disease caused by the *Salmonella paratyphi* organism.

PARAURETHRAL DUCTS Passages for secretions located near the urethra *q.v.*

PAREGORIC 1. A mild derivative of opium. 2. A narcotic containing 4% tincture of opium in combination with camphor. It is used chiefly in the control of diarrhea. 3. A preparation of opium and alcohol *q.v.*

PARENCHYMA 1. An unspecialized, simple cell or tissue. 2. The substance of a gland or solid organ. 3. The distinguishing, functional cells of an organ.

PARENS PATRIAE 1. In law, the concept of the state's guardianship over persons unable to manage their own affairs, e.g., minors. 2. The idea that the state may protect people from themselves, e.g., the requirement of warning labels on packs of cigarettes.

PARENTAL IMAGE The characteristics of a potential mate that remind a person of traits possessed by his or her parent of the opposite sex.

PARENT EFFECTIVENESS TRAINING (PET) A form of parent education centered around the parent engaging in passive and active listening, acknowledgment, and communication openings with the child.

PARENTERAL 1. Administration of a drug by means of injection. 2. Taking a drug other than orally. cf: intravenous; subcutaneous; intramuscular.

PARENTING STYLES Ways of interacting with children by their parents. ~ are measured in the degree of parental control exerted, nurturance, discipline techniques, etc.

PARENT TEACHERS ASSOCIATION (PTA) A national organization composed of parents and teachers that advocates for children and public education.

PARERGASIC Pertaining to psychotic *q.v.* disorders that are characterized by behaviors *q.v.* that are odd or incompetent.

PARESIS 1. An organic mental disease *q.v.* resulting from the invasion of the brain and spinal cord *q.v.* by syphilis *q.v.* 2. A partial paralysis *q.v.* 3. A chronic *q.v.* syphilitic inflammation *q.v.* of the brain and its membranes *q.v.* characterized by progressive mental deterioration and a general paralysis.

PARESTHESIA (PARAESTHESIA) 1. A pathological *q.v.* cutaneous *q.v.* sensation including the feeling of bugs crawling under the skin. 2. A conversion disorder *q.v.* marked by a feeling of tingling or creeping under the skin. 3. An abnormal spontaneous sensation, such as burning, pricking, or numbness.

PARIETAL AREA The wall of any cavity.

PARIETAL LOBES 1. That part of each cerebral hemisphere *q.v.* that lies between the occipital lobe *q.v.* and the central groove *q.v.* 2. That part of the cerebral hemispheres that includes the somatosensory projection area *q.v.*

PARIETAL PLEURA That portion of the pleura *q.v.* lining the inside of the walls of the thoracic cavity *q.v.*

PARITY Pertains to the number of deliveries a woman has had at or beyond the 24th week of gestation *q.v.*

PARKINSONIAN SYMPTOMS The side effects of the phenothiazines *q.v.* that mimic Parkinson's disease *q.v.*, e.g., reduced fine motor control, muscles tremors, blurred vision, and dry mouth.

PARKINSON'S DISEASE 1. A progressive, degenerative disease of the nervous system's *q.v.* motor control center. Characterized by muscles tremors, stiffness, and difficulty moving. 2. Paralysis agitans *q.v.* 3. Parkinsonian symptoms *q.v.* 4. A neurological disorder characterized by involuntary muscle tremors and rigid movements. In advanced stages, the person develops a shuffling gate, with stooped posture and loss of expression. The disease occurs most frequently in persons over 60 years, striking about 1 in 100 persons. The cause is unknown, but scientists have learned that it has to do with a disorder in brain cells that results in the loss of dopamine *q.v.* cf: Levodopa.

PARNATE A commercial preparation of tranylcypromine *q.v.*

PAROCHIAL SCHOOL A school operated and controlled by a particular religious denomination.

PAROLE-EVIDENCE RULE The principle that oral evidence related to matters not contained in a written contract or other instrument is not admissible.

PARONYCHIA An infection of the tissues at one side of a fingernail or a toenail.

PAROREXIA An appetite or craving for peculiar or inappropriate foods.

PAROTID 1. A gland located in front of each ear that produces saliva for the mouth to aid in the digestion of starch. 2. One of three pairs of salivary glands *q.v.* 3. Located near the ear. cf: sublingual; submental.

PAROTITIS 1. Mumps *q.v.* 2. Inflammation and infection of the parotid gland *q.v.*

PAROUS 1. Given birth to. 2. Having had at least one child.

PAROXYSM A sudden attack or recurrence of symptoms.

PARP In epidemiology *q.v.*, population attributable risk percent *q.v.*

PARSIMONY 1. Stinginess. 2. One of the criteria for evaluating the feasibility of theories. A parsimonious theory explains a large set of observations using relatively few explanatory principles.

PARTHENOGENESIS Reproduction by the development of an egg without it being fertilized by a sperm *q.v.*

PARTIAL ANDROGEN INSENSITIVITY A genetic *q.v.* disorder of males in which their bodies have only a partial ability to use androgen *q.v.* At birth, their genitalia *q.v.* are ambiguous. ct: androgen insensitivity syndrome.

PARTIAL EJACULATORY INCOMPETENCE During ejaculation *q.v.*, only seepage of semen *q.v.* occurs and orgasm *q.v.* is void of the pleasurable sensations.

PARTIALISM A type of fetish *q.v.* involving specific parts of the body, such as the breasts or feet. cf: fetishism.

PARTIAL MASTECTOMY The surgical removal of malignant *q.v.* tumors and/or the breast and 2–3 cm of surround tissue, muscle, skin, and fascia. Leaving some of the breast and all auxiliary and inner lymph nodes *q.v.*

PARTIAL REINFORCEMENT 1. Reinforcement *q.v.* that occurs at a rate less often than for every correct response *q.v.* or on every trial. 2. In conditioning *q.v.*, reinforcement that is given intermittently rather than on every trial. 3. A condition in which a response is reinforced only some of the time.

PARTIAL REINFORCEMENT EFFECT The fact that a response *q.v.* is much harder to extinguish when it was acquired during partial rather than continuous reinforcement.

PARTICIPANT OBSERVATION 1. The collection of data while being involved in the phenomenon being studied. 2. A research method in which an investigator joins those who are being studied. Some reveal their true purpose, while others do not.

PARTICIPATIVE APPROACH The strategy of achieving objectives through the involvement of the workers or the students in decision making.

PARTICULATE MATTER 1. Minute, often harmful substances found in tobacco smoke and in polluted air. 2. The solid substances found in a gas. Applied to air pollution, tobacco smoke, etc. cf: particulate pollutants.

PARTICULATE PHASE That portion of tobacco smoke composed of tiny suspended particles. ct: gaseous phase.

PARTICULATE POLLUTANTS 1. Particulate matter *q.v.* 2. A class of air pollutants composed of small solid particles and liquid droplets.

PARTURITION 1. Labor *q.v.* 2. The process of giving birth.

PARTY "HOT" LINE A dedicated telephone line or circuit that serves parties or locations. Although a party line is usually used for emergency or priority traffic, all users have equal priority and may participate in all communications on the circuit.

PASSIONATE LOVE Strong attachment and physical desire.

PASSIVE-AGGRESSIVE PERSONALITY 1. A person who possesses a deep dependency, usually accompanied by deep resentment. There are three forms: (a) passive dependency with helplessness, indecisiveness, and a need to cling to others; (b) passive aggressiveness with an expression of aggression through outing, stubbornness, procrastination, and passive obstructionism; and (c) active aggressiveness with irritability, tantrums, and destructiveness. 2. Passive-aggressive personality disorder *q.v.* Behavior that indirectly resists demands of others by being late, missing appointments, not answering calls, dawdling, and making irrational mistakes.

PASSIVE-AGGRESSIVE PERSONALITY DISORDER 1. Passive-aggressive personality *q.v.* 2. Self-defeating behavior patterns involving such things as procrastination, stubbornness and intentional inefficiency.

PASSIVE-CONGENIAL MARRIAGE A marriage that primarily supports the outside interests of the partners.

PASSIVE DEPENDENCY REACTION 1. A form of passive-aggressive personality *q.v.* 2. An immature reaction characterized by helplessness, indecisiveness, and a tendency to cling to others for protection and support.

PASSIVE EUTHANASIA Indirect euthanasia *q.v.*

PASSIVE IMMUNITY Disease resistance in a person or animal due to the injection of antibodies *q.v.* from another person or animal.

PASSIVE IMMUNIZATION The practice of injecting antibodies *q.v.* directly into the body to confer immunity *q.v.* ct: active immunity.

PASSIVE LEARNING Learning that takes place without the learner being actively involved in the learning experience.

PASSIVE LISTENING A strong nonverbal message that indicates that a person wants to listen. ct: active listening.

PASSIVELY ACQUIRED IMMUNITY A temporary immunity *q.v.* achieved by providing antibodies *q.v.* to a person exposed to a particular pathogen *q.v.*

PASSIVE SMOKING The inhalation of air that is heavily polluted with tobacco smoke from other people's cigarettes.

PASSIVE TRANSPORT A process of diffusion *q.v.* by which substances move from one compartment to another down a concentration gradient *q.v.* and does not require energy.

PASSIVE VOCABULARY All the words a person understands. ct: active vocabulary.

PASSIVITY A characteristic of persons suffering from depression. The inability of a person to act directly on his or her environment.

PASTEURELLA PESTIS The bacterium *q.v.* that causes the bubonic plague *q.v.*

PASTEURELLA TULARENSIS The causative agent of tularemia *q.v.*

PASTEURIZATION Heating a medium to a temperature over a period of time to destroy pathogens *q.v.* There are two methods: (a) the holding method consists of heating the medium to 143°F (62°C) and holding at this temperature for 30 min and (b) the flash method consists of heating the medium to 161°F (72°C) for 15 s.

PATCH TEST A skin test in which small pieces of filter paper or linen soaked in a solution or covered with ointment are applied directly to the skin.

PATELLA 1. The kneecap. 2. A triangular sesamoid *q.v.* bone about 5 cm in diameter, situated at the front of the knee.

PATENT 1. A document that confers a special and exclusive right to manufacture a product. 2. In physiology *q.v.*, open, unobstructed.

PATENT DUCTUS ARTERIOSUS 1. A congenital *q.v.* defect in which the ductus arteriosus *q.v.* fails to close. 2. A congenital defect in which the duct *q.v.* connecting the pulmonary artery *q.v.* to the aorta *q.v.* and serving as a temporary bypass to the lungs during the prenatal *q.v.* period fails to close shortly before or after birth.

PATENT FORAMEN OVALE A congenital defect in which the foramen ovale *q.v.* fails to close.

PATENT MEDICINE 1. A drug that has been patented. 2. A formula that is protected by patent laws and may not be compounded or sold without the specific permission in writing from the patent holder. 3. Generally, over-the-counter drugs *q.v.* 4. Proprietary medicines *q.v.*

PATERNAL 1. Pertaining to the father. 2. A set of chromosomes *q.v.* derived from the sperm *q.v.* in animals and the pollen in plants.

PATH ANALYSIS Based on multiple regression *q.v.* techniques, a causal analysis developed in genetics *q.v.* and economics and now used extensively in sociology *q.v.* The goal is to determine a fit of a particular causal ordering of variables with the relationships that exist in the investigator's data set.

PATHENOGENESIS The origin or the course of development of a disease.

PATHOGEN 1. A microorganism *q.v.* capable of producing an infection *q.v.* in humans. There are four general classes: 1. (a) bacteria, bacillus (rod-shaped); (b) coccus, spherical; (c) spirillum, spiral; (d) rickettsia, small bacteria; (e) virus, ultramicroscopic; 2. fungi, mold and yeast; 3. protozoa, (a) amoeba and (b) plasmodium; 4. metazoan, round worm, tapeworm, and trichinella. 2. An organism capable of eliciting disease symptoms in another organism.

PATHOGENIC Pertaining to the conditions that lead to pathology *q.v.*

PATHOGENIC MODEL The theory that disease is caused by invading organisms.

PATHOLOGICAL Any diseased condition.

PATHOLOGICAL ANXIETY Anxiety *q.v.* so intense that it produces one or more behavioral disorders. ct: normal anxiety.

PATHOLOGICAL DEVIANCE Infrequent, illogical, and antisocial *q.v.* behaviors.

PATHOLOGICAL FRACTURE A fracture *q.v.* in which a specific weakness or destruction of bone caused by some process, such as cancer, is the reason for the break.

PATHOLOGICAL HYPERTENSION Secondary hypertension *q.v.*

PATHOLOGICAL INTOXICATION Severe cerebral *q.v.* and behavioral disturbance in a person whose tolerance *q.v.* to alcohol *q.v.* is extremely low.

PATHOLOGICALLY ORIENTED Disease oriented.

PATHOLOGICAL PERSONALITY TYPES 1. Persons who are neither neurotic *q.v.* nor psychotic *q.v.* but who manage to maintain borderline adjustment that might be compared to an abortive stage in the development of a more severe mental disorder. 2. Borderline neurosis or psychosis.

PATHOLOGICAL PREJUDICE Prejudice *q.v.* attitudes *q.v.* that are part of a person's personality structure. cf: authoritarian personality; endemic prejudice.

PATHOLOGICAL RETARDATION Retardation that results from specific pathologies such as disease, injury, metabolic *q.v.* errors, chromosomal *q.v.* abnormalities, and the like.

PATHOLOGY 1. A medical specialty concerned with the study of the changes in tissues, organs, and cells as a result of disease *q.v.* or other phenomena. 2. A disease or abnormal physical or mental condition. 3. The study of the anatomical *q.v.*, physiological *q.v.*, and psychological deviations resulting from disease.

PATHOLOGY MODEL In psychology, a general conception of mental disorders that holds that 1. one can generally distinguish between symptoms and underlying causes and 2. these causes may be regarded as a form of pathology.

PATIENT ADMISSION PRIVILEGES The rights of physicians to admit patients to certain hospitals.

PATIENT ADVOCATE An attorney, mental health professional, or other person who participates in consent procedures with and for the psychiatric patient.

PATIENT EDUCATION Patient health education *q.v.*

PATIENT HEALTH EDUCATION 1. All of the methods, techniques, and strategies used by the patient health educator *q.v.* to favorably influence the health knowledge, attitudes, and, especially, the behavior of patients recovering from a disease, injury, surgery, or other health episode. 2. Those health experiences designed to influence learning that occurs as a person receives preventive, diagnostic, therapeutic, or rehabilitation services, including experiences that arise from coping with symptoms, referral to sources of information, prevention, diagnosis, and care, and contacts with health providers.

PATIENT HEALTH EDUCATOR A person trained in the methods and techniques of health education *q.v.* as applied to persons who have suffered a disease or disability to educate them on ways of preventing complications or relapse.

PATIENT MEDICATION INSTRUCTIONS Printed information dealing with drugs and their effects. ~ are made available to physicians for distribution to their patients, the goal being to enhance the drug's effectiveness. cf: patient package insert.

PATIENT PACKAGE INSERT (PPI) A leaflet included in a drug package that describes how to use the drug. It includes information about the drug's purposes, hazards, and side effects. cf: patient medication instructions.

PATIENT'S BILL OF RIGHTS A list of 12 standard ethical principles that describe and define considerate and ethical treatment that should be provided in a hospital or nursing home.

PATRIARCHY 1. Control of the family or other groups by the male. 2. A society in which the males control the power structure. ct: matriarchy.

PATRILINEAL 1. A system of tracing descent in which only one of the four grandparents is the direct line of descent. 2. Agnatic descent.

PATRILOCAL 1. A residential system in which the husband brings his wife to live with or near his parents. 2. Virilocal *q.v.*

PATTERNING A specific set or sequence of movement exercises used to treat learning problems.

PATULOUS 1. Being spread wide open. 2. Easily entered.

PAVLOVIAN CONDITIONING Classical conditioning theory *q.v.*

PBI An acronym for protein-bound iodine *q.v.*

PCM An acronym for protein-calorie *q.v.* malnutrition.

PCO_2 Partial pressure of carbon dioxide *q.v.*

PCP 1. Phencyclidine. 2. Also known as angel dust. 3. A synthetic hallucinogen *q.v.* originally used as a general anesthetic, esp. in veterinary medicine. 4. Phencyclidine hydrochloride *q.v.* 5. Pneumocystis carinii pneumonia *q.v.*

PDP An acronym for Personal Development Plan *q.v.*

PDR An acronym for *Physician's Desk Reference*, a listing of most prescription drugs and information concerning these drugs. Updated yearly.

PEAK DAYS That part of the menstrual cycle *q.v.* when a woman is most likely to conceive. Cervical mucous *q.v.* is usually slippery at this time.

PEAK EXPERIENCES 1. Pertains to the experience of good feelings, happiness, and insight. 2. Maslow's term for moments or periods of joy from personal fulfillment or feelings of oneness with the universe.

PEARSON PRODUCT MOMENT CORRELATION COEFFICIENT (*r*) 1. A statistic ranging in value from −1.00 to +1.00. 2. The most common means of denoting a correlational relationship.

PECTIN An complex organic *q.v.* compound present in the intercellular layer and primary wall of plant cells walls.

PECTINASE 1. The enzyme *q.v.* that acts upon pectin *q.v.* 2. Pectase.

PECTINEAL Pertaining to the pubic bone *q.v.*

PECTORAL Pertaining to the chest or breast.

PECTORALIS MUSCLES Muscular tissues attached to the chest wall and to the upper arms. Pectoralis major muscles are the larger muscles, and pectoralis minor muscles are the smaller of the group.

PECTORAL MUSCLES Pectoralis muscles *q.v.*

PEDAGOGY The art, science, and methods of teaching. ~ deals with the principles and methods of formal education *q.v.*

PEDAL Pertaining to the foot.

PEDANTRY Meticulousness.

PEDERASTY 1. Male sexual relations with a boy. 2. Sexual intercourse *q.v.* via the anus *q.v.* cf: pedophilia.

PEDIATRICS A medical specialty concerned with the health of children (usually under the age of 13 years), primarily dealing with the prevention, diagnosis, and treatment of diseases prevalent in children.

PEDICULOCIDE A chemical preparation used to treat lice infestation *q.v.*

PEDICULOSIS 1. Infestation *q.v.* with lice. There are three specific forms: (a) the head louse, *Pediculus humanus capitis*; (b) the body louse, *Pediculus humanus corporis*, and (c) the crab louse, *Phthirus pubis*.

PEDICULOSIS HUMANUS CAPITIS The head louse. Infestation is called pediculosis *q.v.*

PEDICULOSIS HUMANUS CORPORIS The body louse. Infestation is called pediculosis *q.v.*

PEDICULOSIS PUBIS An itchy skin irritation in the genital *q.v.* area caused by infestation and bites of the crab louse *q.v.*

PEDIGREE A table, chart, or diagram representing the ancestral history of an organism, including humans.

PEDIGREE ANALYSIS The pattern of inheritance of a trait among all family members over several generations.

PEDIGREE STUDIES An analysis of inheritance to determine whether a particular trait could be attributed to the transmission of a gene *q.v.* to children within a family.

PEDODONTIA A dental specialty concerned with the diagnosis and treatment of oral and dental conditions of children.

PEDOPHILIA 1. A sexual variance characterized by a person gaining sexual gratification by having sexual relations with children. 2. Child molestation. A relatively rare condition in which sexual arousal is possible only in the presence of children. 3. A condition in an adult who seeks sexual contact with children as a preferred or exclusive method of achieving sexual excitement and gratification. 4. Pedophiliac.

PEEP SHOWS Small booths in pornographic *q.v.* bookstores or similar adult establishments where customers watch short films of hard-core pornography.

PEER APPROACHES Methods that provide an educational environment that encourages a free interchange among learners.

PEER GROUP A social group of equivalent age and status.

PEER-GROUP INFLUENCES The perception of an individual of the importance of the attitudes and values of his or her peers. Adoption of the attitudes and values is seen to boost the person's self-esteem and acceptance by others in the group. cf: peer pressure.

PEER INFLUENCES Pressures exerted upon students by a group of individuals with whom the individuals identify.

PEER PRESSURE The influence one feels from his or her peers to behave in certain ways. ~ changes in complexity and character at various stages in a person's life. cf: peer-group influences.

PEER REVIEW An advisory panel of experts from outside an organization who review research proposals and study results or manuscripts for accuracy and feasibility of the project in question.

PEERS 1. Comembers of a given social category. 2. Peer group *q.v.*

PEG WORD METHOD A mnemonic *q.v.* device that involves associating a new item with a previously learned item.

PEKOE A grade of tea.

PELLAGRA A nutritional deficiency disease resulting from a severe deficiency of niacin *q.v.* ~ is characterized by symptoms of diarrhea, dermatitis, dementia, and, finally, death.

PELLICLE A semirigid membrane surrounding microzoan cells, resulting in a maintenance of cell shape.

PELVIC CAVITY The lowermost portion of the abdominal cavity *q.v.* that contains the rectum *q.v.*, urinary bladder *q.v.*, and in the female, the internal reproductive organs.

PELVIC EXAMINATION 1. An external and internal visual and manual examination whereby the physician evaluates the health of a woman's reproductive organs. 2. An examination of a woman's vagina, cervix, and rectum, performed by a physician or other qualified health professional.

PELVIC INFLAMMATORY DISEASE (PID) 1. Inflammation of the pelvic organs *q.v.* following infection of the urethra *q.v.* or vagina *q.v.* by gonococcus *q.v.* or other organisms. These migrate to infect the cervix *q.v.*, uterus *q.v.*, or fallopian tubes *q.v.*, and other tissues in the abdominal cavity. 2. Infection of the uterus and fallopian tubes. 3. An acute *q.v.* or chronic *q.v.* infection of the peritoneum *q.v.* of the abdominopelvic cavity *q.v.* associated with a variety of symptoms and a potential cause of sterility *q.v.* 4. A generalized infection of the pelvic cavity that results from the spread of an infection through a woman's reproductive organs.

PELVIS A basin or funnel-shaped structure.

PEM An acronym for protein-energy malnutrition *q.v.*

PEMOLINE 1. A stimulant used in ADD *q.v.* with hyperactivity *q.v.* 2. Cylert is a commercial preparation.

PEMPHIGUS A generalized, sometimes fatal, skin disease characterized by recurring crops of large blisters.

PENETRANCE The proportion (in percent) of individuals with a particular gene combination that express the corresponding trait.

PENICILLIN The first of the antibiotic *q.v.* drugs developed by Alexander Fleming in 1929. It is a drug produced by a mold, *Penicillium notatum*. ~ is used in treating several bacteria-caused diseases, e.g., syphilis *q.v.* and gonorrhea *q.v.*

PENICILLINASE An enzyme *q.v.* produced by some bacteria *q.v.* that destroys penicillin *q.v.*

PENILE 1. Pertaining to the male organ of copulation *q.v.* and urination. 2. The penis *q.v.*

PENILE CHORDEE Painful downward curvature of the penis *q.v.* when erect.

PENILE PLETHYMOGRAPH 1. A device for detecting blood flow in the penis *q.v.*, thus recording changes in the size of the penis. 2. A device for recording the level of male sexual arousal.

PENILE PROSTHESIS 1. A penile *q.v.* implant. 2. An inflatable cylinder surgically placed inside the penis *q.v.* and attached to a pumping device that is placed in a man's scrotum *q.v.* Used in cases when the erectile dysfunction *q.v.* is physiologically based.

PENILE SHAFT The body of the penis *q.v.*

PENIS 1. The male organ for copulation *q.v.* 2. The male sex organ that transports semen *q.v.* and urine and becomes erect during sexual excitement for insertion into the vagina *q.v.* during sexual intercourse *q.v.* 3. The structure of the male external genitalia *q.v.* consisting of a root, shaft, and glans.

PENIS CAPTIVUS A condition in humans in which it is alleged that the shaft of the fully introduced penis *q.v.* is tightly encircled by the vagina *q.v.* during coitus *q.v.* and cannot be withdrawn. This condition is not anatomically possible in humans but can be found in the dog.

PENIS ENVY The desire of the female for male sex organs or status. cf: Electra complex; phallic stage.

PENOSCROTAL RAPHE The scar-like line on the underside of the penis *q.v.*, running from the anus *q.v.* to the glans penis *q.v.* The ~ is formed in male prenatal development from the fusion of the urinogenital *q.v.* sinus *q.v.* that closes to form the tubular urethra *q.v.* within the penis.

PENROSE DRAIN A cigarette drain composed of rubber tubing containing a length of absorbent tubing.

PENSION The amount of money paid at regular intervals to a retired employee.

PENTADACTYL Having five digits or fingers.

PENTAZOCINE 1. A narcotic analgesic *q.v.* 2. Talwin is a commercial preparation.

PENTOBARBITAL SODIUM 1. A short-acting barbiturate *q.v.* 2. Nembutal is a commercial preparation.

PENTOSE A monosaccharide *q.v.* containing five carbon atoms *q.v.*, having the chemical formula $(CH_2O)_5$.

PENTOTHAL INTERVIEW Narcotherapy *q.v.*

PEPSIN 1. An enzyme *q.v.* necessary for protein *q.v.* digestion. 2. The primary digestive enzyme produced in the stomach. A proteolytic *q.v.* enzyme.

PEPSINOGEN A substance secreted by the stomach from which pepsin *q.v.* is derived. High levels of ~ in the blood appear to be associated with a predisposition to peptic ulcer *q.v.*

PEPTIC ULCER 1. A ulceration *q.v.* of a part of the gastrointestinal tract *q.v.*, usually the stomach. 2. An open sore seated in the membrane *q.v.* of the stomach or duodenum *q.v.* caused by the action of gastric juice *q.v.* cf: pepsinogen.

PEPTIDE 1. A class of chemicals that form the basis of proteins *q.v.* 2. A group of more than two amino acids linked to the amine group of one and the carboxyl group of another, forming a chain. 3. A breakdown or buildup unit in protein metabolism.

PEPTIDE BOND A covalent bond between two amino acids *q.v.*

PEPTONIZATION Precipitation or digestion of casein *q.v.*

PER An acronym for protein efficiency ratio *q.v.*

PERCEIVED ATTITUDE SIMILARITY The degree to which another person's attitudes *q.v.* are thought to be like one's own.

PERCEIVED SIMILARITY THEORY OF IDENTIFICATION 1. A theory of identification. 2. The theory that children identify with persons whom they perceive as similar to themselves.

PERCENTILE 1. A number corresponding to a score or measure, that is the percentage of the same measure that the score equals or exceeds. 2. Pertaining to a distribution of observations. For example, the 10th percentile is defined as the value below which 10% of the distribution of values will fall. cf: percentile rank.

PERCENTILE RANK The percentage of all the scores in a distribution that lie below a given score. cf: percentile.

PERCEPTION 1. The intermediate level of contact with the internal or external environments. The perceptual area of the brain interprets the impulse as sight, sound taste, smell, or bodily sensation; however, other impulses may be generated and transmitted to other areas of the brain for significance, relationships, and action. What we perceive is not so much dependent upon the sense organ that is stimulated as it is upon the area of the brain that is stimulated. 2. An interpretation of a message as observed by an individual. 3. An intellectual process of becoming aware of exogenous *q.v.* events that stimulate the sense organs and of interpreting their relationships. 4. Receiving impulses through one or more of the sense organs *q.v.*, which results in an intellectual impression or interpretation of the impulse and ultimately a reaction to them. 5. The meaningful interpretation of a stimulation of one of the sense organs and its interpretation. cf: individual perception.

PERCEPTIVE DEAFNESS A type of deafness *q.v.* that involves the auditory *q.v.* nerve, cerebral *q.v.* pathways, or the auditory center of the brain. ct: conductive deafness.

PERCEPTIVENESS The ability to notice happenings.

PERCEPTUAL ABNORMALITY The inability of an individual to interpret internal or external stimuli.

PERCEPTUAL ADAPTATION The gradual adjustment to various distortions of perceptions *q.v.*

PERCEPTUAL CHANGES Changes in sensory *q.v.* awareness.

PERCEPTUAL CONSTANCY The tendency for a person to perceive objects correctly in spite of changes in the proximal stimulus *q.v.* provided by these objects.

PERCEPTUAL DEFENSE 1. The tendency to perceive anxiety-related stimuli less readily than neutral stimuli. 2. The tendency for a person to fail to perceive obscene *q.v.* or otherwise threatening stimuli. 3. Selective perception. 4. The unconscious screening out of, or censoring of, unpleasant or threatening perceptions.

PERCEPTUAL DIFFERENTIATION Learning to perceive features of stimulus *q.v.* patterns that were not perceptible at first.

PERCEPTUAL INVARIANTS Attributes of stimuli *q.v.*, or relationships among stimuli, that remain the same under different conditions.

PERCEPTUAL LEARNING 1. The hypothesis *q.v.* that learning *q.v.* is a matter of developing perceptions *q.v.* or of seeing new relationships. 2. Perception is influenced by learning. 3. Changes in performance or perceptual tasks resulting from experience rather than changes in basic sensory capabilities.

PERCODAN A commercial preparation of oxycodone *q.v.*

PER CURIAM By the court. An opinion with no identification of the author.

PERCUSSION A physician's use of thumping and listening during a medical examination.

PERENNIALISM An educational philosophy that holds that certain truths exist and are universal and unchanging.

PERFORATION The act of piercing through.

PERFORMANCE 1. In psychology, pertaining to that which a child knows offered in response to a direct question. 2. Psychomotor *q.v.* skills or behavior in which a person is engaged. Performance influences cognition *q.v.* and affect *q.v.* 3. Any form of behavior. cf: competence.

PERFORMANCE ANXIETY An apprehension about sexual adequacy that produces anxiety *q.v.* resulting in an inadequate sexual performance *q.v.*

PERFORMANCE-BASED EDUCATION Learning designed to demonstrate actual accomplishment rather than just knowing.

PERFORMANCE CONTRACT In education, an agreement between schools and commercial educational agencies or teachers guaranteeing specified educational results.

PERFORMANCE TEST In intelligence *q.v.* testing, a nonverbal test; a test that requires no language. ct: verbal test.

PERGONAL A drug that induces ovulation *q.v.* by action of FSH *q.v.*

PERIANTH A collective term that includes the calyx *q.v.* and corolla *q.v.*

PERICARDIAL SAC The fibroserous membrane *q.v.* covering the heart.

PERICARDIAL TAMPONADE Acute *q.v.* compression of the heart from the effusion of fluid into the pericardium *q.v.* or from the collection of blood within the pericardium from rupture of the heart or a penetrating injury.

PERICARDITIS Inflammation of the outer covering of the heart (pericardium *q.v.*).

PERICARDIUM The thin outer layer of tissue that encloses or covers the heart.

PERICENTRIC INVERSION An inversion of both arms of a chromosome *q.v.* including the centromere *q.v.*

PERIDONTITIS Inflammation of the periodontal tissues *q.v.*, usually results from localized irritation from deposits of calculus or tartar *q.v.* Other causes are malocclusion *q.v.*, poorly applied restorations, and improperly fitting prosthetics *q.v.* Inflammation of the tissues surrounding a tooth that may lead to tooth loss and a degeneration of the jaw bone.

PERIMETRIUM The external covering of the uterus *q.v.* Sometimes referred to as the serosa *q.v.* This layer of the uterus is very elastic allowing the uterus to accommodate the enlarging embryo *q.v.* and fetus *q.v.*

PERIMYSIUM Covering or binding muscle.

PERINATAL MORTALITY The number of fetal deaths from the 28th week of pregnancy plus the number of deaths in the first week after birth per 100,000 live births.

PERINATAL PERIOD 1. The time from the 28th week of gestation *q.v.* to 1 month following birth. 2. Occurring at or near the time of birth.

PERINEUM 1. The area between the anus *q.v.* and the genitals *q.v.* 2. The area between the thighs, extending from the posterior *q.v.* wall of the vagina *q.v.* to the anus *q.v.* in the female, and from the scrotum *q.v.* to the anus in the male.

PERIOD OF FORMAL OPERATIONS In Piaget's theory, the period from about 11 years on, when genuinely abstract mental operations can be undertaken.

PERIOD OF RECOVERY A stage of an infectious disease *q.v.* when the body has overcome the infectious agent *q.v.* and the body is returning to normal strength and functioning.

PERIOD OF THE OVUM 1. Ovum *q.v.* 2. The period from conception *q.v.* to implantation *q.v.* in the uterus *q.v.*

PERIODONTAL DISEASE Characterized by inflammation and degeneration of any of the structures of the periodontium *q.v.* The most common form is periodontitis *q.v.*

PERIODONTIA 1. A dental specialty concerned with the diagnosis and treatment of conditions of the periodontium *q.v.* 2. The specialized branch of dentistry *q.v.* that is concerned with treating oral conditions of the tissues that surround the teeth.

PERIODONTIUM The supporting structures of the teeth.

PERIOD PREVALENCE In epidemiology *q.v.*, the number of individuals with a specific health outcome at the time period when the count is made. May also be expressed as rate.

PERIOSTEUM The membrane of connective tissue *q.v.* that closely covers all bones.

PERIPHERAL Pertaining to an outside surface.

PERIPHERAL CIRCULATION Blood flow through small vessels surrounded by muscles.

PERIPHERAL NERVOUS SYSTEM 1. Nerves *q.v.* that are located outside the brain and the spinal cord and connect the spinal cord to the effectors *q.v.* and receptors *q.v.* 2. Nerve fibers between the central nervous system *q.v.* and the sense organs, muscles, and glands. cf: central nervous system; autonomic nervous system.

PERIPHERAL ROUTE TO PERSUASION A means of using irrational reasoning in response to persuasive or rational messages.

PERISTALSIS The rhythmic contractions of muscles of the gastrointestinal tract *q.v.* that aid in propelling food and nutrients through the digestive system.

PERITONEAL CAVITY The abdominal cavity *q.v.*

PERITONEAL DIALYSIS A technique for removing impurities from the blood in cases of renal *q.v.* failure, using the person's own peritoneum as the dialyzing *q.v.* membrane. An electrolyte *q.v.* solution is introduced into the peritoneal cavity *q.v.* and removed after a period of time bringing with it the impurities that accumulated as the result of renal failure. It can also be used in cases of poisoning.

PERITONEUM The strong, translucent membrane *q.v.* lining the abdominal cavity *q.v.*

PERITONITIS An inflammation of the peritoneum *q.v.* of the abdominopelvic cavity *q.v.*

PERIVENTRICULAR SYSTEM A group of neurons located in the hypothalamus *q.v.* and thalamus *q.v.* that is the punishment or avoidance center of the nervous system.

PERMANENT CERTIFICATE A certificate issued to a teacher candidate after a required completion of a professional preparation program recognizing full rights as a teacher.

PERMEABILITY 1. The ability of substances to pass through the placental barrier from mother to fetus. 2. The ability to pass through a membrane *q.v.*

PERMEABLE 1. Capable of, or allowing the passage of fluids into or through. 2. Pervious. 3. Porous.

PERMISSIVE Allowing a person to do whatever he or she likes.

PERMISSIVE LEGISLATION Laws that establish the right to carry out a specific action without requiring that it be done.

PERMISSIVE PARENTS Parents who use a minimum of discipline *q.v.*, believing that children should be allowed to develop in their own way without adult interference. ct: authoritative parents; authoritarian parents.

PERMISSIVE THEORY In psychiatry *q.v.* and physiology *q.v.*, the idea that the production of abnormal amounts of norepinephrine *q.v.* and serotonin *q.v.* may be involved in depression *q.v.*

PERMITIL A commercial preparation of fluphenazine *q.v.*

PERNICIOUS Tending to be fatal.

PERNICIOUS ANEMIA 1. A progressive disease in which there is a decrease in the number and an increase in the size of red blood cells, resulting in weakness and gastrointestinal *q.v.* disturbances. 2. A disease caused by a deficiency of cyanocobalamin (vitamin B_{12}) in the diet or of the inability of the body to absorb it.

PERONEUS 1. Peroneal *q.v.* 2. Of or near the fibula *q.v.*

PEROXYACETYL NITRATE (PAN) A toxic substance present in smog *q.v.* that can damage and, under certain conditions, kill plants and irritate the eyes.

PERPHENAZINE 1. An antipsychotic drug *q.v.* 2. Trilafon is a commercial preparation.

PERQUISITES Benefits beyond pay, mainly applied for executives.

PERSECUTION (DELUSION) Characterized by a person falsely believing that other people are enemies who in reality are not. ~ is accompanied by constant fear of bodily harm. cf: delusions.

PERSEVERATION 1. Persistent continuation of a line of thought or activity. 2. Clinically, inappropriate repetition, often found in schizophrenics *q.v.* 3. Continuing a response long after it is no longer appropriate. ct: echolalia.

PERSEVERATIVE ERROR In serial learning *q.v.*, a response that would have been correct had it occurred earlier in the list. ct: anticipatory error.

PERSISTENT OBESITY Obesity *q.v.* that stems from childhood and continues beyond adolescence. ct: transient obesity.

PERSONA The mask or face a person presents to others.

PERSONAL AGENCY The ability a person has to influence events in the physical and social world.

PERSONAL ATTRIBUTES One's physical or mental characteristics. Physical characteristics are (a) physical abilities basic to normal functioning and (b) physical abilities that are generally referred to as talents. Mental attributes are (a) intellectual and functional, (b) emotional functioning, and (c) unusual talents.

PERSONAL CONSTRUCTS The ways in which humans construe, interpret, or attach meaning to experience.

PERSONAL CONTRACT A document that outlines personal health goals and activities that can be evaluated as progress toward achievement is made.

PERSONAL DEVELOPMENT PLAN An analysis of one's strengths and weaknesses with plans to improve one's performance and effectiveness.

PERSONAL EXPECTATIONS The goals a person sets for himself or herself. These goals may be influenced by family, friends, society, culture, etc. ct: social expectations.

PERSONALITY 1. The basic organization of a person's characteristic adjustment to the environment *q.v.* 2. ~ constitutes a person's pattern of living that sets him or her apart from all other persons and how others respond to him or her. 3. ~ is the general pattern or quality of a person's total behavior *q.v.* patterns, as he or she impresses others. 4. All that a person is. 5. The unique pattern of traits that characterizes a person. 6. A person's total reaction to the environment. ct: personality disorder.

PERSONALITY DEVELOPMENT The changes taking place over time in the way that a person feels, thinks, and acts, and in the perceptions *q.v.* he or she communicates to others.

PERSONALITY DISORDER 1. Personality pattern disturbance *q.v.* 2. Character disorder *q.v.* 3. Well-entrenched, maladaptive behavior patterns. 4. A variety of disorders that tend to be long-standing, inflexible, and maladaptive. These impair functioning, but the person does not lose contact with reality.

PERSONALITY EMERGENCE The development of the personality *q.v.* from an obscure condition into a state of well-being recognized by others.

PERSONALITY FACTOR TEST A test developed by Raymond B. Cattell in an attempt to identify and categorize various traits that influence the development of personality *q.v.* Cattell's test included 16 trait factors.

PERSONALITY INVENTORIES 1. Paper and pencil tests of personality that present questions about feelings or customary behavior. 2. A test that indicates whether the subject believes that statements reflect his or her personality traits. 3. A test that measures personality traits that have a bearing on a person's effectiveness in functioning in particular situations. cf: projective techniques.

PERSONALITY PATTERN DISTURBANCES Any of several personality *q.v.* types that can rarely be altered by therapy and tend to decompensate to psychosis *q.v.* under stress *q.v.*: inadequate personality *q.v.*, schizoid personality *q.v.*, cyclothymic personality *q.v.*, and paranoid personality *q.v.*

PERSONALITY STRUCTURE Trait *q.v.*

PERSONALITY TRAIT DISTURBANCE Characterized by immaturity or maladjustment that results in a person being unable to maintain emotional equilibrium and independence under stress *q.v.* There are three forms: (a) emotionally unstable personality *q.v.*, (b) passive-aggressive personality; and (c) compulsive personality *q.v.*

PERSONALITY TRAIT THEORY OF ALCOHOLISM The alcoholic *q.v.* possesses certain traits that are indicative of alcoholism *q.v.*, e.g., feelings of inferiority, low frustration tolerance level, dependency, emotional immaturity, and fearfulness.

PERSONALIZED SYSTEM OF INSTRUCTION (PSI) Keller plan *q.v.*

PERSONAL POWER Power derived from the human relationship that one has with another.

PERSONAL SPACE Characteristic zones of distance that people maintain from one another, depending upon how well they know and like each other.

PERSON-CENTERED SEXUALITY A sexual attraction based on the traits making up the personality of one's partner.

PERSONNEL EVALUATION The evaluation of individual teachers and administrators.

PERSON PERCEPTION 1. Impression formation *q.v.* 2. How a person perceives and describes other people.

PERSPIRE 1. To sweat. 2. To breathe through.

PER STIRPES In law, the principle that property left by a deceased person is equally divided among the children.

PERSUASION STRATEGIES The techniques educators *q.v.* and others use to bring about a change in a person's concept of a particular idea or situation.

PERSUASIVE COMMUNICATION THEORY A theory in which emphasis is placed upon the various techniques used in communications to persuade another person to behave in a certain way. A person's attitudes *q.v.* are influenced or changed by altering his or her opinions or beliefs. cf: information theory.

PERSUASIVE VALUE The influence of decisions of one jurisdiction or area in another jurisdiction.

PERT An acronym for program evaluation and review technique *q.v.*

PERTOFRANE A commercial preparation of desipramine *q.v.*

PERTUSSIS Whooping cough *q.v.*

PERVERSION 1. Sexual deviation. 2. Sexual variance *q.v.* 3. Deviation from normal.

PERVERT A sexual deviate.

PESTICIDE An agent that is used to kill pests.

PESTICIDE RESIDUE A quantity of pesticide *q.v.* remaining on a food product from treatments given to it during its growth or processing.

PET An acronym for parent effectiveness training *q.v.*

PETECHIA Tiny diffuse ecchymotic *q.v.* areas in the skin observed in certain severe diseases.

PETITION 1. A written application to the court for the redress of a wrong or of a grant of a privilege or license. 2. A written request to obtain recognition by the National Labor Relations Board as the official representatives of a group of employees for the purpose of collective bargaining.

PETITIONED HEALTH ASSESSMENT A health assessment *q.v.* conducted at the request of a member of the public. All information pertaining to the petition is presented to a screening committee that ascertains whether there is reasonable basis for conducting a health assessment.

PETITIONER The person who petitions *q.v.* a court. If the case is appealed, this person is referred to as appellant.

PETIT MAL EPILEPSY 1. A type of epilepsy in which the person's seizures are relatively brief and may alter or interrupt consciousness. 2. Petit mal seizures *q.v.* ct: grand mal seizures.

PETIT MAL SEIZURES 1. ~ are associated with epilepsy *q.v.* and usually occur in childhood. They are characterized by a partial loss of consciousness, sometimes accompanied by muscular contractions lasting up to 30 s. 2. Petit mal epilepsy *q.v.* 3. Seizures characterized by periods of inattention with rapid eye movements or head twitching.

PETROUS Rock-like.

PET SCAN 1. Position emission tomography *q.v.* 2. Computer-assisted motion pictures of the brain enhanced by radioactive particles form isotopes *q.v.* that have been injected into the bloodstream.

PETTING 1. Sexual activity that stops short of coitus *q.v.* 2. Necking. 3. Caressing and fondling a sex partner.

PETTY Being overly concerned with unimportant details.

PETULANCE Ill humor.

PEYOTE 1. A small cactus plant found mainly in Mexico and in the Southwest United States. It has the generic name of *Laphaphora williamsii q.v.* and produces alkaloid mescaline *q.v.* that is extracted for its psychoactive *q.v.* effects. 2. A cactus that can be dried and eaten, chewed, or smoked, causing stomach upset and nausea and a variety of LSD *q.v.*-like effects.

PEYRONIE'S DISEASE A condition, usually in men of middle age or older, in which the penis *q.v.* develops a fibrous ridge along its top or sides, causing a curvature during erection *q.v.*

PGHCP An acronym for Primary Grades Health Curriculum Project *q.v.*

pH 1. The chemical symbol for the alkalinity *q.v.* or acidity *q.v.* of a substance. 2. A chemical measure of relative acidity. A pH value of less than 7 is acidic, more than 7 is basic. 3. A pH value of 7 is neither acidic or alkaline (neutral). The pH values can range between 1 (highly acidic) and 14 (highly basic). 4. Hydrogen ion concentration. 5. Negative logarithm of hydrogen ion concentration.

pH (OF THE BODY) Slight alkalinity *q.v.* with a pH between 7.2 and 7.4 for blood. cf: pH.

PHAGE 1. A virus that attacks and destroys bacteria *q.v.* 2. Bacteriophage *q.v.*

PHAGOCYTE A type of white blood cell that attacks and destroys foreign materials such as bacteria *q.v.* through enzymatic *q.v.* action.

PHAGOCYTIC LEUKOCYTES An important component of the immune system *q.v.* Specifically, white blood cells that are capable of engulfing and digesting foreign matter in the blood.

PHAGOCYTOSIS 1. The ingestion and digestion of solid particles by certain white blood cells. 2. The engulfment of particles particularly by cells of the reticuloendothelial system *q.v.* 3. The process by which a segment of a cell membrane forms a small pocket around a bit of solid outside the cell, breaks off from the rest of the membrane, and moves into the cell. ct: pinocytosis.

PHAGOTROPHY The ingestion of food in particulate form.

PHALANGES 1. The 14 small bones of the toes or fingers. 2. Phalanx *q.v.* 3. Finger or toe bones.

PHALANX Phalanges *q.v.*

PHALLIC STAGE According to Freudian psychology *q.v.*, the third psychosexual *q.v.* stage in which sexual pleasure is derived primarily from the genitals *q.v.*, usually the 3rd to 6th year of life. ct: anal stage; oral stage; latency period; genital stage; Oedipus conflict; Electra conflict.

PHALLIC SYMBOL Any object that resembles the erect penis *q.v.*

PHALLIC WORSHIP Worship of images of the penis *q.v.*

PHALLOPLASTY Surgical creation of a structure that resembles a penis *q.v.*

PHALLUS The penis *q.v.*

PHANTASTICA A term describing hallucinogenic drugs *q.v.* that alter perceptions but do not impair real-world interaction.

PHANTASY Fantasy *q.v.*

PHANTOM PAIN Pain that is experienced by some individuals from a missing limb, as if it were still attached.

PHARMACEUTICAL INDUSTRY 1. The industries that are concerned with research for new drugs, improvement of existing drugs, marketing, labeling, and quality control in the manufacturing and distribution of drugs. 2. The composite of manufacturers of drugs and similar products intended as therapeutic agents, preventive agents, or corrective agents.

PHARMACIST 1. A druggist. 2. A person trained in chemistry, toxicology, and related aspects of medicines. 3. One who compounds drugs in accordance with prescriptions *q.v.* from physicians, dentists, and veterinarians.

PHARMACODYNAMIC TOLERANCE 1. The body's attempt to adapt to, accommodate, and oppose the effects produced by drugs. 2. The adaptation of the body's tissues to the effects of drugs so that an increase in drug dosage is required to produce a given effect. 3. The reduced effect of a drug due to an altered tissue response to the drug.

PHARMACOGNOSY 1. The science concerned with the study of the composition, use, and history of drugs derived from plants and animals. 2. An applied science that deals with the biologic, biochemical, and economic features of natural drugs and their constituents. cf: pharmacology.

PHARMACOKINETICS The study of what happens to drugs once they are in the body.

PHARMACOLOGY 1. The science concerned with the nature and action of drugs on biological functions. 2. The branch of science dealing with the effects of chemical agents on living things including medicinal chemistry, experimental therapeutics, and toxicology *q.v.*

PHARMACY 1. The science concerned with the compounding and dispensing of drugs. 2. A drug store.

PHARMOKINETICS The body's attempt to minimize the effects of drugs by increasing its metabolic *q.v.* activity to break down the drugs into inert parts.

PHARYNGEAL Pertaining to the pharynx *q.v.*

PHARYNX 1. The cavity behind the mouth that leads to the larynx *q.v.* 2. The cavity that connects the mouth and the nasal passages with the esophagus *q.v.* 3. The throat.

PHENCYCLIDINE HYDROCHLORIDE 1. PCP. 2. A powerful hallucinogenic *q.v.* drug that is mixed with parsley and smoked. 3. A psychoactive *q.v.* drug that can produce hallucinogenic experiences, as well as being a depressant *q.v.*, anesthetic *q.v.*, analgesic *q.v.*, and psychotomimetic *q.v.* 4. Known in the drug culture as angel dust, peace pill, zombie, and other names. ~ causes profound disorientation, and because of its analgesic effects, causes the user to withstand pain he or she would normally be unable to tolerate.

PHENDIMETRAZINE An amphetamine-like appetite suppressant.

PHENELZINE 1. An MAO *q.v.* inhibitor, used as an antidepressant *q.v.* 2. Nardil is a commercial preparation.

PHENMETRAZINE An amphetamine-like appetite suppressant. 2. Preludin is a commercial preparation.

PHENOBARBITAL 1. A barbiturate *q.v.* 2. A drug used as a hypnotic *q.v.* in nervous insomnia *q.v.* and states of nervous excitement, as a sedative *q.v.* in epilepsy *q.v.*, and to withdraw a person from alcohol dependence.

PHENOCOPY An organism whose phenotype *q.v.* but not its genotype *q.v.* is changed by environmental factors to resemble that of another organism.

PHENOL 1. Carbolic acid *q.v.* 2. Chemical formula C_6H_5OH.

PHENOMENOLOGY 1. In psychology *q.v.*, the application of subjective criteria when evaluating behavioral disorders and their treatment. 2. A philosophy that the phenomena of subjective experience are the bases of behavior and are reflected in how people perceive themselves and the world.

PHENOTHIAZINE 1. The chemical name for a class of major tranquilizers *q.v.* 2. A group of drugs that seem to be effective in alleviating the major symptoms of schizophrenia *q.v.* 3. A class of nonaddictive antipsychotic tranquilizers. cf: chlorpromazine.

PHENOTYPE 1. The expression of inherited traits 2. The overt appearance and behavior of a person regardless of his or her genetic *q.v.* blueprint. 3. The expression of traits resulting from the interaction of an organism's genotype *q.v.* with the environment. ct: genotype.

PHENTERMINE An amphetamine-like appetite suppressant.

PHENYLALANINE One of the essential amino acids *q.v.* present in milk.

PHENYLALANINE HYDROXYLASE An enzyme *q.v.* found in the liver that is essential for metabolizing *q.v.* phenylalanine *q.v.*, an essential amino acid *q.v.*

PHENYLETHYLAMINE A chemical found in chocolate that is similar to amphetamine *q.v.* A person who is in love is said to possess an increased amount of ~.

PHENYLKETONE BODIES Substances formed from the inability of the body to metabolize *q.v.* phenylalanine *q.v.* ~ damage brain cells resulting in mental retardation in infants. cf: phenylketonuria.

PHENYLKETONURIA (PKU) 1. A genetic disease caused by a recessive gene *q.v.* that results in an infant being unable to metabolize *q.v.* phenylalanine *q.v.*, an essential amino acid *q.v.* that is present in milk. It is characterized by the absence of the enzyme *q.v.* phenylalanine hydroxylase *q.v.* that is normally present in the liver. As a result, phenylketone bodies *q.v.* are formed that damage brain cells resulting in mental retardation. ~ can be detected by the Guthrie blood test *q.v.* shortly after birth and, when positive, measures can be taken to prevent the onset of ~. 2. An affliction characterized by mental retardation that is caused by the congenital *q.v.* lack of the enzyme *q.v.* required to convert phenylalanine *q.v.* to tyrosine *q.v.* Phenylpyruvic acid *q.v.* and other phenyl compounds are excreted in the urine. 3. A genetic metabolic disorder that leads to mental retardation unless diet is carefully controlled in early childhood.

PHENYLPROPANOLAMINE (PPA) 1. The active chemical formerly found in most over-the-counter *q.v.* diet products. 2. A drug once used in many nasal and sinus congestion medications.

PHENYLPYRUVIC OLIGOPHRENIA Phenylketonuria *q.v.*

PHENYLTHIOCARBAMIDE (PTC) A substance to which some people are taste blind; an inherited condition.

PHEROMONES 1. An extremely potent sexual attractant secreted by animals. 2. Odor signals that attract sex partners. 3. Special chemicals secreted by many animals that stimulate particular reactions in members of the same species.

PHEUMOENCEPHALOGRAM The result of taking an electroencephalogram *q.v.* after injecting gas into the ventricular spaces of the brain.

PHILIA 1. Love between good friends. 2. Brotherly or sisterly love. 3. The Greek form of love most similar to friendship.

PHILLIPS SCALE 1. Phillips Scale of premorbid adjustment *q.v.* 2. A series of questions that is completed by the researcher from the case history of a schizophrenic *q.v.* and is used to assess premorbid adjustment.

PHILLIPS SCALE OF PREMORBID ADJUSTMENT 1. A scale that assesses the social and sexual adjustment of a person prior to the onset of psychotic symptoms. 2. Phillips Scale *q.v.*

PHILOSOPHY 1. A comprehension of the principles of reality; a body of knowledge that defines the perimeters of life and living. 2. Wisdom of life; of the nature of things. 3. A humanistic discipline that attempts to obtain an informed understanding of reality.

PHILOSOPHY OF EDUCATION 1. An application of philosophical principles to educational programs and practices. 2. Conceptualization of needs, aims, goals, objectives, and practices related to intellectual development through educational processes.

PHILOSOPHY OF HEALTH EDUCATION 1. The beliefs, concepts, attitudes, perceptions, and theory of individual health educators and the profession in general. It sets the boundaries of practice, clarifying the areas of professional concentration. It ties together theory and practice. 2. A person's ~ is subjective *q.v.*, as it is based on the way he or she perceives the factors surrounding it.

PHIMOSIS Tightness of the penile foreskin *q.v.* so that it cannot be drawn back from over the glans *q.v.*

PHI PHENOMENON Apparent motion *q.v.*

PHLEBITIS Inflammation of a vein.

PHLEBOTOMY The surgical opening of a vein for bloodletting.

PHLEGM 1. Thick mucus. 2. One of the four humors suggested by Hippocrates.

PHOBIA 1. An intense, irrational fear of something or a situation. True phobias are neurotic *q.v.* forms of behavior. 2. Persistent and unreal fears of real or imagined objects or situations. 3. One of a group of mental disorders called anxiety disorders *q.v.* that is characterized by an intense fear (Table P-1).

TABLE P-1 PHOBIAS

THE PHOBIC REACTIONS	CHARACTERISTICS OR FEAR OF
Acarophobia	Skin infestation
Acrophobia	Heights
Aerophobia	Fresh air
Agoraphobia	Open spaces; public places; leaving home
Aichmophobia	Pointed objects
Ailurophobia	Cats
Algophobia	Pain (Ponophobia)
Amaxophobia	Wagons
Amychophobia	Being scratched; animal claws
Androphobia	The male sex
Anemophobia	Wind; drafts
Anthrophobia	Society (anthropophobia)
Anthropophobia	Society (anthrophobia)
Aphephobia	Being touched
Apiphobia	Bees; buzzing insects
Arachnophobia	Spiders
Astraphobia (Astrophobia)	Thunder
Ataxophobia	Motor incoordination
Autophobia	Being alone
Automysophobia	Personal uncleanliness
Bacillophobia	Bacteria
Ballistophobia	Missiles
Basiphobia	Walking
Bathophobia	High objects
Batophobia	Heights (acrophobia)
Belonephobia	Needles (aichmophobia)
Bromidrosiphobia	Personal odors
Cainophobia	Anything new
Carcinomatophobia	Tumors
Cardiophobia	Heart disease
Carnophobia	Meat
Catoptrophobia	Mirrors
Cenophobia	New ideas (cainotophobia)
Cherophobia	Gaiety
Cholerophobia	Cholera
Claustrophobia	Closed places
Copraphobia	Filth
Doraphobia	Fur of animals
Eremophobia	Being alone (autophobia)
Ereutophobia	Blushing (erythrophobia)
Ergasiophobia	Responsibility

Ergophobia	Work or working
Erythrophobia	Blushing (ereutophobia)
Gatophobia	Cats (ailurophobia)
Gephyophobia	Water; boats; bridges
Gerotophobia	A hatred for old people
Gymnophobia	Naked body
Gynephobia	Women
Haphephobia	Being touched (aphephobia)
Hematophobia (hemophobia)	Sight of blood
Heterophobia	Sexual contact with members of
Kainophobia (cainotophobia)	New things or situations
Kleptophobia	Stealing
Lyssophobia	Rabies
Maieusiophobia	Childbirth
Merinthophobia	Being tied
Monophobia	Being alone (autophobia)
Mysophobia	Dirt and germs
Mythophobia	Making a false statement
Necrophobia	Dead bodies
Neophobia	The unknown
Nosophobia	Illness
Nudophobia	Being naked
Nyctophobia	Darkness (scotophobia)
Ochlophobia	Crowds
Odontophobia	Dentists
Ombrophobia	Storms or clouds
Ophidiophobia	Snakes
Panophobia	Evil; everything (pantophobia)
Pantophobia	Panophobia
Pharmacophobia	Medicines; drugs
Photophobia	Light
Polyphobia	Many things
Ponophobia	Pain (algophobia)
Psychrophobia	Cold
Pyrophobia	Fire
Rhabdophobia	Punishment (associated with a rod)
Rhypophobia	Fear of the act of defecation or feces
Scotophobia	Darkness (nyctophobia)
Sitophobia	Food
Symbolophobia	Symbolic expression
Syphilophobia	Syphilis
Thanatophobia	Death
Topophobia	A particular locality
Toxicophobia	Being poisoned
Trichophobia	Hair (doraphobia)
Trichopathophobia	Hair on the face
Xenophobia	Strangers
Zoophobia	Animals

PHOBIC DISORDER 1. Anxiety marked by persistent fear of an object, situation, or activity, with the knowledge that the fear is without merit. 2. Phobia *q.v.* 3. An anxiety disorder in which there is intense fear and avoidance of situation or objects that cause the fear.

PHOBIC REACTION A psychoneurotic reaction *q.v.* characterized by irrational fear. cf: phobia.

PHOCOMELIA 1. A congenital defect characterized by stunted extremities at birth. It is the result of pregnant women taking the drug thalidomide *q.v.* during pregnancy. 2. A birth defect *q.v.*

PHONEME 1. A speech sound that functions as a unit in a particular language. 2. An individual sound that is meaningless in itself but is used to make up linguistic utterances. 3. The smallest significant unit of sound in a language.

PHONETICS The branch of linguistics *q.v.* that is concerned with the analysis of the sounds employed in speech.

PHONETIC SYMBOLISM The idea that the sounds of words reflect the attributes of the objects to which the words refer.

PHONOLOGICAL RECODING In reading, translation or recoding from spelling to pronunciation.

PHONOLOGICAL RULES The rules in a language with which sound combinations are allowable and which are not.

PHONOLOGICAL SEGMENTATION The ability to differentiate and recognize phonemes *q.v.* in the flow of speech.

PHONOLOGY The rules in a language that govern the sequence in which phonemes *q.v.* can be arranged. The system of speech sounds that an individual utters.

PHOROMETER An instrument for examining the extrinsic ocular *q.v.* muscles.

PHOROPTOR An instrument used to determine the correct eyeglasses for corrective vision.

PHOSPHATASE TEST A test for the efficiency of pasteurization *q.v.* of milk in which the presence of phenol *q.v.* is determined.

PHOSPHATE ESTERS Compounds formed by combining phosphoric acid with an alcohol *q.v.* cf: ester.

PHOSPHATES Compounds containing phosphorus that can pollute water and cause excessive growth of plant life which, when it decays, reduces water oxygen content that results in a destruction of aquatic life.

PHOSPHATIDYL CHOLINE 1. Lecithin *q.v.* 2. Esters *q.v.* of glycerol *q.v.* that contain two fatty acid *q.v.* molecules and one molecule of phosphoric acid and choline *q.v.* ~ is found in nervous tissue and egg yolk.

PHOSPHATIDYLETHANOLAMINE Cephalin. A phospholipid *q.v.* that is widely distributed in the body, esp. in the brain and spinal cord.

PHOSPHOCREATINE A creatine-phosphoric acid compound that occurs in muscle. ~ is the energy source in muscle contraction. cf: creatinine.

PHOSPHOLIPID 1. A glyceride *q.v.* with fatty acids *q.v.* and a phosphate-containing group. 2. Fat-like substances consisting of glycerol *q.v.*, two fatty acids, a phosphate group, and a nitrogen-containing compound, such as choline *q.v.* (found in the phospholipid, lecithin *q.v.*). cf: lecithin.

PHOSPHORUS A mineral element that is essential in the formation of blood, muscles, and nerves.

PHOSPHORYLATION 1. The addition of phosphate *q.v.* to an organic *q.v.* compound (such as glucose *q.v.*) to form glucose monophosphate. 2. In botany, the process by which high-energy organic phosphate compounds are produced.

PHOTOALLERGY An immune reaction caused by light rays changing medications in the blood to allergic substances.

PHOTOAUTOTROPHIC ORGANISMS Organisms that can manufacture their own basic foods with the energy of light. cf: autotrophic.

PHOTOCHEMICAL Refers to the effect that radiant energy has in producing chemical changes. cf: photochemical smog.

PHOTOCHEMICAL SMOG The chemically uniting of gaseous products in the atmosphere into irritating compounds with the sun's action as a chemical catalyst *q.v.* cf: photochemical.

PHOTOCHROMATIC A term applied to the lens of some eyeglasses that lighten or darken in response to the amount or intensity of ultraviolet light that is present. cf: photogrey.

PHOTOGREY An eyeglass lens that lightens or darkens depending upon the amount of light that is present.

PHOTOMICROGRAPH A photograph of the minute characteristics of a specimen made through a microscope.

PHOTOPERIODISM The response of plants to the relative lengths of day and night.

PHOTOSENSITIVITY A condition in which a person is sensitive to sunlight.

PHOTOSYNTHESIS 1. The production of sugar from carbon dioxide *q.v.* and water in the presence of chlorophyll *q.v.* when exposed to light energy resulting in the release of oxygen. 2. An action of light on chlorophyll molecules that fixates atmospheric carbon dioxide to form phosphorylated *q.v.* 3-carbon sugars.

PHOTOSYNTHETIC UNIT A sheet of 200–300 chlorophyll molecules together with reactive sites at which the light reactions of photosynthesis are completed.

PHOTOTOXICITY A substance that, when consumed or applied to the skin, causes an excessive sunburn when the skin is exposed to the sun.

PHOTOTROPISM A movement in response to one-sided illumination.

PHRASE A sequence of words within a sentence that functions as a unit.

PHRASE STRUCTURE The organization of sentences into phrases *q.v.* consisting of 1. underlying structure *q.v.* and 2. surface structure *q.v.*

PHRENIC Pertaining to the diaphragm *q.v.*

PHRENICECTOMY Resection of the phrenic nerve *q.v.*

PHRENIC NERVE The nerve that activates the diaphragm *q.v.*

PHRENICOTOMY The surgical cutting of the phrenic nerve *q.v.*

PHRENOLOGY A pseudoscience based on the belief that the contours or bumps of the skull are indicative of a person's personality, character, and mental facilities.

PHS An acronym for public health services.

PHTHERIS PUBIS The crab louse. Infestation is called pediculosis *q.v.*

PHTHISIS Tuberculosis *q.v.*

PHYLOGENESIS The development of a species. cf: ontogenesis.

PHYLOGENIC Pertaining to the growth and development of a group or race.

PHYLOGENY The evolutionary history of a species or larger group. ct: ontogeny.

PHYLUM Division *q.v.*

PHYSICAL AGENT A factor in the causation of disease. ~ may be artificially imposed, e.g., air pollutants and radiation, or natural, e.g., sun's rays or temperature variations. Examples are 1. skin cancer from overexposure to the sun's rays or 2. liver cancer from breathing air polluted with asbestos fibers. cf: chemical agent; biological agent.

PHYSICAL ATTRACTIVENESS STEREOTYPE A widely held stereotype *q.v.* that attributes positive characteristics to physically attractive persons.

PHYSICAL ATTRIBUTES 1. Physical characteristics. 2. Physical abilities fundamental for normal functioning and physical abilities that are referred to as talents.

PHYSICAL DEPENDENCE 1. Physiological adaptation *q.v.* of the body to the presence of a drug. In effect, the body develops a continuing need for the drug. Once such dependence has been established, the body reacts with predictable symptoms when the drug is abruptly withdrawn. The nature and severity of withdrawal symptoms *q.v.* depend on the drug being used and the daily dosage level attained. 2. A state of physical need for a drug such that the presence of the drug becomes normal and natural. 3. A state of physical adaptation caused by repetitive drug administration *q.v.*

PHYSICAL DISORDERS Bodily impairments that interfere with one's functioning ability to move, communicate, learn, and/or adequately adjust to changing environmental circumstances.

PHYSICAL ENVIRONMENT One's surroundings that are concrete—the animate and inanimate things that surround a person. ~ includes such things as heat, cold, radiation, atmospheric conditions, water, chemical agents, etc. cf: psychological environment; social environment.

PHYSICAL FITNESS Cardiopulmonary *q.v.* capacity, flexibility, endurance, and strength at levels that are basic to the health and functioning of the body.

PHYSICAL HALF-LIFE The time in which the radioactivity *q.v.* usually associated with a particular isotope *q.v.* is reduced by one-half through radioactive decay.

PHYSICAL POTENTIALS 1. Those human elements that provide a person with unique abilities to perform simple to complex tasks. 2. Inherited capacity to perform physical feats or activities. cf: psychological potentials.

PHYSICAL PRIMARY In vision, a primary color when mixed with other primaries contributes to the production of all visible hues *q.v.* ct: psychological primary.

PHYSICAL PROXIMITY Physical closeness of persons in terms of their places of residence, employment, and recreation.

PHYSICAL THERAPIST A person trained in procedures for rehabilitating diseased or disabled parts of the body, especially the muscles and joints.

PHYSICAL THERAPY 1. The specialized area of treating health conditions by nonmedical, physical means. 2. The treatment of disease or impaired motion through a physical method such as heat, hydrotherapy, massage, exercise, or mechanical devices. cf: rehabilitation therapy.

PHYSICAL WELL-BEING Efficient bodily functioning, resistance to disease, and the physical capacity to respond to varied life events.

PHYSICIAN A person trained and licensed to practice medicine.

PHYSICIAN ASSISTANT A person who performs a number of tasks that were traditionally performed by the physician: taking medical histories, making routine examinations, etc. Training for ~s usually includes a specialized 2-year program. ~ always works under the supervision of a physician.

PHYSICIAN EXTENDERS Various kinds of nurses, nurse midwives, nurse practitioners, and physician's assistants, who provide skilled medical care and many routine services done by physicians.

PHYSICIANS' DESK REFERENCE An annual publication compiled by the pharmaceutical industry providing detailed information on prescription drugs.

PHYSICIAN'S HERALD Caduceus *q.v.*

PHYSICIAN SITE-SPECIFIC TRAINING An ATSDR *q.v.*-designed program to make public health professionals at the state, county, and local levels aware of the possible adverse health outcomes resulting from exposure to hazardous substances released from waste sites.

PHYSIOLOGICAL DRIVES (NEEDS) The need for oxygen, food, water, and elimination. These are influenced by homeostasis *q.v.* and appetite *q.v.*

PHYSIOLOGICAL FITNESS Fitness level in the areas of cardiovascular efficiency, muscular strength and endurance, flexibility, and body composition.

PHYSIOLOGICAL NEEDS Maslow's first set of human needs; also called the basic needs. Essential for survival, the ~ include the need for food, water, rest, elimination, and air.

PHYSIOLOGICAL NYSTAGMUS A continuous tremor *q.v.* of the eyes.

PHYSIOLOGICAL PARADIGM A theoretical view that mental disorders are caused by somatic *q.v.* processes.

PHYSIOLOGICAL PROCESSES The normal functioning of all the systems of the body. cf: physiology.

PHYSIOLOGICAL THEORIES OF ALCOHOLISM Theories that claim that the cause of alcoholism *q.v.* is the result of a biological dysfunction. There are two forms: 1. genetotrophic theory *q.v.* and 2. endocrine theory *q.v.*

PHYSIOLOGICAL ZERO The temperature that is experienced as neither warm nor cold.

PHYSIOLOGIC RACES Subdivisions of a variety, alike in structure, but different in certain physiological, biochemical, or pathological ways.

PHYSIOLOGY 1. The science concerned with the functioning of body cells, organs, tissues, and systems. 2. The study of the functioning of living organisms.

PHYSIOTHERAPY Physical therapy *q.v.*

PHYSIQUE Body build or body type. cf: ectomorphy; endomorphy; mesomorphy.

PHYTATE A phosphate *q.v.*-containing compound found in the outer husk of certain cereals. ~ reduces the absorption of calcium and some other minerals.

PHYTIC ACID A phosphorus *q.v.*-containing organic acid. Phytin is the mixture salt of ~ with calcium and magnesium.

PIAGETIAN THEORY The theory of child development based on the writings of Jean Piaget.

PIA MATER The innermost and most delicate of the three membranes *q.v.* covering the brain and spinal cord.

PICA 1. A craving for nonfood items. 2. A perversion of appetite.

PICK'S DISEASE 1. A form of presenile dementia *q.v.* 2. A progressive atrophy of the frontal *q.v.* and temporal *q.v.* lobes of the brain affecting memory, concentration, and abstract thinking, eventually resulting in psychosis *q.v.* and death.

PICOCURIES A measure of radioactivity.

PICTOGRAM A unit of mass: 10^{-12} g or 10^{-6} μg.

PICTORIAL CUES Distance cues in visual images that include shading, texture, overlay, etc.

PID An acronym for pelvic inflammatory disease *q.v.*

PIDGIN A language that develops when two speech communities attempt to communicate by employing the common features of both languages. Eventually, this new language may become the dominant language in the culture.

PIF An acronym for prolactin-inhibiting factor *q.v.* ~ inhibits the anterior pituitary *q.v.* release of prolactin *q.v.*

PIGMENTATION 1. Coloration of the skin as a result of the presence of a color in the tissues. 2. The coloration of the skin as a result of the secretion of melanin *q.v.* by the melanocytes *q.v.*

PILES Hemorrhoids *q.v.*

PILL 1. A drug in pill, tablet, or capsule form. 2. A medication taken orally. 3. Slang for a chemical contraceptive *q.v.* taken orally. 4. A means of contraception *q.v.* involving the ingestion of synthetic hormones *q.v.* to regulate the menstrual cycle *q.v.* The ~ prevents ovulation *q.v.*

PILL DOCTORS A slang expression for physicians who treat obesity *q.v.* by prescribing drugs to curb appetite or to increase the metabolic rate *q.v.*

PILOCARPINE An alkaloid *q.v.* that stimulates the craniosacral division of the autonomic nervous system *q.v.*

PILOERECTION Hair standing up in response to the cold or to fear.

PILOMOTOR Movement of hair.

PILOT PROGRAM A trial, or test, of a particular program, curriculum, etc., to determine its feasibility on a small scale or with a limited population.

PIMP 1. A man who is supported by one or more prostitutes *q.v.* in exchange for protection, bail money, lawyers, etc. 2. A man who serves as a father, confessor, or business agent for a prostitute.

PIMPLE A small, solid elevation of the skin containing bacteria *q.v.*

PINEAL Shaped like a pinecone.

PINEAL GLAND A gland *q.v.* in the brain that appears to regulate some body biorhythms *q.v.*

PINICILLINASE-PRODUCING NEISSERIA GONORRHEA (PPNG) A strain of gonococci *q.v.* resistant to all forms of penicillin *q.v.*

PIN INDEX A safety attachment on the outlet valve of a gas-filled cylinder.

PINK EYE A highly contagious *q.v.* infection *q.v.* of the eye, usually caused by *staphylococcus q.v.* or *pneumococcus q.v.* bacteria. It is treated with antibiotics *q.v.*

PINOCYTOSIS 1. The process of engulfment of liquid by some animal cells. 2. A process by which a segment of cell membrane *q.v.* forms a small pocket around a bit of fluid outside the cell, breaks off from the rest of the membrane, and moves into the cell. ct: phagocytosis.

PINWORM 1. An intestinal roundworm that causes intense rectal itching. 2. Seat worms. 3. Intestinal infestation with *Enterobius vermicularia.*

PIRIFORMIS Pear-shaped.

P-I-S-A 1. The process of internalization, where P represents perception, I interest, S significance, and A application. Internalization is incomplete unless the learner goes through each phase. 2. A theory of learning proposed by Bedworth and Bedworth in 1978 as a basis for effective health education *q.v.*

PISIFORM Pea-shaped.

PITCH 1. The psychological *q.v.* attribute that depends mainly upon the frequency of the physical stimulus. 2. The intensity of a sound; the highness or lowness of a sound dependent upon the number of vibrations produced. ct: loudness.

PITCH DISORDER A condition where the voice tonal characteristics are abnormal (high, low, or monotone).

PITUITARY GLAND 1. The master gland *q.v.* 2. One of the glands of the endocrine system *q.v.* 3. An endocrine gland located at the base of the hypothalamus *q.v.* and secretes a variety of hormones *q.v.* that regulate the proper functioning of the thyroid *q.v.*, adrenal cortex *q.v.*, gonads *q.v.*, and other endocrine organs.

PITUITARY GONADOTROPINS Hormones *q.v.* produced by the pituitary gland *q.v.* that stimulate the gonads *q.v.*

PIT VIPER 1. A venomous snake that has a hollow, heat-sensitive pit between eye and nostril. 2. Pertaining to the rattlesnake, copperhead, water moccasin, and others.

PKU An acronym for phenylketonuria *q.v.*

PLACEBO 1. In epidemiology *q.v.*, a nontreatment or pseudotreatment used in an experimental study which is believed to be effective by the subject. 2. The use of an inert substance in an experimental study. 3. A pharmacologically inactive substance given to test the true effectiveness of an experimental drug. 4. A therapy, chemical agent, or a manipulation of the environment that affects a person's response because of his or her expectations rather than the true effects of the intervention. 5. A substance that is inert and administered with the hope that it will relieve symptoms. cf: placebo effect.

PLACEBO EFFECT 1. A response to a placebo *q.v.* 2. A response to a treatment that does not result from any pharmacological effect or other direct physical action. 3. An improved status of a person's health that is attributable only to the belief that he or she is being helped by a particular treatment regimen or drug. 4. In psychotherapy *q.v.*, an error introduced by the fact that patients improve as a result of the attention they receive even though they are in the control or placebo group.

PLACEBO PILLS 1. Pills that contain no active ingredients. 2. Placebo *q.v.* cf: placebo effect.

PLACE LEARNING 1. Learning *q.v.* the general location of the goal in any situation. 2. The proposition that mastering a maze is primarily a matter of ~. ct: response learning.

PLACENTA 1. The disk-shaped organ within the uterus *q.v.* through which the exchange of nutrient material and oxygen takes place along with the elimination of waste products from the fetal *q.v.* blood. The ~ becomes the afterbirth when it is expelled following the birth of the child. 2. A spongy structure that grows on the wall of the uterus during pregnancy *q.v.* and through which the fetus is nourished and fetal wastes removed. 3. The cake-like organ that connects the fetus to the uterus by means of the umbilical cord *q.v.* and through which the fetus is fed and waste products are eliminated. 4. In botany, the area of the ovary to which one or more ovules *q.v.* are attached.

PLACENTA PREVIA 1. Low implantation *q.v.* of the blastocyst *q.v.* in the uterus *q.v.* that often results in miscarriage *q.v.* because of premature detachment of the placenta *q.v.* 2. A condition in which the placenta of the unborn child is situated over the cervix *q.v.* making a normal birth impossible.

PLACENTATION In botany *q.v.*, the arrangement of the placentas *q.v.* and ovules *q.v.* within the ovary *q.v.*

PLACE THEORY According to Helmholtz's theory, the physiological *q.v.* condition for pitch *q.v.* perception *q.v.* is in the place on the basilar membrane *q.v.* stimulated by a particular sound. ct: frequency theory.

PLACIDITY EXPLOSIVENESS A central orientation *q.v.* characterized by readiness to react to different situations and whether the reactions tend to be belligerent or calm. cf: emotional expressiveness reserve.

PLAGUE 1. An acute infectious disease characterized by severe prostration, delirium, and diarrhea caused by *Pasteurella pestis*. 2. An infectious epidemic *q.v.* disease caused by a bacterium *q.v.* that is carried by rat fleas. ~ was responsible for millions of deaths during the Middle Ages.

PLAINTIFF The person or persons who bring a legal action by filing a complaint.

PLAN A specific action proposed to facilitate an organization in achieving its objectives.

PLANKTON Small, floating or weakly swimming organisms in a body of water.

PLANNED OBSOLESCENCE A system where the manufacturer makes products that do not last very long, or they create new products to replace those that exist at a rapid pace, forcing the consumer to buy new products sooner.

PLANNED PREGNANCY Conception *q.v.* by choice.

PLANNING 1. The process of establishing priorities, identifying the solutions to existing problems, and allocating resources to achieve objectives. 2. The conscious design of desired future states as described in a plan by its goals *q.v.* and objectives *q.v.* ~ incorporates the description of and selection among alternative means of achieving the goals and objectives, and the conduct of those activities necessary to the design and the activities necessary to assure that the plan is achieved.

PLANTAR The sole of the feet.

PLANT PATHOLOGY The study of plant diseases.

PLAQUE 1. Any patch or flat area. 2. Patches caused by an accumulation of cholesterol *q.v.* and other fatty substances in the inner lining of the artery. 3. Patches on the tongue, cheek, or roof of the mouth associated with tobacco smoke. 4. In dentistry *q.v.*, patches of food and bacterial *q.v.* colonies adhering to the teeth. A major cause of tooth decay and periodontal *q.v.* disease. 5. A bacteria-containing material that can accumulate on teeth. 6. In neurology *q.v.*, certain areas of the brain that have undergone specific form of degeneration. ~s are usually found in persons with Alzheimer's disease *q.v.*, although they are also found to a lesser extent in older persons who are normal. 7. An atheroma *q.v.*

PLASMA 1. The pale yellow liquid portion of the blood consisting of more than 100 constituents including proteins *q.v.*, inorganic salts, gases, waste products, enzymes *q.v.*, and hormones *q.v.* 2. The fluid portion of the blood in which corpuscles *q.v.* are suspended. ~ comprises approximately 60% of the blood. cf: serum.

PLASMA CELLS Derived from B cells, they produce antibodies *q.v.*

PLASMAGENES Self-replicating particles of cytoplasm *q.v.* capable of transmitting traits believed to be responsible for extranuclear inheritance *q.v.*

PLASMA MEMBRANE 1. The membrane *q.v.* that surrounds the cell. It regulates the passage of substances into and out of the cell. 2. A selectively permeable *q.v.* membrane constituting the outermost limit of the cell.

PLASMAPHERESIS A process of filtering the blood.

PLASMODESMA (PL. PLASMODESMATA) Minute cytoplasmic *q.v.* threads that extend through openings in cells, connecting the protoplasts of adjacent cells.

PLASMODIUM A protozoan *q.v.*, some of which cause disease in humans, e.g., malaria *q.v.*

PLASMOLYSIS The shrinking of the protoplasm *q.v.* from the cell wall as a result of outward diffusion of water into a solution with a low diffusion pressure of water.

PLASMOSOME 1. The body within the nucleus *q.v.* of a cell. 2. Nucleolus *q.v.*

PLASTICITY The capacity for being molded or shaped, as in a developmental level where there is a potential for change. cf: human plasticity.

PLASTIC SURGERY A medical specialty concerned with corrective, restorative, or reparative surgery for restoring or improving or repairing deformed or mutilated parts of the body.

PLASTID A body in the cytoplasm *q.v.* of some plants and protozoans *q.v.* Chloroplastids *q.v.* produce chlorophyll *q.v.* involved in photosynthesis *q.v.* Leukoplastids are colorless and are the sites of starch synthesis.

PLATEAU In education, period of no apparent improvement in learning a skill.

PLATEAU PHASE 1. The sexual response *q.v.* phase of sustained arousal. 2. The fully stimulated stage in human sexual response cycle that immediately precedes orgasm *q.v.* 3. The second of four stages of the sexual response cycle described by Masters and Johnson. During this phase, the outer third of the vagina *q.v.* tightens and the clitoris *q.v.* withdraws behind the clitoral hood *q.v.* in females. In males, the diameter of the penis *q.v.* may increase slightly and the size of the testicles *q.v.* may increase. In both genders, there is myotonia *q.v.*, hyperventilation *q.v.*, and tachycardia *q.v.* 4. Plateau stage.

PLATELET ADHESIVENESS The tendency of platelets *q.v.* to clump together, thus enhancing the speed at which blood clots.

PLATELETS A component of blood essential for normal blood coagulation *q.v.*

PLATELET TRANSFUSION A blood transfusion *q.v.* in which red blood cells are removed and the remaining blood, rich in platelets *q.v.*, is transfused.

PLATONIC The close association between two people that does not include a sexual relationship.

PLAY THERAPY A form of psychotherapy *q.v.* used chiefly with children who have emotional problems. The method consists of allowing a child to play with a variety of objects or toys with the intent that the child will reveal sources of his or her emotional problem.

PLEADINGS Formal papers filed in court action in which a complaint by the plaintiff *q.v.* or the defendant is outlined as to what is alleged on one side and admitted to or denied on the other side.

PLEA IN ABATEMENT In law, an objection by the defense as to the time, place, or method of the plaintiff's claim, without disputing the validity of the claim.

PLEASURE CENTERS 1. The areas of the brain where stimulation results in pleasurable sensations. 2. Reward centers.

PLEASURE PRINCIPLE 1. In psychoanalysis *q.v.*, the demand that an instinctual need be immediately gratified regardless of reality. 2. A drive behind human behavior, according to Freud, to maximize sensual pleasure and minimize pain. ct: reality principle.

PLEIOTROPHY 1. A condition in which more than one trait is influenced by a single gene *q.v.* 2. The multiple effects of a single gene on more than one aspect of the phenotype *q.v.*

PLENARY Complete power or jurisdiction over a designated matter.

PLETHYSMOGRAPH An instrument used to determine the amount of blood present or passing through an organ.

PLEURAE 1. Paired, closed sacs that invest nearly the whole surface of the lungs. 2. Tissues that surround the lungs. 3. Pleura.

PLEURAL SPACE The potential space existing between the pleural *q.v.* surfaces.

PLEURISY 1. An inflammation *q.v.* of the lining of the chest cavity and outer surface of the lungs. 2. Inflammation of the pleura *q.v.*

PLEXUS 1. A network of either nerves *q.v.*, blood vessels *q.v.*, or lymphatic vessels *q.v.* 2. A network or tangle. cf: brachial plexus; lumbosacral plexus.

PLICA A fold.

PLUMBISM Lead poisoning.

PLURALISTIC IGNORANCE A situation in which individuals in a group do not know that there are others in the group who share their feelings.

PLUS FACE A facial expression/gesture characterized by raised eyebrows, raised chin, an firmly set neck that, when displayed to another child, typically signals that the face maker will prevail in the encounter.

PLWA An acronym for persons living with AIDS *q.v.*

PMS An acronym for premenstrual syndrome *q.v.*

PNEUMOCYSTIS CARINII PNEUMONIA The most common life-threatening opportunistic infection *q.v.* diagnosed in AIDS *q.v.* patients. ~ is caused by a parasite *q.v.*, *Pneumocystis carinii*.

PNEUMONECTOMY The surgical removal of a lung.

PNEUMONIA 1. A disease of the lungs caused by the pneumococcus *q.v.* organism. 2. An acute infectious disease of the lungs. Symptoms include fever, coughing, and shaking chills. ~ is one of the five leading causes of death among people over 65 years.

PNEUMOTHORAX 1. Air in the pleural cavity *q.v.* 2. An accumulation of air or gas in the pleural cavity usually entering after a wound or an injury causing a penetration to the chest wall or a laceration of the lung. cf: spontaneous pneumothorax.

PNS 1. An acronym for parasympathetic nervous system *q.v.* 2. An acronym for peripheral nervous system *q.v.*

PO_2 Partial pressure of oxygen *q.v.*

POCKET VETO The act of the executive using veto power by leaving a bill unsigned or formally vetoed beyond the adjournment of the legislative body.

PODIATRIST 1. Doctors of Podiatric Medicine (DPM). ~s make devices to correct problems, provide care for nails, prescribe certain drugs, and perform surgery on the foot. 2. A physician who is involved with the diagnosis and treatment of foot problems. cf: podiatry.

PODIATRY The diagnosis and treatment of foot injury or disease. cf: podiatrist.

POIKILOTHERMOPHYTIC Descriptive of organisms that lack a means of maintaining their cytoplasmic temperature at a constant level. ct: homoiothermophytic.

POINT PREVALENCE STUDY Cross-sectional method *q.v.*

POINT SCALE In intelligence *q.v.* testing, a test in which credit is given directly in terms of the number of items passed. ct: age scale.

POINT SOURCE OF POLLUTION Water pollutants *q.v.* from a specific and known source.

POINT TENDERNESS An area of tenderness limited to 2–3 cm in diameter. It can be identified through pain with gentle pressure. ~ can be located in any place of the body as it is usually associated with acute inflammation *q.v.*, as in peritonitis *q.v.*, or disruption of tissue, as in a fracture *q.v.*

POISON 1. Any substance that is toxic *q.v.* 2. Any substance that interferes with the normal functioning of the body. 3. A substance that, when ingested or injected, will result in severe illness or death.

POLAR BODIES In female animals, the smaller cells produced at meiosis *q.v.* that do not develop into ova *q.v.*

POLARITY Positions at the opposite ends of a continuum.

POLARIZATION The process by which attitudes or feelings become more extreme, positive attitudes becoming more favorable, negative attitudes becoming even less favorable.

POLICE POWER Legislative authority granted to law enforcement officials and others to protect the health and welfare of the people through the use of punitive measures.

POLICY 1. A course of action adopted and pursued by a government body or other organization. 2. Any course of action adopted as proper. Health educators *q.v.* can have a significant influence on policy formulation *q.v.*

POLICY FORMULATION Identifying needs, resources, demand, technological alternatives, and maximum potential participation in developing policies that can be supported and authorized by policymakers *q.v.*

POLICYMAKERS Those in the authority structure and the power structure who have the power to influence and establish policy.

POLIOMYELITIS 1. A disease caused by a virus *q.v.* infecting the motor nerves *q.v.* in the spinal cord. 2. Infantile paralysis *q.v.*

POLITICAL BEHAVIORS The actions of institutions, political parties, governments, voters, lobbyists, etc. that serve to regulate and negotiate allocation of resources.

POLITICAL PROCESS The procedures used to initiate and enact legislation.

POLITICAL SOCIALIZATION Socialization *q.v.* of children into the political world in which they live, including the development of attitudes *q.v.* and knowledge about their country, the political process, and government structures and officials.

POLITICS The process of maneuvering to establish public policy.

POLLEN GRAIN The germinated, usually two-celled, microspore *q.v.* of seed plants.

POLLINOSIS 1. Hay fever. 2. Allergy to pollens.

POLLUTANTS Unwanted and undesirable substances within certain segments of the environment *q.v.* ~ may include objects such as litter, chemicals, gases, particles, and combinations of these.

POLLUTION 1. Combining hazardous substances with elements of the environment: air, land, and water. 2. Degradation of the environment; disruption of the ecosystems *q.v.* occurring when the wastes of one organism cannot be scavenged by another organism.

POLONIUM-210 A radioactive *q.v.* substance found in tobacco smoke.

POLYABUSE 1. Abusing more than one drug concurrently. 2. Polydrug use *q.v.*

POLYANDRY A condition in which one woman has more than one husband at one time. ct: polygamy; monogamy.

POLYARTHRITIS Arthritis *q.v.* in many joints at one time; usually acute *q.v.*

POLYCHLORINATED BIPHENYLS 1. Cooling fluids used in electrical capacitors and heat exchange units and are not biodegradable *q.v.* ~ may be associated with a variety of occupational illnesses *q.v.* 2. A class of chlorinated organic *q.v.* compounds similar to DDT.

POLYCYCLIC AROMATIC HYDROCARBONS Chemicals found in tobacco tar that are carcinogenic *q.v.*

POLYCYTHEMIA An abnormal increase in the number of red blood cells in the blood.

POLY DACRON ROPE A specially designed rope made from nonconductive *q.v.* plastic used to manipulate live electrical wires.

POLYDACTYLY A genetic *q.v.* defect characterized by an excessive number of fingers or toes.

POLYDIPSIA Excessive thirst; a symptom of diabetes *q.v.*

POLYDRUG USE The concurrent use of two or more drugs. cf: polyabuse.

POLYGAMY 1. A condition of having more than one husband or wife at one time. 2. The form of marriage in which a spouse of either sex may possess a plurality of mates at the same time. 3. Polyandry *q.v.*, polygyny *q.v.*, and group marriage *q.v.*

POLYGENE One of a series of multiple genes involved in quantitative inheritance *q.v.*

POLYGENETIC MODEL 1. The concept that explains the development of a disorder to a specific group of interacting genes *q.v.* 2. Polygenic *q.v.*

POLYGENIC (INHERITANCE) 1. Inheritance *q.v.* of an attribute whose expression is controlled by many genes *q.v.* or pairs. 2. Polygenetic model *q.v.* 3. Polygenic trait *q.v.* cf: multifactorial inheritance *q.v.*

POLYGENIC TRAIT 1. A trait that is expressed as a result of the action of many genes *q.v.* whose individual effects are not apparent. 2. Polygenic *q.v.*

POLYGRAPH 1. A lie detector. 2. A method of measuring and recording changes in physical reactions that result from emotional stress *q.v.* produced by questions asked by an examiner.

POLYGYNY A condition in which one man is married to more than one woman at the same time.

POLYMASTIA The presence of one or more extra breasts.

POLYMERIZATION A chemical union of two or more molecules of the same kind for forming a new compound having the same elements in the same proportion but of a higher molecular weight and different physical properties.

POLYMERS 1. Large molecules consisting of many smaller molecules that are identical or of several different types. 2. Molecules made up of repeating subunits. 3. Compounds composed of two or more units of the same substance. cf: polymerization.

POLYMICROBIAL The presence of several species of microorganisms *q.v.*

POLYMORPHISM Two or more kind of individuals in a breeding population where the rarer type is maintained by some mechanism other than recurrent mutation *q.v.*

POLYMORPHONUCLEAR Having many-shaped nuclei *q.v.*

POLYMORPHOUSLY PERVERSE Open to any and all forms of sexual stimulation.

POLYNEURITIS 1. An inflammation *q.v.* encompassing many peripheral *q.v.* nerves. 2. A disease of the peripheral nerves.

POLYNEUROPATHY The gradual destruction of nervous system *q.v.* functioning resulting from the influence of alcohol on nerve cells.

POLYNUCLEOTIDE A unit of DNA *q.v.* consisting of four nucleotides *q.v.*

POLYP 1. A stemmed growth that arises from the mucosa and extends into the lumen *q.v.* or opening of any body cavity. 2. Polypus *q.v.*

POLYPEPTIDE 1. A chain of amino acids *q.v.* linked by peptide *q.v.* bonds. 2. A compound containing two or more amino acids and one or more peptide groups.

POLYPHAGIA 1. Excessive craving for food. 2. Hunger; a symptom of diabetes *q.v.*

POLYPHARMACY The use of two or more drugs during the course of treatment for a particular illness.

POLYPLOID More than two sets of chromosomes in one cell. Two sets would be diploid *q.v.*; three sets, triploid *q.v.*; four sets, tetraploid *q.v.*; etc.

POLYPUS Polyp *q.v.*

POLYRIBOSOMES A group of ribosomes *q.v.* working together to synthesize proteins *q.v.*

POLYSACCHARIDES 1. The complex carbohydrates *q.v.*: starches, cellulose, and glycogen. 2. A carbohydrate containing more than 10 monosaccharides *q.v.* 3. A complex carbohydrate *q.v.* 4. A compound of a long chain of glucose *q.v.* units found chiefly in vegetables, fruits, and grains.

POLYSOME A group of ribosomes *q.v.* on a single mRNA *q.v.* molecule *q.v.*

POLYTHELIA The presence of a number of nipples on the breasts.

POLYUNSATURATED FATS Fats derived from vegetables, lean poultry, fish, and cereal. cf: polyunsaturated fatty acids.

POLYUNSATURATED FATTY ACID (PUFA) 1. A fatty acid *q.v.* with two or more double bonds. 2. Fats and oils that have many unsaturated bonds and that tend to be liquid at room temperature. 3. Fats composed of compounds in which multiple hydrogen-bonding positions remain open. cf: polyunsaturated fats.

POLYURIA Excessive excretion of urine *q.v.*

POLYVINAL CHLORIDE A substance used in the manufacture of plaster and is associated with some forms of cancers *q.v.*

PONDIMIN A commercial preparation of fenfluramine *q.v.*

PONS 1. That part of the central nervous system *q.v.* lying between the medulla oblongata *q.v.* and the mesencephalon *q.v.* ventral *q.v.* to the cerebellum *q.v.* 2. The portion of the brain immediately above the medulla oblongata. 3. An area in the brainstem *q.v.* containing nerve fibers connecting the cerebellum with the spinal cord and with the motor areas of the cerebrum. 4. Bridge.

POPLITEAL 1. The area behind the knee joint. 2. Pertaining to the posterior surface of the knee, a lozenge-shaped space at the back of the knee joint.

POPLITEAL ARTERY The contamination of the femoral artery *q.v.* in the popliteal *q.v.* space.

POPPERS A slang term for the inhalant drug, amyl nitrate *q.v.*

POPULATION 1. The number of people in a given geographic area. 2. A group being studied in a research project, from which a sample *q.v.* is drawn. 3. In genetics *q.v.* a group of interbreeding individuals. cf: sample.

POPULATION AT RISK (PAR) 1. In epidemiology *q.v.*, those persons capable of developing a specific health condition. 2. Persons possessing characteristics increasing susceptibility to a health condition.

POPULATION ATTRIBUTABLE RISK PERCENT (PARP) In epidemiology *q.v.*, a measure of the benefit derived by modifying a risk factor *q.v.*

POPULATION GENETICS The branch of genetics *q.v.* that deals with frequencies of alleles *q.v.* in groups of individuals.

POPULATION TRENDS The predictions of population growth or decline.

PORE 1. The site in a cell membrane *q.v.* involved in the transport of a substance across the membrane barrier. 2. The site in the skin through which sweat is excreted from the body.

PORNAE 1. Early Greek women who were hired to provide sexual gratification for men. 2. Greek prostitutes *q.v.*

PORNOGRAPHY Sexually arousing music, art, literature, films, or video. cf: hard-core pornography; soft-core pornography.

PORPHYRIA A disease involving abnormally high blood levels of porphyrin *q.v.*

PORPHYRIN A component of the hemoglobin *q.v.* molecule.

PORTABILITY The mechanism by which an employee can take accumulated health benefits with him or her from one job to another.

PORTAL OF ENTRY In an infectious disease *q.v.*, the means by which the infectious *q.v.* organism enters the body, nose, mouth, skin, etc.

PORTAL VEIN The large vein that collects the blood from the spleen *q.v.* and intestinal tract *q.v.* and carries it to the liver *q.v.*

PORTER–LAWLER MODEL A hypothesis of human motivation *q.v.* that holds that behavior is caused by felt needs, that the strength of the motivation is related to the perceived value of the results of the behavior, and if the person feels that the desired results are probable. The ~ has three additional characteristics: 1. the total value of the reward is determined by both the intrinsic *q.v.* and extrinsic *q.v.* needs of the person at the time the behavior is performed; 2. the effectiveness of the behavior is related to the person's perception of what is required to accomplish the task and his or her ability to perform it; and 3. the person's desire to perform a task is driven by his or her views of the fairness of the rewards to be received once the task is complete.

POSITION DESCRIPTION Also called a job description, it is a detailed outline of a person's responsibilities, authorities, and relationships with other members of the organizational team.

POSITION EFFECT A phenotype *q.v.* that varies depending on the position of a gene *q.v.* or group of genes, in relation to other genes.

POSITION EMISSION TOMOGRAPHY (PET) SCAN A brain imaging technique that uses a radioactive tracer to detect oxygen metabolism *q.v.* in various regions of the brain in order that levels of activity in these regions may be evaluated.

POSITION POWER The inherent power derived by the position a person holds in an organization.

POSITIVE ACCELERATION 1. The curve of progressively increasing returns. 2. Increases in the independent variable *q.v.* lead to larger and larger increases in the dependent variable *q.v.* ct: negative acceleration.

POSITIVE ADDICTION The compelling desire to engage in a health-promoting behavior instead of a health-threatening behavior.

POSITIVE ASSOCIATION In epidemiology *q.v.*, as the amount of a characteristic increases or decreases, the rate of the health condition increases or decreases. ct: negative association.

POSITIVE BIAS The tendency to agree with any persuasive message.

POSITIVE CALORIC BALANCE A state in which the body takes in more calories *q.v.* than it expends.

POSITIVE CONSEQUENCES 1. Pleasant events that occur after a behavior is performed. 2. Rewards.

POSITIVE CORRELATION A correlation *q.v.* in which high measures on one trait are associated with high values on a second trait. ct: negative correlation.

POSITIVE FEEDBACK That part of the feedback system *q.v.* that tends to strengthen the action. ct: negative feedback.

POSITIVE FEEDBACK SYSTEM In sexuality, the enhancement of one erotic stimulus by another.

POSITIVE NORMS Informal group standards that tend to enhance or contribute to organizational productivity.

POSITIVE REINFORCEMENT 1. Pleasurable events following a behavior that tend to reinforce that behavior, leading to an increase in frequency of the behavior. 2. A technique in which the positive aspects of a person's endeavors are rewarded. 3. A form of operant conditioning *q.v.* ct: negative reinforcement.

POSITIVE REINFORCER 1. A reward. 2. An event that increases the strength of the response *q.v.*

POSITIVE RELATIONSHIP A relationship in which increases in the independent variable *q.v.* produce increases in the dependent variable *q.v.* ct: negative relationship. cf: positive correlation.

POSITIVE SIGNS (OF PREGNANCY) The detection of fetal heartbeat, movement, and sonograms of the fetal skeleton. cf: presumptive signs; probable signs.

POSITIVE SOCIAL ACTIONS 1. A type of behavior in which one person does something to benefit another. 2. Prosocial behavior.

POSITIVE SPIKES An EEG *q.v.* pattern from the temporal lobe *q.v.* of the brain of 6–8 cps to 14–16 cps, often found in people with impulsive and aggressive behaviors.

POSITIVE SYMPTOMS In schizophrenia *q.v.* behavior characterized by hallucinations *q.v.* and other bizarre behavioral patterns. ct: negative symptoms.

POSITIVE TRANSFER Transfer in which learning *q.v.* of one skill aids in the learning of a second skill. ct: negative transfer.

POSITIVE TRANSFERENCE Analysis of transference *q.v.*

POSSESSED An ancient term for mental illness *q.v.* based on the belief that the person was possessed by an evil spirit. cf: possession.

POSSESSION The taking over of the mind by evil spirits. cf: possessed.

POST ABSORPTIVE In nutrition, 12 h following the ingestion of food.

POSTADAPTATION A hereditary *q.v.* adaptive change induced by the environment *q.v.*

POST COITAL DOUCHING The insertion of a chemical solution into the vagina *q.v.* following coitus *q.v.* The chemical solution usually contains a spermicide *q.v.* This procedure is generally ineffective as a contraceptive *q.v.* method.

POST COITAL PILL A contraceptive *q.v.* chemical in pill *q.v.* form that is taken the day following sexual intercourse. Also called the morning after pill.

POSTCONCUSSION SYNDROME Symptoms sometimes experienced by an individual who has suffered a concussion *q.v.*, including headaches, anxiety *q.v.*, irritability, and minor cognitive *q.v.* impairment.

POSTCONVENTIONAL LEVEL OF REASONING Kohlberg's third level of development of moral reasoning in which judgments are based on self-accepted moral principles.

POSTERIOR The back or dorsal *q.v.* surface of the body or part. ct: anterior.

POSTERIOR PITUITARY LOBE The section of the pituitary gland *q.v.* that is toward the back or rear. ct: anterior pituitary lobe.

POSTERIOR TIBIAL ARTERY The artery *q.v.* located just posterior *q.v.* to the ankle bone that supplies blood to the foot.

POSTHYPNOTIC SUGGESTION Induced suggestions while hypnotized to be performed by the person following removal from the hypnotic state.

POSTINFERIOR Behind (to the back) and below.

POSTJUCTIONAL RECEPTOR SITE The receptor *q.v.* for a neurotransmitter *q.v.* on the receiving neuron *q.v.*

POSTMARITAL INTERCOURSE Sexual intercourse *q.v.* by a formerly married person.

POSTMARKETING DRUG SURVEILLANCE A system whereby a drug's usefulness and possible side effects are monitored after the drug has been marketed.

POSTMENOPAUSAL YEARS The period in a woman's life after the menses *q.v.* cease.

POSTMORTEM 1. An examination of a body after death. 2. Autopsy *q.v.* 3. Necropsy *q.v.*

POSTNASAL The region behind the nose, toward the back part of the throat.

POSTOPERATIVE Following an operation or surgical procedure.

POSTOVULATORY PHASE The third stage of the menstrual cycle *q.v.* in which the corpus luteum *q.v.* secretes hormones *q.v.*, estrogen *q.v.*, and progesterone *q.v.* that prepare the uterus *q.v.* for the implantation of the fertilized *q.v.* egg.

POSTPARTUM 1. After childbirth. 2. The period of time following the birth of a baby during which the uterus *q.v.* returns to its prepregnancy size.

POSTPARTUM DEPRESSION An emotional low experienced by the mother following childbirth.

POSTPARTUM ILLNESS A mental or emotional state of some women who have recently given birth that is characterized by a hormonal *q.v.* upheaval that results in postpartum depression *q.v.* that may cause bizarre behavior. The behavior may be identified as psychotic *q.v.* with hallucinations *q.v.* and violent urges. This stage is called postpartum psychosis *q.v.* The mother may injure the baby or even kill it. Treatment when administered in time is usually successful and consists of antipsychotic drugs *q.v.* and hormonal therapy.

POSTSECONDARY HEALTH EDUCATION PROGRAM A planned set of health education *q.v.* policies, procedures, activities, and services that are directed toward learners and faculty of colleges and universities.

POSTSYNAPTIC NEURON The neuron *q.v.* on the receiving end of an impulse that responds to the release of a neurotransmitter *q.v.* from the presynaptic neuron *q.v.* that is necessary for the continuance of the impulse through the nerve.

POSTTEST An evaluation instrument that provides the educator with data that are interpreted in terms of the learning that has taken place over a given period of time. A ~ measures learning progress over a given period of time.

POSTTRAUMATIC STRESS DISORDER (PTSD) An anxiety disorder *q.v.*, usually brought about by one or more traumatic events, characterized by a repeated reliving of the event, depression, nightmares, inappropriate social behavior, estrangement from others, and other adjustment problems.

POSTULATE A general term describing a statement that is a premise for a line of reasoning. From that statement, one can deduce more specific propositions.

POSTURAL MUSCLES 1. The muscles that help to maintain posture. 2. The muscles that are active in positioning the body.

POST VACCINAL Following a vaccination *q.v.*, usually referring to some type of reaction.

POTABLE Safe to drink.

POTABLE WATER Water that is fit to drink.

POTASSIUM An alkaline *q.v.* metallic element whose chemical symbol is K (kalium) and that occurs abundantly in nature but always in combination. It is an element that is vital to proper nutrition *q.v.*

POTENCY The amount of a drug that is required to produce a given effect. cf: therapeutic index.

POTENT 1. Having the male capability to perform sexual intercourse *q.v.* 2. Capable of erection *q.v.* 3. Refers to a drug where a small amount produces an effect. ct: impotence.

POTENTIAL 1. Untested ability that may be developed through training, practice, or other activity. 2. In physiology *q.v.*, the difference in electrical charges as found on outer and inner surfaces of cell membranes *q.v.*

POTENTIAL ACTION The difference in electrical charges on the inner and outer surfaces of the cell membrane *q.v.* during impulse conduction *q.v.* The outer surface is negative to the inner surface.

POTENTIAL DIFFERENCE Potential *q.v.*

POTENTIAL ENERGY 1. Energy *q.v.* that is ready to be used. 2. Stored energy. ct: kinetic energy.

POTENTIAL RESTING The difference in electrical charges on the inner and outer surfaces of the cell membrane *q.v.* when it is not conducting impulses. The outer surface is positive to the inner surface.

POTENTIAL STIMULUS The energy present in the environment *q.v.* that would be detected if it came into contact with an appropriate receptor *q.v.* cf: distal stimulus. ct: proximal stimulus; effective stimulus.

POTENTIATED EFFECT 1. The phenomenon whereby the use of one drug intensifies the effect of a second drug. 2. Potentiating drug interaction. cf: potentiation.

POTENTIATION 1. The process of combining two or more drugs resulting in an enhanced reaction. 2. ~ occurs when the action in one drug is enhanced by the presence of another. ~ can be very useful in certain medical procedures; for example, a physician can induce and maintain a specific degree of anesthesia *q.v.* with a small amount of the primary anesthetic *q.v.* agent by using another drug to potentiate the primary anesthetic agent.

POT HEAD A person who is a habitual user of marijuana *q.v.*

POULTICE A hot, soft mulch prepared by wetting powder and placing it on a sore, wound, or inflamed part of the body to soothe it or to draw out poisons.

POVERTY A condition in which a person or family has an income below a governmentally determined level.

POWER 1. In physiology *q.v.*, the speed with which the muscle can apply force. 2. In sociology *q.v.*, the ability to move others to behavior and action, social ~ and political ~. 3. In psychology *q.v.*, holding control over rewards and punishments; a characteristic of models *q.v.* important in observational learning *q.v.* 4. The extent to which an individual can control the actions and/or beliefs of others.

POWER ASSERTION 1. Techniques of parental discipline *q.v.* based on parents' physical power and control of resources. 2. Attempts to control children by physical force or punishment or deprivation of privileges. cf: love withdrawal; induction.

POWER STRUCTURE 1. A group of people in a community whose power often supersedes that of the authority structure *q.v.* and that usually functions for the satisfaction of its own interests. 2. The influential segment of the community.

POWER THEORY OF IDENTIFICATION The theory that children identify with persons who control rewards and punishments, whether the children receive the rewards or punishments.

PPA Phenylpropanolamine *q.v.*

PPI An acronym for patient package insert *q.v.*

PPNG An acronym for penicillinase-producing *Neisseria gonorrhoeae q.v.*

PPO An acronym for preferred provider organization *q.v.*

PRACTICAL SIGNIFICANCE In epidemiology *q.v.*, the existence of significance if the findings have important implications within the conceptual context of the study.

PRACTICE 1. The use of one's knowledge in a particular profession. 2. The ~ of health education is the exercise of one's knowledge and skills of educational theory in the promotion of health, prevention of disease and disability, and the treatment of imbalance among internal physiological conditions.

PRAGMATICS 1. The rules for the appropriate and effective use of language. 2. The use of language in social contexts and the rules that govern such use in communication.

PRAGMATISM A philosophy, particularly promoted by John Dewey, that focuses on the practical application of knowledge.

PRAYER In law, that part of a petition in which a request to the court is sought for the granting of relief.

PRAYER OF MAIMONIDES Formulated in the 12th century by Rabbi Maimon: "Thy eternal providence has appointed me to watch over the life and health of Thy creatures. May the love for my art actuate me at all times; may neither avarice nor miserliness, nor thirst for glory, or for a great reputation engage my mind; for the enemies of truth and philanthropy could easily deceive me and make me forgetful of my lofty aim of doing good to Thy children.

May I never see in the patient anything but a fellow creature in pain.

Grant me strength, time, opportunity always to correct what I have acquired, always to extend its domain; for knowledge is immense and the spirit of man can extend indefinitely to enrich itself daily with new requirements.

Today he can discover his errors of yesterday and tomorrow he can obtain a new light on what he thinks himself sure of today. Oh, God, Thou has appointed me to watch over the life and death of Thy creatures, here am I ready for my vocation and now I turn unto my calling."

PREADAPTATION In genetics *q.v.*, a hereditary adaptation to an environment *q.v.* that the organism is not currently in.

PREADOLESCENCE The second part of the school years according to Sullivan, that begins when children first start to form close friendships marked by sensitivity to the friend as a person. cf: juvenile era.

PRE-AIDS (LYMPHADENOPATHY) SYNDROME A sexually transmitted syndrome *q.v.* that resembles AIDS *q.v.* but is less severe.

PRECANCEROUS LEUKOPLAKIA White patches on the mucous membranes *q.v.* of the mouth that suggest early changes associated with cancer *q.v.* development.

PRECEDE 1. A health education *q.v.* program planning model consisting of seven stages that provides a sequential method for program development. ~ can be used in any setting for any type of program. 2. A model where the predisposing, reinforcing, and enabling factors are considered as part of the program planning process.

PRECEDENCE EFFECT The experience of hearing one sound when two identical sounds are presented laterally, separated by 7–50 ms.

PRECEDENT 1. In law, a decision of the court that is used as the basis for determining the outcome of a like case or similar case that occurs subsequently. 2. That which has been done in the past under similar circumstances.

PRECIPITATE A compound that causes substances in solution to settle out.

PRECIPITATING CAUSE 1. The particular stress *q.v.* that precipitates a disorder. 2. Stress cause and effect.

PRECIPITIN A circulating antibody *q.v.* that functions in the precipitation of homologous antigen *q.v.*

PRECIPITOUS BIRTH A delivery in which the time from the onset of labor *q.v.* until the birth is very short, usually less than 2 h.

PRECLINICAL STUDY A stage in medical education consisting of intensive study in biochemistry, histology, physiology, embryology, and genetics.

PRECOCIOUS 1. Unusually developed. 2. Unusually intelligent.

PRECOCIOUS SEXUALITY The awakening of sexual desire at a prematurely early age.

PRECOITAL FLUID An alkaline *q.v.* fluid secreted by the Cowper's glands *q.v.* that lubricates the urethra and provides a safe environment for the passage of semen *q.v.*

PRECONSCIOUS 1. Thoughts that are temporarily forgotten but can easily be recalled. 2. Preconscious mind (Freudian). cf: conscious; subconscious.

PRECONVENTIONAL LEVEL OF MORAL REASONING Kohlberg's first level of the development of moral reasoning in which actions are judged by their external consequences and the expectation of reward or punishment.

PRECURSOR 1. In chemistry, a substance transformed into another substance by chemical reaction. The ~ for substance x is a compound that is transformed into substance x by chemical reaction. 2. In the metabolic *q.v.* process, a compound that gives rise to the next compound. 3. A chemical ancestor. 4. Something that precedes something else.

PRECYST STAGE The stage immediately preceding cyst *q.v.* formation.

PREDACEOUS Living by preying on other animals.

PREDATOR An animal that preys upon other living animals in order to obtain organic *q.v.* molecules for food.

PREDICTIVE POSTTEST An evaluation instrument used to anticipate future learner competencies. cf: predictive reliability.

PREDICTIVE RELIABILITY Testing in which data are generated indicating a predictable measure of outcome when a particular procedure is used in a real life situation. Particularly useful when a failure of a procedure in real life situations may have significant negative effects.

PREDICTIVE STUDY A study that produces conditional statements from a functional relationship of variables *q.v.*

PREDICTIVE VALIDITY 1. A measure of test's validity *q.v.* based on correlation *q.v.* between the test score and some criterion of behavior the test predicted. 2. Validity established by the capability of a test to predict performance *q.v.* on some future task.

PREDISPOSING CAUSE The factor that lowers the person's stress *q.v.* tolerance and results in a disorder.

PREDISPOSING FACTOR Any characteristic of a person or community that motivates *q.v.* behavior related to health *q.v.*

PREDISPOSITION 1. A latent susceptibility to disease which may be activated under certain environmental conditions. 2. In psychology *q.v.*, the likelihood that a person will develop certain symptoms under given stress *q.v.* conditions. 3. An inclination to respond in a certain way that is either learned or inborn. 4. In abnormal psychology *q.v.*, a factor that lowers the ability of a person to withstand stress and increases the likelihood of pathology *q.v.*

PREECLAMPSIA A toxemia *q.v.* of late pregnancy *q.v.* characterized by hypertension *q.v.* and edema *q.v.* ~ may progress to eclampsia *q.v.*

PREEJACULATORY FLUID In men, a fluid that is secreted by the Cowper's glands *q.v.* that counters the acidity of the urethra *q.v.*

PREFERENCE The act of liking one thing more than another for purely personal reasons.

PREFERENCE METHOD Used to assess the perceptual abilities of preverbal infants, babies are given a choice of two stimuli. Their preference is then evaluated.

PREFERRED PROVIDER ORGANIZATION A prepaid insurance plan or policy in which member hospitals and/or physicians contract with a third-party payer to deliver health services for negotiated fees, generally at a discount.

PREFORMATIONIST One who considers the development of an embryo as merely the growth of a miniature but completely formed individual. cf: homunculus.

PREFORMATION THEORY A discredited biological theory that stated that every sperm cell contains the organism of its kind fully formed and that development consists merely of an increase in size. cf: epigenesis.

PREFRONTAL LOBE The forward part of the frontal lobes *q.v.* of the brain.

PREFRONTAL LOBECTOMY Lobectomy *q.v.*

PREFRONTAL LOBOTOMY 1. A form of psychosurgery *q.v.* involving the severing of the nerves that connect the prefrontal lobe *q.v.* of the brain with the hypothalamus *q.v.* 2. Lobotomy *q.v.* This procedure is rarely used in the United States.

PREGAVID Preceding pregnancy *q.v.*

PREGENERALIZED LEARNING Learning of prejudicial labels and the evaluations attached to them before a person has a clear understanding of what the labels mean.

PREGNANCY 1. The period of fertilization *q.v.* of the egg through the birth of a baby. 2. The time during which the embryo *q.v.* and fetus *q.v.* develop in the uterus *q.v.* 3. The period from conception *q.v.* to birth or abortion *q.v.*

PREGNANT To enlarge. Specifically, the condition following fertilization *q.v.* of the egg through the birth process.

PREHENSION An act of taking hold, seizing, or grasping.

PREJUDICE 1. An attitude that predisposes a person to respond positively or negatively to a person, or group on the basis of social class, race, or category membership. 2. A strong negative attitude. 3. An emotionally toned conception favorable or unfavorable to some person, group, or ideology.

PRELUDIN A commercial preparation of phenmetrazine *q.v.*

PREMACK PRINCIPLE 1. A process whereby learners are allowed to engage in a self-selected activity after they complete the assigned work. 2. Grandma's rule *q.v.*

PREMARITAL INTERCOURSE 1. Coitus *q.v.* before the persons (partners) are married. 2. Premarital sex.

PREMATURE An infant born before full term *q.v.*

PREMATURE BIRTH A birth that occurs after the 6th month of pregnancy, but before the end of the normal term.

PREMATURE EJACULATION 1. The inability of the male to delay ejaculation *q.v.* in order to prolong sexual excitement. 2. Ejaculation prior to, just at, or immediately after intromission *q.v.* 3. Ejaculation praecox *q.v.*

PREMATURE OCCUPATIONAL FORECLOSURE The process of deciding against an occupation before a person has sufficient information or experience to evaluate it objectively and realistically.

PREMATURE WITHDRAWAL Coitus interruptus *q.v.*

PREMEDICAL (SCHOOL OR STUDIES) The stage of medical education that consists chiefly of studies in biology, chemistry, and social sciences.

PREMENSTRUAL SYNDROME (PMS) 1. A group of symptoms that appear to result from an accumulation of fluids during the week or so before menstruation *q.v.* occurs. 2. Discomfort or pain occurring before menstruation. 3. The physical and psychological problems a woman may experience prior to, and sometimes during, menstruation.

PREMENSTRUAL TENSION Stress *q.v.* occurring during the last 7–10 days of the menstrual cycle *q.v.* that is believed due to a change in the processing of sodium in the central nervous system *q.v.* and often accompanied by headache, backache, depression, and irritability.

PREMISES Assumptions upon which means of accomplishing objectives *q.v.* are based.

PREMIUM In insurance, the periodic payment required to maintain a health insurance policy in force.

PREMORAL STAGE The developmental stage in which rules are obeyed to obtain rewards or to avoid punishment.

PREMORBID ADJUSTMENT Referring to mental health, the social and sexual, of an individual before a psychosis *q.v.* is diagnosed. A person with a good premorbid adjustment tends to have been relatively normal in interpersonal and sexual adjustment, while those with poor premorbid adjustment tend to have been inadequate in social and sexual relations.

PREMORBID PERSONALITY According to Maddi, a person who plays social roles well and fulfills his or her social and biological needs but has a feeling of inadequacy and lack of fulfillment and is a candidate for mental illness.

PRENATAL 1. Before birth *q.v.* 2. During pregnancy *q.v.*

PRENATAL CARE The combined efforts of physicians, nurses, and the mother to see that the pregnant woman stays healthy and the unborn child has everything needed to grow and develop.

PRENUPTIAL AGREEMENT An agreement made between two people prior to their marriage describing in detail the division of property, financial, and other assets, should the marriage fail.

PREOPERATIONAL PERIOD 1. The developmental period between ages 2 and 7, characterized by mastery of symbols and the gradual development of the ability to think of more than one thing. 2. In Piaget's theory, the time when children tend to reason in an intuitive, egocentric way. cf: operation.

PREORGASMIC EJACULATION 1. A small amount of fluid involuntarily secreted from the penis *q.v.* during sexual arousal that often contains some sperm *q.v.* 2. Love drop.

PREOVULATORY PHASE The stage of the menstrual cycle *q.v.* that begins with the release of follicle-stimulating hormone *q.v.* from the pituitary gland *q.v.* which stimulates the growth of a follicle *q.v.* in the ovary *q.v.*

PREPARED CHILDBIRTH Childbirth following a series of classes intended to prepare a woman for active participation in the delivery of her child.

PREPARED CHILDBIRTH COURSES Special education courses for expectant couples designed to provide important information on pregnancy, e.g., the birth process and care of the newborn.

PREPAREDNESS 1. The theoretical principle that people are biologically predisposed to respond to particular stimuli more readily than to others. 2. Intersensory associations that are rapidly acquired as a result of an evolutionary development of potential.

PREPATTERN A field of study in which it is believed that regional differentiation is predetermined.

PREPONDERANCE OF EVIDENCE In arbitration or law, the evidence with the greater weight.

PRE-POST CONTROL GROUP DESIGN A research design in which a control group is given the same pre- and posttest as the experimental group but does not receive experimental treatment.

PREPOTENCY The ability of an individual to transmit characteristics to the offspring.

PREPUBESCENCE Pertaining to the period of life just prior to the onset of puberty *q.v.*

PREPUCE 1. The loose skin covering the shaft of the penis *q.v.* or the clitoris *q.v.* 2. The foreskin *q.v.*

PRESBYCUSIS The most common type of hearing loss in people over 65 years. ~ results in a gradual decline in the ability to hear high-pitch sounds or to distinguish consonants in speech which sometimes causes an older person to misinterpret what is being said.

PRESBYOPIA 1. A reduction in the ability to see at close range, due to a gradual loss of elasticity in the lens of the eye which occurs throughout life, but usually does not become apparent until a person reaches the mid-40s. 2. Oldsightedness. 3. Farsightedness of old age.

PRESCRIPTION A written order by a physician, dentist, or veterinarian to the pharmacist *q.v.* for the composition, preparation, or dispensing of a drug to a consumer.

PRESCRIPTION DRUG 1. Drugs or medicines that can legally be dispensed only by a prescription *q.v.* 2. Ethical drug. 3. Legend drug. 4. Drugs whose prescription order is regulated by law to a licensed person.

PRESCRIPTIVE RULES Standards or rules established by authorities about how people ought to speak and write that often fail to conform to the facts related to natural talking and understanding.

PRESCRIPTIVE VALUE ORIENTATION 1. An emphasis on doing good. 2. Rewarding for doing good. 3. Punishment for not doing good. ct: proscriptive value orientation.

PRESENILE Premature old age as judged by physical or mental deterioration.

PRESENILE DEMENTIA An often progressive mental deterioration occurring when the individual is quite young, in the 30s or 40s.

PRESENTATION 1. The presenting part *q.v.* of the fetus *q.v.* 2. The part of the fetus that can be touched through the cervix *q.v.* when an examination is performed immediately before or during labor *q.v.*

PRESENTING PART That part of the body that is born first, usually the head. A headfirst delivery is called cephalic *q.v.* delivery, while a feet first or buttocks first delivery is called a breech *q.v.* delivery.

PRESERVATIVE 1. An additive or preparation used in a food product to prevent microorganisms *q.v.* from growing. 2. A preventive of spoilage.

PRESIDENT'S ADVISORY COMMISSION ON NARCOTIC AND DRUG ABUSE Established by President Kennedy in 1962, the ~ recommended legislation that influenced federal policy and what was to be the Drug Abuse Control Amendments of 1965.

PRESIDENT'S COUNCIL ON PHYSICAL FITNESS AND SPORTS (PCPFS) Established in 1956, the ~ was an outgrowth of the President's Council on Youth Fitness.

PRESSOR A substance that elevates blood pressure.

PRESSORECEPTOR 1. Receptors *q.v.* stimulated by a change in pressure. 2. Baroreceptors *q.v.*

PRESSURE In psychology *q.v.*, a demand made on another person.

PRESSURE-COMPENSATED FLOWMETER An instrument designed to measure the rate of flow of gas from a compressed gas cylinder.

PRESSURE DRESSING A dressing through which enough pressure is applied over a wound to stop the bleeding.

PRESSURE POINTS Areas of the body where pressure can be applied to control arterial *q.v.* bleeding. They are 1. carotid artery for the head and neck, 2. brachial artery for the arm or hand, and 3. femoral artery for the leg or foot.

PRESSURE POINT TECHNIQUE A technique used to stop bleeding by manually applying pressure to key arteries. cf: pressure points.

PRESSURE SPLINTS Inflatable plastic circumferential splints *q.v.* that may be applied to an extremity and inflated to achieve stability after a fracture *q.v.* or suspected fracture.

PRESTIGE SUGGESTION Concurring with a statement because a high-prestige person has approved it.

PRESTRETCHED A situation in which a relaxed muscle is pulled into position of increased tension prior to the start of contraction.

PRESUMPTIVE SIGNS OF PREGNANCY 1. Physical signs that a woman is probably pregnant. 2. Characterized by an absence of menstruation, breast tenderness, frequent urination, etc. cf: probable signs; positive signs.

PRESYMPTOMATIC ATHEROSCLEROTIC HEART DISEASE Narrowing of the coronary arteries *q.v.* but allowing sufficient blood through to the cardiac *q.v.* muscles, even during heavy exercise. There is no symptom *q.v.* of angina pectoris *q.v.* that the disease is present.

PRESYNAPTIC MEMBRANE The area on the proximal *q.v.* side of the synapse *q.v.*

PRESYNAPTIC NEURON The neuron *q.v.* that releases the neurotransmitter *q.v.* into the synapse *q.v.* when stimulated by an impulse. ct: postsynaptic neuron.

PRESYNAPTIC TERMINAL The end bulb *q.v.*

PREVALENCE The number of cases of a disease in existence at a given time and in a particular geographic area or in a given population. cf: incidence; prevalence rate.

PREVALENCE RATE The number of existing cases of a disease at a given place and time per the size of the population. Usually measured in the number of cases per 1,000 in a population.

PREVARICATION A functional characteristic of all languages representing what is not true or real.

PREVENTION In social psychology *q.v.*, primary prevention efforts focus on those measures necessary to reduce new cases of a particular disorder; secondary prevention efforts focus on detecting disorders early and treating effectively; and tertiary efforts focus on reducing the long-term consequences of a disorder through effect treatment.

PREVENTION OF DISEASE 1. Methods taken by each person and by social institutions to prevent the onset of disease. These methods include healthful lifestyles, environments, the use of immunizations, periodic medical examinations, and dental examinations. 2. Protection against disease and disability. cf: secondary prevention; tertiary prevention.

PREVENTION ORIENTATION The conceptualization of changes that can be predicted to result as a consequence of preventive efforts in the form of programs and procedures that preclude the occurrence of particular health problems.

PREVENTION PROFILE A list of eight lifestyle factors that are associated with major effects on a person's health.

PREVENTIVE HEALTH BEHAVIOR 1. Actions taken by a person to prevent the onset of a disease or to delay its onset. 2. Health-directed behavior. ct: health-related behavior.

PREVENTIVE HEALTH CARE Health care directed toward precluding the onset of a health problem.

PREVENTIVE MEDICINE 1. A medical specialty concerned with ways in which diseases can be prevented. 2. Medical and health practice aimed at averting or preventing the occurrence of disease, disability, or premature death. 3. Programs aimed at preventing disease and disability through immunizations, nutrition counseling, health screening, and health education. Usually administered through a department of public health *q.v.* cf: epidemiology.

PRIAPISM 1. A prolonged erection of the penis *q.v.*, lasting more than 4 h, caused by a pathological condition or a drug. 2. A prolonged penile erection not necessarily associated with sexual arousal *q.v.* 3. A state of prolonged erection caused by irritation of the sacral *q.v.* region of the spinal cord *q.v.*

PRIMACY EFFECT In learning or attitude formation, the tendency of the information that is received first to be most important in determining the person's overall view of objects, conditions, issues, or other people.

PRIMACY PRINCIPLE In political socialization *q.v.*, the idea that a person's political orientations are largely determined in childhood with only minor variations in adolescence *q.v.* and adulthood.

PRIMA FACIE 1. At first view, before investigation. 2. A fact presumed to be true unless evidence is provided to the contrary.

PRIMA FACIE CASE In law, a case in which the evidence is so strong that the opposing party can overthrow the evidence only by providing stronger rebutting evidence.

PRIMAL SCENE In psychology *q.v.*, a child's first observation of sexual intercourse *q.v.*

PRIMARY AMENORRHEA A condition in a woman where, by age 18 or older, she has never menstruated *q.v.* cf: secondary amenorrhea.

PRIMARY ANORGASMIA Primary orgasmic dysfunction *q.v.*

PRIMARY CANCER The type of cancer *q.v.* arising from the originating site or organ.

PRIMARY CARE Medical services from a general practitioner *q.v.*, family physician *q.v.*, or internist *q.v.*

PRIMARY CAUSE A condition or cause without which the disorder would not take place.

PRIMARY CUE TO DEPTH An unlearned, biologically determined cue to depth perception. ct: secondary cue to depth.

PRIMARY DEFICIENCY A nutrient deficiency *q.v.* resulting directly from inadequate dietary intake. ct: secondary deficiency.

PRIMARY DEPRESSION Endogenous depression *q.v.*

PRIMARY DESIRE DISORDER Hypoactive sexual desire *q.v.*

PRIMARY DEVIANCE In sociology *q.v.*, behavior that deviates from the norm but that is not used as a basis for self-definition. ct: secondary deviance.

PRIMARY DRIVE An unlearned biological motive *q.v.* ct: acquired drive.

PRIMARY EJACULATORY INCOMPETENCE Ejaculatory incompetence *q.v.*

PRIMARY EMPATHY A form of empathy in which the therapist understands the patient's statements and expressions from his or her phenomenological *q.v.* point of view.

PRIMARY ENDOSPERM NUCLEUS 1. The result of the fusion of the male gamete *q.v.* and the two polar nuclei *q.v.* 2. Triple fusion nucleus.

PRIMARY ERECTILE DYSFUNCTION A condition in which a man has never maintained an erection *q.v.* sufficient to engage in sexual intercourse *q.v.*

PRIMARY EROTIC STIMULI Stimuli that may lead to sexual arousal *q.v.* in the absence of prior learning or experience. ct: secondary erotic stimuli.

PRIMARY GLAUCOMA A condition characterized by the inability of the eyeball to maintain the adsorption and escape of the aqueous humor *q.v.*

PRIMARY GRADES HEALTH CURRICULUM PROJECT (PGHCP) An integrated part of a larger curriculum being taught in the primary grades. It is a companion to the School Health Curriculum Project *q.v.*

PRIMARY GROUP In sociology *q.v.*, the small, informal group with close, personal relationships between members.

PRIMARY HEALTH CARE Health care services provided to people who do not require hospitalization. ct: secondary health care.

PRIMARY HOMOSEXUAL A homosexual *q.v.* who has never responded to heteroerotic *q.v.* stimulation.

PRIMARY IMAGE A projected image, produced by the objective, that is further magnified by the eyepiece.

PRIMARY IMMUNE RESPONSE The production of antibodies *q.v.* 7–10 days after infection *q.v.*

PRIMARY LABELING THEORY The belief that the assignment of labels is a causal factor in abnormal behavior.

PRIMARY LEVEL The early elementary school *q.v.* grades, generally grades kindergarten through grade 3. ct: intermediate level.

PRIMARY LEVEL OF HEALTH Health status *q.v.* measured in terms of wellness. Persons falling within this level are for all practical purposes healthy or well. cf: intermediate level of health; secondary level of health.

PRIMARY MEMORY The retention of the image of an object that persists for a very brief period of time following its presentation. ct: secondary memory.

PRIMARY MENTAL ABILITIES 1. The major components of intelligence *q.v.* postulated on the basis of a factor analysis *q.v.* of performance *q.v.* on intelligence tests. 2. The relativity independent abilities, e.g., verbal comprehension and mathematical abilities., that make up the general intelligence.

PRIMARY NARCISSISM In psychoanalytic theory *q.v.*, the part of the oral stage of psychosexual development *q.v.* in which the ego *q.v.* has not yet differentiated from the id *q.v.*

PRIMARY OOCYTES The cells that have the potential of developing into mature ova *q.v.* during a woman's reproductive life. The average number of ~ is about 2 million in both ovaries *q.v.* cf: oocyte.

PRIMARY ORGASMIC DYSFUNCTION 1. Primary anorgasmia *q.v.* or preorgasm *q.v.* 2. Refers to never having had an orgasm *q.v.*

PRIMARY PREVENTION 1. Maintenance of health. 2. Prevention activities carried out before the person becomes diseased or disabled. 3. Precedes the earliest signs of disease and involves changes in the physical or social environment to reduce the likelihood that the disease can or will occur. Usually, these strategies include health promotion and specific prevention. cf: secondary prevention; tertiary prevention.

PRIMARY PROCESS 1. In Freudian theory *q.v.*, impulses of the id *q.v.* that are pleasure seeking and make no sharp distinction between imagination and reality. 2. One of the id's mechanisms of relieving tension, through the use of the imagination. ct: secondary process.

PRIMARY PROJECTION AREA An area in the brain to which the mental effects of stimulation are conducted directly. ct: diffuse projection.

PRIMARY REINFORCEMENT 1. Reinforcement *q.v.* that depends little or not at all upon previous learning *q.v.* 2. A reward that directly satisfies some needs *q.v.* of the person. ct: secondary reinforcement.

PRIMARY RESPONSE The first response of the immune system *q.v.* to an antigen *q.v.* ct: secondary response.

PRIMARY SEX CHARACTERISTICS 1. Biological traits that differentiate females from males. 2. The internal and external genitalia *q.v.* developed before birth. ct: secondary sex characteristics.

PRIMARY SPERMATOCYTE 1. Spermatocyte *q.v.* 2. The mature spermatogonia *q.v.* that have divided by meiotic *q.v.* division.

PRIMARY SYPHILIS The first stage of syphilis *q.v.* most generally manifested by the appearance of a painless lesion *q.v.*, the chancre *q.v.*

PRIMARY WATER TREATMENT The removal of easily sedimented solid materials by the passage of the water through grit chambers. Some fats, carbohydrates, and proteins may also be removed. ct: secondary water treatment; tertiary water treatment.

PRIMATES The order of animals including humans, apes, and monkeys.

PRIMING Using the environmental stimuli to make a schema salient *q.v.*

PRIMIPARA A woman who is about to deliver a baby for the first time.

PRIMITIVE 1. Pertains to early, less civilized cultures. 2. Not technologically advanced.

PRIMOQUININE A synthetic substitute for quinine *q.v.* used in treating malaria *q.v.*

PRINCIPAL An individual who is the chief administrator of a school.

PRINCIPLE A significant truth that is often stated as a cause-and-effect relationship.

PRINCIPLE OF ACTIVE RESPONDING In programmed learning *q.v.*, the principle that stresses the importance of the learner's performance *q.v.* of the response *q.v.* to be learned.

PRINCIPLE OF IMMEDIATE CONFIRMATION In programmed learning *q.v.*, the principle that stresses the effect of immediate knowledge of the correctness of the response *q.v.*

PRINCIPLE OF SELF-PACING In programmed learning *q.v.*, the principle that emphasizes the importance of allowing the learner to proceed at his or her own pace.

PRINCIPLE OF SMALL STEPS In programmed learning *q.v.*, the principle that emphasizes the importance of leading the learner gradually to a desired goal or level of performance *q.v.*

PRINCIPLE OF SPECIFICITY In fitness training, the concept of training for the component the person wants to improve.

PRINCIPLE OF S-R COMPLEMENTARITY In nonhuman animals, the presumed tendency for a female stimulus pattern to evoke a male response and for the male stimulus pattern to evoke a female response.

PRINCIPLE OF STUDENT TESTING In programmed learning *q.v.*, the principle that stresses the importance of having the student keep a continual evaluation of his or her knowledge.

PRINCIPLE OF SUPPORTIVE RELATIONSHIPS A leadership concept that views all human interaction within an organization should build and maintain a sense of personal worth and the importance of those involved in the interaction.

PRINCIPLE OF THE OBJECTIVE A management principle that maintains that, before any action is initiated, organizational objectives should be clearly determined, understood, and stated.

PRINCIPLES OF COMMUNITY HEALTH EDUCATION Based on the concept that community health education should focus on a particular health problem, risk, or issue, using strategies to prevent the problem or to reduce the risk. As detailed by Green and Anderson, there are 10 broad, but fundamental principles governing educational success: 1. the principle of cumulative learning; a planned sequence of experiences over time; 2. the principle of multiple targets; several causes of a health issue must be addressed; 3. the principle of aggregating educational targets; an accommodation of many and varied personal histories; 4. the principle of participation; involvement of providers and consumers; 5. the principle of situational specificity; educational methods based on an explicit educational diagnosis of the situation; 6. the principle of intermediate targets; health education seldom has an immediate, direct impact on behavior and, therefore, must concern itself with other factors affecting behavior; 7. the principle of multiple methods; no single educational approach can address all of the significant factors influencing behavior; therefore, several approaches should be used as reinforcers; 8. the principle of diversity; educational methods within a particular program should be varied in accordance with the target population; 9. the principle of health promotion; expectations of voluntary change in health behavior; and 10. the principle of administration; any combination of learning designed to facilitate voluntary adaptations conducive to health.

PRION An infectious proteinaceous molecule *q.v.* ~s have some of the properties of viruses and are believed to be agents *q.v.* of such diseases as some encephalopathies *q.v.* and Creutzfeldt–Jakob disease *q.v.*

PRIORITY Alternatives ranked according to value and/or effectiveness.

PRISONER'S DILEMMA 1. A particular arrangement of payoffs in a two-prison situation in which each person has to choose between two alternatives without knowing the other's choice. The payoff structure is so arranged that the optimal strategy for each person depends upon whether he or she can trust the other. When trust is possible, the payoffs for each will be considerably higher than when there is no trust. 2. A laboratory situation designed to facilitate the study of social exchange, esp. exchange in which motive for cooperation and exploitation are simultaneously aroused.

PRIVACY OF INFORMATION ACT OF 1974 An act designed to regulate the gathering and dissemination of information on people.

PRIVATE HEALTH AGENCY A nongovernmental agency usually concerned with a specific health issue. A ~ may be nonprofit incorporated, nonprofit unincorporated, or proprietary. ct: voluntary health agency.

PRIVATE SCHOOLS A school that is controlled by an individual or organization not affiliated with government, usually supported by tuition and fees paid by the student's family and other donations from the public. Normally, they are not funded by tax revenue but may be required to pay tax if they are proprietary schools.

PRIVIES OF PARTIES In law, persons connected to the same issue or action with mutual interest.

PRIVILEGED COMMUNICATION 1. Freedom from the obligation to report to authorities information concerning legal guilt that is revealed by a client or patient during counseling, essentially enjoyed by lawyers, clergy, physicians, and psychologists. 2. Communication in confidence between parties that is protected by law.

PRIZING 1. To be proud of a decision and to make it truly important in life. 2. The second step in the valuing process *q.v.*

PRL 1. An acronym for prolactin *q.v.* 2. A female hormone *q.v.* that stimulates the breasts to produce milk when there is sufficient amounts of estrogen *q.v.* and progesterone *q.v.* present.

PROACTIVE FACILITATION This occurs when past learning allows future learning to become easier. ct: proactive inhibition.

PROACTIVE INHIBITION 1. This occurs when one learning experience causes later ones to be inefficient. 2. A disturbance of recall of some material by other material previously learned. ct: proactive facilitation; retroactive facilitation.

PROACTIVE STRUCTURING Before entering the classroom, planning and preparing for situations that might arise, a characteristic of good classroom management. cf: classroom management.

PROBABILITY In epidemiology *q.v.*, an estimate of the frequency or likelihood of the occurrence of an event.

PROBABILITY SAMPLE 1. In research, a method of random sampling of a population in order that each member of the population has an equal chance of being selected. 2. A sample of the population that matches the characteristics of said population's subgroups.

PROBABILITY THEORY A decision-making strategy used when the outcome of an implemented alternative is not clear.

PROBABLE SIGNS (OF PREGNANCY) A positive pregnancy test plus characteristic changes in the uterus *q.v.* and cervix *q.v.* cf: presumptive signs; positive signs.

PROBAND 1. The person in a genetic *q.v.* investigation who exhibits the diagnosis or trait *q.v.* that is of interest to the investigator. 2. In a pedigree *q.v.* study, the first person in the family to be identified with the trait being investigated.

PROBLEM DRINKING 1. The use of alcohol that results in damage to the drinker, his or her family, or to the greater community. 2. An alcohol use pattern in which a drinker's behavior creates personal difficulties or difficulties for other people.

PROBLEM-SOLVING METHOD 1. A learner-centered method *q.v.* characterized by a series of discoveries by the learners as they proceed to solve a particular health problem. 2. A logical process by means of which data are gathered and reasonable hypotheses are formulated and tested, until the best possible solution is discovered to a given health problem. cf: scientific method; inductive reasoning.

PROBOSCIS A tubular piercing or penetrating accessory organ located at the anterior end of the digestive tract of many small animals.

PROCEDURAL KNOWLEDGE Knowing how to do something. ct: declarative knowledge.

PROCEDURE An established plan that outlines the actions that must be taken to accomplish a particular task.

PROCESSES (HEALTH EDUCATION) 1. Methodologies, techniques, and strategies used to influence teaching and learning that are consistent with known learning principles. 2. All of the cognitive operations applied in the use of the subject matter of health education *q.v.* ct: content.

PROCESS EVALUATION A level of evaluation that focuses on the adequacy of the curriculum and its implementation in the teaching–learning process. cf: formative evaluation. ct: summative evaluation.

PROCESS GOALS Statements of direction or desire that are concerned with how something is achieved rather than what or why it is achieved. ~ emphasize means rather than ends, although the end result is implied.

PROCESS MEDIATION In conflict resolution, the mediator facilitates a process to smooth the process of organization.

PROCESS ORIENTATION TOWARD INTELLIGENCE The tradition of studying intelligence *q.v.* that emphasizes correct answers to questions, IQ tests *q.v.*, and individual differences in intelligence.

PROCESS REACTIVE A process used to distinguish schizophrenics. Process schizophrenics suffer long-term and gradual deterioration prior to the onset of their illness, whereas reactive schizophrenics have a relatively normal history prior to a rapid mental deterioration into schizophrenia. cf: premorbid adjustment.

PROCESS RESEARCH In psychology *q.v.*, research on the psychological mechanisms by which a therapy may bring improvement. ct: outcome research.

PROCHLORPERAZINE 1. A major tranquilizer *q.v.* effective in controlling the symptoms of emotionally disturbed children and for the reduction of nausea that frequently accompanies anxiety *q.v.* 2. An antipsychotic *q.v.* drug. 3. Compazine is a commercial preparation.

PRO-CHOICE A pro-abortion view in which a person supports the right of a woman to choose whether she shall have a baby, esp. after she becomes pregnant. cf: abortion. ct: pro-life.

PROCITITIS Inflammation and infection of the rectum *q.v.*

PROCRASTINATE To put off until some future date.

PROCREATION The producing of offspring; reproduction.

PROCREATIONAL SEX Sexual intercourse *q.v.* solely for the purpose of reproduction. Sometimes advocated as the only acceptable reason for sex.

PROCTECTOMY Excision of the rectum *q.v.*

PROCTOLOGIST A physician who specializes in the diagnosis and treatment of problems associated with the anus *q.v.*, rectum *q.v.*, and colon *q.v.*

PROCTOLOGY A medical specialty concerned with the diagnosis and treatment of diseases of the colon *q.v.* and rectum *q.v.*

PROCTOSCOPE An instrument for examining the rectum *q.v.*

PROCTOSCOPY A rectal *q.v.* examination with a proctoscope *q.v.*

PROCTOSIGMOIDOSCOPY A technique in which an instrument is inserted into the rectum *q.v.* and the sigmoid portion of the colon *q.v.* for examination to detect abnormalities.

PROCURER A person who encourages women to enter the life of prostitution *q.v.*

PRODROMAL Signs indicating the approach of a disease.

PRODROMAL PHASE In psychology *q.v.*, the period before the onset of a mental disorder. A period of deterioration of mental functioning prior to a diagnosable mental illness.

PRODROME 1. The stage of an infectious (communicable) disease *q.v.* at the point when signs and symptoms appear and most diseases are communicable to others. 2. General symptoms of illness before the actual signs of a specific illness.

PRODUCTION DEFICIENCY 1. In education *q.v.*, a failure to employ the strategies and methods that would improve learning and memory. 2. Failure to spontaneously produce a response that could serve as a mediator, even when the child is able to make the response. cf: mediation deficiency; production inefficiency.

PRODUCTION INEFFICIENCY Partial but ineffective use of mediating responses. cf: mediation deficiency; production deficiency.

PROFESSION A career *q.v.*, the practice of which requires an in-depth comprehension of a specific body of knowledge and the abilities to apply this knowledge to a particular area of human need.

PROFESSIONAL CAREERS A broad category of careers *q.v.* that usually requires many years of advanced study in a specialized field.

PROFESSIONALISM 1. The methods, manner, ethics, or spirit of a profession. 2. The practice of engaging in continuing self-education, encouraging research, maintaining high ethical standards, and the willingness to police one's own ranks.

PROFESSIONAL SOCIETIES Organizations consisting of members of a particular profession. These organizations are supported chiefly by dues paid by the membership. Essentially, their function is to promote their profession and to educate the public.

PROFESSIONAL STANDARDS The rules, criteria, and principles *q.v.* that govern a profession *q.v.*

PROFESSIONAL STANDARDS REVIEW ORGANIZATION (PSRO) Established by the U.S. Federal Government in 1972 as part of the Social Security Amendments; designed to review the need, feasibility, and quality of medical and surgical services provided by the Medicare and Medicaid programs. Its name was changed to the Professional Review Organization in the late 1980s. cf: Utilization Review Committee.

PROFOUND MENTAL RETARDATION A limited mental development such that the person's IQ *q.v.* is less than 20. People with ~ require total supervision of their activities.

PROGAMETANGIUM A cell or organ that becomes the gametangium.

PROGENY 1. Offspring of plants or animals. 2. Individuals resulting from a particular mating.

PROGERIA 1. A rare genetic *q.v.* disease in which a person ages prematurely and dies young. 2. Hutchinson–Gilford progeria syndrome. Signs begin to appear in the person after birth, and average life expectancy is approximately 12 years.

PROGESTERONE 1. A female sex hormone *q.v.* associated with maintaining the lining of the uterus *q.v.* when pregnancy *q.v.* occurs. 2. The pregnancy hormone. 3. The hormone that maintains the endometrium *q.v.* to accept a fertilized ovum *q.v.* 4. A female hormone that is involved in the development of the milk-producing glands *q.v.* in the breasts. 5. The hormone produced and released by the corpus luteum *q.v.* during the second half of the ovulatory cycle *q.v.* It is necessary for preparing the lining of the uterus for the implantation of the fertilized *q.v.* egg. ~ is also produced by the placenta *q.v.* during pregnancy. cf: prolactin.

PROGESTIN 1. The hormone *q.v.* progesterone *q.v.* 2. A class of compounds some of which are synthetic and taken orally that are similar to progesterone and used as contraceptives *q.v.* and medicated intrauterine devices *q.v.* 3. Synthetic progesterone. 4. Steroid *q.v.* progestational hormones that are the chemical precursors of androgens *q.v.*

PROGNOSIS 1. A prediction of the outcome of a disease. 2. An estimation as to recovery from a disease as indicated by the symptoms present in the case.

PROGRAM A set of planned activities designed to achieve specified objectives in a given period of time. cf: role delineation.

PROGRAM AIM The overall mission *q.v.* of the health program.

PROGRAM COORDINATION The mutual concerted activities of the elements of an organization or between two or more organizations.

PROGRAM DESIGN The manner in which a program is structured.

PROGRAM EFFECTIVENESS The extent to which program objectives have been achieved as a result of the activities of the program. cf: program.

PROGRAM EFFICIENCY The proportion of resources used in the attainment of specific objectives relative to the total mount of resources expended. cf: program.

PROGRAM EVALUATION The evaluation of the effectiveness of specific programs or elements thereof.

PROGRAM EVALUATION AND REVIEW TECHNIQUE (PERT) 1. A system of management based on identifying the interrelationships between and among a series of actions necessary to achieve a specific goal, depicted in the form of a flow chart showing the time periods necessary to carry out each step or process in the sequence and distinguishing between those steps that are critical to goal achievement and those that contribute to or make the critical steps possible. 2. A scheduling tool illustrating a network of project activities, showing the time necessary to achieve each activity and the sequence to be followed to complete the project.

PROGRAM GUIDE A written document containing an outline of the content and procedures of a program.

PROGRAMMED INSTRUCTION A form of teaching (learning) wherein material to be learned is organized into a series of small steps, called frames, and feedback *q.v.* is supplied after each learner response. cf: programmed learning.

PROGRAMMED LEARNING 1. The presentation of materials to be learned in carefully planned sequences, often with the aid of a computer or other technology. 2. A learning method in which students follow a step-by-step sequence toward a desired objective *q.v.* through written instructions. cf: programmed instruction.

PROGRAM OBJECTIVE A statement of desired outcomes that indicates who is to achieve them, at what time, and to what degree. cf: program; objective; behavioral objective; goal.

PROGRAM/PROJECT OFFICER A person designated by an organization to serve as the official responsible for the scientific, technical, and programmatic aspects of a grant/research project.

PROGRESSIVE DISCIPLINE A series of disciplinary actions, usually beginning with a verbal warning, progressively followed by more severe penalties.

PROGRESSIVE EDUCATION An educational philosophy emphasizing democracy and the importance of creatively meeting the unique needs of individual students and the relationship between school and community.

PROGRESSIVE RELAXATION A system of physical and mental relaxation in which portions of the body are relaxed one by one causing the mind to relax at the same time.

PROGRESSIVE RESISTANCE EXERCISES 1. Muscular strength exercises that use traditional barbells and dumbbells with fixed resistance. 2. A gradual systematic increase of resistance over a period of time.

PROGRESSIVISM An educational philosophy that emphasizes experiences.

PROHIBITION 1. Forbidding a certain act. 2. Laws that forbid the manufacture, sale, or use of alcohol. 3. The period in American history from 1920 to 1933, during which the manufacture, sale, transportation, and importation of potable alcohol was forbidden by law.

PROJECTION 1. A defense mechanism *q.v.* 2. A situation in which the frustrated person attributes to others the undesirable thoughts, actions, and attitudes that he or she has. 3. Seeing one's own traits in others. 4. An ego defense mechanism *q.v.* 5. In Freudian theory *q.v.*, a mechanism for expressing one's own dangerous or hidden thoughts by attributing them to others.

PROJECTION AREAS Regions of the cortex *q.v.* that serve as receiving stations for sensory information or as dispatching stations for motor commands. cf: motor projection areas; sensory projection areas.

PROJECTIVE PLAY Play that a psychologist *q.v.* uses for diagnostic or therapeutic *q.v.* purposes.

PROJECTIVE TECHNIQUES 1. Devices for assessing personality by presenting relatively unstructured stimuli that elicit subjective responses. 2. A psychological *q.v.* assessment tool that employs a set of standard but vague stimuli in hopes that unconscious motivations and fears will be uncovered by the patient's responses to them. cf: projective tests of personality; personality inventories.

PROJECTIVE TESTS OF PERSONALITY Tests allowing relatively free responses to situations, requiring interpretations on the assumption that the nature of the interpretations reveals the important aspects of a person's personality *q.v.* cf: projective techniques.

PROKARYOTIC Cells in some organisms in which hereditary *q.v.* materials are not contained within an organized nucleus *q.v.* but is in constant contact with the cytoplasm *q.v.*

PROLACTIN 1. Lactogenic hormone *q.v.* 2. A hormone secreted by the pituitary gland *q.v.* of women during pregnancy. ~ stimulates the breasts to develop and to produce milk.

PROLAPSE The dropping downward of an internal organ from its normal position.

PROLAPSED CORD A condition whereby the umbilical cord *q.v.* is compressed until the blood supply to the baby is cut off.

PRO-LIFE An antiabortion view in which the person supports the right of a fetus *q.v.* to life. ct: pro-choice; abortion.

PROLIFERATIVE PHASE 1. Preovulatory phase *q.v.* 2. The phase of the menstrual cycle *q.v.* during which the endometrium *q.v.* develops.

PROLIXIN 1. A commercial preparation of phenothiazine *q.v.* 2. One of the major tranquilizers *q.v.* 3. Fluphenazine *q.v.*

PROMISCUITY Nonselective sexual intercourse *q.v.*

PROMISCUOUS 1. Engaging in sexual intercourse *q.v.* with many persons. 2. Engaging in casual sexual relations. 3. Indiscriminate sexual involvement with a number of partners.

PROMOTER A substance that does not in and of itself cause cancer, but that increases the rate of cancer formation when one is exposed to it after being exposed to a carcinogen *q.v.*

PROMOTION OF HEALTH Any and all methods that are intended to enhance individual and societal health. cf: health promotion.

PRONATE To place in a prone *q.v.* position.

PRONATALIST 1. The belief that married couples should have children. 2. A social bias that having children is good and that social influences should be designed to encourage procreation *q.v.*

PRONE 1. Lying flat with the face downward. 2. Lying on the belly.

PRONOUN REVERSAL A speech problem in which a child refers to himself or herself as "he" or "she" and uses "I" or "me" when referring to others.

PRONUCLEUS FEMALE The nucleus *q.v.* of the secondary oocyte *q.v.* containing the maternal contribution of 23 chromosomes *q.v.* At the time of fertilization *q.v.*, it is joined at the center of the ovum by the male pronucleus *q.v.*

PRONUCLEUS MALE Upon penetration into the ovum *q.v.* at the time of conception *q.v.*, the head of the sperm *q.v.*, after its tail separates and disintegrates. It contains the paternal contribution of 23 chromosomes *q.v.*

PROOF (OF ALCOHOL) The percentage of alcohol *q.v.* contained in a beverage expressed in proof. The proof of alcohol is equal to one-half the proof.

PROPAGATED EPIDEMIC A high level of communicable disease *q.v.* that results from the direct or indirect transmission of an agent from one host *q.v.* to another.

PROPHAGE A noninfectious stage of a temperate phage *q.v.* in a bacteria *q.v.* cell.

PROPHASE An early stage in meiosis *q.v.* during which the chromosomes are dispersed throughout the nucleus *q.v.* and are doubled longitudinally.

PROPHYLACTIC 1. Warding off disease. 2. Methods used to prevent the onset of disease. 3. A drug or device used for the prevention of disease.

PROPHYLACTIC ODONTOTOMY The removal of dental fissures *q.v.* to reduce the likelihood of caries *q.v.* from developing.

PROPHYLACTIC TREATMENT A medical treatment that prevents the onset of a disease to which the patient was exposed.

PROPINQUITY Nearness.

PROPINQUITY EFFECT The increase in attraction-based relationships as geographic distance decreases.

PROPORNS Jargon for people who support and are engaged in making pornography *q.v.* available to others.

PROPORTIONAL REASONING A mental process needed to make quantitative comparisons of proportions.

PROPOSITION 1. A significant factor in scientific theory construction. 2. A general term respecting theory building referring to a statement relating to two or more variables in a specific manner.

PROPOSITIONAL LOGIC The logic used to judge the value of arguments that combine propositions, e.g., "if–then" arguments, "both–and" arguments, and "either–or" arguments.

PROPOXYLINE 1. The chemical or generic name *q.v.* for barbiturates *q.v.* 2. A narcotic analgesic *q.v.* 3. Darvon is a commercial name.

PROPRIETARY DRUG 1. Over-the-counter drug. 2. A trademark drug sold directly to the consumer without a prescription *q.v.* 3. A patent medicine. 4. A nonprescription drug. 5. Proprietary medicine *q.v.*

PROPRIETARY HOSPITAL A health and medical facility (hospital) owned and operated by private individuals or corporations as a for-profit organization or as a for-profit investment.

PROPRIETARY MEDICINE 1. Proprietary drug *q.v.* 2. Any chemical or drug used in the treatment of disease that is protected against free competition as to name, product, composition, or process of manufacture by secrecy, patent *q.v.*, copyright, or other means.

PROPRIETARY SCHOOL An educational institution that is privately owned and operated that functions as a for-profit institution and is subject to taxation.

PROPRIOCEPTION 1. The sense of body positioning. 2. An awareness of the body's orientation in space. cf: proprioceptive sense.

PROPRIOCEPTIVE Pertaining to stimuli receptors that are located under the skin, such as in the muscles.

PROPRIOCEPTIVE SENSE The sense of movement and body positioning; derived from an interaction of receptors *q.v.* in the organs, muscles *q.v.*, joints *q.v.*, and the labyrinth *q.v.* of the ear. cf: proprioception.

PROPYL ALCOHOL A type of alcohol *q.v.* used industrially. Unfit for human consumption. ~ has a chemical formula of C_5H_7OH.

PROSCRIPTIVE VALUE ORIENTATION 1. Placing an emphasis on not doing bad. 2. Rewarding for not doing bad. 3. Punishing for doing bad. ct: prescriptive value orientation.

PRO SE In person or on one's own behalf.

PROSENCEPHALON The forebrain *q.v.*

PROSOCIAL BEHAVIOR 1. Forms of behavior that involve understanding the needs and feelings of others, getting along with others, or functioning well in group situations. 2. Socially positive and acceptable behavior. 3. Behavior that is exhibited by altruism *q.v.*, comforting, sharing. Behavior that benefits others. ct: antisocial.

PROSODY The speech features of pitch, loudness, tempo, and rhythm.

PROSPECTIVE PRICING SYSTEM A system of establishing in advance the reimbursement rates for health services.

PROSPECTIVE RESEARCH Research in which the predictor measure is assessed in advance of the outcome.

PROSPECTIVE STUDY In epidemiology *q.v.*, a cohort study *q.v.*

PROSTACYCLIN An anticlotting factor made by blood vessel walls and some other tissues.

PROSTAGLANDIN INDUCTION A method of abortion *q.v.* involving prematurely inducing labor *q.v.* by injecting prostaglandins *q.v.* into the amniotic fluid *q.v.* cf: prostaglandin intrauterine injection.

PROSTAGLANDIN INHIBITORS Drugs that block the production of prostaglandins *q.v.*, thus eliminating the hormonal *q.v.* stimulation of smooth muscles *q.v.*

PROSTAGLANDIN INTRAUTERINE INJECTION The introduction of hormone-like chemicals that, on injection into the amniotic *q.v.* sac, cause uterine muscles to contract and expel the fetus *q.v.* and other contents of the uterus *q.v.* cf: prostaglandin induction.

PROSTAGLANDINS 1. Fatty acids *q.v.* that promote the onset of labor *q.v.* 2. Chemical substances that stimulate smooth muscle contractions. 3. A method of abortion *q.v.* by injection into the amniotic sac *q.v.* 4. Hormones *q.v.* contained in the semen *q.v.* which, when deposited in the vagina *q.v.*, cause the fallopian tubes *q.v.* and uterus *q.v.* to contract. 5. Hormones synthesized in response to cell injury and trigger pain signals. Some drugs, such as aspirin, inhibit the formation of ~. cf: dysmenorrheal; seminal fluid.

PROSTATECTOMY The surgical removal of all or part of the prostate gland *q.v.* The operation is common in older men as the prostate gland often enlarges somewhat and may eventually interfere with urination. Men usually can resume normal sexual activity soon after the surgery.

PROSTATE GLAND 1. A gland *q.v.* that secretes a fluid contributing to the total volume of semen *q.v.* 2. A gland located near the urinary bladder *q.v.* whose secretions make up a large percentage of the volume of semen. 3. The gland in the male that surrounds the urethra *q.v.* and the neck of the urinary bladder *q.v.* 4. A structure of the male internal genitalia *q.v.* that secretes a fluid into the semen prior to ejaculation *q.v.* to aid sperm *q.v.* motility and longer sperm life.

PROSTATIC ACID PHOSPHATASE A fluid secreted by the prostate gland *q.v.*

PROSTATIC FLUID A highly alkaline *q.v.*, watery, milky fluid produced by the prostate gland *q.v.* that constitutes a major portion of the male's semen *q.v.*

PROSTATIC URETHRA The portion of the urethra *q.v.* that passes through the prostate gland *q.v.*

PROSTATITIS Inflammation *q.v.* of the prostate gland *q.v.* ~ is typically a disease of older men.

PROSTHESIS 1. An artificial substitute for a missing body part. 2. Artificial limbs, teeth, and hearing aids, all of which augment or replace lost functions of the body.

PROSTHETIC DEVICE Prosthesis *q.v.* cf: implant.

PROSTHETIC GROUP 1. A nonprotein, organic, chemical group attached to a protein *q.v.*, e.g., heme *q.v.* in the hemoglobin *q.v.* molecule.

PROSTHETICS A branch of surgery involved with the replacement of lost parts of the body by artificial parts.

PROSTHODONTIA A dental specialty concerned with dental prosthetics *q.v.*

PROSTHODONTICS The branch of dentistry *q.v.* concerned with the mechanics of fitting dental appliances, e.g., dentures.

PROSTITUTE A person of either sex, but usually the female, who engages in sexual relations for profit.

PROSTITUTION 1. The practice of selling sexual services. 2. Participating in sexual activity for pay or profit.

PROSTRATION Collapse.

PROTANOPIA Red–green color blindness in which there is, in addition, insensitivity to red.

PROTEASE An enzyme *q.v.* that digests protein *q.v.*

PROTECTION FROM PHYSICAL AND PSYCHOLOGICAL HARM In research, such as psychological studies of volunteers, the ethical principle that requires the volunteers to be able to participate in the study with no risk to their psychological or physical health. This includes guaranteed anonymity and confidentiality.

PROTEIN 1. One of six major classes of nutrients. 2. An organic compound consisting of amino acids *q.v.* linked by peptide *q.v.* bonds. ~s perform a wide variety of structural and functional roles in the body. 3. A complex organic compound consisting of amino acids *q.v.* that contain carbon, hydrogen, oxygen, nitrogen, and (in plant proteins) sulfur. cf: amino acids.

PROTEIN BINDING The process by which a drug binds itself chemically to the protein *q.v.* substances in the plasma *q.v.*

PROTEIN-BOUND IODINE (PBI) The binding of almost all thyroxine *q.v.* in the blood to protein *q.v.* The measure of the amount of ~ is useful as an indicator of the quantity of circulating (in the blood) iodine.

PROTEIN COMPLEMENTARITY The mixing of foods so that all light essential amino acids *q.v.* are ingested in the diet in proper amounts and proportions.

PROTEIN EFFICIENCY RATIO (PER) 1. The biologic method of estimating protein *q.v.* quality. 2. The weight gain per amount of protein consumed.

PROTEIN-ENERGY MALNUTRITION (PEM) A condition caused by an insufficient protein *q.v.* and energy intake characterized by retarded growth, weight loss, and listlessness.

PROTEIN QUALITY A measure of the biological efficiency of dietary protein *q.v.* ~ depends on the amounts and kinds of amino acids *q.v.* contained in the protein.

PROTEINS 1. Organic *q.v.* compounds made up of amino acids *q.v.* 2. One of the major nutrients and constituents of plant and animal cells.

PROTEIN TURNOVER The breakdown and replacement of protein *q.v.* in the body.

PROTEOLYTIC In the chemistry of enzymes *q.v.*, hastening the hydrolysis *q.v.* of proteins *q.v.*

PROTON A positively charged particle located in the nucleus *q.v.* of an atom *q.v.* cf: electron.

PROTOPLASM 1. The essential material of all plant and animal cells. ~ is composed of nucleic acids *q.v.*, proteins *q.v.*, lipids *q.v.*, carbohydrates *q.v.*, and inorganic *q.v.* salts. 2. The living material of the cell.

PROTOPLAST 1. The entire contents of a cell. 2. A unit body of protoplasm *q.v.* 3. The mass of living material within a cell, including the cytoplasm *q.v.* and the nucleus.

PROTOTROPH An organism (bacterium *q.v.*) that grows on a minimal medium.

PROTOTYPE The typical example of a category of meaning.

PROTOZOA Microscopic one-celled animals.

PROTRIPTYLINE 1. A heterocyclic antidepressant *q.v.* 2. Vivactil is a commercial preparation.

PROTUBERANT A part that is prominent beyond a surface.

PROVIRUS The genome *q.v.* of a virus *q.v.* integrated into the chromosome *q.v.* of a host cell and thereby replicated with each division of the host cell.

PROXEMIC RULES The study of special behavior, as in how people maintain interpersonal distance. ~ especially examine the regularities that occur in interpersonal spacing.

PROXIMAL Nearest the trunk or the point of origin. Usually expressed in relation to an extremity, but also any other structure so situated. ct: distal.

PROXIMAL STIMULUS 1. The pattern of physical energies that originates from the distal stimulus *q.v.* and impinges upon a sense organ. 2. The effect of a potential stimulus *q.v.* or distal stimulus *q.v.* upon the receptors *q.v.*

PROXIMATE CAUSE In psychology *q.v.*, explanations of behavior that focus on the immediate etiology *q.v.*

PROXIMODISTAL 1. From near to far. 2. A ~ gradient is evidenced in human physiological development, where maturation proceeds from the head down and from the center out. cf: proximodistal sequence.

PROXIMODISTAL SEQUENCE A sequence of development that proceeds from near the trunk of the body outward to the extremities.

PRP An acronym for psychogenic regional pain *q.v.*

PRUDENT DIET A diet with fat *q.v.* content more than 30%, with a daily intake of not more than 250 mg of cholesterol *q.v.*, protein *q.v.* contributing 15% of the diet, and the rest of the diet in the form of carbohydrates *q.v.*

PRUDISH Extremely or falsely modest.

PRURIENT Lustful or lewd.

PRURIENT INTEREST Extraordinary interest or concern with nudity, sex, or excretion that goes beyond normal curiosity.

PRURITIS Intense itching.

PSA An acronym for prostate-specific antigen *q.v.*

PSEPHOLOGIST A person who specializes in the science of elections.

PSEUDOALLELES Closely linked genes *q.v.* that behave as alleles but can be separable by crossing over *q.v.*

PSEUDOCOMMUNITY A delusional social environment *q.v.* developed or devised by one suffering from paranoia *q.v.*

PSEUDOCYESIS 1. False pregnancy. 2. Pseudopregnancy *q.v.* 3. A hysterical *q.v.* reaction.

PSEUDODEMENTIA A psychological disorder in older people characterized by depression *q.v.* and secondary symptoms or dementia *q.v.*

PSEUDODOMINANCE An apparent dominance of a recessive gene *q.v.* in an area opposite a chromosome *q.v.* deficiency. The recessive gene is expressed because its dominant allele *q.v.* is absent.

PSEUDOEPHEDRINE An OTC *q.v.* sympathomimetic *q.v.* drug.

PSEUDOGLIOMA A benign *q.v.* intraocular *q.v.* disturbance resulting from detachment of the retina *q.v.*

PSEUDOHERMAPHRODISM A condition in which a person has the gonads *q.v.* of one sex and the external genitalia *q.v.* of the other sex. cf: androgenital; testicular feminization; true hermaphrodism syndrome.

PSEUDOHYPERTROPHIC A type of muscular dystrophy *q.v.*

PSEUDOISOCHROMATIC PLATES A test of color vision. The plates contain a color figure embedded in a background of another color.

PSEUDOLALIA Meaningless sounds made by some psychotics *q.v.*

PSEUDOMUTUAL RELATIONSHIP A committed relationship in which the couple persists in maintaining the partnership even though neither is satisfied with it.

PSEUDOPODIA 1. Projections of the cell protoplasm *q.v.* used in effecting movement. 2. Having false feet.

PSEUDOPREGNANCY Pseudocyesis *q.v.*

PSEUDOSCIENTIST 1. A person who invents, misuses, and/or distorts scientific evidence to support a belief or practice. 2. A person who practices a form of health or medical service under false pretenses. cf: quack.

PSEUDOSTIMULATION False stimulation manifested in increased activity, loss of inhibitions, animated feelings, etc. caused by the depressant effect of alcohol or other depressant drug.

PSI 1. An acronym for personalized system of instruction *q.v.* 2. An acronym for pounds per square inch.

PSILOCIN A hallucinogenic *q.v.* drug related to psilocybin *q.v.*

PSILOCYBE MEXICANA A mushroom found chiefly in Mexico and is the source of the psychoactive *q.v.* drug, psilocybin *q.v.*

PSILOCYBIN A psychoactive *q.v.* drug found in the mushroom *Psilocybe mexicana q.v.* When ingested, it causes nausea, relaxation, dilation of the pupils of the eyes, and profound alteration of mood and behavior. When the effects wear off, mental and physical depression are often experienced.

PSITTACOSIS A viral disease *q.v.* of birds transmitted to humans.

PSOAS Pertaining to the loin *q.v.*

PSORIASIS A skin condition characterized by red scaly patches on the scalp, knees, and elbows.

P:S RATIO A comparison of the amount of polyunsaturated *q.v.* and saturated *q.v.* fats consumed on a daily basis. Most experts advocate a ratio of two to three times more polyunsaturated fats than saturated fats.

PSUEDOMYCELIUM A collection of elongated blastocytes *q.v.* that fail to separate and form what resembles mycelium.

PSYCHASTHENIA 1. Obsessive-compulsive reaction *q.v.* 2. Psychasthenic reaction. 3. An emotionally based fatigue in which a person loses the ability to concentrate and is intellectually dull.

PSYCHE 1. The mind. 2. A person's mental life. 3. The conscious and unconscious feelings, thoughts, and attitudes a person possesses. 4. In psychoanalytic theory *q.v.*, the total of the id *q.v.*, ego *q.v.*, and superego *q.v.* including both conscious and unconscious elements.

PSYCHEDELIC 1. A chemical that is purported to expand the consciousness. 2. A chemical that creates altered perceptions of reality, illusions, hallucinations *q.v.*, and strange visions. 3. Drugs that can affect one's perceptions, awareness, and emotions. 4. A drug that can produce a mental state of calmness and intense pleasure.

PSYCHIATRIC EVALUATION Medical, psychological, and sociological data used in the diagnosis *q.v.* of mental disorders.

PSYCHIATRIC NURSE A registered nurse (RN) *q.v.* who has specialized training in nursing services related to psychiatric patients. ~ is generally employed by psychiatric hospitals, outpatient facilities, nursing homes, and mental health clinics.

PSYCHIATRIC SOCIAL WORKER 1. A person who deals with the interpersonal relationships of the patient. 2. Usually concerned with the rehabilitative process and attempts to identify and rectify adverse relationships between the patient and his or her significant others, e.g., family, employer, or close friends. 3. The specialized area of social work *q.v.* primarily concerned with the mentally ill.

PSYCHIATRIC STATUS SCHEDULE A standardized questionnaire in which the interviewer rates the subject's responses based on a predetermined scale of response types.

PSYCHIATRIST 1. A physician who specializes in the diagnosis and treatment of mental and emotional disorders. A ~ may have completed the required training and experience to become Board Eligible *q.v.* or Board Certified *q.v.*

PSYCHIATRY 1. A medical specialty concerned with mental and emotional disorders. 2. The specialized area of medicine dealing with the understanding, diagnosis, treatment, and prevention of mental disorders.

PSYCHIC CHANGES Changes in consciousness or mood.

PSYCHIC CONTACTLESSNESS According to Reich, that state of detachment that comes about when one avoids relating emotionally to others.

PSYCHIC PAIN Anxiety *q.v.*

PSYCHIC STRUCTURES In psychoanalytic theory *q.v.*, hypothesized mental structures that help to explain different aspects of behavior.

PSYCHIC SURGERY A form of fakery using slight-of-hand techniques. A pretense at removing diseased organs by psychic means that leave no wound or require no physical incision. A form of quackery *q.v.*

PSYCHOACTIVE (PSYCHOTROPIC) 1. A drug that affects the functioning of the central nervous system *q.v.* resulting in distortion of the perceptions of reality. 2. Mind-altering drugs. 3. Drugs that affect arousal, mood, and/or information processing.

PSYCHOANALYSIS 1. Developed by Sigmund Freud, as a theory of psychiatric practice and a method of treating mental and emotional disorders. 2. A psychological theory that dreams, emotions, and present behaviors result from repressed, instinctual drives. 3. A type of theory that assumes that all emotional problems are the result of improper psychosexual *q.v.* disorders. 4. A theory of human personality formation whose key assertions include unconscious conflict and psychosexual development. cf: psychoanalytic theory; transference; free association.

PSYCHOANALYST A therapist whose specialty is based on postdoctoral training in psychoanalysis *q.v.* after he or she has earned an MD degree.

PSYCHOANALYTIC Theory or practice of psychoanalysis *q.v.*

PSYCHOANALYTIC MODEL A subcategory of the pathology model *q.v.* that holds that the underlying pathology is a constellation of unconscious conflicts and defenses against anxiety *q.v.*, usually rooted in early childhood; and treatment should involve some form of psychotherapy based on psychoanalytic *q.v.* principles.

PSYCHOANALYTIC THEORY A theory of personality development *q.v.* developed by Sigmund Freud. It was the first major attempt to conceptualize the structure of the personality *q.v.* and to explain the reasons for behavior. ~ is based on the idea that people could be helped to overcome their mental and emotional problems by becoming aware of, and understanding, their unconscious desires and memories. The theory is based on the following premises: 1. All behavior is a result or function of prior stimulation; 2. Each person has a conscious–unconscious dimension—that the mind is made up of three parts—the conscious, preconscious, and subconscious; 3. All behavior is ultimately determined by a set of unconscious drives or instincts. These drives comprise a person's psychic energy and causes a tension that a person seeks to reduce through behaving in a particular manner. Freud hypothesized that the personality is divided into three major components; the id, ego, and superego *qq.v.* In general, personality can be viewed as a composite of biological aspects (id), psychological aspects (ego), and social aspects (superego). Our basic nature is irrational and selfish. Only social prohibitions and rules restrain our instinctive strivings. ~ emphasizes 1. the wholeness of people, 2. the interaction of heredity and experiences upon mental and emotional health; 3. the factors related to learning and intelligence that play a key role in influencing human effectiveness.

PSYCHOANALYTIC THEORY OF ALCOHOLISM Three schools of psychology explain alcoholism using the ~. 1. The Freudian view suggests that alcoholism is caused by unconscious tendencies toward self-destruction, oral fixation, and latent homosexuality; 2. The Adlerian view advances the concept that alcoholism is a symptom of the person's need and struggle for power. 3. The inner conflict view is that alcoholism is a manifestation of a conflict between the drive for dependency an aggressive impulses.

PSYCHOBIOLOGICAL ORIENTATION Orientation toward the study of human development and behavior that emphasizes its roots in both biology *q.v.* and hereditary *q.v.* processes, and in experiences and socialization.

PSYCHOBIOLOGY The broad eclectic approach to human behavior *q.v.*, emphasizing the pluralistic determinants of behavior and the necessity for maintaining a holistic *q.v.* approach.

PSYCHOCATHARSIS Catharsis *q.v.*

PSYCHODRAMA 1. A therapeutic technique used by psychologists, which establishes a secure, nonthreatening environment in which the person can relive some of the painful experiences that are associated with his or her emotional problems. ~ provides the person with free-association and catharsis *q.v.* resulting in insight into why or how the experience contributes to the existing anxiety *q.v.* or emotional state. 2. The use of play acting for diagnostic or treatment purposes. 3. Introduced by Moreno, a kind of group therapy in which patients play out feelings toward significant people and events in their lives.

PSYCHODYNAMIC In psychoanalytic theory *q.v.* relating to the mental and emotional forces that develop in childhood and their effects on later behavior and mental states.

PSYCHODYNAMIC EXPERIENCE The emergence of what heretofore had been in the subconscious allowing for the person to understand and overcome emotional difficulties.

PSYCHODYNAMIC THEORY OF PERSONALITY Any theory of personality *q.v.* that emphasizes motivational *q.v.* dynamics as the foundation of personality. cf: social learning theory.

PSYCHOENERGIZERS Stimulants *q.v.*

PSYCHOGENESIS 1. The development from psychological *q.v.* origins as distinguished from somatic *q.v.* origins. 2. The formation of psychological attributes. ct: organogenesis.

PSYCHOGENIC 1. Reactions that arise from emotional or psychological *q.v.* factors, rather than organic *q.v.* 2. Of psychological origin. ct: somatogenic mental disorders.

PSYCHOGENIC AMNESIA A dissociative disorder *q.v.* in which a person is unable to recall events or information that cannot be explained by normal forgetfulness.

PSYCHOGENIC FUGUE A dissociative disorder *q.v.* in which a person experiences amnesia *q.v.*, relocates to a location, and assumes a new identity.

PSYCHOGENIC ILLNESS An illness resulting from emotional *q.v.* or psychological *q.v.* factors. cf: psychosomatic disorders; psychophysiologic disorders.

PSYCHOGENIC PAIN DISORDER A disorder in which the person experiences intense and prolonged pain with no apparent organic *q.v.* cause.

PSYCHOGENIC PSYCHOSOMATIC DISORDERS Structural and functional disorders *q.v.* resulting from emotional origins.

PSYCHOGENIC REGIONAL PAIN (PRP) A pain signal remotely localized in a field of mental perception or remote localization.

PSYCHOGENIC SHOCK Fainting as a result of transient generalized vasodilation *q.v.* in response to a sudden emotional *q.v.* stimulus *q.v.*

PSYCHOIMMUNOLOGY A field of study focusing on how the stresses of life affect the immune system *q.v.*

PSYCHOLOGICAL Pertaining to the mental and emotional aspects of humans.

PSYCHOLOGICAL ALCOHOL TOLERANCE Characterized by an experienced drinker recognizing the symptoms of intoxication *q.v.* and consciously controls them.

PSYCHOLOGICAL ANDROGYNY 1. The ability of a person to assume masculine or feminine roles without difficulty, self-consciousness, or embarrassment. Reflects the concept that genders *q.v.* do not occupy opposite ends of a single dimension but are two independent dimensions on which any person may be high or low. 2. Possession of instrumental and expressive traits. cf: androgyny.

PSYCHOLOGICAL ANXIETY The symptoms of anxiety *q.v.* that involve a mood of depression and apprehension. cf: somatic anxiety.

PSYCHOLOGICAL APPROACHES TO TREATING ALCOHOLISM Techniques associated with the intrapsychic *q.v.* and interpersonal *q.v.* relationships. Advocates believe that the alcoholic *q.v.* needs the guidance and counseling of professionally trained psychotherapists *q.v.*

PSYCHOLOGICAL ASSESSMENT Psychometric *q.v.* and other personality *q.v.* and behavior *q.v.* assessment data used in the diagnosis of mental and emotional disorders.

PSYCHOLOGICAL AUTOPSY An analysis of a person's suicide *q.v.* through an investigation of letters, emails, and interviews with friends and relatives for the purpose of determining the reasons for the suicide.

PSYCHOLOGICAL DEFICIT The term used to describe performance and other psychological *q.v.* processes that are below those of what is considered normal.

PSYCHOLOGICAL DEPENDENCE 1. An attachment to a drug which results from the drug's ability to satisfy some emotional or personality *q.v.* need of the user. This attachment does not require physical dependence *q.v.*, although a physical dependence may seem to reinforce a psychological dependence. A person may also be psychologically dependent on other substances; for example, food. 2. A condition characterized by a strong desire or craving, leading to repeated used of a drug or other substance in order to fulfill some emotional need. 3. A term used to describe the reason for drug abuse: reliance on a drug in order to cope with various stressful situations, without physiological dependence to it.

PSYCHOLOGICAL ENVIRONMENT 1. The factors that have a direct impact upon one's mental and emotional status and health. 2. That aspect of the environment *q.v.* that influences the stressor *q.v.* factors affecting one's behavior, or those factors that tend to create an atmosphere of security and contentment.

PSYCHOLOGICAL FEEDBACK 1. An evaluation procedure used to keep the educator *q.v.* continuously informed as to the effectiveness of the methodology being used. ~ provides knowledge of results of communications. 2. A process of acquiring knowledge of results whereby the person acquires information concerning the correctness of his or her response. cf: information theory.

PSYCHOLOGICAL HANDICAP Impaired ability resulting from mental or emotional disturbance, resulting in the inability to function adequately on a daily basis.

PSYCHOLOGICAL HEALTH 1. Mental health *q.v.* 2. Emotional and intellectual health *q.v.* 3. According to Maslow, the mature person; one who has gone beyond growth and by means of his or her dynamic inner self *q.v.* has developed a framework of values, a philosophy of life, and decisions that have brought about peak experiences that make living worthwhile along with future hopes, plans, and goals.

PSYCHOLOGICAL NEEDS 1. Needs *q.v.* that are the result of our social environment *q.v.* 2. A sense of security, love, and self-esteem. 3. Emotional needs. 4. The need for love, belongingness, and for self-esteem. 5. The need for social approval.

PSYCHOLOGICAL POTENTIALS Those human elements that enable a person to think, learn, create, initiate, respond, express feelings and emotions, and control the expressions of the physical potential *q.v.* cf: physical potentials.

PSYCHOLOGICAL PRIMARY A sensation that cannot be analyzed into more elementary sensations. ct: physical primary.

PSYCHOLOGICAL RESEARCH ON AGING The scientific investigation of individual characteristics (intellectual ability, personality, attitudes, and behaviors) and social environments (family relationships and work situations) as they influence the way people age.

PSYCHOLOGICAL SELECTIVITY The conscious or unconscious factors influencing perception as to what a person wants to perceive from what a person should perceive.

PSYCHOLOGICAL SET A predisposition to behave or respond in a certain way.

PSYCHOLOGICAL SURGERY 1. A fraudulent practice of some quacks *q.v.* It is a purported technique to perform surgery without cutting into any tissues. Removal of a diseased part of the body by a "mind over matter" approach. 2. Quackery *q.v.*

PSYCHOLOGICAL TEST A standardized procedure designed to measure a person's performance on a specific task.

PSYCHOLOGICAL THEORIES OF ALCOHOLISM Theories that suggest that alcoholism *q.v.* is a symptom of some personality *q.v.* or emotional disorder. Three such theories are 1. psychoanalytic, 2. learning, and 3. personality trait *qq.v.*

PSYCHOLOGIST 1. A nonmedical specialty concerned with psychological testing, evaluation, and diagnosis of emotional problems. 2. A person trained in treating emotional disorders by nonmedical and nonsurgical techniques—group therapy, psychotherapy, etc. *qq.v.* cf: clinical psychologist.

PSYCHOLOGY 1. The study of personality and individual behavior. 2. The profession that studies individual thoughts, feelings, and behaviors. 3. The science of the mind.

PSYCHOMETRIC Pertaining to psychological *q.v.* or mental measurement.

PSYCHOMETRIC APPROACH TO INTELLIGENCE An attempt to understand the nature of intelligence *q.v.* by studying the pattern of results obtained on intelligence tests *q.v.*

PSYCHOMETRICIAN A psychologist *q.v.* trained in the development and administration of standardized tests *q.v.* to measure such things as intelligence *q.v.*, creativity, sociability, etc.

PSYCHOMIMETIC 1. Substances that cause symptoms similar to those of psychosis *q.v.* 2. Psychotomimetic *q.v.*

PSYCHOMOTOR 1. Relating to the psychological *q.v.* basis of voluntary muscular movement. Involving psychological and physical activity.

PSYCHOMOTOR AGITATION Disordered behavior characteristic of unipolar depressive *q.v.* patients.

PSYCHOMOTOR ATTACKS 1. Associated with epilepsy *q.v.* and characterized by a loss of environmental *q.v.* contact, manifested in staggering, purposeless movements, and unintelligible vocal sounds. Confusion often accompanies the attacks that may last from 2 to 3 min following it. 2. Psychomotor *q.v.* epilepsy; a state of disturbed consciousness in which the person may perform various actions for which he or she is later amnesic *q.v.*

PSYCHOMOTOR DOMAIN Includes those aspects of learning through which accumulated knowledge and attitudes are applied to particular life situations. It implies skill development: physical and intellectual. cf: psychomotor objectives.

PSYCHOMOTOR EPILEPSY 1. A loss of consciousness in which a person may appear to be conscious, but is unaware of his or her behavior, or changes in mood, thoughts, or perceptions. 2. Psychomotor attacks *q.v.* 3. A form of epileptic seizure *q.v.*

PSYCHOMOTOR LEARNING The acquisition of motor skills.

PSYCHOMOTOR OBJECTIVES 1. Those objectives *q.v.* that describe physical activities that can be practiced observably and demonstrated directly. 2. Skills. cf: psychomotor domain.

PSYCHOMOTOR RETARDATION Disordered behavior likely to be exhibited by bipolar depressive *q.v.* patients.

PSYCHOMOTOR SEIZURE A seizure *q.v.* characterized by inappropriate behavior such as lip-smacking, and chewing. cf: psychomotor attacks.

PSYCHONEUROSIS Neurosis *q.v.*

PSYCHONEUROTIC DISORDER 1. Behavior *q.v.* pathology *q.v.* in which anxiety *q.v.* plays a part. cf: hysteria; psychasthenia.

PSYCHOPATH A person who commits antisocial acts without a sense of guilt or remorse, and who willingly repeats them.

PSYCHOPATHIC 1. A personality disorder *q.v.* characterized by antisocial *q.v.* reactions. One who possesses little ethical or moral development and find it difficult to adhere to social mores. 2. Sociopath *q.v.* 3. Specific antisocial reactions include (a) inadequate conscience development, (b) irresponsible behavior, (c) establishment of unrealistic goals, (d) lack of feelings of guilt, and (e) defective social relationships. cf: antisocial personality.

PSYCHOPATHIC PERSONALITY Psychopathic *q.v.*

PSYCHOPATHOLOGIST A psychologist, psychiatrist, or biochemist *qq.v.* who conducts research into the nature and causes of mental and emotional disorders.

PSYCHOPATHOLOGY 1. The study of psychological disorders. 2. The science concerned with the causes and nature of abnormal behavior.

PSYCHOPATHY An unusual tendency to rebel against socially exacted standards of behavior.

PSYCHOPHARMACEUTICALS Drugs used in the treatment of mental illness.

PSYCHOPHARMACOLOGY The study of the effects and mechanisms of action of psychoactive drugs *q.v.*

PSYCHOPHYSICAL CORRELATION Pertains to the dependence of some psychological *q.v.* attribute of sensory experience upon a dimension of physical stimulation, e.g., the dependence of brightness on the intensity of visual stimulation.

PSYCHOPHYSICS The science that attempts to relate the characteristics of physical stimuli *q.v.* to the sensory experience they produce.

PSYCHOPHYSIOLOGICAL DYSFUNCTION A general term referring to stress-related diseases. 2. Psychophysiologic disorders *q.v.*

PSYCHOPHYSIOLOGIC DISORDERS 1. Associated with physiological stress *q.v.* resulting in bodily disturbances that are innervated by the autonomic nervous system *q.v.* 2. Psychosomatic disorders *q.v.* 3. Psychophysiologic dysfunction *q.v.* 4. Any physical disorder that is, at least in part, the result of stress. cf: conversion reaction.

PSYCHOPHYSIOLOGY The study of bodily changes that accompany psychological *q.v.* events.

PSYCHOPROPHYLAXIS 1. Mental prevention. 2. A form of prepared childbirth. 3. A concept to reduce the stress *q.v.* and tension of parturition *q.v.* through positive attitude, relaxation of pelvic muscles *q.v.*, and the presence of a supportive coach throughout labor *q.v.* 4. A method of childbirth that stresses relaxation by conditioning reflexes with self-induced signals during uterine *q.v.* contractions.

PSYCHOQUACK An unqualified person who attempts to treat mental illness. cf: quack; charlatan.

PSYCHOSEXUAL DEVELOPMENT In psychoanalytic theory *q.v.*, the description of the progressives stages in the way a child gains his or her main source of pleasure as he or she grows into adulthood, defined by the zone of the body through which this pleasure is derived, and the object toward which this pleasurable feeling is directed. cf: psychosexual stages.

PSYCHOSEXUAL DISORDERS Disorders of sexual functioning caused by psychological *q.v.* factors. These include gender identity disorders *q.v.*, paraphilias *q.v.*, and psychosexual dysfunctions *q.v.*

PSYCHOSEXUAL DYSFUNCTIONS Disorders in which normal sexual response is inhibited in some respect.

PSYCHOSEXUAL STAGES 1. Sigmund Freud's theory of maturation, which consists of five major periods of life: (a) oral stage, (b) anal stage, (c) phallic stage, (d) latency stage, and (e) genital stage. 2. In psychoanalytic theory *q.v.*, important developmental stages that an individual passes through in life corresponding to the area of the body providing maximum erotic gratification. cf: psychosexual development; psychosocial stages.

PSYCHOSEXUAL TRAUMA 1. According to Masters and Johnson, experiences at an earlier stage of life that has adverse effects on present sexual functioning. 2. An extremely disturbing sexual experience.

PSYCHOSIS 1. Mental illness characterized by a loss of touch with reality. 2. A major mental disorder. 3. Any serious mental derangement. ~ replaces the obsolete term insanity *q.v.* 4. A major mental disorder of organic *q.v.* or functional *q.v.* origin in which there is a departure from normal thinking, feeling, and acting characterized by a loss of touch with reality, loss of emotional control, and distortion of perception exemplified by delusions *q.v.* and hallucinations *q.v.* 5. A severe mental disorder that prevents normal functioning. ct: neurosis.

PSYCHOSOCIAL DEVELOPMENT 1. The development of the person in his or her relationships to other people. 2. Stages of personality *q.v.* development as suggested by

Erikson that are characterized by changes in predominant patterns of social interaction. cf: psychosocial stages.

PSYCHOSOCIAL MORATORIUM A period of delay of commitment or a postponement of occupational choice.

PSYCHOSOCIAL STAGES 1. Erik Erikson's psychosocial crises in maturation *q.v.* characterized by a series of eight encounters, one for each stage of development. These encounters contrast a positive success to a corresponding failure as follows: (a) trust versus mistrust; (b) autonomy versus shame and doubt; (c) initiative versus guilt; (d) industry versus inferiority; (e) ego identity versus self-diffusion; (f) intimacy versus isolation; (g) generosity versus self-absorption or stagnation; and (h) integrity versus despair. cf: psychosexual stages.

PSYCHOSOCIAL SYSTEM As defined by Masters and Johnson, the social, cultural, and psychological influences on sexual response *q.v.*

PSYCHOSOMATIC DISORDERS 1. Bodily disturbances emanating from emotional stress *q.v.* 2. A functional *q.v.* disturbance. 3. Psychophysiologic *q.v.* disorders. 4. Illness without apparent physical cause. ct: conversion reaction; hysteria.

PSYCHOSOMATIC MEDICINE That branch of medical practice concerned with the study and treatment of psychosomatic disorders *q.v.*

PSYCHOSURGERY 1. An effective, but rarely used or needed method of relieving some nervous or psychomotor *q.v.* symptoms by serving selected nerve pathways within the brain *q.v.* 2. Any of the various methods of brain surgery for the treatment of mental disorders. cf: lobotomy.

PSYCHOTHERAPY 1. A collective term for all forms of treatment that use psychological *q.v.* rather than somatic *q.v.* means. 2. A means of conversing with one or more clients in which a trained therapist facilitates a greater understanding, objectivity, and maturity in dealing with mental and emotional problems. ct: insight therapy; behavior therapy.

PSYCHOTIC BEHAVIOR Characterized by manifestations of delusions *q.v.*, hallucinations *q.v.*, and exaggerated emotional actions.

PSYCHOTIC BREAKDOWN A radical break with reality, characterized by a major disruption of consciousness, perception, thinking, and social behavior.

PSYCHOTIC DEPRESSIVE REACTION A psychosis *q.v.* characterized by depression *q.v.* and feelings of worthlessness.

PSYCHOTIC EXPERIENCE An experience, often brought on by the use of hallucinogenic *q.v.* drugs, characterized by paranoia *q.v.*, confusion, and depression *q.v.* A bad trip.

PSYCHOTICISM In Eysenck's theory of personality *q.v.*, a dimension referring to the degree of contact with reality.

PSYCHOTIC SYMPTOMS Delusions *q.v.*, hallucinations *q.v.*, and exaggerated and distorted emotional behavior.

PSYCHOTOGENICS Psychedelics *q.v.*

PSYCHOTOMIMETIC 1. Having the power or potential to mimic psychosis *q.v.* 2. Having the potential to produce symptoms of a behavior typical of psychotic behavior *q.v.* Some drugs, the psychedelic drugs, can produce psychotic effects. 3. Psychomimetic. 4. Psychotomimetic drug.

PSYCHOTOMIMETIC DRUG 1. A drug that causes an altered state of consciousness that resembles that of psychosis *q.v.* 2. Psychotomimetic *q.v.* 3. Psychomimetic *q.v.*

PSYCHOTOXIC DRUG Drugs that, depending upon dose level and mode of administration, can produce symptoms of psychosis *q.v.*, anxiety *q.v.*, or significant mood change.

PSYCHOTROPIC DRUGS 1. Drugs that cause mood change. 2. Drugs that affect the mind in one way or another. cf: psychoactive drugs.

PSYCHROPHIL Cold-loving. Refers to organisms that grow at relatively low temperatures.

PTA An acronym for the Parent teacher Association; officially named the National Congress of Parents and Teachers.

PTC An acronym for phenylthiocarbamide *q.v.*

PTERYGOID Wing-shaped.

PTOMAINE POISONING A toxin formed during the decomposition of protein *q.v.* in foods through bacterial *q.v.* action.

PTOMAINES Decomposition products produced by bacterial *q.v.* action on proteins; popularly, but incorrectly believed to cause food poisoning.

PTOSIS 1. A drooping of one or both upper eyelids. 2. An inherited *q.v.* condition in which the nerves to the eyelid muscles do not conduct nervous impulses *q.v.*

PTSD An acronym for posttraumatic stress disorder *q.v.*

PTYALIN 1. An enzyme *q.v.* found in saliva that breaks down starch to simple sugars. 2. Salivary amylase *q.v.*

PUBERTY 1. Pubescence *q.v.* 2. The stage of development in which rapid physical and psychological changes take place. Characterized by the development of reproductive potential and the secondary sex characteristics *q.v.* 3. The age at which the testes *q.v.* of the male and the ovaries *q.v.* of the female begin to function and the person is capable of reproduction, usually beginning at age 12–13.

4. The stage of physical development when reproduction first becomes possible.

PUBERTY PRAECOX Early onset of puberty *q.v.* as a result of a glandular *q.v.* disturbance.

PUBESCENCE Puberty *q.v.*

PUBIC LICE 1. Small insects that infest the genital-rectal region of the body. 2. Tiny organisms that may be transmitted sexually that cause itching and discomfort. ~ live at the roots of pubic hair *q.v.* cf: pediculosis.

PUBIC SYMPHYSIS The joint formed by the union of the bodies of the pubic bones *q.v.* in the median plane, characterized by a thick mass of fibrocartilage *q.v.*

PUBLIC COMMENT An opportunity for the general public to comment on findings or proposed activities.

PUBLIC HEALTH ADVISORY A statement released describing findings of a health issue of significant urgency to require public action. The ~ includes recommended measures to reduce human risk and eliminate or substantially mitigate human exposure to the threat.

PUBLIC HEALTH AGENCY An official, governmental tax supported organization mandated by law for the protection and improvement of the health of the general public. ct: private health agency.

PUBLIC HEALTH EDUCATOR 1. Community health educator *q.v.* 2. A person with professional preparation in public health education *q.v.* including training in the application of selected content from relevant social and behavioral sciences used to influence individual and group learning, mobilization of community health action, and the planning, implementation, and evaluation of health programs.

PUBLIC HEALTH PRACTICE As conceived by Winslow, the science and art of preventing disease, prolonging life, and promoting health and well-being through organized community effort for the sanitation of the environment, the control of communicable infections *q.v.*, the organization of medical and nursing services for the early diagnosis and prevention of disease, the education of the individual in personal health, and the development of the social machinery to assure everyone a standard of living adequate for the maintenance and improvement of health.

PUBLIC HEALTH PRACTICE AND PROGRAM MANAGEMENT A specialized area of public health concerned with the application of knowledge and skills to the planning, implementation, management, and evaluation of activities of health professional disciplines and health problems.

PUBLIC HEALTH PREVENTION MODEL A model for the prevention of health problems that focuses on the host–agent–environment relationship.

PUBLIC HEALTH SERVICES Public health practices that apply the principles of the basic biological, medical, social, and pure sciences in an effort to prevent disease and to promote health. Efforts are directed toward those health issues that are primarily a community responsibility and are carried out by governmental (official) and voluntary health agencies and others concerned with achieving public health goals. These other agencies include the educational community, social services, law enforcement and safety services, and private practitioners.

PUBLIC LAW 94-142 The Education for all Handicapped Children Act. Passed in 1975, this act mandates a free, appropriate public education for all handicapped children.

PUBLIC LAWS Legislation that has been enacted into law.

PUBLIC RELATIONS An enterprise designed to promote positive attitudes toward particular organizations, individuals, and ideas. It is a form of communication with the community.

PUBLIC SCHOOL A school operated publically, under state and federal laws, and funded through local, state, and federal tax dollars. In most cases ~s are operated under policies set by locally elected boards of education *q.v.*

PUBLIC SELF The personality *q.v.* that is presented to others, sometimes in order to mask the real self.

PUBOCOCCYGIAL MUSCLES The muscles surrounding the outer third of the vaginal barrel *q.v.*

PUDENDUM 1. The external genitalia *q.v.*, esp. of the female, which includes the mons pubis *q.v.*, labia majora *q.v.*, the labia minora *q.v.*, and the vestibule of the vagina *q.v.* 2. The vulva *q.v.*

PUDENTAL NERVE The nerve that passes from the external genitalia *q.v.* through the sacral foramen *q.v.* to the spinal cord *q.v.*

PUERPERAL Pertaining to, resulting from, or following childbirth.

PUERPERIUM The period of about 6–8 weeks after labor during which the mother's reproductive organs return to the nonpregnant state.

PUFFERY A form of advertising that uses vague superlatives, exaggerations, or subjective opinions without presenting specific facts.

PULMONARY Pertaining to the lungs and breathing.

PULMONARY ALVEOLI The air sacs of the lungs.

PULMONARY ARTERY The artery *q.v.* extending from the right ventricle *q.v.* of the heart carrying venous blood to the lungs for aeration *q.v.*

PULMONARY CIRCULATION The part of the circulatory system *q.v.* that conveys blood from the heart to the lungs and back to the heart.

PULMONARY CONTUSION A bruise *q.v.* of the pulmonary *q.v.* tissue.

PULMONARY EDEMA An abnormal accumulation of fluid in the pulmonary *q.v.* tissues and air spaces.

PULMONARY EMPHYSEMA A disease, often caused by tobacco *q.v.* smoking or other air pollutants *q.v.*, that results in the inability of the lungs to exchange gases and impair and/or damage the alveolar *q.v.* sacs.

PULMONARY FUNCTION The relative functional health of the pulmonary system *q.v.*

PULMONARY RESUSCITATION A technique of providing artificial ventilation *q.v.* either by mouth to mouth or mouth to nose, or by artificial devices.

PULMONARY STENOSIS A congenital *q.v.* heart defect characterized by obstruction or narrowing of the valve between the right ventricle *q.v.* and the pulmonary artery *q.v.*

PULMONARY VALVE The valve that controls the flow of blood into the pulmonary arteries *q.v.* from the right ventricle *q.v.* of the heart.

PULMONARY VEINS The four veins *q.v.* that return aerated blood from the lungs to the left atrium *q.v.* of the heart.

PULPITIS Characterized by odontalgia *q.v.*, necrosis *q.v.* of the pulp, and inflammation of the periodontal membrane *q.v.* In advanced stages, an abscess *q.v.* will form.

PUNISHMENT 1. A negative experience following a particular behavior resulting in the behavior occurring less frequently. 2. The presentation of an undesirable behavioral consequence and/or removal of a desirable consequence that decrease the likelihood of the behavior continuing. ct: reward.

PUNITIVE (APPROACH TO DISCIPLINE) A situation in which an automatic punishment is imposed for any deviation from accepted standards of behavior.

PUPIL 1. The opening in the center of the iris *q.v.* of the eye for the transmission of light to the retina *q.v.* 2. The opening in the iris of the eye that expands (dilates) and contracts (constricts) to control the amount of light entering the eye.

PURE CULTURE An aggregation of microorganisms *q.v.*, all of one kind, and isolated to prevent contamination with other types of organisms.

PURE LINE A strain of organisms that is relatively pure genetically *q.v.* because of prolonged inbreeding *q.v.* or through other means.

PURE RESEARCH Pertaining to basic research *q.v.*

PURGATIVE 1. An agent that causes evacuation of the intestines *q.v.* 2. A laxative *q.v.*

PURGE 1. The use of vomiting or laxative *q.v.* to remove undigested food from the body. 2. To clear or discharge. 3. To remove.

PURINE 1. The end products of nucleated protein *q.v.* digestion that break down to form uric acid *q.v.* 2. The parent substance of the purine base. Adenine *q.v.* and guanine *q.v.* are the major bases of nucleic acid *q.v.* Other important ~s are xanthine *q.v.* and uric acid *q.v.* 3. A chemical substance present in DNA *q.v.*

PURITAN INFLUENCE In education, the influence of the puritans over the schools of New England during the Colonial period.

PURKINJE PHENOMENON The shift in the relative brightness *q.v.* of colors that occurs with the shift from rod *q.v.* to cone *q.v.* vision.

PURPURA A blood disease characterized by a marked tendency to bleed.

PURULENT Discharging pus *q.v.*

PUS A mixture of white blood cells *q.v.* and cellular debris resulting from an infection *q.v.* and inflammation *q.v.*

PUSTULE A small elevation of the skin containing pus *q.v.*

PUTAMEN The darker outer layer of the lenticular nucleus *q.v.*

PUTRIFICATION Decomposition of organic *q.v.* matter.

P-VALUE In epidemiology *q.v.*, the probability of obtaining a difference between sample estimates as large as the observed difference, given that the null hypothesis *q.v.* is true.

PVO An acronym for private voluntary organization. cf: voluntary health agency; private health agency.

PYELITIS Inflammation *q.v.* of the outlet of the kidney *q.v.* or of the pelvis *q.v.*

PYEMIA A generalized severe blood poisoning.

PYGMALION EFFECT 1. The use of subtle, often unconscious cues *q.v.* to create in others what one expects to find. 2. The tendency for a person who is capable or incapable to act as though he or she is capable or incapable. 3. Self-fulfilling prophecy *q.v.*

PYKNIC A body type identified by Kretschmer whose temperament was supposed to be cyclothymic *q.v.* cf: leptosome.

PYLORIC CAECUM An elongated pouch or diverticulum *q.v.* of the intestine *q.v.*

PYLORUS The opening or valve that lies between the stomach and the duodenum *q.v.*

PYOGENIC Pus-producing.

PYORRHEA 1. A lay term for gum disease. 2. Gingivitis *q.v.* 3. Peridontitis *q.v.* 4. An infection of the periodontal membrane *q.v.* 5. Large discharges of pus *q.v.* associated with severe periodontal disease *q.v.*

PYRAZINE A chemical substance that affects the flavor of tobacco *q.v.* smoke.

PYRENOID Protein *q.v.* granules in the plastids *q.v.* of some algae that serve as centers for starch formation.

PYRETIC Fever or heat producing.

PYRIDOXAL A chemical composition of vitamin B_6 *q.v.*

PYRIDOXAMINE A chemical composition f vitamin B_6 *q.v.*

PYRIDOXINE A chemical composition of vitamin B_6 *q.v.*

PYRIMIDINE The parent substance of several nitrogenous compounds found in nucleic acid *q.v.*, e.g., thymine *q.v.*, uracil *q.v.*, and cytosine *q.v.*

PYROLYSIS 1. Chemical decomposition of matter through the action of heat. 2. A method of waste disposal in which waste is decomposed into charcoal at high temperatures in an oxygen-free chamber. 3. A process using high temperatures and pressure to convert garbage and other wastes into oil and other substances.

PYROMANIA 1. An uncontrollable urge to set fires. 2. A neurosis *q.v.* 3. An obsessive-compulsive reaction *q.v.* 4. A compulsion, often sexually oriented, to set fires.

PYRUVATE A metabolic intermediate formed from glucose *q.v.* in glycolysis *q.v.* and from the deamination *q.v.* of alanine *q.v.*

PYRUVIC ACID A keto acid of 3-carbon atoms. ~ is formed of carbohydrate *q.v.* in aerobic *q.v.* metabolism *q.v.* Pyruvate *q.v.* is the salt or ester *q.v.* of ~.

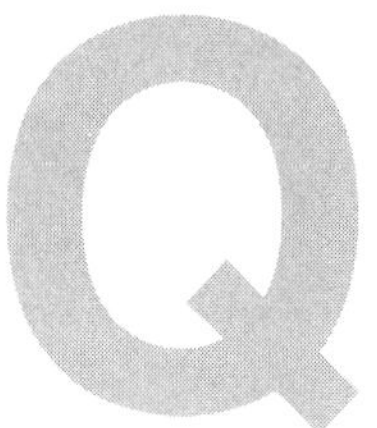

Q.I.D A Latin abbreviation referring to four times a day.

Q FEVER An acute *q.v.* infectious disease *q.v.* caused by a rickettsia *q.v.*, characterized by headaches, fever, malaise, and loss of weight. The disease is transmitted by contaminated dust particles, milk, and through handling animals, e.g., as cows and goats infected with the rickettsial organism. A vaccine *q.v.* is available and the disease is treatable.

Q METHODOLOGY A group of psychometric *q.v.* and statistical *q.v.* procedures that bring about strong analytic potentials. ~ possesses an array of procedures and is a flexible investigative means available to psychologists *q.v.* and educators *q.v.* cf: Q technique; Q sort.

Q SORT 1. In psychology *q.v.*, a personality *q.v.* test used in client-centered therapy *q.v.* or research, in which the person in question categorizes a series of descriptive statements ranging from "very characteristic" to "very uncharacteristic" as they apply to him or her. 2. Generally, a technique used in Q methodology *q.v.* for rank-ordering a set of objects, characteristics, and the like. 3. Unstructured Q sort involves a set of items assembled without specific regard to the variables or factors underlying the items. 4. Structured Q sort involves the variables of a hypothesis *q.v.*, or set of hypotheses, that are built into a set of items along variance design principles.

Q TECHNIQUE 1. A set of procedures used to implement a Q methodology *q.v.* 2. ~ centers particularly in the sorting of decks of cards referred to as Q sorts *q.v.* 3. Chiefly, a sophisticated form of rank-ordering objects and then assigning numerals to subsets of the objects for statistical purposes. ~ uses a rank-order procedure of piles or groups of objects.

QUAALUDES A commercial preparation of methaqualone *q.v.* introduced by the William H. Rorer Company in 1966.

QUACK A person or group of persons who offer fraudulent health services or products for profit. cf: charlatan; quackery.

QUACKERY 1. Any fraudulent misrepresentation in matters concerned with health *q.v.* It may take the form of health services, the use of unproven or useless products, or the manufacture and sale of fraudulent, worthless, or misrepresented products. 2. The marketing of unreliable and ineffective health services, products, or information under the guise of curing disease or improving health.

QUADRANT Pertaining to a specific area of the abdominal *q.v.* wall.

QUADRIPARTITE STRUCTURE A chromosomal *q.v.* ring having four corresponding parts.

QUADRIPLEGIA Paralysis *q.v.* affecting both arms and both legs.

QUADRIVALENT A group of four chromosomes *q.v.* of the same kind in a cell. Resulting from chromosome translocations *q.v.*

QUALITATIVE EVALUATION A grouping of information according to similar characteristics, using words, not numbers, to assess a project.

QUALITATIVE VARIABLE In epidemiology *q.v.*, variety that can be named or classified but cannot be quantified. Nominal variable *q.v.* ct: quantitative variable.

QUALITY 1. The nature, kind, or character of someone or something. 2. The degree of excellence possessed by a person or thing.

QUALITY ASSESSMENT The measurement of success or the degree of excellence as determined by a comparison with accepted standards.

QUALITY OF LIFE The perception by individuals or groups of need satisfaction and the ability to achieve their goals in order to be happy and fulfilled.

QUANTITATIVE EVALUATION A categorization of measurable information according to some standard or quantity.

QUANTITATIVE TRAIT A trait, the characteristics of which can be measured. cf: quantitative variable.

QUANTITATIVE VARIABLE In epidemiology *q.v.*, variables *q.v.* that can be measured. ct: qualitative variable.

QUANTUM MERUIT 1. In law, the implication that the defendant had agreed to pay the plaintiff as much as he or she reasonably deserved for the work performed. 2. The reasonable value of goods and services furnished.

QUARANTINE Used for the first time in 1348. The first ~ law was passed in Marseilles, France, in 1383. Venice imposed a 40-day ~ in 1403. ~ is essentially an attempt at controlling the spread of disease by restricting the freedom of one who has a contagious disease and those who are well but suspected of transmitting it to others. cf: isolation.

QUASI 1. As if. Almost as it were. Analogous to. 2. As if, or almost as it were; e.g., a ~-judicial act of a school board in holding a hearing before dismissing a teacher.

QUASI-EXPERIMENTAL In epidemiology *q.v.*, a research design in which the investigator does not have as much control of the variables *q.v.* as in an experimental design.

QUASI-MEDICAL Having the characteristics of medical use or services, but not generally accepted in modern medical practice.

QUEENS In the gay community, homosexual *q.v.* males who adopt exaggerated feminine behavior.

QUESTION-AND-ANSWER METHOD A teacher or learner-centered method depending upon who is in control of the questioning. It can be a valuable method of motivating two-way communications and in receiving important feedback *q.v.*

QUESTIONNAIRE Survey questions in written form.

QUICKENING Movements of the fetus *q.v.* felt by the mother which usually occurs about the 4th month of pregnancy.

QUID A piece of something to be chewed, e.g., a wad of chewing tobacco *q.v.* in a person's mouth.

QUID PRO QUO 1. Giving one valuable thing for another. 2. Setting a condition for a person to do something in order for an agreement to happen.

QUIET SLEEP 1. Stages 2–4 of sleep during which there are no rapid eye movements and during which the EEG *q.v.* shows progressively less cortical arousal. 2. Non-REM *q.v.* sleep. ct: REM sleep; active sleep.

QUINIDINE A drug derived from cinchona bark that is useful in treating irregularities of the heart beat.

QUININE 1. A white alkaloid *q.v.* sometimes used as an adulterant in street heroin *q.v.* 2. A drug derived from the bark of the cinchona tree, used to treat malaria *q.v.*

QUINSY A severe type of sore throat with abscess *q.v.* formation in the tissues surrounding the tonsil *q.v.*

QUORUM The number of people eligible to vote in a meeting that are required to be in attendance in order to conduct business.

QUO WARRANTO 1. By what authority. 2. A writ to test the claim to a public office.

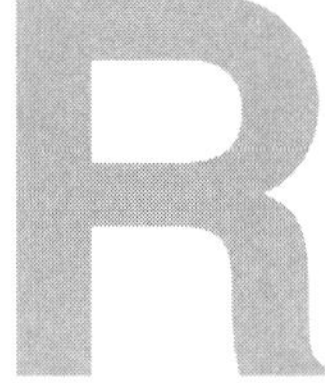

r The statistical symbol for correlation coefficient *q.v.*

RA An acronym for remedial action.

RABBIT FEVER Tularemia *q.v.*

RABIES 1. An infectious *q.v.* disease of the nervous tissue caused by a virus *q.v.* and transmitted through the saliva of a rabid animal. 2. Hydrophobia *q.v.* 3. A disease characterized by excitement, muscular spasms, and later, paralysis and death.

RACE A group of people who differ from others on the basis of physical characteristics.

RACEMOSE In anatomy *q.v.*, shaped like a cluster of grapes.

RACERS A slang expression pertaining to competitive swingers *q.v.*

RACHETIC Suffering from rickets *q.v.*

RACIAL BIAS The degree to which a person's beliefs are influenced on the basis of race *q.v.*

RACIAL DISCRIMINATION Any action or law that limits the ability of a person to function effectively in terms of opportunity, rewards, privileges, etc., based on the person's race.

RACISM Assumptions, beliefs, laws, and behavior that are based on the premise that one race is superior to another.

RAD 1. Roentgen *q.v.* 2. A measure of the dose *q.v.* from ionizing radiation *q.v.* A ~ is equivalent to 100 ergs *q.v.* of energy per gram.

RADIAL ARTERY One of the major arteries *q.v.* of the forearm *q.v.* The pulse *q.v.* of the ~ is palpable *q.v.* at the base of the thumb.

RADIAL HEAD The circular proximal *q.v.* end of the radius *q.v.* allowing the normal rotation motion of the forearm *q.v.* with the ulna *q.v.* as axis.

RADIAL NERVE One of the three major nerves *q.v.* of the arm. The ~ descends at the back of the arm closely applied to the humerus *q.v.* and into the forearm *q.v.* It is ultimately distributed to the skin at the back of the arm, forearm, and hand, the extensor *q.v.* muscles on the back of the arm and forearm, the elbow, joint, and many other joints of the hand.

RADIAL PULSE The pulse *q.v.* taken at the wrist.

RADIANT ENERGY Any energy *q.v.* that is radiated from any source, including electromagnetic waves, radio waves, visible light, X-rays, or nuclear radiation.

RADIATION 1. Rays from the sun, nuclear power, and equipment used in medicine, dentistry, and veterinary medicine. 2. Treatment of disease with various types of radioactive *q.v.* energy. 3. The emission and propagation of energy through space or through a material medium in the form of waves or particles.

RADIATION SICKNESS An illness characterized by fatigue, nausea, weight loss, fever, bleeding from the mouth and gums, hair loss, and immune *q.v.* deficiencies, resulting from overexposure to ionizing *q.v.* radiation. Death can result.

RADIATION THERAPY Treatment for some diseases, e.g., cancer, using a variety of forms of radiation *q.v.*, X-ray, and radioactive isotopes *q.v.*.

RADICAL BEHAVIORISM 1. A belief that assumes that behavior can be understood in its entirety in terms of the environment. 2. A theory of development that holds that all behavior is attributable to classical or operant conditioning *q.v.* cf: behaviorist orientation; neobehaviorism.

RADICAL MASTECTOMY The surgical removal of the breast, lymph nodes *q.v.*, and the underlying muscles. cf: mastectomy; modified mastectomy; lumpectomy.

RADIOACTIVE The emission of particles during the disintegration of the nuclei *q.v.* of radioactive *q.v.* elements. The emissions include alpha particles, beta particles, and gamma rays.

RADIOACTIVE TAG A chemical or drug that bears a radioactive atom (tag) allowing a researcher to follow its behavior in the body.

RADIOACTIVITY The property of spontaneously emitting rays or subatomic particles of matter with the release of large amounts of energy *q.v.*

RADIOIMMUNOASSAY A test whereby the blood of a woman is analyzed to determine whether pregnancy exists.

RADIOISOTOPE 1. A radioactive *q.v.* form of an element. 2. The nucleus of a stable atom when charged by bombarding particles (in a nuclear reactor) becomes radioactive and is labeled or tagged.

RADIOLOGIST A physician *q.v.* specializing in the diagnosis and treatment of disease by means of X-rays or other forms of radioactivity *q.v.*

RADIOLOGY 1. The specialized branch of medicine that deals with roentgen rays *q.v.* and other radiant energy, as used in the diagnosis and treatment of disease. 2. The medical specialty using X-rays, computerized tomography *q.v.* scans, radioactive isotopes *q.v.*, and other similar procedures to diagnose and treat illness.

RADIOPACITY Preventing the passage of X-rays *q.v.*

RADIOPAQUE DYE A dye whose chemical composition absorbs X-rays *q.v.* and allows for an image to be seen on the X-ray film.

RADIORECEPTOR ASSAY TEST A pregnancy *q.v.* test that uses a radioactive *q.v.* substance to determine the presence of human chorionic gonadotropin (HCG) *q.v.* in a serum sample.

RADIO-TRANSLUCENT The ability of any material to allow passage of electric waves or X-rays *q.v.* through it.

RADIUS 1. The bone in the forearm *q.v.* on the side toward the thumb. 2. The bone on the lateral or thumb side of the forearm, so aligned by its head as to describe a circle about the ulna *q.v.* when the hand is rotated. 3. In geometry, the distance from the center of a circle to any point on its circumference. One-half the diameter of a circle.

RALE 1. An abnormal sound that is produced by the lungs by various types of pulmonary *q.v.* diseases. 2. A sound that can be heard in the chest in cases of disease of the lungs or bronchial tubes *q.v.*

RAMUS 1. A branch or branching part. 2. One of the primary divisions of a nerve or blood vessel. 3. A part of an irregularly shaped bone that forms an angle with the main body of the bone.

RANDOM ASSIGNMENT The assignment or selection of subjects in an experiment to either the experimental or the control groups *q.v.* by a random process.

RANDOMIZATION In epidemiology *q.v.*, assigning people to treatment and control groups *q.v.* in an unbiased manner so as to produce groups similar relative to their characteristics. cf: random sample.

RANDOMIZED CLINICAL TRIAL In epidemiology *q.v.*, a clinical trial *q.v.* in which subjects have been randomly assigned to various groups in the study.

RANDOM SAMPLE 1. Sample *q.v.* 2. A subset of a population *q.v.* selected for study so constructed that each member has an equal chance to be picked. 3. In research, a segment of a population selected in such a way as to eliminate bias. 4. Randomness. cf: randomization. ct: stratified sample.

RANDOM SCHEDULE Rewards or punishments are distributed every so often rather than regularly. ct: schedule of reinforcement.

RANGE OF MOTION The distance through which a joint can be moved, measured in degrees.

RAP BOOTHS 1. Jargon for an innovation in prostitution *q.v.* in which a client communicates with a prostitute who serves as a masturbatory *q.v.* aid behind a glass panel. 2. Small booths in which customers can watch and talk to a person who is nude and/or modeling sexual acts.

RAPE Sexual intercourse *q.v.* forced on one person by another. cf: forcible rape; attempted rape; statutory rape.

RAPE, FORCIBLE 1. Sexual intercourse *q.v.* by means of fear, force, or fraud. 2. Forcible sexual intercourse with a person who does not give consent or who offers resistance. ct: statutory rape.

RAPE TRAUMA An acute *q.v.* mental and emotional disorientation following a rape *q.v.* experience.

RAPE TRAUMA SYNDROME (RTS) 1. The emotional consequences that a rape *q.v.* victim experiences. 2. A pattern of response to rape that consists of an acute *q.v.*, disorganized phase followed by a defensive reorganizing process. 3. A set of symptoms exhibited by rape victims that may include fear, anxiety, guilt, shame, excessive sleeping, changes in dietary habits, etc.

RAPID EYE MOVEMENT SLEEP The dream stage of sleep characterized by twitching of the eyes beneath the eyelids. cf: REM sleep.

RAPID-SMOKING TREATMENT An aversive therapy *q.v.* technique (usually unsuccessful) in which the person is directed to smoke at a very rapid pace in order to create an unpleasant experience resulting in a reduced likelihood of further smoking.

RAPPORT Interpersonal relations characterized by a spirit of cooperation, confidence, and harmony.

RAPTURE OF THE DEEP Nitrogen narcosis *q.v.*

RAS 1. An acronym for reticular activating system *q.v.* 2. An acronym for reality-adaptive, supportive therapy *q.v.*

RASH A breaking out on the skin, either localized or generalized.

RAT-BITE FEVER A disease caused by a spirillum bacterium *q.v.* and spread by the bite of a rat.

RATE In epidemiology *q.v.*, a numerical statement of the frequency of an event obtained by dividing the number of persons experiencing the event by the total number capable of experiencing the event and multiplying the quotient by a constant number, such as 1000 or 10,000.

RATING SCALE A device for evaluating oneself or someone else in regard to specific traits *q.v.*

RATIONAL 1. The ability to reason. 2. The ability to choose the most efficient means to a given end.

RATIONAL CONCEPT A relationship between objects rather than the properties of the objects.

RATIONAL EMOTIVE THERAPY APPROACH 1. A method of therapy *q.v.* that assumes that people think irrationally and that this leads to irrational behavior. By encouraging more rational thinking, depression *q.v.* and anxiety *q.v.* can be minimized. 2. A cognitive-restructuring behavior therapy introduced by Albert Ellis. Based on the assumption that a significant amount of inappropriate behavior is based on what people tell themselves. The therapy attempts to alter a person's unrealistic goals.

RATIONALISM A philosophy that asserts that all human thinking must follow certain rules of logic.

RATIONALIZATION 1. A defense mechanism *q.v.* 2. In psychoanalytic theory *q.v.*, a mechanism of defense by means of which unacceptable thoughts or impulses are reinterpreted in more acceptable and thus less anxiety-arousing terms. 3. Establishing good reasons for unacceptable behavior. 4. A defense mechanism in which a reason is invented by the ego *q.v.* to protect itself from confronting the real reason for the action, thought, or emotion.

RATIONAL PSYCHOTHERAPY A psychotherapeutic *q.v.* technique by which the person is encouraged to substitute rational *q.v.* for irrational ideas in an inner dialogue.

RATIO SCALE An interval scale in which there is a true zero point, thus allowing ratio statements. cf: categorical scale; interval scale; ordinal scale.

RAUWOLFIA SERPENTINA Indian snakeroot shrub from which is derived reserpine *q.v.*, the first major tranquilizer used as an antipsychotic *q.v.* drug.

RAW SCORE The first score obtained in grading a test.

RAYNAUD'S DISEASE 1. A psychophysiological *q.v.* disorder in which capillaries, esp. in the fingers and toes, are subject to spasm. The disorder is characterized by cold, moist hands, accompanied by pain and may progress to gangrene *q.v.* 2. Raynaud's phenomenon *q.v.*

RAYNAUD'S PHENOMENON 1. A narrowing of bold vessels in the fingers due to constant heavy vibration. 2. Raynaud's disease *q.v.*

RBC 1. An acronym for red blood cells. 2. Red blood count.

RCRA An acronym for Resource Conservation and Recovery Act of 1976 (amended 1984).

RDA 1. An acronym for recommended daily dietary allowance *q.v.* of nutrients *q.v.* 2. Recommended dietary allowance. 3. Recommended daily allowances recommended by the National Research Council of the National Academy of Sciences *q.v.*

REACTANCE A negative emotional state resulting from a reduction in a person's freedom of choice.

REACTION FORMATION 1. A defense mechanism *q.v.* 2. A process in which dangerous desires are repressed *q.v.* and in which the person consciously advocates the opposed view or attitudes. May be expressed in a physical disturbance. 3. In psychoanalytic theory *q.v.*, a mechanism of defense in which a forbidden impulse is turned into its opposite.

REACTION SENSITIVITY Sensitization or tendency to perceive certain elements of a total situation as a result of acquired attitudes and previous experience.

REACTION TIME The interval between the presentation of a stimulus and the observed response.

REACTION TIME TEST A procedure for determining the interval between the presentation of a stimulus and the beginning of a response.

REACTIVE COPING A form of coping in which the person feels to be at the mercy of events or crises and either fights thoughtlessly or flees. ~ may lead to frustration, tension, fatigue, and stress-induced illnesses or acts of self-indulgence. ct: active coping.

REACTIVE DEPRESSION 1. Neurotic depressive reaction *q.v.* 2. Continued depression *q.v.* in the face of loss or environmental setback.

REACTIVE HYPOGLYCEMIA The lowering of blood glucose *q.v.* levels below normal after the ingestion of large quantities of sugar.

REACTIVE SYMPTOMS The secondary effects of organic *q.v.* brain syndrome. ~ involve changes in emotion, motivation, and behavior that result from the deterioration of cognitive *q.v.* abilities.

REACTIVITY 1. The tendency of a research measurement instrument or the researcher to influence the behavior or results under observation. 2. The phenomenon whereby the object of observation is changed by the very fact that it is being observed.

READINESS 1. In psychology *q.v.*, the developmental level at which a child is able to develop a particular skill. 2. The principle of learning readiness.

READJUSTMENT In education, a movement that emphasizes social usefulness and efficiency. It calls for schools to stress civic training and social responsibility in the curriculum *q.v.*

REAGIN 1. An antibody *q.v.* associated with many diseases. 2. A substance in the blood of those who have syphilis *q.v.* that provides a positive reaction on the Wassermann test *q.v.* 3. An antibody in the blood of persons with an allergy *q.v.* resulting in a positive skin reaction.

REALISM 1. A philosophy *q.v.* that holds that knowledge is derived from perceptual experience, that the physical world assists a person's search for knowledge. 2. In psychology *q.v.*, a philosophy that emphasizes the natural sciences and gaining knowledge through experiences.

REALISTIC LOVE Conjugal love. A type of love *q.v.* that is calm and based on information and interaction with the partner over a number of years. ct: romantic love.

REALITY-ADAPTIVE, SUPPORTIVE (RAS) THERAPY A type of therapy that focuses on the client assuming a productive social role and reestablishing personal relationships.

REALITY ASSUMPTIONS Assumptions that relate to the gratification of needs in light of environmental possibilities, limitations, and dangers.

REALITY: EROTIC, EVERYDAY 1. Erotic reality consists of the way the world is experienced when one is erotically *q.v.* aroused. 2. Everyday reality is the way the world is perceived when one is not erotically aroused.

REALITY PRINCIPLE An awareness of the demands of the environment and adjustment of behavior to meet these demands. ct: pleasure principle.

REALITY TESTING Behavior aimed at testing or exploring the nature of a person's social and physical environment. Often used more specifically to refer to the testing of the limits of permissiveness of a person's social environment.

REALITY THERAPY (RT) William Glasser's method of psychotherapy that seeks to lead people to stop denying the real world and, instead, to accept responsibility for fulfilling their needs for self-esteem *q.v.* and for giving and receiving love.

REAL SELF 1. The true or authentic core of one's personality *q.v.* 2. Pertains to the real or actual feelings, wishes, thoughts, memories, and fantasies that a person experiences without regard to the standards of society. The ~ is a major factor of personality.

REAR ENTRY A coital *q.v.* position in which the female is penetrated by the male from behind her.

REASONING The combining of old habits, knowledge, and concepts to solve a new problem.

REASONING AUTHORITY A person who asserts that something is true with logical explanations or rationale. ct: dogmatic authority.

REBELLION Renunciation of, or opposition to, authority.

REBOUND EFFECT 1. Paradoxical effect. 2. A state of agitation that develops when a person who has been dependent on a depressant drug experiences the opposite effect to that caused by the drug. 3. The reappearance of a drug-suppressed behavior after the drug is discontinued, sometimes to a greater degree than occurred prior to taking the drug. 4. Excessive congestion that results from the overuse of nose drops and nasal sprays.

RECALCITRANT A person who is obstinate in defying authority.

RECALL A task in which some item must be produced from memory. ct: recognition.

RECAPITULATION THEORY The now discredited view that in embryological *q.v.* development each organism goes through the evolutionary history of the species of which it is a member.

RECENCY EFFECT 1. In free recall *q.v.*, the recall superiority of the items at the end of the list compared to those in the middle of the list. 2. In attitude change, the tendency for the most recently received information to take precedence in a person's overall impressions or the object, issue, or person in question. ct: primacy effect.

RECEPTIVE FIELD The retinal *q.v.* area in which visual stimulation affects a particular cell's firing rate.

RECEPTIVE LANGUAGE DISORDERS Difficulty in understanding what others say.

RECEPTORS 1. Specific sites on or within the brain or other organ or cell to which molecules attach in order to produce a particular effect. 2. Specialized structures that respond to various stimuli such as heat, light, cold, and sound. 3. A specific protein *q.v.* on a membrane or in the cytoplasm *q.v.* of a cell with which a drug, a neurotransmitter *q.v.*, or a hormone *q.v.* interacts. 4. A specialized cell that can respond to various physical stimuli. 5. Locations at which neurotransmitters or drugs bind.

RECEPTOR SITE 1. A part of a cell that binds a chemical molecule to exert its biological effect. 2. Specific points within cells where molecules of a specific drug or other chemical fit.

RECEPTOR SITE THEORY The theory *q.v.* that a drug exerts its effect on certain parts of the body because specific receptor *q.v.* cells receive only certain body chemicals or drug molecules that structurally resemble them.

RECESSIVE GENE 1. A unit of heredity *q.v.* that is contrasted to the dominant gene *q.v.* 2. The gene that is masked by the dominant gene when both are paired. 3. The gene that can be expressed only when paired with a second, identical recessive gene. 4. A gene that can be expressed phenotypically *q.v.* only when homozygous *q.v.*

RECIDIVISM 1. The relapse or recurrence of a disease. 2. The return or relapse to a type of behavior, such as drug taking.

RECIPROCAL-ALTRUISM HYPOTHESIS Altruism *q.v.* that is based on the expectation that today's giver will be tomorrow's taker. cf: kin-selection hypothesis; alarm call.

RECIPROCAL CROSSES In genetics *q.v.*, a second cross involving the same strains but carried by sexes opposite to those of the first cross.

RECIPROCAL DETERMINISM In social learning theory *q.v.*, the continuous reciprocal interaction among a person's behavior, personality *q.v.*, and environment *q.v.*

RECIPROCAL INHIBITION The arrangement by which excitation of some neural *q.v.* system is accompanied by inhibition *q.v.* of that system's antagonist *q.v.* cf: reciprocal inhibition psychotherapy.

RECIPROCAL INHIBITION PSYCHOTHERAPY A conditioning *q.v.* approach to habit change using systematic desensitization *q.v.* cf: reciprocal inhibition.

RECIPROCAL INNERVATION The innervations of antagonistic *q.v.* muscles to provide for the relaxation of one muscle as the other contracts.

RECIPROCAL ROLE THEORY OF IDENTIFICATION The theory that sex roles are learned not through identification *q.v.* with same sex models *q.v.* but from persons who interact with boys and girls in role-differentiated ways.

RECIPROCAL STRETCH A flexibility technique whereby a muscle group is isometrically contracted immediately prior to passive stretching of their antagonists takes place.

RECIPROCATE To return feelings and attitudes that are expressed about a person.

RECIPROCITY (NORM) The expectation that good and not harm will be returned to those who have provided benefit.

RECIPROCITY OF PARENT–CHILD RELATIONS Mutual influence between parent and child. In contrast to views that influence is unidirectional from parent to child.

RECITATION METHOD A teacher-centered approach that requires the learner to memorize health facts that are recited to the rest of the class. It has very little value in indicating student comprehension.

RECOGNITION A task in which a stimulus has to be identified as having been previously encountered.

RECOGNITION MEMORY The capacity to discriminate new from old information. An indication of intelligence *q.v.*

RECOGNITION METHOD A method used in the study of retention *q.v.* in which the measure is the number of items recognized as previously learned when correct items are presented along with incorrect items.

RECOMBINANT DNA TECHNIQUES Techniques that involve the isolation of segments of DNA *q.v.* and inserting them into a host cell, which then replicate and are expressed as the host cell multiplies.

RECOMBINATION 1. The formation of new gene combinations as a result of sexual reproduction. 2. The new characteristics that are observed to be different from the traits exhibited by the parents.

RECOMMENDED DIETARY ALLOWANCE (RDA) Standards for the daily intake of certain nutrients: vitamins, minerals, and calories. cf: RDA.

RECOMPENSATION An increase in integration or inner organization. ct: decompensation.

RECOMPRESSION The action of compressing again.

RECOMPRESSION CHAMBER A pressure chamber so designed that air under greater than atmospheric pressure can be administered to a person. The ~ is used in the treatment of the bends *q.v.* and in conditions requiring administration of oxygen under pressure.

RECON 1. The smallest unit of DNA *q.v.* capable of recombination *q.v.* 2. In bacteria, the smallest unit capable of being integrated or replaced in a host chromosome *q.v.* subjected to the transformation process.

RECONDITIONING Conditioning *q.v.* after extinction *q.v.*

RECONSTRUCTION A curricular movement that encourages students to be change agents in society.

RECONSTRUCTIONISM An attempt to form a "perfect society" through teaching techniques associated with experimentalism *q.v.* and existentialism *q.v.*

RECONSTRUCTION METHOD A method of studying retention *q.v.* in which the items are presented in a scrambled order and the subject attempts to put them into correct order.

RECONSTRUCTIVE MAMMAPLASTY Rebuilding of the breast through plastic surgery *q.v.*

RECOVERY PERIOD OF DISEASE 1. The body has overcome the infectious agent *q.v.* and the disease is over, but the person needs time for the body to return to preinfection status. 2. Recovery stage *q.v.*

RECOVERY PULSE RATE The time lapse between the pulse rate at the cessation of physical activity and its return to normal.

RECOVERY STAGE The stage of a disease in which the body's defenses begin to overcome the disease. 2. Recovery period of disease *q.v.*

RECOVERY TIME The period of time it takes for a physiological *q.v.* process to return to its baseline after a response to a stimulus.

RECREATION Any type of activity voluntarily engaged that refreshes the person and is pleasurable.

RECREATIONAL SEX Sexual activity primarily for the pleasure it gives. Emotional involvement and intimacy are purposefully limited. ct: relational sex.

RECRUDESCENCE 1. The recurrence of symptoms following a period when a disease seemed to have been improving. 2. Relapse *q.v.*

RECTAL Pertaining to the rectum *q.v.*

RECTAL SPHINCTER 1. The muscle that controls release of waste material from the rectum *q.v.* 2. The anus *q.v.*

RECTAL TEMPERATURE The body temperature measured by a thermometer inserted into the rectum *q.v.* and retained there for 1 min or more. The ~ is usually 1° higher than oral body temperature.

RECTOCELE A hernia *q.v.* in females in which part of the rectum *q.v.* protrudes into the vagina *q.v.*

RECTUM 1. The lower part of the large intestine *q.v.* terminating at the anus *q.v.* 2. The most distal *q.v.* portion of the large intestine, beginning anterior *q.v.* to the third sacral vertebra *q.v.* as a continuum of the sigmoid colon *q.v.* and ending at the anal canal. 3. The end part of the large intestine through which feces *q.v.* are excreted.

RECURRENCE The return of symptoms of a particular disease, e.g., cancer.

RECYCLE To reuse specific materials.

RED BLOOD CELLS 1. The cells that transport oxygen. ~ contain hemoglobin *q.v.* Most of the hematocrits *q.v.* are ~. 2. Erythrocytes *q.v.*

REDISTRIBUTION In physiology *q.v.*, the process by which a substance, such as a drug, is distributed throughout the body from one area of concentration in order to achieve a uniform concentration systemically.

REDUCED CALORIE (ON FOOD LABELS) A food that must contain one-third less calories than the food it replaces. ct: low calorie.

REDUCED CHOLESTEROL (ON FOOD LABELS) A food that cannot contain more than one-fourth the cholesterol of the food it replaces. ct: low cholesterol.

REDUCING VALVE A device attached to an oxygen container to control the pressure of the oxygen delivered to a person. The ~ reduces the pressure from its very high storage level to one suitable for delivery to the person.

REDUCTION The gain of one or more electrons by an ion *q.v.* or compound by the addition of hydrogen or the removal of oxygen. cf: oxidation.

REDUCTION AD ABSURDUM In law, an interpretation that would lead to results illogical or not intended.

REDUCTION DIVISION 1. Heterotypic division. 2. Meiosis *q.v.* 3. During the process of meiosis, the point at which the maternal and paternal elements of the cell separate.

REDUCTION MAMMOPLASTY Reconstruction of the breast through plastic surgery *q.v.* to reduce its size.

REDUPLICATION One of the ways children simplify language by repeating a single syllable of a word in order to represent the whole word, e.g., "wa-wa" for water.

REFERENCE (DELUSION) Characterized by a person associating great meaning to insignificant events. cf: delusion.

REFERENCE GROUP 1. In social psychology *q.v.*, a group that provides a person with attitudinal and behavioral standards. 2. A group from which a person obtains his or her cues to behavior or attitudes. 3. People against whom a person judges himself or herself.

REFERENTIAL COMMUNICATION Communication that makes reference to objects or situations that cannot be experienced directly.

REFERRAL The sending or recommending of a person to a specialist for further diagnosis and treatment. Applicable to persons with a psychological *q.v.*, sociological *q.v.*, or biological *q.v.* malady.

REFERRED PAIN Pain perceived as coming from an area remote from its actual origin, such as the arm, elbow, or wrist pain felt in angina pectoris *q.v.*, or pain above the clavicle *q.v.* that is common in diaphragmatic pleurisy *q.v.*

REFLECTION A counseling technique whereby feelings are clarified by their restatement by the counselor.

REFLECTIVE TEACHING A concept wherein a teacher critically reflects upon the outcomes of his or her teaching efforts.

REFLEX 1. An automatic, unlearned response that occurs without conscious effort. 2. An inborn action. 3. A simple, stereotyped reaction in response to some stimulus. cf: reflex action.

REFLEX ACTION 1. An automatic response to a stimulus. 2. An automatic reaction during which a nerve impulse is transmitted from a receptor *q.v.* to a nerve center, such as the spinal cord *q.v.*, and outward to the effector *q.v.* without reaching a conscious level.

REFLEX ACTION DISCHARGE The continuation of a reflex action *q.v.* beyond the termination of the stimulus *q.v.*

REFLEX ARC 1. A nerve path chain composed of an incoming sensory neuron *q.v.*, one or more interneurons *q.v.* located in the central nervous system *q.v.*, and an outgoing motor neuron *q.v.* 2. The nervous route used in a reflex action *q.v.* consisting of an afferent nerve *q.v.*, internuncial nerve *q.v.*, and an efferent nerve *q.v.*

REFLEXOGENIC Caused by a reflex *q.v.* action.

REFORM MOVEMENTS OF THE 1980S Educational reforms initiated in the early 1980s in response to several national reports concerning the quality of public education.

REFRACTERY Resistant to ordinary methods of treatment.

REFRACTION 1. The process of determining and then counteracting the optical errors in the eye with eye glasses. 2. The bending of a ray of light as it passes from a medium of one density to one of a different density.

REFRACTIVE PROBLEMS Visual problems that occur when the refractive structures of the eye fail to perform properly so that light rays do not focus on the retina *q.v.*

REFRACTORY ERRORS An incorrect pattern of light ray transmission through the structures of the eye. cf: myopia; hyperopia; astigmatism.

REFRACTORY PERIOD 1. In sexology *q.v.*, a temporary state of psychophysiologic *q.v.* resistance to sexual stimulation immediately following orgasm. 2. That portion of a male's resolution stage *q.v.* during which sexual arousal *q.v.* cannot occur. cf: refractory phase.

REFRACTORY PHASE 1. In physiology *q.v.*, a period following stimulation in which a neuron *q.v.* is less than normally responsive to stimulation. 2. In sexology *q.v.*, a stage in males following orgasm in which further stimulation does not yield further sexual arousal *q.v.* cf: refractory period; relative refractory phase; refractory phase.

REFREEZING A process of internalizing a new behavior by a person. ~ is the third phase of Lewin's process of analysis of change or learning. Unless new attitudes are frozen, individuals, organizations, or communities may easily return to earlier, more familiar forms of behavior.

REGENERATION Replacement or restoration of lost parts.

REGENERATIVE PROCESS Any process that tends to restore the natural function of an organ or tissue.

REGIMEN A regulated scheme of diet, medication, exercise, or other activity designed to achieve certain ends.

REGIMEN SANITATIS A book by Roger of Salerno in the twelfth century. This book was essentially the first publication outlining the "rules for healthful living."

REGISTERED NURSE (RN) A person who has completed the required nursing program in an accredited college and who has passed state board examinations in nursing.

REGISTERED NURSE MIDWIFE A registered nurse *q.v.* who has completed postgraduate education in prenatal care and childbirthing and who is licensed or certified to practice midwifery *q.v.*

REGISTRATION Licensure *q.v.*

REGISTRY OF TOXIC EFFECTS OF CHEMICAL SUBSTANCES (RTECS) An information system that lists both acute *q.v.* and chronic *q.v.* effects of over 100,000 chemicals. It also includes data on skin/eye irritation, carcinogenicity, mutagenicity, and reproductive consequences.

REGRESSION 1. A defense mechanism *q.v.* 2. Retreating to an earlier level of maturity that is perceived as more secure in an attempt to cope with frustration *q.v.* or threatening situations. May be periodic and sporadic or may become severe and frequent. 3. An ego defense mechanism *q.v.* 4. In pathology *q.v.*, improvement in the symptoms of a disease or the subsidence of a disease process.

REGRESSION TO THE MEAN In statistics *q.v.*, pertaining to the measure predicted from another measure on the basis of a correlation *q.v.* less extreme than the measure from which the prediction is made.

REGULATION A rule or order of an agency made under the authority of a statute enacted by the legislature.

REGULATOR GENE 1. A gene *q.v.* that controls the rate of production of another gene. 2. A gene-producing repressor molecule for the control of an operator gene. 3. Regulatory genes *q.v.*

REGULATORY GENES 1. Genes *q.v.* that regulate the activity of other genes through the synthesis *q.v.* of a repressor substance. 2. Regulator gene *q.v.* ct: structural genes.

REGURGITATION 1. A backward flow. 2. Casting up undigested food. 3. Backward flow of blood through a defective valve.

REHABILITATION 1. The restoration to constructive functioning of one who has suffered a disability. 2. A goal of some forms of treatment, which is to teach a person recovering from certain diseases or disabilities how to improve functioning ability despite the presence of a handicapping condition. 3. A return of functioning to a previous level. cf: rehabilitation therapy.

REHABILITATION THERAPY Therapy *q.v.* aimed at restoring or maintaining the greatest possible function and independence of a person. ~ is especially useful to persons who have suffered from stroke *q.v.*, an injury, or disease by helping them recover the maximum use of the affected areas of the body. cf: rehabilitation.

REHFUSS TUBE A fine tube for studying gastric secretion or for nasal feeding.

REINCARNATION A theoretical process of rebirth in some other form of life.

REINFORCED MOTIVATION 1. The arousal of interest in a goal and the learning experience, enhancing the learner's ability to achieve. 2. Awareness of the need or desire. 3. Anticipation of achievement.

REINFORCED TRIAL 1. In classical conditioning *q.v.*, a trial in which the conditioned stimulus *q.v.* is accompanied by the unconditioned stimulus *q.v.* 2. In instrumental conditioning *q.v.*, a trial in which the instrumental response is followed by reward, cessation of punishment, or other reinforcement *q.v.*

REINFORCEMENT 1. In classical conditioning *q.v.*, the procedure by which the unconditioned stimulus *q.v.* is made contingent upon the conditioned stimulus *q.v.* 2. In instrumental conditioning *q.v.*, the procedure by which the instrumental response is made contingent upon some sought-after outcome. 3. The strengthening process that occurs during learning *q.v.* 4. In conditioning, the process of rewarding the learner for making an adequate response. 5. Anything that changes the probability that a particular response will occur. cf: reinforcement schedule. 6. The process of strengthening a behavior by rewarding it or by punishing a different, but related, behavior.

REINFORCEMENT SCHEDULE 1. The sequencing of rewards so that desired responses continue. 2. The rate at which a given response is rewarded or punished. 3. A schedule used to determine when rewards or punishments are given. cf: reinforcement.

REINFORCERS The consequences of a behavior that increase the likelihood that the same response will be made in the future.

REINFORCING FACTOR Any reward or punishment following a particular behavior. cf: reinforcement.

REINFORCING STIMULUS A stimulus *q.v.* that produces reinforcement *q.v.*

REINSTATEMENT A procedure for recovering a memory without having to relearn what is remembered.

REINTEGRATION A condition in which an element of an experience seems to reestablish the whole.

REJECTED SOCIAL STATUS In studies of social status in children's groups, those children who are high on social impact but low on social preference.

REJECTION In immunology *q.v.*, an immune *q.v.* response that causes transplanted organs or tissues to be attacked by the immune system *q.v.* of the body and to destroy the transplanted organ or tissue.

RELAPSE The return of a disease after the beginning of the convalescent *q.v.* period.

RELATIONAL SEX Sexual activity in the context of emotional involvement and intensity. ct: recreational sex.

RELATIONSHIP 1. In psychology *q.v.*, an interpersonal bond of interest, concern, or affection. 2. In statistics *q.v.*, correlation *q.v.*

RELATIVE DEPRIVATION 1. A person's perception of his or her status in comparison with his or her expectations. 2. In a broader sense, the notion that revolutionary activity is most likely to occur when high expectations are dashed.

RELATIVE ODDS In epidemiology *q.v.*, the percentage of cases that were exposed to the presumed condition divided by the percentage of controls that were similarly exposed.

RELATIVE REFRACTORY PHASE A refractory phase *q.v.* in which stronger than normal stimulation produces a nerve impulse. cf: absolutely refractory phase.

RELATIVE RISK In epidemiology *q.v.*, a ratio obtained by dividing the incidence *q.v.* rate of one group by the incidence rate of a second group.

RELATIVE SIZE A secondary cue to depth *q.v.* in which an object producing a smaller retinal image is seen as farther away than an object which is known to be of the same size but produces a larger retinal image.

RELATIVE THEORY A system of rules and principles that guide persons in making value judgments. ~ holds that humans invent values and test them to find which ones best serve society's interests.

RELATIVISM A philosophy *q.v.* that holds that there is a lack of universally valid conclusions as to which perspective on things, life, or events is better.

RELATIVISTIC ETHIC A system of values in which right and wrong are viewed as dependent upon the circumstances that exist at that time. cf: absolutist ethic; hedonistic ethic.

RELAXATION The reduction or relief of tension in the body.

RELAXATION RESPONSE 1. A physiological *q.v.* state of opposition to the fight or flight response *q.v.* of the general adaptation syndrome *q.v.* 2. The physiological opposite of the emergency response *q.v.*, characterized by reduction in metabolic activity and increased feelings of relaxation and calm. 3. A system of exercise designed to enhance a person's ability to relax and reduce vulnerability to stress-related problems.

RELAXATION TRAINING The use of various techniques to produce a state of relaxation or to relieve stress *q.v.* and tension.

RELEASING FACTORS 1. Hormones *q.v.* produced by the hypothalamus *q.v.* that control the release of hormones from the pituitary gland *q.v.* 2. In ethology *q.v.*, stimuli that are genetically *q.v.* programmed to elicit a fixed action pattern *q.v.*

RELEASING HORMONES Hormones *q.v.* produced by the hypothalamus *q.v.* and directed to the pituitary gland *q.v.*

RELEVANT 1. Important to today's society. 2. Connected with the matter at hand.

RELIABILITY 1. In evaluation, the characteristic of a testing instrument that yields consistent results each time it is used. 2. A criterion of assessing the scientific merit of observations. Reliable observations are able to be replicated and agreed on by multiple observers. 3. The consistency with which a test measures what it measures as assessed by the test–retest method *q.v.* cf: validity.

RELIEF 1. In psychology *q.v.*, pertains to a response *q.v.* conditioned to a stimulus *q.v.* associated with the termination or absence of noxious stimulation. 2. In law, legal redress or assistance sought by the complaint.

RELIGION A system of beliefs or worship that tries to interpret or explain the meaning of life and the standards through which people find the good life, sometimes listed as a source of values.

RELIGIOUS AFFILIATED SCHOOL A private school that is controlled by or financed by a particular religious denomination. Except in special circumstances, it is not entitled to tax subsidies or other governmental assistance.

RELOCATION CENTERS Temporary camps set up during World War II by the U.S. government for Japanese-Americans living in this country.

REM 1. Roentgen *q.v.* 2. A unit of the absorbed dose of ionizing radiation *q.v.* that accounts for biological effectiveness. 3. An acronym for rapid eye movement *q.v.*, stage of sleep.

REMEDIATION The development of alternative forms of function to replace those that have been lost or were poorly developed.

REMINISCENCE In psychology *q.v.*, an improvement in performance without practice. ct: spontaneous recovery.

REMISSION 1. The lessening of the severity of an illness or the absence of symptoms of a disease over time. 2. A decrease or disappearance of the symptoms of a disease.

REMITTENT Alternately decreasing and increasing.

REMORSE An emotion characterized by a feeling of distress and a sense of guilt.

REM REBOUND A phenomenon that occurs after a period of drug-induced suppression of REM sleep *q.v.*, where REM cycles reappear more often and longer than normal.

REM SLEEP 1. Rapid eye movement sleep. Dream sleep. 2. A period of desynchronized sleep during which dreams and eye movements occur. 3. Stage 1 sleep or light sleep. cf: active sleep. ct: REM rebound.

RENAISSANCE AND REFORMATION A period in Europe between A.D. 1300 and A.D.1700.

RENAL Having to do with the kidneys *q.v.*

RENAL DISEASE SPECIALIST A physician who specializes in the treatment of kidney diseases.

RENAL DISORDERS Diseases or injuries to the renal system *q.v.*

RENAL SYSTEM Pertaining to the kidneys *q.v.*

RENIN 1. A hormone *q.v.* produced by the kidneys *q.v.*, which is important in regulating normal blood pressure.

RENNET (RENNIN) A partially purified milk-curdling enzyme *q.v.* that is obtained from the glandular layer of the stomach of a calf.

REORGANIZATION The act of legally changing the designation of a school district, changing its boundaries, merging it with another district, etc.

REPEAT DRUGS Drugs that are manufactured with the same pharmaceutical *q.v.* properties as one or more drugs already on the market but are packaged differently.

REPETITION COMPULSION A Freudian concept pertaining to the neurotic compulsion *q.v.* to relive traumatic experiences.

REPETITION MAX (RM) 1. The maximum number of times that an exercise can be repeated within a specified period of time. 2. Maximum repetition *q.v.*

REPETITIONS 1. In weight lifting, the total number of times a weight is lifted within a set. 2. In exercise, the consecutive number of contractions performed during one exercise set. Applied specifically to strength exercises in which implements are used. A set should be repeated three times with suitable rest periods between.

REPLICABILITY In scientific research, the ability of one researcher to duplicate the findings of another. cf: validity; reliability.

REPLICA-PLATING TECHNIQUE A method of transferring bacterial *q.v.* colonies from a master plate.

REPLICATE 1. To repeat. 2. In research, to duplicate an experiment. cf: replicability; replication.

REPLICATION 1. Repetition of an experiment. 2. Duplication of an original experiment to determine whether the same results will be obtained by a different experimenter using different subjects but using identical techniques.

REPLICATION OF FUNCTION In the analysis *q.v.* of brain function, the circumstance in which the same behavior *q.v.* is subserved by more than one brain area.

REPLICON A self-reproducing chromosome-like structure.

REPORTABLE DISEASES Diseases that must be reported by physicians and hospitals in accordance with standards set by the Centers for Disease Control and Prevention *q.v.* They are botulism, brucellosis, chicken pox, diphtheria, infectious encephalitis, infectious hepatitis, gonorrhea, malaria, rubeola, meningococcal infections, mumps, pertussis, poliomyelitis, tetanus, trichinosis, tuberculosis, tularemia, typhoid fever, and typhus fever *qq.v.*

REPRESENTATIONAL THOUGHT In Piaget's theory, thought that is internalized and includes mental representations of prior experiences with objects and events.

REPRESENTATIVE SAMPLE Random sample *q.v.*

REPRESSION 1. Unconsciously preventing a threatening or painful thought from becoming conscious. 2. A defense mechanism *q.v.* 3. In psychoanalytic theory *q.v.*, a mechanism of defense by means of which thoughts, impulses, or memories that give rise to anxiety *q.v.* are pushed out of consciousness. 4. The exclusion of traumatic experiences from memory. 5. A defense mechanism that blocks awareness of impulses and deadens the memory of painful events. ct: suppression.

REPRESSOR MOLECULE A molecule *q.v.* produced by a regulator gene *q.v.*

REPRODUCTION 1. A curricular movement that emphasizes the need to mirror society's values in the public schools. 2. The formation of a new individual by vegetative or sexual methods.

REPRODUCTION METHOD A method of studying retention *q.v.* in which the subject must reproduce materials previously learned.

REPRODUCTIVE BIAS The belief that procreation *q.v.* is the sole purpose and justification of sexual intercourse *q.v.*

REPRODUCTIVE POTENTIAL A male or female who is capable of reproduction. This capability begins in puberty *q.v.* with menarche *q.v.* in the female and ejaculatory *q.v.* functions in the male, providing that ovulation *q.v.* takes place in the female and sperm *q.v.* production is adequate in the male.

REPRODUCTIVE SEXUALITY Sexuality *q.v.* that is centered in the structural, functional, and behavioral aspects of reproduction *q.v.*

REPRODUCTIVE SUCCESS The extent to which organisms are able to produce offspring who survive long enough to pass on their genes *q.v.* to successive generations.

REPRODUCTIVE SYSTEM The body system that consists of all the organs *q.v.* concerned with reproduction *q.v.*

REPULSION 1. The act of pushing or driving back. . 2. The opposite of attraction

RESCUE The freeing of persons from threatening or dangerous situations by prompt and vigorous action. There are three general classes: (a) heavy ~, activity that involves the use of complicated tools, equipment, and procedures; (b) light ~, a ~ activity by simple means and with minimum equipment; and (c) medium ~, a ~ activity using more specialized tools and equipment than are standard in an ambulance.

RESCUE TOOLS Cutting, prying, digging, and pulling tools used to free entrapped persons.

RESEARCH METHOD A learner-centered method *q.v.* that affords the learner an opportunity to develop a research design and to carry it through to a conclusion.

RESECT The surgical cutting away of tissue.

RESEGREGATION A situation following integration in which segregation returns.

RESERPINE 1. A major tranquilizer *q.v.* 2. A drug that reduces the functionality of some neurotransmitters *q.v.* and can produce depression *q.v.*

RESERVOIR 1. A stockpile or pool. 2. A ~ of infection may be a symptomless carrier *q.v.* 3. Any system, fluid, organ, or part of the body that can hold a drug for an extended period of time, allowing for gradual elimination from the body. 4. The place where agents *q.v.* of disease live and multiply.

RESIDENCY Postgraduate medical training that prepares one for practice in a particular specialty of medicine.

RESIDUAL Remaining.

RESIDUAL DISABILITY BENEFITS The benefit paid because of a reduction of earnings resulting from a disability.

RESIDUAL PAIN Pain that persists for 1–4 days after vigorous physical activity.

RESIDUAL PHASE A period following the active phase of schizophrenia *q.v.*, in which motivation, social interaction, and self-care are wanting.

RES IPSA LOQUITUR The thing speaks for itself.

RESISTANCE 1. In weight lifting, the weight to be lifted or the work load. 2. In psychoanalytic theory *q.v.*, the common tendency of a patient to use many kinds of behavior *q.v.* to avoid unpleasant topics. Also, a collective term for the patient's failures to associate freely and say whatever enters his or her mind. 3. The tendency to maintain symptoms and resist treatment or to uncover repressed thoughts or experiences. 4. In disease control, the ability of the body to fight infection through biological activity.

RESISTANCE (TO DISEASE) 1. The general ability of the body to ward off the effects of pathogens *q.v.* 2. Barriers to disease: (a) immune system (general), (b) mechanical (skin and mucous membranes *q.v.*), (c) body secretions, (d) acidity or the alkalinity of fluids, (e) phagocytes (white blood cells), the leukocytes and endothelial cells of the liver, spleen, and lymph nodes *qq.v.* cf: immune system.

RESISTANCE TO EXTINCTION The tendency of a conditioned response *q.v.* to persist in the absence of any reinforcement *q.v.*

RES JUDICATA 1. A matter judicially decided. 2. A matter finally decided by the highest court of competent jurisdiction.

RESOLUTION The subsidence of an inflammatory *q.v.* process.

RESOLUTION PHASE 1. The sexual response phase *q.v.* of loss of arousal. 2. The last stage in the human sexual response cycle during which the sexual system retrogresses to its normal nonexcited state. 3. The fourth stage of the sexual response pattern. cf: excitement phase; orgasmic phase; plateau phase; sexual response cycle.

RESORPTION The withdrawal of a chemical substance from a site in which it had initially been deposited.

RESOURCE GUIDE A listing of all the human and material resources available within the school or community that can be used as an aid in implementing the health program once it is developed.

RESOURCE PERSONS Parents, health providers *q.v.*, and others who can assist teachers, schools, and learners in the promotion of the school health program *q.v.*

RESOURCE THEORY The Foas' model of social exchange. ~ suggests that the set of classes into which the sources of all pleasure-giving activities fall may be limited and that there may be fundamental rules that govern the exchange of activities in the various classes.

RESPIRATION The exchange of gases within the lungs and body cells. (a) Internal respiration is the exchange of carbon dioxide for oxygen by protoplasm *q.v.* (b) External respiration is the entrance of oxygen into the body and the exit of carbon dioxide from the body.

RESPIRATOR A device for maintaining respiration *q.v.* by artificial means.

RESPIRATORY DISEASE A class of infectious diseases *q.v.* characterized by infection of the lungs and related tissues and organs. They generally follow the cycle of incubation, prodrome, fastigium, defervescence, convalescence, and defection *qq.v.*

RESPIRATORY QUOTIENT The ratio of the volume of carbon dioxide exhaled to the amount of oxygen inhaled.

RESPIRATORY SHOCK Shock *q.v.* induced as a result of an insufficient supply of oxygen in the body as a result of an inability to breathe.

RESPIRATORY SYSTEM 1. The lungs and related structures. 2. A system of organs *q.v.*, the function of which is to control the drawing in and breathing out of oxygen and carbon dioxide, respectively.

RESPIRE To breathe in and out.

RESPIROMETER An instrument used to measure carbon dioxide exhaled and oxygen inhaled. cf: respiratory quotient.

RESPONDENT In law, the person against whom legal action is brought, e.g., the noncustodial parent in a child support case.

RESPONDENT PAIN Pain with a definite physical cause. ct: operant pain.

RESPONSE Any measurable reaction.

RESPONSE BIAS A preference for one or another response *q.v.* in a psychophysical *q.v.* experiment, independent of the stimulus *q.v.* situation.

RESPONSE COST An operant conditioning *q.v.* punishment procedure in which misbehavior is fined through already earned reinforcers *q.v.*

RESPONSE DEVIATION A tendency to answer questions in an uncommon way, regardless of their content.

RESPONSE HIERARCHY The ordering of a series of possible responses according to the likelihood of their being elicited by a given stimulus *q.v.*

RESPONSE LEARNING 1. Learning *q.v.* the pattern of movements leading to a goal. 2. The proposition that mastering a maze is primarily a matter of ~. ct: place learning.

RESPONSE MODIFICATION When a response *q.v.* has already been conditioned *q.v.* to a stimulus *q.v.*, a new response can be conditioned to the original stimulus, thereby modifying the original response.

RESPONSE PREVENTION A technique of behavior therapy *q.v.* in which the person is discouraged from making an accustomed response that is used primarily with compulsive *q.v.* rituals.

RESPONSE SET A tendency to respond to test questions in characteristic ways that distort the interpretation of a person's performance *q.v.*

RESPONSE THEORY The theory *q.v.* that certain responses *q.v.* provide reinforcement *q.v.*

RESPONSIBILITY The obligation to perform assigned activity.

RESPONSIBLE DRUG USE The use of any drug in such a way as to minimize the risk of negative consequences of such use.

RESTING METABOLIC RATE (RMR) The metabolism *q.v.* that occurs while a person is at rest.

RESTING PULSE RATE A person's pulse rate *q.v.* while at rest. The normal pulse rate for a person whose fitness *q.v.* average is about 70 beats/min. The less a person is fit, the more likely the resting pulse rate will be higher. A physically fit person usually has a resting pulse rate below 70 beats/min.

RESTORATIVE REHABILITATION Treatments to return a person to his or her predisease or preinjury condition with little or no handicap remaining. cf: supportive rehabilitation; palliative rehabilitation.

RESTORIL A commercial preparation of temazepam *q.v.*

RESTRAIN To prohibit from action, to enjoin.

RESTRAINED-EATING HYPOTHESIS The theory that the oversensitivity of obese persons to external cues is caused by the disinhibition *q.v.* of conscious restraints on eating. cf: externality hypothesis; set-point hypothesis.

RESTRUCTURING A reorganization of a problem, often rather sudden, which seems to be a characteristic of creative thought.

RESUSCITATION 1. Artificial resuscitation *q.v.* 2. The techniques of using assisted breathing to restore adequate ventilation and external cardiac massage to support circulation *q.v.*

RETARDED EJACULATION 1. Ejaculatory incompetence *q.v.* 2. Sexual dysfunction *q.v.* in which a man is aroused but does not ejaculate. 3. A condition in which ejaculation in the vagina *q.v.* occurs only after a lengthy time period and strenuous efforts.

RETENTION 1. The amounts of previously learned material that are remembered. 2. The survival of the memory trace over some interval of time. 3. The ability to recall material previously learned. 4. The inability to void urine *q.v.* or feces *q.v.*

RETENTION PROCESSES In social learning theory *q.v.*, the information remembered from observation that can be replicated at a later time.

RETICULAR 1. Like a net. 2. Netlike.

RETICULAR ACTIVATING SYSTEM (RAS) 1. The system of nerve pathways within the brain that is involved in arousal. 2. A network of nerve cells *q.v.* and fibers extending from the spinal cord *q.v.* to the thalamus *q.v.* that control the level of arousal of the brain.

RETICULAR FORMATION A diffuse neural projection system that, in response to stimulation, arouses the cortex *q.v.*

RETICULOCYTE A young red blood cell *q.v.*

RETICULUM A network.

RETICULUM CELL SARCOMA A form of lymphoma *q.v.*

RETINA 1. The structure of the eye that contains the visual receptors *q.v.* and several layers of neurons *q.v.* farther along the pathway to the brain. 2. The light-sensitive layer in the back of the eye that contains the receptors *q.v.*, rods *q.v.*, and cones *q.v.* for vision. 3. The innermost of the three tunics *q.v.* of the eyeball, supported by the vitreous body against the sclera *q.v.* Its cells are continuous with and for the optic nerve *q.v.*

RETINAL DETACHMENT 1. A condition in which the retina *q.v.* becomes detached from the choroid *q.v.* and sclera *q.v.* 2. A separation of the retina from its pigment layer. It may be partial or complete and results in blindness when not properly reattached. Symptoms include sensation of lights flashing followed by the sensation that a curtain has been placed across the eye.

RETINAL DISPARITY The visual process whereby the two eyes receive slightly different images of the same object, which provides a very sensitive primary cue to depth *q.v.*

RETINAL EXPANSION A dynamic cue that signals when objects are approaching and when they are receding, providing a dynamic cue to depth.

RETINAL HEMORRHAGE Uncontrolled bleeding from vessels within the eye's retina *q.v.*

RETINAL IMAGE The image of an object that is projected on the retina *q.v.* Its size increases with the size of the object and decreases with its distance from the eye.

RETINITIS Inflammation of the retina *q.v.*

RETINITIS PIGMENTOSA A hereditary *q.v.* condition resulting from a break in the choroid *q.v.*

RETINOBLASTOMA A malignant *q.v.* tumor in the retina *q.v.*

RETIREMENT The act of leaving paid employment. The retiree, upon reaching a predetermined age, is usually provided some regular payment such as a pension and/or Social Security payment. cf: flexible retirement; mandatory retirement.

RETRACTOR An instrument used for holding tissues apart during a surgical procedure.

RETREAT, THE Built in England in 1796 and founded on the principles of providing a family environment for the mentally ill patients; there was emphasis on employment and exercise; and the mentally ill were treated more as patients than as inmates. cf: moral treatment movement.

RETRIEVAL The process of searching for some item in memory and finding it. When retrieval fails, this may or may not mean that the relevant memory trace *q.v.* is absent; it simply means that it is inaccessible.

RETRIEVAL CUE A stimulus *q.v.* that helps to retrieve *q.v.* a memory trace *q.v.*

RETROACTIVE AMNESIA 1. A memory deficit suffered after a head injury or concussion in which the person loses memory of some period prior to the injury. 2. Loss of memory for events prior to the person's accident. cf: anterograde amnesia.

RETROACTIVE FACILITATION The review of material or the discovery of new explicit relationships resulting in greater retention of a previous experience. ct: retroactive inhibition.

RETROACTIVE INHIBITION The interference effect that present learning can have on the retention of previously learned material. ct: retroactive facilitation; proactive inhibition.

RETROGRADE EJACULATION A backward ejaculation *q.v.* in males into the posterior urethra *q.v.* and urinary bladder *q.v.* instead of into the anterior urethra and out through the meatus *q.v.* of the penis *q.v.* It occurs in men with multiple sclerosis *q.v.*, diabetes *q.v.*, and some types of prostate *q.v.* surgery.

RETROLENTAL FIBROPLASIA (RLF) Scar tissue behind the lens of the eye, preventing light rays from reaching the retina *q.v.* Caused by the administration of excessive oxygen to premature infants. May result in blindness.

RETROPERITONEAL Behind the peritoneum *q.v.*

RETROSPECTIVE EVALUATION Used to assess how much learning has taken place and what experiences have been significant in establishing the individual's present health behavior. ~ provides information for judging a historical learning perspective.

RETROSPECTIVE RESEARCH DESIGN A method of measuring age-related change by using people's memory of events as data.

RETROSPECTIVE STUDY 1. A study of data from the past. Case–control study *q.v.* 2. Collecting information from people after they have contracted a disease in an attempt to discover the cause of the disease. 3. A method of research that investigates subjects' development, examining their histories by means of records and interviews.

RETROVERSION 1. The tipping of an entire organ backward. 2. Turning backward without flexion or bending of the organ.

RETROVIRUS A class of virus *q.v.* having the ability to transform their own genetic material into DNA *q.v.*, thus incorporating themselves into the genetic *q.v.* structure of an infected cell.

REUPTAKE A process by which a neurotransmitter *q.v.* is removed from a synapse *q.v.* by being taken back up into the cell from which it was released.

REVEALED-DIFFERENCES TECHNIQUE A study of family behavior by observing its members in a laboratory as they try to agree on an answer to a particular question.

REVERSAL DESIGN 1. An experimental design in which behavior is measured during a baseline period, during a period of treatment, during a period in which the baseline conditions are restored, and finally, during a reintroduction of the treatment. 2. A single-subject study in which the effects of treatment on a particular behavior are demonstrated by alternately introducing and withdrawing the treatment program.

REVERSE TOLERANCE An increased sensitivity to a drug the more or longer that it is taken.

REVERSE TRANSCRIPTASE The enzyme *q.v.* used by retroviruses *q.v.* to transform their RNA *q.v.* to DNA *q.v.*

REVERSIBILITY The ability to mentally perform and retrace an action or transformation. cf: operations.

REVERSION 1. A return toward some ancestral type or condition. 2. Atavism *q.v.* 3. The appearance of a trait expressed by a remote ancestor, a throwback.

REVERSION THERAPY Conversion therapy *q.v.*

REVIEW In education *q.v.*, a process of returning to knowledge previously learned, usually for the purpose of understanding relationships and significance to new knowledge to be learned.

REWARD In psychology *q.v.*, any satisfying event or stimulus *q.v.* that reinforces a response when it closely follows that response and increases the likelihood that the subject will respond in like manner again.

REWARD CENTERS Pleasure centers *q.v.*

REWARD TRAINING A form of instrumental conditioning *q.v.* employing a positive reinforcer *q.v.*

REYE'S SYNDROME A rare brain infection in children and adolescents that is more likely to occur as a result of the ingestion of aspirin *q.v.* when the child has a fever along with the flu *q.v.* or chicken pox *q.v.*

RFA (REQUEST FOR APPLICATION) An announcement from a funding source requesting applications for grant awards.

RFP (REQUEST FOR PROPOSALS) An announcement from a funding source for applications that may result in a contract and that describes the specifics of the projects being funded.

RHABDITIFORM A noninfectious *q.v.* feeding larvae found in many roundworms.

RHEUMATIC FEVER An infectious disease *q.v.* caused by a streptococcal *q.v.* infection (usually strep throat). Antibodies *q.v.* produced during the infection can cause inflammation of many body tissues, especially the inner lining of the heart. In addition, the conducting fibers of the heart may be affected, interfering with the transmission of impulses that control the heart beat.

RHEUMATIC HEART DISEASE 1. Damage of the heart valves as a result of rheumatic fever *q.v.* The heart's valves are unable to open and close as they should. 2. A chronic damage to the heart resulting from a streptococcal infection *q.v.* 3. A complication associated with rheumatic fever.

RHEUMATISM Refers to disease in the joints, muscles, bones, and ligaments and includes most forms of arthritis *q.v.*

RHEUMATOID ARTHRITIS 1. A chronic disease of the joints marked by inflammation *q.v.* of the membranes and atrophy *q.v.* of the bones. ~ results in crippling deformities. 2. A chronic *q.v.* systemic disease that involves the joints. ~ is characterized by pain, swelling, and tenderness. It may take the form of adult rheumatoid arthritis or juvenile rheumatoid arthritis.

RHEUMATOLOGY The medical study of rheumatic diseases *q.v.*; the diagnosis and treatment of inflammatory diseases and diseases of the musculoskeletal system *q.v.* cf: arthritis.

RH FACTOR 1. A type of antigen *q.v.* present in a person's blood designated as Rh positive or Rh negative. Incompatibility in parents' Rh factor may adversely affect fetal *q.v.* development. 2. A substance found in most human blood cells; therefore, most people are Rh positive. When a pregnant woman is Rh negative (does not have the Rh factor), her blood may develop antibodies to the fetus' blood.

RH INCOMPATIBILITY A condition in which antibodies *q.v.* form in the blood of a pregnant woman who possesses an Rh-negative blood type, destroying the blood cells of her Rh-positive baby, causing anemia *q.v.*, mental retardation *q.v.*, or fetal death.

RHINENCEPHALON Limbic lobe *q.v.*

RHINITIS Inflammation *q.v.* of the mucous membrane *q.v.* of the nose.

RHINOLOGY The study of disorders of the nose.

RHINOPLASTY The surgical procedure for reshaping the nose.

RHINORRHEA A running nose.

RHINOVIRUS A virus *q.v.* responsible for one form of the common cold.

RH NEGATIVE Having no Rh factor *q.v.* in the blood. ct: Rh positive.

RHODOPSIN A light-sensitive substance found in the rods *q.v.*

RHOGAM 1. The trade name for Rh_o(D) immune globulin. 2. A substance that prevents an Rh-negative *q.v.* woman from developing antibodies to the Rh factor *q.v.* in subsequent embryos *q.v.*

RHOMBENCEPHALON The hindbrain *q.v.*

RHONCHI Loud rales *q.v.*, esp. whistling or snoring sounds produced in the larger bronchi *q.v.* or the trachea *q.v.*

RH POSITIVE Having the Rh factor present in the blood. ct: Rh negative.

RHYTHM 1. A method of birth control in which a couple abstains from intercourse *q.v.* during the days in which the woman is most likely to be fertile *q.v.* 2. A procedure whereby the woman has coitus *q.v.* at times she feels she is least likely to conceive *q.v.* This time is determined by closely monitoring her menstrual cycle *q.v.* cf: rhythm method.

RHYTHMIC PELVIC THRUSTING A pattern of involuntary pelvic movements observed in conjunction with orgasm *q.v.*

RHYTHM METHOD A form of natural birth control *q.v.* involving a woman carefully observing her menstrual cycle to determine the time of ovulation *q.v.* Ovulation indicators may be mittelschmerz *q.v.*, changes in body temperature, changes in the consistency of cervical mucous, and/or spotting.

RHYTIDECTOMY The surgical procedure for a face-lift.

RI An acronym for remedial investigation.

RIB Any one of the paired arches of bone, 12 on either side, that extend from the thoracic vertebrae *q.v.* toward the median *q.v.* line of the trunk. cf: rib cage.

RIB CAGE The thorax *q.v.*

RIBOFLAVIN One of the water-soluble B vitamins *q.v.* ~ was synthesized in 1935 and is necessary for converting energy nutrients *q.v.* into energy needed by the body, and it contributes to healthy skin. A deficiency of ~ in children affects growth, results in the eyes becoming sensitive to light, and may impair vision. ~ assists in the metabolism *q.v.* of carbohydrates *q.v.*, amino acids *q.v.*, and fats.

RIBONUCLEIC ACID (RNA) 1. Similar in structure to deoxyribonucleic acid *q.v.* but with three nitrogenous bases *q.v.*: adenine, cytosine, and guanine *qq.v.* A fourth, uracil *q.v.*, is present, which is complementary to adenine. ~ functions in three capacities as (a) messenger RNA, which embodies the basic pan and order of amino acid *q.v.* molecules for the synthesis of protein within the cell; (b) transfer RNA, which passes out into the cell and, depending upon its nitrogenous base, picks up an amino acid molecule; and (c) ribosomal RNA, which combines with proteins to form the ribosome *q.v.* of the cell. 2. A nucleic acid *q.v.* found in all living cells. A hydrolysin ~ yields adenine, guanine, cytosine, uracil, ribose, and phosphoric acid *q.v.* Hydrolysis takes part in protein synthesis *q.v.* within the cell.

RIBOSE A 5-carbon sugar.

RIBOSOMAL RNA A function of ribonucleic acid *q.v.* ~ combines with proteins to form the ribosomes *q.v.* of cells.

RIBOSOME 1. The site of protein *q.v.* synthesis within a cell. Protein synthesis can take place only when all amino acids *q.v.* are available within the ~ of the cell. 2. Small cellular organelle *q.v.* that is the site for protein synthesis. ~s are found free in cytoplasm *q.v.* and attached to the endoplasmic reticulum *q.v.* 3. A ribonucleic acid *q.v.* containing particles in the cytoplasm *q.v.* of a cell. 4. Submicroscopic granules in the protoplasm *q.v.* They contain RNA and protein and are associated with protein formation.

RICKETS A condition characterized by improper development of bones and teeth resulting from a severe deficiency of vitamin D *q.v.*

RICKETTSIA 1. A microorganism *q.v.* smaller than bacteria *q.v.* but larger than a virus *q.v.* 2. A biological agent *q.v.* responsible for some diseases, such as Rocky Mountain spotted fever *q.v.* ~s are bacteria-like organisms that live inside other living cells. ~s are the cause of typhus fever *q.v.*

RICKETTSIAL POX Transmitted by mites carried by the house mouse.

RIGHT ATRIUM The atrium *q.v.* situated on the right side of the heart.

RIGHT TO REFUSE TREATMENT A legal principle in which a patient may decline to participate in unconventional or risky treatments.

RIGHT TO TREATMENT A legal principle according to which a patient must receive at least minimal treatment, in terms of amount and quality, that will provide a realistic opportunity for meaningful improvement.

RIGHT VENTRICLE The ventricle *q.v.* located on the right side of the heart.

RIGID CONTROL An ego defense mechanism *q.v.* involving reliance upon inner restraints: suppression *q.v.*, repression *q.v.*, and reaction formation *q.v.*

RIGIDITY 1. Extreme muscles tenseness. 2. A condition characterized by continuous and diffuse tension as the limbs are extended.

RIGID SPLINT A splint *q.v.* made from a firm material, either unbending or flexible, to be applied to an injured extremity to prevent motion at the site of a fracture *q.v.* or dislocation *q.v.*

RIGOR A chill.

RIGOR MORTIS Rigidity of the body that occurs after death.

RINGER'S LACTATE 1. A sterile solution of sodium chloride *q.v.*, potassium chloride *q.v.*, and calcium chloride *q.v.* in water for injection. ~ is given as a fluid and electrolyte *q.v.* replenisher by intravenous injection *q.v.*

RINGWORM 1. Tinea *q.v.* 2. A disease caused by a mold *q.v.* (fungus). Transmitted directly or indirectly by the mold or its spores. Characterized by circular vesicles *q.v.* and itching. ~ may occur on the feet (athlete's foot), head, face, or head.

RIPPLE EFFECT The tendency for innocent members of a group to feel threatened by the reprimand directed toward one or more misbehaving persons.

RISK 1. In epidemiology *q.v.*, the probability *q.v.* of a health-related event or outcome. 2. The probability of a negative occurrence as well as its severity.

RISK ASSESSMENT A technique of epidemiological analysis used to identify those specific subgroups within a population that have a higher risk *q.v.* of acquiring a given disease.

RISK BEHAVIOR A lifestyle that tends toward threatening health.

RISK–BENEFIT PRINCIPLE An ethical principle that requires that the potential benefits of research outweigh the risks to participants in the study.

RISK–BENEFIT RATIO A comparison of the value of a drug in treating or preventing morbidity *q.v.* with the hazards of its use, leading to a conclusion to use the drug or to find an alternative.

RISK FACTOR 1. Any activity or genetic *q.v.* trait that makes a person more susceptible or more likely to be exposed to infection, injury, disability, etc. 2. In epidemiology *q.v.*, a characteristic, behavior, or experience that increases the probability *q.v.* of developing a negative health condition. 3. Life styles or environmental conditions that can contribute to the development of some diseases. Behavioral risk factors include smoking, drug abuse, alcohol abuse, tension, and nutritional abuses. Environmental risk factors include polluted air, land, water, occupational health hazards, etc.

RISKY SHIFT The tendency for a group discussion to lead to more risky decisions than if the individuals in the group were making the decisions individually. Shifts toward caution are also possible.

RITALIN A commercial preparation of methylphenidate *q.v.*

RITE OF PASSAGE A ritualized custom of movement from one social class to another.

RITUAL Berne's term for a form of long-term coping that consists of shallow exchanges between people.

RLF An acronym for retrolental fibroplasia *q.v.*

RM An acronym for 1. maximum repetition *q.v.* and 2. repetition max *q.v.*

RMR An acronym for resting metabolic rate *q.v.*

RN An acronym for registered nurse *q.v.*

RNA 1. Ribonucleic acid *q.v.* 2. D-ribose nucleic acid. 3. A group of nucleic acids containing ribose *q.v.* and uracil *q.v.* that are associated with the control of cellular chemical activities.

RNA VIRUSES Viruses *q.v.* that contain RNA *q.v.* as their genetic *q.v.* material.

ROBERT WOOD JOHNSON FOUNDATION Established in 1972 with the objective of improving access to general medical and dental care. Additionally, 1. support for research to make health care arrangements more effective and care more affordable, and 2. support for research, development, and demonstration projects that show promise of helping large numbers of people avoid disabilities and maintain or regain maximum attainable function in their lives.

ROBINSON STRETCHER A split-frame stretcher *q.v.*

ROC CURVE A curve that shows the relationship between hits and false alarms in a detection experiment.

ROCKEFELLER FOUNDATION Chartered in 1913 for the purpose of promoting the well-being of mankind throughout the world. There are five divisions: (a) International Health, (b) Medical Sciences, (c) Natural Sciences, (d) Social Sciences, and (e) Humanities.

ROCKY MOUNTAIN SPOTTED FEVER 1. A disease caused by the bite of a tick that is hosting a rickettsia *q.v.* characterized by chills, fever, pains in muscles and joints, and a reddish purple skin eruption.

ROD–CONE BREAK In a curve of dark adaptation *q.v.*, the sudden increase in sensitivity that occurs after a few minutes. Reflects the transition from primarily cone *q.v.* vision to primarily rod *q.v.* vision.

RODS Visual receptors that respond to lower light intensities and give rise to achromatic *q.v.* sensations. ct: cones.

ROENTGEN 1. A unit of ionizing radiation *q.v.* 2. The international unit of X-ray and gamma radiation *q.v.*

ROENTGENOGRAM A Roentgen-ray photograph.

ROENTGENOLOGIST Radiologist *q.v.*

ROLE 1. In sociology *q.v.*, the behavior *q.v.* expected of a person by reason of membership in a particular group or the actual behavior performed in the fulfillment of a particular position. 2. The set of related responsibilities that depict the nature of the services health educators *q.v.* perform in society (Role Delineation). 3. A prescribed set of behaviors performed by a person, carried out consistently, and supported by the shared perceptions of the performer and others whose behaviors are affected by the role. cf: social role.

ROLE CONFUSION The lack of clear conceptions of sexual and/or occupational roles. cf: role.

ROLE DEFINITION A clearly defined description of the functions of a professional health educator *q.v.*

ROLE DELINEATION The process of clarifying the role performed by health educators *q.v.* through the specification of responsibilities and functions and the identification of requisite skills and knowledge.

ROLE DELINEATION PROJECT 1. Initiated in 1978 by the Bureau of Health Manpower of the U.S. Public Health Service for the purpose of identifying the role and function of health educators *q.v.* The project was subsequently taken over by the National Center for Health Education *q.v.*, identifying the skills and competencies for basic entry-level profession health educators. 2. A project whose purpose it was to define and verify the role of health educators and to develop materials for academic programs preparing health educators, as well as self-assessment tools and continuing education materials for practitioners. cf: role delineation.

ROLE DIFFUSION A wavering uncertain sense of identity.

ROLE MODEL A person who is used as a source of learning about some social role.

ROLE OBSOLESCENCE A condition pertaining to when the social role *q.v.* of a person is no longer of importance to the social group.

ROLE OF HEALTH A mission of health *q.v.* within a person's life cycle *q.v.*

ROLE PLAYING 1. A method of research or therapy *q.v.* in which a person is asked to assume a part or a role. 2. An experimental method used as an alternative to deception. 3. An educational method used in establishing health attitudes *q.v.* and behaviors *q.v.* 4. A training technique that involves acting, performing, and practicing. 5. A form of psychotherapy *q.v.* in which a person acts out a social role *q.v.* other than his or her own or tries out a new role for himself or herself. cf: affective learning.

ROLE SPECIFICATION The identified responsibilities and functions of a professional role *q.v.* which must be carried out through application of identified skills and knowledge. cf: role delineation.

ROLLER DRESSING A strip of rolled up material of variable widths used for bandaging a wound or other open lesion.

ROMAN CULTURE In sexuality *q.v.*, a reference to orgies *q.v.*

ROMANTIC LOVE An intense emotional feeling for another person based on self-constructed illusions *q.v.* about that person, limerance. ~ involves drastic mood swings, palpitations of the heart, and intrusive thinking about the person.

ROMBERG SIGN A tendency to sway when the eyes are closed and the feet are placed close together. The ~ is a diagnostic indication of locomotor ataxia *q.v.*

ROOMING-IN PROGRAM A program in which the mother is allowed to keep her newborn baby in her hospital room most of the day rather than in a hospital nursery.

ROOT 1. In dentistry *q.v.*, the portion of the tooth inferior to the neck and which extends into the jaw bone. 2. In anatomy *q.v.*, the end of the penis *q.v.* at the abdominal *q.v.* wall.

RORSCHACH INKBLOT TEST 1. A projective technique *q.v.* that requires the person to look at inkblots and describe what is seen. 2. The inkblot test, Rorschach Psychodiagnostic Inkblot Test *q.v.*

RORSCHACH PSYCHODIAGNOSTIC INKBLOT TEST A projective test in which the subject interprets 10 inkblots. Patterns of responses are analyzed as indices of anxiety, sexual conflict, hostility, and the like.

ROSENTHAL EFFECT The tendency for the results of an experiment to conform to the researcher's expectations unless safeguards are implemented by minimizing bias.

ROTATION The turning or movement of a body around its axis.

ROTE LEARNING 1. Verbal learning *q.v.* involving fixed mechanical sequences. There may be little or no attention paid to meaning or understanding. 2. Memorizing the sequence of material or events.

ROUGHAGE Dietary fiber *q.v.*

ROUND SHOULDERS A defect in posture in which the tips of the shoulders are drawn forward in front of the gravity line.

ROUTE OF ADMINISTRATION The method by which a drug is introduced into the body.

R-R LAW A law that states the relationship between two items of behavior *q.v.* ct: S-R law.

RT An acronym for reality therapy *q.v.*

RTECS An acronym for Registry of Toxic Effects of Chemical Substances *q.v.*

RTF (RESISTANCE TRANSFER FACTOR) Bacterial episome associated with resistance to certain antibiotics *q.v.*

RTS An acronym for rape trauma syndrome *q.v.*

RU 486 A chemical pill used induce early abortions.

RUBBER A slang expression for a condom *q.v.*

RUBEFACTION A condition of inducing increased blood flow and a redness to the skin, such as with a counterirritant drug.

RUBELLA 1. One form of measles *q.v.* caused by a virus *q.v.* and characterized by fever, skin rash, sore throat, and other symptoms, lasting from about 3 days to 1 week. ~ is most dangerous during the first trimester of pregnancy as it can cause miscarriage *q.v.*, stillbirth, or birth defects *q.v.* The disease can be prevented by inoculating females before they reach childbearing age; however, inoculation must be done at least 3 months prior to pregnancy. 2. German measles. cf: rubeola.

RUBEOLA 1. One form of measles *q.v.* caused by a virus *q.v.* and tends to last for 1–3 weeks. Characterized by nasal discharge, reddened eyes, swollen eyelids, fever, cough, Koplik's spots *q.v.* on the buccal *q.v.* surfaces of the mouth, and a red skin rash. 2. Red or common measles.

RUBIN'S TEST A procedure to check for obstructed fallopian tubes *q.v.* Carbon dioxide is inserted into the uterus *q.v.* to determine whether it passes into the abdomen *q.v.*

RUDIMENT A part or organ that is not fully developed.

RUFFINI CYLINDER A receptor *q.v.* thought to correspond to warmth.

RUGAE Wrinkles or folds.

RULE ETHICS Guiding principles used in all situations to arrive at moral decisions. These principles are believed exhaustive enough to be applicable to all situations.

RULE–ROLE ORIENTATION One of the three major theoretical perspectives in social psychology *q.v.* ~ emphasizes the ways in which shared rules or roles influence behavior over time. cf: behaviorist orientation; cognitive orientation.

RUMINATION 1. Regurgitation. 2. Rechewing of previously swallowed food. 3. Repeatedly dwelling in past events or problems that cannot be changed.

RUPTURE 1. A hernia *q.v.* 2. The tearing apart of tissue. 3. A break in any organ or tissue.

RV An acronym for residual volume.

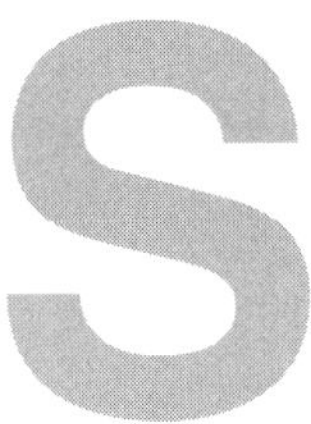

SABBATICAL A leave granted, usually with pay, after a teacher or professor has taught for a certain number of years to conduct research, to write, or to engage in professional development.

SABIN VACCINE A vaccine *q.v.* taken orally to immunize a person against polio *q.v.* cf: Salk vaccine.

SACCULATED ANEURYSM 1. An aneurysm *q.v.* characterized by a bulging on one side of a blood vessel. 2. The formation of a sac on the side of a blood vessel. ct: fusiform aneurysm.

SACCULUS The anterior *q.v.* sac of the membranous labyrinth *q.v.* of the ear.

SACRAL The triangular bone at the lower end of the spine.

SACRAL REGION 1. The lower part of the spinal cord *q.v.* that communicates with the genital area and controls the erection *q.v.* reflex. 2. Sacrum. cf: lumbar.

SACRAL SPINE 1. The finely fused vertebrae *q.v.* that constitute the sacrum *q.v.* 2. A part of the pelvic girdle *q.v.*

SACRAL IDEOLOGY A religious, spiritual view. ct: scientific ideology; secular ideology.

SACROILIAC Pertaining to the joint and ligaments *q.v.* between the sacrum *q.v.* and the ilium *q.v.* An area that is a common site for lower back pain.

SACRUM 1. The base of the spine formed by the fusion of fine vertebrae *q.v.* and located above the coccyx *q.v.* 2. The triangular bone just below the lumbar vertebrae *q.v.* 3. Sacral.

SAD 1. An acronym for seasonal affective disorder (depression) *q.v.* 2. A form of depression that occurs in some people during the fall or winter months, characterized by loss of energy, depression, need for additional sleep, and weight gain.

SADDLE BLOCK 1. A relatively common procedure used in labor *q.v.* to anesthetize the area of the woman's body that would touch a saddle. 2. Spinal block.

SADISM A sexual variance *q.v.* characterized by acts in which sexual pleasure and fulfillment are derived from inflicting physical and/or psychological pain on another person. ct: masochism.

SADOMASOCHISM 1. A combination of sadism *q.v.* and masochism *q.v.*, often involving the acting out of elaborate fantasies. 2. Both giving and receiving physical or psychological pain for sexual satisfaction. cf: sadism; masochism.

SAFE PERIOD The interval of the menstrual cycle *q.v.* when the female is presumably not ovulating *q.v.* cf: rhythm method.

SAFE RESIDUAL The point at which an oxygen cylinder should be replaced to avoid totally depleting its contents. The standard ~ is 200 psi *q.v.*

SAFETY An ever-changing condition in which one attempts to minimize the risks of injury, illness, death, or property damage to maximize success.

SAFETY EDUCATION An attempt to develop the knowledge, attitudes, and skills that will allow an individual to enjoy a maximum level of success with a minimum of risks *q.v.* ct: health education.

SAFETY ENGINEERING Measures taken to increase the safety of the work environment through the design of machinery and the environment itself through the use of protective procedures.

SAFETY NEEDS The need for security, stability, dependency, protection, freedom from fear, anxiety and chaos, and the need for structure, order, law, and limits.

SAFETY SIGNAL A stimulus *q.v.* that has been contingent with the absence of an electric shock, or other negative reinforcer, in a situation in which such shocks are sometimes applied. ct: contingency.

SAGITTAL 1. Like an arrow. 2. Longitudinal.

SALICYLAMIDE A pain-killing drug used to relieve mild pain in rheumatoid *q.v.* conditions or to reduce fever and inflammation *q.v.*

SALICYLATE The class of chemicals that includes aspirin *q.v.*

SALICYLISM 1. A condition caused by the consumption of large doses of aspirin *q.v.* 2. A condition resulting from the consumption of large doses of acetylsalicylic acid *q.v.*, characterized by nausea, vomiting, ringing of the ears, deafness, and headache.

SALINE 1. Containing or pertaining to salt. Saline solution *q.v.* consists of sodium chloride and distilled water, a 0.9% solution of sodium chloride. 2. A method of abortion *q.v.* in which the amniotic sac *q.v.* is filled with saline solution *q.v.* that kills the fetus *q.v.* 3. Saline induction *q.v.*

SALINE ABORTION Saline induction *q.v.*

SALINE CATHARTIC 1. Chemical salts that rush food through the bowels. 2. A laxative *q.v.*

SALINE INDUCTION 1. A form of abortion *q.v.* performed between the 13th and 19th week of pregnancy. It involves the removal of about 200 cc of amniotic fluid *q.v.* and replacing it with a saline solution. Labor is then induced and the fetus *q.v.* is expelled. 2. Saline infusion *q.v.* cf: menstrual extraction; vacuum aspiration; dilation and curettage; hysterotomy.

SALINE INFUSION 1. An abortion *q.v.* procedure used after the sixteenth week of pregnancy in which a strong saline solution *q.v.* is injected into the amniotic sac *q.v.*, triggering expulsion of the fetus *q.v.* 2. Saline induction *q.v.*

SALINE INSTALLATION 1. A means of abortion *q.v.* involving prematurely inducing labor by injecting a saline solution *q.v.* into the amniotic sac *q.v.* 2. Saline induction *q.v.*

SALINE SOLUTION 1. A solution *q.v.* of any salt, but usually referring to sodium chloride *q.v.* 2. A solution of sodium chloride and distilled *q.v.* water equal to 0.9% solution of sodium chloride. The human body fluids consist of 0.85% salt solution.

SALIROMANIA A sexual variance *q.v.* characterized by sexual gratification through damaging or soiling the clothes and/or body of a woman or a representation of a woman. A variance found almost exclusively in men.

SALIVA 1. A digestive *q.v.* secretion of the salivary glands *q.v.* ~ is the first digestive secretion when food is exposed to upon ingestion *q.v.* 2. The clear, alkaline secretion from the glands of the mouth.

SALIVARY AMYLASE The enzyme *q.v.* present in saliva *q.v.* that is necessary for carbohydrate *q.v.* digestion.

SALIVARY GLAND 1. Three pairs of glands *q.v.* in the oral area that secrete saliva *q.v.* 2. The ~s include the parotid *q.v.*, sublingual *q.v.*, and submandibular *q.v.*, as well as numerous small glands in the tongue, lips, cheek, and palate.

SALIVATION An excess secretion of saliva *q.v.*

SALK VACCINE A vaccine given by injection to immunize a person against polio *q.v.* ct: Sabin vaccine.

SALMONELLA 1. A group of bacteria *q.v.* capable of producing gastrointestinal *q.v.* disturbances in humans. 2. An organism associated with food poisoning *q.v.*

SALMONELLA TYPHOSA The causative agent of typhoid fever *q.v.*

SALMONELLA TYPHINURIUM A parasite *q.v.* of rodents and the causative agent of mouse typhoid and of food poisoning *q.v.*

SALMONELLOSIS 1. Infection by one or more of the *Salmonella q.v.* group of bacteria *q.v.* 2. Food poisoning *q.v.* 3. Inflammation of the intestinal tract *q.v.* by infection with *Salmonella*.

SALPETRIERE An insane asylum in France for female lunatics during the eighteenth century. It was here that Philippe Pinel ordered the chains and shackles removed from the patients, thus introducing the moral treatment movement. cf: Bicetre.

SALPINGECTOMY 1. Tubal ligation *q.v.* 2. Surgical removal of a fallopian tube *q.v.* from a woman. 3. A sterilization *q.v.* procedure in which a section of a woman's fallopian tubes are cut and the ends tied off, clamped, or cauterized so that eggs cannot pass down the fallopian tubes to be fertilized *q.v.*

SALPINGITIS Infection of the fallopian tubes *q.v.*

SALPINX 1. Tube. 2. Oviduct *q.v.*

SALTPETER 1. A diuretic *q.v.* ~ has a false reputation of being an anaphrodisiac *q.v.* 2. A common name for potassium nitrate.

SALT SENSITIVE A description of people who overreact to the presence of sodium in the body by retaining fluid resulting in increased blood pressure *q.v.*

SALUTOGENESIS The origin of health *q.v.* as opposed to disease *q.v.*

SALUTOGENIC MODEL A model *q.v.* that locates a person's position on the health/disease continuum.

SALVARSAN An arsenical compound used as a treatment for syphilis *q.v.* before the development of antibiotics *q.v.*

SAM An acronym for Sentence-Analyzing Machinery *q.v.*

SAMPLE 1. In epidemiology *q.v.*, a group of subjects selected for study that represents a larger group or population. 2. A subset of a population having common attributes or characteristics. There are two general forms: (a) random sample *q.v.* and (b) stratified sample *q.v.*

SAMPLE SIZE In epidemiology *q.v.*, the actual number of subjects chosen for study to be representative of a larger population.

SAMPLING VARIABILITY In epidemiology *q.v.*, the differences between the findings for all possible samples from the same or equal populations.

SANDOZ PHARMACEUTICAL COMPANY The first company granted permission by the Food and Drug Administration *q.v.* to conduct research into the possible medical uses of LSD *q.v.*

SANGUINE 1. Abounding in blood. 2. Hopeful.

SANITARY LANDFILL An area where solid waste products are systematically buried.

SANITATION Practices assuring freedom from agents or substances capable of causing damage to health.

SANOREX A commercial preparation of mazindol *q.v.*

SAPHENOUS VEIN The long vein *q.v.* near the inner surface of the thigh. The ~ is often tied off in the treatment of varicose veins *q.v.*

SAPPHIC LOVE Lesbianism *q.v.*

SAPROPHYTE Any organism living on dead or decaying organic *q.v.* matter.

SAPROPHYTIC Obtaining food from nonliving plants or animals.

SARCOLEMMA The cell membrane *q.v.* of muscle fiber *q.v.*

SARCOMA 1. A cancer *q.v.* that arises from connective tissues, muscles, bones, tendons, and ligaments *qq.v.* 2. A malignant *q.v.* tumor *q.v.*

SARCOPLASM The protoplasm *q.v.* of muscles cells.

SARCOPTES SCABIEI The itch mite. The cause of scabies *q.v.*

SAROLE STRETCHER A split-frame stretcher *q.v.*

SARTORIUS 1. Tailor. 2. A long muscle of the thigh. 3. The thigh muscle used to sit cross-legged as a tailor. 4. The longest muscle in the body.

SATIETY CENTER 1. The ventromedial *q.v.* region of the hypothalamus *q.v.* 2. The area of the brain that signals when a person's appetite is satisfied. ct: satiety value.

SATIETY VALUE A food's ability to satisfy feelings of hunger.

SATISFACTION DISORDER A sexual dysfunction *q.v.* in which people do not feel satisfied or pleasured as a result of sexual acts.

SATISFACTION PHASE The feeling of pleasure that accompanies and follows sexual climax. cf: sexual response cycle.

SATURATED FAT 1. Saturated fatty acids *q.v.* 2. A fat made up of compounds in which no further hydrogen bonding can occur. Primarily fats from animal sources. Usually solid at room temperature. ct: unsaturated fat; polyunsaturated fat.

SATURATED FATTY ACIDS Fatty acids *q.v.* whose carbon atoms contain all of the hydrogen possible. They usually come from animal fat sources. They are usually solid at room temperature, and if they come from animal sources, they are often high in cholesterol *q.v.*

SATURATION 1. In psychology *q.v.*, a perceived dimension of visual stimuli *q.v.* that describes the purity of a color, the extent to which it is rich in hue *q.v.* 2. In chemistry *q.v.*, the condition in which a liquid can no longer dissolve a solute *q.v.* at the particular temperature. ct: supersaturation.

SATYRIASIS 1. A male suffering from an uncontrollable urge for sexual gratification. 2. A sexual variance *q.v.* ct: nymphomania.

SAVINGS METHOD 1. A relearning method. 2. A method of studying retention *q.v.* in which the person relearns materials previously learned, and the measure is the amount of time or number of trials saved in relearning.

SCA An acronym for sickle-cell anemia *q.v.*

SCAB A crust formed by the coagulation *q.v.* of blood, pus *q.v.*, serum *q.v.*, or a combination of these on the surface of an ulcer *q.v.*, erosion, or other type of wound *q.v.*

SCABIES A skin infestation caused by the itch mite (*Sarcoptes scabiei q.v.*). Transmitted directly or indirectly, the mite or its eggs. Characterized by itching, with infestation around the waist, armpits, crotch, face, scalp, and arms.

SCALED BEHAVIOR A sequence of incrementally more intimate sexual acts that are followed by people within a particular culture.

SCALING A procedure for assigning value to a subject's responses. cf: categorical scale; interval scale; ordinal scale; ratio scale.

SCAPEGOATING 1. The directing of displaced hostility toward another person or group. 2. The process of blaming less powerful individuals or other targets, because the real cause of the frustration is unavailable or cannot be attacked. cf: displacement.

SCAPEGOAT THEORY The belief that one's own feelings of guilt and suffering can be transferred to some other person or group, thereby relieving oneself of personal stress or pressures.

SCAPULA 1. The flat triangular shaped bone in the back of the shoulder. 2. The shoulder blade.

SCAPULAR SPINE The prominent triangular ridge on the dorsal *q.v.* aspect of the scapula *q.v.*

SCARIFICATION 1. The cutting of the skin, often with multiple cuts, used in bleeding to expel "bad blood" or evil spirits. 2. In botany *q.v.*, the treatment of seeds to break down dormancy through the use of abrasives.

SCARLET FEVER A disease caused by a coccus bacteria *q.v.* (*Hemolytic streptococci q.v.*). Transmitted by direct and indirect contact with an infected person's nasal and throat discharges. Characterized by sore throat (strep throat *q.v.*), fever, nausea, vomiting, flushed cheeks, and sometimes a body rash on the chest and neck.

SCARLATINA Scarlet fever *q.v.*

SCATTER DIAGRAM 1. A graphic representation of a correlation *q.v.* 2. Scatterplot *q.v.*

SCATTERPLOT A graphic representation of the relationship between two variables *q.v.* 2. Scatter diagram *q.v.*

SCAVENGER CELLS Any of a variety of cells that have the capacity to engulf and destroy foreign material and dead tissues.

SCHEDULE OF REINFORCEMENT A rule that determines the occasions when a response is reinforced. cf: fixed-ratio schedule; random schedule.

SCHEDULE I SUBSTANCES Under federal law, substances that have no accepted medical use in the United States; e.g. heroin, LSD, psilocybin *qq.v.*

SCHEDULE II SUBSTANCES Under federal law, substances that have a high potential for abuse with resultant psychological and physical dependence, e.g., morphine, amphetamine, oxycodone *qq.v.* Available only by prescription.

SCHEDULE III SUBSTANCES Drugs considered to have less abuse potential than Schedule II substances. Available by prescription with limited refills.

SCHEDULE IV SUBSTANCES Drugs with less abuse potential than Schedule III substances but available only by prescription.

SCHEDULE V SUBSTANCES Drugs with less abuse potential than Schedule IV substances that may be dispensed by prescription or by requiring a pharmacist to maintain records according to state law.

SCHEMA According to Piaget, a mental pattern.

SCHEME 1. An organizational pattern of behavior or thought. 2. Intellectual structures manifested as recurrent behavior sequences.

SCHICK TEST A test to determine immunity *q.v.* to diphtheria *q.v.*

SCHISTOSOMIASIS A parasitic *q.v.* worm infestation that becomes imbedded in the bladder *q.v.* causing chronic *q.v.* irritation that may result in cancer *q.v.*

SCHIZOAFFECTIVE DISORDER A psychotic *q.v.* disorder in which a person exhibits schizophrenic *q.v.* symptoms accompanied by symptoms of depression or elation.

SCHIZOID PERSONALITY A personality *q.v.* or character disorder characterized by coldness, aloofness, and an avoidance of social contact or emotional closeness. The person is unable to express hostility and fearfulness, avoids competition, and has daydreams of being all-powerful. These people tend to be shy and withdrawn as children and become more introverted, reclusive, and often eccentric at puberty *q.v.*

SCHIZOPHRENIA 1. A psychosis *q.v.* with multidimensional symptoms, such as withdrawal, personality regression, and deterioration of emotional responses. Formerly, for diagnostic purposes, ~ was divided into seven distinct classic types. However, since ~ tends to transit from one type to another during various phases of the psychosis, psychiatrists today are reluctant to use these diagnostic classes. Some forms of ~ manifest symptoms that are gradual, resulting in personality changes characterized by extreme emotionality, lack of interest, and withdrawal. Other forms may manifest symptoms of delusions *q.v.*, silliness, regression, and catatonia *q.v.* 2. A group of mental disorders characterized by disturbances in thinking, mood, and behavior, accompanied by an altered concept of reality and possibly delusions and hallucinations *q.v.* 3. A particular type of psychosis characterized by highly unusual thoughts and behaviors. cf: schizoaffective disorder; schizophreniform disorder; schizophrenia spectrum disorders; brief reactive psychosis.

SCHIZOPHRENIA SPECTRUM DISORDERS Schizophrenia *q.v.* and related personality *q.v.* disorders.

SCHIZOPHRENIFORM DISORDER 1. An acute *q.v.* onset disorder with symptoms identical to those of schizophrenia *q.v.*, but whose duration is usually 2 weeks to 6 months. 2. A mental disorder similar to schizophrenia with a comparatively short duration, accompanied by fear, emotional turmoil, and confusion. Hallucinations *q.v.* are common but do not appear to be caused by stress *q.v.* cf: brief reactive psychosis.

SCHIZOPHRENOGENIC Causing or contributing to the development of schizophrenia *q.v.*

SCHIZOTAXIA According to Meehl, a possibly inherited neurological impairment resulting in an inability to integrate thoughts and emotions, resulting in the inability to cope with stress.

SCHIZOTHYMIC A temperament identified by Kretschmer, characterized by a person who is sensitive, eccentric, and reserved. cf: cyclothymic.

SCHIZOTYPAL PERSONALITY 1. An eccentric person who has unusual thoughts and perceptions, who is often socially isolated and, under stress, may appear psychotic *q.v.* 2. A disorder marked by schizophrenic-like disturbances in perception, thinking, and communicating but does not involve a break from reality.

SCHOOL-BASED CLINICS Programs and facilities that are available on school property to assist students in the areas of birth control, pregnancy, drug abuse, and psychological issues.

SCHOOL-BASED MANAGEMENT A concept of educational reform that advocates that individual schools be involved in decision making and that urges greater teacher participation in school governance.

SCHOOL BONDS A common method of funding a significant, one-time expenditure in a school district, such as a new school building.

SCHOOL/COMMUNITY COMMUNICATIONS A continuous process of informational exchange and direct interaction among all those concerned with health. ~ may take the form of locality development, social planning, and/or social action.

SCHOOL/COMMUNITY HEALTH EDUCATION ADVISORY COMMITTEE Composed of representatives from governmental and voluntary health agencies, civic and service groups, professional health associations, parent groups, and clergy. The ~ identifies health needs of the community, anticipates areas of possible concern in the future, coordinates the health education activities of both the community and the school, and establishes a system of effective communication.

SCHOOL COUNSELOR A professional in a school who provides counseling of students who need mental, emotional, and academic support.

SCHOOL DENTIST A licensed dentist who supervises the school dental health program.

SCHOOL DISTRICT An educational agency that operates public schools and contracts for public school services. A ~ usually operates under policies set by a board of education *q.v.* and carries out local, state, and federal mandates set by law or regulations. cf: local basic administrative unit; local education agency.

SCHOOL FINANCE The ways in which monies are raised, allocated to, and administered by the school district *q.v.*

SCHOOL HEALTH COMMITTEE 1. A representative group of persons from administration, faculty, and students, charged with assessing the school health program *q.v.* and making recommendations for improvement. 2. A fact-finding, recommending, and advisory group. ct: school/community health education advisory committee.

SCHOOL HEALTH CURRICULUM PROJECT Originally called the Berkeley Project, it began in the 1960s as an experimental project focusing on an in-depth study of the heart and circulatory system. It then expanded as an articulated curriculum plan for health education beginning in the primary grades *q.v.* and extending through high school. It is a highly structured plan of instruction for each health area, consisting of uninterrupted instructional phases focusing on each of the body's systems with respect to health and disease.

SCHOOL HEALTH EDUCATION 1. A component of the comprehensive school health program *q.v.* that includes the development, delivery, and evaluation of a planned educational program for learners in preschool through grade 12, for parents, and school staff, designed to positively influence the health knowledge, attitudes, and behaviors of the people involved. 2. All of the planned or unplanned methods, techniques, and strategies used by teachers and health educators to favorably influence the health knowledge, attitudes, and behavior of learners. Its elements include programs for elementary and secondary pupils, teachers, and other school personnel and community resources. 3. The health education process associated with activities planned and conducted under the supervision of school personnel, with involvement of appropriate community health personnel and the use of community resources. 4. Traditionally referred to as "health instruction" and is conceived as including planned instruction, correlated instruction, integrated instruction, and incidental instruction *qq.v.*

SCHOOL HEALTH EDUCATION CURRICULUM 1. The health education curriculum *q.v.* 2. All of the health opportunities affecting learning in the total school curriculum. cf: school health program.

SCHOOL HEALTH EDUCATION All of the planned or unplanned methods, techniques, and strategies health educators *q.v.* use to favorably influence the health knowledge, attitudes, and behaviors of learners.

SCHOOL HEALTH EDUCATION CURRICULUM GUIDE 1. Health education curriculum guide *q.v.* 2. The plan or framework for the health education curriculum *q.v.*

SCHOOL HEALTH EDUCATION STUDY (SHES) Directed by Elena Sliepcevich in 1961, ~ was part of the overall curriculum reforms efforts that resulted from the Sputnik launch by the Soviet Union. The ~ resulted in the conceptual approach to curriculum design *q.v.* in health education.

SCHOOL HEALTH EDUCATOR 1. A practitioner who is professionally prepared in school health education *q.v.*, meets state teaching requirements, and demonstrates competence in the development, delivery, and evaluation of curricula for learners in the school setting that enhance health knowledge, attitudes, problem-solving skills, and behaviors. 2. A person with professional preparation in health education, who is qualified for certification as a health teacher and for participation in the development, improvement, and coordination of school and community health education programs. cf: community health educator.

SCHOOL HEALTH GUIDANCE General assistance given by school health personnel (nurses, health educators, and physicians) to pupils and their parents to help them solve health problems that hinder students' ability to learn. cf: health guidance.

SCHOOL HEALTH PROGRAM 1. Consists of three traditional areas: health education, health services, and healthful school environment *qq.v.* 2. The composite of procedures and activities designed to protect and promote the well-being of student and school personnel. cf: comprehensive health program.

SCHOOL HEALTH SERVICES 1. That part of the comprehensive school health program *q.v.* provided by physicians, nurses, dentists, health educators, allied health personnel, social workers, and teachers to appraise, protect, and promote the health of learners and school personnel. These services are designed to ensure access to and the appropriate use of primary care services to prevent and control communicable diseases, to provide emergency care for injury and other sudden illness, to promote optimum sanitary conditions in a safe environment, and to provide concurrent learning opportunities that are conducive to the maintenance and promotion of individual and community health. 2. A division of the school health program *q.v.* 3. That part of the school health program provided by physicians, nurses, dentists, health educators, social workers, psychologists, and others to appraise, protect, and promote the health of students and school personnel. cf: health services; health and medical services.

SCHOOL NURSE A person trained and certified as a nurse but who functions within school health services *q.v.* Generally, this person does not function in a direct education capacity with the school but does act as a consultant/speaker and provides health counseling.

SCHOOL-NURSE-TEACHER An individual who is trained in both nursing and education and who functions in both health services activities and educational endeavors.

SCHOOL PHOBIA 1. An acute irrational dread of attending school, often accompanied by symptoms of physical illness. 2. An extreme fear of school and matters related to school.

SCHOOL PHYSICIAN A medical doctor who usually functions within the school health services *q.v.* component of the school health program *q.v.* This person may be employed by the school on a full-time or part-time basis. There are some instances where school health services personnel are employed by a city or county health department.

SCHOOL SAFETY PROGRAM Education and environmental procedures to ensure safe living of pupils and staff. The programs consist of the following: (a) teaching pupils how to avoid and cope with hazardous situations, (b) reducing hazardous situations in the school environment, and (c) teaching pupils and staff how to deal with and care for victims of accidents or sudden illness.

SCHOOL SOCIAL WORKER A social worker who works in schools to provide social services to students and their families.

SCHOOLS OF CHOICE A movement in large school districts to provide different types of instruction and/or programs and to permit parents to choose the school that best fits the needs of their children.

SCHOOL SUPERINTENDENT 1. The chief school administrator at the local level, usually appointed by the board of education *q.v.* 2. Superintendent *q.v.*

SCHOOLS WITHOUT WALLS A type of alternative education that stresses the involvement of the total community as a learning resource.

SCIATIC Pertaining to the ischium *q.v.*

SCIATICA Pain in the buttocks, hip, leg, or foot at the site of the great sciatic nerve *q.v.*

SCIATIC NERVE A major collection of nerve fibers arising from the lumbosacral plexus *q.v.* and subserving most sensation of the lower extremity and motion of the leg and foot.

SCIENCE 1. Seeking to establish general laws connecting a number of facts resulting in a possession of knowledge attained through study (research) or practice. 2. A systematically organized body of knowledge. 3. Systemized knowledge based upon observation and experimentation that is aimed at predicting the phenomenon studied.

SCIENTIFIC ASSUMPTION See assumption (scientific) *q.v.*

SCIENTIFIC IDEOLOGY A view of health phenomena from a scientific, clinical viewpoint. Used esp. in relation to sexual phenomena. ct: secular ideology.

SCIENTIFIC MANAGEMENT An approach to management that emphasizes the "one best way" to perform a task.

SCIENTIFIC METHOD 1. Principles and procedures for the systematic pursuit of knowledge, involving collection of data (facts) through observations and experimentation and the formulation and testing of hypotheses. 2. A rational fact-finding method of research to determine empirically the right method or approach. 3. A problem-solving method that follows sequential steps, including observation, formulation of hypotheses, predicting how the consequences of various changes in the system can be predicted, and testing to see if changes in the system yield predicted results.

SCIENTIFIC OBJECTIVITY The state of being unbiased by personal values, beliefs, or expectations in the conduct of scientific research.

SCIENTIFIC RIGOR Strict adherence to a protocol that specifies the experimental treatment in procedural detail.

SCIENTIFIC THEORY 1. An interrelated set of propositions that explain phenomena being examined and that can be tested by making logical predictions based upon them. 2. A conclusion based upon repeated experiments and observations that verify a particular hypothesis. cf: theory. ct: hypothesis; scientific law.

SCIENTOLOGY A mixture of philosophy, psychology, and special counseling techniques, the object of which is to bring the reactive or unconscious mind under control of the analytical or conscious mind.

SCLERA 1. The white, tough, fibrous outer layer of the eye. 2. Greek for hard.

SCLERENCHYMA FIBERS Elongated cells with tapering ends and thick secondary walls, usually nonliving at maturity.

SCLEROSIS 1. A hardening of body tissue, usually as a result of an accumulation of fibrous tissue. 2. Multiple sclerosis *q.v.* is the hardening of small areas throughout various portions of the nervous system *q.v.* cf: sclerotic changes.

SCLEROTIC Scar.

SCLEROTIC CHANGES Thickening or hardening of tissues. cf: sclerosis.

SCOLEX The head of a tapeworm that is adorned with suckers for attachment.

SCOLIOSIS A lateral curvature of the vertebral column *q.v.* ct: lordosis; kyphosis.

SCOOP STRETCHER A split-frame stretcher *q.v.*

SCOPE (OF HEALTH EDUCATION) The entire range of organizing elements considered within the discipline of health education *q.v.* cf: sequence.

SCOPOLAMINE 1. An alkaloid *q.v.* obtained from various plants in the nightshade family. Used medicinally as a sedative-hypnotic *q.v.* 2. An anticholinergic *q.v.*

SCOPTOPHILIA 1. A sexual variance *q.v.* characterized by the person gaining sexual gratification from viewing sexual acts and genitalia *q.v.* 2. Voyeurism *q.v.* 3. Inspectionalism *q.v.* 4. Slang: peeping tom.

SCORE In sexology *q.v.*, jargon for customers of hustlers or pimps *q.v.*

SCORE PROFILE Test profile *q.v.*

SCOTOMA A blind or partially blind area in the field of vision.

SCRATCH TEST A skin test in which a small scratch is made on the skin of the forearm by a small needle wherein a substance is placed to determine the body's reaction to the substance.

SCREENINGS 1. Relatively superficial evaluations of a person's health status designed to identify obvious deviations from normal. 2. A technology designed to select from a large number of people those individuals with signs and symptoms requiring further diagnosis and/or treatment. 3. In employment practices, a process by which applicants for a position are eliminated who do not fit the criteria for the job.

SCREENING TESTS Health screening *q.v.*

SCRIPT 1. A term often used in reference to a written prescription *q.v.* 2. In rule–role theory, the expected sequence of behavior that is appropriate in a particular situation. 3. As proposed by Gagnon and Simon, the differing cultural rules for sexual activities by males and females in the course of sexual development.

SCROTUM 1. A saclike structure of the male that is located externally in the pelvic area and contains the testicles *q.v.* 2. The pouch suspended from the groin that contains the male testicles and their accessory organs. 3. Bag. cf: tunica dartos.

SCUBA Self-contained underwater breathing apparatus used in skin diving.

SCURVY A nutritional deficiency disease resulting from severe and prolonged deprivation of vitamin C. It is characterized by general weakness, loss of appetite, rough and scaly skin with a brown color, spongy gums, and hemorrhages.

SCUTULA Concretions of serous secretions and debris that form at scalp level around hairs infected with *Trichophyton schoenleinii.*

SD 1. In statistics, standard deviation *q.v.* 2. In physiology, systolic *q.v.* discharge.

SDA An acronym for specific dynamic action.

SDE An acronym for specific dynamic effect *q.v.*

SDS 1. An acronym for Supplementary Data System *q.v.* 2. An acronym for a radical political group during the 1960s and 1970s: Student for a Democratic Society.

SEAT WORMS Pinworms *q.v.*

SEA-EPOCH-ENVI PROJECT An acronym for Southeastern Association for Education Physicians in Occupational Health and the Environment *q.v.*

SEBACEOUS GLAND A small gland in the skin that secretes oil, which helps to keep the skin soft.

SEBORRHEA An excessive discharge from the sebaceous glands *q.v.* that forms greasy scales or hard, cheesy-like plugs on the body.

SEBORRHEIC DERMATITIS 1. An irritation to the scalp caused by excess oil secreted by glands at the hair roots. 2. A disease caused by overactive oil glands and characterized by greasy scales on the body.

SEBUM 1. A secretion of fatty material from the sebaceous glands *q.v.* 2. A thick, semifluid substance composed of fat and epithelia debris from the cells of the skin. 3. Latin for tallow.

SECONAL A commercial preparation of one of the barbiturates *q.v.* Developed in 1930.

SECONDARY AMENORRHEA A condition in which a woman has ceased menstruating *q.v.* but had previously menstruated at least once. cf: primary amenorrhea.

SECONDARY ANORGASMIA Secondary orgasmic dysfunction *q.v.*

SECONDARY ASSOCIATION In epidemiology *q.v.*, relationships produced by confounding variables *q.v.* Indirect association *q.v.*

SECONDARY BACTERIAL INFECTION A bacterial *q.v.* infection that develops as a consequence of a primary infection *q.v.*

SECONDARY CARE Medical care involving a visit to a specialist. ct: primary care.

SECONDARY CAUSE The factor that contributes to a disorder but, in and of itself, would not have produced it. ct: primary cause.

SECONDARY CUE TO DEPTH A cue to depth perception that depends upon previous experience. ct: primary cue to depth.

SECONDARY DEFICIENCY A nutrient deficiency *q.v.* caused by some factor other than inadequate ingestion of nutrients *q.v.*, e.g., malabsorption. ct: primary deficiency.

SECONDARY DERESSION Exogenous depression *q.v.*

SECONDARY DESIRE DISORDER Hypoactive sexual desire.

SECONDARY DEVIANCE A sociological term for behavior that deviates from the norm and that is used as a basis for self-definition. ct: primary deviance.

SECONDARY DISPOSITION A peripheral trait of personality *q.v.* that appears in a limited number of situations.

SECONDARY EJACULATORY INCOMPETENCE Ejaculatory incompetence *q.v.* that occurs after a man achieves successful ejaculation.

SECONDARY ERECTILE DYSFUNCTION A condition in which a man is unable to achieve or maintain an erection long enough to engage in successful sexual intercourse although he has been able to perform adequately in the past. ct: primary erectile dysfunction.

SECONDARY EROTIC STIMULI Learned or conditioned stimuli *q.v.* that influence sexual motivation and behavior. ct: primary erotic stimuli.

SECONDARY HEALTH CARE Services associated with hospitalization. ct: primary health care.

SECONDARY HOMOSEXUAL A homosexual *q.v.* who has had heterosexual *q.v.* contacts but who has learned to prefer homosexual activity.

SECONDARY HYPERTENSION High blood pressure *q.v.* that results from a specific cause or pathological condition. ct: essential hypertension.

SECONDARY IMMUNE RESPONSE After repeated exposure to an antigen *q.v.*, an accelerated production of antibodies *q.v.*

SECONDARY IMPOTENCE 1. Impotence *q.v.* 2. A sexual dysfunction *q.v.* in which a man who has previously been able to achieve an erection is now unable to do so in some or all sexual encounters.

SECONDARY INFECTION An infection *q.v.* occurring in someone already suffering from an infection or from a wound that becomes secondarily infected after the wound was inflicted.

SECONDARY LABELING THEORY The hypothesis that the labeling of an individual can stigmatize the person in question, resulting in a limitation in learning, recovery, or rehabilitation. ct: primary labeling theory.

SECONDARY LEVEL OF HEALTH 1. A level of health characterized by people who have contracted conditions that when left untreated will result in disability or death. 2. Health status *q.v.* measured in terms of severe and permanent conditions. Persons falling within this level of health have developed progressive or permanent diseases or disabilities. ct: primary level of health; intermediate level of health.

SECONDARY MEMORY Long-term memory *q.v.* ct: primary memory.

SECONDARY OOCYTE Oocyte *q.v.*

SECONDARY ORGASMIC DYSFUNCTION A woman who has experienced orgasm *q.v.* in the past but is unable to do so at the present time.

SECONDARY PREVENTION 1. Measures taken after a disease exists to prevent further complications or new cases from occurring. ~ strategies include screening, case finding, diagnosis, and treatment. 2. Identifies diseases at their earliest stages and initiates appropriate treatment to limit the course and consequences of the disease. ct: primary prevention; tertiary prevention.

SECONDARY PROCESS 1. In Freudian theory *q.v.*, behavior *q.v.* that is reality oriented and under the control of the ego *q.v.* 2. Reality-based decision-making and problem-solving activities of the ego. ct: primary process.

SECONDARY REINFORCEMENT 1. Learned reinforcement *q.v.* 2. A reward that does not directly satisfy any need but has come to be satisfying in itself, usually as an association with a primary reinforcement *q.v.* 3. A reinforce paired with a primary reinforce designed to influence behavior after the primary reinforce is no longer provided.

SECONDARY RESPONSE A stronger response of the immune system *q.v.* following the invasion of an antigen *q.v.* into the body. ct: primary response.

SECONDARY SCHOOLS Schools that provide education to older students, usually in grades 9–12 or 10–12.

SECONDARY SEX CHARACTERISTICS The appearance of traits during adolescence *q.v.* that are typical for the mature sex of the person as male or female. Traits include larger breasts in the female, and facial and body hair and deeper voice in the male.

SECONDARY SPERMATOCYTE 1. Spermatocyte *q.v.* 2. The product of the second division of the mature spermatogonia *q.v.*, which will divide into spermatids *q.v.*

SECONDARY SYPHILIS The second stage of syphilis *q.v.* ct: primary syphilis; tertiary stage of syphilis.

SECONDARY WATER TREATMENT The removal of up to 90% of suspended organic matter from sewage water by the use of trickling filters or activated sludge aeration tanks where bacterial action breaks down most of the organic matter. ct: primary water treatment; tertiary water treatment.

SECOND-ORDER CHANGE 1. Change from outside the group that results in movement of the group to a higher logical type. 2. Change from one way of behaving to another way of behaving.

SECOND WIND A sudden relief from the symptoms of exhaustion, such as breathlessness, muscle fatigue, and rapid pulse.

SECRETAGOGUE 1. Causing secretion *q.v.* 2. That which stimulates an organ capable of secretion to secrete.

SECRETARY OF EDUCATION A cabinet level official in charge of the United States Department of Education *q.v.*

SECRETE 1. To separate from the blood or a gland. .2. To form a secretion

SECRETOR A person with a water-soluble form of antigen A or B, in which the antigen may be detected in body fluids as well as on the erythrocytes *q.v.*

SECRETORY CELLS Specialized cells within the breast that will, upon stimulation from specific hormones *q.v.*, produce milk.

SECRETORY PHASE The postovulatory phase *q.v.* The second half of the menstrual cycle *q.v.*

SECTOR THERAPY A type of goal-limited psychotherapy *q.v.* using associative anamnesis *q.v.* as a therapeutic *q.v.* technique for keeping the therapy focused on a particular problem area.

SECULAR DECLINE HYPOTHESIS The theory that the onset of menstruation has been occurring at an increasingly earlier age over the past century and a half.

SECULAR IDEOLOGY A world view of sexual phenomena. cf: sacred ideology; scientific ideology.

SECULAR TREND 1. In epidemiology *q.v.*, the trend over a period of time. 2. In social psychology *q.v.*, a systematic change in some characteristics of a population that is due to social changes rather than genetic *q.v.* changes.

SECURITY 1. One of the basic needs *q.v.* 2. The maintenance of conditions necessary to need gratification. 3. An inner feeling of safety.

SECURITY NEEDS Maslow's second set of human needs *q.v.* reflecting the human desire to keep free from physical harm.

SECURITY OPERATIONS According to Sullivan, behavior that one exhibits in order to remain safe in the opinions of others.

SEDATIVE 1. A drug that calms a person without inducing sleep. 2. A psychoactive drug that decreases excitation and anxiety as part of its general depressant effect. Higher doses may produce a hypnotic *q.v.* effect. 3. An agent that quiets nervous excitement. ~s are designated according to the part of the body or the specific organ upon which their specific action is directed: cardiac ~, cerebral ~, respiratory ~, etc.

SEDATIVE-HYPNOTIC 1. A drug that either induces sedation or sleep, depending upon dosage. 2. A class of central nervous system depressants *q.v.* that in large doses produce sleep. 3. In central nervous system *q.v.* depression, the chronic use of which could lead to a deterioration of psychomotor *q.v.* functioning, disturbed sleep patterns, and physiological *q.v.* problems.

SEDATIVISM A chemical dependence on sedative-hypnotic *q.v.* drugs, particularly barbiturates *q.v.*, minor tranquilizers *q.v.*, and ethyl alcohol *q.v.*

SEDENTARY 1. Referring to a lifestyle of those individuals who spend much of their time in passive work and recreation. 2. Inactive.

SEDIMENTATION 1. The settling out of solution. 2. A precipitate that has separated and settled out. cf: Erythrocyte Sedimentation Rate.

SEDIMENTS Fine particles of soil that are washed into a body of water, become suspended, and eventually settle to the bottom.

SEDUCTION Luring a person into sexual intercourse *q.v.* without the use of force.

SEGREGATION 1. In sociology *q.v.*, a clustering of people or activities based upon the sharing or presence of common activities or characteristics. 2. In genetics *q.v.*, the separation of chromosomes *q.v.* from different parents at meiosis *q.v.* 3. Separation of allelic genes *q.v.* when gametes *q.v.* are produced. 4. The separation of the paternal from the maternal chromosomes at meiosis, and the consequent separation of alleles and their phenotypic differences as observed in the offspring. Mendel's first principle of inheritance. 5. In psychology *q.v.*, a defense mechanism *q.v.* in which thoughts are made into groupings that have no basis in logic.

SEICUS An acronym for Sex Education and Information Council of the United States *q.v.*

SELF-REPORT BIAS A bias *q.v.* introduced into the results of a study due to either the participants' desire to appear normal or memory lapses.

SEX EDUCATION AND INFORMATION COUNCIL OF THE UNITED STATES (SEICUS) An organization dedicated to improving sex education in the United States.

SEIZURE 1. Petite mal and grand mal seizure *qq.v.* 2. A sudden violent attack. 3. An attack or the sudden onset of a disease, or of certain symptoms. 4. A convulsion *q.v.* 5. A cluster of behaviors that occurs in response to abnormal neurochemical *q.v.* activity in the brain. 6. In labor–management relations, a partial or total government takeover and operation of a business enterprise during a labor dispute.

SELECTION 1. In epidemiology *q.v.*, factors that influence the composition of the populations being studied so as to confuse comparisons between groups. 2. The isolation and preservation from a population of individuals with certain characteristics. ~ may be natural or artificial.

SELECTION PRESSURE The effectiveness of the environment *q.v.* in changing the frequency of alleles *q.v.* in a population.

SELECTIVE ABSTRACTION The tendency to overemphasize one detail out of context and ignore other important features of a situation.

SELECTIVE BREEDING 1. The method of study of genetic *q.v.* factors in which subjects with specific characteristics are mated together for the purposes of studying the transmission of these characteristics to the offspring. 2. A controlled breeding program in which mating pairs are selected on the basis of a shared phenotypic *q.v.* trait.

SELECTIVE EXPOSURE A way of obtaining information in which a person attends to data that support his or her choice or preference and overlooks data to the contrary.

SELECTIVE LEARNING Trial and error learning *q.v.* in which the subjects learn to select the correct response from among many possible responses.

SELECTIVE MORTALITY A possible confounding factor in longitudinal *q.v.* research in which less healthy people in a sample are more likely to dropout.

SELECTIVE SCREENING A health-screening *q.v.* procedure conducted on persons who are at high risk for contracting a specific health condition.

SELECTIVE SEXUAL BEHAVIOR 1. Minimizing the number of one's different sexual partners. 2. Avoiding sexual practices that carry a high risk of contracting a sexually transmitted disease *q.v.*

SELECTIVE SURVIVAL In epidemiology *q.v.*, the result of differences between those who die and those who live. Those who survive can have characteristics related to maintaining life that confound retrospective studies *q.v.* of health conditions causing mortality *q.v.*

SELF 1. A perception and awareness of one's own personality *q.v.* 2. Ego *q.v.* 3. The integrating core of the personality that mediates between needs *q.v.* and reality. 4. An individual's feelings about his or her own value as a person, formed early in life in the parent–child relationship.

SELF-ACCEPTED MORAL PRINCIPLES Moral behavior selected by a person as opposed to socially imposed moral and ethical codes or standards.

SELF-ACTUALIZATION 1. The highest level of personality *q.v.* development. A self-actualized *q.v.* person recognizes his or her roles in life and uses personal strengths and attributes to the fullest. 2. Development of one's potentialities. 3. Self-fulfillment *q.v.*

SELF-ACTUALIZATION NEEDS 1. The ways a person actually behaves according to the ways in which he or she is fitted to behave. 2. The need for emotional and spiritual growth. 3. Maslow's fifth set of human needs, including the desire to maximize potential.

SELF-ACTUALIZATION THEORY (OF PERSONALITY DEVELOPMENT) An inherent nature to pass through a sequential series of stages, progressing toward higher levels of motivation and organization. The most prominent of these are Carl Roger's self-theory; Abraham Maslow's self-actualization theory; and Rollo May's, Paul Tillich's, and Erich Fromm's existential theories.

SELF-ACTUALIZING The ongoing process of realizing one's potential.

SELF-ALIENATION A process of conflict between what a person is and what his or her real self is. ~ can occur when a person's self is markedly incompatible with the real self.

SELF-ANALYSIS Autognosis *q.v.* cf: introspection *q.v.*

SELF-CARE 1. Self-help. 2. A concept of health care stressing that persons can manage many of their own health problems when given sufficient instruction and appropriate medications. It teaches how and when to use self-treatment techniques and when to seek professional help.

SELF-CARE MOVEMENT The trend toward persons taking increasing responsibility for prevention or management of their own health needs and conditions.

SELF-CENTEREDNESS Egocentrism *q.v.*

SELF-CONCEPT 1. The idea, understanding, and feeling one has about himself or herself. 2. The impression a person forms about himself or herself, consisting of ideas, attitudes, and beliefs, usually in comparison to others. cf: authentic self. ct: self-esteem.

SELF-CONFESSION Autognosis *q.v.* cf: introspection.

SELF-CONTAINED AIR MASK A complete unit for delivery of air to a rescuer when entering contaminated areas. The unit has a tight-fitting mask, controls, and an air supply.

SELF-CONTAINED CLASSROOM A classroom organization wherein students remain in the same room with the same teacher all day.

SELF-DIRECTED LEARNING A method closely akin to individualized learning *q.v.* Its primary purpose is to provide a means for learners not only to proceed at their own pace but to offer a variety of learning options under the guidance of a teacher. It is a learner-centered *q.v.* approach.

SELF-DISCLOSURE The revelation of oneself to another.

SELF-DEVALUATION The lowered feelings of worth and self-esteem *q.v.*

SELF-DIFFERENTIATION The degree to which a person achieves a sense of unique identity apart from the group or other people.

SELF-EFFICACY 1. A feeling that a person has that he or she can successfully achieve a particular goal. 2. Agency *q.v.* 3. Personal agency *q.v.*

SELF-ESTEEM 1. The confidence and satisfaction one has of himself or herself. 2. A feeling of personal worth. ct: self-concept.

SELF-EVALUATION 1. The way in which a person views himself or herself. 2. A person's sense of worth or adequacy.

SELF-FULFILLING PROPHECY 1. Acting in ways that tend to make one's expectations come true. 2. Merton's term for a belief, that when put into action, causes the belief to come true. 3. Pygmalion effect *q.v.* 4. In research, the phenomenon in which the experimenter conveys an expectation that directly influences the subject's behavior.

SELF-FULFILLING PROPHECY EFFECT When children's performance matches what someone expects of them.

SELF-FULFILLMENT Self-actualization *q.v.*

SELF-HANDICAPPING The process by which a person who is threatened with failure makes tasks more difficult in order to have an excuse for failing.

SELF-HELP Self-care *q.v.*

SELF-HELP GROUP Individuals with a common problem who come together periodically to assist each other in dealing with the problem.

SELF-IDEAL Ego-ideal *q.v.*

SELF-IDENTITY 1. Self-concept *q.v.* 2. Self-esteem *q.v.*

SELF-IMAGE 1. Self-concept *q.v.* 2. Self-esteem *q.v.*

SELF-INSIGHT Understanding oneself. Self-esteem *q.v.* cf: self-concept.

SELF-INSTRUCTIONAL DEVICE A term used to include instructional materials that can be used by the student.

SELF-INVENTORIES Instruments designed to require the learners to provide information about themselves.

SELF-LIMITING CONDITION 1. A disease condition, usually of minor nature, that tends to run its course to recovery without treatment. 2. Capable of not progressing beyond a specific point. Self-correcting.

SELF-MEDICATION 1. Purchasing, using, administering drugs to oneself without the advice of a physician, dentist, or pharmacist. 2. The practice of treating oneself with medications for the relief of symptoms, usually associated with minor diseases or disorders.

SELF-MONITORING 1. Snyder's concept summarizing the key factors that influence a person's ability to manage social relationships. 2. In behavioral assessment *q.v.*, a procedure in which the individual observes and reports certain aspects of his or her own behavior, thoughts, or emotions.

SELF-PERCEPTION THEORY The assertion that people do not know themselves directly, but rather infer their own states and dispositions by an attribution process analogous to that they use when trying to explain the behavior of other persons. cf: attribution theory.

SELF-PSYCHOLOGY Kohut's variant of psychoanalysis *q.v.*, in which the focus is on the development of a person's self-worth from acceptance and nurturance by key figures in childhood.

SELF-RECRIMINATION 1. Self-condemnation and blame. 2. Accepting one's fault or guilt.

SELF-SERVING BIAS The tendency to see oneself as the cause of one's success but to attribute failure to external sources.

SELF-SUFFICIENCY The capability of mating one's needs within the context of existing environmental circumstances. The quality of one's health influences ~.

SELF-THEORY The personality theory *q.v.* that uses the self-concept *q.v.* as the integrating core of personality *q.v.* organization and function.

SELF-UNDERSTANDING 1. Self-concept *q.v.* 2. Self-insight *q.v.*

SELLA TURCICA 1. A saddle-like prominence on the upper surface of the sphenoid bone in which the hypophysis lies. 2. Turkish saddle. 3. A saddle-shaped depression in the sphenoid bone *q.v.*

SEMANS' TECHNIQUE A method developed by Semans for treating premature ejaculation *q.v.* in which the male signals his partner to stop stimulation when he feels the urge to ejaculate and signals when it is time to resume stimulation.

SEMANTIC DIFFERENTIAL 1. A self-report inventory requiring the respondent to rate each concept in one of seven positions between a number of polar objectives. 2. An instrument based on the scales designed by Osgood, Suci, and Tannenbaum as a means of measuring attitudes toward specific concepts.

SEMANTIC FEATURE The smallest significant unit of meaning within a word. cf: semantic memory; semantics.

SEMANTIC GENERALIZATION A form of mediated generalization *q.v.* that occurs because of similarity in meaning between the original conditioned stimulus *q.v.* and the new test stimulus *q.v.*

SEMANTIC INTEGRATION Incorporation of new information into the context of what a person already knows.

SEMANTIC MEMORY 1. Memory as knowing. 2. The entire body of meaningful information a person knows. 3. The component of generic memory *q.v.* that concerns the meaning of words and concepts. cf: long-term memory; semantic feature; semantics.

SEMANTIC RECODING In reading, the process of translation from spelling to meanings.

SEMANTIC RULES Rules in grammar that have to do with meaning.

SEMANTICS The organization of meaning in language. cf: semantic features; semantic memory.

SEMEIOLOGY Symptomatology *q.v.*

SEMEN 1. The product of the male reproductive organs consisting of spermatozoa *q.v.* and fluid secretions from the prostate gland *q.v.* and other reproductive glands. 2. Seminal fluid *q.v.* 3. Seminal emission *q.v.* 4. Latin for seed.

SEMEN ANALYSIS Testing the ejaculate *q.v.* for the number of sperm *q.v.*, the sperm's mobility, and the amount of fructose. The purpose of ~ is to determine the cause of infertility *q.v.*

SEMICIRCULAR CANAL Curved tubular canals in the inner ear that are concerned with equilibrium.

SEMICONSCIOUS Partly conscious *q.v.*

SEMILUNAR Half-moon shaped.

SEMILUNAR VALVE A half-moon shaped valve located in the main arteries that prevents blood from flowing back into the heart ventricles *q.v.*

SEMINAL DUCT Vas deferens *q.v.*

SEMINAL EMISSION Seminal fluid *q.v.*

SEMINAL FLUID Male reproductive fluid consisting of sperm *q.v.* and secretions from the seminal vesicles *q.v.* and prostate gland *q.v.* It is ejaculated through the penis *q.v.* upon reaching orgasm *q.v.*

SEMINAL VESICLE 1. A male gland *q.v.* located at the superior end of the vas deferens *q.v.*, the primary source of the fluid of the semen *q.v.* 2. Secondary male sex organ, a pair of sacs located on both sides of the urinary bladder *q.v.* that contribute substances and fluid to the ejaculate *q.v.* 3. Two pouches in the male, on each side of the prostate *q.v.*, behind the urinary bladder, that are attached to and open into the sperm ducts *q.v.* 4. A part of the male's internal genitalia *q.v.* that secrete nutrients to help sperm become motile.

SEMINIFEROUS TUBULES A network of tubelike structures in the testicles *q.v.* in which sperm *q.v.* development takes place.

SEMIOTIC FUNCTION 1. The ability to represent aspects of one's experiences either in private images or in public codes. 2. Symbolic functions.

SELECT SENATE COMMITTEE ON NUTRITION AND HUMAN NEEDS In 1977, the ~ released its report on the dietary goals *q.v.* for the United States.

SENATE A legislative body, usually the upper house of a legislature.

SENESCENCE 1. Aging and the deterioration of the body resulting from growing old. 2. The normal process of growing old, a process that occurs continuously at every biological level: cellular, tissue, organs, systems, and organism.

SENILE DEMENTIA 1. An outdated term for dementia *q.v.* Previously, dementia was thought to be part of the normal aging process, but today we know that most people do not become demented as they grow older and that dementia, when it occurs, is due to some specific disease process. 2. Deterioration of the central nervous system *q.v.* in old age. 3. A disorder brought on by progressive deterioration of the brain, marked by memory loss, inability to think abstractly, poor personal hygiene, and disorientation.

SENILE PLAQUES Spherical formations consisting mostly of degenerated brain cells that impede circulation in the brain arteries *q.v.*, caused by cerebral arteriosclerosis *q.v.*

SENILE PSYCHOSIS A mental illness usually occurring in old age and caused by cerebral atherosclerosis *q.v.* or arteriosclerosis *q.v.* impairing the flow of blood to the brain. cf: senility.

SENILITY 1. An obsolete term referring to abnormal deterioration in the mental functions of old people. 2. The deterioration of mental processes, especially as related to senescence *q.v.* 3. Senile psychosis *q.v.*

SENIOR CENTER A community facility for the elderly. ~s provide a variety of activities for their members, including any combination of recreational, educational, cultural, or social events. Some centers offer nutritious meals and limited health care services.

SENSATE FOCUS 1. A series of touching exercises for couples in sex therapy to teach nonverbal communication and reduce sexual anxiety. 2. Pleasuring. 3. A therapeutic technique emphasizing the sense of touch in which bodily surfaces are gently, manually explored by self or partner to reestablish the sensual reactions of childhood. 4. Sex exercise for couples in which they engage in nongenital touching.

SENSATION 1. The primitive experiences that the senses give. 2. The conscious experience of a sensory event, such as touch, sight, smell, and sound.

SENSE OF WELL-BEING A subjective, positive feeling resulting from an assessment of the progress being made in controlling the course that life is taking.

SENSE ORGANS Nerve endings that receive stimuli and transmit impulses to the brain for interpretation (perception *q.v.*). There are five such ~: 1. touch, temperature, pressure, pain; 2. smell, odors; 3. taste; 4. sight; and 5. hearing.

SENSITIVE PERIOD 1. A period of development when a form of behavior occurs most readily. 2. A period of development when an organism is particularly susceptible to the effects of specific experiences. ct: critical periods.

SENSITIVITY In epidemiology *q.v.*, related to tests of validity *q.v.* The percent of all cases that are identified correctly. ct: specificity.

SENSITIVITY (ENCOUNTER) GROUP A small group of people who spend a period of time together both for therapy and for educational experiences. Participants are encouraged to examine their interpersonal functioning and their overlooked or repressed feelings about themselves and others.

SENSITIVITY TRAINING 1. The process of learning to be increasingly sensitive to a stimulus *q.v.*, often the feelings and emotions of others. 2. A group-behavior approach in which participants learn about themselves and how to relate to others.

SENSITIZATION The development of allergic *q.v.* reactions to particular products or substances.

SENSOR An acronym for Sentinel Event Notification System for Occupational Risks.

SENSORIMOTOR PERIOD 1. A developmental period from birth to 2 years of age, characterized by learning through the senses and motor activities. 2. Piaget's first major period of intellectual growth. cf: object constancy.

SENSORINEURAL DEAFNESS Perception deafness *q.v.*

SENSORINEURAL HEARING LOSS 1. A hearing loss resulting from an abnormal sense organ (inner ear) and a damaged auditory nerve. 2. Perception deafness *q.v.*

SENSOR RECEPTORS Structures in the nervous system *q.v.* found in the eyes, ears, nose, and skin that transmit messages to the brain relative to environmental conditions or stimuli.

SENSORY ADAPTATION The decline in sensitivity found in most sensory systems after continuous exposure to the same stimulus.

SENSORY-AWARENESS PROCEDURES Techniques that help people tune into their feelings and sensations, e.g., sensate focus *q.v.*, in order to open new ways of experiencing and expressing.

SENSORY CODING The process by which the nervous system *q.v.* translates various aspects of the stimulus into dimensions of a person's sensory experience.

SENSORY DEPRIVATION 1. An experimental procedure in which the person experiences markedly reduced stimulation for a relatively long period of time. 2. The restriction of sensory stimulation below the level required for normal functioning of the central nervous system *q.v.*

SENSORY DIVISION That part of the peripheral nervous system *q.v.* that transmits messages from receptors *q.v.* toward the central nervous system *q.v.*

SENSORY MODALITIES Vision, hearing, taste, touch, and smell. The pathways for stimuli to register in the brain.

SENSORIMOTOR INTELLIGENCE According to Piaget, intelligence during the first 2 years of life that consists chiefly of sensations and motor impulses with, at first, little in the way of internalized representations.

SENSORY NERVE A peripheral nerve *q.v.* that conducts impulses from a sense organ to the central nervous system *q.v.*

SENSORY PROJECTION AREAS One aspect of projection areas *q.v.* ct: motor projection areas.

SENSORY RECEPTORS The receiving sites at which stimuli enter the body. Sensory modalities *q.v.*

SENSORY REGISTERS 1. A system of memory storage in which material is held for a second or so in its original, unprocessed, sensory form. 2. The memory structure that holds information for possible processing. cf: long-term memory; short-term memory.

SENSORY SEIZURE A seizure *q.v.* that is characterized by visual, auditory, gustatory, olfactory, or emotional *qq.v.* sensations.

SENSORY STORE 1. According to the Atkinson and Shiffrin model of memory, a store that retains raw information for a very brief period of time. The first stage of information processing.

SENSORY THRESHOLD The least physical stimulus to which an individual responds.

SENSUAL Pertaining to any effects on the senses. A term implying a broader concept than sexual.

SENTENCE-COMPLETION TEST 1. In psychology *q.v.*, a form of projective technique *q.v.* using incomplete sentences that the person must complete. 2. In education *q.v.*, the use of sentences that must be correctly completed by the insertion of accurate information in the form of a word or phrase. 3. A test of knowledge recall.

SEPARATION An arrangement by which a husband and wife live apart and separately by mutual agreement. May be a prelude to divorce *q.v.*

SEPARATION ANXIETY DISORDER A disorder in which a child feels intense fear and apprehension when away from someone on whom he or she is dependent. Some believe ~ may be a factor in the cause of school phobia *q.v.*

SEPSIS 1. The presence of various forms of pus-forming or other pathological *q.v.* organisms, or their toxins, in the blood or tissue. 2. Bacteriological *q.v.* process of decay.

SEPTAL DEFECT A heart defect in which there is an unnatural opening in the wall of the tissue that divides the heart into right and left sides.

SEPTAL REGION A triangular double membrane *q.v.* separating anterior horns of lateral ventricles *q.v.* of the brain.

SEPTATE Pertaining to a hymen *q.v.*

SEPTATE HYMEN A hymen *q.v.* with two or more openings.

SEPTICEMIA Blood poisoning brought about by the presence of microorganisms multiplying in the blood.

SEPTIC SHOCK Shock *q.v.* developing in the presence of, and as a result of, severe infection *q.v.*

SEPTIC TANK A reservoir in a sewage disposal system where bacterial digestion liquefies solid waste. cf: cesspool.

SEPTUM A dividing wall or membrane *q.v.*, as in the wall that separates the nostrils.

SEQUELAE 1. Symptoms of a disorder that remain as the aftereffect of the disorder, e.g., paralysis following poliomyelitis *q.v.* 2. A lesion or infection following or caused by an attack of a disease.

SEQUENCE A plan for the ordering of organizing elements either vertically or horizontally for any one course or sequence. cf: scope.

SEQUENTIAL MULTIPLE ANALYSIS COMPUTER (SMAC) Analysis of biochemicals in the blood by use of a computer.

SEQUENTIAL PILL A chemical contraceptive *q.v.* The first 15 pills taken in any given menstrual cycle *q.v.* contain synthetic estrogen *q.v.*, the remaining five or six contain both estrogen and progestogen *q.v.* The estrogen inhibits ovulation *q.v.*, while the progestogen prepares the uterus *q.v.* for a menstrual flow.

SEQUESTRUM A fragment of bone that separates as the result of infection or injury.

SERAX A commercial preparation of oxazepam *q.v.*

SERENTIL A commercial preparation of mesoridazine *q.v.*

SERIAL ANTICIPATION METHOD A method of rote learning *q.v.* employing a serial list in which the person must respond with the next item on the list. cf: serial learning.

SERIAL LEARNING The learning *q.v.* of a list. cf: serial anticipation learning.

SERIAL MONOGAMY The practice of limiting one's serious relationships to one partner at a time, in contrast to staying with one partner permanently. cf: serial polygamy.

SERIAL POLYGAMY Being married to only one person at a time but repeatedly divorcing and remarrying. cf: serial monogamy.

SERIAL POSITION CURVE A graph showing the ease of learning *q.v.* each item in a serial list. cf: serial learning.

SERIAL POSITION EFFECT The tendency to remember items at the beginning and at the end of a long list better than those items in the middle of the list.

SERIAL TRANSMISSION The passing of information from one individual to another through a series of intermediaries.

SERIATION 1. The process of arranging a series of objects in order of their value on a single dimension. 2. The ability to construct a series mentally and then to reason about their relations. Usually occurs in the concrete operational period *q.v.* of development.

SERNYL An obsolete commercial preparation of phencyclidine (PCP) *q.v.*

SEROCONVERSION The development of antibodies *q.v.* to a particular virus *q.v.*

SEROLOGIC STUDY A comparison of the serum *q.v.* of individuals.

SEROLOGIC TEST Laboratory test made on serum *q.v.*

SEROLOGY The study of antigen *q.v.* and antibody *q.v.* reactions in blood serum tests *q.v.*

SEROPOSITIVE Producing a positive reaction to antibody tests for human immunodeficiency virus (HIV) *q.v.*

SEROSA 1. Perimetrium *q.v.* layer of the uterus *q.v.* 2. The outermost layer of most organs, usually continuous with the lining of the body cavities. 3. A thin membrane *q.v.* having the capability to exude plasma *q.v.* in response to injury and to absorb material in solution *q.v.*

SEROUS CAVITY A large lymph *q.v.* space.

SEROTONIN 1. A neurotransmitter *q.v.* found primarily in the upper brainstem *q.v.* ~ may prevent overreaction to various stimuli and regulate the release of hypothalamic hormones *q.v.* that in turn regulate the pituitary's *q.v.* release of gonadotropins *q.v.* 2. A neurotransmitter, the disturbance of which results in depression *q.v.* and mania *q.v.*

SERRATUS Saw toothed.

SERTOLI CELLS Supporting elongated cells of the seminiferous tubules *q.v.* that nourish spermatids *q.v.*

SERUM 1. The clear portion of any fluid from an animal's body that remains after the solid particles have been separated out. Blood serum *q.v.* is the clear, straw-colored liquid that remains after blood has clotted. 2. The plasma from which fibrinogen *q.v.* has been removed.

SERUM CHOLESTEROL The cholesterol *q.v.* in the blood that may contribute to cardiovascular disease *q.v.* cf: serum cholesterol level.

SERUM CHOLESTEROL LEVEL The amount of cholesterol *q.v.* present in a given amount of blood serum *q.v.* Typically measured in μg/ml.

SERUM HEPATITIS An acute infection of the liver caused by a virus *q.v.* Transmitted by contaminated blood during transfusion, medical instruments, or drug abusers using contaminated equipment. Characterization and symptoms similar to infectious hepatitis *q.v.*

SERUM LIPID ANALYSIS The analysis of fat substances in the bloodstream, which includes cholesterol *q.v.* levels and triglyceride *q.v.* measurements.

SERVICE A specific unit of health care provided to a particular population.

SERVICE BENEFIT A contract benefit that is paid directly to the provider of hospital or medical care for health services rendered.

SES An acronym for socioeconomic status *q.v.*

SESAMOID 1. A small nodular bone embedded within a tendon *q.v.* or joint capsule. 2. Shaped like a sesame seed.

SET 1. In exercise and weight lifting, the number of repetitions *q.v.* done consecutively without resting. 2. The psychological *q.v.* makeup or behavior of an individual. 3. The total internal environment *q.v.* of an individual. 4. Readiness to respond. cf: mental set.

SET-POINT 1. A general term for the level at which negative feedback *q.v.* tries to maintain the system. 2. The weight range that is natural to a person's body, which, according to the set point theory, the body strives to maintain itself by adjusting its metabolic rate *q.v.* cf: set-point hypothesis.

SET-POINT HYPOTHESIS The theory that different persons have different set-points *q.v.* for weight.

SETS Groups of muscular repetitions performed for a particular movement or exercise.

SETTING The total external environment of an individual. In relation to drug use, the physical surroundings in which a drug is taken.

SETTINGS The variety of organizational entities in which health educators *q.v.* are found working.

SEVERE MENTAL RETARDATION Mental development measured by IQ tests *q.v.* at a level of between 20 and

34. At this level, individuals are unable to care for themselves and engage in very limited communication, and are listless and inactive.

SEVERE AND PROFOUND MULTIPLE DISORDERS A description of those individuals who exhibit physical, sensory, intellectual, and/or social and interpersonal performance deficits beyond three standard deviations from the norm. These deficits are evident in all environmental settings.

SEVERITY RATE In industrial safety, the number of days lost due to accidents per million hours worked.

SEWAGE TREATMENT The process of handling sewage to safely return it to the environment. The process consists of 1. preliminary treatment to remove solid particles, 2. primary treatment to create a substance void of free oxygen to allow anaerobic bacteria *q.v.* to digest all organic materials, 3. secondary treatment to allow the effluent to come into contact with air so that aerobic bacteria *q.v.* can oxidize *q.v.* putrescible *q.v.* material, 4. chlorination *q.v.* to decontaminate *q.v.* the effluent, and 5. final disposal of the liquid end product, usually into a large body of water.

SEX Male or female, gender. Also used to mean coitus *q.v.*

SEX-AGGRESSION DEFUSION RAPIST A rapist *q.v.* for whom sexual and aggressive acts have become fused. Violence becomes necessary to attain the desired level of sexual excitement.

SEX-CHANGE SURGERY A type of surgery in which the existing genitalia *q.v.* is removed and a substitute set of genitalia is constructed of the opposite sex. Performed on those who are transsexuals *q.v.*

SEX CHROMOSOMES 1. X and Y chromosomes *q.v.* 2. Chromosomes that are involved in the determination of gender. ct: autosomal chromosomes.

SEX DRIVE The desire for sexual expression.

SEX EDUCATION 1. The formal and informal learning about the biological, sociological, psychological, spiritual, and interpersonal aspects of human sexuality. 2. Educational activities designed to increase the sexual knowledge of learners and to help them make sexually related decisions.

SEX FLUSH 1. A rash that develops in some women during sexual arousal *q.v.* as a result of vasocongestion *q.v.* of blood vessels near the surface of the skin. It begins at the abdomen, spreading to the throat, neck, and finally to the breasts. 2. A skin response to increasing sexual tension that begins in the plateau phase *q.v.* 3. Macropapular *q.v.*

SEX GLAND 1. A gonad *q.v.* 2. The testicles *q.v.* in the male and the ovaries *q.v.* in the female. 3. A structure of the endocrine system *q.v.*

SEX GUILT A sense of guilt resulting from the violation of personal standards or of proper sexual behavior.

SEX HORMONE A substance secreted by the sex glands *q.v.* directly into the bloodstream.

SEX-INFLUENCED TRAITS Those genetic traits *q.v.* in which the dominant expression depends on the sex of the individual. cf: sex-linked trait.

SEXISM 1. Prejudice and discrimination based upon one's gender *q.v.* 2. The systematic degradation and domination of women based upon the belief that being male is superior to being female.

SEX-LIMITED TRAIT A trait that expresses itself only in one gender *q.v.* even though either gender may carry genes *q.v.* for the trait.

SEX LINKAGE 1. An association or linkage of a hereditary *q.v.* character with sex. 2. The gene *q.v.* for a particular trait is in a sex chromosome *q.v.*

SEX-LINKED DISORDERS Inherited *q.v.* physical problems that are carried on sex chromosomes *q.v.*

SEX-LINKED PREPOTENCY The presumed tendency for both male and female animals to be more responsive to the opposite-gender patterns of stimulation than to same-gender patterns of stimulation based upon differences in brain mechanisms and hormone *q.v.* secretions.

SEX-LINKED TRAIT 1. A trait that is determined by a gene *q.v.* on one of the sex chromosomes *q.v.* 2. Sex-limited *q.v.*

SEX MOSAIC Gynandromorph *q.v.*

SEX OFFENDER A person who commits an act designated by law as a sex offense and, therefore, a crime.

SEXOLOGY According to Knox, a body of knowledge concerned with the differentiation and dimorphism of sex and the erotosexual pair bonding of partners.

SEX ORGANS 1. The organs *q.v.* used in sexual intercourse *q.v.*: the male penis *q.v.* and the female vagina *q.v.* 2. In botany *q.v.*, the archegonia *q.v.* and antheridia *q.v.*

SEXOSOPHY The philosophy, principles, and knowledge that people have about their own personally experienced erotosexuality and that of other people, singly or collectively.

SEX RATIO The number of males in a population per each 100 females.

SEX REASSIGNMENT OPERATION A surgical procedure designed to remove the external genitalia *q.v.* and replace them with genitalia appropriate to those of the opposite sex.

SEX REVERSAL 1. A change in the characteristics of an individual from male to female or vice versa. 2. Transexualism *q.v.*

SEX ROLE A set of expected gender-specific behaviors.

SEX ROLE FLEXIBILITY The willingness and ability to engage in a variety of activities, perform them at will, and feel good about doing them regardless of how they are sex typed.

SEX ROLE IDENTITY A sense of oneself as masculine or feminine, possessing attributes prescribed by sex role standards. cf: sexual identity.

SEX ROLE LEARNING The process of learning the socially accepted pattern of sex behavior.

SEX ROLE STEREOTYPE 1. A culture's fixed beliefs about which jobs, rights, and privileges are appropriate to each sex. 2. A cluster of sociocultural beliefs regarding the characteristics and proper behavior of each sex. cf: sex role identity.

SEX-SKIN The labia minora *q.v.* in the female, which shows a discoloration response in the plateau phase *q.v.* of the sexual response cycle *q.v.*

SEX STEREOTYPE A highly distorted and standardized view of gender roles *q.v.*

SEX STEROIDS A name for a group of compounds including sex hormones *q.v.* with estrogenic *q.v.* and androgenic *q.v.* properties.

SEX THERAPIST A member of a recognized profession who has training and experience in helping persons with sexual dysfunctions *q.v.*

SEX THERAPY A variety of approaches that seek directly to change the sexual behavior of dysfunctional couples by reducing performance anxiety *q.v.* and teaching sexual skills.

SEX-TYPED BEHAVIOR Behavior *q.v.* considered appropriate for one sex but not the other.

SEXUAL ABUSE 1. Sexual acts that are negatively sanctioned by society. 2. Unwanted sexual acts or sexual advances imposed or forced on another person.

SEXUAL ACT, PURPOSES OF There are four chief purposes of coitus *q.v.* and related sexual activity: 1. to reproduce, 2. to demonstrate affection for another person, 3. to provide sexual pleasure and satisfaction for one's partner, and 4. to provide sexual pleasure and satisfaction for oneself.

SEXUAL-AIM RAPIST A rapist *q.v.* who is largely motivated by sexual desires.

SEXUAL ANESTHESIA A hysterical *q.v.* conversion *q.v.* neurosis *q.v.* causing a woman to feel nothing when sexual stimulation is attempted. cf: frigidity.

SEXUAL APATHY Inhibited sexual desire *q.v.*

SEXUAL AROUSAL A variety of physiological *q.v.* changes and psychological *q.v.* reactions that accompany lovemaking, including intercourse *q.v.* In the female, characterized by the vagina *q.v.* becoming lubricated, the barrel darkens in color, the inner two-thirds of the barrel increases in length and width, the clitoris *q.v.* becomes erect and increases in diameter. A sex flush *q.v.* may also occur. In the male, the most apparent characteristic is penile *q.v.* erection. Some may experience a sex flush. There is vasocongestion *q.v.* of the scrotum *q.v.*, and the testicles *q.v.* are drawn closer to the body. Both males and females experience an increase in pulse rate and an increase in blood pressure and deeper respiration. Sexual arousal culminates in orgasm *q.v.* There are four basic phases to ~: 1. excitement phase, characterized by vasocongestion of the genitals and breasts, vaginal lubrication, rapid breathing, increased pulse rate, and other physiological changes; 2. the plateau phase, characterized by maintenance of sexual arousal and building of excitement; 3. the orgasmic phase, characterized by muscle spasms (ejaculation in the male) and an increase in the rate of breathing and a rise in blood pressure; 4. the resolution phase, characterized by a gradual return to the pre-excitement phase of sexual arousal. There is refractory period in males following orgasm in which it is difficult for further stimulation to result in heightened arousal.

SEXUAL AVERSION An extreme negative reaction to sexual activity.

SEXUAL CONTINUUM A range of sexual attraction with infinite degrees falling between the two extremes of exclusive homosexual *q.v.* attraction to exclusive heterosexual *q.v.* attraction.

SEXUAL DEVELOPMENT There are three general stages of ~: 1. conception *q.v.* determines the sex of the embryo/fetus but is not recognized until the genitals *q.v.* appear during fetal development; 2. puberty *q.v.*, when the secondary sex characteristics *q.v.* begin to appear; and 3. the stage of reproductive potential, menarche *q.v.* for the female and the production of sperm for the male. cf: biochemistry of sex.

SEXUAL DEVIATE A person who manifests sexually pathological *q.v.* behavior. cf: sexual variant.

SEXUAL DEVIATION Sexual variance *q.v.*

SEXUAL DIFFERENTIATION The development of male or female genitalia *q.v.* in the womb *q.v.* signaled by the presence or absence of a Y chromosome *q.v.*

SEXUAL DIMORPHISM The structural and functional differences between the sexes.

SEXUAL DYSFUNCTION 1. The inability to engage in or to enjoy sexual encounters. 2. A specific disorder of coital *q.v.* performance.

SEXUAL FANTASY 1. Erotic *q.v.* thoughts that produce sexual arousal *q.v.* 2. Fantasies or daydreams with sexual themes or overtones.

SEXUAL FULFILLMENT The state of being satisfied with one's sex life and sexual relationships.

SEXUAL HARASSMENT Any action by a person of either sex that involves the use of sex or sexuality of the other to impose restrictions on that person. Usually applied to activities in the workplace.

SEXUAL IDENTITY 1. A sense of oneself as male or female, generally established before 3 years. 2. A person's commitment to heterosexual *q.v.*, homosexual *q.v.*, or bisexual *q.v.* behavior. cf: gender identity.

SEXUAL INADEQUACY Any degree of sexual response *q.v.* that is not sufficient over a protracted period of time. Frequent or total inability to achieve orgasm *q.v.*

SEXUAL INTERCOURSE 1. Coitus *q.v.* 2. The insertion of the penis *q.v.* into the vagina *q.v.*

SEXUALITY 1. One's personality traits related to being masculine or feminine. 2. All of the human feelings, attitudes, and actions that people attach to their own or other's biological sex.

SEXUAL JEALOUSY A felt threat from an outsider to an important relationship resulting in feelings of anger and fear.

SEXUALLY TRANSMITTED DISEASES (STD) 1. Those infectious diseases contracted through intimate sexual contact, including candidiasis, chancroid, gonorrhea, granuloma inguinale, herpes, lymphogranuloma venereum, syphilis, and acquired immune deficiency syndrome (AIDS) *qq.v.* 2. The venereal diseases *q.v.* 3. Social diseases. 4. Infections or infestations passed from person to person by sexual contact.

SEXUAL MORAL VALUES The worth assigned to those behaviors, conduct, or relationships concerned with proper sexual activities.

SEXUAL MOTIVATION 1. Sex drive *q.v.* 2. The arrangement of one's environment so that one can approach erotic stimuli or create them in fantasy.

SEXUAL OBJECT PREFERENCE A person's preference concerning the nature of a sexual partner.

SEXUAL ORIENTATION 1. The gender to whom a person is attracted. 2. A person's choice of sexual partners. cf: gender identity; gender role; sexual preference.

SEXUAL ORIENTATION DISTURBANCE An outdated term for ego-dystonic homosexuality.

SEXUAL OUTLET Any of a variety of ways by which sexual tension is released through orgasm *q.v.*

SEXUAL PREFERENCE A person's choice of sexual partner by choice of homosexuality, heterosexuality, or bisexuality *qq.v.* cf: sexual orientation.

SEXUAL PSYCHOPATH Most generally, a person exhibiting compulsive, repetitive, and/or bizarre sexual behavior. A legal label that allows for people to be given jail sentences and implies that they are a menace to society.

SEXUAL REPRODUCTION 1. The process by which half of the genes *q.v.* of each parent organism combine to create a new individual. 2. The fusion of gametes *q.v.* followed by meiosis *q.v.* and recombination *q.v.* at some point in the life cycle. ct: asexual reproduction; sexual selection.

SEXUAL RESPONSE 1. Sexual capacity as determined by one's genetic *q.v.* potentials and learned experiences. Learned experiences are associated with a person's total psychosocial *q.v.* capacity and emotional makeup. 2. Related to stimuli *q.v.* that bring about a reaction. These stimuli act upon a person's erogenous zones *q.v.* resulting in a sexual arousal *q.v.*

SEXUAL RESPONSE CYCLE 1. The four stages through which a person passes when responding to sexual stimulation: the excitement phase, the plateau phase, the orgasmic phase, and the resolution phase *qq.v.* 2. The general pattern of sexual arousal building to an orgasm *q.v.* as described by Masters and Johnson.

SEXUAL SCRIPT 1. Learned behaviors and expectations related to sexual arousal *q.v.*, values, and appropriateness. 2. Shared interpretations and expected behaviors in a social situation. 3. The framework and context within which people interpret sexual events. 4. Rules people have for guiding their actions in sexual situations.

SEXUAL SELECTION The nonrandom choice of a mate among animals that reproduce sexually. cf: natural selection; sexual reproduction.

SEXUAL UNRESPONSIVENESS 1. Frigidity *q.v.* 2. Sexual dysfunction *q.v.* 3. Impotence *q.v.* 4. A sexual dysfunction causing a person to experience little or no erotic *q.v.* pleasure from sexual stimulation.

SEXUAL VALUES Social rules about sexuality and how it is expressed.

SEXUAL VALUE SYSTEM As defined by Masters and Johnson, the activities that an individual holds to be acceptable and necessary in a sexual relationship.

SEXUAL VARIANCE 1. Those sex acts engaged in by adults that vary from penile–vaginal intercourse *q.v.* This does not include foreplay or past coital *q.v.* activities related to the total love making, nor does it include homosexual activity. 2. Deviant sexual acts that are engaged in solely for one's personal gratification at the expense of another person. 3. Sexual variation *q.v.* 4. Paraphilia *q.v.*

SEXUAL VARIANT 1. One or more sex acts that deviate from the norm. 2. A person who engages in sexual acts exclusive of penile/vaginal intercourse.

SEXUAL VARIATION 1. Any sexual activity that a person prefers or is compulsively attracted to as a substitute for heterosexual *q.v.* activity. 2. Sexual variance *q.v.*

SEXUAL VICTIMIZATION Sexual abuse *q.v.* of children, family members, or subordinates by a person in a position of power.

S FACTORS OF INTELLIGENCE Specific factors unique to a particular intellectual task. cf: g factor of intelligence.

SHA An acronym for State Health Agencies.

SHADOW 1. In psychology *q.v.*, the hidden and unconscious parts of the mind. 2. According to Jung, hidden personality components that are often projected onto others. 3. Our unconscious aspect made up of anima, our feminine aspect, and animus, our masculine aspect.

SHADOW AREA A dead spot in a communicating area where radio or telephone contact is difficult or impossible to achieve.

SHAFT 1. The long, slender body of the penis *q.v.* 2. The body of the penis composed of three cylindrical parts and a network of blood vessels, which are encircled by a band of fibrous tissue and covered by skin. cf: glans penis; root.

SHAMANS 1. Pertaining to teachers, doctors, and health professionals who use magic in their professional practice. 2. One who practices shamanism. cf: quack.

SHAME AVERSION THERAPY Cognitive restructuring *q.v.*

SHAPE CONSTANCY The tendency to perceive the shape of objects as more or less the same despite the fact that the retinal *q.v.* image of these objects changes in shape as a person changes the angle orientation from which they are viewed. cf: size constancy.

SHAPING 1. In operant conditioning *q.v.*, reinforcing responses that are successively closer approximations of the desired behavior. 2. The process of providing reinforcers to alter a child's behavior into appropriate forms. 3. Rewarding small accomplishments toward a desired goal.

SHARERS In regard to sexual activity, swingers *q.v.* who maintain their marriages by sharing their adultery *q.v.* by reciprocating sex acts.

SHCP An acronym for School Health Curriculum Project *q.v.*

SHEATH 1. In anatomy *q.v.*, the inner lining of the vagina *q.v.* 2. Condom *q.v.*

SHELs An acronym for significant human exposure levels *q.v.*

SHELF LIFE The period of time during which a drug is expected to remain stable and effective if stored properly.

SHELL SHOCK 1. A term used in World War I for what is now referred to as posttraumatic stress disorder *q.v.* It was originally believed to be caused by sudden atmospheric changes from nearby explosions. 2. Battle fatigue.

SHELL TEMPERATURE The temperature of the extremities and surface of the body. ct: core temperature.

SHELTERED WORKSHOP A workshop where the mentally retarded or other handicapped persons can become involved in constructive and productive work in the community *q.v.*

SHES An acronym for School Health Education Study *q.v.*

SHIATSU Finger pressure message used to relieve muscular tension.

SHIGELLA DYSENTERIAE The microscopic organism that causes bacillary dysentery *q.v.*

SHIGELLOSIS Bacillary dysentery *q.v.*

SHINGLES 1. A viral infection affecting the nerve endings of the skin. 2. A skin condition characterized by blisters that erupt on the skin in a band or over a large area of the body. 3. Herpes zoster *q.v.*

SHIVERING Trembling of the body from cold or fear or other emotional state.

SHOCK 1. A condition that results because the blood tends to pool in the blood vessels in the viscera *q.v.* depriving the brain of needed blood and oxygen. Usually follows some physical or emotional trauma *q.v.* 2. The disruption of blood circulation because the blood pressure is inadequate to force the blood through the vital organs and tissues. This may happen after a serious blood loss. 3. A potentially fatal condition of diminished and inadequate circulation. 4. A profound collapse of many vital body functions evident during acute intoxication *q.v.* and other serious health emergencies. 5. ~ is generally classified according to cause or effect, e.g., anaphylactic ~, cardiogenic ~, hemorrhagic ~, hypovolemic ~, insulin ~, metabolic ~, neurogenic ~, psychogenic ~, respiratory ~, and septic ~ *qq.v.*

SHOCK REACTION A transient personality *q.v.* decompensation *q.v.* in the face of sudden, acute stress *q.v.*

SHOCK THERAPY A form of therapy *q.v.* for mental illness employing convulsions produced by electric shock or a drug. cf: insulin shock therapy; electroconvulsive shock therapy.

SHORT-TERM MEMORY (STM) 1. A memory system that keeps material for intervals of a minute or so, that has a small storage capacity, and that holds material in relatively less processed form than long-term memory *q.v.* 2. Working memory. cf: sensory register.

SHORT-TERM MEMORY STORE According to the Atkinson and Shiffrin model, the store that holds information being processed at the moment. The ~ is limited in size, and without practice, and retention is only about 30 s.

SHOULDER BLADE Scapula *q.v.*

SHOULDER GIRDLE The encircling bony structure supporting the upper limbs and comprising the scapula *q.v.* and the clavicle *q.v.* and their central attachments.

SHOULDER JOINT A ball-and-socket joint *q.v.* between the head of the humerus *q.v.* and the glenoid fossa *q.v.* of the scapula *q.v.*

SHOW A small discharge of blood and mucus from the cervix *q.v.* that indicates birth is imminent.

SHPDA An acronym for State Health Planning and Development Agency.

SHUNT A passageway between two blood vessels or between two sides of the heart.

SIAMESE TWINS 1. An outdated term describing identical twins *q.v.* that have not been completely separated at birth. 2. Conjoined twins.

SIBLINGS Genetically *q.v.*, brothers and sisters from the same parents.

SIBLING STATUS The place where a person is located in the sibling *q.v.* structure of the family.

SIB-MATING (CROSSING OF SIBLINGS) Matings involving two or more individuals of the same parentage, brother–sister mating.

SICKLE-CELL ANEMIA (SCA) 1. A genetic blood defect. 2. A recessive gene hereditary *q.v.* blood disease. Characterized by sickle-shaped red blood cells instead of the normal round, donut-shaped cells. 3. An inherited disease of the blood in which hemoglobin *q.v.* is altered. cf: sickle-cell anemia trait.

SICKLE-CELL ANEMIA TRAIT A genetic condition in which a person has inherited one recessive defective gene *q.v.* and one normal gene. The person is not clinically sick but can pass the sick-cell anemia (disease) onto his or her offspring. However, the person may experience mild symptoms under severe environmental conditions. cf: sickle-cell anemia.

SICKLEDEX TEST A laboratory test to diagnose sickle-cell anemia trait *q.v.*

SICK-ROLE BEHAVIOR As defined by SOPHE, that which occurs after the appearance of a symptom of illness or disease. ct: health behavior; illness behavior.

SIDE-BY-SIDE A coital *q.v.* position in which the partners are positioned facing each other while lying on their sides.

SIDE EFFECT 1. A reaction to a drug that does not contribute to its intended purpose and may result in complications. 2. An unwanted or undesirable reaction. 3. A given drug may have many actions on the body. Usually, one or two of the more prominent actions will be medically useful. The others may be considered ~s. 4. Adverse effect. cf: main effect.

SIDEROPHILIN Transferrin *q.v.*

SIDESTREAM SMOKE 1. Smoke inhaled from the burning tobacco products or others. 2. The smoke from the burning end of a cigarette, containing higher amounts of ammonia, carbon dioxide, nicotine, and other substances than that inhaled by the smoker.

SIDS An acronym for sudden infant death syndrome *q.v.*

SIGMOID 1. The S-shaped terminal section of the descending colon *q.v.* 2. ~ colon.

SIGMOID COLON The terminal division of the large intestine *q.v.* that makes several turns resembling the letter S and terminating at the rectum *q.v.*

SIGMOIDOSCOPE An instrument consisting of a hollow tube that can be passed through the anus *q.v.* into the rectum *q.v.* and the lower part of the large intestine *q.v.* for diagnosis of conditions within these organs.

SIGMOIDOSCOPY Examination of the colon *q.v.* immediately above the rectum *q.v.* by the use of a sigmoidoscope *q.v.*

SIGN (OF DISEASE) An observable indication that something is wrong with a part of the body, e.g., rash, bleeding. ct: symptom.

SIGNAL-DETECTION THEORY A theory that asserts that the observers who are asked to detect the presence or absence of a stimulus *q.v.* try to decide whether an internal sensory experience should be attributed to background noise or to a signal added to background noise.

SIGNIFICANT DIFFERENCE 1. In statistics, a difference that is unlikely to have occurred by chance. 2. Statistical significance *q.v.*

SIGNIFICANT HUMAN EXPOSURE LEVELS (SHELs) A health risk-assessment tool used to assist the health assessor in making determinations about human health risks by defining exposure levels believed to cause adverse health effects.

SIGNIFICANT OTHERS Persons in one's life who have an influence upon the way one behaves: spouse, children, close friends and relatives, and coworkers.

SILICOSIS A pulmonary disease caused by the inhalation of finely powdered silica or quartz.

SIMILARITY EFFECT The tendency for people who are similar to become attracted to each other.

SIMON–BINET SCALE Albert Binet and Thomas Simon were the first to develop a measurement of intelligence *q.v.* in 1905. ~ is an intelligence quotient *q.v.* scale or measurement.

SIMPLE CARBOHYDRATE 1. A sugar that is composed of one or two sugar molecules. 2. A carbohydrate *q.v.* that is composed of short molecular chains containing few saccharide *q.v.* units. 3. The simple sugars *q.v.* ct: complex carbohydrate.

SIMPLE FRACTURE A bone that is broken but does not protrude through the skin. ct: compound fracture.

SIMPLE MASTECTOMY Surgical removal of the breast tissue only.

SIMPLE PHOBIA An irrational fear caused by a specific object or situation.

SIMPLE SCHIZOPHRENIA Schizophrenia *q.v.* in which the chief symptoms *q.v.* are apathy and withdrawal.

SIMPLE SUGARS 1. Simple carbohydrates *q.v.* 2. Chemicals that are an intermediate step between carbohydrate and glucose *q.v.*

SIMPLEX TYPE 1 1. Herpes *q.v.* 2. Cold sore or fever blister. ct: simplex type 2.

SIMPLEX TYPE 2 1. Genital herpes *q.v.* 2. A sexually transmitted disease *q.v.* 3. A disease characterized by painful blisters on the genitals *q.v.*, thighs, and buttocks. It may also cause central nervous system *q.v.* infection in infants born to infected mothers. ~ has been linked to the development of cervical cancer *q.v.*

SIMULTANEOUS ORGASM Two partners engaging in sexual activity and reaching orgasm *q.v.* at the same time.

SIMULTANEOUS PAIRING Forward pairing *q.v.* and backward pairing *q.v.*

SINEQUIN A commercial preparation for doxepin *q.v.*

SINGLEHOOD A state of not being married.

SINGLE STANDARD Within a particular culture *q.v.*, the application of one standard of behavior for members of both sexes. ct: double standard.

SINGLE-SUBJECT EXPERIMENTAL DESIGN 1. A design for research in which one subject is studied under a variety of variables. 2. Single-subject studies *q.v.*

SINGLE-SUBJECT STUDIES 1. In research, an approach that involves taking objective and reliable measures of a person's behavior under varied conditions. 2. Single-subject experimental design *q.v.*

SINOATRIAL NODE 1. SA node. 2. Pacemaker *q.v.* 3. A small mass of specialized cells in the right upper chamber of the heart that gives rise to electrical impulses that initiate contractions of the cardiac *q.v.* muscle. 4. A region in the right atrium *q.v.* of the heart that regulates heartbeat.

SINSEMILLA 1. A seedless variety of high-potency marijuana *q.v.* 2. A technique of marijuana production in which unpollinated female plants are used which contain high levels of THC *q.v.*

SINUS 1. A channel for the passage of blood. 2. A hollow in a bone or other tissue. 3. One of the cavities connecting with the nose. 4. A suppurating cavity. 5. Air spaces within a bone structure. There are two frontal sinuses (in the frontal lobe of the skull), one above each eye, and two maxillary sinuses, one under each eye of the maxillary bone *q.v.* (upper jaw). cf: sinus cavities.

SINUS CAVITIES Sinus *q.v.* with the skull and facial bones that connect with the nasal cavities through a shared mucous membrane *q.v.*

SINUSITIS Irritation or inflammation of the sinuses *q.v.*

SINUSOID A blood space in certain organs, such as the spleen *q.v.* or liver *q.v.*

SITE-SPECIFIC SURVEILLANCE The systematic collection, analysis, and interpretation of health data from persons residing near hazardous waste sites.

SITUATION The combination and interaction of two or more variables.

SITUATIONAL DETERMINANTS The environmental *q.v.* conditions that precede and follow a particular behavior, being a primary focus of behavioral assessment *q.v.*

SITUATIONAL HOMOSEXUALITY Homosexual *q.v.* behavior that takes place in sex-segregated situations, such as prisons, boarding schools, the military, and the like.

SITUATIONAL MORALITY A moral standard based upon what seems right in the immediate situation.

SITUATIONAL ORGASMIC DYSFUNCTION A condition in which a woman has never experienced an orgasm *q.v.* during sexual intercourse *q.v.* with a particular partner or in a specific situation.

SITUATIONAL TEST A test that measures performance in a simulated life situation.

SITUATION AND BEHAVIOR ANALOGUES In research, studies of the conditions that will induce symptoms similar to minor psychopathology *q.v.* in humans.

SITUATION ETHICS A belief that no one set of rules or principles can be applicable to all situations. Each specific situation must be analyzed to determine which ethical *q.v.* principles are applicable.

SITUATIONISM 1. Decision making on the basis of the context of a particular situation, not on the basis of a prescribed set of laws or codes of action. 2. The view that human behavior is largely determined by the characteristics of the situation rather than those of the person. ct: trait theory.

SIX-MAN STRETCHER PASS A method of transporting an injured person on a litter *q.v.* over rough terrain. It consists of passing a stretcher *q.v.* by six persons in two parallel rows, the last two persons in line proceeding ahead each time as the stretcher passes them.

SIXTY-NINE 1. Simultaneous cunnilingus *q.v.* and fellatio *q.v.* 2. Two partners simultaneously stimulating each other's genitalia *q.v.* orally.

SIX WARNING SIGNS OF KIDNEY DISEASE The ~ are as follows: 1. burning or difficulty during urination *q.v.*, 2. frequent urination especially at night, 3. passage of bloody-appearing urine, 4. puffiness around the eyes, swelling of hands and feet, especially in children, 5. pain in the small of the back, and 6. high blood pressure.

SIZE CONSTANCY The tendency to perceive the size of objects as more or less the same despite the fact that the retinal image of these objects change in size whenever we change the distance from which we view them. cf: shape constancy; unconscious interference.

SIZE-UP The rapid gathering of facts and analyzing of the details of the incident or accident immediately upon arrival at the scene.

SKAGGS–ROBINSON HYPOTHESIS The hypothesis *q.v.* that retroactive inhibition *q.v.* is greatest when there is an intermediate degree of similarity between original and interpolated learning *q.v.*

SKELETAL AGE Age as determined through a comparison of a person's bone development relative to norms for people of the same age.

SKELETAL (VOLUNTARY) MUSCLE 1. One of the muscles that is attached to bone and is under voluntary control. 2. Striated muscle *q.v.* attached to and moving the bones.

SKELETAL SYSTEM Those organs, functioning in unity, that are associated with movement, protections of other organs, and stability. The ~ consists of the bones, joints, and ligaments, and is closely associated with the muscular system *q.v.*

SKELETON The framework of the body consisting of the bones. In humans, there are 206 whole bones that make up the skeletal system *q.v.* (Table S-1).

SKENE'S GLANDS Small glands *q.v.* just inside the urethral *q.v.* opening in females, believed to develop from the same embryonic *q.v.* tissue as the male prostate gland *q.v.* and responsible for emitting fluid from the urethra during orgasm *q.v.*

SKEW Role distortion within families of schizophrenics *q.v.* resulting from domination of the family system by one parent.

SKEWED CURVE An asymmetrical frequency distribution *q.v.* in which the range of scores on one side of the mode *q.v.* is greater than on the other side.

SKEWING In research, the displacing of frequencies up or down, usually within a normal curve *q.v.*

SKILL Job-related behavior necessary to perform activities.

SKILLED NURSING FACILITY A health care center that provides rehabilitative services and full 24-h nursing from registered nurses and LPNs *q.v.* for convalescent patients. Patients are under the supervision of a physician, and the facility has a transfer agreement with a nearby hospital. Services may be covered by both Medicare *q.v.* and Medicaid *q.v.* cf: domiciliary care facility; intermediate care facility.

SKILL-RELATED STRESS Perceived stress *q.v.* that occurs when a person is uncertain whether he or she has skills to do the task.

SKIN 1. The body's first line of defense against disease. ~ prevents organisms and disease-producing substances from entering the body. The ~ is sometimes referred to as the body's 10th system and is sometimes referred to as an organ. 2. The outer integument *q.v.* of the body consisting of the dermis *q.v.* and the epidermis *q.v.* and resting upon the subcutaneous *q.v.* tissue. The ~ contains various sensory *q.v.* and regulatory mechanisms. 3. The integumentary system *q.v.*

SKIN CANCER A malignancy *q.v.* of the skin *q.v.* ~ is the most common, but most preventable, of all cancers *q.v.* Most common in geographic areas in which people are excessively exposed to the sun's ultraviolet rays.

SKINFOLD CALIPERS An instrument used to measure thickness of a skinfold in various parts of the body to assess obesity *q.v.*

SKINFOLD MEASURES A procedure to estimate total body fat by measuring the thickness of a fold of two layers of skin and the fatty tissue attached.

SKINFOLD THICKNESS An index of body fat accumulation determined by measuring the thickness of a fold of skin.

SKINNER BOX A device developed by B.F. Skinner to study operant conditioning *q.v.*

TABLE S-1 TABLE OF BONES

THE AXIAL SKELETON (80)[a]		THE APPENDICULAR SKELETON (126)[a]	
General Description	Bone[a]	General Description	Bone[a]
1. Skull (29)		1. Upper Extremity (64)	
a. Cranium (8)	Frontal, parietal (2), occipital, ethmoid, temporal (2), sphenoid	a. Shoulder girdle (14)	Clavicle(2)
			Scapula (2)
		b. Arm (2)	Humerus (2)
b. Face (14)	Maxilla (2), zygomatic (2), lacrimal (2), nasal (2), inferior nasal concha (2), palatine (2), vomer, mandible	c. Forearm (4)	Ulna (2)
			Radius (2)
		d. Hand (54)	Carpals (16)
			a. Scaphoid navicular (2)
			b. Lunate (2)
c. Neck	Hyoid[b]		c. Triquetrum (2)
d. Ear (6)	Auditory ossicles (6)		d. Pisiform (2)
	1. Malleus (2)		e. Greater multangular (2) (trapezium)
	2. Incus (2)		f. Lesser multangular (2) (trapezoid)
	3. Stapes (2)		g. Captitate (2)
2. Vertebral column (26)	Cervical vertebrae (7), thoracic vertebrae (12), lumbar vertebrae (5), sacrum, and coccyx		h. Hamate (2)
3. Thorax	Sternum, true ribs(vertebrosternal) (14), false ribs (10)—vertebrochondral(6), and free ribs (vertebral) (4)		Metacarpals (10)
			Phalanges (28)
			a. Proximal (10)
			b. Middle (10)
			c. Distal (8)
		2. Lower extremity (62)	
		a. Pelvic girdle (2)	Innominate or os coxae (2)
		b. Thigh (2)	Femur (2)
		c. Knee (2)	Patella (2)
		d. Leg (4)	Tibia (2)
		e. Foot (52)	Fibula (2)
			Tarsals (14)
			a. Calcaneus (2)
			b. Talus (2)
			c. Navicular (2)
			d. First, second, and third cunei-forms (6)
			e. Cuboid (2)
			Metatarsals (10)
			Phalanges (28)
			a. Proximal (10)
			b. Middle (8)
			c. Distal (10)

The human skeleton has four chief functions: 1. support, 2. protection, 3. movement, and 4. hemopoiesis. It is composed of bones, cartilages, and joints. The skeleton is divided into two main parts: 1. the axial skeleton and 2. the appendicular skeleton. There are 206 individual bones.

[a]The figures in parentheses indicate the number of each bone listed.

[b]This bone is neither a part of the face nor technically a part of the cranium but is located in the neck where it is suspended.

SLEEPER EFFECT 1. The increased power of a low credibility source in influencing an audience after a period of time has elapsed. 2. In child development, patterns of parent/early child interaction that correlate more highly with the child's later behavior as an adult than with the child's behavior during growth.

SKIN-POPPING The subcutaneous *q.v.* injection of a drug.

SKIN TEST A tuberculin *q.v.* test to determine whether a person has had previous contact with the tuberculosis bacillus *q.v.*

SKULL The bones of the head when taken collectively.

SLEEP AID Usually referring to an over-the-counter medication used to produce mild sedation *q.v.* Such ~s often contain antihistamines *q.v.* to produce drowsiness.

SLEEPING PILL A drug in pill form that induces sleep.

SLEEPING SICKNESS Encephalitis lethargica *q.v.*

SLIDING SCALE In relation to health and medical care, a method of payment for services in which a person's fees are scaled according to income level.

SLING AND SWATHE A bandage in which the arm is placed in a sling and is bound to the chest by a swathe bandage *q.v.*

SLOUGH To separate from the living tissue.

SLOW BRAIN WAVES The theta rhythm recorded by an EEG *q.v.* from the subcortical parts of the brain and the delta rhythm, normally recorded during deep sleep. Sometimes recorded in awake sociopaths *q.v.*

SLOW-TO-WARM-UP CHILDREN Children whose temperament patterns include initial withdrawal from new situations, slow adaptability, and mild intensity of reaction.

SLOW-TWITCH FIBERS . A type of muscle cell especially suited for aerobic *q.v.* activities. 2. The type of muscle fibers *q.v.* used during repetitive endurance *q.v.* activities.

SLOW WAVE SLEEP The stage of sleep characterized by minimal dream activity.

SLUDGING The clumping of blood cells in the capillaries causing minor hemorrhaging, often as a result of excessive, chronic alcohol use.

SLUM 1. Crowded and squalid neighborhood within a city community. 2. Ghetto.

SMALL INTESTINE See intestine *q.v.*

SMALLPOX The first disease ever eradicated through human effort on a worldwide basis. The World Health Organization *q.v.* announced in 1979 that no diagnosed case had been found for over 2 years. No subsequent cases have been diagnosed since outside of the laboratory setting. The success of the eradication rests upon the development of a vaccine *q.v.* by Edward Jenner in 1798. ~ is characterized by a severe viral *q.v.* infection that results in skin eruptions, fever, malaise, and frequently, death. Immunity *q.v.* is complete in over 97% of the people who were immunized.

SMALL TALK A superficial form of conversation that allows people to seek common ground to determine whether they will pursue a relationship.

SMAZE A form of air pollution *q.v.* that is a combination of smoke, haze, and other pollutants. cf: smog.

SMEGMA 1. A foul smelling substance secreted by glands *q.v.* at the tip of the penis *q.v.* or around the clitoris *q.v.* 2. A cellular discharge that accumulates beneath the clitoral hood *q.v.* and the foreskin *q.v.* of an uncircumcised penis.

SMOG 1. Air pollution *q.v.* composed of a combination of smoke, photochemical *q.v.* compounds, and fog. 2. Air pollution by chemicals, smoke, particles, and dust suspended in fog. 3. A form of air pollution that may occur as either sulfur dioxide smog (high levels of sulfur dioxide and ozone combined with particulate matter *q.v.* and fog) or photochemical smog *q.v.* (the result of the interaction of sunlight, temperature inversion *q.v.*, and exhaust emissions from automobiles). cf: smaze.

SMOKELESS TOBACCO 1. Tobacco *q.v.* products that are chewed or sucked rather than burned or smoked. 2. Snuff, chewing tobacco.

SMOKERS' BRONCHITIS An inflammation of the lining of the bronchioles *q.v.* as a result of tobacco smoke.

SMOKING Inhaling the smoke from tobacco *q.v.* Also, inhaling the smoke from marijuana *q.v.* and opium *q.v.*

SMOKING CESSATION 1. The act of stopping smoking *q.v.* behavior. 2. To quit the smoking habit.

SMOKING-RELATED DISEASES Smoking *q.v.* causes or contributes to the development of many diseases including lung cancer and several other forms of cancer, emphysema, stroke, coronary heart disease, and chronic bronchitis *qq.v.*

SMOOTH MUSCLE 1. The muscles found in the arteries *q.v.*, veins *q.v.*, and hollow organs such as the stomach. 2. Muscles that line the walls of all hollow viscera *q.v.*, except the heart. ct: cardiac muscle; striated muscle.

SMR In epidemiology *q.v.*, an acronym for standardized mortality ratio *q.v.*

SMSA An acronym for standard metropolitan statistical area *q.v.*

SNELLEN EYE TEST A visual acuity test using graduated sizes of the letters of the alphabet for a visual distance of 20 ft. cf: STYCAR; illiterate E.

SNORKEL A tube housing an air intake and exhaust pipe that can be used for breathing under water when one end is projected above the water surface.

SNORTING A method of taking drugs in which a fine powder preparation containing the drug is sniffed into the nose, allowing the drug to be absorbed through the mucous membranes lining the nasal cavity.

SNOW BLINDNESS Obscured vision caused by sunlight reflected from snow.

SNS An acronym for sympathetic nervous system *q.v.*

SNUFF Powdered tobacco introduced to the body through inhalation.

SNUFF DIPPING The placing of snuff *q.v.* between the gum and the cheek where absorption of the nicotine *q.v.* occurs through the mucous membranes *q.v.*

SOBRIETY Behavior that excludes the use of intoxicating drugs, esp. alcohol.

SOCIAL Pertaining to the relationship and interaction of one person with others, with one group with other groups.

SOCIAL ACCOMMODATION Learning how others differ from oneself and how to deal with such differences. ~ occurs esp. rapidly during the school years.

SOCIAL ACTION One of the major approaches used to create change at the community level. ~ emphasizes task and process goals *q.v.* Objectives usually entail the modification of policies of formal organizations.

SOCIAL ANONYMITY The state of being unrecognized as an individual by society.

SOCIAL APPROACHES TO TREATING ALCOHOLISM Includes small and large group interactions and are represented by halfway houses *q.v.*, the day and night hospitals *q.v.*, voluntary agencies, e.g. alcoholic anonymous, and rehabilitation centers.

SOCIAL AUDIT The process of measuring the social responsibility activities of an organization.

SOCIAL CHANGE The process of affecting change through altering the structure and function of a social system involving individual and group learning.

SOCIAL CLASS 1. A grouping of people on a dimension of social prestige. Often perceived as ranging from upper-upper to lower-lower. 2. A category of people within a stratified society who share similar characteristics, such as socioeconomic status.

SOCIAL CLIMATE SCALE An instrument used to assess a specific environment involving several factors, such as personal relationships, person development, and environmental quality.

SOCIAL COGNITION A person's knowledge and understanding or person's social relationships and social institutions.

SOCIAL COMPARISON 1. A process of reducing the uncertainty about a person's beliefs and attitudes by comparing them to those of others. 2. The comparison of oneself to others and in so doing discover the proper "labels" for oneself.

SOCIAL CONSCIOUSNESS Awareness of civic and social issues and the willingness to act for social improvement.

SOCIAL CONTROL In sociology *q.v.*, the process or means whereby a social system enforces its norms.

SOCIAL DESIRABILITY In the completion of personality inventories *q.v.*, the tendency of the subject to give the responses he or she considers to be the socially acceptable answer. cf: social desirability effect; social desirability response set.

SOCIAL DESIRABILITY EFFECT 1. Social desirability *q.v.* 2. A change or response bias attributable to being observed and wanting to do the right thing.

SOCIAL DESIRABILITY RESPONSE SET The tendency to respond to questionnaire items in ways that are socially acceptable. cf: social desirability.

SOCIAL DEVIANCE Extreme and persistent behavior that is offensive or harmful to others.

SOCIAL DIAGNOSIS The assessment of social problems, such as economics, work, unemployment, criminal behavior, etc., measured in both objective and subjective terms.

SOCIAL DISTANCING A concept that demonstrates how each person has varying levels of intimacy with others.

SOCIAL DRINKER A person who uses alcohol *q.v.* for the purpose of enhancing the quality of his or her social interactions. cf: social drinking.

SOCIAL DRINKING The use of alcohol *q.v.* in ways that are socially acceptable and that enhances interpersonal interactions.

SOCIAL DRUG Any chemical substance used to enhance social interactions. Used primarily to describe alcohol *q.v.* or marijuana *q.v.*

SOCIAL ECOLOGY The relationships of one's physical system to the social context. cf: ecology.

SOCIAL ENVIRONMENT 1. Related to socioeconomic factors, political and other social institutions associated with one's way of life. 2. A general concept in social psychology *q.v.* pertaining to the many important social factors in the environment *q.v.*

SOCIAL EXPECTATIONS Goals or behavior patterns set by a culture or society. ct: personal expectations.

SOCIAL FACILITATION The improvement in performance resulting from social interaction.

SOCIAL FEEDBACK The exchange of error-reducing information among members of a group.

SOCIAL HEALTH The degree to which a person interacts effectively with the social environment *q.v.*

SOCIAL IMPACT THEORY 1. Latane's theory that the impact people have on others in a variety of situations is determined by the number of influence sources, the strength of the sources, and the closeness of the sources to the target. 2. The amount of influence or effect a person has on a group.

SOCIAL INDICATORS 1. Measurements of various criteria that indicate the character of a society over time. 2. A factor, the change of which, is expected to reflect a change in the quality of life.

SOCIAL INFLUENCE Pressure that changes behavior or attitudes in the direction of the prevailing patterns of a culture. cf: compliance; conformity; obedience.

SOCIALIZATION 1. The process through which persons learn the values, beliefs, and behavior patterns of the social group. 2. The changes in a person resulting from social influence.

SOCIAL LEARNING THEORY 1. The application of learning theory *q.v.* principles to personality *q.v.* and social development with emphasis on observational learning *q.v.* and reinforcement *q.v.* 2. ~ is used to explain how people learn to behave and is based upon four principles: (a) drive, (b) cue, (c) response, and (d) reward. 3. An extension of general learning theory that emphasizes the role of imitation and observation in human learning. 4. Modeling *q.v.* 5. The process of learning resulting from the observation of the experiences of others. 6. There is a continuous, reciprocal interaction among the person's behavior, other personal factors, and environmental consequences of behavior. 7. Reciprocal determinism. 8. An approach that stresses learning by observing others who serve as models for a child's behavior. The effect of the model may be to allow learning by imitation and may be to show a child whether a response he or she already knows should or should not be performed. ct: psychodynamic theory.

SOCIALIZATION 1. Introduction to the norms that a society has for its members. 2. Learning to accept the social behaviors expected in the group. 3. The process whereby a child acquires the patterns of behavior characteristic of the society. 4. The process by which one's behavior is shaped by other members of the society. The ways in which children acquire the knowledge of the standards and rules required to function effectively in society.

SOCIALIZED MEDICINE 1. A health policy and program for the people or certain segments of the population directed, authorized, and administered by the government. 2. Government-controlled medical practice and health care.

SOCIALIZED SUBCULTURAL DELINQUENCY The adoption of values or behaviors by a subculture that is considered deviant by the society as a whole.

SOCIALIZING AGENT Any person or institution that shapes a person's values and behavior.

SOCIAL LOAFING One who fails to contribute to a group but benefits from the contribution of others.

SOCIAL LUBRICANT Any product that, when taken internally, enhances the quality of social relationships. cf: social drinking.

SOCIALLY APPROVED DRUG USE The collectively viewed appropriateness of certain drug use based upon the drug's legality, how the drug was obtained, the purpose for the drug's use, and the type of person using the drug.

SOCIAL MOBILITY The movement of a person from one social class *q.v.* to another.

SOCIAL NEEDS Maslow's third set of human needs, including a desire to belong and the desire for friendship, companionship, and love.

SOCIAL PATHOLOGY 1. Abnormal patterns of social organization, attitudes, or behavior. 2. Undesirable social conditions that tend to produce pathology *q.v.* in a person.

SOCIAL PHOBIA 1. The irrational fear of interaction with others. 2. A collection of fears linked to the presence of others.

SOCIAL PLANNING Approaches used to create change at the community level. ~ emphasizes the solution to substantive social problems, e.g., poverty, unemployment, and disease.

SOCIAL PREFERENCE In studies of social status, the degree to which children prefer to be with a given child or not.

SOCIAL PRESSURE 1. The desire to go along with or rebel against others. 2. The influence of a social group upon the behavior of an individual.

SOCIAL PROBLEM A situation that a significant number of people believe to be a problem, consisting of objective as well as subjective components.

SOCIAL PROCESS The form or characteristics that interaction *q.v.* takes, interaction being a master process.

SOCIAL PSYCHOLOGY 1. A discipline devoted to the scientific study of human interactions and its psychological bases. 2. A scientific field that is based in both sociology *q.v.* and psychology *q.v.* and stresses understanding the ways in which the social system affects the individual and his or her interaction with others.

SOCIAL REFERENCING The use of emotional expressions of others to resolve the meaning of ambiguous situations.

SOCIAL REPRESENTATION The body of shared beliefs constituting the truths of a given culture or social group.

SOCIAL RESPONSIBILITY NORM A generally accepted norm *q.v.* that persons should be generous to or help others, by which children may judge others regardless of whether they behave according to the norm themselves.

SOCIAL ROLE The particular place or function of a person within a group.

SOCIAL SECURITY 1. A retirement or senior citizens' income guaranteed by the passage of the Social Security Act of 1935 and its subsequent amendments. 2. A national insurance program that provides income to workers when they retire or are disabled and to dependent survivors when a worker dies. Retirement *q.v.* payments are based upon workers' earnings during employment.

SOCIAL SELF Pertains to what a person would like others to think he or she is.

SOCIAL SERVICES Services designed to help persons with problems that concern housing, transportation, meals, recreation, child support, and family support and relations.

SOCIAL SKILLS The ability to successfully interact with others while maintaining physical, social, and emotional well-being.

SOCIAL SKILL TRAINING 1. Used in the treatment of sex offenders. This procedure teaches the person how to initiate and maintain socially appropriate relationships as an alternative to the undesirable behavior. 2. A type of behavior therapy *q.v.* to teach people how to meet others, how to communicate effectively, and how to improve their overall relations with people.

SOCIAL STIMULUS VALUE The characteristics that influence the way others respond.

SOCIAL STRATIFICATION A ranking of social status and the roles of each status in the social system. Such ranking may be referred to as a social class or a social caste, depending upon whether one's status is based upon achievement or upon an ascription at birth.

SOCIAL SUPPORT 1. Personal relationships that may be relied upon for emotional or material support in times of need. 2. The giving of aid, comfort, or meaning to another person's life.

SOCIAL SYSTEM An interrelated set of status and roles within a society. A ~ may involve the society as a whole and its institutions, or with individuals and small group interactions.

SOCIAL SYSTEM MODEL A school of psychology *q.v.* that holds that abnormal behavior is the result of distortions in the social relations experienced by an individual.

SOCIAL WELL-BEING 1. A sense of being comfortable and able to interact with other people in a variety of social situations. 2. Desirable relations with others and adaptation to the social environment *q.v.*

SOCIAL-WITHDRAWAL DISORDER A disorder characterized by extreme shyness, especially among children, exhibited by never being able to warm up to others even after prolonged exposure to them. They also do not join in group activities and tend to avoid crowded places.

SOCIAL WORKER A person trained in psychology and sociology who is concerned with emotional problems related to a person's interactions with others.

SOCIETY 1. A self-sufficient grouping of people who have a common culture and that has continuity from one generation to another. 2. A stable, relatively cooperative group of people with organized patterns of relationships. A ~ structure is seen in humans, nonhuman primates, and other social animals.

SOCIETY FOR PUBLIC HEALTH EDUCATION (SOPHE) Founded in 1950 and originally called the Society of Public Health Educators. A professional society whose members are largely health educators but which also serves the professional needs of other health professionals. ~ has been a driving force in the credentialing of health educators and for the accreditation of health education professional preparation programs. ~ is also responsible for the publication of journals and monographs related to health education.

SOCIOBIOLOGY 1. A subcategory of biology *q.v.* that attempts to trace social behavior to genetically *q.v.* based predispositions, an approach that has led to some controversy when extended to humans. 2. The study of the biological basis for social behavior in humans and other animals.

SOCIOECONOMIC STATUS (SES) 1. A classification of a population into strata on the basis of income, residence, occupation, or education. 2. The position of a person on the social and economic scale in the community *q.v.*

SOCIOGENIC 1. Originating from social (psychosocial) need, expectations, and aspirations. 2. Stemming from social and cultural mores. 3. Originating with society. cf: sociogenic motive.

SOCIOGENIC MOTIVE A motive originating from social expectations or social aspirations.

SOCIOGRAM 1. A visual representation of the social preferences of members of a group. 2. A diagram showing which children in a group are chosen by others based upon sociometric techniques *q.v.* 3. A sociometric diagram illustrating the personal feelings of members of a group with respect to who in the group socialize with each other.

SOCIOLOGICAL THEORIES OF ALCOHOLISM Concerned with the variations in cultural attitudes and values that may be related to alcoholism *q.v.* There are two types of theories: 1. the cultural theory *q.v.* and 2. the deviant behavior theory *q.v.*

SOCIOLOGY The science that studies human societies. ~ has some overlap with cultural anthropology *q.v.*, political science *q.v.*, economics, and psychology *q.v.*

SOCIOMETRIC TECHNIQUE 1. A means of determining popularity by asking learners to reveal which classmates they like best. 2. Methods for studying a person's social standing among peers.

SOCIOMETRY An analytical tool used to determine what informal groups exist within an organization and their memberships.

SOCIOPATH 1. A person without a conscious *q.v.* 2. A person with an antisocial personality *q.v.* 3. An individual who displays repetitive, impulsive, and purposeless antisocial behavior. This behavior is accompanied by emotional indifference and with guilt. cf: sociopathic personality disturbance.

SOCIOPATHIC PERSONALITY DISTURBANCE 1. A condition in which a person is unable to cope or conform to prevailing social standards. 2. A lack of social responsibility. Conditions include (a) antisocial behavior, (b) dissocial behavior, (c) sexual deviation, and (d) addiction to alcohol or other drugs *qq.v.* 3. A character disorder *q.v.* 4. A person whose behavior *q.v.* reflects no influence by the usual social conventions. cf: sociopath.

SOCIOTHERAPY Treatment of the interpersonal aspects of a person's life situation.

SOCRATIC METHOD A way of teaching that centers on the use of questions by the teacher to lead students to certain conclusions.

SODIUM 1. A chemical element. 2. A chief component of salt. 3. A component of table salt with the chemical formula NaCl.

SODIUM AMYTAL A barbiturate *q.v.* sometimes used in psychotherapy *q.v.* to produce a state of relaxation and suggestibility.

SODIUM FLUORIDE A compound used to fluoridate a water supply to help prevent tooth decay. cf: fluoridation.

SODIUM HYDROXIDE A caustic soda soluble in water and used externally as a caustic.

SODIUM NITRATE ~ along with or in place of sodium nitrite is added to meats to inhibit the growth of *Clostridium bacterium* *q.v.* organisms.

SODIUM NITRITE See sodium nitrate.

SODIUM PENTOTHAL A barbiturate *q.v.* cf: sodium amytal.

SODOMY 1. A paraphilia *q.v.* variously defined by law to include sexual intercourse *q.v.* with animals, and mouth/genital *q.v.* or anal *q.v.* contact between humans. 2. Anal intercourse between two males. 3. Named after the Biblical city of Sodom, the practice of anal intercourse. 4. Any "unnatural sex act" as defined by law. cf: zoophilia; bestiality; fellatio; cunnilingus.

SOFT CHANCRE Chancroid *q.v.*

SOFT-CORE PORNOGRAPHY Depictions of nudity or sexual acts without penetration. ct: hard-core pornography.

SOFT TISSUE The nonbony and noncartilaginous tissue of the body.

SOFT WATER Water that is low in mineral content. ct: hard water.

SOIXANTE-NEUF 1. Sexual stimulation by simultaneous cunnilingus *q.v.* and fellatio *q.v.* 2. Slang—sixty-nine.

SOL A colloid in liquid suspension, resembling a solution.

SOLAR HEAT Warmth originating from the sun. cf: greenhouse effect.

SOLDIER'S DISEASE Morphine *q.v.* addiction stemming from the use of morphine during the American Civil War.

SOLEUS 1. Pertaining to the sole. 2. A muscle in the leg shaped like the sole of a shoe.

SOLID WASTES Material generally occurring in a solid state and deemed useless. There are three general classes: 1. trash discarded by households and businesses, much of which is recyclable, and is usually dumped into landfills and covered with earth; 2. excrement eliminated through the large intestine *q.v.*; and 3. Hazardous waste, comprising solids containing materials toxic to life, including radioactive materials.

SOLO PRACTICE 1. A medical practice consisting of one physician in one office. 2. A physician who maintains a practice of medicine by himself or herself but may consult with other physicians from time to time. Such physicians often also have hospital privileges.

SOLVENT 1. A substance in which another substance is dissolved (the solute *q.v.*). 2. Dissolving, producing a solution.

SOLUTE A substance dissolved in another substance (the solvent *q.v.*).

SOLUTION 1. A dosage form in which the drug is dissolved in a liquid. 2. A homogenous mixture of two or more substances.

SOMA The totality of an organism's physical makeup.

SOMA CELLS The cells that make up the body, as contrasted the germ cells *q.v.* that are capable of reproducing the organism. cf: somatic cells.

SOMATIC 1. In anatomy *q.v.*, relating to the trunk. 2. The wall of the body cavity. 3. Pertaining to the body.

SOMATIC ANXIETY Anxiety *q.v.* that involves respiratory *q.v.*, gastrointestinal *q.v.*, and autonomic *q.v.* symptoms. ct: psychological anxiety.

SOMATIC CELLS See soma cells.

SOMATIC DAMAGE 1. Cell damage. 2. Damage to some physical part of the body.

SOMATIC DEPRESSION A type of depression *q.v.* characterized by sleep disturbances, significant fluctuations in weight or appetites, and a variety of other physical complaints that may be interpreted as being hypochondriacal *q.v.*

SOMATIC NERVE One of the nerves *q.v.* of sensation or motion.

SOMATIC SYSTEM 1. Part of the nervous system *q.v.* that controls voluntary, skeletal muscles *q.v.* 2. That part of the peripheral nervous system *q.v.* that innervates body parts under voluntary control.

SOMATIC THERAPIES A collective term for any treatment of mental disorders by means of some organic *q.v.* manipulation, drug administration, any form of surgery, and convulsive treatments.

SOMATIC WEAKNESS The vulnerability of a particular organ or body part to a particular psychophysiological disorder *q.v.*

SOMATIZATION DISORDER 1. A somatoform disorder *q.v.* in which a person seeks medical help for physical symptoms that have no observable physical cause. 2. Briquet's syndrome *q.v.* cf: hypochondriasis.

SOMATOGENESIS The development from physical origins as opposed to psychological origins. ct: psychogenesis.

SOMATOFORM DISORDERS Disorders in which physical symptoms suggest a physiological cause but which present no evidence of same; therefore, they are believed to be psychologically based. cf: somatization disorder; conversion disorder; psychogenic pain disorder; hypochondriasis.

SOMATOGENIC MENTAL DISORDERS Mental disorders *q.v.* that are produced by an organic *q.v.* cause. ct: psychogenic illness.

SOMATOGENIC PSYCHOSOMATIC DISORDER An illness caused by stress *q.v.* lowering a person's immunity *q.v.* or resistance to pathogens *q.v.*

SOMATOPLASM The nonreproductive material comprising the body of an organism in contrast to germplasm *q.v.*

SOMATOPSYCHOLOGICAL Of the body and mind.

SOMATOSENSORY PROJECTION AREA That part of the cerebral cortex *q.v.* that receive impulses *q.v.* for skin sensations.

SOMATOTONIA 1. The desire for power, delight in physical activity, and an indifference to people. 2. A mesomorphy *q.v.* body type. 3. A tendency toward action rather than thought and introvert behavior. ct: viscerotonic; cerebrotonia.

SOMATOTONIC The temperament originally assumed to be associated with a mesomorphic *q.v.* body type.

SOMATOTROPIN A growth hormone *q.v.* produced by the anterior pituitary gland *q.v.* ~ triggers the growth spurt of adolescence *q.v.*

SOMATOTYPE 1. Refers to body shape or types. 2. Sheldon's classification of body types each of which can be identified with a corresponding personality *q.v.* type: endomorphy, mesomorphy, and ectomorphy *qq.v.*

SOMNAMBULISM Sleepwalking.

SOMPA An acronym for the System of Multicultural Pluralistic Assessment, developed by Mercer and Lewis in 1977.

SONOGRAM 1. A live video image of the fetus *q.v.* resulting from an ultrasound scan that is used to determine the sex of the fetus and to assist in determining its health. 2. An image derived from bouncing sound waves off an object and used for medical diagnoses.

SOPHE An acronym for Society for Public Health Education *q.v.*

SOPOR A commercial preparation for methaqualone *q.v.*

SOPORIFIC A drug that produces deep sleep.

S-O-R MODEL A theory of cognition *q.v.* expanding on the S-R theories *q.v.* to include O—the organism and its perceptions, past experiences, abilities, and desires.

SORBITOL A substance produced by hydrogenating dextrose *q.v.*, one-half to three-fourths as sweet as sucrose *q.v.* Excessive consumption will cause a laxative *q.v.* effect.

SORC An acronym for four sets of variables that are the focus of behavioral assessment *q.v.*: situational determinants, organismic variables, overt responses, and reinforcement contingencies.

SORORATE The marriage custom that holds that when a sister dies, the surviving sister will marry the widower.

SOUL KISSING 1. A French kiss *q.v.* 2. The touching of tongues during a kiss.

SOUND ASSIMILATION One of the ways young children simplify the phonology *q.v.* of language. It involves changing one of the sounds of a word to make it more like another sound.

SOUND DELETION A way of simplifying phonology *q.v.*, used by children and involves deleting a syllable from a word to make it easier to say.

SOUND SUBSTITUTION A means of simplifying the phonology *q.v.* of a language by substituting a sound that is easy to produce for one that is difficult.

SOUND WAVES Successive pressure variations in the air that vary in amplitude and wave length.

SOURCE The object, person, or substance from which an infectious agent *q.v.* passes to a host *q.v.*

SOURCE/ENCODER That person involved in interpersonal communication who originates and encodes information that is to be shared with others.

SOURCE OF MESSAGE The place from which communications originate. It may originate from the physical environment *q.v.*, learning resources *q.v.*, the teacher, or the individual's thought processes. It is a component of information theory *q.v.*

SOURCE TRAIT A basic trait of personality *q.v.* reflected in a variety of more superficial surface traits *q.v.*

SOUR GRAPES MECHANISM A form of rationalization *q.v.* in which the person denies the pain of frustration *q.v.* by concluding that what he or she wanted is not worth having.

SOUTHEASTERN ASSOCIATION FOR EDUCATION PHYSICIANS IN OCCUPATIONAL HEALTH AND THE ENVIRONMENT A project cosponsored by ATSDR *q.v.* and the National Institute for Occupational Safety and Health *q.v.* The primary goal of the ~ project is the development and implementation of curricula that will improve the ability of primary care physicians *q.v.* to properly diagnose illness and effectively treat patients who have occupational or environmentally related diseases or injuries.

SOVEREIGN IMMUNITY 1. Above all else, in that an organization or individual cannot be held liable for wrongdoing. 2. Independent and not subject regulation.

SPACED PRACTICE Practice with relatively long pauses between trials. ct: massed practice.

SPANISH FLY A drug widely purported to be an aphrodisiac *q.v.* that is derived from the beetle *Cantharis vesicatoria*. When ingested, the substance causes inflammation of the genitourinary tract *q.v.* and possibly erection *q.v.* in males. Excessive doses may cause violent illness and death.

SPAN OF ATTENTION The number of items a person can comprehend in a single glance.

SPASM An intense, involuntary, usually painful contraction of a muscle or group of muscles.

SPASMODIC DYSMENORRHEAL The presence of cramping, pain, in the lower abdomen *q.v.* and nausea at the beginning of the menstrual cycle *q.v.*

SPASTICITY 1. A marked hypertonicity *q.v.* or continual over-contraction of muscles, causing stiffness, awkwardness, and motor incoordination. 2. A type of cerebral palsy *q.v.* in which movement is restricted by contraction of the muscles. 3. Involuntary contractions of various muscle groups.

SPATIAL MAZE A maze in which there is a definite and continuous route from start to goal. ct: temporal maze.

SPATIAL ORIENTATION Concept of distance, direction, and positions of objects in space.

SPATIAL SUMMATION Two or more impulses from spatially separated neurons *q.v.* arriving at a synapse *q.v.* at the same time and strength, firing the succeeding neuron when neither impulse alone is strong enough.

SPATULA A small, spoon-shaped instrument used during a medical examination. The ~ is used to scrape a tiny amount of tissue from the cervix *q.v.* that is used for a Pap smear *q.v.*

SPEARMAN'S THEORY OF GENERAL INTELLIGENCE Based upon factor analysis *q.v.* studies that ascribe intelligence test performance to one underlying factor, general intelligence (g), which is tapped by all students, and a large number of specific skills that depend on abilities specific to each subtest.

SPECIAL ACTION OFFICE FOR DRUG ABUSE PREVENTION Established in the Executive Office of the President of the United States. ~ was provided with more than one billion dollars by the Congress in 1972 through 1975. The bill gave the director authority to establish a National Institute on Drug Abuse within the National Institute of Mental Health, National Advisory Council for Drug Abuse Prevention, and a National Drug Abuse Training Center.

SPECIAL EDUCATION Special programs developed for the education of children with disabilities.

SPECIALIST 1. A person whose occupation is defined within narrow limits. 2. A person who specializes in a particular area of knowledge or practice.

SPECIALIZED CELLS Cells that have particular and unique functions within the body: red blood cells, white blood cells, muscles cells, bone cells, etc.

SPECIAL RISK INSURANCE A special policy covering special hazards.

SPECIAL SYMPTOM REACTION A condition in which one symptom is identified indicating a personality or character disorder *q.v.* These special symptoms include stuttering, nail biting, enuresis *q.v.*, tics, narcolepsy *q.v.*, and learning difficulties.

SPECIES 1. A group of closely related individuals. 2. A unit of classification. 3. A basic category in the classification of plants or animals below the genus level and above the variety or subspecies level.

SPECIFIC ATTITUDES THEORY The hypothesis that certain attitudes *q.v.* are associated with certain psychophysiological disorders *q.v.*

SPECIFIC DEATH RATE The number of deaths from any one cause per 100,000 population.

SPECIFIC DEVELOPMENTAL DISORDERS 1. Delays in the development of language and articulation, the ability to read and to do arithmetic, and skills that are related to maturation. ~ may extend into adulthood. 2. Learning disabilities *q.v.*

SPECIFIC DYNAMIC EFFECT (SDE) The increase in metabolic rate *q.v.* observed after the digestion, absorption, and metabolism *qq.v.* of food.

SPECIFIC EFFECTS The effects of drugs that depend upon the amount and type of the drugs taken.

SPECIFIC FACTOR In the factor analysis *q.v.* of intelligence *q.v.*, a skill that is specific to a particular kind of test. ct: general factor.

SPECIFIC GRAVITY An object's dry weight divided by the weight of water. Used to determine the percentage of fat in a person's body.

SPECIFIC IMMUNE MECHANISM A part of the immune system *q.v.* that is activated when a specific organism or foreign substance enters the body. ct: nonspecific immune mechanism.

SPECIFICITY 1. A training concept that fitness components can be increased for very specific tasks or functions. 2. The concept that the physiological *q.v.* effects of training are unique to the exercise or sport one is involved in and do not necessarily fully condition the body for different sports or exercises. 3. The property of an antibody *q.v.* that enables it to recognize and combat only one type of foreign substance or organism. 4. In epidemiology *q.v.*, related to tests of validity *q.v.* The percent of all true noncases that are identified correctly. ct: sensitivity.

SPECIFIC MORTALITY RATE The number of deaths for a specific cause per 100,000 population.

SPECIFIC REACTION THEORY The hypothesis that an individual develops a given psychophysiological *q.v.* disorder because of the innate tendency of the autonomic system *q.v.* to respond in a particular way to stress *q.v.*

SPECIES-TYPICAL BEHAVIOR A term that should be substituted for the term instinct *q.v.* to avoid the misleading implication that some behaviors are predetermined and not subject to the developmental process.

SPECIMEN 1. A sample. 2. A small amount of body fluid to be examined, frequently, a ~ of urine *q.v.* or feces *q.v.*

SPECTATOR ATTITUDE 1. A response to one's feelings of sexual inadequacy in which the individual observes his or her own sexual performance rather than partaking in the act unselfconsciously. 2. Spectatoring *q.v.* 3. Spectator role *q.v.*

SPECTATORING 1. In sexology *q.v.*, a psychological process wherein a person becomes a spectator to his or her own sexual performance, characterized by monitoring and evaluating the performance. 2. Self-awareness during sexual relations that interferes with sexual response *q.v.* 3. Spectator attitude *q.v.* 4. Spectator role *q.v.* 5. A form of sexual dysfunction *q.v.* in that, by focusing on one's own sexual performance, it inhibits pleasure and sexual responsiveness.

SPECTATOR ROLE 1. As described by Masters and Johnson, a pattern of behavior in which the individual's own performance inhibits his or her own sexual response. 2. Spectatoring *q.v.* 3. Spectator attitude *q.v.*

SPECTRUM 1. In regard to AIDS *q.v.*, a range of factors associated with HIV *q.v.* infection or a range of outcomes. 2. The range of physical stimuli *q.v.* to which a receptor *q.v.* responds. Most often used in relation to visual stimuli.

SPECULUM 1. A tubular instrument used to look into an opening of the body, such as the nose or ear. 2. A metal instrument that is inserted into the vagina *q.v.* to hold the walls apart, allowing for examination of the vagina *q.v.* and cervix *q.v.*

SPEECH The audible production of language.

SPEECH DISORDERS Speech behavior that is sufficiently abnormal to attract attention, interfere with communication, or to interfere with the communication for either the speaker or the listener.

SPEED RUNS Refers to prolonged use of methamphetamine, usually injected, followed by long periods of what is called a "crash."

SPERM 1. The male reproductive cell that fertilizes the ovum *q.v.* 2. The cell from the male that carries half of the chromosomes *q.v.* necessary for reproduction.

SPERMATIC CORD 1. The cord extending from the abdomen *q.v.* to the testis *q.v.* and comprising the vas deferens *q.v.*, testicular artery *q.v.*, and nerves. 2. The structure in males by which the testicle is suspended and contains the sperm ducts *q.v.*, nerves, and veins.

SPERMATIDS 1. The four cells formed by the meiotic *q.v.* divisions in spermatogenesis *q.v.* ~ become mature spermatozoa *q.v.* 2. The product of the third and last division of the male germ cell *q.v.* that matures into spermatozoa.

SPERMATOCELE A soft swelling on either side of the scrotum *q.v.*, the result of an intrascrotal cyst *q.v.*

SPERMATOCYTE The cell that undergoes two meiotic *q.v.* divisions to form four spermatids *q.v.*

SPERMATOGENESIS 1. The manufacture of sperm *q.v.* in the male. 2. The process of sperm production. ct: oogenesis.

SPERMATAGONIUM Primitive male germ cells *q.v.* that mature into primary spermatocytes *q.v.*

SPERMATOZOA 1. Spermatozoon *q.v.* 2. The mature male germ cell *q.v.*

SPERMATOZOON 1. Spermatozoa *q.v.* 2. A mature male germ cell *q.v.* 3. A mature sperm *q.v.*

SPERM BANK A center where a man's semen *q.v.* may be frozen and stored for later use in artificial insemination *q.v.*

SPERM DUCT 1. The tube in males that conveys the sperm *q.v.* from the epididymis *q.v.* to the seminal vesicles *q.v.* and urethra *q.v.* 2. The vas deferens *q.v.*

SPERMICIDAL CREAM (JELLY) 1. A chemical used to kill sperm *q.v.* 2. A chemical contraceptive *q.v.*

SPERMICIDAL SUPPOSITORY A spermicide *q.v.* in suppository form that effervesces or dissolves when it comes in contact with the moisture and warmth of the vagina *q.v.*

SPERMICIDE 1. A chemical capable of killing sperm *q.v.* 2. A cream, jelly, foam, or suppository that is placed in the vagina to kill sperm to prevent pregnancy.

SPERM SEPARATION METHOD A method of gender selection in which X-bearing and Y-bearing sperm *q.v.* are separated and the woman is artificially inseminated *q.v.* with the desired sperm.

SPERM VIABILITY The ability of a sperm *q.v.* cell to swim quickly toward the ovum *q.v.* and fertilize *q.v.* it.

SPF An acronym for sun protection factor *q.v.*

SPHENOID Wedge shaped.

SPHINCTER A ringlike muscle that controls a natural orifice *q.v.*

SPHINCTER MUSCLE A muscle that encircles a duct *q.v.*, tube, or opening in such a way that contraction constricts the opening.

SPHYGMOMANOMETER An instrument used to measure blood pressure *q.v.*

SPINA BIFIDA A developmental defect of the spinal column *q.v.*

SPINA BIFIDA CYSTICA A malformation of the spinal column *q.v.* in which a tumorlike sack is produced on the infant's back.

SPINA BIFIDA MENINGOCELE A cystic swelling or tumorlike sack that contains spinal fluid but no nerve tissue *q.v.*

SPINA BIFIDA OCCULATA A mild form of spina bifida *q.v.* in which there is an oblique slit in one or several of the vertebral *q.v.* structures.

SPINAL BLOCK 1. Saddle block *q.v.* 2. A common type of anesthesia *q.v.* administered during childbirth in which only the lower half of the body is anesthetized, leaving the woman conscious during the birth process.

SPINAL CANAL A bony channel formed by the vertebral bodies and neural arches that contains and protects the spinal cord *q.v.*

SPINAL CORD The cord of nervous tissue *q.v.* extending from the brain through the length of the spinal canal *q.v.* Paired motor *q.v.* and sensory *q.v.* nerves branch off from the ~.

SPINAL CORD INJURY An injury in which the spinal cord *q.v.* is traumatized or transected.

SPINAL NERVES Nerves arising from the spinal cord *q.v.* There are 31 pairs of ~.

SPINAL TAP Lumbar puncture *q.v.*

SPINDLE A fibrous-appearing structure associated with the chromosomes *q.v.* in mitosis *q.v.*

SPINDLE FIBERS A group of fibers that extends from the centromeres *q.v.* of the chromosomes *q.v.* to the poles of the spindle in a dividing cell.

SPINE 1. In anatomy *q.v.*, the backbone; the vertebrae *q.v.* 2. In botany *q.v.*, a sharp-pointed woody structure, usually modified from a leaf.

SPINEBOARD A wooden or metal device primarily used for extraction and transportation of victims with actual or suspected spinal injuries. May also serve as a litter *q.v.* and can be used to raise or lower victims or to provide rigid support during cardiac compression.

SPINGOMYELIN A group of phospholipids *q.v.* found in the brain, spinal cord, and kidney *qq.v.* On hydrolysis *q.v.*, ~ yields phosphoric acid, choline *q.v.*, sphingosine, and a fatty acid *q.v.*

SPIRAL FRACTURE A fracture *q.v.* in which the line of break runs obliquely up one side of the bone.

SPIREME A stage in mitosis *q.v.* at which the chromatin *q.v.* material of the nucleus *q.v.* appears in the form of a skein of filaments.

SPIRILLA One of the three classes of bacteria *q.v.* cf: spirillum. ct: bacilli; cocci.

SPIRILLUM A spiral- or corkscrew-shaped bacterium *q.v.*

SPIRITUAL WELL-BEING The possession of an inner strength or energy that includes aspirations, ideals, and the motivation to direct everyday life activities.

SPIROCHETE A bacteria *q.v.* of the class spirilla *q.v.* It is corkscrew in shape and is responsible for syphilis *q.v.* infection, among others.

SPLANCHNIC Pertaining to the viscera *q.v.*

SPLEEN A large organ situated under the ribs in the upper left side of the abdomen *q.v.* The ~ functions in the normal destruction of old red blood cells.

SPLENECTOMY The surgical removal of the spleen *q.v.*

SPLENOMEGALY Enlargement of the spleen *q.v.*

SPLINT A device to immobilize an injured part. There are generally two types of ~s: traction *q.v.* and rigid *q.v.*

SPLIT BRAIN A condition in which the corpus callosum *q.v.* and some other fibers are cut so that the two cerebral hemispheres *q.v.* are isolated.

SPLIT-FRAME STRETCHER A carrying device for the injured that is divided longitudinally, slipped beneath the injured from each side, and locked at each end, thus providing an extraction device and litter *q.v.*

SPLIT HALF METHOD A method of establishing reliability *q.v.* in which performance *q.v.* is paired on two halves of the same test.

SPONDYLITIS OF ADOLESCENCE A form of rheumatoid arthritis *q.v.* that affects the entire body rather than isolated joints or areas.

SPONGE Related to sexuality *q.v.*, a soft, pliable, plastic device containing spermicide *q.v.* that is inserted into the vagina *q.v.* before intercourse to prevent sperm *q.v.* from entering the uterus *q.v.*

SPONGY BODY The lower cylinder of erectile tissue of the penis *q.v.* that extends the length of the penile shaft *q.v.* ct: cavernous bodies.

SPONTANEOUS ABORTION 1. Miscarriage. 2. Expulsion of the embryo/fetus *q.v.* without deliberate effort. Reasons for ~ are (a) lack of one of the sex hormones *q.v.*, (b) genetic defects *q.v.* present in the embryo, (c) abnormal placental *q.v.* development, (d) poor implantation of the fertilized egg, and (e) congenital *q.v.* defects present. 3. Naturally occurring termination of pregnancy.

SPONTANEOUS AGGRESSIVE MOLESTER A molester who attacks a child sexually as a target of opportunity, rather than as a deliberately planned assault.

SPONTANEOUS COMBUSTION Under certain circumstances, material begins to burn without an external source of fire or heat.

SPONTANEOUS ERECTION The stiffening and enlargement of the penis *q.v.* without a sexual stimulus. Relatively common in adolescent males.

SPONTANEOUS HUMAN COMBUSTION An extremely rare, theoretical phenomenon characterized by the incineration of the body by a chemical interaction within the body's physiology or biochemistry.

SPONTANEOUS MUTATION A mutation *q.v.* whose cause is unknown.

SPONTANEOUS PNEUMOTHORAX A pneumothorax *q.v.* occurring from disease of the lung. Not the result of trauma.

SPONTANEOUS RECOVERY 1. An increase in the tendency to perform an extinguished response after a time interval in which neither the conditioned stimulus *q.v.* nor the unconditioned stimulus *q.v.* are presented. 2. Spontaneous remission *q.v.* 3. After extinction *q.v.*, an improvement in performance *q.v.* after a lapse of time. 4. Improvement of a patient's condition with little or no therapeutic intervention.

SPONTANEOUS REMISSION An event or phenomenon characterized by recovery from an illness without treatment or apparent cause.

SPORADIC Occurring only occasionally.

SPOROZOITE A motile, infective stage of plasmodium, injected into the bloodstream by mosquitoes.

SPOTTED FEVERS Fevers characterized by spots on the skin. ~ are carried by ticks.

SPOTTING Breakthrough bleeding *q.v.*

SPRAIN An injury to ligaments, tendons, or muscles by hyperextension or stretching.

SPRUE A chronic *q.v.* disease caused by the imperfect absorption of nutrients from the small intestine *q.v.* ~ is characterized by diarrhea *q.v.*, subnormal body weight, and sensations of fatigue.

SPURIOUS In epidemiology *q.v.*, artifactual *q.v.* When applied to associations, they are not real but rather false relationships produced by methodological errors or confounding variables *q.v.*

SPUTUM Mucus-based material that can be expectorated *q.v.* from the lungs and air passages. ~ usually results from disease of the air passages.

SQUAMOUS Scaly or platelike.

SQUAMOUS CELL CANCER 1. Squamous cell carcinoma. 2. A type of skin cancer *q.v.*

SQUEEZE TECHNIQUE A method used in the treatment of premature ejaculation *q.v.* The procedure involves squeezing the penis *q.v.* below the coronal ridge *q.v.* just before ejaculation takes place so that the male will lose his urge to ejaculate. cf: basilar squeeze technique; stop–start technique.

SQUELCH A system for removing objectionable background noise from a public address system or radio speaker.

S-R LAW A law that states the dependence of behavior upon antecedent conditions. ct: R-R law.

S-R PSYCHOLOGISTS 1. Psychologists *q.v.* who emphasize the role of stimulus/response connections in learning. 2. Associationists *q.v.*

S-R THEORY 1. The hypothesis *q.v.* that learning consists of the formation of connections between stimuli *q.v.* and responses. 2. S-R learning theories. ct: cognitive psychology.

S-SHAPED FUNCTION A function that begins with positive acceleration *q.v.* and then shifts to negative acceleration.

ST An acronym for slow-twitch fibers *q.v.*

STABLE EMOTIONS Controlled and appropriate emotional responses that do not cause disproportionate discomfort or unwise behavior.

STABILIMETER A device for measuring the activities of an infant.

STABILITY-LABILITY A means of classifying responsiveness of the autonomic nervous system *q.v.* Labile individuals are those who respond to a wide range of stimuli resulting in autonomic arousal. Stable individuals are not as easily aroused.

STABILIZED IMAGE An image on the retina *q.v.* presented in a way to eliminate the small movements usually produced by physiological nystagmus *q.v.* cf: stabilized image technique.

STABILIZED IMAGE TECHNIQUE A process by which the retina *q.v.* receives a stationary image even though the eye is moving. cf: stabilized image.

STABLE ANGINA Pain of angina pectoris *q.v.* that is felt only once in a while and as a result of a significant increase in the work of the heart. ct: unstable angina.

STAFF People whose functions are advisory and supportive in nature and who contribute to the efficiency and maintenance of an organization.

STAFF DEVELOPMENT A process of ongoing education for teachers or other members of an organization provided by professional organizations or schools.

STAGE OF EXHAUSTION The final stage of the general adaptation syndrome *q.v.* in which there is a physiological *q.v.* collapse.

STAGE OF RESISTANCE The second stage of the general adaptation syndrome *q.v.* in which the person temporarily compensates for stress *q.v.*

STAGES OF DYING Five predictable, but not universally applicable, psychological stages through which a person passes during the course of a terminal illness. These stages have been identified as denial, anger, bargaining, depression, and acceptance.

STAGGERED MONOGAMY A marital form in which a person mates with just one other person at a time, but may end one relationship to form another.

STAGING A procedure in which a variety of diagnostic tests are performed (X-rays, blood tests, body scans, urinalysis, etc.) to ascertain the extent of a disease beyond an initial diagnosis.

STAMINA The ability to mobilize energy to maintain movement over an extended period of time.

STANDARD The level of performance established to serve as a model for evaluating the performance of an individual or organization.

STANDARD DEVIATION (SD) 1. A measure of the variability of a frequency distribution *q.v.* that is the square root of the variance. 2. The most commonly used measure of variability. cf: variance.

STANDARD ERROR A measure of variation of a population of means.

STANDARD ERROR OF THE MEASUREMENT The standard deviation *q.v.* of the distribution of scores theoretically associated by correlation with a single score. In predicting a score from this latter score, it is possible to describe a hypothetical distribution of predicted scores.

STANDARD ERROR OF THE MEAN 1. A measure of the variability of the mean *q.v.* whose value depends both upon the standard deviation *q.v.* of the distribution and upon the number of cases in the sample *q.v.* 2. The standard deviation of frequency distribution *q.v.* of means that would be obtained in theory from a series of samples all selected in the same way.

STANDARDIZATION In test construction, the process of trying the test out on a sample *q.v.* to establish standard methods of administration, scoring, and interpretation.

STANDARDIZATION GROUP The group against which a person's test score is evaluated.

STANDARDIZED MORTALITY RATIO (SMR) In epidemiology *q.v.*, the ratio of observed events to those expected if standard rates are applied to the study populations. Usually the figure used in indirect adjustments *q.v.*

STANDARDIZED TEST 1. Based upon the norms of a large population. It is best used to verify strengths and weaknesses of a program and to justify what is being done. 2. A test prepared for nationwide use by establishing norms *q.v.* by presenting a carefully selected set of test items to a representative sample of learners. 3. A test that is norm-referenced *q.v.* and has specific standards for administration so scores can be compared. 4. A test whose validity *q.v.* and reliability *q.v.* have been established by means of statistical procedures.

STANDARD OF IDENTITY An official formula or recipe established by the Food and Drug Administration *q.v.* that specifies the ingredients that must be contained in certain foods in order for those products to carry a particular name on their labels.

STANDARD METROPOLITAN STATISTICAL AREA (SMSA) 1. A county or a group of contiguous counties containing at least one city of 50,000 or more inhabitants. 2. A community *q.v.*

STANDARD POPULATION In epidemiology *q.v.*, an arbitrary distribution of a characteristic is used as a common standard for two groups when comparing their rates.

STANDARDS Translation of functions into specific tasks and measurements that distinguish among various levels of performance.

STANDARD SCORE 1. *Z*-score *q.v.* 2. A score that is expressed as a deviation from the mean *q.v.* in standard deviation *q.v.* units, which allows a comparison of scores drawn from different distributions.

STANFORD-BINET TEST 1. An intelligence *q.v.* test that compares a subject's performance in developmentally graded tasks to a chronological norm. 2. The American version of the mental age scale developed by Binet and Simon in France. ~ was developed by psychologists at Stanford University.

STANINE A score that indicates a learner's position in a distribution divided into nine one-half standard deviation *q.v.* units.

STAPES 1. One of the three bones of the middle ear *q.v.* that transmits sound vibrations from the ear drum to the inner ear *q.v.* 2. Stirrup. cf: malleus; incus; cochlea.

STAPHYLOCOCCUS 1. A spherical bacterium *q.v.* occurring in grapelike clusters. 2. A group of germs found constantly on the skin and is the most common agent in wound infections *q.v.*

STAPHYLOCOCCUS AUREUS A disease-producing bacterium *q.v.* that can contaminate food.

STARCH 1. A complex carbohydrate *q.v.* 2. Found in plants, a group of nutrients *q.v.* essential in the human diet. 3. A polysaccharide *q.v.* A compound of long-chain glucose elements. 4. A carbohydrate, insoluble in water, converted to soluble forms by enzymes *q.v.*

STARCH PHOSPHORYLASE An enzyme *q.v.* that converts starch *q.v.* to glucose phosphate *q.v.*

STARCH SYNTHETASE The primary enzyme *q.v.* concerned in starch *q.v.* synthesis in plants.

STARE DECISIS 1. A legal doctrine whereby prior decision of courts are followed under similar fact. 2. The principle that when a court has made a decision regarding a legal principle, it is the law until changed by a competent authority.

STARS SOCIAL STATUS In studies of social status, those children who are high in both social preference *q.v.* and social impact *q.v.*

STARTLE REACTION A sudden, involuntary motor reaction to unexpected stimuli *q.v.* as a result of a state of hypersensitivity *q.v.*

STASIS Stagnation or congestion of blood in a restricted area.

STAT 1. An expression used in hospitals or other health care facilities to indicate urgency. 2. Immediately. 3. Right away.

STATE AID Funding provided to school districts out of tax revenue raised by the state.

STATE-BASED SURVEILLANCE SYSTEMS A means by which to link a variety of diverse databases used by state health departments for purposes such as mandatory registration of vital events or municipal water testing.

STATE BOARD EXAMINATION An examination administered by a State Board of Examiners as required for state licensure in a medical, dental, paramedical, or other profession requiring a license or certificate to practice.

STATE DEPARTMENT OF EDUCATION A unit within state government that governs the operation of public and private schools of the state and ensures compliance with state and federal education laws.

STATE-DEPENDENT LEARNING The phenomenon whereby an organism shows the effects of learning that took place in a special condition, better than in the ordinary condition in which learning usually occurs.

STATE-DEPENDENT MEMORY 1. A phenomenon that partly explains the unreliability of retrospective studies. 2. A phenomenon in which a person is more able to remember an event if he or she is in the same state as when the event occurred.

STATE-DEPENDENT PHENOMENON A behavior triggered by the emotional state of an individual.

STATIC CONTRACTION Isometric contraction *q.v.*

STATIC FLEXIBILITY EXERCISES Exercises in which a position is held steady for a period of time at an extreme range of motion.

STATISTIC 1. A value based on a sample of a population from which estimates for the entire population may be drawn. 2. A systematic arrangement and description of data *q.v.* 3. A science of inferring generalities from specific observations.

STATISTICAL CONCEPT A concept *q.v.* derived from mathematics and associated with probability *q.v.*

STATISTICAL CORRELATION The amount of relationship between two or more sets of data *q.v.* cf: positive correlation; negative correlation.

STATISTICALLY SIGNIFICANT An indication that the relationship examined is not due to chance or the effect of sampling.

STATISTICAL MODEL OF HEALTH The use of morbidity and mortality rates *qq.v.* as criteria for determining health status *q.v.* ct: medical model of health; holistic model of health.

STATISTICAL REGRESSION The tendency for extreme scores to become less extreme with retesting because chance variation leads to a broader range of scores on the original test.

STATISTICAL RELATIVITY A method of labeling that defines deviance based on the frequency of a behavior or characteristic. An average frequency is calculated and a person's status is compared with that average.

STATISTICAL STRUCTURE OF LANGUAGE A method of describing language in terms of the relative frequencies of sounds and combinations of sounds.

STATISTICAL TEST OF SIGNIFICANCE In epidemiology *q.v.*, methods of determining the probability *q.v.* that estimates of population parameters *q.v.* are different because of sampling variability *q.v.* only.

STATISTICS The science concerned with the collection, analysis, interpretation, and presentation of large amounts of data.

STATOCYSTS Organs of equilibrium.

STATUS 1. In sociology *q.v.*, a person's position in social space, or prestige and esteem that a person commands. 2. The rights and duties related to a position with a socially assigned amount of prestige. 3. The positioning of importance of a group member in relation to other members of the group.

STATUS ENVY THEORY OF IDENTIFICATION The theory that children identify with persons whose status they envy.

STATUS EPILEPTICUS A condition in which one major attack of epilepsy *q.v.* succeeds another with little or no intermission.

STATUS ORGASMUS A sustained orgasmic response experiences by some women that lasts 20 or more seconds.

STATUTORY RAPE 1. Voluntary sexual intercourse with a person who is under the age of consent. 2. Nonviolent voluntary sexual intercourse between an adult and a minor who is under the age of consent. cf: age of consent. ct: rape.

STAYING POWER The ability to remain on a weight reduction regimen in the face of temptations to discontinue dieting.

ST. BONIFACE, HOSPITAL OF A mental hospital located in Florence, Italy, where Vincenzo Chiarugi introduced the moral treatment movement *q.v.* in the late 1700s.

STD An acronym for sexually transmitted disease *q.v.*

STEADY STATE 1. In biochemistry *q.v.*, the situation that exists when the rate of elimination of a drug from the body equals the rate of intake of the drug. 2. In exercise, a condition in which the oxygen demand of an activity is exactly equal to the oxygen intake. 3. A situation when the population has reached births and deaths in perfect balance. 4. Zero population growth (ZPG) *q.v.*

STEARIC ACID A saturated fatty acid *q.v.* composed of 18 carbon atoms.

STEATORRHEA Excess lipid *q.v.* in the feces *q.v.* May be caused by any of several factors that impair fat digestion and absorption.

STEIN–LEVENTHAL SYNDROME 1. Reproductive malfunction in women. 2. A syndrome *q.v.* of endocrine *q.v.* origin that involves ovarian cysts *q.v.*, amenorrhea *q.v.*, and infertility *q.v.*

ST. ELIZABETH HOSPITAL The first national mental hospital erected in Washington, DC, in 1852.

STELAZINE 1. A commercial preparation of the major tranquilizers *q.v.* 2. A commercial preparation of phenothiazine *q.v.* 3. A commercial preparation of trifluoperazine *q.v.*

STEM CELLS Cells that can become any specialized cell in the body. ~ may be embryonic, present in bone marrow, or other tissues of the body.

STENOSIS 1. A narrowing or stricture of an opening. 2. Mitral stenosis *q.v.* or aortic stenosis *q.v.* indicate narrowing of those valves. 3. A narrowing in a vessel or valve that impedes the normal passage of blood.

STEP ALLELISM The concept of a series of alleles *q.v.* with graded effects on the same trait *q.v.*

STEPPINGSTONE THEORY The belief that the use of one drug leads to the use of more dangerous drugs. cf: gateway drugs.

STEP TEST A submaximal exercise that measures the heart rate recovery after stepping on and off a bench for 3 min.

STEREOGNOSIS Awareness of the shape of an object by means of touch.

STEREOTYPE 1. A preconceived, prejudiced view of the members of a particular group. 2. A socially derived category into which people are placed solely on the basis of their group identification.

STEREOTYPED MOVEMENT DISORDERS 1. Conditions that are characterized by abnormal gross motor behaviors. 2. Tics *q.v.*

STERILE 1. Aseptic or free from all living microorganisms *q.v.* and their spores *q.v.* 2. Not fertile *q.v.*

STERILITY 1. The absence of sex cells and, therefore, the inability to reproduce. 2. The inability to produce offspring. cf: infertility.

STERILIZATION 1. Rendering the male or female incapable of impregnation or conceiving. 2. Generally, a permanent birth control technique that surgically disrupts the normal passage of ova *q.v.* or sperm *q.v.* 3. The process of killing or removing all living things. cf: vasectomy; laparoscopy; culdoscopy.

STERILIZE 1. To render sterile *q.v.* or free from microorganism *q.v.* contamination *q.v.* 2. To render an organism unable to reproduce *q.v.*

STERNOCLAVICULAR JOINT The articulation *q.v.* between the clavicle *q.v.*, the sternum *q.v.*, and the cartilage *q.v.* of the first rib with an articular disc, subdividing the joint into two cavities *q.v.*

STERNOCLEIDOMASTOID MUSCLE The large muscle that is easily felt at the side of the neck attached to the mastoid bone *q.v.* at the top and the sternum *q.v.* at the bottom.

STERNUM 1. The breastbone. 2. The longitudinal bone plate forming in the middle of the anterior *q.v.* wall of the thorax *q.v.*, articulating above with the clavicles *q.v.* and along the sides with cartilages *q.v.* of the first seven ribs.

STEROID HORMONE 1. A chemical that suppresses the immune system *q.v.* 2. Hormones *q.v.* secreted by the gonads *q.v.* and the adrenal glands *q.v.*, some of which influence sexual behavior *q.v.* cf: estradiol; gonadal hormones; testosterone.

STEROL An alcohol *q.v.* of high molecular *q.v.* weight, such as cholesterol *q.v.* and ergosterol *q.v.*

STETHOSCOPE An instrument used to listen to the heart and lungs actions.

STEWARDSHIP The acceptance of responsibility for the wise use and protection of the earth's natural resources.

STH An acronym for somatotropic (somatotropin) hormone *q.v.*

STILLBIRTH 1. The neonate *q.v.* being born dead. 2. Perinatal mortality *q.v.* 3. Birth of a dead fetus.

STIMULANT 1. A drug that speeds up the activities of the central nervous system *q.v.* 2. A drug that increases alertness and motor activity, reduces fatigue, and increases wakefulness. 3. Any of several drugs that act on the central nervous system producing excitation, alertness, and wakefulness. Medical uses include treatment for mild depression, overweight, hyperactivity *q.v.*, and narcolepsy *q.v.* cf: caffeine; amphetamine; cocaine.

STIMULATION Increase in the rate of functional activity, speeding up of the central nervous system *q.v.* function.

STIMULATION THEORY The theory *q.v.* that reinforcement *q.v.* is a matter of stimulation *q.v.*

STIMULUS 1. Anything in the environment *q.v.* that an organism can detect and respond to. 2. Any antecedent or cause of behavior *q.v.* 3. Environmental energy *q.v.* cf: distal stimulus; proximal stimulus; effective stimulus; potential stimulus.

STIMULUS GENERALIZATION 1. A similar reaction to a variety of stimuli *q.v.* 2. In classical conditioning *q.v.*, the tendency to respond to stimuli other than the original conditioned stimulus *q.v.* 3. In instrumental conditioning *q.v.* a response to stimuli other than the original discriminative stimulus *q.v.* 4. The spread of a conditioned response to some stimulus similar to, but not identical with, the conditioned stimulus.

STIMULUS/RESPONSE BIT A conceptual unit consisting of sensory input to a person and the response that input produces.

STIMULUS-RESPONSE THEORY S-R theory *q.v.*

STIPULATION 1. A particular provision in an agreement. 2. An agreement between counsel concerning issues before the court.

STM An acronym for short-term memory *q.v.*

STOIC Capable of enduring pain and discomfort while remaining calm.

STOMACH The expansion of the alimentary canal *q.v.* between the esophagus *q.v.* and the duodenum *q.v.*

STOMACH MEDICINE A slang expression for drugs used or intended for gastrointestinal *q.v.* disturbances, e.g., antacids.

STOMATITIS Inflammation of mouth tissues.

STOOL Feces *q.v.*

STOP–START TECHNIQUE Treatment for premature ejaculation *q.v.* in which stimulation is ceased just prior to ejaculation, then resumed once the urge to ejaculate dissipates. cf: squeeze technique.

STORAGE FAT 1. Excessive reserves of body fat. 2. Adipose *q.v.* tissue. ct: essential fat.

STORE-FRONT CLINIC Usually, a small health services program located in a neighborhood for the ready access of residents.

STORGE 1. The love between children, parents, and grandparents. 2. The Greek form of love, most similar to attachment.

STOVE-IN CHEST Flail chest *q.v.*

STP Also known as DOM, a synthetic hallucinogen *q.v.* chemically related to methamphetamine *q.v.* It is said that ~ was named after the fuel additive, "scientifically treated petroleum," but also may have been named by Timothy Leary and stands for "serenity, tranquility, and peace."

STRABISMUS 1. A visual condition characterized by one eye not maintaining a parallel relationship with the other eye because one or more of the ocular muscles is paralyzed. It results in blurred vision, headache, and diplopia *q.v.* If left untreated, blindness in the weak eye will result. 2. Cross-eye.

STRADDLE LOAD A method of placing a victim on a long spineboard *q.v.* by straddling both board and victim and sliding him or her onto it.

STRAIGHT Heterosexual *q.v.*

STRAIN 1. In genetics *q.v.*, a population of animals produced through a prolonged inbreeding *q.v.* program resulting in little genetic variability. 2. In anatomy *q.v.*, a wrenching injury to ligaments *q.v.* supporting a joint *q.v.* cf: sprain.

STRAMONIUM ALKALOIDS Atropine-like drugs *q.v.* derived from jimson weed.

STRANGER ANXIETY 1. The species-specific response of human infants to strangers, esp. in the period from 8 to 10 months of age. 2. Fear of unfamiliar people.

STRANGULATION 1. Choking. 2. The cutting off of circulation to an organ or tissue by compression.

STRATEGIES 1. A combination of methods planned to complement, supplement, and reinforce each other in the learning process. 2. A broad, general plan developed to reach long-range objectives. 3. Implies techniques used to maneuver the learner into a position in which learning will occur more readily. It is a component of methodology *q.v.*

STRATIFIED SAMPLE 1. Sample *q.v.* 2. A subset of a population selected for study so constructed that every relevant subgroup is randomly sampled in proportion to its size. ct: random sample.

STRATOSPHERE The earth's atmosphere above 35,000 ft. ct: troposphere.

STRATUM Layer.

STREET VALUE The theoretical value of an amount of a particular drug sold in small quantities on the street.

STREETWALKER 1. A prostitute *q.v.* who generally practices her or his trade on city streets. 2. A prostitute who solicits clients by roaming the streets.

STRENGTH 1. The amount of force a muscle produces when it contracts. 2. The basic muscular force required for movement. cf: muscular strength.

STREPHOSYMBOLIA Literally twisted symbols. Usually involves reversals and mirror reading or writing.

STREPTOCOCCIOSIS A general term pertaining to all diseases caused by streptococci *q.v.* bacteria.

STREPTOCOCCUS 1. A bacterium *q.v.* that is the cause of strep throat and other diseases. 2. A group of germs responsible for virulent *q.v.* infections, including blood poisoning.

STREPTOCOCCUS ALBUS A bacterium *q.v.* found on the skin. It is believed to be associated with acne *q.v.*

STRESS 1. Physical or emotional tension caused by environmental forces, tending to produce health problems if severe or chronic and not beneficially dealt with. 2. The response of an organism to demands made of it by its internal and external environment. 3. Physiological and psychological state of imbalance caused by the body's response to an unanticipated, disruptive, or stimulating event. 4. An extreme, prolonged disruption of mind/body harmony. 5. Any condition impinging on the person that requires adjustive reactions. 6. Any situation in which the body's homeostatic *q.v.* balance is disturbed.

STRESS FRACTURE A small crack in a bone's surface, generally occurs in the feet, legs, or hands.

STRESS-INOCULATING TRAINING A therapeutic technique in which the person learns how to cope with stressors *q.v.* in a clinic setting in order to deal with stressors that present themselves in the future.

STRESS INTERVIEW An interview of a person under simulated stress *q.v.* conditions.

STRESSORS 1. Stimuli that produce stress *q.v.* 2. Factors or events, real or imagined, that elicit a state of stress. 3. Any condition that elicits the specific psychological *q.v.* and physiological *q.v.* responses characteristic of stress. 4. Any demand that gives rise to a coping response. 5. Any psychological or physiological condition that disturbs one's homeostatic *q.v.* balance.

STRESS TEST An examination and analysis of heart/lung function while the body is undergoing physical exercise, generally accomplished when a person walks or runs on a treadmill device while being monitored by a cardiograph *q.v.*

STRESS TOLERANCE 1. Frustration tolerance *q.v.* 2. The nature, degree, and duration of stress *q.v.* that a person can tolerate without undergoing serious personality decompensation *q.v.*

STRETCHER A device enabling two persons to lift and carry a victim in a lying down position. Several forms of ~s include the following: ambulance ~, army ~, basket ~, Robinson ~, Sarole ~, scoop ~, split-form ~, and Stokes basket.

STRETCHER LASH A method for using a rope to secure an injured person to a stretcher *q.v.* for the purpose of raising or lowering him or her from heights or depths or for transporting over rough terrain.

STRETCHING In exercise, the movement of a body part through the full range of motion in order to maintain or improve its flexibility.

STRETCH REFLEX The reflex contraction of a muscle in response to a sudden stretch of the muscle beyond its normal length. Serves to protect the muscle from overstretching.

STRIATED Marked with parallel lines.

STRIATED MUSCLE 1. The skeletal muscles *q.v.* 2. The muscles that are responsible for voluntary movement. ct: cardiac muscle; smooth muscle.

STRICTURE The abnormal narrowing of a canal, duct *q.v.*, or passage.

STRIDOR Noisy, labored breathing.

STROBOSCOPE A device that turns a light on and off in very rapid and controllable flashes.

STROKE 1. A cerebral accident *q.v.* 2. Death of brain cells resulting from a lack of blood to a portion of the brain. ~ may result in speech impairment, loss of memory, mental disturbances, and impaired motor functioning. In extreme cases, death may result. Cause is cerebral thrombosis *q.v.* or cerebral hemorrhage *q.v.* 3. The condition resulting from a blood clot lodging in a vessel in the brain. 4. Any obstruction or rupture of arteries *q.v.* in the brain resulting in brain damage or death.

STROKE VOLUME 1. The amount of blood pumped by the heart with each beat. 2. The volume of blood squeezed from the left ventricle *q.v.* during a heart beat by contraction of the ventricular musculature.

STRONTIUM-90 A radioactive *q.v.* element found in fallout from atomic or nuclear explosions.

STROOP EFFECT A marked decrease in the speed of naming the colors in which various color names are presented when the colors and names are different. An example of automatization *q.v.*

STRUCTURAL DEFECTS Genetic defects *q.v.* affecting the body parts, size, and shape.

STRUCTURAL DIFFERENTIATION The organization and specialization of tissues and organs within the body of the developing organism.

STRUCTURAL GENE 1. A gene in operon *q.v.* directing polypeptide *q.v.* synthesis. 2. A gene that controls actual protein *q.v.* by determining the amino acid *q.v.* sequence. cf: operator gene; regulator gene.

STRUCTURALISM A school of psychology *q.v.* based on the study of the effects of specific stimuli on the sensory experience.

STRUCTURAL PRINCIPLES OF LANGUAGE Rules that describe principles according to how native speakers of the language actually arrange their words in sentences. Sentences formed according to these principles are called well-form or grammatical. ct: prescriptive rules.

STRUCTURAL THEORY A Freudian theory that identifies the three parts of the human psyche: the id, ego, and superego *qq.v.*

STRUCTURE In sociology *q.v.*, the stable, patterned features of a social system.

STRUCTURED ANSWER TEST An objectively scorable instrument by means of which the learner indicates an answer to each test item by checking the best or correct choice among several alternatives presented.

STRUCTURED CLASSROOM Traditional classroom *q.v.*

STRUCTURE OF COMMUNICATION The typical pattern of communication *q.v.* adopted by a group in order to function.

STRUCTURES D'ENSEMBLE Literally, structures of the whole. Piaget's term for hypothetical holistic structures that are available to children in each level of development. Each period is characterized by a unique ~.

STRYCHNINE 1. A poison that stimulates the central nervous system *q.v.* 2. An alkaloid *q.v.* from seeds of Strychnos nux-vomica, an extremely potent stimulant *q.v.* of the central nervous system.

STUDENT An individual for whom educational programs are directed under the jurisdiction of a school, school system, or other educational institution.

STUDENT-CENTERED CURRICULUM A curriculum organization in which learning activities are centered on the individual student and his or her interests.

S-TUBE An oropharyngeal airway *q.v.* shaped like an S that can be used to prevent a victim's tongue from obstructing the airway while artificial ventilation *q.v.* is being given through the device.

STUDENT ROLE A set of behaviors required of students in classrooms by most teachers.

STUDY GROUP 1. The unit that receives the treatment being tested in a study. 2. Experimental group *q.v.* ct: control group.

STUFFING TECHNIQUE A procedure whereby the penis *q.v.* is stuffed into the vagina *q.v.* Used chiefly by elderly men who have soft erections *q.v.* and by men with spinal cord injuries.

STUPOR 1. A condition characterized by lethargy and unresponsiveness, with partial or complete unconsciousness. 2. A state of suspended or diminished sensibility.

STURM UND DRANG German for "storm and stress." An outdated term describing the characteristics of adolescence in favor of one that views adolescence as a series of smoother, more gradual changes.

STUTTERING 1. Stammering. 2. A speech disorder characterized by blocking and repetition of the initial sounds of words.

ST. VITUS DANCE 1. A hysterical *q.v.* chorea *q.v.* common during the Middle Ages. 2. Involuntary and uncontrollable muscular twitching of the face and limbs. 3. Sydenham's chorea.

STY A condition that results when the glands surrounding roots of eyelashes become infected, usually by *Staphylococcus* *q.v.* bacterium *q.v.*

STYCAR 1. An acronym for Sheridan's test for young children and retardates. 2. An eye examination chart using the letters H, O, T, and V, which are to be matched on a screen with the same letters on a card held by the person being tested. cf: Snellen eye test; illiterate E.

SUBACUTE A disease with characteristics of acute *q.v.* and chronic *q.v.* symptoms.

SUBARACHNOID Situated or occurring beneath the arachnoid *q.v.*

SUBCLAVIAN ARTERY The large artery *q.v.* just under the collarbone that supplies blood to the main artery of the arm, head, neck, and axilla *q.v.* through its branches.

SUBCLINICAL The presence of a disease but without signs of symptoms.

SUBCLINICAL DEFICIENCY A deficiency of a substance so mild that the deficiency is not recognized by ordinary visual clinical means.

SUBCONSCIOUS 1. Unconscious thoughts that have been repressed *q.v.* 2. Thoughts that are brought to the awareness only with great difficulty, if at all. 3. ~ is a term no longer in common use. cf: conscious; preconscious.

SUBCONSCIOUS MIND A Freudian concept of one of the parts of the mind. cf: subconscious.

SUBCORTICAL STRUCTURES Structures of the brain lying under the cortex *q.v.*

SUBCULTURE A distinctive culture *q.v.* within the framework of a larger culture.

SUBCUTANEOUS 1. Under the skin. 2. An injection just beneath the skin. 3. An injection in which the needle penetrates about 0.5 in beneath the surface of the skin, but does not penetrate a muscle or enter a vein.

SUBCUTANEOUS EMPHYSEMA The presence of gas or air in the subcutaneous *q.v.* tissues of the body.

SUBCUTANEOUS FAT Fat deposited in the adipose *q.v.* tissue immediately under the skin's surface. ~ constitutes approximately 80% of the body's stored fat.

SUBCUTANEOUS INJECTION A hypodermic *q.v.* injection of drugs or other fluids just beneath the surface of the skin. cf: subcutaneous.

SUBCUTANEOUS MASTECTOMY Surgical removal of the internal breast tissue, leaving the skin and preserving the nipple, if possible.

SUBDURAL HEMATOMA 1. Hemorrhaging and swelling of the arachnoid *q.v.* torn by a fractured bone of the skull. 2. A collection of blood or clots caused by a laceration *q.v.* or rupture *q.v.* of a meningeal *q.v.* vessel lying between the dura mater *q.v.* and the arachnoid.

SUBFAMILY A married couple with or without children, living with a person or couple who maintains the household. The most common example is a married couple living in the home of the husband's or wife's parents.

SUBINTENTIONAL DEATH 1. A death that is believed to have been caused in some measure by a person's unconscious desires. 2. The behavior of individuals who play an unconscious role in their own death through repeated high-risk behaviors.

SUBJECT ANALOGUES Research studies in which animals are used to broaden the researcher's range of options when it comes to inducing stress or testing drugs, etc., and to giving the researcher greater control over conditions.

SUBJECT-CENTERED CURRICULUM A curriculum *q.v.* in which content and activities are organized around a particular subject.

SUBJECTIVE DISTRESS Experiences of excessive and inhibiting fearfulness, depression, agitation, or other disturbing emotion *q.v.*

SUBJECTIVE INSTRUMENT A test instrument that requires the scorer to be trained, experienced, and skilled in the responses expected from the use of the test. Scoring is based on the judgment of the scorer.

SUBJECTIVE MORAL REASONING 1. In moral judgment, judging an act as good or bad on the basis of the person's intentions. 2. According to Piaget, a judgment of guilt based on the intentions of the wrongdoer and not simply the degree of damage done. ct: objective moral reasoning.

SUBJECTIVE TEST INSTRUMENT A test that requires the scorer to be trained, experienced, and skilled in the responses expected from the use of the instrument. Scoring is based on the judgment of the scorer. ct: objective test instrument.

SUBJECTIVE THEORY One of the major systems of rules and principles that guide persons in making value judgments. ~ claims that values are chosen by each person as a matter of personal preference.

SUBJECTIVISM A philosophy that our knowledge is produced by own minds, that the external world is either denied or viewed as unimportant.

SUBJECT MATTER Topical content, such as facts, theories, controversies, and ideas appropriate to the needs, interests, and developmental levels of the learner.

SUBLETHAL GENE A lethal gene *q.v.* with delayed effect. The gene, in proper combination with other elements of heredity *q.v.* or environmental factors, kills its possessor in infancy, childhood, or adulthood.

SUBLIMATION 1. A defense mechanism *q.v.* that involves the acceptance of a substitute goal that provides a socially acceptable outlet of expression, most typically associated with an undesirable sexual urge. 2. Redirection of sexual energy. 3. Conversion of a person's unacceptable impulses into socially acceptable outlets.

SUBLIMAZE A commercial preparation of fentanyl *q.v.*

SUBLIMINAL 1. Below the threshold of consciousness *q.v.* a stimulus *q.v.* is present, but the person is unaware of its presence. 2. A stimulus too weak to produce a response, below the normal threshold of consciousness.

SUBLIMINAL ADVERTISING Advertising that stimulates a person's unconsciousness *q.v.* cf: subliminal perception.

SUBLIMINAL PERCEPTION The assumed fact that stimuli below the absolute threshold *q.v.* have an effect on perception *q.v.*

SUBLINGUAL Under the tongue.

SUBLUXATION A purported malalignment of the vertebral column *q.v.* or other joint.

SUBMENTAL Under the chin.

SUBORDINATION In sociology, the placing of a group or class in a lower rank relative to another group.

SUBPOENA The process of commanding a witness to appear and testify before a judicial or other official body.

SUBSTANCE ABUSE 1. Drug abuse characterized by impairment in occupational or social functioning caused by a pattern of long-term pathological use. 2. Repeated episodes of drug misuse that places the individual and others at heightened risk and is often the result of a compulsion to misuse one or more drugs.

SUBSTANCE DEPENDENCE A form of substance use that involves a physiological *q.v.* dependence on the drug and a withdrawal syndrome *q.v.* should drug use be suddenly terminated for an extended period of time.

SUBSTANCE-INDUCED ORGANIC MENTAL DISORDER A physical disorder that is a direct result of a substance's physiological *q.v.* effects on the central nervous system *q.v.*

SUBSTANCE P A peptide *q.v.* found in nerves *q.v.* that transmits pain signals.

SUBSTANCE-SPECIFIC RESEARCH Studies to determine whether adequate information on the health effects of each listed substance is available. The purpose of the ~ program is to supply the informational needs of the agency regarding health assessments.

SUBSTANCE ABUSE DISORDERS Disorders in which drugs such as alcohol *q.v.* and cocaine *q.v.* are abused to such an extent that behavior becomes pathologically impaired, social and occupational functioning are disrupted, and control of abstinence becomes impossible.

SUBSTERNAL Beneath the sternum *q.v.*

SUBSTITUTE BEHAVIOR Any behavior *q.v.* that provides indirect or symbolic satisfaction of a need *q.v.*

SUBSTITUTE (ON FOOD LABELS) A substance in a food that is often an imitation of another food substance, nutritionally equivalent to the real substance that the substitute is imitating.

SUBSTITUTION 1. A defense mechanism *q.v.* 2. The process of accepting new goals, but with no change in the quality of conscious desire.

SUBTRACTIVE COLOR MIXTURE 1. Mixing colors by subtracting one set of wavelengths from another set. 2. Mixture of pigments. ct: additive mixture.

SUBSTRATE 1. Any substance on which an enzyme *q.v.* acts chemically. 2. The "reactant" portion of any biochemical reaction *q.v.* 3. Any substance used as a nutrient by a microorganism *q.v.*

SUBTROCHANTRIC AREA The area below the trochanter *q.v.*

SUBUNIT VACCINE A vaccine *q.v.* that uses only one component of an infectious agent *q.v.* rather than the whole agent in order to stimulate an immune response *q.v.*

SUCCESSIVE APPROXIMATIONS A method of training in which successively more nearly exact performances *q.v.* of the correct response *q.v.* are required.

SUCCINYLCHOLINE A muscle relaxant used to prevent bone fractures during electroconvulsive *q.v.* therapy.

SUCCORANT Needing aid or help.

SUCKING CHEST WOUND A wound *q.v.* of the chest wall through which air passes into and out of the pleural *q.v.* space with each respiration *q.v.*

SUCRASE 1. An enzyme *q.v.* that hydrolyzes *q.v.* sucrose *q.v.* into glucose and fructose *qq.v.* 2. Invertase *q.v.*

SUCROSE 1. Table sugar. 2. A disaccharide *q.v.* produced by a combination of glucose and fructose *qq.v.* 3. A plant sugar. 4. A molecule of glucose and a molecule of fructose chemically bonded together.

SUCTION ABORTION 1. Vacuum curettage *q.v.* 2. Suction curettage *q.v.* 3. Vacuum aspiration *q.v.* 4. A method of therapeutic or elective abortion *q.v.* usually performed up to the 12th week of pregnancy that involves removal of the fetus via suction through a large tube that is inserted into the uterus *q.v.*

SUCTION CATHETERS Hollow semiflexible tubes of varying diameter that are used to aspirate material from within the pharynx *q.v.*, trachea *q.v.*, and upper bronchi *q.v.*

SUCTION CURETTAGE 1. Vacuum aspiration *q.v.* 2. Suction abortion *q.v.*

SUCTION LIPTECTOMY A surgical technique involving the insertion of a tube into fat tissue whereby the tissue is removed by suction. The procedure is generally used on people who have excess deposits of adipose *q.v.* tissue in specific areas of the body, e.g., the hips.

SUDDEN CARDIAC DEATH An acute *q.v.* coronary *q.v.* attack that results in death within 24 h.

SUDDEN DEATH The death of a victim of coronary heart attack *q.v.* within 24 h after the appearance of symptoms.

SUDDEN INFANT DEATH SYNDROME (SIDS) 1. Also called crib death. 2. The sudden and unexplained death of an infant apparently associated with apnea *q.v.*

SUDORIFEROUS Secreting sweat.

SUFFOCATE 1. To impede respiration *q.v.* 2. To suffer from need of oxygen. 3. To be unable to breathe. cf: asphyxiation.

SUFFOCATION A lack of oxygen getting into the lungs. May be caused by a blockage of the windpipe, pressure on the chest, or insufficient supply of oxygen in the air being breathed. cf: asphyxiation.

SUGAR 1. An edible form of carbohydrate *q.v.* used as an energy source in the body. 2. A simple form of carbohydrate. cf: starch.

SUGAR ADDICTION A misnomer since there is no evidence that sugar *q.v.* intake results in addictive physiological *q.v.* changes in the body. The term is usually applied to persons who consume large quantities of refined sugar products beyond the amount needed by the body as a ready source of energy.

SUGAR-FREE OR SUGARLESS (ON FOOD LABELS) Said foods cannot contain sucrose *q.v.*, but may have such sweeteners as honey, corn syrup, fructose *q.v.*, sorbitol *q.v.*, or mannitol.

SUICIDAL INTENT SCALE A technique used to assess the seriousness of suicide intent. The scale attempts to objectively assess the circumstances related to the attempt.

SUICIDE A self-destructive act. The ninth leading cause of death for all ages. The second leading cause of death among those 18–24 years of age. Many attempts at ~ are planned, deliberate acts of aggression or hostility toward oneself. Often the act is essentially a reaction to a crisis of despair or despondency and represents a dramatic appeal for help or to attract attention, to spite other, or to submit oneself to trial by ordeal.

SUICIDE CLUSTERS Communities in which suicide *q.v.* rates are significantly higher than the national average.

SUICIDE OBSERVATION 1. Suicide watch. 2. A precautionary, continuous observation by medical and nursing staff of those considered to be at severe risk of suicide *q.v.*

SULCUS 1. A shallow furrow in the cerebral cortex *q.v.* separating adjacent convolutions. 2. Furrow or groove.

SULFA DRUGS Drugs *q.v.* that contain the crystalline compound, sulfanilamide *q.v.*

SULFONAMIDE Derivative of sulfanilic acid.

SULFANILAMIDE A type of antibiotic *q.v.*

SULFUR Chemical symbol is S. A chemical element that is found in the essential amino acid, methionine *q.v.*, and in the vitamins, thiamin and biotin *qq.v.*

SULFUR DIOXIDE A gaseous byproduct (SO_2) of the combination of any organic substance containing sulfur *q.v.*

SULFURIC ACID 1. A colorless, nearly odorless, heavy, oily, corrosive liquid containing 96% absolute acid *q.v.* Used occasionally as a caustic. 2. H_2SO_4 is the chemical formula of ~.

SUMMARY Immediate, without full proceeding, as in summary judgment.

SUMMATION The addition of the intensities of nerve impulses so that the combined effect is strong enough to cross a synapse *q.v.*

SUMMATION TONE A third tone sometimes heard when two tones are sounded together. Its pitch *q.v.* is that which corresponds to the total of the two component frequencies. ct: difference tone.

SUMMATIVE EVALUATION 1. In education, using tests to establish how well a learner has met the objectives of a unit or to determine a final grade. 2. In research, an evaluation of the outcomes of a particular study. ct: formative evaluation.

SUN PROTECTION FACTOR (SPF) A number indicating the degree of protection provided by a sunscreen product against the ultraviolet rays of the sun.

SUNSTROKE 1. Failure of the body's heat regulation system resulting in a body temperature of 105°F or higher. 2. A condition due to prolonged exposure to the sun characterized by coma *q.v.* and a high body temperature. 3. Heatstroke *q.v.*

SUPEREGO 1. One's moral code. 2. The conscious *q.v.* It has two components: the ego ideal and the conscious *qq.v.* 3. In Freudian psychology, the component of personality concerned with morality or conscious. 4. The higher social mores and values, the moral conscience and self-critical nature of a person. 5. A set of reaction patterns within the ego that represent the internalized rules of society and that control the ego by instilling guilt.

SUPERFICIAL On the surface. Cursory. Not thorough.

SUPERFUND Another name for the Comprehensive Environmental Response, Compensation, and Liability Act of 1980 *q.v.* that created ATSDR *q.v.*

SUPERINCISION 1. Removal of the foreskin *q.v.* from the penis plus cutting of the shaft of the penis *q.v.* 2. Circumcision *q.v.*

SUPERINTENDENT 1. The chief school administrative officer in local school districts. 2. School superintendent.

SUPERIOR Above, in relation to another body structure. ct: inferior.

SUPERIOR VENA CAVA 1. The body's largest vein *q.v.* 2. The vessel that conveys blood from the upper body regions back to the right atrium *q.v.* of the heart.

SUPERMALE 1. A male possessing the XYY chromosomal *q.v.* structure. 2. Males with an extra Y chromosome.

SUPERNUTRITION Any dietary regimen of specialized foods and nutritional supplements *q.v.* designed to increase the quality of body functioning. Used frequently by athletes. Usually not necessary or effective.

SUPERORDINATE GOALS Goals that can be achieved only by working together as a group.

SUPERSATURATION In chemistry *q.v.*, the condition in which a solvent *q.v.* has dissolved a greater quantity of a solute *q.v.* than it is capable of at a particular temperature.

SUPINATE To turn the palm of the hand upward. ct: pronate.

SUPINE POSITION 1. Lying on the back. 2. Turning of the forearm so that the palm of the hand faces upward.

SUPPLEMENTARY FACTORS Factors that modify a more fundamental factor.

SUPPLEMENTAL SECURITY INCOME (SSI) A national program that provides supplemental payments to older persons who already receive public assistance. The program's aim is to raise the incomes of these people to the poverty threshold.

SUPPLEMENTARY DATA SYSTEM (SDS) A voluntary program in which participating states code accident and injury cases from workers' compensation agencies. The information is provided to the Bureau of Labor Statistics for the development of a database to identify when occupational health and safety problems exist.

SUPPLEMENTARY HEALTH INSURANCE Medigap insurance *q.v.*

SUPPLENESS The quality of muscles and joints that permits a full range of movement.

SUPPLY REDUCTION A strategy for reducing drug abuse by lowering or restricting the supply of legal drugs and eliminating the supply of illegal drugs.

SUPPORTIVE REHABILITATION Treatments aimed at returning a person to a state of self-sufficiency even though a permanent disability has resulted from a disease or injury.

SUPPORTIVE THERAPY Psychotherapy *q.v.* consisting of emotional support and reassurance, esp. for people with sexual dysfunction *q.v.*

SUPPOSITORY A drug product that is administered by insertion into a body opening, usually the rectum or vagina, where it melts to release its active ingredients.

SUPPRESSION 1. A conscious effort to forget an event or experience. 2. The forcible and intentional expulsion of unpleasant thoughts from consciousness *q.v.* 3. Conscious inhibition of desires or impulses. ct: repression.

SUPPRESSOR T CELLS A subset of T cells that carry the T8 marker and turn off antibody *q.v.* production and other immune *q.v.* responses.

SUPPURATION The formation of pus *q.v.* in a wound.

SUPERCLAVICULAR NODES Lymph nodes *q.v.* located above the clavicle *q.v.* or collar bone.

SUPRACONDYLAR FRACTURE A fracture *q.v.* of the distal *q.v.* end of the humerus *q.v.*

SURFACE CONTACT According to Levinger, a stage of a relationship in which people seek common ground and test mutual attraction.

SURFACE STRUCTURE The phrase *q.v.* organization of sentences as they are spoken or written. cf: phrase structure. ct: underlying structure.

SURFACE TRAIT A relatively superficial *q.v.* and modifiable trait of the personality *q.v.* ct: source trait.

SURGERY 1. A medical specialty concerned with the operative treatment of diseases. 2. A treatment method characterized by cutting into the body to correct a malfunction or malformation, or to remove a diseased tissue or organ, or part of a tissue or organ. ~ may involve organ transplants *q.v.*, implants *q.v.*, and prosthetic *q.v.* attachments. A general surgeon is qualified to perform many common operations but most specialized in one area of the body.

SURGICAL INSURANCE A policy that pays for surgical procedures usually when conducted in a hospital setting. There are usually deductible and exclusion clauses.

SURROGATE 1. A substitute. 2. A person who takes the place and role of another person, e.g., a ~ mother, a ~ sex partner.

SURVEILLANCE 1. The process of accumulating information about the incidence *q.v.* and prevalence *q.v.* of disease in a particular area. 2. The secret watching of suspected individuals, places, objects, etc., to obtain information on suspected criminal activity.

SURVEILLANCE ACTIVITY Those activities which evaluate exposure or trends in adverse health effects over a specified period of time. ~ addresses the ongoing systematic collection, analysis, and interpretation of health data in the process of describing and monitoring a health event. Data obtained through surveillance are very important for appropriate decisions regarding the planning, evaluation, or implementation of public health interventions.

SURVEY A research technique in which subjects are asked questions about their behavior, attitudes, or intentions related to a particular subject.

SURVEY RESEARCH Research in which a representative sample of a population *q.v.* is asked a series of questions regarding their behavior, attitudes, or beliefs.

SURVIVAL RATE Refers to the percentage of people who live a set period of time after a surgical procedure or the diagnosis of disease, as opposed to the percentage of those who die.

SURVIVAL SKILLS 1. A set of skills that are necessary to survive in today's society. A ~ curriculum *q.v.* may center on the development of these skills. 2. Life skills curriculum.

SUSCEPTIBLE A person with no specific resistance to a disease or condition.

SUSCEPTIBLE HOST A person not possessing sufficient resistance against a particular organism to prevent contracting an infection *q.v.* when exposed to the organism.

SUSPENSION A dosage form in which particles of an insoluble drug are suspended in a liquid.

SUTURE A thread composed of catgut, silk, cotton, or other material used for sewing any two structures together in the course of a surgical procedure.

SV An acronym for stroke volume.

SW An acronym for slow wave sleep *q.v.*

SWATHE BANDAGE A bandage *q.v.* that passes around the chest, splinting an injured arm to the chest.

SWEATING PHENOMENON The appearance of tiny droplets of fluid in the walls of the vagina *q.v.* early in the excitement phase *q.v.* of the sexual response cycle *q.v.*

SWIMMER'S EAR A nonemergency condition that results from inflammation *q.v.* in the external ear canal created by the growth of infecting *q.v.* organisms, usually contracted during swimming.

SWINGING Mate swapping *q.v.*

SWS An acronym for slow wave sleep *q.v.*

SYLLABARY A writing system in which the symbols stand for syllables of words.

SYLLABIC STRUCTURE 1. Babbling *q.v.* 2. Consisting of a consonant plus a vowel structure. Common in infants *q.v.* at about 6 months of age.

SYLLABUS 1. Enumeration of course objectives with an outline of major topics. 2. A presentation of the material necessary for a comprehensive view of the whole subject, often in outline form.

SYLLOGISM 1. A form of deductive reasoning *q.v.* 2. An analysis of reasoning consisting of a major premise, minor premise, and a conclusion which logically follows. Conclusions may be inaccurate when premises are inaccurate.

SYMBIONT An organism living in intimate association with another dissimilar organism.

SYMBIOSIS 1. In biology *q.v.*, the living together of two or more dissimilar organisms. Includes parasitism *q.v.* if only one of the organisms benefit and mutualism *q.v.* if all of the organisms benefit. 2. In psychology *q.v.*, a parent–child relationship in which there is extreme parental interference, preventing the child from developing a sense of autonomy. 3. An association of two or more organisms living together for mutual benefit.

SYMBIOTIC A relationship of two or more living things contributing to each other's existence. cf: parasite.

SYMBIOTIC PSYCHOSIS A disorder of childhood marked by extreme reluctance of the child to be separated from his or her mother and by panic attacks.

SYMBOL An image, object, or activity that is used to represent something else, e.g., a phallic ~.

SYMBOLIC FUNCTION Semiotic function *q.v.*

SYMBOLIC LOSS In psychoanalytic theory *q.v.*, the unconscious interpretation by the ego *q.v.* of an event as a total loss such as suffered in the death of a loved one.

SYMBOLIC REPRESENTATION An abstract representation as in verbal learning or problem solving.

SYMBOLISM A representation of one idea or object by another. cf: symbol.

SYMBOLIZATION 1. A phobia *q.v.* of symbols. 2. Extreme fear of something that is unconsciously related to an unpleasant experience. 3. Fear of symbolic expression. 4. Symbolophobia.

SYMMETRIGENIC FISSION Binary longitudinal fission *q.v.* with duplication of cell organelles *q.v.* preceding fission.

SYMPATHECTOMY A surgical procedure that interrupts some part of the sympathetic nervous system *q.v.*

SYMPATHETIC A division of the autonomic nervous system *q.v.* stimulated by emotional *q.v.* states. ct: parasympathetic nervous system.

SYMPATHETIC NERVE One of the nerves *q.v.* of the sympathetic portion of the autonomic nervous system *q.v.*

SYMPATHETIC NERVOUS SYSTEM 1. A part of the autonomic nervous system *q.v.* that tends to speed up actions of various organs. 2. A division of the autonomic nervous system that innervates the viscera *q.v.* and prepares it for vigorous physical and psychological arousal 3. The thoracolumbar nervous system *q.v.* ct: parasympathetic nervous system.

SYMPATHETIC PREGNANCY A condition in which a father experiences some of the symptoms of pregnancy encountered by the mother.

SYMPATHISM An ego defense mechanism *q.v.* by means of which a person achieves the sympathy of others by relating to them his or her difficulties.

SYMPATHOADRENAL An agent having effects similar to those of adrenal *q.v.* function.

SYMPATHOLYTIC DRUG A drug that acts on the sympathetic nervous system *q.v.* to lower blood pressure directly.

SYMPATHOMIMETIC 1. A substance that produces a reduction or relief of nasal congestion. 2. A drug that acts on the sympathetic nervous system *q.v.* and has adrenergic *q.v.* effects. 3. A drug that acts on the postjunctional receptor sites for norepinephrine and epinephrine *qq.v.* 4. Any drug that stimulates the sympathetic nervous system, e.g., amphetamine *q.v.*

SYMPHYSIS Greek for growing together.

SYMPHYSIS PUBIS 1. The hair-covered mound in the female that is anterior *q.v.* to the external genitalia *q.v.* 2. The articulation between the pubic bones *q.v.* in the lower abdomen *q.v.* 3. The firm fibrocartilaginous joint between the two pubic bones.

SYMPOSIUM 1. A gathering of people for the purpose of intellectual discussion and exchange relative to a specific topic, issue, or problem. 2. A drinking party.

SYMPTO-THERMAL METHOD A rhythm method *q.v.* of contraception *q.v.* that combines the techniques of observing basal body temperature and cervical mucus *q.v.* consistency to determine when a woman ovulates *q.v.*

SYMPTOM 1. A measurable indication that the body or mind is reacting to a foreign substance or agent or experience. 2. An indication felt by a person that something is wrong with the functioning of a part of the body, e.g., fever, nausea. An observable physical or psychological manifestation of a disease, often occurring in a patterned group of symptoms to constitute a syndrome *q.v.* 4. The subjective evidence of a person's condition as opposed to a sign *q.v.*

SYMPTOMATIC Presenting symptoms *q.v.* of a known disease condition.

SYMPTOMATIC ALCOHOLISM Overindulgence in the use of alcohol *q.v.*

SYMPTOMATIC TREATMENT Treatment designed to alleviate the overt manifestations of a person's illness without recognizing or dealing with the causes of that illness.

SYMPTOMATOLOGY 1. The science concerned with indications, symptoms, and signs of a disease or other condition. 2. Semeiology *q.v.*

SYMPTOM SEVERITY A parameter of classification referring to the degree of variation from the norm.

SYNANON A therapeutic community in which residents, typically drug addicts, learn to take responsibility for and change their behavior.

SYNAPSE 1. In neurology and anatomy *qq.v.*, junction or meeting place between two nerve cells *q.v.* 2. A space or junction where the presynaptic membrane of an axon *q.v.* is in proximity to the dendrites *q.v.* and the cell body of another neuron *q.v.* 3. In genetics *q.v.*, a pairing of homologous chromosomes *q.v.*

SYNAPSIS A conjunction of pairs of homologous chromosomes *q.v.* of maternal and paternal origin, respectively.

SYNAPTIC CLEFT The space between two neurons *q.v.* at which a nervous impulse passes from one neuron to another.

SYNAPTIC JUNCTION Synapse *q.v.*

SYNAPTIC VESICLE A membrane-enclosed sac of neurotransmitter *q.v.* found in the end bulb of a neuron *q.v.*

SYNCOPE 1. Fainting *q.v.* 2. Temporary loss of consciousness resulting from cerebral *q.v.* anemia *q.v.*

SYNCYTIUM An undivided mass of protoplasm *q.v.* containing several nuclei *q.v.*

SYNDROME 1. A group of signs and symptoms *q.v.* of a disorder that are characteristic of the disorder. 2. All of the signs and symptoms associated with a disease.

SYNERGISM The interaction of two drugs that produces an effect greater than the total effect of each drug acting individually.

SYNERGIST A drug that, when combined with another drug, produces effects greater than those when the drugs are taken separately. cf: additive effect; potentiation.

SYNESTHESIS 1. The sensation created from the use of certain drugs causing a person to "see sounds" or "hear colors." 2. A drug effect in which there is a mingling of the senses. 3. Experiencing the stimuli to one sensory modality which in turn is appropriate to another sensory modality.

SYNGAMY The union of the gametes *q.v.* in fertilization *q.v.*

SYNOVIA 1. The viscid fluid of a joint or similar cavity. 2. Synovial fluid *q.v.* 3. A clear viscid fluid the function of which is to lubricate a joint. 4. Literally, with egg.

SYNOVIAL Of, or pertaining to, or secreting synovia *q.v.*

SYNOVIAL CELLS Cells that produce the lubricating fluid required for smooth function of the joints.

SYNOVIAL FLUID Synovia *q.v.*

SYNOVITIS Inflammation of the membrane *q.v.* lining a joint.

SYNOVIUM The lining membrane *q.v.* of a joint cavity.

SYNTAX The order and way in which words and sequences of words are combined into phrases, clauses, and sentences.

SYNTHESIS 1. The development of more complex chemical structures from their simpler components. 2. The formation of chemical compounds.

SYNTHETIC A substance formed by a chemical reaction in a laboratory.

SYNTHETIC CONVENTIONAL STAGE The stage of faith development generally associated with adolescence *q.v.* in which one lives within the constructs formulated by others for the individual.

SYNTHETIC MEDIUM A chemically defined medium in which the exact chemistry of each component is known.

SYNTHETIC NARCOTICS A subgroup of narcotic *q.v.* drugs manufactured in the laboratory as opposed to derivation from plants or animals.

SYNTHETIC OPIATES 1. Opiate-like drugs that are not by-products of the oriental poppy plant. 2. Drugs that are manufactured in the laboratory that have similar effects as natural opiates *q.v.*

SYPHILIS 1. A chronic sexually transmitted disease *q.v.* caused by the spirochete *q.v.*, *Treponema pallidum q.v.* It may attack any organ of the body when left untreated. Its transmission is through intimate sexual contact by an infected mother to her unborn baby (congenital syphilis) or through blood transfusion with infected blood. ~ has three stages when left untreated: 1. The primary stage, or acute stage, characterized by a chancre *q.v.* at the point of infection. 2. The secondary stage characterized by fever, skin eruptions, and headache, followed by a latency period when there are no symptoms. However, during the period, the disease is invading muscle and nerve tissue. 3. The tertiary stage characterized by a variety of symptoms depending upon the organs or tissues that are involved. Treatment is by the use of penicillin *q.v.*

SYRINGOMYELIA The existence of abnormal cavities filled with fluid in the substance of the spinal cord *q.v.*

SYRUP OF IPECAC A drug that will induce vomiting. cf: ipecac.

SYSTEM 1. In sociology *q.v.*, according to Bever, an orderly arrangement of components that are interrelated and act and interact to perform some task or function in a particular environment *q.v.* 2. A unit of interacting personalities *q.v.*, which has persistence in time and which has a physical and cultural base that sustains it. 3. A way of thinking about a human problem. The elements of a ~ are environment, inputs within the system, and outputs from the system. 4. In anatomy *q.v.*, a group of organs that function as a unit to achieve a particular physiological *q.v.* goal. The body's systems are nervous, muscular, skeletal, endocrine, digestive, reproductive, excretory, integumentary, circulatory, and respiratory *qq.v.*

SYSTEMATIC DESENSITIZATION 1. Behavior therapy *q.v.* 2. The step-by-step process of assisting to learn to reduce a fear reaction or other negative response to a stimulus. 3. A form of behavior therapy in which a person is gradually exposed to increasingly more fearful situations until each situation has lost its threat. cf: implosive therapy; operant conditioning.

SYSTEMATIC RATIONAL RESTRUCTURING A type of rational-emotive therapy *q.v.* in which the patient imagines of series of increasingly threatening situations while talking about them in a more realistic, diffusing fashion.

SYSTEMIZED DELUSION A set of highly organized mistaken beliefs that have become the dominant focus of a paranoid *q.v.* patient's life.

SYSTEMIC Spread throughout the body. Affecting, generally, all body systems.

SYSTEMIC CIRCULATION The part of the circulatory system *q.v.* that supplies all parts of the body with oxygenated blood and returns the oxygen-deficient blood to the heart.

SYSTEMIC ILLNESS 1. Diseases that affect many systems or every system of the body. 2. A disease that becomes generalized in the body. ct: local illness.

SYSTEM OF MULTICULTURAL PLURALISTIC ASSESSMENT SOMPA *q.v.*

SYSTEMS MODEL OF EVALUATION The ~ views organizations as pursuing other functions besides the achievement of predetermined goals. These functions include the acquisition of resources, coordination of subunits, and adaptation of the organization to its environment. The model is concerned with measuring the ability of an organization to establish itself as a social unit that is capable of achieving a goal.

SYSTOLE The contraction of the heart in each heartbeat. ct: diastole. cf: systolic blood pressure.

SYSTOLIC BLOOD PRESSURE The pressure exerted on the arterial walls when the ventricles *q.v.* of the heart contract. It is the higher of the two numbers recorded as the blood pressure; e.g., 100/70. ct: diastolic blood pressure.

SYZYGY Celestial alignment. A phenomenon in which the Sun, Earth, and Moon are in exact alignment—a straight line.

T

TA An acronym for transactional analysis *q.v.*

TABES A gradual and progressive wasting in any chronic *q.v.* disease.

TABES DORSALIS 1. Locomotor ataxia *q.v.* 2. Degeneration of the posterior *q.v.* columns of the spinal cord *q.v.*

TABLE OF SPECIFICATIONS A chart of types and numbers of test items to be included in an examination to ensure thorough and systematic coverage of a unit of study.

TABLE WINE A beverage made from fermented *q.v.* fruit juice with an alcohol content of 9% to 12%. ct: fortified wine.

TABOCA A Y-shaped pipe used for smoking by early American Indians.

TABOO An absolute prohibition based on religion, cultural mores, tradition, social usage, or superstition.

TABULA RASA The view of the developing child associated with British empiricist, John Locke, in which the child's mind is a blank slate to be written on by experience.

TACHISTOSCOPE A device for presenting stimuli *q.v.* for brief, controllable periods of time.

TACHYCARDIA 1. Abnormally fast heartbeat, generally more than 100 beats per minute. 2. Rapid heartbeat, such as from stress or stimulant *q.v.* drugs. 3. A racing of the heartbeat often associated with high levels of stress *q.v.*

TACHYPHYLAXIS A rapid tolerance to a potential toxic dose of a drug *q.v.* shortly after receiving smaller doses.

TACTIC A method or approach used as a part of a strategy *q.v.*

TACTILE Pertaining to the sense of touch.

T'AI CHI CH'WAN Chinese exercises that are designed to produce physical and mental harmony.

TALUS The most superior of the tarsal *q.v.* bones and the one that articulates *q.v.* with the tibia *q.v.* and fibula *q.v.* to form the ankle joint.

TALWIN A commercial preparation of pentazocine *q.v.*

TAMPON A vaginal plug made of material that absorbs menstrual flow *q.v.*

TAMPONADE A general term indicating compress. cf: cardiac tamponade.

T-ANTIGEN SKIN TEST A procedure to diagnose breast cancer *q.v.* in which a patient's skin is tested for the presence of T antigen, suspected to be present only in the membranes *q.v.* of women with breast cancer.

TAPEWORM 1. A metazoan, pathogenic *q.v.* to humans. 2. An animal pathogen. 3. A parasitic *q.v.* flatworm that absorbs food from the intestinal tract where it normally attaches itself. 4. An intestinal cestode worm. 5. A flat, tape-like parasite composed of segments that attaches to the wall of intestines. There are two types: (a) *Taenia solium*, the pork ~; and (b) *Taenia saginata*; the beef ~.

TAR 1. The condensate of a gas such as tobacco *q.v.* smoke. Composed of a variety of chemicals, some of which may be carcinogenic *q.v.* or cocarcinogenic *q.v.* 2. Particulate matter in cigarette smoke containing polycyclic hydrocarbons, phenols, cresols, agricultural chemicals, and other compounds. 3. The yellowish, brown residue of tobacco smoke.

TARACTIN A commercial preparation of a major tranquilizer *q.v.*, phenothiazine *q.v.*

TARANTISM 1. Wild dancing mania *q.v.*, prevalent in the thirteenth century in Western Europe; supposedly caused by the bite of a tarantula. 2. A nervous condition characterized by stupor, melancholy, and uncontrollable dancing mania.

TARAXEIN 1. A substance derived from blood of schizophrenics *q.v.*, which, when injected into the veins of subjects, produced psychotic *q.v.* symptoms. 2. A protein *q.v.* in the blood serum *q.v.* of schizophrenics asserted to be responsible for their psychoses *q.v.*

TARDIVE DYSKINESIA 1. A long-term side effect of major tranquilizers *q.v.*, characterized by the inability to control the lips and tongue. 2. Irreversible symptoms of neurological *q.v.* damage that results from sustained intake of phenothiazines *q.v.*

TARGET BEHAVIOR The type of activity to be shaped through the use of behavior modification *q.v.*

TARGET HEART RATE (THR) 1. The number of times per minute that the heart must contract to produce a training effect *q.v.* 2. A heart rate 60% to 70% greater than that of the resting rate that must be maintained during exercise to produce a training effect.

TARGET ORGAN A body organ whose metabolic *q.v.* function responds to a hormone *q.v.* in a specific way.

TARGET PULSE RATE A heart rate above the resting rate but less than the maximum rate. cf: maximum pulse rate.

TARGET SEEKING A concept developed by James Tanner, which holds that a mechanism monitors the growth of individuals, and if the person's growth deviates from a normal pattern, the mechanism kicks in that helps get growth back on target.

TARSAL Pertaining to a tarsus *q.v.*

TARSAL BONE One of the seven bones of the ankle.

TARSAL PLATE The firm framework of connective tissue *q.v.* that gives shape to the upper eyelid.

TARSUS 1. The ankle joint. 2. The root of the foot or instep. 3. The fibrous plates giving solidity to and form the edges of the eyelids. Sometimes referred to as tarsal cartilages *q.v.*

TASK ANALYSIS A description of the elements or components of a task or skill.

TASK FORCE ON ALCOHOL AND HEALTH With passage of the Comprehensive Alcohol Abuse and Alcoholism Prevention, Treatment and Rehabilitation Act of 1970, a task force was authorized to study the problems associated with alcohol abuse and alcoholism. On February 18, 1972, the first report, *Alcohol and Health*, was issued. The three major findings were as follows: 1. alcohol is the most abused drug in the United States and can impair health; 2. the abuse of alcohol can lead to alcoholism; and 3. alcoholism is not a crime, it is an illness or disease and, therefore, the criminal law is not an appropriate device for preventing or controlling it.

TASK GOALS Statements of desired outcomes that emphasize concern for what is to be done and focus upon achievement of objectives.

TASK ORIENTATION The achievement attitude *q.v.* toward a task. ct: ego orientation.

TASK-ORIENTED REACTION A realistic rather than ego-defensive mechanism *q.v.* to dealing with stress *q.v.*

TASTE BUDS The receptor *q.v.* organs for taste.

TAT An acronym for Thematic Apperception Test *q.v.*

TAXONOMIES A classification of learning levels or thinking levels. Some classifications, such as Bloom's, are hierarchical.

TAXONOMY 1. A classification system. 2. A comprehensive classification scheme *q.v.* 3. The science of classification of plants and animals into categories according to their natural relationships.

TAXONOMY OF EDUCATIONAL OBJECTIVES A scheme classifying educational objectives *q.v.* according to six levels of cognition, from lowest to highest in complexity, wherein the ability to demonstrate skill in each level presupposes and depend upon achievement of those preceding it in the hierarchy: (a) knowledge, (b) comprehension, (c) application, (d) analysis, (e) synthesis, and (f) evaluation.

TAYLOR MANIFEST ANXIETY SCALE An instrument comprising 50 items drawn from the MMPI *q.v.* as a self-reporting mechanism to assess anxiety *q.v.*

TAY–SACHS DISEASE Characterized by a lack of the enzyme *q.v.* hexosaminidase A (Hex A), which is essential for the body to properly use lipids *q.v.* The lipids tend to accumulate in the cells, especially brain cells, resulting in their destruction and eventually death. ~ is a genetic *q.v.* disease within the group known as inborn errors of metabolism *q.v.* ~ is a single-gene recessive hereditary *q.v.* defect.

T CELL A specialized lymphocyte *q.v.* that, upon exposure to an antigen *q.v.*, releases chemicals that have localized effects that, collectively, are called cell-mediated immunity *q.v.* cf: T lymphocyte.

TD Tetanus and diphtheria toxoid *q.v.* cf: DPT.

TEACHABLE MOMENTS A term and process coined by J.B. Nash. The concept stresses the importance of teachers to take advantage of current situations, many of them being unplanned, to teach pupils.

TEACHER AIDE A lay person who assists teachers with clerical work, library duties, noninstructional supervision, etc. cf: paraprofessional.

TEACHER-CENTERED CURRICULUM GUIDE Describes what teachers will be doing to affect pupil learning. ct: learner-centered curriculum guide.

TEACHER-CENTERED METHODS Teacher-dominated approaches to teaching/learning. ct: learner-centered methods.

TEACHER CERTIFICATION The set of legal requirements established by each state to ensure that a person is qualified to teach.

TEACHER CONTRACTS Fixed terms of employment and compensation for teachers. ~ are established by authority of local boards of education *q.v.*

TEACHER CORPS A federally funded program that encourages teachers and student teachers to work in disadvantaged areas while attending courses and seminars dealing with the special problems they encounter.

TEACHER EDUCATION Academic programs that prepare prospective teachers with content and pedagogy *q.v.* in education. cf: teacher preparation programs.

TEACHER EFFECTIVENESS A professional movement designed to study and understand the necessary skills and conditions associated with successful teaching.

TEACHER EMPOWERMENT A school environment designed to enable teachers to actively determine the structure of the educational system. cf: teacher power.

TEACHER INDUCTION A gradual process of orientating and mentoring teachers into the public education system.

TEACHER POWER Associated with organized groups of teachers that advocate for the improvement of education. cf: teacher empowerment.

TEACHER PRACTITIONER The role assumed by a teacher when enthusiastically committed to a particular educational method or technique. ct: teacher theorist.

TEACHER PREPARATION PROGRAMS Departments, schools, and institutions of higher education that confer degrees in education.

TEACHER ROLE The set of behaviors generally expected of one who is a teacher.

TEACHER'S ROLE DEFINITION What teachers perceive as their function in the classroom and their expectations about their ability to carry out that role.

TEACHERS' UNIONS Organizations of teachers that lobby on behalf of the education profession at the state and federal levels, organize at the local levels to ensure the fair employment practices of school districts, and negotiate for teacher contracts.

TEACHER TESTING A program of testing teachers' basic skills, begun in Arkansas in the early 1980s. The concept of such testing rapidly spread throughout the country and is now a requirement in most states as a certification *q.v.* requirement.

TEACHER THEORIST The role assumed by a teacher when evaluating the effectiveness of various educational and instructional techniques. ct: teacher practitioner.

TEACHING HOSPITAL A hospital *q.v.* in which preprofessional students and graduates receive clinical experience. ∼s are affiliated with one or more medical schools.

TEACHING/LEARNING TEAMS A group of teachers and/or learners who implement and conduct the health education program. Such groups also facilitate an interdisciplinary approach to health education.

TEACHING METHODS 1. Those planned approaches or procedures that the teacher intends to employ to most effectively influence the learners by favorably affecting their comprehension of a new situation or influencing further their comprehension of a familiar situation. 2. A process that involves the reasonable ordering or balancing of the elements of an educational function, purposes, nature of the learner, materials of instruction, and total teaching and learning situation. ct: learning methods; teaching strategies technique.

TEACHING NURSING HOME A nursing home affiliated with a university medical school or medical center. In addition to the teaching function of the ∼, it conducts research on the chronic health problems that often lead older persons to be institutionalized, e.g., dementia, incontinence, loss of mobility, depression, and sleep disorders.

TEACHING STRATEGIES Techniques *q.v.* used by the teacher to motivate or manipulate learning. cf: learning strategies. cf: teaching methods.

TEACHING STYLES Methods and techniques used by a teacher based on his or her personality, philosophy, and mindset to influence learning, classroom management, and the like.

TEACHING TECHNIQUES Procedures or activities used for facilitating the attainment of instructional objectives *q.v.* ct: teaching methods; teaching strategies.

TEAM TEACHING Teachers of several disciplines, e.g., health education, social studies, and science, meet to plan various ways in which each discipline contributes to an understanding of a particular health issue. Teachers of each discipline follow through on the health issue as it pertains to their specific discipline.

TEAROOM A slang term referring to a men's public toilet where men meet for fast, impersonal sex.

TECHNIQUE The manner in which a teaching or learning method is performed.

TECHNOLOGY 1. The application of chemical, biological, and physical information and development to industry, business, education, government, and others. 2. A replacement of manual efforts with mechanics. 3. New ideas, inventions, techniques, and methods to increase the efficiency of productivity.

TEENAGE HEALTH-TEACHING MODELS (THTM) Designed as a smaller version of traditional health education *q.v.* units, ∼ provide for greater flexibility. ∼ is a health education curriculum *q.v.* composed of 16 modules, each consisting of 4–15 h of instructional time. The modules are arranged so that they can be presented independently or as a part of a larger curriculum design.

~ were developed in 1982 by the Education Development Center, Inc., of Newton, MA.

TEETOTALER A person who does not drink alcoholic beverages.

TEGMENTUM Part of the brainstem *q.v.* that covers the posterior surface of the cerebral *q.v.* peduncles and the pons *q.v.*

TELEGONY The alleged appearance in the offspring of characteristics derived from a previous sire or mate of the female.

TELEKINESIS The apparent production of motion in objects without physical means.

TELEMETRY The measurement of diagnostic signs by electrical instruments and the transmission of them, esp. by radio, to a distant place for recording. Used for electrocardiograph *q.v.* signals.

TELENCEPHALON The anterior portion of the brain *q.v.* cf: diencephalon.

TELEOLOGY The use of design, purpose, or utility as an explanation of any natural phenomenon.

TELEPHONE HOT LINE A direct, dedicated telephone circuit that connects two or more points for instant communication.

TELOGEN EFFLUVIUM Loss of hair resulting from crash diets, infections, fever, or chemotherapy.

TELOPHASE The final phase of mitosis *q.v.*

TEMPERAMENT 1. The behavioral style that indicates a person's approach to living. 2. A characteristic level of reactivity and energy, often thought to be based on constitutional factors. 3. A person's characteristic style of behavior.

TEMPERANCE 1. A moderation or restraint in some behavior. 2. With reference to alcohol *q.v.* consumption, moderation in drinking. ct: prohibition (Table T-1).

TEMPERATE PHAGE A phage (virus) *q.v.* that invades but does not destroy the host (bacterial) *q.v.* cell. cf: virulent phage.

TEMPERATURE INVERSION A phenomenon in which a layer of cool air is trapped under a layer of warm air. Pollutants *q.v.* also become trapped and are subjected to the action of sunlight, which produces additional pollutants

TEMPERATURE METHOD A periodic abstinence *q.v.* method of birth control *q.v.* that relies on the correlation between body temperature and the ovulation *q.v.* process to determine a woman's safe period or infertility days in her menstrual cycle *q.v.*

TEMPLATE 1. A pattern or mold. 2. In genetics *q.v.*, the DNA *q.v.* stores coded information and acts as a model or ~ for information that is taken by messenger RNA *q.v.*

TABLE T-1 TEMPERANCE MOVEMENTS IN THE UNITED STATES

1826—The American Society for the Promotion of Temperance was formed.

1826—The first national convention of temperance was held in Philadelphia, and the United States Temperance Union was formed.

1836—The United States Temperance Union became the American Temperance Union.

1840—The Washingtonian Movement began. The Washington Temperance Society crusaded for total abstinence, and as a result, institutions for treating alcoholism were established in Boston in 1857.

1841—The Independent Order of Bechabites was formed.

1842—The Order of the Sons of Temperance was formed.

1851—The Order of Good Templars was formed. Maine passed the first prohibition law. This law remained in effect until its repeal in 1933.

1854—*Ten Nights in a Bar-Room* was published.

1874—The Women's Christian Temperance Union was formed.

1893—The American Anti-Saloon League was founded. This was probably the most aggressive of all of the prohibition groups.

1907—Georgia and Alabama passed prohibition legislation. Alabama repealed its prohibition law in 1911 and reinstated it in 1915.

1908—North Carolina became a dry state.

1912—West Virginia passed prohibition legislation.

1913—The Webb-Kenyon Act was passed. This bill was vetoed by President Taft, but overridden by Congress.

1914—Virginia, Arizona, Colorado, Oregon, and Washington passed prohibition legislation.

1915—Arkansas, Alabama, and South Carolina passed prohibition legislation.

1917—The 18th amendment to the United States Constitution was passed by Congress.

1919—Three-fourths of the states ratified the 18th Amendment and the Volstead Act was passed by Congress. Only Connecticut and Rhode Island did not ratify the 18th Amendment. President Wilson vetoed the act but it was overridden by Congress on October 28.

1933—The 18th Amendment was repealed by the ratification of the 21st Amendment to the Constitution.

1966—Mississippi repealed its state prohibition. This was the last dry state to go wet.

TEMPORAL ARTERY The arteries *q.v.* located on either side of the face in front of the ear supplying blood to the scalp *q.v.*

TEMPORAL LOBE 1. A lobe in each cerebral hemisphere *q.v.* that includes the auditory projection area *q.v.* 2. The portion of the brain located beneath the temples. 3. A large area in each cerebral hemisphere situated below the lateral sulcus *q.v.* and in front of the occipital lobe *q.v.* that contains primary auditory *q.v.* projections and association areas and general association areas.

TEMPORAL MAZE A maze in which an organism must respond differently to the same portion of the maze, depending on previous behavior *q.v.* ct: spatial maze.

TEMPORAL SUMMATION A form of summation *q.v.* in which two impulses arriving at a synapse *q.v.* in very rapid succession add in strength and cross it. ct: spatial summation.

TEMPORARY MANDIBULAR JOINT DYSFUNCTION (TMJ) A condition of the jaw characterized by pain and clicking in the jaw. Pain may also radiate to the neck and other parts of the head.

TEMPOROMANDIBULAR JOINT 1. Mandibular joint *q.v.* 2. The articulation *q.v.* between the head of the mandible *q.v.* and the mandibular fossa *q.v.* and articular tubercle of the temporal bone *q.v.*

TENDON 1. A cord or band of strong, white fibrous tissue that connects a muscle to a bone or other structure. 2. Connective tissue *q.v.* that attaches muscle to the periosteum *q.v.* of bone.

TENDONITIS Inflammation of tendons *q.v.*

TENEMENT A squalid apartment building, usually defined as one in which several, unrelated families share the same facilities, such as the bathroom.

TENESMUS 1. Ineffectual and painful straining to urinate *q.v.* or defecate *q.v.* 2. A painful spasm of the anal sphincter *q.v.* with an urgent desire to evacuate the bowel or urinary bladder *q.v.* 3. Involuntary straining with passage of very little fecal matter or urine.

TENOSYNOVITIS 1. Inflammation and swelling of tendons *q.v.* 2. Inflammation of a tendon sheath.

TENSION 1. Stress *q.v.* 2. A condition arising out of the mobilization of psychobiological *q.v.* resources to meet a threat. ~ involves an increase in muscle tonus and other emergency physiological *q.v.* Psychologically *q.v.*, ~ is characterized by feelings of stress *q.v.*, uneasiness, and anxiety *q.v.*

TENSION HEADACHE A headache caused by a persistent contraction of the muscles in the neck and scalp.

TENSION OF OBLIGATION An uncomfortable psychological *q.v.* state occurring when a person receives benefit from another and feels a need to reciprocate.

TENSION PNEUMOTHORAX A condition that develops when air is continually pumped into the chest cage outside the lung and is unable to escape. ~ is associated with compression of the lung and heart.

TENSION-REDUCTION THEORY The theory *q.v.* that reinforcement *q.v.* consists in the reduction of a need *q.v.* or drive *q.v.*

TENTING The expansion of the vagina *q.v.* during intercourse.

TENUATE A commercial preparation of diethylpropion *q.v.*

TENURE An employee benefit that makes it difficult to terminate the employment of someone, often provided to teachers after several years of successful teaching experience.

TEPANIL A commercial preparation of diethylpropion *q.v.*

TERATA 1. Fetal monsters. 2. Neonates *q.v.* that have the features of a monster. 3. Extreme genetic *q.v.* or congenital *q.v.* anomalies.

TERATOGEN An agent that interferes with the normal development of the fetus *q.v.*

TERATOGENESIS The production of a deformity or other anomaly in the developing fetus *q.v.*

TERATOGENIC Damage to the fetus *q.v.*

TERATOGENIC DRUGS Drugs that, if taken by a woman who is pregnant, can interfere with crucial stages of a baby's prenatal development and are thus associated with some birth defects.

TERATOLOGY 1. That division of embryology *q.v.* and pathology *q.v.* that deals with abnormal development and congenital *q.v.* malformation. 2. The study of terata *q.v.*

TERM 1. The completion of a pregnancy. 2. The point at which the fetus *q.v.* has the maximum chance for extrauterine *q.v.* survival, generally 37–42 weeks of gestation *q.v.*

TERMINAL Pertaining to or occurring at the end.

TERMINAL BEHAVIOR The desired result preselected by an experimenter or programmer who intends to shape behavior by applying operant conditioning *q.v.* techniques.

TERMINAL GOAL (OBJECTIVE) The ultimate end result of the learning process. When all terminal goals have been achieved, the aim *q.v.* of health education has been accomplished.

TERMINAL HAIR Course, long hair that grows as eyebrows, beard, and hair on the top of the head and other places where there are large visible hairs.

TERMINALIZATION The repelling movement of the centromeres *q.v.* of bivalents *q.v.* that tend to move the chiasmata toward the ends of the centromeres, thereby reducing the chances of crossing over *q.v.*

TERMINAL OXIDATION The transfer of electrons and hydrogen ions *q.v.* to oxygen, forming H_2O in respiration *q.v.*

TERMINAL STAGE The final stage of advanced cancer *q.v.* when only palliative *q.v.* care is possible.

TERM LIFE POLICY 1. A life insurance policy that does not build cash value, but has much lower premiums than whole life policies *q.v.* 2. An insurance policy that is in force for a specified time period but may be renewable.

TERPENEX Hydrocarbons *q.v.* obtained from plants.

TERRAMYCIN A commercial preparation of the antibiotics *q.v.*

TERRITORY In ethology *q.v.*, a region a particular animal stakes out as its own. The ~ holder is usually a male, but in some species the ~ is held by a mating pair or group.

TERTIARY HEALTH CARE 1. Those services involved in posthospitalization care. 2. Medical care involving advanced equipment and procedures. ct: primary health care; secondary health care.

TERTIARY PREVENTION 1. Controlling the progress of a disease and rehabilitating a person. 2. The third level of prevention. Efforts directed at those with advanced stages of illness and aimed at preventing the recurrence of the illness. 3. The maintenance of appropriate treatment through its full course to complete rehabilitation *q.v.* and returning the person to optimal health *q.v.*, thereby minimizing the likelihood of recurrence. ct: primary prevention; secondary prevention.

TERTIARY STAGE OF SYPHILIS The final stage of the syphilis *q.v.* infection characterized by a variety of symptoms depending upon the organs and tissues involved. When the brain is involved, an organic *q.v.* mental illness *q.v.*, general paresis *q.v.* results. Syphilis *q.v.* is treated with penicillin *q.v.* or other antibiotics *q.v.*

TERTIARY WATER TREATMENT The purification of water by using chemicals to remove phosphates and other compounds, and electrodialysis to remove dissolved salts. ct: primary water treatment; secondary water treatment.

TESTABILITY The extent to which a hypothesis is amenable to systematic scientific study.

TESTATOR A person who has made a will.

TEST CROSS A cross of a dominant with a homozygous recessive *q.v.* to determine whether the dominant is homozygous or heterozygous *q.v.* Used as a test for linkage.

TESTES 1. Testicles *q.v.* 2. The male gonads *q.v.*

TESTICLES 1. Testes *q.v.* 2. The male gonads *q.v.* that normally produce sperm *q.v.* and sex hormones *q.v.*

TESTICLE SELF-EXAMINATION A procedure whereby men can detect abnormalities in their testicles *q.v.* when preformed every 6–8 weeks.

TESTICULAR FEMINIZATION SYNDROME 1. A condition in which a person has the external genitals *q.v.* of a female, but the internal organs of a male. 2. Androgen *q.v.* insensitivity syndrome *q.v.* 3. An inherited condition in which tissues are insensitive to the effects of testosterone *q.v.* The person is born with a 46-XY chromosome *q.v.* pattern but with female genitals.

TESTIMONIAL 1. A claim by the user of a product or procedure that it is effective. 2. A personal opinion of a product or service.

TESTING PLAY A form of play that allows children to test their physical skills, emotional reactions, and ability to cope with different situations.

TESTIS The male gonad *q.v.* that produces spermatozoa *q.v.* and testosterone *q.v.* (pl. testes, testicles).

TESTOSTERONE 1. Male reproductive hormone *q.v.* secreted by the seminiferous tubules *q.v.* and is responsible for the development of the secondary sex characteristics *q.v.* Increased levels of ~ inhibit the anterior pituitary gland *q.v.* 2. The principal androgen *q.v.* produced by the testes *q.v.*, which is responsible for the development of secondary sex characteristics in the male and sex drive in both sexes. ~ is also produced by the adrenal cortex *q.v.* and the ovaries *q.v.* 3. The male hormone responsible for the maintenance of muscle mass and bone tissue in the adult male.

TEST PROFILE A graphic indication of a person's performance on several components of a test. This is frequently useful for guidance or clinical evaluation as it indicates which abilities or traits are relatively high or low for that person.

TEST-RETEST METHOD A method of establishing reliability *q.v.* that involves giving the test twice to the same sample *q.v.* of persons.

TEST TUBE BABY 1. A misnomer. 2. The process of fertilizing *q.v.* an egg in the laboratory and later transplanting it in the uterus *q.v.* of a woman. 3. Test tube fertilization *q.v.*

TEST TUBE FERTILIZATION 1. In vitro *q.v.* fertilization *q.v.* 2. A procedure in which an egg is removed from a ripe follicle *q.v.* and fertilized *q.v.* by a sperm *q.v.* cell in a culture dish. The fertilized egg is allowed to grow and divide for about 2 days and is inserted into the woman's uterus *q.v.* where it becomes implanted *q.v.*

TETANUS 1. Lockjaw. 2. A disease caused by the *Clostridium tetani* bacteria, which release a poison that attacks the central nervous system *q.v.*

TETANY A condition characterized by sharp bending (flexion) of the wrist and ankle joints, muscle twitching, cramps, and convulsions. Inadequate calcium in the blood causes irritability of the nerves and muscles so that they respond to a stimulus *q.v.* with greater sensitivity and force than is normal.

TETRACYCLINE An antibiotic *q.v.*

TETRAD A group of four spores formed from a spore mother cell after meiosis *q.v.*

TETRAHYDROCANNABINOL 1. THC. 2. Delta-9 tetrahydrocannabinol. 3. The active ingredient in marijuana *q.v.*

TETRAIODOTHYRONINE Thyroxine *q.v.*

TETRALOGY OF FALLOT A combination of congenital *q.v.* defects that include an enlarged right ventricle *q.v.* of the heart, overriding aorta *q.v.* and pulmonary valve stenosis *q.v.* that prevents the blood from receiving sufficient oxygen.

TETRAPLOID Twice the usual number (diploid *q.v.*) of chromosomes *q.v.*

TEXTBOOK 1. A publication of a specific educational discipline that contains the standard information and logical order of learning related to the subject matter. 2. A reference. A guide to learning. A learning resource.

TEXTBOOK CENSORSHIP The process employed by some groups for determining which textbooks meet their standard, and forcing states or school districts to reject others that may not present the groups' views on a subject as they would like.

TEXTBOOK METHOD A teacher-centered approach *q.v.* in which the student reads aloud or silently a specific text assignment. This is usually repeated until the whole textbook has been read.

TEXTURED VEGETABLE PROTEIN A processed protein *q.v.* derived from soybeans, often formulated to appear as familiar meat products.

TEXTURE GRADIENT A distance cue *q.v.* based on changes in surface texture, which depends upon the distance of the observer.

TFR An acronym for total fertility rate *q.v.*

TFS An acronym for testicular feminization syndrome *q.v.*

T GROUP An intensive group interaction that emphasizes human relations skills.

TH An acronym for thyrotropic hormone *q.v.*

THALAMUS 1. A pair of egg-shaped masses of nuclei *q.v.* on the walls of the diencephalon *q.v.* The ~ serves as an integrating center that relays excitation to the sensory projection areas *q.v.* of the cerebral cortex *q.v.* 2. A portion of the forebrain *q.v.* where sensations such as pain are interpreted and relayed to appropriate areas of the cerebral cortex. 3. The region of the brain that integrates sensory and motor *q.v.* responses.

THALASEMIA A genetic *q.v.* defect characterized by anemia that varies in intensity according to the inheritance pattern but may be fatal. Particularly centered in populations of Mediterranean or Southeast Asian descent.

THALIDAMIDE A drug originally prescribed to pregnant women to prevent miscarriages *q.v.* and linked to phocomelia *q.v.* Still in use in some countries for treatment of other medical conditions.

THALLOPHYTE A thallus *q.v.* plant, algae, bacteria, of fungi *qq.v.*

THALLUS A type of plant body that is undifferentiated into root, stem, or leaf.

THANATOLOGIST A person who studies factors surrounding life and death. cf: thanatology.

THANATOLOGY 1. The study of death. ~ is concerned with the multitude of issues raised by death and prolonging life. These issues are related to philosophy, law, theology, the social sciences, literature, and history. 2. ~ is concerned with issues of life as well as issues of death, with the societal impact advanced technology has on the prolongation of life, organ transplants, medicological, and ethical issues. ~ is concerned with death and birth, genetic *q.v.* engineering, and all of the issues related to who shall live and who shall die.

THANATOPHOBIA An irrational fear of death.

THANATOS 1. An unconscious urge toward death. The powerful and destructive death force. 2. In psychoanalytic theory *q.v.*, the death instinct that is the second of the two basic instincts within the id *q.v.*, the other being Eros.

THC An acronym for delta 9-tetrahydrocannabinol *q.v.*

THEA SINENSIS The plant from which tea leaves are derived. cf: caffeine.

THEMATIC APPERCEPTION TEST (TAT) A projective technique *q.v.* in which persons are shown a set of pictures and asked to write a story about each in which the subjects will project into the story his or her deepest concerns.

THEMATIC APPROACH In education *q.v.*, the use of an integrating theme that serves to integrate various aspects of the curriculum *q.v.*

THEOBROMA CACAO 1. Cocoa. 2. The plant from which cocoa is derived.

THEOBROMINE 1. An alkaloid *q.v.* resembling caffeine *q.v.*, prepared from the dried seed of the Theobroma cacao *q.v.* or made synthetically. 2. A mild stimulant, similar to caffeine.

THEOPHYLLINE A mild stimulant found in tea. Also used to treat asthma *q.v.*

THEORETICAL EFFECTIVENESS Pertaining to the failure rate of contraceptives *q.v.* when used as directed. ct: use effectiveness.

THEORETICAL FAILURE RATE The failure rate of a contraceptive *q.v.* method when it is used correctly. ct: actual failure rate.

THEORETICAL LAW OF EFFECT The theory *q.v.* that reward is necessary for learning to take place.

THEORIES OF LEARNING Concerned with the principles and descriptions of the ways in which learning *q.v.* takes place. cf: learning; connectionist theory; cognitive theory.

THEORIES OF PERSONALITY DEVELOPMENT Factors that influence the development of personality *q.v.* have motivated the establishment of a variety of theories, which include the following: 1. analytic, 2. body type, 3. existential, 4. individual, 5. psychoanalytic, 6. self-actualization, and 7. trait *qq.v.*

THEORY 1. A set of interacting, interlocking, or independent principles designed to account for a wide range of observations or facts. 2. A set of principles, forming an organized structure, used to explain the facts of a science *q.v.*

THEORY OF LOGICAL TYPES 1. Used by Watzlawick to explain change from outside the group. ~ involves a process by which a class or group moves to a higher logical level. 2. A change of a change.

THEORY X A set of negative assumptions about the nature of people.

THEORY Y A set of positive assumptions about the nature of people.

THEORY Z The premise that managers who use either Theory X or Theory Y *qq.v.* can be successful depending upon the circumstances in their particular situation.

THERAPEUTIC Pertaining to treatment or healing.

THERAPEUTIC ABORTION 1. An abortion *q.v.* that is legal under state law. 2. An abortion performed when abnormal conditions threaten the well-being of the mother or the unborn child.

THERAPEUTIC AGENT A drug used for treating or preventing disease, or to maintain health.

THERAPEUTIC COMMUNITY 1. A residential treatment approach to those with drug abuse or other addiction problems consisting of group therapy *q.v.*, educational sessions, medical services, etc. 2. A special hospital-type milieu that encourages patients to function within a range of social norms. 3. The concept that many influences in a person's environment may contribute to the cure of mental illnesses.

THERAPEUTIC INDEX 1. An assessment of the relative safety of drugs. The ratio between the median lethal dose and the median effective dose of a drug used for a particular effect. 2. The relative margin of safety of a particular drug. The dose required to produce a toxic effect *q.v.* divided by the dose required to produce a therapeutic effect *q.v.* ct: effective dose; lethal dose.

THERAPEUTIC LEVEL The concentration of a drug in the body in a quantity that is effective for accomplishing the desired results.

THERAPEUTIC RATIO Therapeutic index *q.v.*

THERAPEUTICS The science concerned with medicinal substances that have curative potentials. ct: pharmacognosy; materia medica; toxicology.

THERAPY 1. Treatment. 2. The application of techniques designed to heal.

THERIACA 1. The shotgun approach to prescribing medicines. 2. The practice of prescribing a number of drugs with the hope that one would be effective.

THERMAL Pertaining to or characterized by heat.

THERMAL CONDUCTIVITY The power to transmit or convey heat.

THERMAL INVERSION A weather condition in which a layer of warm, stable air forms above a cooler, polluted layer, inhibiting dispersal of pollutants *q.v.*

THERMAL POLLUTION The addition of heat to a natural body of water sufficient to damage the aquatic ecosystem *q.v.*

THERMOGRAPHY 1. A diagnostic technique using heat waves to detect breast cancer *q.v.* in its early developmental stages. 2. A picture showing heat variations in the body or a specific part of the body.

THERMOLABILE Inactivated or destroyed by high temperatures.

THERMOMETER, CLINICAL An instrument for measuring the temperature of the body. There are two types: 1. oral and 2. rectal. The ~ was developed in 1611.

THERMOPHILIC 1. Heat-loving. 2. Organisms that grow at relatively high temperatures.

THERMOSTABLE Unaffected by relatively high temperatures.

THERMOTACTIC OPTIMUM The temperature that determines direction.

THERMOTAXIS The regulation of body temperature.

THETA RHYTHM Slow brain waves *q.v.*

THIAMINE 1. A water-soluble vitamin *q.v.* discovered in 1926. Essential for carbohydrate *q.v.* metabolism *q.v.* Severe deficiency of ~ results in the disease beriberi *q.v.* 2. One of the vitamin B complex *q.v.* group.

THIGH That portion of the lower extremity between the hip and knee.

THIGMONASTY A nastic movement in response to touch.

THIGMOTROPISM A growth movement as a result of contact with a solid object.

THIORIDAZINE An antipsychotic *q.v.* drug. Mellaril is the commercial preparation.

THIOTHIXENE An antipsychotic *q.v.* drug. Navane is the commercial preparation.

THIRD-PARTY PAYER A payment service other than the patient or provider.

THIRD-VARIABLE PROBLEM The difficulty with correlational research on two subjects or variables *q.v.* when their relationship may be attributable to a third factor.

THIRD WORLD 1. Those nations that lack significant economic development. 2. Developing nations. 3. Underdeveloped nations.

THIRTY (30) DOUBLINGS The time required for the cells of a particular tissue to undertake 30 reproductive divisions. ~ is thought to be the time required for a cancerous *q.v.* process to be clinically observable.

THOMAS SPLINT A rigid splint *q.v.* made either of metal or plastic that can provide support for and a steady longitudinal pull on a lower extremity. When traction is applied through the foot and ankle hitch, contraction is applied against the ischial tuberosity *q.v.* Rigid bars extend the length of the splint, the upper end is curved, and the leg fits within the framework or is supported by it.

THORACIC Pertaining to the thorax *q.v.* or chest cavity.

THORACIC CAGE The chest.

THORACIC CAVITY The space within the thoracic *q.v.* walls bounded below by the diaphragm *q.v.* and above by the neck.

THORACIC SPINE The vertebrae *q.v.*, usually 12 in number, between the cervical spine *q.v.* and the lumbar spine *q.v.*

THORACOLUMBAR NERVOUS SYSTEM The sympathetic nervous system *q.v.*

THORACOTOMY The surgical opening of the chest wall.

THORAX 1. The chest. 2. That portion of the body above the diaphragm *q.v.* and within the rib cage.

THORAZINE Chlorpromazine *q.v.*, one of the phenothiazines *q.v.*; an antipsychotic drug *q.v.*

THOUGHT DISORDER A symptom of schizophrenia *q.v.*, characterized by incoherence, loose associations, and distortion of concrete reasoning.

THR An acronym for target heart rate *q.v.*

THREADY PULSE A pulse *q.v.* that is weak and scarcely perceptible. A ~ is characteristic of the pulse when a person is in shock *q.v.*

THREAT The perception of imagined or real danger to the self *q.v.*

THREE DIMENSIONS OF HEALTH The major areas of health in which specific strengths or limitations are found: physical, social, and psychological. ct: five dimensions of health; dimensions of health.

THREE-MAN LIFT A method in which a number of persons may lift and move an injured person smoothly.

THREE-POINT SUSPENSION The distribution of the weight of an injured person while being moved, the trunk, buttocks, and legs are separately supported.

THREONINE An essential amino acid *q.v.*

THRESHOLD Some value a stimulus *q.v.* must reach to produce a response.

THRESHOLD DOSE The least amount of drug that produces a given effect.

THRESHOLD LEVEL A level of a substance below which the risk of harm is greatly diminished or absent.

THRESHOLD TRAIT A trait *q.v.* that can be judged to be present or absent. ct: quantitative trait.

THROMBECTOMY The surgical removal of a blood clot *q.v.* from a blood vessel.

THROMBIN 1. Fibrin *q.v.* ferment. 2. ~ converts fibrinogen *q.v.* into fibrin.

THROMBOCYTES The platelets *q.v.* of the blood. Essential for normal blood clotting *q.v.*

THROMBOCYTOPENIA Lack of platelets *q.v.* in the blood.

THROMBOEMBOLISM Obstruction of a blood vessel by a blood clot *q.v.*, often the result of a clot moving from its site of origin to a smaller vessel, where it causes the obstruction.

THROMBOSIS 1. A blood clot that becomes trapped in an artery *q.v.* or vein *q.v.* causing an occlusion *q.v.* 2. The blockage of a blood vessel as a result of the formation of a blood clot within the vessel itself. ct: cerebral thrombosis; coronary thrombosis; embolism.

THROMBUS A blood clot *q.v.* that forms inside a blood vessel.

THRUSH 1. A disease usually of infants, but also adults, characterized by whitish spots in the mouth, or in female adults, in the vagina *q.v.* It is caused by the fungus *Candida albicans* *q.v.* 2. An infection in the throat caused by oral-genital *q.v.* contact.

THTM An acronym for Teenage Health-Teaching Modules *q.v.*

THYMINE 1. One of the four nitrogenous bases *q.v.* in nucleic acid *q.v.* 2. A pyrimidine base *q.v.* found in DNA *q.v.* The others are adenine, cytosine, and guanine *qq.v.*

THYMOSIN A hormone *q.v.* secreted by the thymus gland *q.v.* that may be important in the aging process.

THYMUS GLAND A two-lobed ductless gland *q.v.* located behind the upper part of the sternum *q.v.* and extending into the neck. The ~ is fairly large in childhood but usually shrinks by adulthood. The ~ is structured like a lymph node *q.v.* and contains lymphatic follicles. It may play a role in immune *q.v.* reactions.

THYROCALCITONIN Calcitonin *q.v.*

THYROID CARTILAGE The largest of the cartilages *q.v.* of the larynx *q.v.*

THYROIDECTOMY Partial or total excision of the thyroid gland *q.v.*

THYROID GLAND The endocrine gland *q.v.* situated in the neck that secretes thyroid hormone *q.v.*, which regulates many body functions including maintenance of reproductive function, metabolism, intelligence, and physical growth.

THYROXIN 1. A hormone *q.v.* produced by the thyroid gland *q.v.* that is necessary for proper metabolism *q.v.* 2. A hormone secreted by the thyroid gland that helps to regulate the activity level of adults and the growth, development, and intelligence of infants. 3. An iodine-containing hormone secreted by the thyroid gland that plays a role in carbohydrate *q.v.* metabolism, regulating activity, and influencing infants' growth, development, and intelligence.

TIA An acronym for transient ischemic attack *q.v.*

TIBIA 1. The larger of the two bones of the leg. 2. The shin bone.

TIC Intermittent twitching, usually of facial muscles, associated with a disguised emotional disturbance.

TICK A blood-sucking parasite *q.v.* that may carry disease to humans as well as other animals.

T.I.D A Latin abbreviation pertaining to three times a day.

TIMBRE The quality of sounds that enables people to distinguish one kind of sound from another. ~ depends upon the set of overtones *q.v.* associated with the fundamental tones *q.v.*

TIME ACTION FUNCTION The relationship between the time elapsed since a drug was taken and the intensity of a drug effect. ct: dose–response relationship.

TIME COMPETENCE The ability to tie past experiences to future goals while being fully in the present moment.

TIME-OF-MEASUREMENT EFFECTS In longitudinal research *q.v.*, the effects of particular events on the variable being studied at a particular point during the study.

TIME-OUT A punishment procedure in operant conditioning *q.v.* in which the subject is temporarily removed from a setting where reinforcers can be obtained.

TIME SAMPLING A method of studying social behavior by observing a child for a few seconds and then classifying actions into categories.

TIME STRUCTURING Berne's term for a kind of long-term coping that ranges from withdrawal to intimacy.

TIMING-PLUS-DOUCHE A method of gender selection relying on the acidity or alkalinity of the vaginal *q.v.* environment and the timing of intercourse *q.v.* and ovulation *q.v.*

TINCTURE An alcoholic or hydroalcoholic solution of a drug or other chemical substance.

TINDAL A brand name for acetophenazine *q.v.*

TINEA 1. Ringworm. 2. A disease caused by a fungus (mold) *q.v.* 3. *Tinea corporis q.v.* 4. *Tinea pedis q.v.*

TINEA CORPORIS Ringworm of the body. ct: *Tinea pedis.*

TINEA CRURIS A fungus infection causing irritation to the skin of the genital *q.v.* area.

TINEA PEDIS Athlete's foot. ct: *Tinea corporis.*

TINNITUS A relatively continuous ringing sound in the head with no apparent external source.

TISSUE 1. An aggregation of cells of the same type contributing to the functioning purpose of the ~. 2. A group of cells of generally similar origin and function.

TISSUE CULTURE The growth of cells from plants or animals in sterile media, often to be used in research or the diagnosis of disease.

TISSUE FLUID Body fluid that fills the spaces between the cells.

TITER Level or amount.

TITLE XVIII Amendment to the Social Security Act authorizing Medicare *q.v.*

TITLE XIX Amendment to the Social Security Act authorizing Medicaid *q.v.*

TITRATION The process of determining a particular level of a drug within the body that will achieve a desired effect. Done by frequently administering small doses of a drug until the desired effect is achieved.

T LYMPHOCYTES 1. T cell *q.v.* 2. Small, circulating white blood cells that, in the presence of specific antigens *q.v.*, form small sensitized lymphocytes *q.v.*, the basic components of the body's cellular immunity *q.v.* cf: B lymphocyte.

TM An acronym for transcendental meditation.

TMJ An acronym for temporary mandibular joint dysfunction *q.v.*

TMR An acronym for total metabolic rate *q.v.*

TOBACCO A plant, *Nicotiana tabacum*, consisting of cellulose, starches, proteins, sugars, alkaloids, hydrocarbons, phenols, fatty acids, isoprenoids, sterols, and a number of inorganic minerals, also found in many other plants. However, ~ also contains nicotine, nornicotine, myosmine, and anabasine not found in other plants.

TOBACCO ADDITIVES Tobacco substitutes added to cigarettes during their manufacture to enhance flavor or to facilitate processes.

TOBACCO AMBLYOPIA 1. A condition characterized by a dimness of vision. 2. A syndrome *q.v.* of visual failure including the loss of visual acuity *q.v.* and color perception, related to nutritional deficiencies or the body's inability to detoxify cyanide found in tobacco smoke.

TOFRANIL A commercial preparation of imipramine *q.v.*

TOKEN ECONOMY 1. An arrangement for operant *q.v.* behavior modification in hospital settings. Certain responses are reinforced with tokens that can be exchanged for desirable items. 2. In education *q.v.*, reinforcing learners through the use of behavior modification *q.v.* procedures by supplying tokens that can be traded for some reward.

TOLERANCE 1. The adaptation *q.v.* of the body to a drug resulting in the need for a larger dosage to create the desired reaction. 2. A central nervous system *q.v.* adaptation to a particular drug or chemical. 3. An immunity to the effects of a drug acquired through continued use.

TOLERATION METHOD A method of breaking habits by presenting the controlling stimulus *q.v.* in gradually increasing intensities.

TOMOGRAPHY A noninvasive technique designed to show detailed images of internal structures in a selected plane of the body.

TONIC 1. In psychology *q.v.* and physiology *q.v.*, pertaining to muscle tension or contraction. 2. In physiology, muscle tone. 3. In medicine, a substance that restores or refreshes.

TONIC-NECK REFLEX In infants a postural reflex *q.v.*, which is characterized by limb extension to the side to which the head is turned and limb flexion in the opposite direction.

TONIC PHASE The state of rigid muscular tension *q.v.* and suspended breathing, as in a grand mal epileptic *q.v.* attack.

TONOMETRY The measurement of tension *q.v.* or pressure.

TONOPLAST The membrane *q.v.* surrounding an intracellular vacuole *q.v.*

TONSILLECTOMY The surgical removal of the tonsils *q.v.*

TONSILS A collection of lymphoid *q.v.* tissue located at the sides of the throat behind the nose and on the back of the tongue.

TONUS Continued, partial contraction of a muscle.

TOOTH DECAY 1. Dental cavity. 2. Dental carie *q.v.* caused by the formation of dental plaque *q.v.* on a susceptible tooth. ~ begins on the external surfaces of a tooth. No single bacteria *q.v.* has been implicated in the etiology *q.v.*, rather, several bacteria are believed to be responsible, such as *Lactobacillus acidophilus q.v.* and streptococcal *q.v.* bacteria.

TOOTH TRANSPLANT Transplanting a tooth from one position in the jaw to another or from one person to another.

TOP-DOWN PROCESSES Processes in form recognition that begin with higher units and then work down to smaller units. ct: bottom-up processes.

TOPECTOMY A type of brain surgery in the treatment of certain cases of chronic mental illnesses that do not respond to other types of therapy *q.v.* ~ involves the removal of circumscribed areas of brain tissue.

TOPICAL 1. Pertaining to the surface of the skin. 2. To apply topically. ~ medications normally affect only the area to which they are applied, although some ~ medications may be absorbed into the bloodstream causing a systemic *q.v.* effect.

TOPICAL APPLICATION 1. Local application. 2. Placing a substance directly on the surface of the skin.

TOPICAL USE OF A DRUG A drug that is applied to the surface area of a body part. cf: topical.

TOPV An acronym for trivalent oral polio virus vaccine *q.v.*

TORT A legal wrong committed against a person, his or her reputation, and the property of another, independent of contract. cf: tort law.

TORTICOLLIS 1. Wryneck. 2. A contracted state of the cervical muscles producing twisting of the neck and an unnatural position of the head.

TORT LAW Civil liability laws governing acts or failure to act by which a person injures another person or property or reputation either directly or indirectly.

TOTAL EXPENDITURES PER PUPIL IN AVERAGE DAILY ATTENDANCE All expenditures that are allocable to per pupil costs divided by average daily attendance. Used to calculate the amount of state aid *q.v.* received by school districts.

TOTAL FERTILITY RATE (TFR) The average number of children a woman would have if she bore children throughout her child-bearing years, age 15 through 44 years, at the same rate of those ages in a given year. ct: fertility rate.

TOTAL IMMEDIATE ANCESTRAL LONGEVITY (TIAL) The sum of the ages of death of both parents and all four grandparents of a given individual. It will fall somewhere between 100 and 600 years. Developed by Raymond Pearl.

TOTALITARIANISM A form of government in which the state controls all phases of the people's lives.

TOTAL MARRIAGE A marriage in which the needs and goals of each partner are assigned a lower priority for the good of the partnership. ct: vital marriage.

TOTAL MASTECTOMY Simple mastectomy *q.v.*

TOTAL MOTHER PERSON A composite score that summarizes several of a mother's traits *q.v.* Used to determine the effect of mothering upon the adjustment of her child.

TOTAL PERSON A holistic *q.v.* view of a person, incorporating the dynamic interplay of physical, emotional, social, intellectual, and spiritual factors. cf: dimensions of health.

TOTAL PUSH In psychology *q.v.*, a type of therapy *q.v.* in which all treatment procedures—medical, psychological, and sociological—are coordinated into a total therapeutic regimen.

TOTIPOTENT CELL An undifferentiated cell that when separated from others develops into a complete embryo *q.v.*

TOURETTE'S SYNDROME 1. A convulsive tic *q.v.* associated with a lack of motor coordination, incoherent grunts, and involuntary swearing and coprolalia *q.v.* 2. Gilles de la Tourette's syndrome.

TOURNIQUET A strap device sometimes used to control severe bleeding of an arm or leg.

TOXEMIA 1. A serious condition occurring in pregnant women characterized by high blood pressure *q.v.*, excess fluids in the tissues, and albumin *q.v.* in the urine. 2. Toxemia of pregnancy *q.v.* 3. Any condition in which the blood contains toxic *q.v.* substances. 4. A pathological condition resulting from poison in the blood.

TOXEMIA OF PREGNANCY A pathologic condition occurring in pregnant women and characterized by excessive vomiting, hypertension, albuminuria *q.v.*, and edema. It may progress to eclampsia *q.v.*

TOXIC 1. Poisonous. 2. Harmful. 3. Destructive. 4. Deadly. cf: toxicology.

TOXIC DELIRIA 1. A psychosis *q.v.* 2. A severe disturbance in cerebral *q.v.* functioning resulting from toxins *q.v.* 3. A coma *q.v.* or delirium caused by poisons entering the body.

TOXIC DOSE The quantity or level of a substance that produces a poisonous effect.

TOXIC EFFECTS The poisonous effects of any substance taken into the body or applied topically. With drugs, the margin between the dosage that produces beneficial effects or ~ varies greatly. Moreover, this margin will vary with the person taking the drug.

TOXICITY 1. The quality of being poisonous. 2. The degree to which a substance is poisonous. Such effects may be acute *q.v.* or chronic *q.v.*

TOXICOLOGIST A person trained in the field of toxicology *q.v.*

TOXICOLOGY 1. The science that is concerned with the nature and effects of poisons. 2. The study of poisons. 3. The study of toxic *q.v.* substances.

TOXIC PSYCHOSIS A severe mental disturbance induced by a poisonous substance.

TOXIC REACTION A disruption in the functioning of one or more parts of the body caused by a toxic *q.v.* substance.

TOXIC SHOCK SYNDROME (TSS) 1. A rare group of symptoms in women characterized by vomiting, fever, diarrhea, a skin rash, and a rapid decrease in blood pressure and shock *q.v.* A bacterium *q.v.* is suspected as the cause and whose growth may be enhanced by the use of tampons *q.v.* 2. A condition in which the bacteria, *Staphylococcus aureus*, *q.v.* produces a poison that is released into the bloodstream. Absorbent tampons are thought to produce a favorable environment for the growth of these bacteria. 3. A potentially fatal condition resulting from the proliferation of certain bacteria in the vagina that enter the general blood circulation.

TOXIC SYNDROME A result of the use of high doses of stimulant drugs, characterized by tremors, irritation, hostility, and panic.

TOXIC WASTE Industrial chemicals and by-products that are poisonous, corrosive, reactive, radioactive, or ignitable. When dumped in landfills, they may seep into and pollute groundwater *q.v.*

TOXINS Poisonous substances, a term often used to refer to substances produced by microorganisms *q.v.*, either through their metabolic activity or through their death and decomposition.

TOXOID An attenuated *q.v.* microorganism *q.v.* that has lost its toxic *q.v.* qualities while retaining its ability to stimulate the production of antitoxins *q.v.* Used to establish a temporary immunity *q.v.*

TOXOPLASMA GONDII 1. A parasite *q.v.* that causes brain inflammation, called toxoplasmosis *q.v.*, in AIDS patients. 2. A protozoan *q.v.* transmitted to humans from domesticated cats and capable of causing severe fetal *q.v.* damage when contracted during pregnancy.

TOXOPLASMOSIS 1. A disease with symptoms similar to mononucleosis *q.v.* that can affect a pregnant woman and her unborn child. It may be contracted by consuming inadequately cooked meat or by poor personal hygiene. 2. An infection caused by a protozoa *q.v.* carried in raw meat and fecal *q.v.* material.

TPI An acronym for Treponema pallidum Immobilization Test *q.v.*

TPN An acronym for triphosphopyridine nucleotide *q.v.*

TRABECULA 1. A septum *q.v.* that extends into an organ from its wall or capsule. 2. A fibrous cord of connective tissue *q.v.*

TRACE CONSOLIDATION HYPOTHESIS The hypothesis *q.v.* that newly acquired memory traces *q.v.* undergo a gradual change that makes them more and more resistant to any disturbance.

TRACE ELEMENTS 1. The nutrients *q.v.* that the body needs in very small amounts. 2. Micronutrients *q.v.* 3. Minerals needed by the body in amounts of 0.01 g or less each day.

TRACE MINERALS See trace elements.

TRACHEA 1. The windpipe. 2. The main trunk for air passing to and from the lungs.

TRACHEOSTOMY TUBE A tube used to keep a tracheotomy *q.v.* open.

TRACHEOTOMY (TRACHEOSTOMY) An opening made surgically in the trachea to create an airway in cases of respiratory obstruction.

TRACHOMA A contagious disease of the conjunctivas *q.v.* It is related to psittacosis *q.v.* and lymphogranuloma venereum *q.v.* It is characterized by conjunctival congestion, swelling of the eyelids, and may involve the entire cornea *q.v.* It is the leading cause of blindness on a worldwide basis.

TRACKING In education *q.v.*, the practice of placing students according to their ability level in relatively homogeneous classes.

TRACT A bundle of axons *q.v.* located within the central nervous system *q.v.*

TRACTION The act of pulling.

TRADITIONAL CLASSROOM A classroom based on the philosophy that children learn best when materials are presented to them in an organized, structured way. Lesson plans, materials, space, and objectives are determined by the teacher and follow a standard format for all students. ct: open classroom.

TRADITIONAL EDUCATION A system of education based upon progressive grading, self-contained classrooms, and lessons conducted by certified teachers. ct: open education.

TRADITIONAL SEX TYPING Showing high acceptance of behaviors traditionally stereotyped as appropriate for one's own sex and low self-acceptance of sex role behaviors stereotyped as appropriate for the opposite sex.

TRAFFICKING The unauthorized manufacture, distribution, or possession with intent to distribute any drug.

TRAIL-MAKING TEST A test designed to reveal the individual's capacity to scan and integrate information under the pressure of time.

TRAINABLE CHILD The noneducable child capable of developing useful skills of one type or another. cf: educable child.

TRAINING In exercise, repeated activities that are highly sports specific. ct: exercise prescription.

TRAINING EFFECT 1. The point at which regular exercise produces positive changes in the body. 2. The significant, positive effect that exercise has on the heart, lungs, and blood vessels.

TRAIT 1. A characteristic of personality *q.v.* 2. An enduring attribute of a person that is manifested in a variety of situations. 3. A somatic *q.v.* characteristic or predisposition *q.v.* to respond in a particular way.

TRAIT THEORY OF PERSONALITY DEVELOPMENT 1. One's personality *q.v.* and behavior are influenced by consistent behavioral characteristics (traits *q.v.*). 2. The view that people differ in regard to a number of underlying attributes that partially determine behavior and that are presumed to be essentially consistent from time to time and from situation to situation. cf: Personality Factor Test; situationism.

TRANCE 1. A sleeplike state in which the range of consciousness is limited and voluntary activities are suspended. 2. A deep hypnotic *q.v.* state.

TRANCE LOGIC A way of thinking while under hypnosis *q.v.* that allows a person to accept as real situations and images that would be unreal without hypnosis.

TRANQUILIZERS 1. A group of drugs that produce a calming effect without resulting in drowsiness or sleep. ~ are further classified as major ~ and minor ~ *qq.v.* 2. Sedatives *q.v.* 3. Used to control psychotic *q.v.* symptoms and reduce anxiety *q.v.* and tension.

TRANSACTIONAL ANALYSIS (TA) 1. A form of therapy *q.v.* in which an individual becomes aware of his or her ability to control his or her own fate, thinks independently, and makes rational decisions. 2. An interpersonal therapy in which a person learns to manage the interaction between "parent," "child," and "adult" ego states.

TRANSACTIONAL THOUGHT DISORDER A form of communication deviance in which there is a pattern of ambiguous, incomplete communication.

TRANS ARRANGEMENT Repulsion *q.v.*

TRANSCELLULAR FLUID Together with interstitial fluid *q.v.*, accounts for 80% of all extracellular fluid *q.v.* in the body.

TRANSCEND To go beyond the ordinary or normal limits of something.

TRANSCENDENTAL MEDITATION™ 1. A regimen designed to develop the will power and control of the psyche so that the whole body can function in a more integrated and orderly manner. 2. A form of self-hypnosis *q.v.* 3. An activity focused on intense concentration.

TRANSCENDERS Self-actualized *q.v.* people who have achieved a quality of being ordinarily associated with higher levels of spiritual growth.

TRANSCONFIGURATION A configuration of two linked genes *q.v.*, with one dominant allele *q.v.* of one pair on the same homologue *q.v.* as the recessive allele of the second pair.

TRANSCRIPTION 1. Encoding of mRNA *q.v.* by DNA *q.v.* 2. The copying of the genetic message of DNA into RNA so that the information can be used.

TRANSDUCTION 1. The process by which a receptor *q.v.* translates some physical stimulus *q.v.* to give rise to an action potential in another neuron *q.v.* 2. Genetic *q.v.* recombination in bacteria *q.v.* mediated by a bacteriophage *q.v.*

TRANSDUCTION, SPECIALIZED Transduction *q.v.* by bacteriophage *q.v.* that carry only a specific portion of bacterial chromosome *q.v.*

TRANSFERENCE 1. In psychoanalysis *q.v.*, the patient's tendency to transfer emotional reactions that were originally directed to his or her own parents and to redirect them toward the analyst. 2. The close emotional attachment of the patient in psychoanalysis *q.v.* to the analyst. 3. A patient's directing of emotions at the analyst who represents someone of importance in the patient's past.

TRANSFERENCE NEUROSIS A phase of psychoanalysis *q.v.* in which the patient reacts to the analyst as if he or she were the patient's parent. Such an event enables the analyst and patient to examine deep conflicts that may have been repressed *q.v.* prior to this phase of treatment.

TRANSFER OF LEARNING The influence the learning of one task has upon the learning or performance of another task. cf: transfer of training.

TRANSFER OF TRAINING The effect of having learned one task on learning another. When learning the first task helps in learning the second, the transfer is called positive. When it impedes in learning the second, the transfer is said to be negative. cf: transfer of learning.

TRANSFERRIN 1. An iron-binding protein *q.v.* in the blood that transports iron. 2. Beta globulin *q.v.* cf: globulin.

TRANSFER RNA 1. A type of RNA *q.v.* that unites with specific amino acids *q.v.* and aligns them to messenger RNA *q.v.* in the formation of polypeptides *q.v.* 2. A type of RNA that transports amino acids to the ribosome *q.v.*, where they are assembled into proteins *q.v.*

TRANS FORM Certain atoms *q.v.* or groups of atoms relative to a double bond between two carbon atoms on opposite sides of the molecule *q.v.*

TRANSFORMATION A genetic *q.v.* recombination in bacteria *q.v.* brought about by adding foreign DNA *q.v.* to a culture.

TRANSFORMED CELLS 1. Cells that have been changed by a carcinogenic *q.v.* substance; however, the cells are not yet cancer *q.v.* cells. 2. Precancerous *q.v.*

TRANSFUSION The introduction of whole blood or blood cellular components directly into the bloodstream.

TRANSGENDERISM A social movement assert and advocate the rights of people who are transgender.

TRANSGENDERIST A person who identifies strongly with the opposite sex and may cross-dress, yet does not wish to undergo transsexual surgery. cf: transsexualism.

TRANSIENT ERECTILE DYSFUNCTION Erectile dysfunction *q.v.*

TRANSIENT ISCHEMIC ATTACK (TIA) . A temporary spasm of a cerebral artery *q.v.* that produces symptoms similar to those of a minor stroke *q.v.* ~ is often a forewarning of a true cerebrovascular accident *q.v.* 2. "Little strokes."

TRANSIENT OBESITY Obesity *q.v.* that occurs during preadolescence that disappears following maturity. ct: persistent obesity.

TRANSIENT SITUATIONAL PERSONALITY DISORDERS An acute *q.v.* symptom response to an overwhelming situation in a basically stable personality *q.v.*

TRANSILLUMINATION A method of detecting breast cancer *q.v.* in which light is passed through breast tissues to detect and differentiate between cysts *q.v.* and malignant tumors *q.v.*

TRANSITION PREPHASE The first of two prephases to the sexual response cycle *q.v.* during which a person makes the transition from a nonsexual to a sexual physiologic *q.v.* state.

TRANSITORY ISCHEMIC ATTACK (TIA) Transient ischemic attack *q.v.*

TRANSKETOLASE An enzyme *q.v.* that uses thiamin *q.v.* pyrophosphate as a coenzyme *q.v.* ~ brings about the transfer of a 2-carbon unit from sugar to aldoses.

TRANSLATION The production of protein *q.v.* from RNA *q.v.*

TRANSLOCATION 1. A chromosomal *q.v.* malfunctioning characterized by a portion of a chromosome from one group to, in effect, create a new chromosome. 2. The change in position of a segment of a chromosome to another part of the same chromosome or to a different chromosome. cf: Down syndrome.

TRANSMISSION The conveyance of disease from one person to another.

TRANSMISSION OF INFECTIOUS DISEASES Infectious diseases *q.v.* may be transmitted from person to person in one of two ways: 1. indirect contact (airborne, water and food borne, vector borne *qq.v.*) and 2. direct contact.

TRANSMITTER OF MESSAGE Changes information into a form that can be easily conveyed from the source to the destination. A component of information theory *q.v.*

TRANSORBITAL LOBOTOMY Lobotomy *q.v.*

TRANSPIRE To breathe across.

TRANSPIRATION The giving off of water through the leaves of plants.

TRANSPLANTATION 1. The stage of cancer *q.v.* during which cancer cells move into different parts of the body. 2. Metastasis *q.v.*

TRANSPOSITION The phenomenon whereby visual and auditory *q.v.* patterns remain the same even though the parts of which they are composed are changed. Having learned to discriminate two stimuli *q.v.*, the person responds to a new pair of stimuli as though the original learning *q.v.* had consisted of the learning of a relationship.

TRANSSEXUAL A person who feels trapped in the body of the wrong gender *q.v.* Some ~s have reversed core gender identities. cf: transsexualism.

TRANSSEXUALISM 1. A surgical and psychological procedure to alter the obvious sex of a person. 2. Changing sexes from male to female or from female to male. 3. A condition in which a person is severely uncomfortable with his or her gender *q.v.* In some instances, it is possible to make one's physiological gender compatible with one's psychological gender through surgery and medication. 4. The condition of believing that one is trapped in the body of the opposite sex. ct: transvestism. cf: sex reversal; transgenderism.

TRANSUDATION The passing of a fluid through a membrane *q.v.*, esp. the lubrication in the vagina *q.v.* during sexual arousal.

TRANSURETHRAL RESECTION 1. A surgical procedure involving the insertion of an instrument into the urethra *q.v.* to relieve pressure exerted by an enlarged prostate gland *q.v.* 2. Removal, by surgical means, of portions of the prostate gland through the urethra.

TRANSVERSE COLON That division of the large intestine *q.v.* that crosses the abdomen *q.v.*, located between the ascending colon *q.v.* and the descending colon *q.v.*

TRANSVERSE FISSION The cleavage of the cytoplasm *q.v.* horizontally across the middle of the cell following nuclear division, resulting in more or less equal daughter cells.

TRANSVERSE FRACTURE A fracture *q.v.* whose line forms a right angle with the axis of the bone.

TRANSVERSE POSITION 1. In childbirth, when the baby lies across the uterus *q.v.* and a shoulder or arm will first be seen at the opening of the vagina *q.v.* A cesarean section *q.v.* is often necessary if the baby cannot be turned. 2. Transverse presentation *q.v.*

TRANSVERSE PRESENTATION Transverse position *q.v.*

TRANSVESTITE 1. A person who dresses in the clothing of the opposite sex. 2. Cross-dressing *q.v.* cf: transvestism.

TRANSVESTISM A sexual variance *q.v.* characterized by emotional and/or sexual gratification derived from dressing in clothes of the opposite sex. It is usually not accompanied by a homosexual *q.v.* preference. cf: transvestite.

TRANXENE A commercial preparation of chlorazepate *q.v.*

TRANYLCYPROMINE An MAO *q.v.* inhibitor used as an antidepressant *q.v.* Parnate is a commercial preparation.

TRAUMA 1. A wound or injury of either a psychological *q.v.* or a physiological *q.v.* nature. 2. A severe physical or psychological injury caused by an external force having lasting effect.

TRAUMATIC Pertaining to a wound or injury.

TRAUMATIC ASPHYXIA Asphyxia *q.v.* occurring as a result of sudden or severe compression of the throat *q.v.* or upper abdomen *q.v.* or both.

TRAUMATIC DISEASE An illness caused by external factors, such as poison, a blow, or stress *q.v.*

TRAUMATIC EMPHYSEMA Emphysema *q.v.* occurring as a result of trauma *q.v.*

TRAUMATIC ENCEPHALOPATHY A syndrome caused by repeated injuries to the brain, marked by slurred speech, unsteady gait, and sometimes, psychotic *q.v.* symptoms.

TRAUMATIC NEUROSIS Shock reaction *q.v.*

TRAZODONE A heterocyclic antidepressant *q.v.* Desyrel is the brand name.

TREATMENT The management and care of a person for the purpose of combating disease or disability.

TREATMENT BIAS The tendency of treatment for physiological *q.v.* or psychological *q.v.* diseases to be treated differently depending upon the patient's social class, race, gender, or ability to pay.

TREATMENT MODALITIES The variety of forms of therapy *q.v.* available to correct a disease, dysfunction, or malfunction. They include chemotherapy, electronic therapy, psychotherapy, social interactions, and surgery *qq.v.*

TREMATODE A parasitic *q.v.* worm, fluke.

TREMOR 1. An abnormal trembling or shaking of a body part. 2. Involuntary quivering of one or more voluntary muscles *q.v.*, usually confined to one area of the body.

TREMULOUSNESS Trembling of parts of the body, esp. the hands.

TRENCH FOOT 1. A chronic *q.v.* condition of cold injury affecting the feet of a person obliged to stand for long periods of time in cold water, snow, or mud. 2. A vascular injury of the feet.

TRENCH MOUTH Vincent's disease *q.v.*

TREND CORRELATION A statistical technique that assumes that a change in the dependent variable *q.v.* can be predicted or measured by the change that occurs in the independent variable(s) *q.v.*

TREND LINE An indicator of changes in the character of a given phenomenon over time.

TREPHINE (TREPAN) A small crown saw used in surgery, esp. of the skull.

TREPHINING To operate with a trephine *q.v.* for the purpose of cutting a small hole in the head.

TREPONEMA PALLIDUM A spirochete bacterium *q.v.* responsible for syphilis *q.v.*

TREPONEMA PALLIDUM IMMOBILIZATION TEST (TPI) 1. Nelson's specific test using living treponemas mixed with the serum *q.v.* of a person immune to syphilis *q.v.* The organism becomes fixed in the presence of compliment. 2. A test for confirming a biological false-positive reaction.

TREXAN A commercial preparation of naltrexone *q.v.*

TRIAGE The sorting or selection of injured to determine the priority of care to be rendered to each.

TRIAL AND ERROR LEARNING Attempts to solve a problem by trying out alternative solutions or possibilities and discarding those that prove to be unsatisfactory.

TRIAL MARRIAGE A relationship in which a man and a woman live together before making a final decision to marry.

TRIANGULAR BANDAGE A piece of cloth in the shape of a right-angled triangle and used as a sling for the arm.

TRIANGULAR SYSTEM A psychoanalytic *q.v.* concept proposing that a male homosexual's *q.v.* parents consist of an intimate and controlling mother and a detached, rejecting father.

TRIAZOLAM A benzodiazepine *q.v.* hypnotic *q.v.* Halcion is the brand name.

TRICARBOXYLIC ACID CYCLE 1. Krebs cycle *q.v.* 2. Citric acid cycle.

TRICEPS 1. The large muscle at the back of the upper arm. 2. A muscle having three points of origin.

TRICHINELLA 1. A metazoan, pathogenic *q.v.* to humans. 2. An animal pathogen. 3. A parasite *q.v.* that occurs in pigs and infects humans through the ingestion of improperly cooked pork.

TRICHINELLA SPIRALIS A small, round parasitic *q.v.* worm that causes trichinosis *q.v.*

TRICHINOSIS A disease caused by a metazoan (trichinella *q.v.*) that is ingested in insufficiently cooked pork containing encysted larvae.

TRICHLOROACETALDEHYDE 1. Chloral hydrate *q.v.* 2. Mickey Finn *q.v.*

TRICHLOROETHYLENE A substance used in dry-cleaning agents and may be associated with certain diseases.

TRICHOLOGIST A person who specializes in hair.

TRICHOMONAS VAGINALIS 1. A protozoan *q.v.* causing vaginal *q.v.* or other genital *q.v.* infections. 2. A one-celled parasite *q.v.* that can infect the urogenital *q.v.* tract. 3. A protozoan responsible for trichomoniasis *q.v.*

TRICHOMONAS VAGINITIS 1. An infection of the vagina *q.v.* caused by bacteria (*Trichomonas vaginalis q.v.*). 2. A frothy, thin, greenish or yellowish gray, foul-smelling discharge causing burning and itching. 3. Trichomoniasis *q.v.*

TRICHOMONIASIS A relatively common and chronic *q.v.* disease of the female characterized by vaginitis *q.v.* and a rather profuse, yellowish discharge. In the male, the disease usually infects the prostate, seminal vesicles, and urethra *qq.v.* It is caused by the protozoan *q.v.*, *Trichomonas vaginalis q.v.*

TRICHOTILLOMANIA The twirling or plucking at segments of hair resulting in trauma to the hair follicles *q.v.* causing patches of baldness.

TRICHROMATIC COLOR VISION 1. Color vision. 2. Normal color vision in which all visible hues *q.v.* can be reproduced by appropriate mixtures of three primary colors.

TRICK Vernacular for trichomoniasis *q.v.*

TRICK VOCABULARY The use of language without respect to meaning.

TRICUSPID VALVE A three-cusp valve that regulates blood flow between the right atrium *q.v.* and the right ventricle *q.v.* of the heart.

TRICYCLIC Refers to a group of chemicals used in treating depression *q.v.*

TRICYCLIC ANTIDEPRESSANTS 1. Drugs used to treat bipolar and unipolar depression *q.v.*, believed to regulate neurotransmitters *q.v.* at the synapses *q.v.* in the brain. 2. Tricyclic compounds *q.v.*

TRICYCLIC COMPOUNDS 1. Drugs used to elevate moods and to treat certain types of depression *q.v.* 2. Tricyclic antidepressants *q.v.* 3. Tricyclic drug *q.v.*

TRICYCLIC DRUG 1. One of the group of antidepressants *q.v.*, called tricyclic because of its chemical structure, that interferes with the reuptake of norepinephrine *q.v.* and serotonin *q.v.* by a neuron *q.v.* after it has fired. 2. Tricyclic compounds *q.v.*

TRIFLUOPERAZINE An antipsychotic *q.v.* drug. Stelazine is the brand name.

TRIFLUPROMAZINE An antipsychotic *q.v.* drug. Vesprin is the brand name.

TRIGLYCERIDE 1. A glycerol *q.v.* ester *q.v.* containing three fatty acids *q.v.* 2. Types of lipid *q.v.* molecules that are specialized for storing energy. 3. Body fat that is stored economically in the adipose *q.v.* tissues in the form of three attached fatty acids.

TRIGONE A triangular area of the interior of the urinary bladder *q.v.*, between the opening of the ureters *q.v.* and the orifice *q.v.* of the urethra *q.v.*

TRIHEXYPHENIDYL An anticholinergic *q.v.* used to control extrapyramidal *q.v.* symptoms. Artane is the brand name.

TRIHYBRID The offspring from homozygous *q.v.* parents differing in 3 pairs of genes *q.v.*

TRILAFON 1. A commercial preparation of one of the major tranquilizers *q.v.* 2. A commercial preparation of phenothiazine *q.v.* 3. A brand name of perphenazine *q.v.*

TRIMESTER A period of 3 months, applied to the pregnancy period.

TRIOXIDE An oxide containing three oxygen atoms.

TRIP An slang term referring to a hallucinogenic *q.v.* experience.

TRIPHOSPHOPYRIDINE NUCLEOTIDE (TPN) Nicotinamide adenine dinucleotide phosphate *q.v.*

TRIPLEGIA Paralysis *q.v.* involving three appendages. ct: paraplegia; quadriplegia.

TRIPLET A group of three consecutive DNA *q.v.* nucleotides containing information for a specific amino acid *q.v.* in polypeptide *q.v.* synthesis.

TRIPLOID An organism with three genomes *q.v.* or sets of chromosomes *q.v.*

TRISMUS A spasm of the muscles of the jaw. Commonly associated with tetanus *q.v.*

TRISOMY The presence of an additional third chromosome *q.v.* of a particular chromosome pair. ~ is caused by improper splitting (nondisjunction) of the cell nucleus *q.v.* during cell division *q.v.* cf: trisomy 21; Down's syndrome.

TRISOMY 21. Down's syndrome *q.v.*

TRISTEARIN A triglyceride *q.v.* of stearic acid *q.v.*

TRNA (SOLUBLE, ADAPTER, TRANSFER) A molecule transferring amino acid *q.v.* to ribosome *q.v.* associated with an mRNA molecule *q.v.*

TROCHANTER Either of the two bony prominences developed from independent centers near the upper extremity of the femur *q.v.* below the femoral neck. The greater ~ *q.v.* and the lesser ~*q.v.*

TROCHLEAR Pertaining to a pulley.

TROILISM 1. A sexual variance *q.v.* in which three people participate in a series of sexual activities. 2. Having sexual relations with another person while a third person watches.

TROPHIC Pertaining to nutrition *q.v.*

TROPHIC LEVEL A step in the movement of energy through an ecosystem *q.v.*

TROPHOBLASTIC CELLS A layer of cells attaching the fertilized ovum *q.v.* to the uterine *q.v.* wall and supplying nutrition to the embryo *q.v.* cf: trophoblasts.

TROPHOBLASTS A layer of cells that develop over the surface of the blastocyst *q.v.* and help in the ovum's *q.v.* adherence to the uterine *q.v.* wall. ~ plus other cells eventually form the placenta *q.v.* cf: trophoblastic cells.

TROPHOTROPIC That which is tranquil, restorative, or nurturing. cf: ergotropic.

TROPIC Having to do with a turning or change.

TROPISM The automatic directing of an organism toward or away from a source of stimulus.

TROPOSPHERE That part of the atmosphere located between the earth's surface and the stratosphere *q.v.* In this stratum, convective disturbances occur, clouds form, and the temperature decreases with an increase in altitude.

TRUE HERMAPHRODITES Persons born with the gonads *q.v.* of both sexes. ct: pseudohermaphrodism.

TRUE NEGATIVES In epidemiology *q.v.*, related to tests of validity labeling noncases or the absence of characteristics correctly. ct: true positives.

TRUE POSITIVES In epidemiology *q.v.*, related to tests of validity, labeling cases, or characteristics correctly. ct: true negatives.

TRUNCATED DISTRIBUTION A distribution *q.v.* that covers less than the complete range of scores.

TRUNK The body, excluding the head and extremities.

TRUTH IN TESTING A movement to require publishers of standardized tests *q.v.* to permit examination of scoring keys and answer sheets.

TRUTH SERUM 1. Drugs, usually depressants *q.v.*, that increase the likelihood that a person will talk without inhibition. Used in psychotherapy *q.v.* or interrogation. 2. Sodium pentothal *q.v.*

TRYPTAMINERGIC A neuron that is activated by the neurotransmitter *q.v.*, serotonin (5-hydroxytryptamine) *q.v.*

TRYPTOPHAN 1. An essential amino acid *q.v.* 2. A precursor of niacin *q.v.*

TS AND BLUES A mixture of pentazocine, a narcotic analgesic *q.v.*, and tripelennamine, an antihistamine *q.v.*, and used as a heroin *q.v.* substitute.

T SCORE A measure for how far a raw score is from the mean *q.v.* in numerical terms, calculated by using a mean of 50 and a standard deviation *q.v.* of 10.

TSETSE FLY The carrier of the African sleeping sickness organism.

TSH An acronym for thyroid-stimulating hormone *q.v.*

TSS An acronym for toxic shock syndrome *q.v.*

T TEST A statistical test to determine whether a difference is significant *q.v.*

TUBAL LIGATION 1. A surgical procedure to tie off the fallopian tubes *q.v.* so that sperm and egg cannot meet. 2. A surgical technique for rendering a woman unable to conceive *q.v.* 3. A form of sterilization *q.v.* 4. A contraceptive *q.v.* technique.

TUBAL PATENCY TEST The projection of dye through the fallopian tubes *q.v.* to determine there is a blockage.

TUBAL PREGNANCY A type of displaced or ectopic *q.v.* pregnancy in which the embryo *q.v.* fails to descend into the uterus *q.v.* and, instead, develops in the fallopian tube *q.v.*

TUBAL STERILIZATION 1. Tubal ligation *q.v.* 2. A method of severing the oviducts *q.v.* to prevent ova *q.v.* from reaching the uterus or to prevent sperm *q.v.* from reaching the ova.

TUBE FEEDING The feeding of a person by inserting a flexible tube through the nostril into the throat and pouring liquid nutrients directly into the esophagus *q.v.*

TUBERCLE 1. A fibrous capsule that walls off the destructive action of tubercle bacilli *q.v.* in living tissue. 2. In tuberculosis *q.v.*, a nodule in the tissues produced by the tubercle bacillus and is the characteristic lesion *q.v.* of tuberculosis.

TUBERCULOSIS 1. A disease of the lung caused by the presence of *Mycobacterium tuberculosis* *q.v.* 2. Phthisis *q.v.*

TUBERCULOSIS AND RESPIRATORY DISEASE ASSOCIATION The former name of the American Lung Association *q.v.*

TUBEROSITY A broad eminence on a bone.

TUBULE (KIDNEY) The structure connecting a glomerulus *q.v.* with the pelvis.

TUINAL A commercial preparation of a barbiturate *q.v.* Amobarbital and Secobarbital combination.

TULAREMIA 1. Rabbit fever. 2. A disease transmitted from rodents that have been bitten by an insect infected with *Pasteurella tularensis* or by direct contact. 3. Deer fly fever.

TUMESCENCE 1. The process of swelling or of being swollen. 2. Engorgement with blood. ct: detumescence.

TUMOR 1. A neoplasm *q.v.* 2. ~s may be benign *q.v.* or malignant *q.v.* 3. An abnormal mass of tissue that grows more rapidly than normal. 4. Lesion *q.v.*

TUMOR INITIATOR 1. A chemical that stimulates the growth of a tumor *q.v.* 2. A chemical that may cause certain cells to become tumorous. 3. Tumor promoters *q.v.* cf: carcinogen; cocarcinogen.

TUMOR PROMOTERS 1. Tumor initiators *q.v.* 2. Substances that enhance the development of cancer *q.v.* cells without actually causing genetic *q.v.* changes.

TUMOR VIRUS Any virus *q.v.* that can produce a cancer *q.v.* in an organism.

TUNIC 1. An investing membrane. 2. A sheath.

TUNICA DARTOS In the scrotum *q.v.*, the inner layer of smooth muscle *q.v.* that contracts during arousal, strenuous exercise, or exposure to the cold.

TURBINADO SUGAR Common in some commercial establishments as a substitute for raw sugar, partially refined to remove impurities and some of the molasses.

TURBINATE Shaped like a cone, scroll, or spiral.

TURGOR 1. The condition of being swollen or congested. 2. The swollen condition of a cell caused by internal water pressure.

TURGOR PRESSURE The pressure within a cell that causes turgor *q.v.*

TURNER'S SYNDROME 1. A genetic *q.v.* abnormality affecting females in which one of the sex-determining pair of chromosomes *q.v.* is missing, leaving a total of 45 rather than 46 chromosomes. Symptoms of ~ include incomplete development of the ovaries, short stature, and webbing of the neck. 2. A condition in which a female has only one sex chromosome (XO) rather than two (XX). The result is abnormal development of the ovaries *q.v.*, failure to menstruate *q.v.*, and infertility *q.v.*

TWILIGHT STATE A state of disordered consciousness in which a person performs purposeful acts for which he or she is later amnesic *q.v.* cf: psychomotor epilepsy.

TWIN METHOD A research strategy in behavior genetics *q.v.* in which behavioral patterns of monozygotic and dizygotic *qq.v.* twins are compared.

TWINS Two individuals from the same birth. May be monozygotic *q.v.* (identical) or dizygotic *q.v.* (fraternal).

TWIN STUDIES 1. A method of testing genetic *q.v.* influences by comparing identical and fraternal twins. 2. Studies comparing monozygotic *q.v.* and dizygotic *q.v.* twins and their families in order to gain insight into the relative importance of heredity *q.v.* and environment *q.v.* in creating individual differences.

TWISTING Writing a new insurance policy rather than renewing an old one.

TWO-DISEASE THEORY An explanation of mood disorders that proposes that there are two types of depressive illnesses, one caused by functional deficits of norepinephrine *q.v.* and the other by functional deficits of serotonin *q.v.*

TWO-FACTOR THEORY 1. A theory of learning that makes the assumption that classical and instrumental learning *qq.v.* are different with respect to the principle of reinforcement *q.v.* 2. Mowrer's theory of avoidance learning according to which (a) fear is attached to a neutral stimulus *q.v.* by pairing it with a noxious unconditioned stimulus *q.v.* and (b) a person learns to escape fear elicited by the conditioned stimulus *q.v.*, thereby avoiding the unconditioned stimulus.

TWO-FACTOR THEORY OF EMOTION According to Schachter, a person's emotional experience requires generalized physical arousal followed by a cognitive *q.v.* label for the arousal.

TWO-STEP PROCEDURE Breast biopsy *q.v.* followed by breast surgery within hours or days.

TYLECTOMY 1. The surgical removal of a cancerous tumor *q.v.* or lesion *q.v.* and a portion of adjacent tissue. 2. Literally, within the region or territory. 3. A form of mastectomy *q.v.* cf: lumpectomy.

TYLOMA Calluses.

TYMPANIC MEMBRANE 1. Ear drum. 2. A thin tissue that separates the external ear *q.v.* from the middle ear *q.v.* The ~ vibrates from sound waves and in turn vibrates the malleus, incus, and stapes bones *qq.v.*, which stimulate nerve endings in the inner ear *q.v.* sending nervous impulses to the brain to be interpreted.

TYMPANUM 1. The membrane separating the outer and middle ear *qq.v.* 2. The ear drum. 3. The tympanic membrane *q.v.* 4. The cavity of the middle ear. 5. Drum.

TYNDALLIZATION A sterilization process carried out on three consecutive days by exposure to moist steam at 100°C.

TYPE 1 DIABETES MELLITUS 1. A form of diabetes *q.v.* generally seen for the first time in childhood or adolescence. 2. Juvenile onset diabetes *q.v.* 3. Insulin-dependent diabetes *q.v.* ct: type 2 diabetes mellitus.

TYPE 2 DIABETES MELLITUS 1. Noninsulin-dependent diabetes *q.v.* 2. A form of diabetes traditionally seen for the first time in persons over 35 years. Now, increasingly seen in younger people largely because of increasing rates of obesity *q.v.* 3. Adult onset diabetes *q.v.* ct: type 1 diabetes mellitus.

TYPE A BEHAVIOR Exhibited by people who are competitive, rushed, aggressive, and overcommitted to their work. ct: type B behavior. cf: type A personality.

TYPE A PERSONALITY 1. A predisposition to some diseases, e.g., coronary heart disease *q.v.* 2. A person who possesses personality traits characterized by compulsion, neatness, perfection, and the like. 3. A person with type A behavior.

TYPE B BEHAVIOR Characterized by people who are relaxed, relatively free of pressure, and not overly aggressive. ct: type A behavior. cf: type B personality.

TYPE B PERSONALITY A person who is relaxed, patient, noncompetitive, and who has lower risk of coronary heart disease *q.v.* than those with type A personality.

TYPE I ERROR In epidemiology *q.v.*, rejection of the null hypothesis *q.v.* that is really true. ct: Type II error.

TYPE II ERROR In epidemiology *q.v.*, failure to reject a null hypothesis *q.v.* that is really false. ct: Type I error.

TYPE THEORY In personality theory *q.v.*, any position that views people as members of categories rather than as points on a set of dimensions.

TYPHOID FEVER A contagious disease transmitted through water, milk, and food containing *Salmonella typhosa* bacteria *q.v.*

TYPHUS FEVER 1. An acute *q.v.* infectious disease *q.v.* transmitted by lice and fleas. 2. A rickettsial *q.v.* disease marked by high fever, stupor alternating with delirium, intense headache, and a dark red rash.

TYROSINE A nonessential amino acid *q.v.* ~ spares the essential amino acid phenylalanine *q.v.*

TYROSINELESS A strain of bacteria *q.v.* not capable of synthesizing *q.v.* the amino acid *q.v.* tyrosine *q.v.*

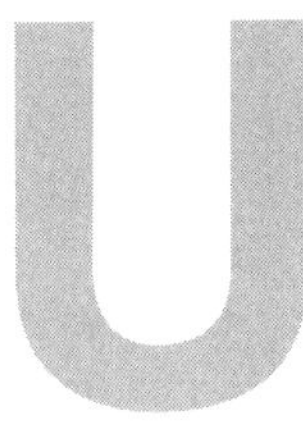

UCR An acronym for unconditioned response *q.v.*

UCS An acronym for unconditioned stimulus *q.v.*

UHF 1. Ultrahigh frequency. 2. The radio frequencies between 300 and 3000 MHz.

ULCER 1. A break in skin or mucous membrane *q.v.* accompanied by tissue disintegration. 2. Any break or sore on the skin surface or on internal tissues that line the body. cf: decubitus ulcer; peptic ulcer.

ULCERATION The formation of an ulcer *q.v.*; a lesion *q.v.* on the surface of the skin or a mucous membrane *q.v.* caused by a loss of tissue, often with inflammation *q.v.*

ULCERATIVE COLITIS Inflammation *q.v.* of the mucous *q.v.* lining of the large intestine (colon) *q.v.*

ULNA The larger of the two bones of the forearm *q.v.* on the little finger side of the arm.

ULNAR ARTERY The major artery *q.v.* of the forearm *q.v.*, on the side opposite the thumb.

ULTIMATE CAUSE Explanations of behavior that focus on why a particular behavior increased reproductive success during the process of evolution *q.v.*

ULTIMATE ENVIRONMENT An abstract concept pertaining to a set of conditions in which a person comfortably understands himself or herself and others and the natural world.

ULTRADIAN RHYTHM A fixed pattern of changes in basic body processes occurring in 90–100 min cycles.

ULTRASONOGRAPHY The visualization of deep structures of the body through the recording of high-frequency sound waves directed into tissues. cf: ultrasound device.

ULTRASOUND 1. High-intensity sound waves used to create an image of internal body structures. 2. ~ waves used to elevate the internal temperature of cancer *q.v.* cells for the purpose of killing these cells.

ULTRASOUND DEVICE A mechanism that transforms electrical energy into sound energy for use in diagnosis, surgery, dental care, and other therapeutic procedures. cf: ultrasonography.

ULTRASOUND SCAN A procedure whereby sound waves are used to project an image on a video screen to aid the physician during amniocentesis *q.v.* and other diagnostic procedures during pregnancy. cf: ultrasound device.

ULTRA VIRES 1. In law, outside the power of an individual or body. 2. Beyond the scope of authority.

UMBILICAL CLAMP A device, usually of plastic, used to compress the umbilical cord *q.v.*, allowing it to be cut without endangering the mother and neonate *q.v.* from blood loss.

UMBILICAL CORD 1. The flexible cord connecting the fetus *q.v.* and the placenta *q.v.*, containing the umbilical blood vessels, and that carries nutrients to the fetus and waste from the fetus through the placental wall. 2. The lifeline between the mother and the fetus that contains two arteries *q.v.* and one vein *q.v.* Food, oxygen, and nutrients go to the fetus through the arteries, and waste is returned to the mother through the vein.

UMBILICUS 1. Navel. 2. Belly button. 3. A small depression in the abdominal *q.v.* wall marking the point where the fetus *q.v.* was attached to the umbilical cord *q.v.*

UNBALANCED DIET A diet lacking adequate representation of nutrients essential for body functioning. ct: balanced diet.

UNCERTAINTY CONDITION A state in which multiple variables make behavior unpredictable. ct: complete certainty conditions.

UNCOMMON FOODS Foods introduced into a weight reduction diet that a person finds unfamiliar and perhaps unappetizing.

UNCONDITIONAL POSITIVE REGARD According to Rogers, an essential characteristic of a client-centered therapist *q.v.*, who needs to be totally accepted by the client, in order for him or her to adequately evaluate the client's behavior in relation to progress toward self-actualization *q.v.*

UNCONDITIONED REFLEX Unconditioned response *q.v.*

UNCONDITIONED RESPONSE (UR) 1. The reaction (response) that is made to the unconditioned stimulus *q.v.* in classical conditioning *q.v.* An example is an inborn reflex. 2. In classical conditioning, the response that is elicited by the UCS without prior training. ct: conditioned response; conditioned stimulus.

UNCONDITIONED STIMULUS (UCS) 1. The activator (stimulus) that elicits the unconditioned response *q.v.* in classical conditioning *q.v.* 2. In classical conditioning, the stimulus that elicits the UR and the presentation of which acts as reinforcement *q.v.* ct: conditioned response; conditioned stimulus.

UNCONSCIOUS 1. Subconscious *q.v.* 2. A lack of awareness. 3. In Freudian psychology *q.v.*, that portion of the psyche that is a storehouse of repressed *q.v.* or forgotten memories and desires that are not directly accessible to consciousness but may be brought into consciousness when ego *q.v.* restraints are removed. 4. Not conscious.

UNCONSCIOUS ACTION Behavior in which a person is experiences no sensory awareness.

UNCONSCIOUS INTERFERENCE A process to explain certain perceptual phenomena such as size constancy *q.v.* An object is perceived to be in the distance and is, therefore, unconsciously perceived as larger than it appears to be retinally *q.v.* cf: shape constancy.

UNCONSCIOUS MIND Subconscious mind.

UNCONSCIOUS MOTIVATION Motivation *q.v.* for a person's behavior of which he or she is not aware.

UNCONSUMMATED Characterized by not having had coitus *q.v.*

UNDERCONTROLLED In reference to childhood disorders, problem behavior that creates trouble for others, e.g., disobedience and aggressiveness.

UNDEREXTENSION A child's tendency to limit the meaning of words to fewer referents than would an adult.

UNDERLYING STRUCTURE The phrase organization that describes the meaning of parts of a sentence. cf: phrase structure. ct: surface structure.

UNDERNUTRITION 1. A condition resulting from insufficient food. 2. The lack of nutrients *q.v.* in the diet.

UNDERSTEER A term describing the handling characteristics of a vehicle that has the center of gravity located forward of the center of the vehicle making steering more difficult.

UNDERWEIGHT A deficiency of more than 10% under one's desirable weight.

UNDESCENDED TESTICLE 1. Failure of a testicle *q.v.* to descend into the scrotum *q.v.* 2. A developmental defect in males in which the testicles fail to descend into the scrotum. 3. Cryptorchidism *q.v.*

UNDIFFERENTIATED SEX TYPING Showing how acceptance for behaviors stereotyped *q.v.* as appropriate for either sex.

UNDOING 1. Atonement *q.v.* 2. An ego defense mechanism *q.v.* by means of which the person performs activities designed to atone for his or her misdeeds, thereby undoing them.

UNDULANT FEVER 1. Brucellosis *q.v.* 2. An infectious disease *q.v.* marked by alternating latent *q.v.* periods and attacks of fever, swelling of the joints, pain, and weakness; it is spread by contaminated milk.

UNFOUNDED 1. Without a sound basis in fact. 2. Applied by law enforcement agencies to a reported case when it believes that a report is groundless. 3. In scientific research *q.v.*, a term describing a case when no significant evidence to support a conclusion is apparent.

UNFREEZING The first phase of Lewin's three-part process of change. Learning *q.v.* occurs when a person can make an informed choice of whether to change an existing behavior. The learning, or change, process that leads to an informed choice is based on ~ previous attitudes, beliefs, and behaviors and creating receptivity to new knowledge that may provide the basis for the development of new ideas. Once ~ has occurred, individuals are able to experiment with alternative attitudes and behaviors that they may then adopt.

UNGRADED SCHOOLS Schools in which students' progress is based on their ability rather than their chronological age.

UNICELLULAR Composed of a single cell.

UNIFORM DONOR CARD A card or document that indicates that specific organs are to be donated for research or to persons who need organ transplants.

UNINSURABLE RISK A person not acceptable for insurance coverage because he or she is an excessive risk.

UNION SHOP A company or other workplace that operates under a contract between a union and management. New employees are required to join the union within a specified period of time.

UNIPARTITE STRUCTURES (CHROMOSOMES) Single units.

UNIPOLAR AFFECTIVE DISORDER 1. An affective disorder *q.v.* in which there is no sudden or dramatic swings between emotional extremes. 2. Extreme mania *q.v.* or extreme depression *q.v.*, usually for extended periods of time.

UNIPOLAR DEPRESSION 1. A term applied to an individual who has experienced episodes of clinical depression *q.v.* but not mania *q.v.* 2. A mood disorder characterized by periods of severe depression.

UNIQUENESSES AND COMPETENCIES Those functional traits that make a person recognizably different from other persons. cf: personality; ideographic characteristics. ct: nomothetic.

UNIT 1. An organization of curriculum *q.v.* implying a unity or wholeness. 2. A basic building block of curriculum development or organization. Usually consists of title; goals and objectives; content outline; strategies, techniques, activities; summary and evaluation; and available resources to be used.

UNIT APPROACH A curricular framework in which a program or subject is divided into various segments or building blocks of study.

UNITED STATES BUREAU OF THE CENSUS Census Bureau.

UNITED STATES CONSUMER PRODUCT SAFETY COMMISSION Established as a result of the passage of the Consumer Product Safety Act of 1972 *q.v.* The Commission is concerned with reducing injuries associated with consumer products used in the home, schools, and recreational areas. Its authority was expanded by enactment of the Federal Hazardous Substance Act, Flammable Fabrics Act, Poison Prevention Packaging Act, and Refrigerator Safety Act. The ∼'s jurisdiction does not include foods, drugs, cosmetics, medical devices, and other products that come under authority of other federal agencies.

UNITED STATES DEPARTMENT OF HEALTH, EDUCATION, AND WELFARE Now the United States Department of Health and Human Services.

UNITED STATES PHARMACOPEIA (USP) A publication listing standard drug formulas.

UNITED STATES POSTAL SERVICE Among other functions, the ∼ protects health consumers from the use of the mails for fraudulent purposes.

UNITED STATES PUBLIC HEALTH SERVICE (USPHS) The chief federal agency responsible for the health of the United States. ∼ consists of six major subdivisions: Alcohol, Drug abuse, and Mental Health Administration; Centers for Disease Control and Prevention; Food and Drug Administration; Health Resources Administration; Health Services Administration; and the National Institutes of Health. The major functions of the ∼ are 1. to assist states and communities with the development of health resources and to improve the development of education of health professionals; 2. to assist in the improvement of the delivery of public health services; 3. to conduct and support research in the medical and other health sciences; 4. to protect the nation against the importation and use of unsafe drugs and other potential health hazards; and 5. to protect against the spread of communicable diseases.

UNITED STATES TEMPERANCE UNION Formed in 1833, an organization designed to educate the public and exert political pressure to minimize the adverse effects of beverage alcohol. See Table T-1.

UNIT OF LEARNING An organized set of topics, methods, and activities designed to present to the learner experiences that enhance learning.

UNIVALENT An unpaired chromosome *q.v.* at meiosis *q.v.*

UNIVERSAL ANTIDOTE An antidote *q.v.* composed of one part strong tea, two parts crumbled brown toast, and one part milk of magnesia.

UNIVERSAL DRESSING A large, 9″ × 36″ dressing of multilayered material that can be used open, folded, or rolled to cover most wounds, to pad splints, or to form a cervical collar.

UNIVERSAL EMERGENCY TELEPHONE NUMBER A master telephone number, 911, that in most areas may be called in case of any kind of emergency.

UNIVERSAL VARIABLES 1. In epidemiology *q.v.*, effect modifiers *q.v.* 2. Characteristics that in nature generally modify or change many health conditions or events and need to be considered when comparing groups.

UNIVERSITY OF SALERNO A medical school, one of the first, founded in 1150 in honor of Roger of Salerno.

UNLAWFUL INTERCOURSE Statutory rape *q.v.*

UNOBTRUSIVE MEASURE A means of gathering information about a subject's behavior without his or her knowledge. An ∼ does not change the behavior being observed.

UNPROVEN METHODS OF CANCER CONTROL A variety of purported cancer treatments or cures that have little or no scientific evidence of their effectiveness.

UNRELATED SUBFAMILY A group of two or more people who are related to each other by birth, marriage, or adoption but are not related to the householder.

UNSALTED; SALT FREE; WITHOUT SALT ADDED (ON FOOD LABELS) No salt added during processing, but salt may be present that occurs naturally or from other ingredients. cf: low sodium.

UNSATURATED FATTY ACIDS Fatty acids *q.v.* whose carbon atoms lack two or more hydrogen atoms. They are usually liquid at room temperature and come from vegetable products. ∼ contain no cholesterol *q.v.* ct: saturated fatty acids.

UNSOCIALIZED-AGGRESSIVE DELINQUENCY Juvenile behavior whose adult counterpart is sociopathic *q.v.* behavior.

UNSTABLE ANGINA Pain of angina pectoris *q.v.* when there is a pronounced occlusion *q.v.* of an artery in the heart. The pain is often frequent and severe. This may be a forewarning of a possible myocardial infarction *q.v.* ct: stable angina.

UNWEIGHTED AVERAGE In epidemiology *q.v.*, providing equal weight to each component on the average. ct: weighted average.

UPTAKE The process by which a cell expends energy to increase the concentration of certain chemicals within itself, e.g., precursor substances taken in by a neuron *q.v.* that will be synthesized *q.v.* into neurotransmitters *q.v.*

URACIL A pyrimidine base found in RNA *q.v.* but not in DNA *q.v.* The DNA uracil is replaced by thymine *q.v.*

URATE 1. A combination of uric acid *q.v.* with a base. 2. A salt of uric acid.

URBANIZE To change from rural to urban in characteristic.

UREA The chief end product of protein *q.v.* metabolism *q.v.* and one of the chief nitrogenous constituents in urine *q.v.*

UREMIA 1. The presence of urinary constituents in the blood. Symptoms include nausea, vomiting, headache, vertigo, and coma. 2. The retention of excessive waste products of metabolism *q.v.* in the blood and the toxic *q.v.* condition produced thereby. Usually a result of failure of normal kidney *q.v.* function.

URETER 1. The tube that connects the kidneys *q.v.* with the urinary bladder *q.v.* through which urine *q.v.* is transported. 2. The fibromuscular tube that conveys urine from the urinary bladder to the outside.

URETHRA 1. The tube that runs from the urinary bladder *q.v.* to the penis *q.v.* in the male and to the vulva *q.v.* in the female through which urine *q.v.* is excreted from the body. 2. In the female, the duct that carries urine from the urinary bladder to the outside of the body. In the male, the ~ has the additional function of carrying the semen *q.v.* during ejaculation *q.v.*

URETHRAL BULB An enlarged section of the urethra *q.v.* at the base of the penis *q.v.* in which semen *q.v.* collects prior to ejaculation *q.v.*, causing sensations of ejaculatory inevitability *q.v.*

URETHRAL OPENING The meatus *q.v.* of the urethra *q.v.*

URETHRITIS Inflammation *q.v.* of the urethra *q.v.*

URETHROCELE 1. In women, a protrusion of the urethra *q.v.* through the vaginal *q.v.* wall. 2. A hernia *q.v.*

URIC ACID A nitrogenous end product of purine *q.v.* metabolism *q.v.* ~ is present in the blood and excreted in the urine *q.v.* An accumulation of ~ may contribute to the development of gout *q.v.*

URINALYSIS An analysis of the urine *q.v.* to determine how the kidneys *q.v.* are functioning and the health of other organs.

URINARY BLADDER Located in the pelvis *q.v.*; it is a storage sac for urine *q.v.*

URINARY BLADDER CANCER A malignancy *q.v.* of the urinary bladder *q.v.*

URINARY STRESS INCONTINENCE Discharge of urine from the urethra *q.v.* due to physical straining.

URINARY SYSTEM The organs *q.v.* concerned in the formation and voiding of urine *q.v.* The system consists of the kidneys, ureters, urinary bladder, and urethra *qq.v.*

URINE Liquid waste that has been removed from the blood by the kidneys *q.v.* and transported to the urinary bladder *q.v.* by the ureters *q.v.*

UROGENITAL 1. The urinary *q.v.* and genital *q.v.* systems. 2. Relating to the urinary and reproductive system *q.v.* taken collectively.

UROGENITAL FOLDS 1. Undifferentiated tissue within the embryo *q.v.* from which the penile urethra *q.v.* or the labia minora *q.v.* develop. 2. Part of the rudimentary genitals *q.v.* of the male and female embryo. The presence or absence of androgen *q.v.* determines whether the genitals develop into male or female organs, respectively.

UROLOGIST A medical specialist who treats diseases and disorders of the urinary tract *q.v.* of both sexes and of the genital *q.v.* tract of the male.

UROLOGY A medical specialty concerned with the diagnosis and treatment of diseases and disorders of the kidneys *q.v.*, urinary bladder *q.v.*, and related structures, and the male reproductive organs. ct: gynecology.

URTICARIA 1. An allergic *q.v.* condition characterized by itching wheals. 2. Hives *q.v.* 3. An eruption of the skin marked by elevated patches and severe itching.

URUSHOIL An oily resin responsible for the skin reaction caused by poison ivy, poison oak, and poison sumac.

USE EFFECTIVENESS Pertaining to the failure rate of contraceptives *q.v.* when adherence to prescribed instruction is unknown. ct: theoretical effectiveness.

USP An acronym for United States Pharmacopeia *q.v.*

USRDA See RDA.

U.S. RECOMMENDED DAILY DIETARY ALLOWANCES Governmental recommendations for daily intake of carbohydrates, proteins, fats, and seven important vitamins and minerals *qq.v.* They must appear on food labels indicating the percentage of the USRDA *q.v.* per serving.

UTERINE Pertaining to the uterus *q.v.*

UTERINE CANCER 1. Malignancy *q.v.* of the uterus *q.v.* 2. Cancer that involves the tissues of the uterus. 3. Cancer of the endometrium *q.v.*

UTERINE PERFORATION Penetration by a foreign object through the uterine *q.v.* wall.

UTERINE SOUFFLÉ A rushing sound in the uterus *q.v.* due to maternal blood filling the placenta *q.v.*, blood vessels, and spaces.

UTERINE TUBE The fallopian tube *q.v.* that extends from each ovary *q.v.* to the uterus *q.v.*

UTERUS 1. The womb. 2. The hollow, muscular organ that is the prenatal *q.v.* environment for the embryo and fetus *qq.v.* 3. A pear-shaped structure in the pelvic cavity *q.v.* consisting of the body, fundus *q.v.*, isthmus *q.v.*, and cervical uteri *q.v.*

UTILITARIANISM The philosophy that the good is determined by what is beneficial to the greatest number of people.

UTILIZATION REVIEW COMMITTEE A committee charged with the review of health care utilization, effectiveness, and cost.

UTRICLE Little sac.

UVULA 1. The small cylinder-like mass that hangs down from the center of the soft palate *q.v.* 2. Latin for a little grape.

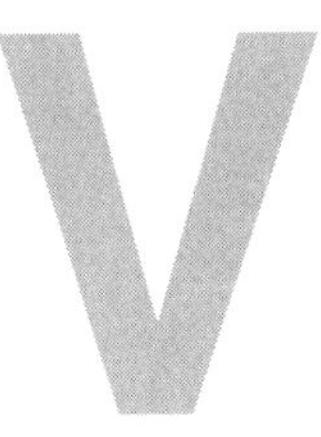

V Variance *q.v.*

VACATE 1. In law, annul. 2. To render an act void, as to set aside a judgment.

VACCINATION A medical procedure through which specially prepared antigens *q.v.* are introduced into the body for the purpose of activating the immune system *q.v.*

VACCINE A substance that prevents infection *q.v.* or establishes immunity *q.v.* to a disease *q.v.*

VACILLATE 1. To waver or fluctuate between two or more alternatives. 2. The inability to make a decision.

VACUOLE A cavity within the protoplasm *q.v.* of a cell containing a solution *q.v.* of sugars, pigments, etc., together with colloidal *q.v.* materials.

VACUOLE MEMBRANE The innermost layer of the cytoplasm, the tonoplast *q.v.*

VACUUM ACTIVITY Instinctive *q.v.* activity that occurs in the absence of a characteristic releasing stimuli *q.v.*

VACUUM ASPIRATION 1. Suction curettage *q.v.* 2. The use of a suction pump in which the embryo *q.v.* and other products of pregnancy *q.v.* are sucked out of the uterus *q.v.* cf: dilation and curettage; saline induction; menstrual extraction; hysterotomy.

VACUUM CURETTAGE Vacuum aspiration *q.v.*

VAGINA 1. The canal in the female that extends from the vulva *q.v.* to the cervix uteri *q.v.* The ~ provides the place for the penis *q.v.* during coitus *q.v.* and serves as the passageway for the fetus *q.v.* at birth and provides an exit for the menstrual flow *q.v.* 2. Sheath.

VAGINAL ASPIRATION 1. Suction curettage *q.v.* 2. A method of induced abortion *q.v.* in which the contents of the uterus are removed by suction with an electric pump.

VAGINAL BARREL The vaginal *q.v.* cavity in women.

VAGINAL DOUCHE A stream of water, or other liquid, directed into the vagina *q.v.* for sanitary, hygienic, or medical purposes.

VAGINAL INTROITUS The vaginal *q.v.* entrance.

VAGINAL LIP STIMULATION A method of stimulating the penis *q.v.* and vulva *q.v.* by rubbing the penis up and down the vaginal *q.v.* lips of the female.

VAGINAL LUBRICATION A clear fluid that appears on the walls of the vaginal barrel *q.v.* within a few seconds after the onset of sexual stimulation.

VAGINAL OPENING Introitus *q.v.*

VAGINAL ORGASM An ambiguous term referring to an orgasm *q.v.* achieved by vaginal *q.v.* stimulation without clitoral *q.v.* stimulation in women.

VAGINAL PLETHYSMORGRAPH A device for recording the amount of blood in the walls of the vagina *q.v.*, providing an indication of the level of sexual arousal *q.v.*

VAGINAL RING A form of hormonal contraception *q.v.* in which a ring, containing progestin *q.v.* and estrogen *q.v.*, is placed at the cervix *q.v.* to prevent ovulation *q.v.* and implantation *q.v.* of a fertilized egg.

VAGINAL SPERMICIDES Nonprescription foams, creams, or jellies that prevent conception by killing sperm *q.v.* before they reach the egg.

VAGINAL SUPPOSITORY A chemical device that is inserted into the vagina *q.v.* prior to sexual intercourse *q.v.* where it effervesces and serves as a spermicidal agent *q.v.*

VAGINISMUS 1. A condition in which the muscles at the entrance of the vagina *q.v.* contract, making intromission *q.v.* painful and nearly impossible. 2. Involuntary, spasmodic contractions of the vaginal muscles. 3. A sexual dysfunction *q.v.* 4. Painful spasmodic contractions of the outer third of the vaginal barrel *q.v.*, making insertion of the penis *q.v.* difficult, if not impossible.

VAGINITIS Inflammation *q.v.* of the vagina *q.v.*, usually resulting from infection *q.v.*

VAGINOPLASTY Surgical creation of a vagina *q.v.*

VAGUS Latin for wandering.

VAGUS NERVE The 10th cranial nerve *q.v.* that serves the larynx, lungs, heart, esophagus, stomach, and most of the abdominal viscera *qq.v.*

VALENCE In expectancy theory of motivation *q.v.*, the perceived attractiveness of an outcome.

VALENCE SHELL The outer ring of an atom *q.v.* that contains those electrons *q.v.* involved in reactions with other atoms.

VALIDATE A procedure in determining whether a test measures the qualities, criteria, predictions, or correlations that it is intended to measure.

VALIDITY 1. The term applied to a test that measures what it is intended to measure. 2. The accuracy and soundness of a person's perceptions. 3. Scientific accuracy. 4. The extent to which experimental results can be attributed to the manipulation of the independent variable *q.v.* cf: construct validity; predictive validity.

VALINE An essential amino acid *q.v.*

VALIUM 1. A commercial preparation of diazepam *q.v.* 2. One of the commercial preparations of minor tranquilizers *q.v.*

VALUE 1. Things, behaviors, or qualities that have worth to persons. 2. A preference shared within a community. 3. An object or idea that a person freely chooses from two or more alternatives.

VALUE ASSUMPTION Any assumption as to the nature of right and wrong or good and bad.

VALUE CONFLICTS Differing or opposing thoughts and actions that a person sometimes finds when he or she reexamines his or her values.

VALUE HIERARCHY Reflective of the ranking, in order of importance, that a group or community places upon its values *q.v.*

VALUE JUDGMENT 1. A statement as to how one ought to behave in a community under particular circumstances. 2. A decision or opinion based on an object or idea that has worth to a person. He or she reaches his or her decision only after studying the information and carefully considering the alternatives.

VALUES 1. One's beliefs about moral, ethical, and social relationships. 2. That which a group feels ought to be desired from which societal norms or standards of behavior are constructed. 3. Standards that guide conduct. cf: value.

VALUES CLARIFICATION 1. The teaching/learning method dealing with techniques that help learners clarify their ethical, moral, and social relationships. 2. The teaching method that encourages decision making based on the recognition of one's values. 3. In drug education, a type of affective *q.v.* education that encourages students to recognize their own values in hopes of discouraging inappropriate drug use. 4. Techniques of humanistic education *q.v.* designed to help students to choose, prize, and act on their beliefs.

VALUES INDICATORS Inferences of values *q.v.* made from the goals, purposes, aspirations, etc., of a community, as opposed to the values themselves.

VALVE A structure that permits flow of fluid in one dirsection only.

VALVULAR PULMONARY STENOSIS A heart defect characterized by the fusing of the leaflets of the valve *q.v.* at the entrance of the pulmonary artery *q.v.* causing a reduction of the flow of blood from the right ventricle *q.v.* to the lungs.

VARIABILITY 1. The tendency of scores in a frequency distribution *q.v.* to scatter away from the central value. 2. Differences among scores. cf: central tendency; standard deviation; variance.

VARIABLE (PL. VARIABLES) 1. A concept defined so that its magnitude can be measured. 2. A dependent variable *q.v.* is that which the researcher is trying to explain. 3. An independent variable *q.v.* is that which has an effect on the dependent variable. It is the cause of change. 4. Factors in a research project that are capable of changing when acted upon by an outside force. 5. Things or conditions that affect other things or conditions. 6. A factor or condition that is systematically varied in an experiment. cf: dependent variable; independent variable.

VARIABLE BEHAVIOR A conscious, calculated reaction resulting from one's experience. ct: invariable behavior; adaptive behavior.

VARIABLE INTERVAL SCHEDULE In conditioning *q.v.*, reinforcement *q.v.* supplied after sporadic or unpredictable intervals of time. ct: variable ratio schedule.

VARIABLE RATIO SCHEDULE In conditioning *q.v.*, reinforcement *q.v.* supplied according to a variable pattern of responses *q.v.* ct: variable interval schedule.

VARIABLE RESISTANCE Resistance that varies in proportion to the force exerted.

VARIANCE (V) 1. A measure of variability *q.v.* of a frequency distribution *q.v.* ~ is computed by finding the difference between each score and the mean *q.v.*, squaring the result, adding all the squared deviations obtained in this manner, and dividing it by the number of cases. 2. The square of the standard deviation *q.v.*

VARIANT Different from the statistical average.

VARIATION In anatomy *q.v.* and physiology *q.v.*, differences between individuals of the same species caused by either environmental or hereditary factors.

VARICELLA Chicken pox *q.v.*

VARICELLA-ZOSTER VIRUS The organism that causes chicken pox and herpes zoster *q.v.*

VARICOCELE 1. A swelling or enlargement of the veins *q.v.* in the spermatic cord *q.v.* 2. A varicose vein *q.v.* in a male's spermatic veins that can cause infertility *q.v.*

VARICOSE 1. Pertaining to unnatural swelling of a vein *q.v.* 2. Varicosis *q.v.* 3. Abnormally swollen or dilated.

VARICOSE VEINS 1. A condition caused by defective valves *q.v.* in the veins *q.v.*, usually in the legs. 2. Varicosis *q.v.* 3. Abnormally lengthened, dilated veins in the legs. 4. ~ develop from heavy pressure of blood against the walls of veins usually after many years. While there are several types of ~, the most common one develops in the calves just under the skin surface. These veins sometimes look prominent but only rarely cause a problem.

VARICOSITY Varicose vein *q.v.*

VARIETY A subdivision of a species *q.v.*

VARIOLA Smallpox *q.v.*

VAS 1. Vessel. 2. Duct *q.v.*

VASA EFFERENTIA The duct *q.v.* through which sperm *q.v.* produced in the seminiferous tubules *q.v.* travel to the epididymis *q.v.*

VASA VASORIUM The small nutrient arteries in the walls of the larger blood vessels.

VASCULAR Pertaining to blood vessels.

VASCULAR SYSTEM The tubular blood-conducting network of the body composed of arteries, veins, and capillaries *qq.v.*

VAS DEFERENS A tube in the male reproductive system *q.v.* that passes from the epididymis *q.v.* into the abdominal cavity *q.v.*: the seminal vesicles *q.v.* cf: vasa efferentia.

VASECTOMY 1. Sterilization *q.v.* of the male by a surgical procedure that removes a small section of the sperm duct *q.v.* sealing the ends by clipping, tying, or cauterizing with an electrode. 2. A method of contraception *q.v.* in which the vasa efferentia *q.v.* are closed to prevent sperm *q.v.* from being ejaculated *q.v.*

VASIFORM Having the appearance of a vessel.

VASOCONGESTION 1. Swelling, especially of erectile tissues *q.v.* 2. Engorgement of blood vessels, as a primary response to sexual arousal. cf: vasodilation. ct: vasoconstriction.

VASOCONSTRICTION 1. Narrowing of a blood vessel. 2. The constriction of the capillaries *q.v.* brought about by activation of the sympathetic *q.v.* division of the autonomic nervous system *q.v.* in response to excessive cold or stress *q.v.* ct: vasodilation; vasocongestion.

VASOCONSTRICTOR An agent or compound that acts to decrease the caliber of blood vessels. cf: vasoconstriction. ct: vasodilation.

VASODILATION 1. Widening of the blood vessels causing increased volume of flow in those vessels. 2. The dilation *q.v.* of the capillaries *q.v.* brought about by activation of the parasympathetic *q.v.* division of the autonomic nervous system *q.v.* in response to excessive heat. ct: vasoconstriction.

VASOMOTOR Pertaining to the walls of the blood vessels.

VASOSPASM Sudden decrease in the size of a blood vessel.

VAS SCLEROSING Male sterilization *q.v.* wherein the vas deferens *q.v.* is blocked, preventing passage of sperm *q.v.*

VASTUS 1. Wide. 2. Of great size.

VC An acronym for vital capacity.

VD An acronym for venereal diseases *q.v.*

VDRL An acronym for Venereal Disease Research Laboratory *q.v.*

VECTOR 1. An organism that carries disease agents *q.v.*, e.g., the anopheles mosquito is the vector for malaria *q.v.* 2. A biological or physical vehicle that carries an agent to a host *q.v.* 3. An organism that transmits a disease from one host to another.

VECTOR-BORNE DISEASE 1. A class of infectious diseases *q.v.* that are transmitted by an intermediate host, usually an insect. 2. Insect-borne diseases.

VEGAN 1. A strict vegetarian *q.v.* 2. A person who eats no animal products at all.

VEGAN DIET A strict vegetarian *q.v.* diet that excludes all animal products.

VEGETABLE 1. A plant. 2. A herbaceous plant cultivated for its edible parts. 3. A plant used for human nutrition. 4. Any edible part of a plant that is not formed from a matured ovary or its associated parts.

VEGETARIAN 1. A person who eats only foods from plant sources. 2. A person who does not eat foods from animal sources. cf: vegan.

VEGETARIANISM The practice of consuming a diet consisting exclusively of plant foods or plant products.

VEGETATIVE In psychology *q.v.*, withdrawn or deteriorated to the point where the person leads a passive, vegetable-like existence.

VEINS Blood vessels that return oxygen-depleted blood from the body to the heart.

VELLUS HAIR Very fine hair that covers all of the body.

VEL NON In law, or not.

VENA CAVA 1. The principle vein *q.v.* returning blood to the right atrium *q.v.* 2. Superior and inferior ~.

VENA COMITARIS A deep vein *q.v.* following the same course as its corresponding artery *q.v.*

VENEREAL Pertaining to sexual intercourse *q.v.*

VENEREAL DISEASE (VD) Diseases that are chiefly transmitted through intimate sexual contact. Also called sexually transmitted diseases *q.v.* or sexually transmitted infections.

VENEREAL DISEASE RESEARCH LABORATORY Engaged in tests to measure syphilis *q.v.* antibodies or reagin. Conducts tests to detect syphilis infection.

VENEREAL WARTS 1. Benign tumors *q.v.* that may result from a viral infection *q.v.* Growth is encouraged in moist parts of the body. Infection can spread on oneself or be transmitted to others. 2. Condylomata acuminatum *q.v.* 3. Viral warts of the genital *q.v.* and anogenital *q.v.* areas.

VENIPUNCTURE The puncture of a vein *q.v.*

VENOM A poisonous fluid secreted by some snakes, spiders, or scorpions.

VENOUS Pertaining to a vein *q.v.* or to the veins.

VENOUS BLOOD Unoxygenated blood transmitted from the body in veins *q.v.* and carried back to the heart.

VENOUS STASIS The pooling of blood in enlarged veins *q.v.*

VENTILATION 1. In physiology *q.v.*, the movement of air into and out of the lungs, measured in liters per minute (lpm). 2. In ecology *q.v.*, air movement intended to dissipate or replace foul air. 3. In psychology *q.v.*, airing of grievances and other emotionally significant feelings through the verbal medium of expression.

VENTRAL 1. Pertaining to the belly. 2. Describing a position toward the belly. 3. Anterior *q.v.* 4. Front. ct: dorsal; posterior.

VENTRICLE 1. A small cavity. 2. One of the lower chambers of the heart. 3. The chambers of the heart that pump blood to the lungs (right ventricle) and throughout the body (left ventricle).

VENTRICULAR FIBRILLATION An arrhythmia *q.v.* in which the walls of the ventricle *q.v.* of the heart quiver rather than beat regularly. This causes an interruption of the flow of blood and lack of oxygen to the brain, possibly resulting in death.

VENTROMEDIAL REGION OF THE HYPOTHALAMUS An area in the hypothalamus *q.v.* that is said to be a satiety center as in an antagonistic *q.v.* relation to a hunger center (the lateral hypothalamus).

VENTURI MASK A breathing unit designed to provide a specific concentration of oxygen through a delivery tube connected to a standard face mask.

VENULES 1. The small veins *q.v.* 2. Any of the small vessels that collect blood from the capillary *q.v.* plexi and join to form veins.

VERBAL COMMUNICATION The sharing of ideas through speech.

VERBAL CONDITIONING The instrumental modification of verbal responses *q.v.* by making reward contingent upon the utterance of particular verbalizations.

VERBAL TEST A test that requires the use of language. ct: performance test; written test.

VERBIGERATION Prolonged and monotonous repetition of meaningless words and phrases.

VERICOSIS 1. A condition characterized by a swelling of a vein *q.v.* 2. Varicose *q.v.* veins.

VERIFIABILITY An essential property of statements in science *q.v.* Statements are verifiable when they can be subject to empirical test.

VERMIFORM Worm-shaped.

VERMIFORM APPENDIX A vestigial organ *q.v.* located at the beginning of the large intestine *q.v.*

VERNIX CASEOSA 1. The cheese-like protective substance covering the skin of the fetus *q.v.* 2. A whitish, pasty substance made up of shed fetal *q.v.* cells that protects the skin of the fetus in the uterine *q.v.* environment.

VERONAL A commercial preparation of one of the barbiturates *q.v.*

VERRUCA A wart.

VERTEBRA 1. A spinal bone. 2. Any of the 34 bones of the spinal column *q.v.* that consists of the 7 cervical; coccygeal, comprising 3–5 rudimentary vertebrae that form the coccyx *q.v.*; the 5 vertebrae of the lumbar *q.v.* region; 5 fused vertebrae of the sacral *q.v.* region; and 12 thoracic *q.v.* vertebrae.

VERTEBRAL ARCH 1. A posterior projection from a vertebra *q.v.* 2. Neural *q.v.* arch.

VERTEBRAL BODY The round, solid bone forming the front part of each vertebra *q.v.*

VERTEBRAL SPINE 1. The posterior *q.v.* projection of each vertebra *q.v.* 2. Spinous process.

VERTEBRATE An animal having a vertebral column or backbone.

VERTEX PRESENTATION In childbirth, when the crown of the head is seen first at the opening of the vagina *q.v.*

VERTICAL CURRICULUM FORMAT The most conventional curricular organization or arrangement. Basically, it is composed of topic, objectives, content outline, activities, and resources. cf: horizontal curriculum format.

VERTICAL DECALAGE Across different periods of intellectual growth, successive rediscovery of the same principle at each new stage of thinking. cf: horizontal decalage.

VERTICAL ENRICHMENT The teacher instructs learners who complete assignments faster than classmates to do more difficult or advanced assignments. ct: horizontal enrichment.

VERTIGO 1. A hallucination *q.v.* or sensation that one's environment is revolving around him or her or that the person is revolving around the environment. 2. Dizziness.

VERUMONTANUM A small mound in men in the portion of the urethra *q.v.* passing through the prostate *q.v.*, which contains openings of the ejaculatory ducts *q.v.*

VERY LOW SODIUM On food labels, 35 mg or less per serving. cf: low sodium.

VESICLE 1. A small watery lesion *q.v.* produced by the skin. 2. Swollen end of a sporangiophore or conidiophores. 3. A papule *q.v.* 4. Fluid-filled blister-like eruptions on the skin or mucous membranes *q.v.*

VESPRIN 1. A commercial preparation of phenothiazine *q.v.* 2. A major tranquilizer *q.v.*, triflupromazine *q.v.*

VESSEL 1. In anatomy *q.v.*, a tubelike structure that carries blood to the heart, from the capillaries *q.v.* 2. In botany *q.v.*, a tubelike structure of the xylem *q.v.*

VESSEL ELEMENT One of the cells composing a vessel *q.v.*

VESTED Fixed, accrued, not subject to any contingency.

VESTED RIGHT A right completely defined and settled that cannot be cancelled or impaired.

VESTIBULAR BULBS Muscles *q.v.* located beneath the bulbocavernosus *q.v.* muscles on both sides of the vaginal *q.v.* opening.

VESTIBULAR MECHANISM A structure of the inner ear *q.v.* containing three semicircular canals filled with fluid. The ~ assists the person in maintaining equilibrium.

VESTIBULAR SENSES A set of receptors *q.v.* that provide information about the orientation and movements of the head, located in the semicircular canals *q.v.* and the vestibular sacs *q.v.* of the inner ear *q.v.*

VESTIBULE 1. A long, narrow depression of the vulva *q.v.* that contains the urethral *q.v.* and vaginal *q.v.* openings. 2. The area surrounding the vaginal and urethral opening.

VESTIGIAL A small or imperfectly developed bodily part or organ that remains from one more fully developed in an earlier stage of the person, or in a past generation, or in closely related forms.

VESTIGIAL ORGAN An organ no longer serving a useful purpose in the body.

VESTIGIAL REFLEXES Reflexes *q.v.* present at birth but which disappear after the first few months of life.

VHF 1. An acronym for very high frequency. 2. Radio frequencies between 30 and 300 megahertz (MHz).

VIABILITY The degree of capability to live and develop normally.

VIABLE In embryology *q.v.*, a fetus *q.v.* capable of living outside of the mother.

VIBRATOR A device that produces pleasurable sensations when placed on or near the genital *q.v.* region. Sometimes used as a sex aid. cf: dildo.

VICARIOUS CONDITIONING 1. Learning *q.v.* through observation. 2. Observing the reactions of others to particular stimuli *q.v.*

VICARIOUS FUNCTIONING When, following the destruction of a brain area that normally subserves some function, that function is first lost and then reappears, the assumption is that some other area of the brain has vicariously taken over control of that function.

VICARIOUS LIVING An attempt to evade efforts toward self-fulfillment by repressing one's own individuality and identifying with some hero or ideal.

VICARIOUSLY FORMED STIMULI Erotic stimuli that originate in a person's imagination.

VICARIOUS MENSTRUATION A phenomenon of extragenital bleeding occurring during the menstrual flow *q.v.* in which bleeding may take place from the nose or other body structure. cf: menstruation.

VICARIOUS REINFORCEMENT Seeing someone else rewarded or punished for a behavior resulting in a tendency to behave accordingly.

VICIOUS CIRCLE In psychology *q.v.*, a sort of chain reaction in which the person reacts to an unhealthful defensive reaction in trying to solve his or her problems, which only serves to complicate the problem and make it more difficult to solve.

VICTIM-PRECIPITATED HOMICIDES Instances in which the actions of an individual contribute to his or her death, e.g., engaging in high-risk behavior, and provoking aggressive behavior in others.

VICTORIAN ERA The period during which Queen Victoria was the monarch of England (1837–1901).

VILLI Small, fingerlike projections that line the small intestine *q.v.* ~ function in the absorption of nutrients into the bloodstream.

VILLUS A hairlike projection.

VINCENT'S DISEASE 1. Trench mouth. 2. Necrotizing ulcerative gingivitis *q.v.* 3. An acute *q.v.* or chronic *q.v.* infection of the gingivae *q.v.* Characterized by redness, swelling, pain, and ulceration of the gums. It may involve other tissues of the mouth and throat. ~ is not contagious. ~ is caused by the bacterium *Borrelia vincentii q.v.*

VINELAND ADAPTIVE BEHAVIOR SCALE 1. An instrument designed to measure the levels and quantities of age-appropriate, socially adaptive behaviors in children. 2. Vineland Scale of Social Maturity *q.v.*

VINELAND SCALE OF SOCIAL MATURITY 1. A scale measuring the child's level of appropriate, socially adaptive behavior. 2. Vineland Adaptive Behavior Scale *q.v.*

VIRAL HEPATITIS Hepatitis A *q.v.*

VIRAL INCLUSION Aggregations of viral *q.v.* material within a cell.

VIRAL SHEDDING Discharge of viral *q.v.* particles from a skin lesion *q.v.*

VIRGIN Someone who has never engaged in sexual intercourse *q.v.*

VIRGIN BIRTH Parthenogenesis *q.v.*

VIRGINITY The physical state of a girl or woman before first sexual intercourse *q.v.* or coitus *q.v.*

VIRICIDE An agent that destroys a virus *q.v.*

VIRILISM Accentuation of masculine *q.v.* secondary sex characteristics *q.v.*, esp. in women or boys, caused by overactivity of the adrenal cortex *q.v.*

VIRION A single virus *q.v.* particle or unit.

VIROLOGY The science that deals with the study of viruses *q.v.*

VIRTUAL 1. In anatomy *q.v.*, appearing to be present but not really so. 2. Potential, but not actual.

VIRTUAL IMAGE An image of the object seen by the eye that appears to originate at the surface of the object but is formed as a visual extension of the light waves from below the object.

VIRULENCE The ability of an organism to sicken or kill its host *q.v.*

VIRULENT PHAGE A phage (virus *q.v.*) that destroys the host (bacterial *q.v.*) cell. cf: temperate phage.

VIRUS 1. A chemical substance that has characteristics of a living organism. 2. An agent of disease. 3. An ultramicroscopic agent *q.v.* that is characterized by a lack of metabolism *q.v.* and that proliferates only in living healthy host *q.v.* cells. 4. An ultramicroscopic particle consisting of a core of DNA *q.v.* or RNA *q.v.* contained within a protein *q.v.* coat. All ~es are intracellular parasites *q.v.* 5. An infectious nucleoprotein *q.v.* considered to be subliving. They multiply only within living, infected host cells.

VISCERA The internal organs of the body.

VISCERAL 1. Refers to the internal organs, such as stomach, intestines, etc. 2. The large internal organs of the body that appear in any of the three great body cavities, esp. in the abdominal cavity *q.v.*

VISCERAL PLEURA The portion of the pleura *q.v.* covering the lungs.

VISCERATONIA 1. An endomorphic *q.v.* body type. 2. Love of food and comfort, sociable and in need of affsection. 3. The personality *q.v.* type associated with gluttonous, comfort-loving, and extroverted behavior. ct: cerebrotonia; somatatonia; somatotype.

VISCEROPTOSIS Abdominal paunch.

VISCEROTONIC The temperament originally assumed to be associated with an endomorphic *q.v.* body type.

VISCOSITY The state of being sticky.

VISCUS An organ of the body.

VISUAL ACUITY The sharpness or clearness of vision.

VISUAL CLIFF 1. A device for assessing depth perception *q.v.* in young organisms. ~ consists of a glass surface that extends over an apparently deep side and an apparently shallow side. 2. A device used to indicate whether infants can interpret visual cues that signal a drop-off.

VISUAL DISCRIMINATION The act of distinguishing one visual stimulus from another.

VISUAL DISORDER A dysfunction of the eyes, optic nerve *q.v.*, or perceptual center of the brain.

VISUAL PERCEPTION AREA An area in the temporal lobe *q.v.* of the cerebral cortex *q.v.* where visual stimuli are interpreted.

VISUAL PURPLE A pigment formed in the retina *q.v.* of the eye by the action of light on rhodopsin *q.v.*

VISUAL SCREENING A health screening *q.v.* procedure to detect the presence of visual problems.

VITAL BALANCE According to Menninger, the principle of homeostasis *q.v.* as applied to mental health *q.v.*

VITALISM The doctrine that the functions of a living organism are due to a vital principal force distinct from physical forces.

VITAL MARRIAGE A marriage *q.v.* in which the needs and goals of the individual, as well as the needs of the marital union, are given priority. ct: total marriage.

VITAL SIGNS 1. Indicators of life: heart and pulse rate, respiration, blood pressure, pupil reflex (and other reflexes), brain activity, and body temperature. 2. The observable physical signs by which the physical state of a person can be determined.

VITAL STATISTICS 1. Records of life and death. 2. Records of births, diseases, deaths, and other human activities.

VITAMIN A A vitamin *q.v.* essential for (a) preventing night blindness, (b) promoting growth in children, (c) maintaining normal mucous secretions of the mucous membranes *q.v.*, (d) healthy skin, and (e) adequate tear secretions of the eyes. Rich food sources are leafy green vegetables and yellow vegetables, dairy products, eggs, and meats. Excessive amounts of ~ can result in serious health problems called hypervitaminosis *q.v.* ~ is a fat-soluble vitamin *q.v.*

VITAMIN B A complex of vitamins *q.v.* with similarities. The B vitamins are thiamin, riboflavin, niacin, B_6, pantothenic acid, biotin, folacin, and cobalamin *qq.v.* They are water soluble *q.v.*

VITAMIN B_6 A water-soluble vitamin *q.v.* consisting of three chemical compounds: pyridoxine, pyridoxal, and pyridoxamine *qq.v.* Pyridoxine was synthesized in 1939 and is particularly important for protein *q.v.* metabolism *q.v.* Severe deficiency, although rare, results in convulsions, loss of weight, irritability, depression, and anemia. Women who use oral contraceptives *q.v.* may need to increase their intake of ~ as the metabolism of the essential amino acid *q.v.* tryptophan is impaired.

VITAMIN B_{12} Cobalamin *q.v.*

VITAMIN B_{17} Proponents of Laetrile *q.v.* claim that it is a vitamin rather than a drug. Nutritionists are unable to identify any vitamin known as B-17. Probably a hoax.

VITAMIN C Ascorbic acid *q.v.*

VITAMIN D 1. A vitamin occurring in the body as ~ or provitamin. Provitamin D is a form of cholesterol occurring in animals and ergosterol in plants and is changed to vitamin D upon exposure to ultraviolet light *q.v.* 2. Also know as the sunshine vitamin. 3. The function of ~ is for efficient use of calcium and phosphorus. ~ is a fat-soluble vitamin *q.v.* whose absorption is facilitated through the intestinal membrane *q.v.* A severe deficiency of ~ results in improper development of bones and teeth and the development of rickets *q.v.* ~ was discovered in 1932.

VITAMIN-DEPENDENCY ILLNESS A disease characterized by the need for higher than normal amounts of a particular vitamin *q.v.*

VITAMIN E A vitamin that is easily supplied by eating a relatively normal diet. It is found in such foods as vegetable oils, many vegetables, grain products, meats, fish, poultry, eggs, fruits, and nuts. ~ is a fat-soluble vitamin.

VITAMIN K A fat-soluble vitamin *q.v.* Its chief function is to aid in the coagulation of blood by promoting the formation of prothrombin. A deficiency of ~ results in hemorrhaging *q.v.*, especially in infants born prematurely. Excessive amounts may result in the break down of red blood cells in infants.

VITAMIN P Bioflavonoids *q.v.*

VITAMINS Organic *q.v.* compounds essential in very small amounts for promoting growth and maintaining life. They are abundant in the foods available to people. ~ act as catalysts *q.v.* as they interact with each other and with other nutrients *q.v.* They are categorized according to their solubility in water or fats (Table V-1).

VITAMIN SUPPLEMENTS Synthetic preparations of vitamins *q.v.* to be ingested in addition to the quantities obtained in the normal daily diet.

VITELLINE MEMBRANE The membrane *q.v.* forming the surface layer of the egg.

VITILIGO An abnormality of the skin characterized by a loss of pigment, producing white patches surrounded by pigmented borders. cf: leukoderma.

VITREOUS HUMOR 1. A jellylike fluid in the after chamber of the eye. 2. A viscous *q.v.* substance contained within the globe of the eye giving support to its form.

VIVACTIL A commercial preparation of protriptyline *q.v.*

VIVIPAROUS Bringing forth living young.

VO_2 1. Volume of oxygen. 2. Oxygen consumption.

VOCAL CORDS A fold of mucous membrane *q.v.* in the larynx *q.v.* forming the inferior *q.v.* boundary of the ventricle *q.v.* of the larynx. ~ are activated by air passing over them, and their vibrations produce sound which is the voice.

VOCATIONAL EDUCATION Educational programs designed to prepare persons for a career.

VOCATIONAL REHABILITATION Training handicapped individuals to enable them to perform meaningful work.

VOCATIONAL THERAPY A form of treatment for training a person (often handicapped or emotionally disturbed) in some skills that may make it possible to obtain a job.

VOCATIONAL TRAINING The learning of a skill or trade necessary to a certain career *q.v.*

VOCS An acronym for volatile organic compounds *q.v.*

VOICE BOX The larynx *q.v.*

VOICE DISORDER Abnormal acoustic qualities in a person's speech, characterized by differences in pitch, loudness, or quality in comparison with others of the same age and gender.

VOID 1. In law, having no effect. 2. Having no legal force or binding effect.

VOLAR 1. Pertaining to the palm of the hand or the sole of the foot. 2. Palmar. 3. Plantar.

VOLATILE A liquid that changes rapidly and easily into a vapor, as in the case of the evaporation of gasoline, alcohol, or ether.

VOLATILE CHEMICAL An easily vaporized substance capable of dissolving another substance. ~s produce a state of intoxication *q.v.* when inhaled.

VOLATILE ORGANIC COMPOUNDS Substances containing carbon, hydrogen, and oxygen that easily become vapors or gases.

TABLE V-1 TABLE OF VITAMINS

WATER SOLUBLE	DIETARY SOURCES	PHYSIOLOGY
Thiamin (B_1)	Breads and cereals, veal, beef, lamb, chicken breast, calf's liver, eggs, nuts, beans, potatoes, milk, green vegetables	1. Generates energy by reacting with carbohydrates, fats, and amino acids. 2. Metabolism of nucleic acids. 3. Aids in converting tryptophan to niacin. 4. Plays a role in nerve functioning. RDA: 1.0–1.5 mg
Riboflavin (B_2)	Dairy products, beef, veal, pork, lamb, chicken breast, calf's liver, fish, eggs, nuts, beans, breads and cereals, green and yellow vegetables	1. Releasing of energy from carbohydrates, fats, and proteins. 2. Plays a role in the synthesis of corticosteroids and the production of red blood cells. RDA: 1.2–1.7 mg
Niacin	Beef, pork, veal, lamb, chicken breast, turkey, calf's liver, fish, eggs, beans, nuts, breads and cereals, green vegetables, potatoes	1. Releasing energy and oxidation of glucose, amino acids, and fats. 2. Synthesis of fatty acids and cholesterol. RDA: 13–19 mg
Biotin	Egg yolk, milk, organ meats, cereals, legumes, nuts	1. Fatty acid synthesis and cholesterol. 2. Protein and carbohydrate metabolism. 3. Antibody formation. 4. Synthesis of pancreatic amylase. RDA: Probably 100–200 μg
Pantothenic acid (B_3)	Organ meats, grains, eggs, yeast	Fatty acid synthesis. RDA: 4–7 mg
Folacin	Green vegetables, liver, fish, poultry, meats, legumes	1. Metabolism of certain amino acids. 2. Synthesis of the nucleotide bases of nucleic acids. 3. Formation of thymine necessary for red blood cells. RDA: 400 μg
Cobalamin (B_{12})	Liver, sea foods, meats, eggs, milk	1. A coenzyme of all cell activities. 2. Formation of thymine necessary for red blood cells. 3. Nervous system functioning. 4. Carbohydrate metabolism. 5. Formation and maintenance of myelin. 6. Metabolism of some fatty acids. RDA: 3 μg
Pyridoxine (B_6)	Meats, bananas, grains, lima beans, cabbage, potatoes, spinach, milk, avocadoes	1. Coenzyme in the synthesis and breakdown of amino acids. 2. Formation of hemoglobin. 3. Plays a role in converting tryptophan to niacin. RDA: 1.8–2.2 mg
Ascorbic acid (C)	Citrus fruits, broccoli, strawberries, cabbage, tomatoes, potatoes	1. Formation of collagen. 2. Necessary for healing wounds and burns. 3. Enhances the absorption of iron.
FAT SOLUBLE	DIETARY SOURCES	PHYSIOLOGY
Retinol (alcohol), Retinal (aldehyde), and Retinoic acid (Vitamin A)	Liver, egg yolk, dairy products, sweet potatoes, winter squash, green vegetables, carrots, broccoli, cantelope, apricots	1. Carotenes serve as the precursors of vitamin A. 2. Important in the maintenance of vision, esp. night vision. 3. Maintenance of epithelial tissues and synthesis of mucus. 4. Normal growth and development of bones and teeth. RDA[a]: 800–1000 RE[b] (4000–5000 IU)
Vitamin D	Fortified milk, eggs, cheese, butter, fish, ultraviolet rays of the sun converts plant egosterol to ergocalciferol (vitamin D_2) in the human body	1. Increases the absorption of calcium and phosphorus. 2. Aids in bone formation. 3. Aids in the synthesis of calcium-binding protein. 4. Enhances mineralization in bones. 5. Stimulates the release of calcium and phosphorus from bone to blood. RDA: 5.0–7.5 μg
Tocopherol (vitamin E)	Vegetable oils, green vegetables, wheat germ, yellow corn	1. Aids in the synthesis of heme. 2. Prevents the oxidation of polyunsaturated fats, vitamin A, and some enzymes. 3. Increases the stability of cellular and intracellular membranes. 4. May slow cell aging processes. RDA: 8–10 mg
Vitamin K	Green vegetables, liver, eggs, dairy products	Essential for blood clotting. RDA: 70–140 μg

[a] RDA, recommended daily allowance.

[b] Retinol equivalent (1 IU = 0.3 μg of retinol).

VOLATILE PHENOLS Chemicals found in tobacco smoke and may contribute to a variety of diseases associated with cigarette smoking.

VOLUME RECEPTORS Receptors *q.v.* that help to control water intake by responding to the total volume of fluids in the body. cf: osmoreceptors.

VOLUMINOUS Having a great volume or bulk.

VOLUNTARY 1. Pertaining to or acting in obedience to the will. 2. To consciously act.

VOLUNTARY HEALTH AGENCY 1. An organization concerned with some aspect of health and is supported by donations and endowments and is operated by unpaid volunteers and paid professional people. 2. Any nonprofit association organized on a national, state, or local level composed of lay and professional persons who are dedicated to the prevention, alleviation, and cure of a particular health condition or conditions. cf: nongovernmental organization. ct: governmental health agency.

VOLUNTARY HOSPITAL A public facility (hospital) owned and operated on a nonprofit basis.

VOLUNTARY MEDICAL CARE PLAN A plan in which the person voluntarily subscribes for partial or total medical and hospital expenses. Usually, these plans are based on a prepayment schedule whereby a person pays a certain amount each month, whether he or she is well or ill.

VOLUNTARY MUSCLES 1. Made up of striated *q.v.* muscle cells. 2. Those nearly 300 muscles of the body that are controlled more or less by one's volition. They are also called skeletal muscles *q.v.* 3. The muscles of movement of the body parts: arms, legs, fingers, etc.

VOLUNTARY ORGANIZATION See voluntary health organization.

VOLUNTARY RESIDENT-TRACKING SYSTEM (VRTS) An organization composed of residents within a given area whose purpose it is to identify the present and past residents who have been exposed to air contaminants emanating from a landfill.

VOLVULUS A twisting of the intestine *q.v.* causing obstruction.

VOMER 1. Plowshare. 2. The plow-shaped bone that forms the lower and posterior *q.v.* portion of the nasal septum *q.v.*

VOMITUS Vomited matter.

VOODOO DEATH The demise of a person in a primitive culture who violates tribal laws or who is cursed by a witch doctor.

VOUCHER In education, a means of financing schools whereby funds are provided to parents who then purchase education for their children in any public or private school.

VOYEURISM 1. A sexual variance *q.v.* characterized by a person gaining sexual pleasure from viewing nudes. 2. A state in which a person becomes sexually excited and derives sexual pleasure from watching others who are naked, undressing, or engaging in sexual activity. 3. A peeping Tom. cf: scoptophilia.

VROOM EXPECTANCY MODEL A model of motivation *q.v.* that hypothesizes that the strength of needs *q.v.* and motivation depends upon the degree of desire to perform a behavior.

VRTS An acronym for Voluntary Resident-Tracking System *q.v.*

VULNERABILITY The capability of being hurt or affected in some way.

VULVA 1. The external genital *q.v.* region of the female. 2. That region of the external genital organs of the female that includes the labia *q.v.*, mons pubis *q.v.*, clitoris *q.v.*, and the vestibule *q.v.* of the vagina *q.v.*

VULVAL TISSUES Tissues surrounding the vaginal *q.v.* opening. cf: vulva.

VULVOVAGINITIS Inflammation of the vulva *q.v.* and vagina *q.v.*

V-Z An acronym for varicella-zoster virus *q.v.*

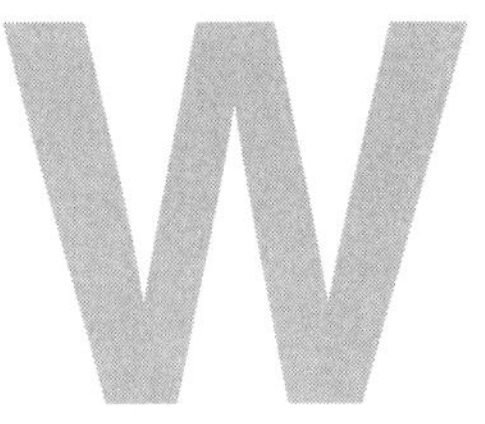

WAIS-R An acronym for Wechsler Adult Intelligence Scale-Revised *q.v.*

WAIVE In law, to renounce or abandon a right.

WAIVER 1. An amendment to a regular insurance policy that exempts from coverage certain disabilities normally covered by such a policy. 2. In law, intentional and voluntary relinquishment of a known right.

WARM-GLOW EFFECT The tendency for a person to behave in an altruistic, magnanimous manner immediately after being made to feel good about himself or herself.

WARM-UP 1. The first phase of any exercise prescription *q.v.* 2. The preparation of the body for vigorous physical activity through stretching, calisthenics, or running in order to raise core body temperature.

WAR NEUROSIS Combat reaction *q.v.*

WARNING LIGHTS Flashing lights that serve as a signal of some sort of emergency or hazard.

WARNING SIGNAL An intermittent audible sound of varying tone made by a siren or other device to alert others to the emergency vehicle so that the way may be cleared.

WARNING SIGNS OF CANCER The American Cancer Society *q.v.* for many years has promoted the educational concept that each person should be aware of the early signs of cancers and to take immediate action should one or more appear. These warning signs are as follows: 1. change in bowel or bladder habits; 2. a sore that does not heal; 3. unusual bleeding or discharge from any body opening; 4. thickening or lump in the breast or elsewhere on the body; 5. indigestion or difficulty in swallowing; 6. obvious change in a wart or mole—color, size, etc.; 7. nagging cough or hoarseness.

WART 1. A cauliflower-like overgrowth of epidermal cells. 2. A virus-induced skin lesion *q.v.* resulting in local overgrowth of cells.

WASSERMANN TEST A blood test used to determine whether or not a person has syphilis *q.v.*

WATER Chemical formula is H_2O. The human body is mostly ∼, and it is necessary for all the chemical reactions that take place within the body. When ∼ balance is not maintained, one of two reactions may occur: 1. edema *q.v.* or 2. dehydration *q.v.*

WATER-ABSORBING POWER OF THE CELL The ability of the cell to absorb water because the diffusion *q.v.* pressure of water within the cell is lower than the diffusion pressure of pure water.

WATER CYCLE The constant circulation of water between the atmosphere, the earth's surface, and the water table.

WATER INTOXICATION A potentially fatal condition caused by an intake of fluid that exceeds the maximum rate of urinary flow.

WATER POLLUTION Pollution *q.v.* of lakes, oceans, rivers, and streams from open dumps, improperly disposed of industrial wastes, contaminated rain, temperature, sewage disposal plants, and surface water drainage.

WATER-SOLUBLE VITAMINS The groups of vitamins *q.v.* identified as C and B complex and are soluble in water. ct: fat-soluble vitamins.

WAX A lipid *q.v.* with a high melting point, composed of esters *q.v.* of fatty acids *q.v.* with an alcohol *q.v.* or other glycerol *q.v.*

WAXY FLEXIBILITY A characteristic of a catatonic *q.v.* state in which a patient's limbs can be moved into a variety of positions where they are maintained for unusually long periods of time.

WBC 1. An acronym for white blood cells. 2. White blood count.

WEAPONS EFFECT A state in which the mere presence of weapons increases the likelihood of violent or aggressive behavior.

WEBER'S LAW The observation that the size of the difference threshold *q.v.* is proportional to the intensity of the standard stimulus *q.v.*

WEB OF CAUSATION An illustration or map of those hypothesized relationships that are believed to exist between a health problem and the environmental, host, or agent factors that have caused the health problem to appear.

WECHSLER ADULT INTELLIGENCE SCALE-REVISED (WAIS-R) 1. A revised version of the original

Wechsler–Bellevue Intelligence Scale, which is a standardized test *q.v.* for measuring adult intelligence *q.v.* 2. A test that yields a verbal score, a performance score, and a full-scale IQ *q.v.* with a mean *q.v.* of 100 and a standard deviation *q.v.* of 15.

WECHSLER INTELLIGENCE SCALE FOR CHILDREN-REVISED (WISC-R) 1. A standardized test *q.v.* of intelligence appropriate for children from 6 to 17 years. 2. An intelligence test for children that provides separate subtest scores in individual areas, as well as overall verbal and performance scores and an intelligence quotient *q.v.*

WECHSLER PRESCHOOL–PRIMARY SCALE OF INTELLIGENCE (WPPSI) 1. A standardized test of intelligence *q.v.* of children from 4 to 6.5 years. 2. An intelligence test for preschool- and primary school-aged children, yielding scores for individual areas as well as overall verbal and performance scores and an IQ *q.v.* score.

WEIGHT CONTROL The process of controlling one's weight through proper nutrition *q.v.* and exercise.

WEIGHTED AVERAGE In epidemiology *q.v.*, the providing of different weights to each component of the average. ct: unweighted average.

WEIGHTED PUPIL METHOD A method of state funding of education based on the needs of the types of students in a district.

WEIGHTED VEST A specially designed garment that contains compartments to hold varying amounts of weight.

WEIGHTLESSNESS The absence of downward pressure that is normally caused by the pull of gravity. In space, the gravitational pull of the earth is counterbalanced by the centrifugal force imparted to the spaceship by its initial rocket blast.

WEIL'S DISEASE Leptospirosis *q.v.*; spread by the urine *q.v.* of rats.

WELL-BEING CENTER 1. A basic unit of the health care delivery system *q.v.* organized to provide people with learning opportunities with respect to their health. 2. A place where people learn about health behaviors and issues that result in the ill health of populations and organize themselves to solve health problems.

WELLNESS An abstract concept that relates to the development of health-related behaviors *q.v.* involving exercise, nutrition, meditation, stress control *qq.v.*, etc.

WELLNESS BEHAVIOR Daily activities that tend toward the prevention of ill health and the promotion of optimal health *q.v.* cf: health-related behavior; health-directed behavior.

WELLNESS CENTERS Units within hospitals or clinics that provide a wide range of rehabilitation, disease prevention, and health enhancement programs.

WEN 1. A lump on the body. 2. A subcutaneous *q.v.* cyst *q.v.*

WERNICKE'S AREA 1. The superior temporal convolution *q.v.* 2. Wernicke's center, the auditory language center, located in the posterior part of the superior temporal convolution. cf: aphasia. ct: Broca's area.

WERNICKE'S DISEASE 1. Wernicke's syndrome *q.v.* 2. A chronic brain disorder caused by a severe deficiency of B-complex vitamins *q.v.*, characterized by unsteady gait, partial paralysis *q.v.* of the eye muscles, confusion, and drowsiness. Lesions *q.v.* are also presented in the pons, cerebellum, and mammillary bodies *qq.v.*

WERNICKE'S SYNDROME 1. Characterized by eye muscles paralysis, clouding of consciousness, poor coordination, and a sense of indifference. It is associated with abnormal metabolic *q.v.* action in cells, chronic alcohol use, and a severe deficiency of thiamin *q.v.* ~ was first described by Carl Wernicke in 1881. 2. Wernicke's disease *q.v.*

WET DREAM 1. Slang for nocturnal emission *q.v.* 2. Ejaculation *q.v.* of seminal fluid *q.v.* during sleep, beginning in adolescence, as androgen *q.v.* levels increase.

WET SUIT A close fitting body covering made of rubber, used by underwater divers or people exposed for extended periods to cold water.

WHEAL A swelling on the skin produced by a sting, an injection, an external force, or an internal reaction.

WHEEZING Breathing with difficulty and noisily.

WHITE CORPUSCLES 1. Disease-fighting bodies in the blood. 2. Leukocytes *q.v.*

WHITE MATTER The neural tissue *q.v.*, esp. of the brain and spinal cord, consisting of nerve fibers.

WHITE NOISE Noise composed of sounds of all frequencies.

WHITLOW Felon *q.v.*

WHOLE-GRAIN FLOUR 1. Flour made from grain that has undergone only minimal processing. 2. Flour containing essentially all of its original nutrients *q.v.*

WHOLE LIFE POLICY A life insurance policy that has a fixed premium that accumulates a cash value over a period of time and is in force for the life of the insured as long as premiums are paid.

WHOOPING COUGH 1. Pertussis *q.v.* 2. A disease caused by a bacillus *q.v.*

WHORE–MADONNA COMPLEX A conflict in which a person perceives women as either pure or sluttish but cannot believe that a decent woman would have sexual urges.

WILD TYPE 1. In genetics *q.v.*, the customary or usual phenotype *q.v.* used as a standard for comparison. 2. The best adapted phenotype in a given environment.

WILL A legal document that describes how a person wishes his or her estate to be disposed of following death.

WIND-CHILL FACTOR A factor taking into account the relationship of wind velocity to thermometer temperature of the air in determining the effect on living organisms.

WINDPIPE The trachea *q.v.*

WINE An alcoholic beverage containing 10% to 14% alcohol by volume that is made from fermenting *q.v.* the juice of grapes or other fruits.

WINE COOLER A beverage made from mixing wine with a fruit-based soft drink.

WISC-R An acronym for Wechsler Intelligence Scale for Children-Revised *q.v.*

WISH FULFILLMENT IN DREAMS The latent dream *q.v.* that represents the person's hidden desires. cf: Freud's theory of dreams.

WITHDRAWAL 1. Withdrawal syndrome *q.v.* 2. The phenomenon that occurs when a person who is physically dependent *q.v.* on a drug stops taking the drug. Symptoms include nausea, dizziness, chills, runny nose, and itching. 3. Abstinence syndrome. 4. In psychology *q.v.*, intellectual, emotional, or physical retreat. 5. Coitus interruptus *q.v.*

WITHDRAWAL EFFECTS Opponent-process theory of motivation *q.v.*

WITHDRAWAL SYMPTOMS 1. Abstinence syndrome consisting of physical functioning and behavior observed after a person is denied a drug. Symptoms may include nausea, insomnia, tremors vomiting, cramps, elevated blood pressure, anxiety, convulsions, and depression. 2. A negative physical and psychological response when a dependent person suddenly stops taking a drug. 3. The physical and psychological response resulting from the sudden and prolonged abstinence from a drug. cf: substance dependence; withdrawal syndrome.

WITHDRAWAL SYNDROME The combination of physical and psychological symptoms *q.v.* that appear when an addicting drug *q.v.* is denied. cf: withdrawal symptoms.

WITHIN-GROUP HERITABILITY The extent to which variation within groups is attributable to genetic *q.v.* factors. cf: between-group heritability; heritability.

WITHITNESS An attribute of good classroom managers characterized by alertness to what happens throughout the classroom, helping to prevent disciplinary incidents. cf: classroom management.

WITHOUT PREJUDICE In law, no rights or privileges will be considered waived or lost.

WOLFFIAN DUCTS 1. The primitive genital ducts *q.v.* that, under hormonal *q.v.* influence, evolve into male genitalia *q.v.* 2. Ducts that are present in the human embryo *q.v.* during the 7th through 12th week of prenatal development. 3. The initial embryonic structures from which the internal male genitalia develops. cf: Mullerian ducts.

WOMAN YEAR A means of measuring the effectiveness of contraceptives *q.v.* in which women use one means of contraception exclusively for a period of 1 year. The number of pregnancies that occur during that year determine the rate per ~.

WOMB The uterus *q.v.*

WOOLY MAMMOTH In psychoanalytic theory *q.v.*, a metaphor to describe conflicts housed in the unconscious *q.v.* making them inaccessible to examination.

WORD ASSOCIATION TEST A test sometimes used for personality *q.v.* diagnosis in which a person gives the first word that comes to mind in response *q.v.* to a series of stimulus *q.v.* words.

WORD HASH 1. Jumbles or incoherent use of words by a psychotic *q.v.* or disoriented person. 2. Word salad *q.v.*

WORD SALAD 1. Word hash *q.v.* 2. The incoherent use of language by some psychotic *q.v.* or disoriented people, rendering effective communication with them impossible.

WORKAHOLIC A misnomer. An erroneously coined term to take the place of the acceptable term, ergomania *q.v.* Based on a misrepresentation and misconception about alcohol *q.v.*

WORK HYPERTROPHY The concept that our body becomes increasingly capable of sustained exercise as a result of training.

WORKING MEMORY 1. Short-term memory *q.v.* 2. Memory that emphasizes that the information in short-term memory is not just being stored, it is being processed.

WORKING THROUGH 1. Confronting and dealing with a problem situation until satisfactory adjustments are achieved and firmly established. 2. A growth influence in the direction of maturity *q.v.* 3. In psychoanalysis *q.v.*, an arduous, time-consuming process through which the patient confronts conflicts repeatedly until the problems are adequately resolved.

WORK INJURY REPORT (WIR) SURVEY PROGRAM Attempts to find causal data concerning specific problem areas that are identified by SDS *q.v.*

WORKLOAD The amount of weight used in performing a particular exercise.

WORK RESPONSES Answers to questions that are attempts to respond in some relevant way.

WORRY Persistent, undue concern about a past behavior or about an anticipated happening.

WPPSI An acronym for Wechsler Preschool–Primary Scale of Intelligence *q.v.*

WRECKING BAR A short metal bar, chisel-shaped on both ends, one end of which is a half circle, used to effect forceful entry to release victims trapped in a vehicle or other enclosure.

WRINKLES A condition caused by atrophy *q.v.* of elastic tissue changes in the skin. Some ~ develop in the normal course of aging, but severe wrinkling comes from repeated exposure to the sun. No cream, oil, or facial exercise can permanently smooth or remove ~. Only cosmetic surgery can produce a long-lasting effect on the appearance of ~.

WRIST The region of articulation *q.v.* between the forearm and hand.

WRIT IN VACATION In law, a court order issued during intermission of court session.

WRIT OF ERROR In law, a situation in which an appellate court orders a lower court to submit a record of an action on which the lower court has based its decision, so that the appellate court may examine the alleged errors of the lower court.

WRY NECK 1. Torticollis *q.v.* 2. A pulling of the neck to one side by spasm of the neck muscles.

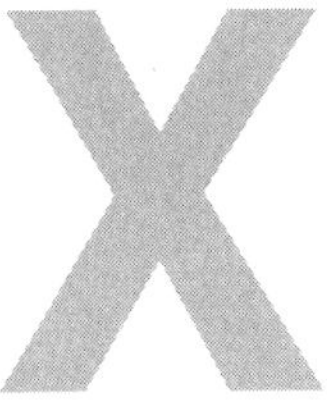

XANAX The commercial preparation of alprazolam *q.v.*

XANTHINE 1. A nitrogenous extractive contained in muscles tissue, liver, spleen, pancreas *qq.v.*, and other organs and in the urine *q.v.*, formed during the metabolism *q.v.* of nucleoproteins *q.v.* It is acted upon by certain enzymes *q.v.* to form uric acid *q.v.* and is excreted in the urine. 2. The class of chemicals that includes caffeine, theobromine, and theophylline *qq.v.*

XANTHOMA A small yellow plaque *q.v.* in the skin due to a fat deposit.

XANTHURENIC ACID A metabolite *q.v.* of tryptophan *q.v.* ~ is found in normal urine *q.v.*, but appears in increased amounts in cases of vitamin B_6 *q.v.* deficiency.

X-AXIS 1. Abscissa. 2. The horizontal axis on a graph, usually representing the independent variable *q.v.* ct: y-axis.

X CHROMOSOME 1. A sex-determining chromosome *q.v.* present in all of a female's ova *q.v.* and in one-half of a male's sperm *q.v.* The fertilization *q.v.* of an ovum by a sperm having an ~ will result in the conception of a female (XX chromosome). 2. A chromosome associated with sex determination. In most animals, the female has two ~s, and the male has one ~. ct: Y chromosome.

XENON-WASHOUT BLOOD FLOW TEST 1. A test of blood flow to the male genitals *q.v.* to diagnose erectile dysfunction *q.v.* 2. Infusion cavernosography.

XERODERMA Excessive dryness of the skin.

XEROPHTHALMIA 1. Excessive dryness of the conjunctiva *q.v.* 2. A disease of the eyes resulting from a deficiency of vitamin A *q.v.* in which the conjunctiva becomes inflamed and atrophied *q.v.*

XERORADIOGRAPHY 1. A diagnostic technique to detect breast cancer *q.v.* in its early developmental stages. 2. An X-ray examination in which the results are recorded in the form of a picture image on paper. cf: mammography; thermography.

XEROSIS An abnormal dryness, as in conjunctiva *q.v.* or skin.

XEROSTOMIA Dry mouth. ~ may be caused by disease, some medications, radiation therapy, or aging. The condition may be treated by the administration of a saline substitute.

XIPHOID 1. The smallest and most dependent part of the breast bone. 2. Xiphoid process. 3. Sword-shaped.

X-LINKED GENE A gene known to be located on the X chromosome *q.v.*

X-RAY Electromagnetic radiation.

XYLETOL A sugar alcohol *q.v.* made from birch trees, with sweetness equal to that of sucrose *q.v.* and caloric values the same as glucose *q.v.* No longer used in the United States.

XYY A rare chromosomal *q.v.* abnormality in men. Long suspected as a cause of a strong predisposition for violence.

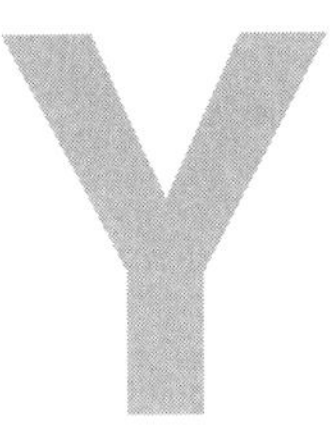

YANG One of the two opposing forces in eastern philosophy associated with the earth, heat, brightness, activity, and masculinity. ct: yin.

YAWS 1. A treponemal *q.v.* disease causing infirmity *q.v.* 2. A tropical disease caused by a spirochete *q.v.*, characterized by skin eruptions.

Y-AXIS 1. Ordinate. 2. The vertical axis on a graph, usually representing the dependent variable *q.v.* ct: *x*-axis.

Y CHROMOSOME 1. A sex-determining chromosome *q.v.* present in one-half of a male's sperm *q.v.* The fertilization *q.v.* of an ovum *q.v.* by a sperm having a ~ will result in a male (XY chromosome). 2. The mate to the X chromosome *q.v.* in the male of most animal species. The ~ carries genes that influence maleness.

YEAST A single-celled plant responsible for the fermentation *q.v.* of plant products. cf: fungus.

YEAST INFECTION 1. In sexology *q.v.*, a vaginal *q.v.* infection caused by *Candida albicans*, often transmitted sexually. 2. Generally, any invasion of fungi *q.v.* in the body resulting in an adverse reaction or disruption of function.

YELLOW FEVER A viral *q.v.* disease transmitted to humans by the bite of a specific mosquito, the *Aedes aegypti*.

YEN A craving or desire for drugs or foods.

YEN ASLEEP A drowsy but restless state during a drug withdrawal period.

YEN HOOK An instrument used in opium *q.v.* smoking.

YEN SHEE Opium *q.v.* ash.

YEN SHEE SUEY Opium *q.v.* wine.

YIN One of the two opposing forces in eastern philosophy associated with the moon, water, coldness, darkness, passivity, and femininity. ct: yang.

YIN AND YANG In certain Asian philosophies, the opposing forces that, when in balance, produce healthful harmony in people and in nature.

YOGA 1. Union. 2. The discipline by which a person attains unity with the "supreme being" or "absolute." 3. A system of exercises used to achieve mental and physical control. 4. A discipline by which a person seeks to attain a state of health and well-being by achieving union with the supreme spirit.

YOGURT 1. Whole milk with varying amounts of added milk solids. 2. Curdled milk containing lactic acid.

YOHIMBINE An alkaloid *q.v.* from the bark of an African tree that is thought by some to have aphrodisiac *q.v.* properties.

YOKED CONTROL An experimental method in which the control subject receives the same treatment as the experimental subject on the same schedule. Usually, the two subjects are run at the same time and the experimental subject's reactions control the events presented to the control subject.

YOUNG ADULT YEARS 1. That segment of the life cycle *q.v.* from ages 18 to 22. 2. A transitional period between adolescence and adulthood.

YOUNG–HELMHOLTZ THEORY A theory of color vision that assumes three types of cones *q.v.*, usually assumed to be maximally responsive to red, green, and blue.

YOUTH REBELLION A general concept referring to the tendency of the young to assert their independence from their parents and to form their identity. ~ may be characterized by a rejection of parental and social values, use of psychoactive drugs *q.v.*, delinquent behavior, etc.

Z

ZEIGARNIK EFFECT The tendency to remember incomplete tasks better than completed ones.

ZEITGEIST The German word for the trends of thought and feeling characteristic of a culture at a particular time.

ZEN MACROBIOTIC DIETS Developed by George Ohsawa in the early 1960s. Based on the misconception that human diseases were unnecessary and could be prevented by diets consisting of unpolished brown rice. Some of the diets included some kinds of vegetables. Nutritionists claim that strict adherence to the Zen diets will result in severe malnutrition in the form of scurvy, anemia, hypoproteinemia, and emaciation *qq.v.*

ZERO CONTRACT According to Levinger, a stage prior to a relationship in which a couple is unaware of one another.

ZERO POPULATION GROWTH (ZPG) The point at which the number of births equals the number of deaths in a given population.

ZONA PELLUCIDA 1. The coating of the human ovum *q.v.* 2. The jellylike material surrounding the mature egg.

ZOOGAMETE Motile isogamete *q.v.*

ZOOGLEA A translucent, gelatin-like film that adheres to the teeth and surrounding mucous membrane *q.v.*

ZOOPHILIA 1. Bestiality *q.v.* 2. A form of sexual variance *q.v.*

ZOOPLANKTON Microscopic aquatic animals.

ZOOSPORANGIUM Spore *q.v.* mother cell in which motile asexual *q.v.* spores are formed by mitosis *q.v.* via cleavage of the cytoplasm *q.v.*

ZOOSPORE A motile spore *q.v.* found among algae *q.v.* and fungi *q.v.*

ZPG An acronym for zero population growth *q.v.*

Z-SCORE 1. Standard score *q.v.* 2. A number that expresses the distance of a particular score (X) above or below the mean *q.v.* (M) in units of standard deviation *q.v.* 3. How far a raw score is from the mean in standard deviation units.

ZYGOMA 1. The cheekbone. 2. Yoke.

ZYGOMATIC PROCESS OF THE FRONTAL BONE The massive projection of the frontal bone *q.v.* that joins the zygomatic bone to form the lateral margin of the orbit *q.v.*

ZYGOMATIC PROCESS OF THE MAXILLA The rough projection from the maxilla *q.v.* that articulates *q.v.* with the zygomatic bone.

ZYGOMORPHIC Irregular.

ZYGONEMA A stage in meiosis *q.v.* during which synapsis *q.v.* occurs.

ZYGOTE 1. The fertilized *q.v.* egg. The moment a sperm *q.v.* enters the egg it becomes a ~. 2. A single cell resulting from the union of two germ cells *q.v.* at conception *q.v.* 3. The cell produced by the union of two mature gametes *q.v.* in reproduction.

Bibliography

Ackernecht, E. H. (1965). *History and Geography of the Most Important Diseases*. New York: Hafner Publishing Company, Inc.

Allegrante, J. P. (Ed.). (1981). *Health Promotion Monographs, No. 1*. New York: Teachers College, Columbia University.

Allegrante, J. P., & Sleet, D. (Eds.). (2004). *Derryberry's Educating for Health: A Foundation for Contemporary Health Education Practice*. New York: John Wiley & Sons.

American Alliance for Health, Physical Education, Recreation and Dance. (2007). *National Health Education Standards: Achieving Excellence*. Retrieved May 31, 2008, from www.aahperd.org/aahe/pdf_files/standards.pdf.

American Psychiatric Association. (1969). *A Psychiatric Glossary* (3rd ed.). Washington, DC: American Psychiatric Association.

Anderson, C. L. (1968). *School Health Practice* (4th ed.). St. Louis, MO: The C.V. Mosby Company.

Anderson, C. L., & Creswell, W. H. (1976). *School Health Practice* (6th ed.). St. Louis, MO: The C.V. Mosby Company.

Anthony, C. P., & Kolthoff, N. J. (1975). *Textbook of Anatomy and Physiology* (9th ed.). St. Louis, MO: The C.V. Mosby Company.

Asimov, I. (1964). *A Short History of Biology*. Garden City, NY: The Natural History Press.

Ballard, J., & Timmermann, T. (1976). *Strategies for Humanistic Education*. Amherst, MA: Mandala Books.

Barr, H. H., & Cortese, P. A. (1990). "Report of the 1990 Joint Committee on Health on Health Education Terminology." Washington, DC: The Association for the Advancement of Health Education/American Alliance for Health, Physical Education, Recreation and Dance.

Bartley, S. H. (Ed.) (1977). *Essentials of Life and Health* (2nd ed.). New York: CRM, Random House.

Baker, N. (Oct.–Nov., 1968). "Human rights in 1968." *World Health: The Magazine of the World Health Organization*.

Bandura, A. (1977). *Social Learning Theory*. Englewood Cliffs, NJ: Prentice-Hall, Inc.

Bates, I. J., & Winder, A. E. (1984). *Introduction to Health Education*. Palo Alto, CA: Mayfield.

Baurer, W. W., & Schaller, W. E. (1965). *Your Health Today* (2nd ed.). New York: Harper & Row Publishers.

Becker, H., & Hill, R. (Eds.). (1948). *Family, Marriage, and Parenthood*. Boston: D.C. Heath.

Bedworth, D. A. (2007). *Defensive Driving for Health Care Workers*. Delmar, NY: Cengage Publishers.

Bedworth, A. E., & Bedworth, D. A. (1982). *Health for Human Effectiveness*. Englewood Cliffs, NJ: Prentice-Hall.

Bedworth, A. E., & D'Elia, J. A. (1973). *Basics of Drug Education*. Farmingdale, NY: Baywood.

Bedworth, D. A., & Bedworth, A. E. (1976). *Health Education: A Process for Human Effectiveness*. New York: Harper & Row, Publishers.

Bedworth, D. A., & Bedworth, A. E. (1992). *The Profession and Practice of Health Education*. Dubuque, IA: Wm. C. Brown Publishers.

Beggs, D. W., & Buffie, E. G. (1967). *Nongraded Schools In Action*. Bloomington, IN: Indiana University Press.

Bersoff, D. N. (1976). "Child Advocacy: The next step." *New York University Education Quarterly*. New York: New York University Press.

Bever, D. L. (1984). *Safety: A Personal Focus*. St. Louis, MO: Times Mirror/Mosby College Publishing.

Black, H. (1967). *The American Schoolbook* . New York: William M. Morrow, Inc.

Blair, G. M., James, R. S., & Simpson, R. H. (1968). *Educational Psychology* (3rd ed.). New York: Macmillan.

Bloom, B. et al. (1956). *Taxonomy of Educational Objectives, Handbook I: Cognitive Domain*. New York: David McKay Co.

Blum, R., Bloom, E., & Garfield, E. (1976). *Drug Education: Results and Recommendations*. Lexington, MA: D.C. Heath and Company.

Biehler, R., & Snowman, J. (1982). *Psychology Applied to Teaching* (4th ed.). New York: Houghton Mifflin Co.

Brill, L., & Lieberman, L. (1969). *Alcohol and Addiction*. Boston, MA: Little, Brown and Company.

Brown, B. F. (1963). *The Ungraded High School*. Englewood Cliffs, NJ: Prentice-Hall.

Bruess, C. E., & Tevis, B. (1985). *Decisions for Health*. Belmont, CA: Wadsworth.

Bucher, C. A., Olsen, E. A., & Willgoose, C. E. (1967). *The Foundations of Health*. New York: Appleton-Century-Crofts.

Bugelski, B. R. (1956). *The Psychology of Learning*. New York: Henry Holt.

Bugelski, B. R. (1971). *The Psychology of Learning Applied to Teaching.* Indianapolis, IN: Bobbs-Merrill.

Burrup, P. E. (1967). *The Teacher and the Public School System* (2nd ed.). New York: Harper & Row.

Burt, J. J., & Miller, B. T. (1972). *Personal Health Behavior in Today's Society.* Philadelphia, PA: W. B. Saunders.

Byler, R. V. (Ed.). (1969). *Teach Us What We Want to Know.* New York: Mental Health Materials Center, Inc.

Byer, C. O., Shainberg, L. W., and Jones, K. L. (1988). *Dimensions of Human Sexuality.* Dubuque, IA: Wm. C. Brown Publishers.

Byrd, O. E. (1964). *School Health Administration.* Philadelphia, PA: W. B. Saunders.

Carrol, C. R. (1985). *Drugs in Modern Society.* Dubuque, IA: W. C. Brown.

Cashman, J. (1966). *The LSD Story.* Greenwich, CN: Fawcett.

Certo, S. C. (1983). *Principles of Modern Management* (2nd ed.). Dubuque, IA: W. C. Brown.

Cirese, S. (1977). *Quest: A Search for Self.* New York: Holt, Rinehart and Winston.

Clayton, P. J. (1975). "The Funeral Director and Bereavement." In Margolis, O. et al. (Eds.) *Grief and the Meaning of the Funeral.* New York: MSS Information Corporation.

Cleary, H., Kichen, J. M., & Ensor, P. G. (1985). *Advancing Health Through Education.* Palo Alto, CA: Mayfield.

Cockrum, E. L., & McCauley, W. J. (1965). *Zoology.* Philadelphia, PA: W. B. Saunders.

Cohen, S. (1969). *The Drug Dilemma.* New York: McGraw-Hill.

Cole, W. E., & Cox, R. L. (1968). *Social Foundations of Education.* New York: American Book Company.

Coleman, J. C. (1964). *Abnormal Psychology and Modern Life* (3rd ed.). Chicago, IL: Scott, Foresman.

Corkrum, E. L., & McCauley, W. J. (1965). *Zoology.* Philadelphia, PA: W. B. Saunders.

Cornacchia, H. J., & Barrett, S. (1985). *Consumer Health: A Guide to Intelligent Decisions.* St. Louis: Times Mirror/Mosby.

Cornacchia, H. J., Staton, W. M., & Irwin, L. W. (1970). *Health in Elementary Schools* (3rd ed.). St. Louis, MO: C. V. Mosby.

Corry, J. M., & Cimbolic, P. (1985). *Drugs: Facts, Alternatives, Decisions.* Belmont, CA: Wadsworth.

Cox, F. D. (1978). *Human Intimacy: Marriage, the Family and Its Meaning.* St. Paul, MN: West.

Crane, D. P. (1979). *Personnel: The Management of Human Resources* (2nd ed.). Belmont, CA: Wadsworth.

Creswell, W. H., Newman, I. M., & Anderson, C. L. (1985). *School Health Practice* (8th ed.). St. Louis, MO: Times Mirror/Mosby.

Dale, E. (1946). *Audiovisual Methods in Teaching.* New York: Holt, Rinehart and Winston.

Davison, G. C., & Meale, J. M. (1986). *Abnormal Psychology: An Experimental Clinical Approach* (4th ed.). New York: John Wiley & Sons.

DeBold, R. C., & Leaf, R. C. (Eds.). (1967). *LSD: Man & Society.* Middletown, CT: Wesleyan University Press.

Denny, N. W., & Quadagno, D. (1988). *Human Sexuality.* St. Louis, MO: Times Mirror/Mosby.

Deutsch, A. (1937). *The Mentally Ill in America: A History of Their Care and Treatment from Colonial Times.* New York: Doubleday, Doran & Co.

Deutsch, R. M. (1976). *Realities of Nutrition.* Palo Alto, CA: Bull.

deVries, H. A. (1979). *Health Science: A Positive Approach.* Santa Monica, CA: Goodyear.

Dewey, J. (1933). *How We Think.* Boston, MA: D. C. Heath.

DiMatteo, M. R. (1991). *The Psychology of Health, Illness, and Medical Care: An Individual Perspective.* Pacific Grove, CA: Brooks/Cole.

Dintiman, G. B. et al. (1984). *Developing Lifetime Fitness.* St. Paul, MN: West.

Donatelle, R. J. (2008). *Access to Health* (10th ed.). San Francisco, CA: Pearson Education.

Dorland's Illustrated Medical Dictionary (24th ed.). (1967). Philadelphia, PA: W. B. Saunders.

Dubos, R. (1965). *Man Adapting.* New Haven, CT: Yale University Press.

Edlin, G., & Golanty, E. (1985). *Health & Wellness: A Holistic Approach* (2nd ed.). Boston, MA: Science Books International.

Editors of Consumer Guide. (1985). *The New Prescription Drug Reference Guide.* Skokie, IL: Publications International.

Edwards, G. (1972). *Reaching Out: The Prevention of Drug Abuse Through Increased Human Interaction.* Garden City, NY: Innovative Designs for Educational Action, Inc.

Edwards, G., Russell, M. A. H., Hawks, D., & MacCafferty, M. (Eds.). (1976). *Drugs and Drug Dependence* . Lexington, MA: Saxon House/Lexington Books, Heath.

Eichenlaub, J. E. (1962). *College Health.* New York: Macmillan.

Ehrenreich, B., & Ehrenreich, J. (1970). *The American Health Empire.* New York: Vintage.

Elder, C. A. (1972). *Making Value Judgments: Decisions for Today.* Columbus, OH: Merrill.

Elzey, F. T. (1966). *A Programmed Introduction to Statistics.* Belmont, CA: Brooks/Cole.

Eschleman, J. R. (1985). *The Family: An Introduction.* Boston, MA: Allyn and Bacon.

Flora, R. R., & Land, T. A. (1982). *Health Behaviors.* St. Paul, MN: West.

Florio, A. E., Alles, W. F., & Stafford, G. T., *Safety Education* (4th ed.). New York: McGraw-Hill.

Frobisher, M. (1944). *Fundamentals of Bacteriology* (3rd ed.). Philadelphia, PA: W. B. Saunders

Galea, R. P., Lewis B., & Baker, L. A. (Eds.). (1988). *AIDS and IV Drug Abusers: Current Perspectives.* Owing Mills, MD: National Health Publishing.

Galli, N. (1978). *Foundations and Principles of Health Education.* New York: Wiley.

Galton, F. (1909). *Essays in Eugenics.* London: The Eugenics Education Society.

Gardner, E. J. (1968). *Principles of Genetics* (3rd ed.). New York: John Wiley & Sons.

Garrett, H. E. (1951). *Great Experiments in Psychology* (3rd ed.). New York: Appleton-Century-Crofts.

Gearhart, B. R. (1973). *Learning Disabilities: Educational Strategies.* St. Louis, MO: C. V. Mosby.

Gergen, K. J., & Gergen, M. M. (1986). *Social Psychology* (2nd ed.). New York: Springer.

Gerth, H., & Mills, C. W. (1953). *Character and Social Structure: The Psychology of Social Institutions.* New York: Harcourt, Brace.

Gleitman, H. (1986). *Psychology* (2nd ed.). New York: W. W. Horton & Company.

Goerke, L. S., & Stebbins, E. L. (1968). *Mustard's Introduction to Public Health* (5th ed.). New York: Macmillan.

Goldstein, B. (1976). *Human Sexuality.* New York: McGraw-Hill.

Goldstein, M., Baker, B. L., & Jamison, K. R. (1986). *Abnormal Psychology* (2nd ed.). Boston, MA: Little, Brown.

Good, C. V., & Merkel, W. R. (Eds.). (1959). *Dictionary of Education* (2nd ed.). New York: McGraw-Hill.

Gordon, T., & Burch, N. (1974). *T. E. T.: Teacher Effectiveness Training.* New York: Peter H. Wyden.

Gould, L. C., Walker, A. L., Crane, L. E. & Lidz, C. W. (1974). *Connections: Notes from the Heroin World.* New Haven, CT: Yale University Press.

Gove, P. B. (Ed.). (1976). *Webster's Third New International Dictionary of the English Language: Unabridged.* Springfield, MA: G. & C. Merriam.

Green, L. W., & Anderson, C. L. (1982). *Community Health* (4th ed.). St. Louis, MO: Mosby.

Green, L. W., Kreuter, M. W., Deeds, S. G., & Partridge, K. B. (1980). *Health Education Planning: A Diagnostic Approach.* Palo Alto, CA: Mayfield.

Greenberg, J. S. (2001). *The Code of Ethics for the Health Education Profession: A Case Study Book.* Boston, MA: Jones and Bartlett.

Greenberg, J. S., & Pargman, D. (1986). *Physical Fitness: A Wellness Approach.* Englewood Cliffs, NJ: Prentice-Hall.

Greenberg, J. S., Bruess, C. E., & Sands, D. W. (1986). *Sexuality: Insights and Issues.* Dubuque, IA: Wm. C. Brown.

Greene, W. H., & Simons-Morton, B. G. (1984). *Introduction to Health Education*. New York: Macmillan.

Greisheimer, E. M. (1945). *Physiology and Anatomy.* Philadelphia, PA: Lippincott.

Grinspoon, L. (1971). *Marijuana Reconsidered.* Cambridge, MA: Harvard University Press.

Grout, R. E. (1963). *Health Teaching in Schools* (4th ed.). Philadelphia: W. B. Saunders.

Haag, J. H. (1965). *Health Education for Young Adults.* Austin, TX: Steck-Vaughn.

Hanlon, J. J. (1969). *Principles of Public Health Administration.* St. Louis, MO: C. V. Mosby.

Hanlon, J. J. (1974). *Public Health Administration and Practice* (6th ed.). St. Louis, MO: C. V. Mosby.

Hannan, T. H. (1975). *The Economics of Methadone Maintenance.* Lexington, MA: D. C. Heath.

Hardman, M. L., Drew, C. J., & Egan, M. W. (1987): *Human Exceptionality: Social, School, and Family* (2nd ed). Newton, MA: Allyn and Bacon.

Hart, C. L., Ray, O. S. & Ksir, C. J. (2006). *Drugs, Society, and Human Behavior* (12th ed.). New York: McGraw-Hill.

Haynes, K. S., & Mickelson, J. S. (1986). *Affecting Change: Social Workers in the Political Arena.* White Plains, NY: Longman.

Health in Schools: Twentieth Yearbook. (1951). Washington, DC: American Association of School Administrators.

Heidenreich, C. A. (1967). *Personality and Social Adjustment.* Dubuque, IA: Wm. C. Brown.

Hein, F. V., & Farnsworth, D. L. (1965). *Living: A College Text in Health Education* (4th ed.). Atlanta, GA: Scott, Foresman.

Hellman, A. D. (1975). *Laws Against Marijuana.* Urbana, IL: University of Illinois Press.

Henry, M. A., & Beasley, W. W. (1972). *Supervising Student Teachers the Professional Way.* Terra Haute, IN: Sycamore Press.

Hilgard, E. R., Atkinson, R. C., & Atkinson, R. L. (1971). *Introduction to Psychology* (5th ed.). New York: Harcourt, Brace, Jovanovich.

Hochbaum, G. M. (1976). "At The Threshold of a New Era." *Health Education*. 7(4), 2–5.

Horman, R. E., & Fox, A. M. (Eds.). (1970). *Drug Awareness.* New York: Avon Books.

Hubbard, W. N. Jr. (1970). "Health Knowledge." In B. Jones (Ed.). *The Health of Americans.* Englewood Cliffs, NJ: Prentice-Hall.

Hughes, P. H. (1977). *Behind the Wall of Respect: Community Experiments in Heroin Addiction Control.* Chicago, IL: The University of Chicago Press.

Hyde, M. O. (1968). *Mind Drugs.* New York: McGraw-Hill.

Initial Role Delineation for Health Education. (1980). San Francisco, CA: The National Center for Health Education.

Irwin, L. W., & Mayshark, C. (1964). *Health Education in Secondary Schools.* St. Louis, MO: C. V. Mosby.

Irwin, L. W., Humphrey, J. H., and Johnson, W. R. (1956). *Methods and Materials In School Health Education.* St. Louis, MO: C. V. Mosby.

Jacobson, P. B., Reaves, W. C., & Logsdon, J. D. (1963). *The Effective School Principle.* Englewood Cliffs, NJ: Prentice-Hall.

Jenne, F. H., & Greene, W. H. (1976). *Turner's School Health and Health Education* (7th ed.). St. Louis, MO: C. V. Mosby.

Johansen, J. H., Collins, H. W., & Johnson, J. A. (1982). *American Education: An Introduction to Teaching* (4th ed.). Dubuque, IA: Wm. C. Brown.

Johns, E. B., Sutton, W. C., & Webster, L. E. (1966). *Health for Effective Living* (4th ed.). New York: McGraw-Hill.

Johnson, J. A., et al. (1991). *Introduction to the Foundations of American Education* (8th ed.). Needham Heights, MA: Allyn and Bacon.

Joint Committee on Health Education Terminology. (1973). *Health Education Monographs* (No. 33). San Francisco, CA: SOPHE, Inc.

Joint Committee on Health Education Terminology. (1990). "Report of the 1990 Joint Committee on Health Education terminology." *Journal of Health Education.* 22(2), 97–208.

Jones, H. B., & Jones, H. C. (1977). *Sensual Drugs: Deprivation and Rehabilitation of the Mind.* Cambridge, MA: Cambridge University Press.

Jones, K. L., Shainberg, L. W., & Byer, C. O. (1985). *Health Science* (5th ed.). New York: Harper & Row.

Jones, K. L., Shainberg, L. W., & Byer, C. O. (1986). *Dimensions: A Changing Concept of Health.* New York: Harper & Row.

Jones-Witters, P., & Witters, W. (1983). *Drugs and Society: A Biological Perspective.* Belmont, CA: Wadsworth.

Keller, M., & McCormick, M. (1968). *A Dictionary of Words About Alcohol.* New Brunswick, NJ: Rutgers Center of Alcohol Studies.

Kendler, H. H. (1963). *Basic Psychology.* New York: Appleton Century Crofts.

Kerlinger, F. N. (1964). *Foundations of Behavioral Research: Educational and Psychological Inquiry.* New York: Holt, Rinehart and Winston.

Kilander, H. F. (1965). *Health for Modern Living* (2nd ed.). Englewood Cliffs, NJ: Prentice-Hall.

Kilander, H. F. (1968). *School Health Education* (2nd ed.). Toronto, ON: Collier-Macmillan.

Kimble, G. A., & Garmezy, N. (1963). *Principles of General Psychology* (2nd ed.). New York: The Ronald Press.

Kime, R. E., Schlaadt, R. G., & Tritsch, L. E. (1977). *Health Instruction: An Action Approach.* Englewood Cliffs, NJ: Prentice-Hall.

Klausmeier, H. J., & Goodwin, W. (1966). *Learning and Human Abilities* (2nd ed.). New York: Harper & Row.

Knox, D. (1984). *Human Sexuality: The Search for Understanding.* St. Paul, MN: West.

Koopman, G. R. (1966). *Curriculum Development.* New York: The Center for Applied Research in Education.

Krathwohl, D. R. (1993). *Methods of Educational and Social Science Research: An Integrated Approach.* White Plains, NY: Longman.

Krathwohl, D. R., et al. (1964). *Taxonomy of Educational Goals: Handbook II: Affective Domain.* New York: David McKay Co.

Kreutler, P. A. (1980). *Nutrition in Perspective.* Englewood Cliffs, NJ: Prentice-Hall.

Kubler-Ross, E. (1969). *On Death and Dying.* New York: Macmillan.

Laurie, P. (1967). *Drugs: Medical, Psychological and Social Tacts.* Baltimore, MD: Penguin.

Lang, R. W. (1974). *The Politics of Drugs.* Lexington, MA: D. C. Heath.

Langton, C. V., Allen, R. L., & Wexler, P. (1961). *School Health Organization and Services.* New York: The Ronald Press.

LaPlace, J. (1987). *Health* (5th ed.). Englewood Cliffs, NJ: Prentice-Hall.

Last, J. M. (Ed.). (2007). *A Dictionary of Public Health.* New York: Oxford University Press.

Levy, M. R., Digman, M., & Shirreffs, J. H. (1984). *Life & Health* (4th ed.). New York: Random House.

Liebert, R. M., & Spiegler, M. D. (1982). *Personality: Strategies and Issues.* Homewood, IL: The Dorsey Press.

Light, P. K. (1975). *Let the Children Speak: A Psychological Study of Young Teenagers and Drugs.* Lexington, MA: D. C. Heath.

Lindesmith, A. R. (1968). *Addiction and Opiates.* Chicago: Aldine Publishing.

Lingeman, R. R. (1969). *Drugs from A to Z: A Dictionary.* New York: McGraw-Hill.

Liska, K. (1981). *Drugs and the Human Body.* New York: Macmillan.

Louria, D. B. (1968). *The Drug Scene.* New York: McGraw-Hill.

Louria, D. B. (1971). *Overcoming Drugs: A Program for Action.* New York: McGraw-Hill.

Longstreth, L. E. (1968). *Psychological Dimensions of the Child.* New York: Ronald Press.

MacDougal, M. S., & Hegner, R. (1943). *Biology: The Science of Life.* New York: McGraw-Hill.

Maslow, A. H. (1970). *Motivation and Personality.* New York: Harper & Row.

Masters, W. H., & Johnson, V. E., & Kolodny, R. C. (1982). *Human Sexuality.* Boston, MA: Little, Brown.

Mayshark, C. E., Shaw, D. D., & Best, W. H. (1967). *Administration of School Health Programs: Its Theory and Practice.* St. Louis, MO: C. V. Mosby.

McCary, J. L., & Copeland, D. R. (Eds.). (1976). *Modern View of Human Sexuality.* Chicago, IL: Science Research Associates.

McCary, J. L., & McCary, S. P. (1982). *McCary's Human Sexuality* (4th ed.). Belmont, CA: Wadsworth.

McGraw, K. O. (1987). *Developmental Psychology.* New York: Harcourt, Brace, Jovanovich.

McKenzie, J. F., Pinger, R. R., & Kotecki, J. E. (2005). *An Introduction to Community Health* (5th ed.). Sudbury, MA: Jones & Bartlett.

Means, R. K. (1975). *Historical Perspectives on School Health.* Thorofare, NJ: Charles B. Slack.

Meredith, F. L. (1946). *Hygiene* (4th ed.). Philadelphia, PA: Blakiston.

Merrill, R. M., & Timmreck, T. C. (2006). *Introduction to Epidemiology* (4th ed.). Sudbury, MA: Jones and Bartlett.

Merson, M. H., Black, R. E., & Mills, A. J. (2006). *International Public Health: Diseases, Programs, Systems, and Policies* (2nd ed.). Sudbury, MA: Jones and Bartlett.

Milio, N. (1975). *The Care of Health in Communities.* New York: Macmillan.

Miller, B. F., & Burt, J. J. (1972). *Good Health: Personal and Community* (3rd ed.). Philadelphia, PA: W. B. Saunders.

Miller. D. K., & Allen, T. E. (1986). *Fitness: A Lifetime Commitment* (3rd ed.). Edina, MN: Burgess.

Miller, M. M. (1975). *Evaluating Community Treatment Programs: Tools, Techniques and a Case Study.* Lexington, MA: D. C. Heath.

Miller, V. (1965). *The Public Administration of American School Systems.* New York: Macmillan.

Moehlman, A. B. (1940). *School Administration: Its Development, Principles and Future in the United States.* New York: Houghton Mifflin.

Moore, M. H. (1977). *Being the Best.* Lexington, MA: D. C. Heath.

Moss, B. R., Southworth, W. H., & Reichert, J. L. (Eds.). (1961). *Health Education: A Guide for Teachers and a Text for Teacher Education* (5th ed.). Washington, DC: National Education Association of the United States.

Mustard, H. S., & Stebbins, E. L. (1959). *An Introduction to Public Health* (4th ed.). New York: Macmillan.

National Cancer Institute. (1980). *Breast Cancer Digest.* Bethesda, MD: United States Public Health Service.

National Committee on School Health Policies. (1966). *Suggested School Health Policies* (5th ed.). Joint Committee on Health Problems in Education of the NEA and AMA. Chicago, IL: American Medical Association.

The National Health Assembly. (1949). *America's Health: A Report to the Nation.* New York: Harper and Brothers.

Newman, W. H., & Summer, Jr., C. E. (1961). *The Process of Management.* Englewood Cliffs, NJ: Prentice-Hall.

Nolte, M. C., & Linn, J. P. (1963). *School Law for Teachers.* Danville, IL: The Interstate Printers & Publishers.

Novick, L. F., & Mays, G. P. (2001). *Public Health Administration: Principles for Population-Based Management.* Gaithersburg, MD: Aspen.

Oberteuffer, D., & Beyrer, M. K. (1966). *School Health Education: A Textbook for Teachers, Nurses, and Other Professional Personnel* (4th ed.). New York: Harper & Row.

Oberteuffer, D., Harrelson, O. A., & Pollock, M. B. (1972). *School Health Education* (5th ed.). New York: Harper & Row.

Ogburn, W. F., & Nimkoff, M. F. (1946). *Sociology.* New York: Houghton Mifflin.

O'Neill, N., & O'Neill, G. (1972). *Open Marriage: A New Life Style For Couples.* New York: Evans Publishing.

Payne, W. A., & Hahn, D. B. (1986). *Understanding Your Health.* St. Louis, MO: Times Mirror/Mosby.

Perlman, H., & Jaszi, P. (1976). *Legal Issues in Addiction Diversion.* Lexington, MA: D. C. Heath.

Phares, E. J. (1979). *Clinical Psychology: Concepts, Methods, and Profession* (Rev.). Homewood, IL: Dorsey Press.

Pollock, M. B., & Middleton, K. (1984). *Elementary School Health Instruction.* St. Louis, MO: Times Mirror/Mosby.

Pollock, M. B., & Oberteuffer, D. (1974). *Health Science and the Young Child.* New York: Harper & Row.

Powers, G. P., & Baskin, W. (1969). *Sex Education: Issues and Directives.* New York: Philosophical Library.

Price, J. H., Galli, N., & Slenker, S. (1985). *Consumer Health: Contemporary Issues and Choices.* Dubuque, IA: Wm. C. Brown.

Rachin, R. L., & Czajkoski, E. H. (1975). *Drug Abuse Control.* Lexington, MA: D. C. Heath.

Rathbone, F. S., & Rathbone, E. T. (1971). *Health and the Nature of Man.* New York: McGraw-Hill.

Rathus, S. A. (1983). *Human Sexuality.* New York: Holt, Rinehart and Winston.

Read, D. A., & Greene, W. H. (1975). *Creative Teaching in Health.* New York: Macmillan.

Read, D. A., & Stoll, W. (1973). *The Concept of Health* (2nd ed.). Boston, MA: Holbrook Press.

Reed-Flora, R., & Lang, T. A. (1982). *Health Behaviors.* St. Paul, MN: West.

Reid, J. G., & Thomson, J. M. (1985). *Exercise Prescription for Fitness.* Englewood Cliffs, NJ: Prentice-Hall.

Reiss, I. (1986). *Journey Into Sexuality: An Exploratory Voyage.* Englewood Cliffs, NJ: Prentice-Hall.

Reutter, Jr., E. E., & Hamilton, R. R. (1976). *The Law of Public Education* (2nd ed.). Mineola, NY: The Foundation Press.

Rich, J. M. (1978). *Innovations in Education: Reformers and Their Critics* (2nd ed.). Boston, MA: Allyn and Bacon.

Ridenour, N. (1961). *Mental Health in the United States: A Fifty-Year History.* Cambridge, MA: Harvard University Press.

Rogers, C. R. (1967). "The Interpersonal Relationship in the Facilitation of Learning." In *Humanizing Education: The Person in the Process.* Washington, DC: Association for Supervision and Curriculum Development, NEA.

Rosebury, T. (1973). *Microbes and Moral: The Strange Story of Venereal Disease.* New York: Ballantine Books.

Rosenfeld, A. H. (1976). *The Archeology of Affect.* Washington, DC: DHEW.

Ross, H. S. (1976). "Redefining the Future of Health Education." *Health Education.* 7(4), 5.

Ross, H. S., & Mico, P. R. (1980). *Theory and Practice of Health Education.* Palo Alto, CA: Mayfield.

Rubinson, L., & Alles, W. F. (1984). *Health Education: Foundations for the Future.* St. Louis, MO: Times Mirror/Mosby.

Ruch, F. L. (1967). *Psychology and Life.* Glenview, IL: Scott, Foresman.

Russell, R. D. (1975). *Health Education* (6th ed.). Washington, DC: National Education Association.

Sagan, C. (2006). *The Varieties of Scientific Experience: A Personal View of the Search for God.* New York: Penguin.

Sagan, C., & Druyan, A. (1992). *Shadows of Forgotten Ancestors: A Search For Who We Are.* New York: Random House.

Saylor, J. G. (1966). *Curriculum Planning for Modern Schools.* New York: Holt, Rinehart and Winston.

Scientific American Editors (1973). *Life and Death and Medicine: A Scientific American Book.* San Francisco: W.H. Freeman.

Schaller, W. E., & Carroll, C. R. (1976). *Health, Quackery & the Consumer.* Philadelphia, PA: W. B. Saunders.

School Health Education Study. (1967). *Health Education: A Conceptual Approach to Curriculum Design.* St. Paul, MN: 3M Education Press.

Scott, G. D., & Carlo, M. W. (1974). *On Becoming a Health Educator.* Dubuque, IA: Wm. C. Brown.

Selye, H. (1956). *The Stress of Life.* New York: McGraw-Hill.

Shain, M., Riddell, W., & Kilty, H. L. (1977). *Influence, Choice, and Drugs.* Lexington, MA: D. C. Heath.

Shipley, R. R., & Plonsky, C. G. (1980). *Consumer Health: Protecting Your Health and Money.* New York: Harper & Row.

Simon, S. B., Howe, L., & Kirschbaum, H. (1972). *Values-Clarification: A Handbook of Practical Strategies for Teachers and Students.* New York: Hart.

Sinacore, J. S. (1974). *Health: A Quality of Life* (2nd ed.). New York: Macmillan.

Skinner, B. F. (1974). *About Behaviorism.* New York: Alfred A. Knopf.

Smillie, W. G. (1958). *Preventive Medicine and Public Health* (2nd ed.). New York: Macmillan.

Smith, R. L. (1960). *The Health Hucksters.* New York: Crowell.

Smith, T. E. C. (1987). *Introduction to Education.* St. Paul, MN: West.

Smolensky, J., & Bonvechio, L. R. (1966). *Principles of School Health.* Boston, MA: D. C. Heath.

Smolensky, J., & Haar, F. B. (1961). *Principles of Community Health.* Philadelphia, PA: W. B. Saunders.

Solleder, M. K. (1969). *Evaluation Instruments in Health Education.* Washington, DC: The American Association for Health, Physical Education, and Recreation.

Solomon, D. (Ed.). (1966). *The Marijuana Papers.* New York: The New American Library.

Sorenson, H., & Malm, M. (1957). *Psychology for Living.* New York: McGraw-Hill.

Sorochan, W. D. (1981). *Promoting Your Health.* New York: Wiley.

Sorochan, W. D., & Bender, S. J. (1975). *Teaching Elementary Health Science.* Reading, MA: Addison-Wesley.

Stine, G. J. (1993). *Acquired Immune Deficiency Syndrome.* Englewood Cliffs, NJ: Prentice-Hall.

Stone, D. B., O'Reilly, L. B., & Brown, J. D. (1976). *Elementary School Health Education: Ecological Perspectives.* Dubuque, IA: Wm. C. Brown.

Strasser, M. K., Aaron, J. E., & Bohn, R. C. (1981). *Fundamentals of Safety Education* (3rd ed.). New York: Macmillan.

Strommen, E. A., McKinney, J. P., & Fitzgerald, H. E. (1983). *Developmental Psychology: The School-Aged Child* (2nd ed.). Homewood, IL: The Dorsey Press.

Sumption, M. R., & Engstrom, Y. (1966). *School-Community Relations.* New York: McGraw-Hill.

Tanner, D. (1972). *Using Behavior Objectives in the Classroom.* New York: Macmillan.

Thygerson, A. L. (1982). *The First Aid Book.* Englewood Cliffs, NJ: Prentice-Hall.

Turner, C. E. (1959). *Personal and Community Health* (11th ed.). St. Louis, MO: C. V. Mosby.

Turner, C. E., Sellery, C. M., & Smith, S. L. (1961). *School Health and Health Education.* St. Louis, MO: C. V. Mosby.

Tyler, V. E., Brady, L. R., & Robbers, J. E. (1976). *Pharmacognosy* (7th ed.). Philadelphia, PA: Lea & Febiger.

U.S. Department of Health, Education and Welfare. (1973). *The Report of the President's Committee on Health Education.* Washington, DC: USDHEW.

U.S. Department of Health and Human Services. (1979). *Healthy People: The Surgeon General's Report on Health Promotion and Disease Prevention.* Washington, DC: USDHHS.

U.S. Department of Health and Human Services. (1980). *Promoting Health, Preventing Disease: Objectives for the Nation.* Washington, DC: USDHHS.

U.S. Department of Health and Human Services. (1984). *Proceedings of Prospects for a Healthier America: Achieving the Nation's Health Promotion Objectives.* Washington, DC: USDHHS.

U. S. Department of Health and Human Services. (2000). *Healthy People 2010: Understanding and Improving Health.* Washington, DC: USDHHS.

Ware, M. C., & Remmlein, M. K. (1979). *School Law* (4th ed.). Danville, IL: The Interstate Printers and Publishers.

Warga, R. G. (1974). *Personal Awareness: A Psychology of Adjustment.* New York: Houghton Mifflin.

Weisfeld, V. D. *A Century of Science: 1884–1984.* Saranac Lake, NY: Trudeau Institute, Inc., Biomedical Research Laboratories.

Whaley, R. (1982). *Health.* Englewood Cliffs, NJ: Prentice-Hall.

Wilcox, S. G., & Sutton, M. (1985). *Understanding Death and Dying: An Interdisciplinary Approach* (3rd ed.). Palo Alto, CA: Mayfield.

Wilhelms, F. T. (1967). "Humanizing Via the Curriculum." In Guper, R. R. (Ed.). *Humanizing Education: The Person in the Process.* Washington, DC: Association for Supervision and Curriculum Development, NEA.

Willgoose, C. E. (1969). *Health Education in the Elementary School* (3rd ed.). Philadelphia, PA: W. B. Saunders.

Williams, J. B. (Ed.). (1967). *Narcotics and Hallucinogens: A Handbook Revised.* Beverly Hills, CA: Glencoe.

Williams, J. B. (1974). *Narcotics and Drug Dependence.* Beverly Hills, CA: Glencoe.

Wilson, C. Z., & Loomis, W. E. (1967). *Botany* (4th ed.). New York: Holt, Rinehart and Winston.

Wilson, C. C. (Ed.). (1953). *School Health Services.* Washington, DC: National Education Association.

Wilson, C. C. (Ed.). (1957). *Healthful School Living.* Washington, DC: National Education Association.

Wilson, E. D., Fisher, K. H., & Fuqua, M. E. (1975). *Principles of Nutrition.* New York: John Wiley & Sons.

Wright, J. R., & Thornton, Jr., J. W. (1963). *Secondary School Curriculum.* Columbus, OH: Charles E. Merrill.

Witters, P. J., & Witters, W. L. (1983). *Drugs and Society: A Biological Perspective.* Monterey, CA: Wadsworth.

Zahorte, M. W. (1990). *School Law: Cases and Concepts* (3rd ed.). Englewood Cliffs, NJ: Prentice-Hall.

Zuria, Z., Friedman, S., & Rose, M. D. (1987). *Human Sexuality.* New York: John Wiley & Sons.

Zusman, J., & Wurster, C. R. (1975). *Program Evaluation: Alcohol, Drug Abuse, and Mental Health Services.* Lexington, MA: D. C. Heath.